Pediatric Kidney Disease

Franz Schaefer • Larry A. Greenbaum
Editors

Pediatric Kidney Disease

Third Edition

Volume I

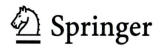

Editors
Franz Schaefer
Division of Pediatric Nephrology
Heidelberg University
Heidelberg, Germany

Larry A. Greenbaum
Emory School of Medicine
Emory University
Atlanta, GA, USA

Previously published as COMPREHENSIVE PEDIATRIC NEPHROLOGY with Elsevier, The Netherlands, 2008

Springer-Verlag Berlin Heidelberg 2016
ISBN 978-3-031-11664-3   ISBN 978-3-031-11665-0   (eBook)
https://doi.org/10.1007/978-3-031-11665-0

© The Editor(s) (if applicable) and The Author(s), under exclusive license to Springer Nature Switzerland AG 2008, 2016, 2023
This work is subject to copyright. All rights are solely and exclusively licensed by the Publisher, whether the whole or part of the material is concerned, specifically the rights of translation, reprinting, reuse of illustrations, recitation, broadcasting, reproduction on microfilms or in any other physical way, and transmission or information storage and retrieval, electronic adaptation, computer software, or by similar or dissimilar methodology now known or hereafter developed. The use of general descriptive names, registered names, trademarks, service marks, etc. in this publication does not imply, even in the absence of a specific statement, that such names are exempt from the relevant protective laws and regulations and therefore free for general use.
The publisher, the authors, and the editors are safe to assume that the advice and information in this book are believed to be true and accurate at the date of publication. Neither the publisher nor the authors or the editors give a warranty, expressed or implied, with respect to the material contained herein or for any errors or omissions that may have been made. The publisher remains neutral with regard to jurisdictional claims in published maps and institutional affiliations.

This Springer imprint is published by the registered company Springer Nature Switzerland AG
The registered company address is: Gewerbestrasse 11, 6330 Cham, Switzerland

Preface

We are delighted to welcome you to the new edition of Pediatric Kidney Disease. As in the previous versions of this textbook, our goal has been to bridge the gap between multivolume "library-level" books and numerous pocket handbooks available in our specialty. We hope that Pediatric Kidney Disease will continue to be the standard textbook for reference to busy clinicians, who need to obtain an up-to-date, easy-to-read, review of virtually all kidney disorders that occur in children.

Following a critical review of the previous edition and the downloadable figures of each chapter, the table of contents was revised to optimally reflect the needs and expectations of our readers. One-third of the chapters were written by new authors. For chapters with unchanged authorship, each author was asked to thoroughly update the materials, which has resulted in extensive revisions of most chapters. A number of new topics have been included, such as metabolic disorders affecting the kidney, pediatric kidney tumors, sickle cell nephropathy, diabetic kidney disease, and strategic choices in kidney replacement therapy.

For all chapters, we have requested the authors to ensure the relevance and clinical usefulness of their chapter for busy pediatric and pediatric nephrology clinicians as well as the multidisciplinary team members. We hope that the included material and its presentation are of value and will contribute to the expansion of knowledge in the field of pediatric nephrology.

Heidelberg, Germany
Atlanta, GA, USA

Franz Schaefer
Larry A. Greenbaum

Contents

Volume I

Part I Investigative Techniques in Pediatric Nephrology

1 Antenatal Assessment of Kidney Morphology and Function 3
Khalid Ismaili, Benedetta D. Chiodini, Marie Cassart, and Karim Khelif

2 Laboratory Evaluation of Renal Disease in Childhood 37
Damien Noone and Valérie Langlois

3 Imaging and Radiological Interventions in the Pediatric Urinary Tract 69
Bernarda Viteri, Seth Vatsky, Amy Farkas, Mohamed Elsingergy, Richard D. Bellah, and Erum A. Hartung

4 Molecular Diagnosis of Genetic Diseases of the Kidney: Primer for Pediatric Nephrologists 119
Aoife Waters and Mathieu Lemaire

5 Tools for Kidney Tissue Analysis 171
Anette Melk

Part II Disorders of Kidney Development

6 Functional Development of the Nephron 189
Aoife Waters

7 Structural Development of the Kidney 217
Melissa Anslow and Jacqueline Ho

8 Disorders of Kidney Formation 257
Norman D. Rosenblum and Indra R. Gupta

Part III Ciliopathies

9 Ciliopathies: Their Role in Pediatric Kidney Disease 289
Miriam Schmidts and Philip L. Beales

vii

10 Polycystic Kidney Disease: ADPKD and ARPKD 317
Max Christoph Liebau, Djalila Mekahli, and Carsten Bergmann

11 Nephronophthisis and Autosomal Dominant Tubulointerstitial Kidney Disease (ADTKD) 349
Jens König and Heymut Omran

Part IV   Glomerular Disorders

12 Hematuria and Proteinuria 373
Hui-Kim Yap and Perry Yew-Weng Lau

13 Steroid Sensitive Nephrotic Syndrome 405
Elisabeth M. Hodson, Deirdre Hahn, Stephen I. Alexander, Nicole Graf, and Hugh McCarthy

14 Steroid Resistant Nephrotic Syndrome 443
Rasheed Gbadegesin, Keisha Gibson, and Kimberly Reidy

15 Hereditary Nephrotic Syndrome 471
Stefanie Weber

16 Alport Syndrome and Other Type IV Collagen Disorders 493
Michelle N. Rheault and Rachel Lennon

17 IgA Nephropathy 509
Rosanna Coppo and Licia Peruzzi

18 Membranous Nephropathy 531
Myda Khalid and Laurence H. Beck Jr

19 Postinfectious and Infectious Glomerulopathies 555
Velibor Tasic and Mignon McCulloch

20 Rapidly Progressive Glomerulonephritis 575
Shina Menon and Arvind Bagga

Part V   Complement Disorders

21 The Role of Complement in Kidney Disease 593
Michael Kirschfink and Christoph Licht

22 Atypical Hemolytic Uremic Syndrome 605
Michal Malina, Veronique Fremeaux-Bacchi, and Sally Johnson

23 C3 Glomerulopathies 641
Christoph Licht, Marina Vivarelli, Magdalena Riedl Khursigara, and Patrick D. Walker

Part VI   The Kidney and Systemic Disease

24   Postinfectious Hemolytic Uremic Syndrome 667
Martin Bitzan and Anne-Laure Lapeyraque

25   Renal Vasculitis in Children 707
Mojca Zajc Avramovič, Tadej Avčin, and Marina Vivarelli

26   Lupus Nephritis 737
Stephen D. Marks, Matko Marlais, and Kjell Tullus

**27   IgA Vasculitis Nephritis (Henoch-Schönlein
Purpura Nephritis)** 765
Jae Il Shin

28   Metabolic Disorders Affecting the Kidney 783
Aude Servais, Olivia Boyer, Myriam Dao,
and Friederike Hörster

29   Primary Hyperoxaluria 795
Bodo B. Beck, Cristina Martin-Higueras, and Bernd Hoppe

30   Cystinosis 821
Elena Levtchenko, Leo Monnens, and Aude Servais

31   The Kidney in Sickle Cell Disease 849
Jeffrey Lebensburger and Cristin Kaspar

32   Diabetic Kidney Disease 865
Allison B. Dart

33   Disordered Hemostasis and Renal Disorders 877
Sara Rodriguez-Lopez, Verna Yiu, Stephanie Carlin,
and Leonardo R. Brandão

Volume II

Part VII   Renal Tubular Disorders

**34   Differential Diagnosis and Management of Fluid,
Electrolyte and Acid-Base Disorders** 905
Giacomo D. Simonetti, Sebastiano A. G. Lava,
Gregorio P. Milani, and Mario G. Bianchetti

**35   Renal Fanconi Syndromes and Other Proximal
Tubular Disorders** 967
Detlef Bockenhauer and Robert Kleta

36   Bartter-, Gitelman-, and Related Syndromes 991
Siegfried Waldegger, Karl Peter Schlingmann,
and Martin Konrad

37   Disorders of Calcium and Magnesium Metabolism 1007
Karl Peter Schlingmann and Martin Konrad

38 Disorders of Phosphorus Metabolism 1047
Dieter Haffner and Siegfried Waldegger

39 Renal Tubular Acidosis 1071
R. Todd Alexander and Detlef Bockenhauer

40 Diabetes Insipidus 1095
Detlef Bockenhauer and Daniel G. Bichet

Part VIII Renal Neoplasia and Tubulointerstitial Disease

41 Pediatric Renal Tumors 1115
Kathryn S. Sutton and Andrew L. Hong

42 Tubulointerstitial Nephritis in Children 1141
Priya S. Verghese, Kera E. Luckritz, and Allison A. Eddy

Part IX Urinary Tract Disorders

43 Diagnosis and Management of Urinary Tract Infections 1171
Ian K. Hewitt and Giovanni Montini

44 Vesicoureteral Reflux 1193
Ranjiv Mathews, Tiffany L. Damm, and Sverker Hansson

45 Obstructive Uropathies 1211
Benedetta D. Chiodini, Khalid Ismaili, David A. Diamond,
and Michael P. Kurtz

46 Renal Calculi 1221
Larisa Kovacevic and Paul Goodyer

47 Voiding Disorders in Children 1245
Johan Vande Walle and Søren Rittig

Part X Hypertension

**48 Hypertension: Epidemiology, Evaluation, and
Blood Pressure Monitoring** 1283
Ian Macumber and Andrew M. South

49 Renovascular Hypertension in Children 1317
Agnes Trautmann and Kjell Tullus

50 Renal Hypertension: Etiology and Management 1337
Elke Wühl and Franz Schaefer

Part XI Acute Kidney Injury and Neonatal Nephrology

**51 Acute Kidney Injury: Pathophysiology,
Diagnosis and Prevention** 1365
Prasad Devarajan

52 Management of Pediatric Acute Kidney Injury 1413
Lyndsay A. Harshman, Patrick D. Brophy,
and Jordan M. Symons

53 Neonatal Kidney Dysfunction 1437
Isabella Guzzo, Stefano Picca, and David Askenazi

Part XII Chronic Kidney Disease

54 Demographics of CKD and ESRD in Children 1471
Julien Hogan and Karlijn J. van Stralen

**55 Progression of Chronic Kidney Disease and
Nephroprotective Therapy** 1483
Elke Wühl and Franz Schaefer

56 Growth and Puberty in Chronic Kidney Disease 1517
Dieter Haffner and Lesley Rees

57 Neurodevelopment in Chronic Kidney Disease 1553
Rebecca J. Johnson and Lyndsay A. Harshman

58 Nutritional Challenges in Pediatric Kidney Disease 1577
Rayna Levitt and Caitlin E. Carter

59 Anemia in Chronic Renal Disease 1603
Larry A. Greenbaum

**60 Disorders of Bone Mineral Metabolism in Chronic
Kidney Disease** 1631
Claus Peter Schmitt and Rukshana C. Shroff

**61 Cardiovascular Disease in Pediatric Chronic
Kidney Disease** 1669
Anke Doyon and Mark Mitsnefes

62 Ethical Issues in End Stage Kidney Disease 1703
Aaron Wightman and Michael Freeman

**63 Psychosocial Issues in Children with Chronic
Kidney Disease** 1719
Amy J. Kogon and Stephen R. Hooper

Part XIII Kidney Replacement Therapy

**64 Initiation of Kidney Replacement Therapy:
Strategic Choices and Preparation** 1747
Jérôme Harambat and Iona Madden

65 Management of Peritoneal Dialysis in Children 1769
Alicia M. Neu, Bradley A. Warady, and Franz Schaefer

66 Management of Hemodialysis in Children 1805
Daljit K. Hothi, Rukshana C. Shroff, and Benjamin Laskin

67 Immunosuppression in Pediatric Kidney Transplantation 1849
Burkhard Tönshoff, Anette Melk, and Britta Höcker

68 Non-Infectious Post-Transplant Complications: Disease Recurrence and Rejection 1887
Lyndsay A. Harshman, Sharon M. Bartosh, and Stephen D. Marks

69 Prevention and Treatment of Infectious Complications in Pediatric Renal Transplant Recipients 1919
Jodi M. Smith, Sarah J. Kizilbash, and Vikas R. Dharnidharka

70 Long-Term Outcome of Kidney Failure in Children 1937
Jaap W. Groothoff

Part XIV Drugs and Toxins

71 Drug Use, Dosing, and Toxicity in Kidney Disease 1965
Matthias Schwab, Simon U. Jaeger, and Guido Filler

72 Complementary Therapies for Renal Diseases 1987
Cecilia Bukutu and Sunita Vohra

73 Environmental Nephrotoxins 2019
Jie Ding and Ruth A. Etzel

Index 2039

Part I

Investigative Techniques in Pediatric Nephrology

Antenatal Assessment of Kidney Morphology and Function

1

Khalid Ismaili, Benedetta D. Chiodini, Marie Cassart, and Karim Khelif

Introduction

Due to high patient expectations and demand, obstetrical two-dimensional (2D) ultrasound (US) is now a routine component of the care of pregnant women in most Western countries. In Europe, three sonographic examinations are performed, one in each trimester [1]. In other countries, including the United States and Canada, only one second-mid-trimester examination is performed routinely, with first-trimester or third-trimester examinations performed in case of specific indications [2]. Assessment of the fetal genitourinary tract is part of every routine fetal US examination. Congenital abnormalities of the kidney and urinary tract (CAKUT) make up one of the largest groups of congenital anomalies amenable to neonatal care, affecting 0.2–2% of all newborns [1]. Moreover, dramatic changes have occurred in the management of these children, and nowadays, CAKUTs are mostly found in asymptomatic infants and the treatment applied is mainly preventive with a low rate of surgical procedures performed during the last decade [3]. Also, the antenatal detection and postnatal follow-up have brought new insights into the natural history of many CAKUTs [4, 5].

Fetal Imaging Methods

Ultrasound is the first line imaging technique used in antenatal diagnosis. It has now been nearly four decades since its first use to evaluate the fetus and it is presently accepted as a safe and noninvasive imaging modality. The transducers most commonly used are curvilinear sector transducers (3–8 MHz), which have good penetration of the sound beam and allow for a visualization of the whole fetus. Higher frequency linear transducers (5–10 MHz) or transvaginal probes are used to achieve high resolution scans in near fields. The transducers most frequently used in daily clinical practice are multifrequency probes which allow for harmonic, three-dimensional and Doppler flow imaging. *3D imaging* is mostly used for the study of the face and vertebral column [6], the other organs are well depicted by C

K. Ismaili (✉) · B. D. Chiodini
Department of Pediatric Nephrology, Hôpital Universitaire des Enfants—Reine Fabiola, Université Libre de Bruxelles, Brussels, Belgium
e-mail: khalid.ismaili@huderf.be; benedetta.chiodini@huderf.be

M. Cassart
Department of Fetal and Pediatric Imaging, Ixelles Hospital—Iris South, Brussels, Belgium
e-mail: mcassart@his-izz.be

K. Khelif
Department of Pediatric Urology, Hôpital Universitaire des Enfants—Reine Fabiola, Université Libre de Bruxelles, Brussels, Belgium
e-mail: karim.khelif@huderf.be

© The Author(s), under exclusive license to Springer Nature Switzerland AG 2023
F. Schaefer, L. A. Greenbaum (eds.), *Pediatric Kidney Disease*,
https://doi.org/10.1007/978-3-031-11665-0_1

imaging. Hence, 3D imaging is currently not routinely performed for urinary tract and kidney diseases. *Doppler imaging* is useful to evaluate the vascularization of the organs and the fetal well-being [2].

MR imaging of the fetus is a more recent technique. The examinations are performed on 1.5–3 T magnets. Although no deleterious effects on the fetus have been demonstrated to date [7], MR imaging is generally avoided during organogenesis in the first trimester. *MR imaging* is mostly performed in order to establish a more precise diagnosis where US cannot completely depict the suspected malformation or anomaly. The advantages of MR imaging are the larger field of view and the better contrast resolution which allow for a better characterization of the anatomy of the organs. The indications mostly concern the brain but it is presently extended to the fetal digestive and urinary tracts in specific indications [8]. Depending on local practice, sedation can be given to the mother before the examination to reduce fetal movement. Contrast media are not currently used due to the lack of data concerning potential side effects in pregnant women and fetuses [9]. Fast sequences (20 s) are performed in different planes and can be repeated in case of fetal movements. In urinary tract and kidney diseases the indications of fetal MR imaging are closely circumscribed; they will be illustrated in the next paragraphs.

The Normal Urinary Tract

Bladder

Urine starts to be produced during the ninth week of fetal life. At that time, the urine is collected in the bladder, which can be visualized as a fluid-filled structure within the fetal pelvis. During the second and third trimester, the fetus normally fills and partially or completely empties the bladder approximately every 25 min and the cycle can be monitored during the sonographic examination [10]. The bladder can easily be located by its outline of umbilical arteries, which are identifiable on color Doppler.

Kidneys

Endovaginal probes can be used to visualize fetal anatomic structures earlier than with transabdominal US. Thus, the fetal kidneys can be seen at around 11 weeks endovaginally and around 12–15 weeks with transabdominal probes. During the first trimester, the kidneys appear as hyperechoic oval structures at both sides of the spine (their hyperechogenicity can be compared with that of the liver or spleen) [11]. This echogenicity will progressively decrease and during the third trimester the cortical echogenicity will always be less than that of the liver or spleen. In parallel with the decrease of echogenicity, corticomedullary differentiation will appear at about 14–15 weeks. It should always be visible in fetuses older than 18 weeks (Fig. 1.1). Prominent pyramids should not be misinterpreted as calyceal dilatation.

Growth of the fetal kidneys can be evaluated throughout pregnancy. As a rule, a normal kidney grows at about 1.1 mm per week of gestation.

Evidence of Normally Functioning Urinary Tract

Besides visualization of the bladder and normal kidneys, assessment of the urinary tract should include an evaluation of the amniotic fluid volume. After 14–15 weeks, two thirds of the amniotic fluid is produced by fetal urination and one third by pulmonary fluid. A normal volume of

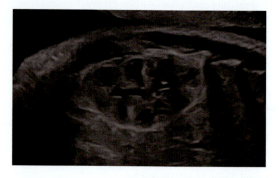

Fig. 1.1 Normal third trimester fetal kidney. Sagittal US scan of the kidney with clear visibility of the corticomedullary differentiation

amniotic fluid is required for the proper development of the fetal lungs. This can be confirmed by measuring thoracic diameters or thoracic circumference [12].

Ultrasound Findings as Evidence of Abnormal Fetal Kidney and Urinary Tract

Abnormal US appearance of the kidneys as a pathophysiological base of CAKUT have been described extensively [13, 14]. Anomalies of the urinary system detected in utero are numerous; they can include anomalies of the kidney itself, of the collecting system, of the bladder and of the urethra. In addition, they can be isolated or in association with other systems. Therefore, the sonographic examination should be as meticulous as possible in order to visualize the associated features. These findings, among others, will determine the prognosis.

Abnormal Renal Number

Renal agenesis refers to the complete absence of one or both kidneys without identifiable rudimentary tissue [15].

Bilateral renal agenesis is part of Potter's syndrome and is incompatible with extrauterine life. The diagnosis is based on the absence of renal structure and the presence of oligohydramnios after 15 weeks of gestation. Pulmonary hypoplasia is invariably associated and leads to death from respiratory failure soon after birth. In this context, enlarged globular adrenals should not be mistaken for kidneys [16]. The use of color Doppler may help demonstrate the absence of renal arteries and subsequently confirm the diagnosis [17].

Unilateral renal agenesis is more common (1 in 500 pregnancies), usually asymptomatic and incidentally detected. This situation usually has no significant consequence on postnatal life as long as the solitary kidney shows compensatory hypertrophy [18]. The pathogenesis of renal agenesis is mostly due to a failure of the formation of the metanephros. In addition, interruption in vascular supply and regression of a multicystic dysplastic kidney (MCDK) may also lead to renal agenesis in the fetal period [19]. An investigation after birth is necessary to confirm the status of the remnant kidney and to look for possible associated anomalies such as hearing deficits, ear pits, coloboma, cleft lip or palate, single umbilical artery, syndactyly, microphallus, cryptorchidism, duplicated Mullerian structures, and ectopic ureteral insertion [18, 20]. In the long term, blood pressure and urinalysis should be monitored, in order to detect high blood pressure and/or microalbuminuria due to compensatory glomerular hyperfiltration. Children with congenital injury to the solitary kidney are at higher risk of adverse outcome, with a median time to chronic kidney disease of 14.8 years [21].

Abnormal Location of Kidney

Ectopic kidney, especially in the pelvic area, is part of the differential diagnosis of the "empty renal fossa" in the fetus and may represent 42% of these cases [18]. The diagnosis of horseshoe or crossed fused kidneys can also be assessed in utero through the demonstration of renal parenchyme crossing the midline in horseshoe kidney (Fig. 1.2) or attached to the lower pole of the normally positioned contralateral kidney, i.e. crossed fused renal ectopia [22]. An ectopic kidney is usually small and somewhat malrotated with numerous small blood vessels and associated ureteric anomalies. Ectopic kidneys may be asymptomatic, but complications such as ureteral obstruction, infection, and calculi are common [23]. Therefore, at birth, the anomaly has to be confirmed by US or by MRI and a voiding cystourethrography (VCUG) may be useful in complex cases.

Abnormal Renal Echogenicity

Hyperechogenicity of the fetal kidney is defined by comparison with the adjacent liver or spleen. This is difficult to assess in the first and second

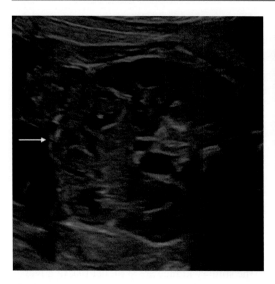

Fig. 1.2 Horseshoe kidney. Axial US scan on the fetal abdomen showing the parenchymal bridge crossing the midline (arrow)

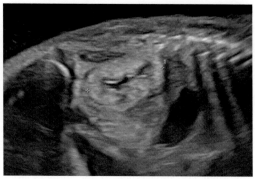

Fig. 1.3 Hyperechoic undifferentiated kidney. Sagittal US scan of the left kidney of a fetus with post natal diagnosis of nephrocalcinosis

trimester as the kidney is "physiologically" hyperechoic (or isoechoic at the end of the second trimester). It is easier to characterize after 28–32 weeks as the renal cortex by that time should be hypoechoic compared to the liver and spleen [11]. Increased echogenicity of the renal parenchyma is nonspecific and occurs as a response to different changes in renal tissue [24]. Interstitial infiltration, sclerosis and multiple microscopic cortical and medullary cysts may account for hyperechogenicity even in the absence of macrocysts. The detection of hyperechoic kidneys represents a difficult diagnostic challenge and generates significant parental anxiety due to the uncertain prognosis [25, 26]. The differential diagnosis must be based on kidney size, corticomedullary differentiation, the presence of macrocysts, the degree of dilatation of the collecting system and the amount of amniotic fluid [27]. The diagnosis must also take into account the familial history, the presence of associated anomalies and/or aberrant karyotype and genetic diseases [25]. Metabolic disorders should also be added to the long list of causes of hyperechoic kidneys in children (Fig. 1.3): tyrosinemia, galactosemia, fructosemia, mitochondrial disorders, glutaric aciduria, carnitine palmitoyltransferase II deficiency, congenital disorders of glycosylation, and peroxisomal disorders can all be accompanied by hyperechoic kidneys [28].

So far, the outcome of fetal hyperechoic kidneys can only be accurately predicted in severe cases with significant oligohydramnios [26, 27]. For some patients, the characteristic US patterns will appear after birth or even later. A follow-up is therefore mandatory. It should be stressed that some cases remain unsolved and have to be considered as normal variants [25, 27]. Table 1.1 provides information on the spectrum of renal disorders associated with fetal hyperechoic kidneys.

Abnormal Renal Size

Measurements of the kidneys must be systematic whenever an anomaly of the urinary tract or amniotic fluid volume is suspected. It is therefore important to have standards for renal size and volume measurements covering the complete gestational age range, because renal pathology often presents late in pregnancy [31]. Small kidneys most often correspond to hypodysplasia or damaged kidneys from obstructive uropathy or high-grade vesicoureteral reflux (VUR) [32, 33]. Enlarged kidneys may be related to urinary tract dilatation, renal cystic diseases or tumoral involvement.

1 Antenatal Assessment of Kidney Morphology and Function

Table 1.1 Conditions associated with hyperechoic kidneys on prenatal ultrasound

	Kidney size	Amniotic fluid volume	Renal cysts	Collecting system	Associated abnormalities	Inheritance	Alternative prenatal diagnosis
Obstruction	−2 to 0 SD	Normal or reduced	Cortical <1 cm	Dilated	No	Sporadic	MRI
Renal vein thrombosis	0 to 2 SD	Normal	No	Not seen	Thrombus in the inferior vena cava	Sporadic	Doppler
ARPKD	2 to 4 SD	Reduced	Small medullary	Not seen	Lung hypoplasia	AR	Genetics
ADPKD	0 to 2 SD	Normal or reduced	Subcapsular and medullar	Not seen	No	AD	Genetics
Glomerulocystic dysplasia	0 to 2 SD	Variable	Small cortical	Not seen	Variable if syndromic	Variable	Genetics (*HNF1B/TCF2*)
Bardet-Biedl syndrome	2 to 4 SD	Variable	No or medullary	Not seen	Polydactyly	AR	Genetics
Beckwith-Wiedeman syndrome	2 SD	Normal or increased	No or medullary	±	Macrosome, omphalocele	AD or dysomy	Genetics
Perlman syndrome	2 SD	Normal or reduced	No	±	Macrosome	AR	–
Infantile Hypercalcemia [29]	0 SD	Normal	No	Not seen	No	AR	Genetics SLC34A1
17q12 microdeletion syndrome [30]	Enlarged	Reduced or elevated	No or multicystic	Not seen	No	Sporadic	Microarray CGH
Normal variant	0 to 2 SD	Normal or increased	No	±	No	Sporadic	–

ARPKD autosomal recessive polycystic kidney disease, *ADPKD* autosomal dominant polycystic kidney disease, *AD* autosomal dominant, *AR* autosomal recessive, *MRI* magnetic resonance imaging, *HNF-1β* hepatocyte nuclear factor-1β

Urinary Tract Dilatation

Fetal renal pelvis dilatation is a frequent abnormality that has been observed in 4.5% of pregnancies [34]. Pyelectasis is defined as dilatation of the renal pelvis whereas pelvicaliectasis and hydronephrosis include dilatation of calyces. In practice, these terms are interchanged and used as descriptions of a dilated renal collecting system regardless of the etiology [35].

The third-trimester threshold value for the anteroposterior (AP) renal pelvis diameter of 7 mm is certainly the best prenatal criterion both for the screening of urinary tract dilatation and for the selection of patients needing postnatal investigation [35, 36].

There are several theories that account for the visibility of the renal pelvis during pregnancy. The distension of the urinary collecting system may be simply a dynamic and physiologic process [37]. The size of the fetal renal collecting system is highly variable over a 2-h period [38]. The tendency of renal pelvis dilatation to resolve spontaneously is supported by normal postnatal renal appearances reported in 36–80% of cases followed up after birth [39, 40]. However, prenatally detected renal pelvis dilatation may be an indicator of significant urinary tract pathologies [41]. The likelihood of having a clinically significant uropathy is directly proportional to the severity of the hydronephrosis [35]. A summary of the literature describing the postnatal uronephropathies found in neonates who presented with fetal renal pelvis dilatation is given in Table 1.2. The incidence and type of pathology varies considerably between studies, reflecting the differences in prenatal criteria and the variability in postnatal assessment. The two main pathologies found are pelviureteric junction stenosis and VUR. US is the first examination to perform after birth [46]. In babies diagnosed in utero with renal pelvis dilatation, the presence of persistent renal pelvis dilatation or other ultrasonographic abnormalities (such as calyceal or ureteral dilatation, pelvic or ureteral wall thickening and absence of the corticomedullary differentiation) and signs of renal dysplasia (such as small kidney, thinned or hyperechoic cortex or cortical cysts) should determine the need for further investigations [47, 48]. In cases when the urinary tract appears normal on neonatal US examinations, no further evaluation is needed [39]. Based on our own experience [34, 39, 49, 50], we propose an algorithm for a rational postnatal imaging strategy (Fig. 1.4). Using this algorithm, we found that very few abnormal cases escaped the work up and that the risk of complications was very low.

Renal Cysts

Renal cystic diseases should be suspected not only in the case of obvious macrocysts but also in the case of hyperechoic kidneys [51]. Cysts may be present in one or both kidneys. Their origin may be genetic, and they may occur as an isolated anomaly or part of a syndrome. Familial history is of a great importance for the diagnosis [51].

Obstructive renal dysplasia and MCDK are the most common entities in which macrocysts can be detected. Obstructive renal dysplasia is associated with urinary tract obstruction that may have resolved at the time of diagnosis, leaving the cystic sequelae behind as the unique evidence that a urinary flow impairment ever existed [11]. In this condition, the cysts measure less than 1 cm and are located within the hyperechoic cortex (Fig. 1.5) [51]. MCDK is discussed further under Renal Causes of Fetal Renal Abnormalities in this chapter. Although rare, isolated cortical cysts may be seen in utero. They may persist after birth or regress spontaneously [52].

The most frequent genetically transmitted cystic renal diseases are the autosomal dominant polycystic kidney diseases and abnormalities of the hepatocyte nuclear factor-1β (HNF1B) encoded by the *TCF2* gene [53]. HNF1B diseases are typically associated with bilateral cortical renal microcysts as well as other renal parenchymal abnormalities including MCDK and renal dysplasia [53]. HNF1B plays an important role in the early phases of kidney development [54]. Both the type and the severity of the renal disease are variable in children with HNF1B mutations. Their

Table 1.2 Incidence of uro-nephropathies in neonates with antenatally diagnosed renal pelvis dilatation

Authors	Year	Threshold value of renal pelvis (mm)	Total	Abnormal (%)	UPJS (%)	VUR (%)	Megaureter (%)	Mild dilatation (%)	Duplex kidney (%)	Other (%)	(%) Undergoing surgery
Dudley [42]	1997	5	100	64	3	12	3	43	4	7	3
Jaswon [43]	1999	5	104	45	4	22		8		4	1
Ismaili et al. [39]	2004	4–7	213	39	13	11	7	18[a]	5	3	3
Bouzada [44]	2004	5	100	57	30	2	2		1		11
Vasconcelos [45]	2019	5	624		18	8	6	40	3		26

UPJS uretero-pelvic junction stenosis, *VUR* vesicoureteral reflux

[a] In this study mild and transient dilatations were considered as non-significant findings

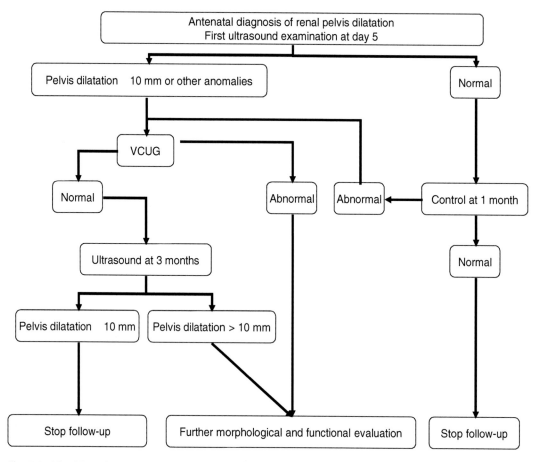

Fig. 1.4 Algorithm of a rational postnatal imaging strategy in infants with fetal renal pelvis dilatation

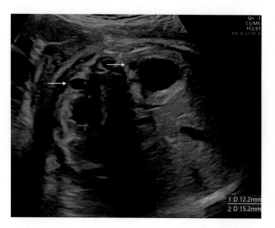

Fig. 1.5 Bilateral obstructive cystic nephropathy. Axial slice on the dilated renal pelvis with hyperechoic and cystic parenchyma (arrows)

range from severe prenatal renal failure to normal renal function in adulthood. There is no obvious correlation between the type of mutation and the type and/or severity of renal disease. Furthermore, the inter- and intrafamilial variability of the phenotype in patients who harbor the same mutation is high, making genetic counseling particularly difficult in these families [55]. Cystic kidneys are also part of many syndromes (Tables 1.1 and 1.3) with many associated anomalies that are sometimes typical of the underlying pathology.

Renal Tumors

Fetal renal tumors occur only rarely. Mesoblastic nephroma represents the most common congenital renal neoplasm [65]. It is a solitary hamartoma with a usually benign course. Mesoblastic nephroma appears as a large, solitary, predominantly solid, retroperitoneal mass arising and not

1 Antenatal Assessment of Kidney Morphology and Function

Table 1.3 Syndromes with cystic renal disease

	Renal cysts	Associated abnormalities	Inheritance	Reference
Meckel-Gruber syndrome	Medullary	Encephalocele, brain/cardiac anomalies, hepatic ductal dysplasia, cleft lip/palate, polydactyly	AR	[56]
Trisomy 9	Medullary	Mental retardation, intrauterine growth retardation, cardiac anomalies, joint contractures, prominent nose, sloping forehead	Chromosomal	[57]
Trisomy 13	Medullary	Mental retardation, intrauterine growth retardation, cardiac anomalies, cleft lip/palate, polydactyly	Chromosomal	[57]
Trisomy 18	Medullary	Mental retardation, intrauterine growth retardation, cardiac anomalies, small face, micrognathia, overlapping digits	Chromosomal	[57]
Bardet-Biedl syndrome	No or medullary	Polysyndactyly, obesity, mental retardation, pigmented retinopathy, hypogonadism	AR	[58]
Zellweger syndrome	Medullary	Hypotonia, seizures, failure to thrive, distinctive face, hepatosplenomegaly	AR	[59]
Ivemark syndrome	No or medullary	Polysplenia, complex heart disease, midline anomalies, situs inversus	Sporadic, AR	[60]
Beckwith-Wiedeman syndrome	Medullary	Overgrowth, macroglossia, omphalocele, hepatoblastoma, Wilm's tumor	Sporadic, AD	[61]
Jeune's syndrome	Medullary	Narrow chest, short limbs, polydactyly, periglomerular fibrosis	AR	[62]
Tuberous sclerosis	Medullary	Mental retardation, seizures, facial angiofibroma, angiomyolipoma, hypopigmented spots, cardiac rhabdomyomas, cerebral hamartomas	AD	[63]
Alagille syndrome	Renal dysplasia with or without cysts	Cholestasis, peripheral pulmonic stenosis, characteristic face	AD	[64]

AD autosomal dominant, *AR* autosomal recessive

separable from the adjacent kidney. It does not have a well-defined capsule and may sometimes appear as a partially cystic tumor [11]. In case of a tumor with multiple cysts, a MCDK should be considered first. Mesoblastic nephroma frequently coexists with polyhydramnios although the reason for this association remains unclear [65]. Fetal Wilm's tumor is exceptionally rare and may be indistinguishable from mesoblastic nephroma on imaging [66]. Another differential diagnosis is nephroblastomatosis, which appears either as hyperechoic nodule(s) or as a diffusely enlarged hyperechoic kidney [67]. Renal tumors have to be differentiated from adrenal tumors and intra-abdominal sequestrations [68].

Bladder Abnormalities

On fetal US examinations, the bladder should always be seen from the tenth week of gestation.

Nonvisualization of the bladder in the setting of oligohydramnios is highly suspicious of a bilateral severe renal abnormality with decreased urine production. It is important to carefully analyze the kidneys in order to exclude agenesis or dysplasia associated with poor outcome.

Nonvisualization of the bladder with an otherwise normal sonogram (kidneys and amniotic fluid) may be due to physiologic bladder emptying cycle in the fetus. Normal repletion should be checked within the following 20 min. Persistent non visualized bladder can be due to its inability to store urine, for example in cases of bladder or cloacal extrophy [69]. In this context, no bladder is seen between the two umbilical arteries. Bladder extrophy or cloacal malformations represent a diagnostic challenge on US, and MRI may help to define the pelvic anatomy of the fetus [70].

Enlarged bladder in the first trimester has a poor prognosis. Most of the cases are secondary to urethral atresia or stenosis, some are part of a syndrome (such as Prune Belly), or associated with chromosomal anomalies. Later in pregnancy, megabladder is defined as a cephalo-caudal diameter superior to 3 cm in the second trimester and to 5 cm in the third trimester. Megabladders are mainly due to outflow obstruction or to a major bilateral reflux [71]. It is often difficult to make a clear distinction between both abnormalities, as they may be associated. An irregular and thickened bladder wall is suggestive of an outflow obstruction. Megacystis-microcolon hypoperistalsis (MMH) syndrome is another differential diagnosis that carries a very poor prognosis [72]. It can be excluded by MRI during the third trimester because the colon is well visualized at that time.

Assessment of Fetal Renal Function

In utero, excretion of nitrogenous waste products and regulation of fetal fluid and electrolytes balance as well as acid-base homeostasis are maintained by the interaction of the placenta and maternal blood [73]. Thus, the placenta functions as an in vivo dialysis unit. Several parameters have been used in the evaluation of renal function in fetal life. However, since fetal homeostasis depends on the integrity of the placenta, it is very difficult to assess the functional status of the fetal kidney. Furthermore, changes in the volume or composition of fetal urine may in many instances reflect the condition of the placenta rather than the condition of the fetal kidney [74]. However, exact diagnosis of the renal abnormalities and accurate prediction of the renal function after birth are important tasks, because during parental counseling parents often want to know if their child will have renal failure and whether or not surgery or other aggressive therapies will be performed. Therefore, in addition to using fetal renal sonography to determine potential fetal renal anatomical abnormalities, it is important to assess function as accurately as possible.

Amniotic Fluid Volume

During the first trimester of gestation the placenta (chorion and amniotic membrane) is the principal source of amniotic fluid, while after 15 weeks the volume of amniotic fluid is maintained by fetal urine production. Therefore, the assessment of the quantity of amniotic fluid after 15 weeks constitutes the initial step in the evaluation of the fetal urinary tract. Abnormal amounts of amniotic fluid must alert the sonographer to search meticulously for renal and urinary tract anomalies [75]. Assessing amniotic fluid volume is difficult and mostly subjective. However, the four-quadrant sum of amniotic fluid pockets (amniotic fluid index) provides a reproducible method for assessing amniotic fluid volume with interobserver and intraobserver variation of 3–7% [76].

Various cut-off criteria have been suggested for definition of oligohydramnios by amniotic fluid index, including less than 3rd percentile [77], or 5th percentile for gestational age [76]. Oligohydramnios of any cause typically compresses and twists the fetus, thus leading to a recurrent pattern of abnormalities that has been called the oligohydramnios sequence [12]. Oligohydramnios may be caused by decreased production of fetal urine from bilateral renal agenesis or dysplasia, or by reduced egress of urine into the amniotic fluid due to urinary obstruction [78]. Other causes may be fetal death, growth retardation, rupture of the membranes, or post-term gestation (Table 1.4).

In cases of bilateral obstructive uropathy, the evaluation of amniotic fluid by the amniotic fluid index seems to be the most reproducible and inexpensive method to predict renal function after birth [79]. An amniotic fluid index less than the 5th percentile is generally associated with an adverse perinatal outcome [76, 79]. Yet, an amniotic fluid index between the 5th and 25th percentiles should be considered as a warning sign since it may be a subtle indication of renal impairment, especially early in gestation when ultrasonographic signs of renal dysplasia may not be present and when fetal urinalysis is not available [79].

Table 1.4 Causes of oligohydramnios and polyhydramnios

	Origin	Pathologies
Oligohydramnios	Uronephropathy	Bilateral renal agenesis
		Bilateral renal dysplasia
		Autosomal recessive polycystic kidney disease
		Bilateral obstructive uropathy
		Bilateral high-grade reflux
		Bladder outlet obstruction
	Other	Premature rupture of membranes
		Placental insufficiency
		Fetal death
		Fetal growth retardation
		Twin-to-twin transfusion (twin donor)
		Maternal drug intake: prostaglandin synthase inhibitors, angiotensin-converting enzyme inhibitors, cocaine
		Postmaturity syndrome
Polyhydramnios	Uronephropathy	Renal tumors, especially mesoblastic nephroma
		Bartter syndrome
		Congenital nephrotic syndrome
		Alloimmune glomerulonephritis
	Other	Maternal diabetes
		Maternal drug intake: lithium
		Multiple gestations
		Twin-to-twin transfusion (twin recipient)
		Fetal infections: rubella, cytomegalovirus, toxoplasmosis
		Fetal gastrointestinal obstructions: esophageal atresia, duodenal atresia, gastroschisis
		Fetal compressive pulmonary disorders: diaphragmatic hernia, pleural effusions, cystic adenomatoid malformations, narrow thoracic cage
		Neuro-muscular conditions: anencephaly, myotonic dystrophy
		Cardiac anomalies
		Hematologic anomalies (fetal anemia)
		Hydrops fetalis
		Fetal chromosome abnormalities: trisomy 21, trisomy 18, trisomy 13
		Syndromic conditions: Beckwith-Wiedeman syndrome, achondroplasia
		No evident cause

Finally, one of the most devastating consequences of oligohydramnios, especially before 24 week's gestation, is pulmonary hypoplasia [80]. Traditional explanations suggest that oligohydramnios causes pulmonary hypoplasia either by compression of the fetal thorax [80] or by encouraging lung liquid loss via the trachea [81]. However, since several morphogenetic pathways governing renal development are shared with lung organogenesis, this sequence is put into question. Some reports suggest that abnormal lung dysplasia may precede the advent of oligohydramnios in fetuses with intrinsic defects of renal parenchymal development [82].

Polyhydramnios, also referred to as hydramnios, is defined as a high level of amniotic fluid. Because the normal values for amniotic fluid volumes increase during pregnancy, this definition will depend on the gestational age of the fetus. During the last 2 months of pregnancy, polyhydramnios usually refers to amniotic fluid volumes greater than 1700–1900 mL. Severe cases are associated with much greater fluid volume excesses. The two major causes of polyhydramnios are reduced fetal swallowing or absorption of amniotic fluid and increased fetal urination (Table 1.4). Increased fetal urination is typically observed in maternal diabetes mellitus, but it may be associated with fetal renal diseases as mesoblastic nephroma [65], Bartter syndrome [83], congenital nephrotic syndrome [84] and alloimmune glomerulonephritis [85].

Fetal Urine Biochemical Markers

The healthy fetus produces hypotonic urine. In case of kidney damage, proximal tubular function is harmed and urine osmolality increases. Fetal urine biochemistry was first introduced four decades ago as an additional test to improve prediction of renal function after birth [86]. Thereafter, investigators started to establish gestational age-dependent reference ranges for various biochemical parameters of fetal urine [87]. Rapidly, two important pitfalls emerged in this area of research. Initially, biochemical markers were analyzed either from amniotic fluid or bladder sampling based on the debatable assumption that both liquids have nearly identical composition. Subsequently, a practice has emerged whereby reference ranges are only taken from bladder or fetal urinary tract sampling. The second pitfall involved the pertinence of the use of urinary solutes that are filtered by the glomerulus and reabsorbed by the tubules. These solutes express a tubular damage rather than a compromised GFR and it is therefore questionable if they can accurately predict renal function.

Fetal urine biochemistry is currently used especially in dilated uropathies because of technical difficulties of sampling fetal urines from a nondilated urinary tract, as seen in the majority of nephropathies. β2-microglobulin is the most widely used fetal urinary marker, although other compounds such as calcium, chloride and sodium may also be of interest; prognostic values of these markers are outlined in Table 1.5. Most fetal urine studies agree on some points [88, 89]: (1) fetuses with renal damage (dysplasia) show increased urinary solute concentrations; (2) a combination of β2-microglobulin and cystatin C or chloride exhibits better accuracy than the measurement of any single electrolyte; (3) the predictive accuracy of the proposed parameters is, however, far from perfect.

Novel approaches to fetal urine biochemistry such as proteomics and metabolomics may yield novel markers that may improve the usefulness of this technique in the near future [95]. The ongoing European ANTENATAL study was designed to validate a fetal urine peptide signature proposed by Buffin-Meyer in order to predict postnatal renal function in fetuses with posterior urethral valves [96, 97]. The final results are expected in 2023.

Fetal Blood Sampling

Fetal blood sampling poses probably greater risks than urine sampling, but it allows a more accurate evaluation of fetal glomerular filtration rate (GFR) [94, 98, 99]. In the fetus, creatinine cannot be used as a marker of GFR because it crosses the placenta and is cleared by the mother. This is not the case for α1-microglobulin, β2-microglobulin and cystatin C, which have been used to predict renal function in uropathies and nephropathies (Table 1.6). This technique may be helpful, especially in cases where fetal urine is difficult to sample. It is however unlikely that fetal serum

Table 1.5 Fetal urine biochemical markers of postnatal prognosis

	Normal limits [90]	Good prognosis [91–93]	Moderate renal failure at age 1 year [94]	Poor prognosis (neonatal death or termination of pregnancy) [92–94]
Na⁺	75–100 mmol/L	<100 mmol/L	59 mmol/L (54–65)	121 mmol/L (100–140)
Ca²⁺	2 mmol/L		2 mmol/L (1.5–2.5)	2 mmol/L (1.5–2.5)
Cl⁻		<90 mmol/L	57 mmol/L (52–62)	98 mmol/L (85–111)
β2 microglobulin	<4 mg/L	<6 mg/L	6.8 mg/L (4.2–9.4)	19.5 mg/L (11–28)
Cystatin C		<1 mg/L	0.47 mg/L (0.05–4.75)	4.1 mg/L (0.45–13.1)
Protein		0.22 g/L (0.09–0.97)		0.28 g/L (0.06–13.5)
Osmolarity	<200 mOsm/L	<210 mOsm/L		

1 Antenatal Assessment of Kidney Morphology and Function

Table 1.6 Fetal serum biochemical markers of postnatal prognosis

	Controls [98]	Bilateral hypoplasia and dysplasia [99]	Bilateral uropathies [100]
Outcome		Good prognosis	Postnatal renal failure
β2-microglobulin	4.28 mg/L (2.95–6.61)	3.2 mg/L (1.5–3.7)	5.3 mg/L (3.5–7.2)
Cystatin C	1.67 mg/L (1.12–2.06)	1.43 mg/L (1.09–1.86)	1.95 mg/L (1.56–4.60)
α1-microglobulin			60.5 mg/L (31.8–90.1)

α1-microglobulin, β2-microglobulin and cystatin C will overcome the limitations associated with fetal urinalysis [98]. The only clinical useful information emerging from the studies performed to date is that fetal serum β2-microglobulin remains the best marker of renal function; however its helpfulness is questionable outside extreme values (less than 3.5 mg/L good outcome; more than 5 mg/L poor outcome) [100].

Ultrasound-Guided Renal Biopsies

Ultrasound-guided renal biopsy would theoretically allow precise definition of the extent of renal damage in obstructed and primarily dysplastic kidneys [101]. However, this is an invasive procedure with a high rate of failure in obtaining an adequate sample [94]. Furthermore, a focal needle aspiration is not representative of the whole kidney parenchyma since renal dysplasia is patchily distributed.

Specific Renal and Urinary Tract Pathologies

Causes of fetal abnormalities of the kidney and urinary tract may be considered as prerenal, renal and postrenal.

Pre-renal Causes of Fetal Renal Abnormalities

Intrauterine Growth Restriction (IUGR)

Intrauterine growth restriction (IUGR) complicates up to 10% of all pregnancies. It is associated with a perinatal mortality rate that is six to ten times higher when compared to normally grown fetuses and is the second most important cause of perinatal death after preterm delivery. The cause of IUGR is multifactorial. Worldwide, maternal nutritional deficiencies and inadequate utero-placental perfusion are among the most common causes of IUGR.

IUGR caused by placental insufficiency is often associated with oligohydramnios due to reduced urine production rate in these fetuses. This phenomenon is probably due to chronic hypoxemia that leads to the brain-sparing redistribution of oxygenated blood away from non-vital peripheral organs such as the kidneys [73]. As a consequence, fetal renal medullary hyperechogenicity may develop between the 24th and the 37th weeks of gestation due to tubular blockage caused by Tamm-Horsfall protein precipitation, and may be a sign of hypoxic renal insufficiency [102]. IUGR complicated by renal medullary hyperechogenicity suggests a more serious state, because these fetuses have a higher risk of pathological postnatal clinical outcome, such as neonatal mortality (8%), fetal distress leading to cesarean section (36%), transfer to intensive care unit (64%), and perinatal infection (24%) [102]. IUGR not only leads to a low birth weight but it might also reprogram nephrogenesis, which results in a low nephron endowment. According to the hyperfiltration hypothesis, this reduction in renal mass is supposed to lead to glomerular hyperfiltration and hypertension in remnant nephrons with subsequent glomerular injury with proteinuria, systemic hypertension and glomerulosclerosis in adult age [103].

Renal Vein Thrombosis

Renal vein thrombosis is the most common vascular condition in the newborn kidney and represents 0.5/1000 of admissions to neonatal intensive care units [104]. Factors predisposing a neonate to renal vein thrombosis include dehydration, sepsis, birth asphyxia, maternal diabetes, polycythemia and the presence of indwelling umbilical venous catheter [104]. In addition, prothrombotic abnormalities may be present in more than 40% of these babies, such as Protein C or S deficiency, Factor V Leiden mutation, Lupus anticoagulant and Antithrombin III deficiency [105].

Renal vein thrombosis may also occur in utero. However, the origin of the thrombosis is not always obvious. Sonographically, the fetal kidney appears somewhat enlarged; the cortex may appear hyperechoic and without corticomedullary differentiation (Fig. 1.6a). Pathognomonic vascular streaks may be visible in the interlobar areas. Thrombus in the inferior vena cava is a common association [11]. Color Doppler US may be used in addition to grey-scale examination in the assessment of renal vein thrombosis. In the early stages of renal vein thrombosis, intrarenal and renal venous flow and pulsatility may be absent and renal arterial diastolic flow may be decreased, with a raised resistive index. Collateral vessels develop very rapidly (Fig. 1.6b) and in most cases there are no consequences on further renal development [106]. After birth, the hyperechoic streaks and the thrombus are calcified. This feature helps differentiate antenatal from postnatal onset of the renal vein thrombosis [106].

The Twin-To-Twin Transfusion Syndrome

The twin-to-twin transfusion syndrome complicates 10–15% of monochorionic twin pregnancies [107]. The etiology of this condition is thought to result from an unbalanced fetal blood supply through the placental vascular shunts, with the larger twin being the recipient and the smaller twin the donor [108]. The twin-to-twin transfusion syndrome is defined by the existence of a oligo-polyhydramnios sequence (that is, the deepest vertical pool being 2 cm or less in the donor's sac and 8 cm or more in the recipient's sac) [107]. Additional phenotypic features in the donor include a small or nonvisible bladder and abnormal umbilical artery Doppler with absent or reverse end-diastolic frequencies. In addition to the neonatal complications of growth restriction, up to 30% of donors have renal failure and/or renal tubular dysgenesis due to the chronic renal hypoperfusion state in utero [107]. In the recipient, confirmatory features include large bladder, cardiac hypertrophy and eventually hydrops. Risk of renal failure in the recipient twin is considerably smaller than in the donor twin. This can be seen as one fetus dying and vascular resistance dropping significantly to cause reversed blood transfusion from the recipient twin to the dead fetus, resulting in hypovolemia and anemia in the live fetus [109].

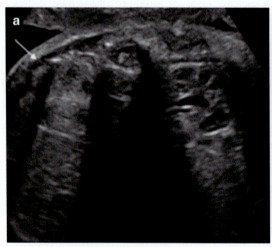
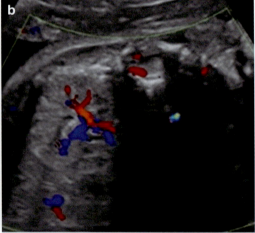

Fig. 1.6 Right renal vein thrombosis. (**a**) Axial US scan showing differences of size and echogenicity of both kidneys. The right kidney is enlarged and hyperechoic (arrow). (**b**) Axial US scan showing normal renal arterial and venous flow on the right kidney attesting of rapid revascularisation

Maternal Alcohol/Drug Intake

Mother's alcohol and/or drug consumption can in certain cases affect fetal kidney function or cause congenital kidney anomalies.

Alcohol

Based on both animal and human studies, it has been suggested that children with fetal alcohol syndrome (FAS) should be screened for renal anomalies [110]. The kidneys of children exposed prenatally to ethanol (with or without FAS) were smaller as compared to children with no evidence of alcohol exposure in utero [110]. Recent studies from Portugal have found an association between alcohol consumption during pregnancy and a decreased kidney function later in childhood, especially in overweight school-children [111].

Renin-Angiotensin System (RAS) Antagonists

Administration of angiotensin converting enzyme inhibitors (ACEIs) and angiotensin type I receptor blockers (ARBs) can severely affect renal development and function at any gestational age. RAS inhibitors lead to tubular dysgenesis, oligohydramnios, growth restriction, neonatal anuria and stillbirth [112–115]. In one study almost 9% of children exposed to ACEIs during the first trimester (but not later in pregnancy) showed major congenital anomalies (cardiovascular, central nervous system and renal malformations) at a rate 2.7 times that among unexposed infants [113]. The renal anomalies are thought to be caused both directly by antagonism of the fetal intrarenal renin-angiotensin system and indirectly by fetoplacental ischemia resulting from maternal hypotension and a drop of fetal-placental blood flow [73]. Pregnancies exposed to RAS blockers and complicated by oligohydramnios are associated with the highest rate of adverse pregnancy outcomes. Combined monitoring of amniotic fluid volume evaluation and fetal serum β2-microglobulin may be helpful in the management of these pregnancies [116].

Nonsteroidal Antiinflammatory Drugs (NSAID)

Cyclooxygenase type 1 (COX-1) inhibitors such as indomethacin, the most common NSAID used as a tocolytic, definitely reduce urine output and may lead to oligohydramnios and renal dysfunction [73]. It was hoped that cyclooxygenase type 2 (COX-2) inhibitors would target COX-2 activity and potentially spare COX-1-specific fetal side effects. However, COX-2 expression is higher in fetal as compared to adult kidneys and may even occur constitutively in fetal kidney tissue [73]. Sulindac and nimesulide administration has therefore been linked both to constriction of the ductus arteriosus and oligohydramnios [117].

Cocaine

Maternal cocaine use adversely influences fetal renal function by hypoperfusion and thus influences the fetal renin-angiotensin system. It is also associated with oligohydramnios as well as other fetal vascular complications leading to higher renal artery resistance index and a significant decrease in urine output [118]. However, and contradicting a widely held belief [119], a prospective, large-scale, blinded, systematic evaluation for congenital anomalies in prenatally cocaine-exposed children did not identify any increase in the number or consistent pattern of genitourinary tract malformations [120].

Immunosuppressive Medications During Pregnancy

Historically, physicians discouraged pregnancy in female kidney transplant recipients, due to concerns for maternal, graft, and fetal health [121]. Nevertheless, a large number of women with transplanted organs have completed pregnancies [122]. Although some immunosuppressants such as corticosteroids, cyclosporine and azathioprine have been shown to be teratogenic in animals, case reports and registry records have not identified any consistent malformation patterns in children of allograft recipients [123–126] (Table 1.7). On the contrary, the use of mycophenolate mofetil (MMF) during pregnancy has been

Table 1.7 In utero malformations caused by the exposure to immunosuppressive drugs used in kidney transplant recipients

Immunosuppressive drugs	Congenital malformations	References
Corticosteroids	In animals: increased risk of cleft palate. In humans: no increased prevalence of congenital malformations even at high doses.	[123]
Calcineurin inhibitors	In animals: skeletal retardation in cyclosporine exposure. In humans: no increased prevalence of congenital malformations.	[124, 125]
Azathioprine	In animals: various congenital malformations. In humans: safe in pregnant women.	[126]
Mycophenolic acid	In animals: wide range of teratogenic and fetotoxic effects; high miscarriage rate. In humans: congenital malformation prevalence of 26% (orofacial defects, hypoplastic nails, short fifth finger, corpus callosum agenesis, myelomeningocele, hydronephrosis, atrial septal defect, and tracheo-esophageal atresia).	[127–129]
Rapamicin inhibitors (mTOR)	In animals: high risk of intra-uterine growth retardation, impaired skeletal ossification, and miscarriage. In humans: few studies, no congenital malformations reported.	[130]
ATG	No data available	[131]
Basiliximab	No data available	[131]
Rituximab	No data available	[131]
Belatacept	No data available	[131]

clearly associated with teratogenicity in humans [127–129] (Table 1.7). Therefore, European best practice guidelines recommend that women receiving MMF switch to another drug and wait at least 6 weeks before attempting to conceive [131, 132].

Primary Congenital Kidney Anomalies

CAKUT is the most common cause of pediatric kidney failure [133]. CAKUT is highly heterogeneous, and the etiologic factors are not completely understood. These conditions are genetically variable and encompass a wide range of anatomical defects, such as renal agenesis, renal hypodysplasia, pelviureteric junction stenosis, and VUR. Mutations in genes causing syndromic disorders, such as *HNF1B* and *PAX2* mutations, are detected in only 5–10% of cases [134]. Familial forms of nonsyndromic disease have also been reported [135], further supporting a genetic determination such as *ACTA2* and *CHRM3* genes in Prune belly syndrome, *HPSE2* and *LRIG2* genes in Ochoa syndrome, among many others (Table 1.8). However, owing to locus heterogeneity and small pedigree size, the genetic cause of most familial or sporadic cases remains unknown [135].

Multicystic Dysplastic Kidney (MCDK)

These kidneys contain bizarrely shaped tubules surrounded by a stroma, that includes undifferentiated and metaplastic cells (for example, smooth muscle and cartilage). According to Liebeschuetz [155] the prevalence of MCDK is about 1 in 2400 live births, which is higher than other reports [156]. MCDK is usually unilateral and presents a typical US pattern: multiple noncommunicating cysts of varying size and nonmedial location of the largest cyst, absence of normal renal sinus echoes, and absence of normal renal parenchyma [157]. MCDK may also develop in the upper part of a duplex system or be located in an ectopic position. Unilateral isolated MCDK carries a good prognosis but careful examination of the contralateral kidney is essential because there is a high incidence of associated pathologies, many of which may not be detected until birth [158]. These associated malformations include ectopic ureteral insertions more commonly in the semi-

1 Antenatal Assessment of Kidney Morphology and Function

Table 1.8 Genes implicated in urinary tract malformations

Urinary tract malformation	Genes implicated	Mutated protein
Bladder extrophy	ISL1 [136]	Transcription factor potentially involved in formation of the bladder and urethra
Branchio-oto-renal syndrome	EYA1 [137]	Transcriptional co-activator required for eye morphogenesis
	SIX1 [138]	Homeobox protein similar to EYA gene product
Campomelic dysplasia (sex reversal, megaureter)	SOX9 [139]	Transcription factor modulating smooth muscle in the ureter
Diverse kidney malformations	TCF2 [140]	Transcription factor widely expressed in renal tract epithelia
Megaureter	TBX18 [141]	Transcription factor affecting ureter morphogenesis
	TSHZ3 [142]	Transcription factor modulating smooth muscle
Primary VUR, Ehler-Danlos	TNXB [143]	Extracellular matrix protein found in the urinary tract
Posterior urethral valves	BNC2 [144]	Basonuclin 2, a zinc finger containing protein implicated in epithelial maturation
Prune belly syndrome, megacystis microcolon intestinal hypoperistalsis	ACTA2 [145]	Smooth muscle contractile protein
	ACTG2 [146]	Smooth muscle contractile protein γ2-actin
	CHRM3 [147]	M3, the main acetylcholine receptor in detrusor smooth muscle
	MYH11 [148]	Smooth muscle contractile protein called myosin heavy chain 11
	MYLK [149]	Myosin light chain kinase modifying myosin in smooth muscle cells
	MYOCD [150]	Transcription-related protein needed for the expression of smooth muscle contractile proteins

Table 1.8 (continued)

Urinary tract malformation	Genes implicated	Mutated protein
Renal hypodysplasia, primary VUR	NRIP1 [151]	Nuclear receptor transcriptional cofactor that modulates retinoic acid transcriptional activity
Small kidneys, VUR, optic nerves malformation	PAX2 [152]	Transcription factor widely expressed in the developing ureter and kidney
Urofacial-Ochoa syndrome	HPSE2 [153]	Heparanase 2, a protein probably modulating growth factor signaling in bladder nerves
	LRIG2 [154]	Leucine-rich-repeats and immunoglobulin-like-domains 2 probably modulating growth factor signaling in bladder nerves

nal glands in boys and (hemi)vagina in girls. These ectopic insertions should be searched in utero but are more obvious after birth. An early diagnosis has a relevant clinical impact and leads to better management of the children and planning of further surgery in symptomatic cases [159]. The distinction between MCDK and cystic renal dysplasia associated with urinary tract obstruction may be difficult, especially in the absence of hydronephrosis. This distinction, although helpful in terms of diagnosis, may be somewhat artificial in terms of prognosis, since in either case, the affected kidney has no or minimal functional capacity.

Autosomal Recessive Polycystic Kidney Disease (ARPKD)

ARPKD belongs to the family of cilia-related disorders, has an incidence of 1 in 20,000 live births and may cause fetal and neonatal death in severe cases [160, 161]. Mutations in the PKHD1 fibrocystin gene are usually demonstrated in this disease [162]. Yet, since some patients survive the neonatal period with few or slight symptoms, different combinations of PKHD1 gene mutations and its resulting changes in the fibrocystin/

polyductin protein structure may at least partially explain the phenotypic variance [163]. The disease is characterized by marked elongation of the collecting tubules that expand into multiple small cysts. The cystic dilatation of the tubules is variable and predominates in the medulla. The outer cortex is spared since it contains no tubules. The classical in utero pattern of ARPKD includes markedly enlarged (+4 SD) hyperechoic kidneys without corticomedullary differentiation (Fig. 1.7). This appearance can be observed in the second trimester. The patterns may evolve and the size of the kidneys may continuously increase during the third trimester. Oligohydramnios and lung hypoplasia may be present, and therefore the prognosis is extremely poor.

Another presentation of ARPKD is of reversed corticomedullary differentiation with large kidneys (+2 to +4 SD). This finding is probably related to increased interfaces within the medullae and to the presence of material within the dilated tubules [164]. It is an important observation since there are few other causes of reversed corticomedullary differentiation. Liver involvement, typical of the condition, is usually impossible to demonstrate in utero. The differential diagnosis includes the glomerulocystic type of autosomal dominant polycystic kidney disease,

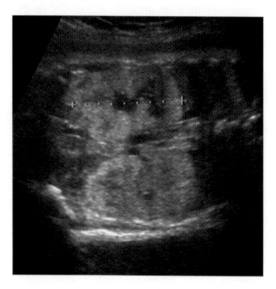

Fig. 1.7 Autosomal recessive polycystic kidney disease. Third trimester-coronal scan through the kidneys that appear large (+3 SD), and hyperechoic

Bardet-Biedl syndrome in which polydactyly is present [58] and other rare entities such as bilateral renal tumors, medullary sponge kidney, bilateral nephroblastomatosis, Finnish-type congenital nephrotic syndrome, medullary cystic disease, or congenital metabolic diseases (that is, glycogen storage disease or tyrosinosis). Oligohydramnios and absence of urine within the bladder would suggest ARPKD over all these rare entities.

Autosomal Dominant Polycystic Kidney Disease (ADPKD)

ADPKD is a common hereditary kidney disease, with 1/1000 people carrying the mutation. The pathological abnormality consists of a cystic dilatation of all parts of the nephron, which causes the kidneys to enlarge while the cortex and medulla become replaced by cysts, thus leading to end-stage renal failure [164, 165].

There are two major types of ADPKD: type I is caused by mutations in the *PKD1* gene on chromosome 16p13.3 and accounts for 85–90% of cases [164], and type II is caused by mutations in the *PKD2* gene on chromosome 4q21-22 and accounts for 10–15% of cases [165]. Other ciliopathy genes are likely to be involved since some obvious cases have none of these mutations. Although the age of clinical onset of this disorder is typically in the third to fifth decade of life, early manifestations during childhood or young adult age are now well described [166]. It is however unknown whether early diagnosis of ADPKD can enable earlier management and improve outcomes [167].

There may be different presentations in utero. In most cases, the kidneys are not grossly enlarged, but the corticomedullary differentiation is increased due to cortical hyperechogenicity. In this type of ADPKD, cysts are unusual in utero; they will develop after birth. Markedly enlarged kidneys resembling ARPKD are another pattern that can be encountered in utero and suggests either the homozygous presentation of ADPKD or the glomerulocystic type of ADPKD [168]. In these presentations of the disease renal failure may be already present in utero or at birth [163].

Renal Hypoplasia and Dysplasia

Renal dysplasia refers to abnormal differentiation or organization of cells in the renal parenchyma and is characterized histologically by the presence of primitive ducts and nests of metaplastic cartilage [32, 33]. Hypoplasia is a reduction of the number of nephrons in small kidneys (below −2 SD) (Fig. 1.8) [33]. Hypoplasia may coexist with dysplasia and the diagnosis is inferred from the hyperechoic appearance on US caused by the lack of normal renal parenchyma and structurally abnormal small kidneys [32, 33]. As in most cases the diagnosis is made by US examination, the spectrum of renal dysplasia includes inherited or congenital causes of renal hypoplasia, renal adysplasia, cystic dysplasia, oligomeganephronic hypoplasia, reflux nephropathy and obstructive renal dysplasia [32]. Cases with oligohydramnios have the poorest outcome [169].

A number of developmental genes have been implicated in the pathogenesis of hypodysplastic kidneys [134]: *EYA1* and *SIX1* causing autosomal dominant branchio-oto-renal syndrome [137, 138], *HNF1B/TCF2* associated with autosomal dominant renal cysts and diabetes syndrome [140, 170], and *PAX2* causing autosomal dominant renal-coloboma syndrome [152].

After birth, the prognosis depends on the residual renal function at 6 months of age. Infants with a GFR below 15 mL/min per 1.73 m² are at high risk to require early renal replacement therapy [32].

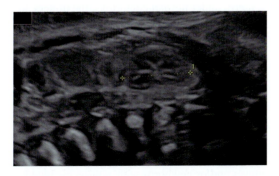

Fig. 1.8 Unilateral renal hypoplasia. Sagittal US scan through a small-sized right kidney: 18 mm at 31 weeks: between calipers

Congenital Nephrotic Syndrome

Congenital nephrotic syndrome (CNS) is defined as proteinuria leading to clinical symptoms in the first 3 months after birth. Infantile nephrotic syndrome manifests later, in the first year of life. However, these definitions are arbitrary as the time of onset ranges from fetal life to few years of age [171]. Moreover, CNS is a heterogeneous group of genetic disorders with variable clinical presentations and progression to end-stage renal failure [172, 173]. In a recent cohort study on renal transplanted infants weighing ±15 kg, CNS represented 35% of cases [174].

Congenital nephrotic syndrome of the Finnish type (CNF) is characterized by autosomal recessive inheritance and is caused by mutations in the nephrin gene (*NPHS1*) [175]. Most infants are born prematurely, with low birth weight for gestational age. The placenta is enlarged, weighing more than 25% of newborn weight. Edema is present at birth or appears within a few days due to severe nephrotic syndrome. In utero, the observation of hydrops fetalis and increased nuchal translucency reflects massive proteinuria [176, 177]. Most of the α-fetoprotein measured in the amniotic fluid is produced by fetal urine [178]. CNF should be suspected in front of an α-fetoprotein concentration exceeding 250–500 mg/L (mean normal values: 16.3 mg/L at 15 weeks of gestation; 8.1 mg/L at 20 weeks of gestation) [179].

Other cases of prenatally diagnosed congenital nephrotic syndrome have been reported, including Podocin gene (*NPHS2*) mutations [180], Pierson syndrome [181, 182], *PLCE1* gene mutations [183], secondary nephrotic syndrome due to CMV or other intrauterine infections [184] and massive proteinuria in offsprings of mothers with homozygous deficiency for the metallomembrane endopeptidase [85].

Postrenal Causes of Fetal Renal Abnormalities

Dilatations of the renal pelvis, calyces and ureters are the principal signs of impaired urinary flow on antenatal ultrasound scanning.

Pelvicoureteric Junction Stenosis

Pelvicoureteric junction stenosis occurs in 13% of children with antenatally diagnosed renal pelvis dilatation [39] and is characterized by obstruction at the level of the junction between the renal pelvis and the ureter. The anatomical basis for obstruction includes intrinsic stenosis/valves, peripelvic fibrosis, or crossing vessels. Sonographic diagnosis depends on the demonstration of a dilated renal pelvis in the absence of any dilatation of ureter or bladder. It should be particularly suspected when severe (greater than 15 mm) dilatation is seen, when the cavities appear round shaped and in the presence of a perirenal urinoma [35, 185] (Fig. 1.9). The anomaly is twice as common on the left side and twice as common in boys than in girls [186]. Prognosis may be poor in bilateral cases associated with oligohydramnios and hyperechoic parenchyma. The postnatal management of these children still remains a controversial topic among the nephro-urologic community [187]. It involves close monitoring of both sonomorphological and functional criteria assessed by radionuclide renogram including renal transit limited to the cortical area, differential function and output function (drainage pattern) [188–191]. Importantly, while the wait-and-see approach has gained wide acceptance, the decision to follow up those neonates conservatively requires some level of vigilance and clear parental consent and cooperation in order to avoid any evitable complications including renal functional deterioration [192].

Vesicoureteric Reflux (VUR)

VUR is defined as the retrograde flow of urine from the bladder upward within the ureter, sometimes extending into the renal pelvis, calyces and collecting ducts. Fetal renal pelvis dilatation can signal the presence of VUR in 11% [39] to 30% [193] of cases with the lower figure being more realistic. Making a precise diagnosis of VUR in utero is difficult. However, intermittent renal collecting system dilatation during real-time scanning (Fig. 1.10) or pelvicaliceal wall thickening are sonographic criteria highly suggestive of this diagnosis [194]. Although some children with high-grade, prenatally diagnosed VUR may have associated renal dysplasia [5, 194], VUR related to fetal renal pelvis dilatation was found in a large and prospective study to be of low-grade in 74% of cases with a high rate of 2-year spontaneous resolution (91%) [5]. Furthermore, in the absence of infections, reflux is not per se associated with progressive kidney injury [5]. The systematic use of VCUG in those babies is therefore questionable, especially since parents are frequently reluctant to consent to an invasive and uncomfortable examination for their child [195].

Uretero-Vesical Junction Obstruction (Megaureter)

In utero, under normal conditions, the ureters are not visualized. Megaureter should be suspected in the presence of a serpentine fluid-filled structure with or without dilatation of the renal pelvis and calices (Fig. 1.11). The ureter may be dilated because of obstruction at the level of the junction between the ureter and the bladder or as a result of nonobstructive causes including high-grade reflux. The differential diagnosis relies on VCUG. Megaureter could also be encountered in fetuses and/or newborns with neurogenic bladder or posterior urethral valves. In those cases, specific treatment strategies should be directed

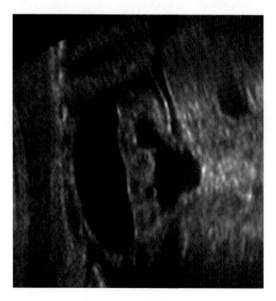

Fig. 1.9 Pelvicaliceal dilatation and perirenal urinoma in a fetus with pelviureteric junction stenosis. Coronal US scan through the right fetal kidney

1 Antenatal Assessment of Kidney Morphology and Function

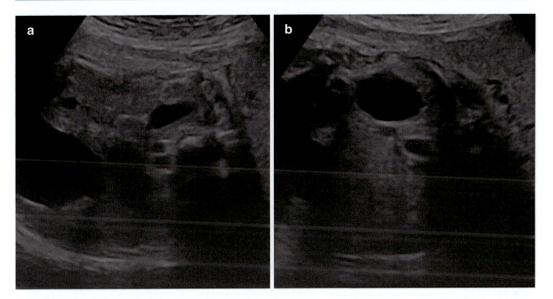

Fig. 1.10 (**a** and **b**) Fetal vesicoureteral reflux. Transverse scans of the fetal abdomen. Intermittent renal collecting system dilatation during the same antenatal ultrasound examination only visible in figure **b**, due to vesicoureteral reflux

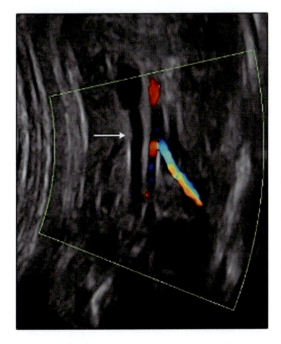

Fig. 1.11 Megaureter. Coronal scan of the fetal abdomen showing a fluid-filled structure (arrows) laterally to the aorta corresponding to a dilated ureter

toward the underlying condition. Prognosis of primary megaureter is generally good since most cases resolve spontaneously between ages 12 and 36 months [196]. However, in children with high-grade hydronephrosis, or a retrovesical ureteral diameter of greater than 1 cm, the condition may resolve slowly and may require surgery [196].

Duplex Kidneys

Duplication of the renal collecting system is characterized by the presence of a kidney having two pelvic structures with two ureters that may be completely or partially separated [197]. Most cases with non-dilated cavities have no renal impairment and should be considered as normal variants [4]. However, a proportion of duplex kidneys may be associated with significant pathology, usually due to the presence of VUR or obstruction. Fetal urinary tract dilatations are related to complicated renal duplication in 4.7% of cases [39]. VUR usually involves only the lower pole ureter in 90% of cases. Compared to single-system reflux, duplex system VUR tends to be of a higher grade with a high incidence of lower pole dysplasia [198]. Obstructive ureteroceles are associated with the upper pole ureter in 80% of cases, although obstruction of the upper pole may also occur secondary to an ectopic insertion or an isolated vesicoureteric junction obstruction (Fig. 1.12a) [198, 199]. In utero, duplex kidneys are highly suspected in the presence of two separate noncommunicating renal

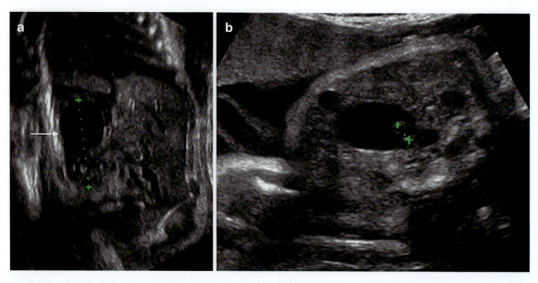

Fig. 1.12 (a) Fetal duplex kidney with dilatation of the upper pole (arrow). Sagittal US scan through the fetal kidney. (b) Fetal bladder with ureterocele (between crosses). Axial US scan through the fetal bladder

pelves, dilated ureters, cystic structures within one pole, and echogenic cyst in the bladder, representing ureterocele (Fig. 1.12b) [199, 200]. After birth, the classical radiological workup of abnormal duplex kidneys is based on US and VCUG [4]. Most people agree that the surgical approach to complicated duplex systems is largely predicated on the function of the affected renal moiety and the presence or absence of function [4].

Bladder Outlet Obstruction

When bladder obstruction is suspected in the first trimester, the most common causes are Prune Belly syndrome or fibrourethral stenosis, which is mainly associated with chromosomal and multiple congenital anomalies and carries a very poor prognosis [201]. In the second trimester, the most common cause of lower urinary tract obstruction in male fetuses is posterior urethral valves, which are tissue leaflets fanning distally from the prostatic urethra to the external urinary sphincter. The failure of the bladder to empty during an extended examination and the presence of abnormal kidneys and oligohydramnios must raise suspicion of posterior urethral valves. On occasion a megabladder with a thickened wall may be seen (Fig. 1.13a), and the dilated posterior urethra may take the aspect of a keyhole (Fig. 1.13b). In extreme cases in utero bladder rupture may be observed with extravasation of urine resulting in urinary ascites. This phenomenon was thought to be a protective pop-off mechanism, although recent reports provided evidence against this hypothesis [202].

In many cases there is only a partial obstruction, and amniotic fluid volume can be maintained throughout pregnancy. In some cases, spontaneous rupture of valves appears to occur in utero with the reappearance of cyclical emptying of the bladder. The most reliable prognostic indicators of poor renal functional status are presentation before 24 weeks, oligohydramnios, increased cortical echogenicity, and the absence of corticomedullary differentiation [203, 204].

The prognosis in severe cases is often relatively easy to predict, and perinatal death will occur secondary to pulmonary hypoplasia and renal failure [204]. The renal parenchymal lesions may be secondary to the obstruction but also to associated high-grade reflux. In partial obstruction, however, the outcome is less predictable, and late morbidity most commonly takes the form of end-stage renal failure, which affects 15–30% of individuals some time in childhood [205]. Once the prognosis has been determined

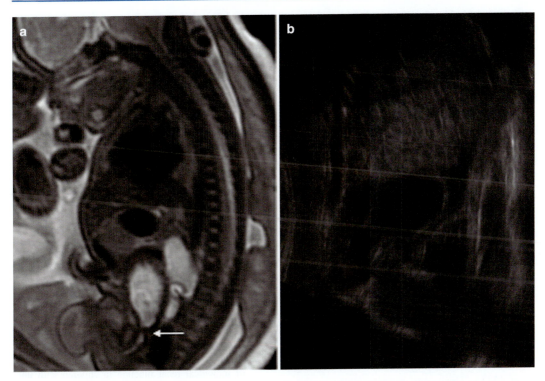

Fig. 1.13 (**a**) Fetal urethral valve with thickened bladder wall. Posterior urethral dilatation (arrow). Sagittal MR image on the fetal pelvis. (**b**) Megabladder. Third trimester scan. Huge enlargement of the fetal bladder due to posterior urethral valves. The key-hole sign is present

as accurately as possible, management of these cases should be performed in a fetal medicine and pediatric surgery reference center. In each new case, the great variability of presentation makes participation of different specialists necessary in the difficult decision-making process. Various options should be considered, including in utero follow-up with planned postnatal management (sustained medical treatment or palliative care), termination of pregnancy, and occasionally, in utero therapy [50].

Fetal Intervention for Lower Urinary Tract Obstruction

There was considerable interest in fetal intervention for obstructive uropathies in the 1980s and 1990s, which was revolutionary at that time. In utero intervention was thought to improve neonatal outcome by restoring amniotic fluid levels, thereby allowing normal pulmonary maturation and eventual renal function [206, 207]. A variety of in utero therapeutic approaches to bladder outflow obstruction have been tried. Expectably, the open surgical technique of **fetal vesicostomy** was not free of risks and has been abandoned due to significant fetal loss, premature uterine contractions and maternal morbidity [206, 207].

Direct endoscopic ablation of urethral valves is a more recent technique and requires the introduction of an endoscope into the fetal bladder, leading to ablation of the valves either by laser, saline irrigation or mechanical disruption using guide wire [208]. Direct visualization of the valves, however, is difficult, and it may be hard to avoid damage to surrounding tissues.

Vesicoamniotic shunting is performed under US guidance using a pigtail shunt, which when inserted leaves one end in the fetal bladder and the other in the amniotic space. This technique, which was first reported in 1982 [209], is preferred to bladder drainage by serial vesicocentesis. A previous systematic review to assess the effectiveness of bladder drainage (vesico amniotic shunting or vesicocentesis) showed that fetal bladder drainage increased survival [210]. However, the studies identified in this systematic review were small, heterogeneous, observational, and non-randomized trials and so the potential for bias in these results was substantial. In addition, using survival alone as a marker of efficacy in these patients was misleading, since most of the survivors were left with significant renal morbidity. End-stage renal failure was present in 40% of those children who survived [90]. After decades of absence of serious clinical research, Rachel Morris and colleagues orchestrated and published in *The Lancet* in 2013 the results of the PLUTO (Percutaneous vesicoamniotic shunting in Lower Urinary Tract Obstruction) trial, in which fetuses with fetal lower urinary tract obstruction were randomly assigned to either vesicoamniotic shunting or conservative management [211]. Thirty-one women with singleton pregnancies complicated by lower urinary tract obstruction were included in the trial, with 16 allocated to the vesicoamniotic shunt group and 15 to the conservative management group. Unfortunately, the trial was stopped early because of poor recruitment after only about 20% of the planned 150 pregnancies were randomly assigned during a 4-year period. Although the results of PLUTO results have to be interpreted with caution due to the premature termination of the study and the small number of patients [212], postnatal survival was three-times higher in the fetuses receiving vesicoamniotic shunting. However, only two of seven shunted survivors had normal renal function at age 1 year. These results suggest that the chance of newborn babies to survive with normal renal function is very low irrespective of whether or not vesicoamniotic shunting is done. These findings are in line with results from studies in animals, which have shown that renal damage occurs rapidly after the onset of obstruction and might be only partly reversible [213].

In conclusion, the evidence available so far suggests that intrauterine shunting of an obstructed urinary tract will improve perinatal survival but does not carry any advantage with regards to the rescue of postnatal kidney function and long-term renal survival.

References

1. Wiesel A, Queisser-Luft A, Clementi M, Bianca S, Stoll C, The EUROSCAN Study Group. Prenatal detection of congenital renal malformation by fetal ultrasonographic examination: an analysis of 709 030 births in 12 European countries. Eur J Med Genet. 2005;48:131–44.
2. Gagnon A, Wilson RD, Allen VM, Audibert F, Blight C, Brock JA, Désilets VA, Johnson JA, Langlois S, Murphy-Kaulbeck L, Wyatt P, Society of Obstetricians and Gynaecologists of Canada. Evaluation of prenatally diagnosed structural congenital anomalies. J Obstet Gynaecol Can. 2009;31:875–81.
3. Capello SA, Kogan BA, Giorgi LJ, Kaufman RP. Prenatal ultrasound has led to earlier detection and repair of ureteropelvic junction obstruction. J Urol. 2005;174:1425–8.
4. Ismaili K, Hall M, Ham H, Piepsz A. Evolution of individual renal function in children with unilateral complex renal duplication. J Pediatr. 2005;147:208–12.
5. Ismaili K, Hall M, Piepsz A, Wissing KM, Collier F, Schulman C, Avni FE. Primary vesicoureteral reflux detected among neonates with a history of fetal renal pelvis dilatation: a prospective clinical and imaging study. J Pediatr. 2006;148:222–7.
6. Gonçalves LF, Espinoza J, Kusanovic JP, Lee W, Nien JK, Santolaya-Forgas J, Mari G, Treadwell MC, Romero R. Applications of 2D matrix array for 3D and 4D examination of the fetus: a pictorial essay. J Ultrasound Med. 2006;25:745–55.
7. Michel SC, Rake A, Keller TM, Huch R, König V, Seifert B, Marincek B, Kubik-Huch RA. Fetal cardiographic monitoring in 1.5 T MR imaging. Am J Roentgenol. 2003;180:1159–64.
8. Cassart M. Fetal body imaging, when is MRI indicated? J Belg Soc Radiol. 2017;101(Suppl 1):3.
9. Lum M, Tsiouris AJ. MRI safety considerations during pregnancy. Clin Imaging. 2020;62:69–75.
10. Lee SM, Jun JK, Lee EJ, Lee JH, Park CW, Park JS, Syn HC. Measurement of fetal urine production to differentiate causes of increased amniotic fluid volume. Ultrasound Obstet Gynecol. 2010;36:191–5.
11. Avni FE, Garel L, Hall M, Rypens F. Perinatal approach in anomalies of the urinary tract, adrenals and genital system. In: Avni FE, editor. Perinatal imaging. From ultrasound to MR imaging. Berlin: Springer; 2002. p. 153–96.
12. Thomas IF, Smith DW. Oligohydramnios: cause of the non renal features of Potter's syndrome including pulmonary hypoplasia. J Pediatr. 1974;84:811–5.

13. Cuckow PM, Nyirady P, Winyard PJ. Normal and abnormal development of the urogenital tract. Prenat Diagn. 2001;21:908–16.
14. Avni FE, Cos T, Cassart M, Massez A, Donner C, Ismaili K, Hall M. Evolution of fetal ultrasonography. Eur Radiol. 2007;17:419–31.
15. Stonebrook E, Hoff M, Spencer JD. Congenital anomalies of the kidney and urinary tract: a clinical review. Curr Treat Options Pediatr. 2019;5:223–35.
16. Oh KY, Holznagel DE, Ameli JR, Sohaey R. Prenatal diagnosis of renal developmental anomalies associated with an empty renal fossa. Ultrasound Q. 2010;26:233–40.
17. Sepulveda W, Staggianis KD, Flack NJ, Fisk NM. Accuracy of prenatal diagnosis of renal agenesis with color flow imaging in severe second-trimester oligohydramnios. Am J Obstet Gynecol. 1995;173:1788–92.
18. Chow JS, Benson CB, Lebowitz RL. The clinical significance of an empty renal fossa on prenatal sonography. J Ultrasound Med. 2005;24:1049–54.
19. Mesrobian HG, Rushton HG, Bulas D. Unilateral renal agenesis may result from in utero regression of multicystic renal dysplasia. J Urol. 1993;150:793–4.
20. Toka HR, Toka O, Hariri A, Nguyen HT. Congenital anomalies of kidney and urinary tract. Semin Nephrol. 2010;30:374–86.
21. Westland R, Kurvers RA, van Wijk JA, Schreuder MF. Risk factors for renal injury in children with a solitary functioning kidney. Pediatrics. 2013;131:e478–85.
22. Jeanty P, Romero R, Kepple D, Stoney D, Coggins T, Fleischer AC. Prenatal diagnoses in unilateral empty renal fossa. J Ultrasound Med. 1990;9:651–4.
23. Zajicek M, Perlman S, Dekel B, Lahav E, Lotan D, Lotan D, Achiron R, Gilboa Y. Crossed ectopic kidney: prenatal diagnosis and postnatal follow-up. Prenat Diagn. 2017;37:712–5.
24. Chaumoitre K, Brun M, Cassart M, Maugey-Laulom B, Eurin D, Didier F, Avni EF. Differential diagnosis of fetal hyperechogenic cystic kidneys unrelated to renal tract anomalies: a multicenter study. Ultrasound Obstet Gynecol. 2006;28:911–7.
25. Yulia A, Napolitano R, Aiman A, Desai D, Johal N, Whitten M, Ushakov F, Pandya PP, Winyard PJD. Perinatal and infant outcome in prenatally diagnosed hyperechogenic kidneys. Ultrasound Obstet Gynecol. 2020; https://doi.org/10.1002/uog.22121. Online ahead of print.
26. Tsatsaris V, Gagnadoux MF, Aubry MC, Gubler MC, Dumez Y, Dommergues M. Prenatal diagnosis of bilateral isolated fetal hyperechogenic kidneys. Is it possible to predict long term outcome? BJOG. 2002;109:1388–93.
27. Mashiach R, Davidovits M, Eisenstein B, Kidron D, Kovo M, Shalev J, Merlob P, Verdimon D, Efrat Z, Meizner I. Fetal hyperechogenic kidney with normal amniotic fluid volume: a diagnostic dilemma. Prenat Diagn. 2005;25:553–8.
28. Hertz-Pannier L, Déchaux M, Sinico M, Emond S, Cormier-Daire V, Saudubray JM, Brunelle F, Niaudet P, Seta N, de Lonlay P. Congenital disorders of glycosylation type I: a rare but new cause of hyperechoic kidneys in infants and children due to early microcystic changes. Pediatr Radiol. 2006;36:108–14.
29. Hureaux M, Molin A, Jay N, Saliou AH, Spaggiari E, Salomon R, Benachi A, Vargas-Poussou R, Heidet L. Prenatal hyperechogenic kidneys in three cases of infantile hypercalcemia associated with *SLC34A1* mutations. Pediatr Nephrol. 2018;33:1723–9.
30. Jones GE, Mousa HA, Rowley H, Houtman P, Vasudevan PC. Should we offer prenatal testing for 17q12 microdeletion syndrome to all cases with prenatally diagnosed echogenic kidneys? Prenatal findings in two families with 17q12 microdeletion syndrome and review of the literature. Prenat Diagn. 2015;35:1336–41.
31. van Vuuren SH, Damen-Elias HA, Stigter RH, van der Doef R, Goldschmeding R, de Jong TP, Westers P, Visser GH, Pistorius LR. Size and volume charts of fetal kidney, renal pelvis and adrenal gland. Ultrasound Obstet Gynecol. 2012;40:659–64.
32. Ismaili K, Schurmans T, Wissing M, Hall M, Van Aelst C, Janssen F. Early prognostic factors of infants with chronic renal failure caused by renal dysplasia. Pediatr Nephrol. 2001;16:260–4.
33. Winyard P, Chitty L. Dysplastic and polycystic kidneys: diagnosis, associations and management. Prenat Diagn. 2001;21:924–35.
34. Ismaili K, Hall M, Donner C, Thomas D, Vermeylen D, Avni FE. Results of systematic screening for minor degrees of fetal renal pelvis dilatation in an unselected population. Am J Obstet Gynecol. 2003;188:242–6.
35. Ismaili K, Hall M, Piepsz A, Alexander M, Schulman C, Avni FE. Insights into the pathogenesis and natural history of fetuses with renal pelvis dilatation. Eur Urol. 2005;48:207–14.
36. Herthelius M, Axelsson R, Lidefelt KJ. Antenatally detected urinary tract dilatation: a 12–15-year follow-up. Pediatr Nephrol. 2020;35:2129–35.
37. Sherer DM. Is fetal hydronephrosis overdiagnosed? Ultrasound Obstet Gynecol. 2000;16:601–6.
38. Persutte WH, Hussey M, Chyu J, Hobbins JC. Striking findings concerning the variability in the measurement of the fetal renal collecting system. Ultrasound Obstet Gynecol. 2000;15:186–90.
39. Ismaili K, Avni FE, Wissing KM, Hall M. Long-term clinical outcome of infants with mild and moderate fetal pyelectasis: validation of neonatal ultrasound as a screening tool to detect significant nephro-uropathies. J Pediatr. 2004;144:759–65.
40. Sairam S, Al-Habib A, Sasson S, Thilaganathan B. Natural history of fetal hydronephrosis diagnosed on mid-trimester ultrasound. Ultrasound Obstet Gynecol. 2001;17:191–6.
41. Nguyen HT, Benson CB, Bromley B, Campbell JB, Chow J, Coleman B, Cooper C, Crino J, Darge K,

Herndon CD, Odibo AO, Somers MJ, Stein DR. The Society for Fetal Urology consensus statement on the evaluation and management of antenatal hydronephrosis. J Pediatr Urol. 2014;10:982–98.

42. Dudley JA, Haworth JM, McGraw ME, Frank JD, Tizzard EJ. Clinical relevance and implications of antenatal hydronephrosis. Arch Dis Child. 1997;76:F31–4.

43. Jaswon MS, Dibble L, Puri S, Davis J, Young J, Dave R, Morgan H. Prospective study of outcome in antenatally diagnosed renal pelvis dilatation. Arch Dis Child. 1999;80:F135–8.

44. Bouzada MC, Oliveira EA, Pereira AK, Leite HV, Rodrigues AM, Fagundes LA, Gonçalves RP, Parreiras RL. Diagnostic accuracy of fetal renal pelvis anteroposterior diameter as a predictor of uropathy: a prospective study. Ultrasound Obstet Gynecol. 2004;24:745–9.

45. Vasconcelos MA, Oliveira EA, Simões E, Silva AC, Dias CS, Mak RH, Fonseca CC, Campos APM, Steyerberg EW, Vergouwe Y. A predictive model of postnatal surgical intervention in children with prenatally detected congenital anomalies of the kidney and urinary tract. Front Pediatr. 2019;7:120.

46. De Bruyn R, Gordon I. Postnatal investigation of fetal renal disease. Prenat Diagn. 2001;21:984–91.

47. Ismaili K, Avni FE, Hall M. Results of systematic voiding cystourethrography in infants with antenatally diagnosed renal pelvis dilation. J Pediatr. 2002;141:21–4.

48. Moorthy I, Joshi N, Cook JV, Warren M. Antenatal hydronephrosis: negative predictive value of normal postnatal ultrasound, a 5-year study. Clin Radiol. 2003;58:964–70.

49. Avni EF, Ayadi K, Rypens F, Hall M, Schulman CC. Can careful ultrasound examination of the urinary tract exclude vesicoureteric reflux in the neonate? Br J Radiol. 1997;70:977–82.

50. Chiodini B, Ghassemi M, Khelif K, Ismaili K. Clinical outcome of children with antenatally diagnosed hydronephrosis. Front Pediatr. 2019;7:103.

51. Gimpel C, Avni EF, Breysem L, Burgmaier K, Caroli A, Cetiner M, Haffner D, Hartung EA, Franke D, König J, Liebau MC, Mekahli D, Ong ACM, Pape L, Titieni A, Torra R, Winyard PJD, Schaefer F. Imaging of kidney cysts and cystic kidney diseases in children: an International Working Group Consensus Statement. Radiology. 2019;290:769–82.

52. Blazer S, Zimmer EZ, Blumenfeld Z, Zelikovic I, Bronshtein M. Natural history of fetal simple cysts detected early in pregnancy. J Urol. 1999;162:812–4.

53. Decramer S, Parant O, Beaufils S, Clauin S, Guillou C, Kessler S, Aziza J, Bandin F, Schanstra JP, Bellanné-Chantelot C. Anomalies of the *TCF2* gene are the main cause of fetal bilateral hyperechogenic kidneys. J Am Soc Nephrol. 2007;18:923–33.

54. Coffinier C, Thepot D, Babinet C, Yaniv M, Barra J. Essential role for the hemeoprotein vHNF1/HNF1beta in visceral endoderm differentiation. Development. 1999;126:4785–94.

55. Heidet L, Decramer S, Pawtowski A, Morinière V, Bandin F, Knebelmann B, Lebre AS, Faguer S, Guigonis V, Antignac C, Salomon R. Spectrum of HNF1B mutations in a large cohort of patients who harbor renal diseases. Clin J Am Soc Nephrol. 2010;5:1079–90.

56. Logan CV, Abdel-Hamed Z, Johnson CA. Molecular genetics and pathogenic mechanisms for the severe ciliopathies: insights into neurodevelopment and pathogenesis of neural tube defects. Mol Neurobiol. 2011;43:12–26.

57. Jones KL. Smith's recognizable patterns of human malformation. 5th ed. Philadelphia: WB Saunders; 1997.

58. Cassart M, Eurin D, Didier F, Guibaud L, Avni EF. Antenatal renal sonographic anomalies and postnatal follow-up of renal involvement in Bardet-Biedl syndrome. Ultrasound Obstet Gynecol. 2004;24:51–4.

59. Waterham HR, Ebberink MS. Genetics and molecular basis of human peroxisome biogenesis disorders. Biochim Biophys Acta. 2012;1822:1430–41.

60. Larson RS, Rudoloff MA, Liapis H, Manes JL, Davila R, Kissane J. The Ivemark syndrome: prenatal diagnosis of an uncommon cystic renal lesion with heterogeneous associations. Pediatr Nephrol. 1995;9:594–8.

61. Soejima H, Higashimoto K. Epigenetic and genetic alterations of the imprinting disorder Beckwith-Wiedemann syndrome and related disorders. J Hum Genet. 2013;58:402–9.

62. Baujat G, Huber C, El Hokayem J, Caumes R, Do Ngoc Thanh C, David A, Delezoide AL, Dieux-Coeslier A, Estournet B, Francannet C, Kayirangwa H, Lacaille F, Le Bourgeois M, Martinovic J, Salomon R, Sigaudy S, Malan V, Munnich A, Le Merrer M, Le Quan Sang KH, Cormier-Daire V. Asphyxiating thoracic dysplasia: clinical and molecular review of 39 families. J Med Genet. 2013;50:91–8.

63. Dabora SL, Jozwiak S, Franz DN, Roberts PS, Nieto A, Chung J, Choy YS, Reeve MP, Thiele E, Egelhoff JC, Kasprzyk-Obara J, Domanska-Pakiela D, Kwiatkowski DJ. Mutational analysis in a cohort of 224 tuberous sclerosis patients indicates increased severity of *TSC2*, compared with *TSC1*, disease in multiple organs. Am J Hum Genet. 2001;68:64–80.

64. Kamath BM, Podkameni G, Hutchinson AL, Leonard LD, Gerfen J, Krantz ID, Piccoli DA, Spinner NB, Loomes KM, Meyers K. Renal anomalies in Alagille syndrome: a disease-defining feature. Am J Med Genet A. 2012;158A:85–9.

65. Leclair MD, El-Ghoneimi A, Audry G, Ravasse P, Moscovici J, Heloury Y. French pediatric urology study group. The outcome of prenatally diagnosed renal tumors. J Urol. 2005;173:186–9.

66. Powis M. Neonatal renal tumours. Early Hum Dev. 2010;86:607–12.

67. Ambrosino MM, Hernanz-Schulman M, Horii SC, Raghavendra BN, Genieser NB. Prenatal diagnosis of nephroblastomatosis in two siblings. J Ultrasound Med. 1990;9:49–51.

68. Daneman A, Baunin C, Lobo E, Pracros JP, Avni F, Toi A, Metreweli C, Ho SS, Moore L. Disappearing suprarenal masses in fetuses and infants. Pediatr Radiol. 1997;27:675–81.

69. Wilcox DT, Chitty LS. Non visualisations of fetal bladder: aetiology and management. Prenat Diagn. 2001;21:977–83.

70. Martin C, Darnell A, Duran C, Bermudez P, Mellado F, Rigol S. Magnetic resonance imaging of the intra uterine fetal genito-urinary tract. In: Abdominal imaging. New York: Springer-Verlag; 2004.

71. Pinette M, Blackstone J, Wax J, Cartin A. Enlarged fetal bladder: differential diagnosis and outcomes. J Clin Ultrasound. 2003;31:328–34.

72. Muller F, Dreux S, Vaast P, Dumez Y, Nisand I, Ville Y, Boulot P, Guibourdenche J, The Study Group of the French Fetal Medicine Society. Prenatal diagnosis of megacystis-microcolon-intestinal hypoperistalsis syndrome: contribution of amniotic fluid digestive enzyme essay and fetal urinalysis. Prenat Diagn. 2005;25:203–9.

73. Vanderheyden T, Kumar S, Fisk NM. Fetal renal impairment. Semin Neonatol. 2003;8:279–89.

74. Spitzer A. The current approach to the assessment of fetal renal function: fact or fiction? Pediatr Nephrol. 1996;10:230–5.

75. Hobbins JC, Romero R, Grannum P, Berkovitz RL, Cullen M, Mahony M. Antenatal diagnosis of renal anomalies with ultrasound. I. Obstructive uropathy. Am J Obstet Gynecol. 1984;148:868–77.

76. Moore TR, Cayle JE. The amniotic fluid index in normal human pregnancy. Am J Obstet Gynecol. 1990;162:1168–73.

77. Owen J, Albert PS, Buck Louis GM, Fuchs KM, Grobman WA, Kim S, D'Alton ME, Wapner R, Wing DA, Grantz KL. A contemporary amniotic fluid volume chart for the United States: the NICHD fetal growth studies-singletons. Am J Obstet Gynecol. 2019;221(67):e1–67.e12.

78. Loos S, Kemper MJ. Causes of oligohydramniosis: impact on prenatal counseling and postnatal outcome. Pediatr Nephrol. 2018;33:541–5.

79. Zaccara A, Giorlandino C, Mobili L, Brizzi C, Bilancioni E, Capolupo I, Capitanucci ML, De Genaro M. Amniotic fluid index and fetal bladder outlet obstruction. Do we really need more? J Urol. 2005;174:1657–60.

80. Peters CA, Reid LM, Docimo S, Luetic T, Carr M, Retik AB, Mandell J. The role of the kidney in lung growth and maturation in the setting of obstructive uropathy and oligohydramnios. J Urol. 1991;146:597–600.

81. Laudy JA, Wladimiroff JW. The fetal lung. 1: developmental aspects. Ultrasound Obstet Gynecol. 2000;16:284–90.

82. Smith NP, Losty PD, Connell MG, Meyer U, Jesudason EC. Abnormal lung development precedes oligohydramnios in transgenic murine model of renal dysgenesis. J Urol. 2006;175:783–6.

83. Brochard K, Boyer O, Blanchard A, Loirat C, Niaudet P, Macher MA, Deschenes G, Bensman A, Decramer S, Cochat P, Morin D, Broux F, Caillez M, Guyot C, Novo R, Jeunemaître X, Vargas-Poussou R. Phenotype-genotype correlation in antenatal and neonatal variants of Bartter syndrome. Nephrol Dial Transplant. 2009;24:1455–64.

84. Männikkö M, Kestilä M, Lenkkeri U, Alakurtti H, Holmberg C, Leisti J, Salonen R, Aula P, Mustonen A, Peltonen L, Tryggvason K. Improved prenatal diagnosis of the congenital nephrotic syndrome of the Finnish type based on DNA analysis. Kidney Int. 1997;51:868–72.

85. Nortier J, Debiec H, Tournay Y, Mougenot B, Noel JC, Deschodt-Lackman MM, Janssen F, Ronco P. Neonatal disease in neutral endopeptidase alloimmunization: lessons for immunological monitoring. Pediatr Nephrol. 2005;21:1399–405.

86. Glick PL, Harrisson MR, Golbus MS, Adzick NS, Filly RA, Callen PW, Mahony PS. Management of the fetus with congenital hydronephrosis. II: prognosis criteria and selection for treatment. J Pediatr Surg. 1985;20:376–87.

87. Burghard R, Pallacks R, Gordjani N, Leititis JU, Hackeloer BJ, Brandis M. Microproteins in amniotic fluid as an index of changes in fetal renal function during development. Pediatr Nephrol. 1997;1:574–80.

88. Nicolini U, Spelzini F. Invasive assessment of fetal renal abnormalities: urinalysis, fetal blood sampling and biopsy. Prenat Diagn. 2001;21:964–9.

89. Dreux S, Rosenblatt J, Moussy-Durandy A, Patin F, Favre R, Lortat-Jacob S, El Ghoneimi A, Oury JF, Deschenes G, Ville Y, Heidet L, Muller F. Urine biochemistry to predict long-term outcomes in fetuses with posterior urethral valves. Prenat Diagn. 2018;38:964–70.

90. Coplen DE. Prenatal intervention for hydronephrosis. J Urol. 1997;157:2270–7.

91. Crombleholme TM, Harrisson MR, Golbus MS, Longaker MT, Langer JC, Callen PW, Anderson RL, Goldstein RB, Filly RA. Fetal intervention in obstructive uropathy: prognostic indicators and efficacy of intervention. Am J Obstet Gynecol. 1990;162:1239–44.

92. Muller F, Bernard MA, Benkirane A, Ngo S, Lortat-Jacob S, Oury JF, Dommergues M. Fetal urine cystatine C as a predictor of postnatal renal function in bilateral uropathies. Clin Chem. 1999;45:2292–3.

93. Abdennadher W, Chalouhi G, Dreux S, Rosenblatt J, Favre R, Guimiot F, Salomon LJ, Oury JF, Ville Y, Muller F. Fetal urine biochemistry at 13-23 weeks of gestation in lower urinary tract obstruction: criteria for in-utero treatment. Ultrasound Obstet Gynecol. 2015;46:306–11.

94. Muller F, Dommergues M, Mandelbrot L, Aubry MC, Nihoul-Féketé C, Dumez Y. Fetal urinary biochemistry predicts postnatal renal function in children with bilateral obstructive uropathies. Obstet Gynecol. 1993;82:813–20.

95. Klein J, Lacroix C, Caubet C, Siwy J, Zürbig P, Dakna M, Muller F, Breuil B, Stalmach A, Mullen W, Mischak H, Bandin F, Monsarrat B, Bascands JL, Decramer S, Schanstra JP. Fetal urinary peptides to predict postnatal outcome of renal disease in fetuses with posterior urethral valves (PUV). Sci Transl Med. 2013;5:198ra106.

96. Buffin-Meyer B, Klein J, Breuil B, Muller F, Moulos P, Groussolles M, Bouali O, Bascands JL, Decramer S, Schanstra JP. Combination of the fetal urinary metabolome and peptidome for the prediction of postnatal renal outcome in fetuses with PUV. J Proteome. 2018;184:1–9.

97. Buffin-Meyer B, Klein J, van der Zanden LFM, Levtchenko E, Moulos P, Lounis N, Conte-Auriol F, Hindryckx A, Wühl E, Persico N, Oepkes D, Schreuder MF, Tkaczyk M, Ariceta G, Fossum M, Parvex P, Feitz W, Olsen H, Montini G, Decramer S, Schanstra JP, Antenatal Consortium. The ANTENATAL multicentre study to predict postnatal renal outcome in fetuses with posterior urethral valves: objectives and design. Clin Kidney J. 2019;13:371–9.

98. Bökenkamp A, Dieterich C, Dressler F, Mühlhaus K, Gembruch U, Bald R, Kirschstein M. Fetal serum concentrations of cystatin C and β2-microglobulin as predictors of postnatal kidney function. Am J Obstet Gynecol. 2001;185:468–75.

99. Muller F, Dreux S, Audibert F, Chabaud JJ, Rousseau T, D'Hervé D, Dumez Y, Ngo S, Gubler MC, Dommergues M. Fetal serum β2-microglobulin and cystatin C in the prediction of post-natal renal function in bilateral hypoplasia and hyperechogenic enlarged kidneys. Prenat Diagn. 2004;24:327–32.

100. Nguyen C, Dreux S, Heidet L, Czerkiewicz I, Salomon LJ, Guimiot F, Schmitz T, Tsatsaris V, Boulot P, Rousseau T, Muller F. Fetal serum α-1 microglobulin for renal function assessment: comparison with β2-microglobulin and cystatin C. Prenat Diagn. 2013;33:775–81.

101. Bunduki V, Saldanha LB, Sadek L, Miguelez J, Myiyadahira S, Zugaib M. Fetal renal biopsies in obstructive uropathy: feasibility and clinical correlations—preliminary results. Prenat Diagn. 1998;18:101–9.

102. Suranyi A, Retz C, Rigo J, Schaaps JP, Foidart JM. Fetal renal hyperechogenicity in intrauterine growth retardation: importance and outcome. Pediatr Nephrol. 2001;16:575–80.

103. Schreuder MF, Nauta J. Prenatal programming of nephron number and blood pressure. Kidney Int. 2007;72:265–8.

104. Schmidt B, Andrew M. Neonatal thrombosis: report of a prospective Canadian and International Registry. Pediatrics. 1995;96:939–43.

105. Marks SD, Massicotte P, Steele BT, Matsell DG, Filler G, Shah PS, Perlman M, Rosenblum ND, Shah VS. Neonatal renal venous thrombosis: clinical outcomes and prevalence of prothrombotic disorders. J Pediatr. 2005;146:811–6.

106. Lalmand B, Avni EF, Nasr A, Katelbant P, Struyven J. Perinatal renal vein thrombosis: US demonstration. J Ultrasound Med. 1990;9:437–42.

107. Wee LY, Fisk NM. The twin-twin transfusion syndrome. Semin Neonatol. 2002;7:187–202.

108. Talbert DG, Bajoria R, Sepulveda W, Bower S, Fisk NM. Hydrostatic and osmotic pressure gradients produce manifestations of fetofetal transfusion syndrome in a computerized model of monochorial twin pregnancy. Am J Obstet Gynecol. 1996;174:598–608.

109. Chiang MC, Lien R, Chao AS, Chou YH, Chen YJ. Clinical consequences of twin-to-twin transfusion. Eur J Pediatr. 2003;162:68–71.

110. Taylor CL, Jones KL, Jones MC, Kaplan GW. Incidence of renal anomalies in children prenatally exposed to ethanol. Pediatrics. 1994;94:209–12.

111. Correia-Costa L, Schaefer F, Afonso AC, Correia S, Guimarães JT, Guerra A, Barros H, Azevedo A. Prenatal alcohol exposure affects renal function in overweight schoolchildren: birth cohort analysis. Pediatr Nephrol. 2020;35:695–702.

112. Sedman AB, Kershaw DB, Bunchman TE. Recognition and management of angiotensin converting enzyme inhibitor fetopathy. Pediatr Nephrol. 1995;9:382–5.

113. Cooper WO, Hernandez-Diaz S, Arbogast PG, Dudley JA, Dyer S, Gideon PS, Hall K, Ray WA. Major congenital malformations after first-trimester exposure to ACE inhibitors. N Engl J Med. 2006;354:2443–51.

114. Lambot MA, Vermeylen D, Noel JC. Angiotensin-II-receptor inhibition in pregnancy. Lancet. 2001;357:1619–20.

115. Alwan S, Polifka JE, Friedman JM. Angiotensin II receptor antagonist treatment during pregnancy. Birth Defects Res. 2005;73:123–30.

116. Spaggiari E, Heidet L, Grange G, Guimiot F, Dreux S, Delezoide AL, Renin-Angiotensin System Blockers Study Group, Muller F. Prognosis and outcome of pregnancies exposed to renin-angiotensin system blockers. Prenat Diagn. 2012;32:1071–6.

117. Loudon JA, Groom KM, Bennett PR. Prostaglandin inhibitors in preterm labour. Best Pract Clin Obstet Gynecol. 2003;17:731–44.

118. Mitra SC, Ganesh V, Apuzzio JJ. Effect of maternal cocaine abuse on renal arterial flow and urine output in the fetus. Am J Obstet Gynecol. 1994;171:1556–9.

119. Greenfield SP, Rutigliano E, Steinhardt G, Elder JS. Genitourinary tract malformations and maternal cocaine abuse. Urology. 1991;37:455–9.

120. Behnke M, Eyler FD, Garvan CW, Wobie K. The search for congenital malformations in newborns with fetal cocaine exposure. Pediatrics. 2001;107:E74.

121. Pregnancy and renal disease. Lancet. 1975;2:801–2.
122. McKay DB, Josephson MA. Pregnancy in recipients of solid organs—effects on mother and child. N Engl J Med. 2006;354:1281–93.
123. Carmichael SL, Shaw GM, Ma C, Werler MM, Rasmussen SA, Lammer EJ, National Birth Defects Prevention Study. Maternal corticosteroid use and orofacial clefts. Am J Obstet Gynecol. 2007;197(585):e1–585.e7.
124. Mason RJ, Thomson AW, Whiting PH, Gray ES, Brown PA, Catto GR, Simpson JG. Cyclosporine-induced fetotoxicity in the rat. Transplantation. 1985;39:9–12.
125. Farley DE, Shelby J, Alexander D, Scott JR. The effect of two new immunosuppressive agents, FK506 and didemnin B, in murine pregnancy. Transplantation. 1991;52:106–10.
126. Cleary BJ, Källén B. Early pregnancy azathioprine use and pregnancy outcomes. Birth Defects Res A Clin Mol Teratol. 2009;85:647–54.
127. Moritz MJ, Constantinescu S, Coscia LA, Armenti D. Mycophenolate and pregnancy: teratology principles and national transplantation pregnancy registry experience. Am J Transplant. 2017;17:581–2.
128. Hoeltzenbein M, Elefant E, Vial T, Finkel-Pekarsky V, Stephens S, Clementi M, Allignol A, Weber-Schoendorfer C, Schaefer C. Teratogenicity of mycophenolate confirmed in a prospective study of the European Network of Teratology Information Services. Am J Med Genet A. 2012;158A:588–96.
129. Anderka MT, Lin AE, Abuelo DN, Mitchell AA, Rasmussen SA. Reviewing the evidence for mycophenolate mofetil as a new teratogen: case report and review of the literature. Am J Med Genet A. 2009;149A:1241–8.
130. Veroux M, Corona D, Veroux P. Pregnancy under everolimus-based immunosuppression. Transpl Int. 2011;24:e115–7.
131. Chandra A, Midtvedt K, Asberg A, Elde IA. Immunosuppression and reproductive health after kidney transplantation. Transplantation. 2019;103:e325–33.
132. EBPG Expert Group in Renal Transplantation. European best practice guidelines for renal transplantation. Section IV.10. Long-term management of the transplant recipient—pregnancy in renal transplant recipients. Nephrol Dial Transplant. 2002;17(suppl 4):50–5.
133. Mong Hiep TT, Ismaili K, Collart F, Van Damme-Lombaerts R, Godefroid N, Ghuysen MS, Van Hoeck K, Raes A, Janssen F, Robert A. Clinical characteristics and outcomes of children with stage 3-5 chronic kidney disease. Pediatr Nephrol. 2010;25:935–40.
134. Weber S, Morinière V, Knüppel T, Charbit M, Dusek J, Ghiggeri GM, Jankauskiené A, Mir S, Montini G, Peco-Antic A, Wühl E, Zurowska AM, Mehls O, Antignac C, Schaefer F, Salomon R. Prevalence of mutations in renal developmental genes in children with renal hypodysplasia: results of the ESCAPE study. J Am Soc Nephrol. 2006;17:2864–70.

135. Woolf AS, Lopes FM, Ranjzad P, Roberts NA. Congenital disorders of the human urinary tract: recent insights from genetic and molecular studies. Front Pediatr. 2019;7:136.
136. Zhang R, Knapp M, Suzuki K, Kajioka D, Schmidt JM, Winkler J, Yilmaz Ö, Pleschka M, Cao J, Kockum CC, Barker G, Holmdahl G, Beaman G, Keene D, Woolf AS, Cervellione RM, Cheng W, Wilkins S, Gearhart JP, Sirchia F, Di Grazia M, Ebert AK, Rösch W, Ellinger J, Jenetzky E, Zwink N, Feitz WF, Marcelis C, Schumacher J, Martinón-Torres F, Hibberd ML, Khor CC, Heilmann-Heimbach S, Barth S, Boyadjiev SA, Brusco A, Ludwig M, Newman W, Nordenskjöld A, Yamada G, Odermatt B, Reutter H. ISL1 is a major susceptibility gene for classic bladder exstrophy and a regulator of urinary tract development. Sci Rep. 2017;7:42170.
137. Abdelhak S, Kalatzis V, Heilig R, Compain S, Samson D, Vincent C, Levi-Acobas F, Cruaud C, Le Merrer M, Mathieu M, König R, Vigneron J, Weissenbach J, Petit C, Weil D. Clustering of mutations responsible for branchio-oto-renal (BOR) syndrome in the eyes absent homologous region (eyaHR) of EYA1. Hum Mol Genet. 1997;6:2247–55.
138. Ruf RG, Xu PX, Silvius D, Otto EA, Beekmann F, Muerb UT, Kumar S, Neuhaus TJ, Kemper MJ, Raymond RM Jr, Brophy PD, Berkman J, Gattas M, Hyland V, Ruf EM, Schwartz C, Chang EH, Smith RJ, Stratakis CA, Weil D, Petit C, Hildebrandt F. SIX1 mutations cause branchio-oto-renal syndrome by disruption of EYA1-SIX1-DNA complexes. Proc Natl Acad Sci U S A. 2004;101:8090–5.
139. Meyer J, Südbeck P, Held M, Wagner T, Schmitz ML, Bricarelli FD, Eggermont E, Friedrich U, Haas OA, Kobelt A, Leroy JG, Van Maldergem L, Michel E, Mitulla B, Pfeiffer RA, Schinzel A, Schmidt H, Scherer G. Mutational analysis of the SOX9 gene in campomelic dysplasia and autosomal sex reversal: lack of genotype/phenotype correlations. Hum Mol Genet. 1997;6:91–8.
140. Kolatsi-Joannou M, Bingham C, Ellard S, Bulman MP, Allen LI, Hattersley AT, Woolf AS. Hepatocyte nuclear factor-1beta: a new kindred with renal cysts and diabetes and gene expression in normal human development. J Am Soc Nephrol. 2001;12:2175–80.
141. Vivante A, Kleppa MJ, Schulz J, Kohl S, Sharma A, Chen J, Shril S, Hwang DY, Weiss AC, Kaminski MM, Shukrun R, Kemper MJ, Lehnhardt A, Beetz R, Sanna-Cherchi S, Verbitsky M, Gharavi AG, Stuart HM, Feather SA, Goodship JA, Goodship TH, Woolf AS, Westra SJ, Doody DP, Bauer SB, Lee RS, Adam RM, Lu W, Reutter HM, Kehinde EO, Mancini EJ, Lifton RP, Tasic V, Lienkamp SS, Jüppner H, Kispert A, Hildebrandt F. Mutations in TBX18 cause dominant urinary tract malformations via transcriptional dysregulation of ureter development. Am J Hum Genet. 2015;97:291–301.
142. Jenkins D, Caubit X, Dimovski A, Matevska N, Lye CM, Cabuk F, Gucev Z, Tasic V, Fasano L, Woolf AS. Analysis of TSHZ2 and TSHZ3 genes

143. Gbadegesin RA, Brophy PD, Adeyemo A, Hall G, Gupta IR, Hains D, Bartkowiak B, Rabinovich CE, Chandrasekharappa S, Homstad A, Westreich K, Wu G, Liu Y, Holanda D, Clarke J, Lavin P, Selim A, Miller S, Wiener JS, Ross SS, Foreman J, Rotimi C, Winn MP. *TNXB* mutations can cause vesicoureteral reflux. J Am Soc Nephrol. 2013;24:1313–22.

144. Kolvenbach CM, Dworschak GC, Frese S, Japp AS, Schuster P, Wenzlitschke N, Yilmaz Ö, Lopes FM, Pryalukhin A, Schierbaum L, van der Zanden LFM, Kause F, Schneider R, Taranta-Janusz K, Szczepańska M, Pawlaczyk K, Newman WG, Beaman GM, Stuart HM, Cervellione RM, Feitz WFJ, van Rooij IALM, Schreuder MF, Steffens M, Weber S, Merz WM, Feldkötter M, Hoppe B, Thiele H, Altmüller J, Berg C, Kristiansen G, Ludwig M, Reutter H, Woolf AS, Hildebrandt F, Grote P, Zaniew M, Odermatt B, Hilger AC. Rare variants in *BNC2* are implicated in autosomal-dominant congenital lower urinary-tract obstruction. Am J Hum Genet. 2017;104:994–1006.

145. Richer J, Milewicz DM, Gow R, de Nanassy J, Maharajh G, Miller E, Oppenheimer L, Weiler G, O'Connor M. R179H mutation in *ACTA2* expanding the phenotype to include prune-belly sequence and skin manifestations. Am J Med Genet A. 2012;158A:664–8.

146. Thorson W, Diaz-Horta O, Foster J 2nd, Spiliopoulos M, Quintero R, Farooq A, Blanton S, Tekin M. De novo *ACTG2* mutations cause congenital distended bladder, microcolon, and intestinal hypoperistalsis. Hum Genet. 2007;133:737–42.

147. Weber S, Thiele H, Mir S, Toliat MR, Sozeri B, Reutter H, Draaken M, Ludwig M, Altmüller J, Frommolt P, Stuart HM, Ranjzad P, Hanley NA, Jennings R, Newman WG, Wilcox DT, Thiel U, Schlingmann KP, Beetz R, Hoyer PF, Konrad M, Schaefer F, Nürnberg P, Woolf AS. Muscarinic acetylcholine receptor M3 mutation causes urinary bladder disease and a prune-belly-like syndrome. Am J Hum Genet. 2011;89:668–74.

148. Gauthier J, Ouled Amar Bencheikh B, Hamdan FF, Harrison SM, Baker LA, Couture F, Thiffault I, Ouazzani R, Samuels ME, Mitchell GA, Rouleau GA, Michaud JL, Soucy JF. A homozygous loss-of-function variant in *MYH11* in a case with megacystis-microcolon-intestinal hypoperistalsis syndrome. Eur J Hum Genet. 2015;23:1266–8.

149. Halim D, Brosens E, Muller F, Wangler MF, Beaudet AL, Lupski JR, Akdemir ZHC, Doukas M, Stoop HJ, de Graaf BM, Brouwer RWW, van Ijcken WFJ, Oury JF, Rosenblatt J, Burns AJ, Tibboel D, Hofstra RMW, Alves MM. Loss of function variants in *MYLK* cause recessive megacystis microcolon intestinal hypoperistalsis syndrome. Am J Hum Genet. 2017;101:123–9.

150. Boghossian NS, Sicko RJ, Giannakou A, Dimopoulos A, Caggana M, Tsai MY, Yeung EH, Pankratz N, Cole BR, Romitti PA, Browne ML, Fan R, Liu A, Kay DM, Mills JL. Rare copy number variants identified in prune belly syndrome. Eur J Med Genet. 2018;61:145–51.

151. Vivante A, Mann N, Yonath H, Weiss AC, Getwan M, Kaminski MM, Bohnenpoll T, Teyssier C, Chen J, Shril S, van der Ven AT, Ityel H, Schmidt JM, Widmeier E, Bauer SB, Sanna-Cherchi S, Gharavi AG, Lu W, Magen D, Shukrun R, Lifton RP, Tasic V, Stanescu HC, Cavaillès V, Kleta R, Anikster Y, Dekel B, Kispert A, Lienkamp SS, Hildebrandt F. A dominant mutation in nuclear receptor interacting protein 1 causes urinary tract malformations *via* dysregulation of retinoic acid signaling. J Am Soc Nephrol. 2017;28:2364–76.

152. Sanyanusin P, Schimmenti LA, McNoe LA, Ward TA, Pierpont ME, Sullivan MJ, Dobyns WB, Eccles MR. Mutation of the *PAX2* gene in a family with optic nerve colobomas, renal anomalies and vesico-ureteral reflux. Nat Genet. 1995;9:358–64.

153. Daly SB, Urquhart JE, Hilton E, McKenzie EA, Kammerer RA, Lewis M, Kerr B, Stuart H, Donnai D, Long DA, Burgu B, Aydogdu O, Derbent M, Garcia-Minaur S, Reardon W, Gener B, Shalev S, Smith R, Woolf AS, Black GC, Newman WG. Mutations in *HPSE2* cause urofacial syndrome. Am J Hum Genet. 2010;86:963–9.

154. Stuart HM, Roberts NA, Burgu B, Daly SB, Urquhart JE, Bhaskar S, Dickerson JE, Mermerkaya M, Silay MS, Lewis MA, Olondriz MB, Gener B, Beetz C, Varga RE, Gülpınar O, Süer E, Soygür T, Ozçakar ZB, Yalçınkaya F, Kavaz A, Bulum B, Gücük A, Yue WW, Erdogan F, Berry A, Hanley NA, McKenzie EA, Hilton EN, Woolf AS, Newman WG. *LRIG2* mutations cause urofacial syndrome. Am J Hum Genet. 2013;92:259–64.

155. Liebeschuetz S, Thomas R. Unilateral multicystic dysplastic kidney (letter). Arch Dis Child. 1997;77:369.

156. James CA, Watson AR, Twining P, Rance CH. Antenatally detected urinary tract abnormalities: changing incidence and management. Eur J Pediatr. 1998;157:508–11.

157. Scala C, McDonnell S, Murphy F, Leone Roberti Maggiore U, Khalil A, Bhide A, Thilaganathan B, Papageorghiou AT. Diagnostic accuracy of midtrimester antenatal ultrasound for multicystic dysplastic kidneys. Ultrasound Obstet Gynecol. 2017;50:464–9.

158. Ismaili K, Avni FE, Alexander M, Schulman C, Collier F, Hall M. Routine voiding cystourethrography is of no value in neonates with unilateral multicystic dysplastic kidney. J Pediatr. 2005;146:759–63.

159. Cassart M, Majoub N, Irtan S, Joannic JM, Ducou le Pointe H, Blondiaux E, Garel C. Prenatal evaluation and postnatal follow-up of ureteral ectopic insertion

in multicystic dysplastic kidneys. Fetal Diagn Ther. 2019;45:373–80.

160. Erger F, Brüchle NO, Gembruch U, Zerres K. Prenatal ultrasound, genotype, and outcome in a large cohort of prenatally affected patients with autosomal-recessive polycystic kidney disease and other hereditary cystic kidney diseases. Arch Gynecol Obstet. 2017;295:897–906.

161. Bergmann C. Early and severe polycystic kidney disease and related ciliopathies: an emerging field of interest. Nephron. 2019;142:50–60.

162. Ward CJ, Hogan MC, Rossetti S, Walker D, Sneddon T, Wang X, Kubly V, Cunningham JM, Bacallao R, Ishibashi M, Milliner DS, Torres VE, Harris PC. The gene mutated in autosomal recessive polycystic kidney disease encodes a large, receptor-like protein. Nat Genet. 2002;30:259–69.

163. Büscher R, Büscher AK, Weber S, Mohr J, Hegen B, Vester U, Hoyer PF. Clinical manifestations of autosomal recessive polycystic kidney disease (ARPKD): kidney-related and non-kidney-related phenotypes. Pediatr Nephrol. 2014;29:1915–25.

164. Wilson PD. Polycystic kidney disease. N Engl J Med. 2004;350:151–64.

165. Mochizuki T, Wu G, Hayashi T, Xenophontos SL, Veldhuisen B, Saris JJ, Reynolds DM, Cai Y, Gabow PA, Pierides A, Kimberling WJ, Breuning MH, Deltas CC, Peters DJ, Somlo S. *PKD2*, a gene for polycystic kidney disease that encodes an integral membrane protein. Science. 1996;272:1339–42.

166. Gimpel C, Bergmann C, Bockenhauer D, Breysem L, Cadnapaphornchai MA, Cetiner M, Dudley J, Emma F, Konrad M, Harris T, Harris PC, König J, Liebau MC, Marlais M, Mekahli D, Metcalfe AM, Oh J, Perrone RD, Sinha MD, Titieni A, Torra R, Weber S, Winyard PJD, Schaefer F. International consensus statement on the diagnosis and management of autosomal dominant polycystic kidney disease in children and young people. Nat Rev Nephrol. 2019;15:713–26.

167. Janssens P, Jouret F, Bammens B, Liebau MC, Schaefer F, Dandurand A, Perrone RD, Müller RU, Pao CS, Mekahli D. Implications of early diagnosis of autosomal dominant polycystic kidney disease: a post hoc analysis of the TEMPO 3:4 trial. Sci Rep. 2020;10:4294.

168. Garel J, Lefebvre M, Cassart M, Della Valle V, Guilbaud L, Jouannic JM, Ducou le Pointe H, Blondiaux E, Garel C. Prenatal ultrasonography of autosomal dominant polycystic kidney disease mimicking recessive type: case series. Pediatr Radiol. 2019;49:906–12.

169. Avni EF, Thoua Y, Van Gansbeke D, Matos C, Didier F, Droulez P, Schulman CC. The development of hypodysplastic kidney. Radiology. 1985;164:123–5.

170. Bingham C, Bulman MP, Ellard S, Allen LI, Lipkin GW, Hoff WG, Woolf AS, Rizzoni G, Novelli G, Nicholls AJ, Hattersley AT. Mutations in the hepatocyte nuclear factor-1beta gene are associated with familial hypoplastic glomerulocystic kidney disease. Am J Hum Genet. 2001;68:219–24.

171. Ismaili K, Pawtowski A, Boyer O, Wissing KM, Janssen F, Hall M. Genetic forms of nephrotic syndrome: a single-center experience in Brussels. Pediatr Nephrol. 2009;24:287–94.

172. Hölttä T, Jalanko H. Congenital nephrotic syndrome: is early aggressive treatment needed? Yes. Pediatr Nephrol. 2020;35:1985–90.

173. Bérody S, Heidet L, Gribouval O, Harambat J, Niaudet P, Baudouin V, Bacchetta J, Boudaillez B, Dehennault M, de Parscau L, Dunand O, Flodrops H, Fila M, Garnier A, Louillet F, Macher MA, May A, Merieau E, Monceaux F, Pietrement C, Rousset-Rouvière C, Roussey G, Taque S, Tenenbaum J, Ulinski T, Vieux R, Zaloszyc A, Morinière V, Salomon R, Boyer O. Treatment and outcome of congenital nephrotic syndrome. Nephrol Dial Transplant. 2019;34:458–67.

174. Chiodini B, Herman J, Lolin K, Adams B, Hennaut E, Lingier P, Mikhalski D, Schurmans T, Knops N, Wissing KM, Abramowicz D, Ismaili K. Outcomes of kidney transplantations in children weighing 15 kilograms or less: a retrospective cohort study. Transpl Int. 2018;31:720–8.

175. Kestilä M, Lenkkeri U, Lamerdin J, McCready P, Putaala H, Ruotsalainen V, Morita T, Nissinen M, Herva R, Kashtan CE, Peltonen L, Holmberg C, Olsen A, Tryggvason K. Positionally cloned gene for a novel glomerular protein—nephrin—is mutated in congenital nephrotic syndrome. Mol Cell. 1998;1:575–82.

176. Huttunen NP. Congenital nephrotic syndrome of Finnish type. Study of 75 cases. Arch Dis Child. 1976;51:344–8.

177. Souka AP, Skentou H, Geerts L, Bower S, Nicolaides KH. Congenital nephrotic syndrome presenting with increase nuchal translucency in the first trimester. Prenat Diagn. 2002;22:93–5.

178. Rapola J. Why is congenital nephrotic syndrome associated with a rise in the concentration of alpha-fetoprotein in the amniotic fluid? Pediatr Nephrol. 1990;4:206.

179. Pagana K, Pagana TJ, editors. Mosby's manual of diagnostic and laboratory tests. 5th ed. St. Louis, MO: Elsevier; 2014.

180. Weber S, Gribouval O, Esquivel EL, Morinière V, Tête MJ, Legendre C, Niaudet P, Antignac C. *NPHS2* mutation analysis shows genetic heterogeneity of steroid-resistant nephrotic syndrome and low post-transplant recurrence. Kidney Int. 2004;66:571–9.

181. Mark K, Reis A, Zenker M. Prenatal findings in four consecutive pregnancies with fetal Pierson syndrome, a newly defined congenital nephrosis syndrome. Prenat Diagn. 2006;26:262–6.

182. Zenker M, Aigner T, Wendler O, Tralau T, Müntefering H, Fenski R, Pitz S, Schumacher V, Royer-Pokora B, Wühl E, Cochat P, Bouvier R, Kraus C, Mark K, Madlon H, Dötch J, Rascher W, Maruniak-Chudek I, Lennert T, Neumann LM, Reis A. Human laminin beta 2 deficiency causes congenital nephrosis with mesangial sclerosis and distinct eye abnormalities. Hum Mol Genet. 2004;13:2625–32.

183. Boyer O, Benoit G, Gribouval O, Nevo F, Pawtowski A, Bilge I, Bircan Z, Deschênes G, Guay-Woodford LM, Hall M, Macher MA, Soulami K, Stefanidis CJ, Weiss R, Loirat C, Gubler MC, Antignac C. Mutational analysis of the *PLCE1* gene in steroid resistant nephrotic syndrome. J Med Genet. 2010;47:445–52.

184. Besbas N, Bayrakci US, Kale G, Cengiz AB, Akcoren Z, Akinci D, Kilic I, Bakkaloglu A. Cytomegalovirus-related congenital nephrotic syndrome with diffuse mesangial sclerosis. Pediatr Nephrol. 2006;21:740–2.

185. Coplen DE, Austin PF, Yan Y, Blanco VM, Dicke JM. The magnitude of fetal renal pelvic dilatation can identify obstructive postnatal hydronephrosis, and direct postnatal evaluation and management. J Urol. 2006;176:724–7.

186. Johnston JH, Evans JP, Glassberg KI, Shapiro SR. Pelvic hydronephrosis in children: a review of 219 personal cases. J Urol. 1977;117:97–101.

187. Ismaili K, Avni FE, Wissing KM, Piepsz A, Aubert D, Cochat P, Hall M. Current management of infants with fetal renal pelvis dilatation: a survey by French-speaking pediatric nephrologists and urologists. Pediatr Nephrol. 2004;19:966–71.

188. Ismaili K, Piepsz A. The antenatally detected pelviureteric junction stenosis: advances in renography and stategy of management. Pediatr Radiol. 2013;43:428–35.

189. Duong HP, Piepsz A, Khelif K, Collier F, de Man K, Damry N, Janssen F, Hall M, Ismaili K. Transverse comparisons between ultrasound and radionuclide parameters in children with presumed antenatally detected pelvi-ureteric junction obstruction. Eur J Nucl Med Mol Imaging. 2015;42:940–6.

190. Onen A. Grading of hydronephrosis: an ongoing challenge. Front Pediatr. 2020;8:458.

191. Duong HP, Piepsz A, Collier F, Khelif K, Christophe C, Cassart M, Janssen F, Hall M, Ismaili K. Predicting the clinical outcome of antenatally detected unilateral pelviureteric junction stenosis. Urology. 2013;82:691–6.

192. Passoni NM, Peters CA. Managing ureteropelvic junction obstruction in the young infant. Front Pediatr. 2020;8:242.

193. Grazioli S, Parvex P, Merlini L, Combescure C, Girardin E. Antenatal and postnatal ultrasound in the evaluation of the risk of vesicoureteral reflux. Pediatr Nephrol. 2010;25:1687–92.

194. Garin EH, Campos A, Homsy Y. Primary vesicoureteral reflux: review of current concepts. Pediatr Nephrol. 1998;12:249–56.

195. Ismaili K, Avni F, Piepsz A, Collier F, Schulman C, Hall M. Vesicoureteric reflux in children. Eur Urol Suppl. 2006;4:129–40.

196. McLellan DL, Retik AB, Bauer SB, Diamond DA, Atala A, Mandell J, Lebowitz RL, Borer JG, Peters CA. Rate and predictors of spontaneous resolution of prenatally diagnosed nonrefluxing Megaureter. J Urol. 2002;168:2177–80.

197. Whitten SM, Wilcox DT. Duplex systems. Prenat Diagn. 2001;21:952–7.

198. Peppas DS, Skoog SJ, Canning DA, Belman AB. Nonsurgical management of primary vesicoureteric reflux in complete ureteral duplication. Is it justified? J Urol. 1991;146:1594–5.

199. Avni FE, Dacher JN, Stallenberg B, Collier F, Hall M, Schulman CC. Renal duplications: the impact of perinatal US on diagnosis and management. Eur Urol. 1991;20:43–8.

200. Decter RM. Renal duplication and fusion anomalies. Pediatr Clin N Am. 1997;44:1323–41.

201. Jouannic JM, Hyett JA, Pandya PP, Gulbis B, Rodeck CH, Jauniaux E. Perinatal outcome in fetuses with megacystis in the first half of pregnancy. Prenat Diag. 2003;23:340–4.

202. Spaggiari E, Dreux S, Czerkiewicz I, Favre R, Schmitz T, Guimiot F, Laurichesse Delmas H, Verspyck E, Oury JF, Ville Y, Muller F. Fetal obstructive uropathy complicated by urinary ascites: outcome and prognostic value of fetal serum β-2-microglobulin. Ultrasound Obstet Gynecol. 2013;41:185–9.

203. Hochart V, Lahoche A, Priso RH, Houfflin-Debarge V, Bassil A, Sharma D, Behal H, Avni FE. Posterior urethral valves: are neonatal imaging findings predictive of renal function during early childhood? Pediatr Radiol. 2016;46:1418–23.

204. Fontanella F, van Scheltema PNA, Duin L, Cohen-Overbeek TE, Pajkrt E, Bekker MN, Willekes C, Oepkes D, Bilardo CM. Antenatal staging of congenital lower urinary tract obstruction. Ultrasound Obstet Gynecol. 2019;53:520–4.

205. Dinneen MD, Duffy PG. Posterior urethral valves. Br J Urol. 1996;78:275–81.

206. Holmes N, Harrison MR, Baskin LS. Fetal surgery for posterior urethral valves: long term postnatal outcomes. Pediatrics. 2001;108:36–42.

207. Quintero RA, Hume R, Smith C, Johnson MP, Cotton DB, Romero R, Evans M. Percutaneous fetal cystoscopy and endoscopic fulguration of posterior urethral valves. Am J Obstet Gynecol. 1995;172:206–9.

208. Agarwal SK, Fisk NM. In utero therapy for lower urinary tract obstruction. Prenat Diagn. 2001;21:970–6.

209. Golbus MS, Harrison MR, Filly RA. In utero treatment of urinary tract obstruction. Am J Obstet Gynecol. 1982;142:383–8.

210. Clark TJ, Martin WL, Divakaran TG, Whittle MJ, Kilby MD, Khan KS. Prenatal bladder drainage in the management of fetal lower urinary tract obstruction: a systematic review and meta-analysis. Obstet Gynecol. 2003;102:367–82.

211. Morris RK, Malin GL, Quinlan-Jones E, Middleton LJ, Hemming K, Burke D, Daniels JP, Khan KS, Deeks J, Kilby MD, For the Percutaneous Vesicoamniotic Shunting in Lower Urinary Tract Obstruction (PLUTO) Collaborative Group. Percutaneous vesicoamniotic shunting versus conservative management for fetal lower urinary tract obstruction (PLUTO): a randomised trial. Lancet. 2013;382:1496–506.

212. Van Mieghem T, Ryan G. The PLUTO trial: a missed opportunity (comment). Lancet. 2013;382:1471–3.

213. Kitagawa H, Pringle KC, Koike J. Vesicoamniotic shunt for complete urinary tract obstruction is partially effective. J Pediatr Surg. 2006;41:394–402.

Laboratory Evaluation of Renal Disease in Childhood

2

Damien Noone and Valérie Langlois

Assessment of the Urine

Urinalysis

The American Academy of Pediatrics stopped recommending routine yearly urinalysis as a screening tool for chronic kidney disease (CKD) in otherwise healthy school-aged children over a decade ago [1]. Nonetheless, the value of the urinalysis in the evaluation of kidney disease should not be underestimated in certain patient populations. Important information can be learned from this simple, quick, inexpensive test when used in the appropriate setting. Commercially available reagent strips can be used to screen the urine for pH, specific gravity (SG), protein, blood, glucose, ketones, leukocytes, and nitrates. Urine specimens should be fresh and clean-voided midstream in older children. If analysis cannot be done within 4 h, then the sample needs a preservative and/or to be stored at 4 °C or lower (−20 or −80 °C) to maintain the integrity and prevent degradation of the specimen. The variations in pH and osmolality of the urine can cause particles within the urine to lyse. Various preservatives can be used, e.g., boric acid (changes urinary pH), sodium azide (to prevent bacterial overgrowth),

D. Noone (✉) · V. Langlois
Division of Nephrology, Department of Paediatrics,
The Hospital for Sick Children, Toronto, ON, Canada
e-mail: damien.noone@sickkids.ca;
valerie.langlois@sickkids.ca

formaldehyde (causes false positive leucocyte esterase), mercury salts and chlorhexidine [2].

Depending on urine concentration, the urine color varies from pale yellow to amber. Red or tea colored urine suggests the presence of blood, hemoglobin, myoglobin, porphyrin, non-pathologic pigments (beets, food color) or certain medications. Blue to green is suggestive of the presence of biliverdin or Pseudomonas infection.

The urine is normally clear, but can be cloudy in the presence of leukocytes, epithelial cells, bacteria, or precipitation of amorphous phosphate or urate. Unusual urine odor can lead to the diagnosis of rare metabolic disorders such as maple syrup urine disease (maple syrup odor), phenylketonuria (musty odor) or hypermethioninemia (fishy odor).

SG reflects the urinary concentrating and diluting capability of the kidney. In normal conditions, it reflects the patient's hydration status. However, with abnormal kidneys, a very low SG may represent a concentrating defect. It may be useful in distinguishing pre-renal states from intrinsic renal disease. SG usually ranges from 1:001 to 1:035 and can be measured using a urinometer or a refractometer, but more commonly using the reagent strips. The reagent strip test is based on pKa change of polyelectrolytes in relation to ionic concentration [3].

Urinary pH usually ranges from 5.0 to 8.5 depending on the acid-base balance of the body and can be estimated using the reagent test strip.

© The Author(s), under exclusive license to Springer Nature Switzerland AG 2023
F. Schaefer, L. A. Greenbaum (eds.), *Pediatric Kidney Disease*,
https://doi.org/10.1007/978-3-031-11665-0_2

However, precise measurements need to be obtained using a pH meter with a glass electrode, particularly when <5.5 or >7.5. Urinary pH is important in the diagnosis of renal tubular acidosis and monitoring the treatment for prevention of urinary stones.

Glucose is not usually present in the urine. Glucose is freely filtered at the glomerulus and reabsorbed in the proximal tubule via a sodium-coupled active transport mechanism. Glucosuria can be seen when the serum glucose is above the renal threshold, or due to isolated renal glucosuria or generalized proximal tubular dysfunction (Fanconi syndrome). Normal values for maximal tubular glucose reabsorption (TmG) in children vary from 254 to 401 mg/min/1.73 m^2 [4]. Reagent test strips are usually impregnated with the enzyme glucose oxidase and only detect glucose. Other sugars can be detected by the copper reduction test such as Clinitest Tablet (Ames Co.). A false negative glucose can occur with high dose vitamin C and in the setting of elevated ketones [2].

Ketone bodies are formed during the catabolism of fatty acids and include acetoacetic acid, β-hydroxybutyric acid, and acetone. Most reagent strips for ketones are based on a color reaction with sodium nitroprusside and are sensitive for acetoacetic acid but will not detect β-hydroxybutyric acid or acetone.

Strip tests detect leukocyte esterase, an enzyme found in neutrophils. Nitrites indicate the presence of bacteria capable of reducing dietary nitrate, such as *Escherichia coli*, *Enterobacter*, *Citrobacter*, *Klebsiella*, and *Proteus* species. A positive urinalysis for both leucocytes and nitrites is suggestive of bacteriuria or a urinary tract infection (UTI), and if both are negative then a UTI is unlikely. If either are positive, then a further confirmatory urine culture is required [5, 6]. Samples should be processed rapidly to avoid degradation of esterases and false negative results [7]. For children under the age of two, urinalysis is less reliable for the diagnosis of UTI [6]. For infants less than one year of age, microscopic presence of moderate bacteria and >10 white cells/high powered field is more accurate in diagnosing a UTI [6]. An alkaline pH or the

ingestion of beets can cause a false positive leukocyte esterase and there may be a false negative in the setting of high urinary glucose, protein or with antibiotics. There may be a false negative nitrite when the urine SG is high, with ascorbic acid ingestion (reducing agent), if the child eats insufficient fruits and vegetables to provide the nitrate substrate in the urine or if the incubation time is too short due to urinary frequency [2, 8]. The accuracy of urinary nitrites in the diagnosis of UTIs in those under age 2 years has been recently called into question; they miss UTIs in about 75% of young children [8].

Hematuria is defined as the presence of >5 red blood cells (RBCs) per high power field in centrifuged urine. The presence of RBCs can only be confirmed by microscopic evaluation of fresh urine. Reagent strips detect RBCs, myoglobin, and hemoglobin because all contain a heme moiety. As with nitrite detection, ascorbic acid can cause a false-negative due to it being a strong reducing agent. The supernatant of a centrifuged urine containing red blood cells will be clear yellow as opposed to being pink if the urine contains hemoglobin or myoglobin. The morphology of the cells can help determine their origin. The presence of dysmorphic red blood cells suggests glomerular hematuria.

Urine Microscopy

"…the ghosts of dead patients that haunt us do not ask why we did not employ the latest fad of clinical investigation. They ask us, why did you not test my urine?"—Sir Robert Grieve Hutchison (1871–1960) [9].

Microscopic evaluation of fresh urine (within 1–2 h) is extremely valuable in the evaluation of renal disease. Ideally, 10 mL of urine is centrifuged at 1500 rpm for 5 min, and about 9.5 mL is decanted off. The remainder is gently agitated; a single drop is placed on a glass slide; and a cover slip is added. The urine sediment is examined at low (×10) and high (×40) magnification for the presence of casts, cells, and crystals. Although hyaline (containing primarily uromodulin) and granular casts can be seen in normal states, cellular casts are pathologic. Granular casts contain degraded cell lysosomes and other debris from degenerated renal tubular epithelial cells and typically reflect tubular injury or acute tubular necrosis. Red blood cell casts are pathognomonic of glomerular disease and white blood cell (WBC) casts can be seen with pyelonephritis or post-infectious glomerulonephritis [10].

Crystals are rarely seen in fresh urine but appear after the urine stands for a period. Uric acid, calcium oxalate, amorphous urate, cystine, tyrosine, leucine, and cholesterol crystals are usually found in acid urine. Uric acid and calcium oxalate crystal can be seen in normal and pathological conditions. Amorphous urate crystals are of no clinical significance. Cystine, tyrosine, leucine, and cholesterol crystals are always relevant. Cystine crystals (colorless and hexagonal) are present in patients with cystinuria, leucine crystals can be associated with maple syrup urine disease, methionine malabsorption syndrome and severe liver disease. Tyrosine crystals also occur in severe liver disease, tyrosinosis, and methionine malabsorption syndrome. The presence of cholesterol crystals can indicate excessive tissue breakdown, or nephritic or nephrotic syndrome [3]. Triple phosphate, calcium carbonate, ammonium biurate, amorphous phosphates and calcium phosphate crystals are usually found in alkaline urine. Calcium carbonate and amorphous phosphate are of no clinical significance [10]. Many drugs are associated with crystalluria, including acyclovir, amoxicillin, atazanavir, ciprofloxacin, methotrexate, sulfadiazine, triamterene and vitamin C [10].

The association of urinary eosinophils with acute interstitial nephritis (AIN) was first reported by Galpin et al. [11] and became widely accepted as supportive of a diagnosis of AIN. Hansel's stain replaced Wright's stain, the latter being ineffective when urine pH was <7, and the former revealing the bright red granules of eosinophils. However, eosinophiluria may be seen in a variety of conditions, including prostatitis, cystitis, and glomerulonephritis, limiting the sensitivity and positive predictive value of the test. Compared to the gold standard of kidney biopsy, eosinophiluria lacks sensitivity and specificity, and can-

not distinguish AIN from acute tubular necrosis. Hence, it really has no diagnostic utility [12].

Automated microscopy that uses laminar flow digital imaging technology can classify and count cells (RBCs, WBCs and epithelial cells) and particulate matter (bacteria, yeasts and crystals) in uncentrifuged urine. Urine particle flow cytometers can quantify cells more accurately than manual urine microscopy [13].

Urinary Protein Excretion

In the normal state, most of the filtered low molecular weight (MW) proteins (MW < 40,000) are reabsorbed in the proximal tubules. Proteins of higher MW, such as albumin (MW = 60,000), are not usually filtered. Tamm Horsfall proteins are secreted by the tubular cells in the ascending thick limb of the loop of Henle and are the main protein found in normal urine.

In disease states, increased amount of protein can be found in the urine and may reflect damage in the glomerular barrier (glomerular proteinuria) or impaired tubular reabsorption (tubular proteinuria). In glomerular proteinuria, albumin, which is not usually present, is the dominant protein. β2-microglobulin, α-1-microglobulin, and retinol-binding protein are markers of tubular proteinuria.

Proteinuria can vary by age, sex, ethnicity and body mass index [14, 15]. In the first month of life, proteinuria is 4–5 times higher than in older infants, perhaps reflecting the evolving maturity of the tubules, and the 90th percentile for urinary albumin/creatinine ratio (UACR) in the neonatal period was reported as 17.5 (90% Confidence Interval 7.1–79.7) mg/mmol in one study [16]. Normative ranges for UACR at different ages are presented in Table 1 [17].

The 2012 KDIGO Clinical Practice Guideline for the evaluation and management of CKD recommends, in order of preference, a UACR, a urine protein/creatinine ratio (UPCR), reagent strip urinalysis for total protein with automated reading and, finally, a reagent strip with manual reading for assessment of proteinuria. All should ideally be done on an early morning urine specimen [18]. It is not usually necessary to obtain a timed urine collection. A standard urine dipstick can be used to detect increased total urine proteins and albumin-specific dipsticks are acceptable to detect microalbuminuria. Microalbuminuria refers to albumin excretion above the normal range, but below the level of detection of the standard urine dipstick. UACR or UPCR ratio should be done within 3 months of a positive dipstick to confirm albuminuria or proteinuria, respectively. Post-pubertal children with diabetes of 5 or more years' duration should have urine albumin measured by albumin-specific dipstick or UACR, and this should be performed annually [19, 20].

Urine dipstick can provide an estimate of proteinuria and is most sensitive for albumin. False positive dipstick can be the result of prolonged immersion of the reagent strip, alkaline urine (pH > 7.5), presence of pyuria, bacteriuria or mucoprotein and penicillin [21]. A false negative can occur in very dilute urine [2].

Twenty-four-hour urine collections have long been the gold standard for quantification of urine protein excretion. The adequacy of the collection is verified by quantifying the total creatinine content of the sample, which should be about 15–20 mg/kg in females and 20–25 mg/kg in males [22]. However, collection in young children often requires catheterization and is not practical. First morning urine for UPCR is generally accepted as being valid in the assessment of proteinuria in children [18]. A recent study confirmed that UPCR is positively correlated with 24-h urine protein in children, and the cutoff of UPCR <0.2 g/g corresponds to normal protein excretion and the cutoff UPCR ≥2 g/g is nephrotic-range proteinuria [23].

Twenty-four-hour urine protein excretion of <4 and >40 $mg/m^2/h$ is normal and nephrotic-range proteinuria, respectively. Normal urinary albumin excretion is between 30–300 mg/day on a 24-h collection, 20–200 µg/min in an overnight collection and 3–30 mg/mmol on a first morning urine sample (Table 2) [24]. There can be significant diurnal variation in proteinuria in children and adolescents that is generally not considered pathological and resolves by adulthood. Orthostatic proteinuria is defined as an elevated protein excretion in the upright position, but normal excretion in the recumbent position. It can be assessed on a split 24-h urinary protein assessment [22]. Previous studies reported an incidence of 2–5% [22]; however, a study using 24-h total urinary protein excretion found a much higher incidence of 19.8% in a cohort of 91 children [25]. The original studies had used dipstick analysis [22], spot UPCR [26] or timed collections of less than 24 h [25, 27].

In 2006, Mori et al. [28] measured the UPCR in a cohort of Japanese children with urinary tract abnormalities or glomerular disorders and found that it varies according to body size and composition, reflecting muscle mass. They suggested that evaluation of UPCR should also consider body height, because as height and therefore muscle mass (denominator) increases, the ratio will decrease. A normative range for urinary protein excretion for the different sexes and as height and body surface area increases remains to be defined [28]. Kim et al. [29] proposed urine protein-to-

Table 1 Mean urinary albumin excretion, expressed as a albumin/creatinine ratio [17]

Age	Spot urine (mg/mmol)
Neonates	5.24
1–3 months	5.01
4–6 months	4.06
7–23 months	1.76
2–4 years old	1.34
3–19 years old	3

Table 2 Reference values for urinary protein excretion [19]

	24 Hour collection ($mg/m^2/h$)	24 Hour Collection ($mg/m^2/day$)	Spot urine protein/creatinine (mg/mg)	Spot urine protein/creatinine (mg/mmol)
Normal range				
6–24 months	<4	<150	<0.5	<50
>24 months		<150	<0.2	<20
Nephrotic	>40	>3 g/1.73 m^2/day	>2	>200

osmolality ratio as an alternative test to 24-h urinary protein excretion. Urinary protein-to-osmolality corrects for hydration status, can be used in children with decreased muscle mass, and has now been validated in two further pediatric populations against both spot UPCR and 24-h urinary protein excretion [30, 31]. In children, a spot urinary protein-to-osmolality ratio above 0.33 and 1.75 mg/L/mOsm/kg represents abnormal proteinuria and nephrotic-range proteinuria, respectively [31].

Standard urine dipstick tests are primarily sensitive to detect albumin. Screening for low MW protein can be done by the sulfosalicylic acid test. The addition of sulfosalicylic acid to the supernatant of centrifuged urine will cause cloudiness in the presence of any protein in the urine. A negative reagent strip test with a positive sulfosalicylic acid test is suggestive of low MW proteinuria. Urine protein electrophoresis can confirm the diagnosis. A false positive sulfosalicylic acid test can be produced by radiographic contrast, penicillin, cephalosporins, sulfonamide metabolites and high uric acid concentration [21].

Assessment of Renal Function

Glomerular Filtration

Glomerular filtration rate (GFR) is the most commonly used measure of kidney function and is used to classify various stages of CKD (Table 3) [18]. It can be quantified by measuring the clear-

Table 3 NKF-K/DIGO 2012 Classification of the stages of chronic kidney disease in children greater than 2 years of age [38]

Stage	Description	GFR (mL/min/ 1.73 m²)
1	Kidney damage with normal or increased GFR	>90
2	Kidney damage with mild reduction of GFR	60–89
3a	Moderate reduction of GFR	45–59
3b	Moderate to severe decrease of GFR	30–44
4	Severe reduction of GFR	15–29
5	Kidney failure	<15

ance rate of a substance from the plasma. The substance can be endogenous or exogenous. It is often referred to as the "marker". Different markers such as inulin, creatinine, iothalamate, iohexol, ethylenediaminetetraacetic acid (EDTA) and diethylenetriamine pentaacetic acid (DTPA) are available. The ideal marker must have a stable plasma concentration, should be filtered, but not reabsorbed, secreted, synthesized or metabolized by the kidney so that the amount filtered equals the amount excreted.

The renal clearance of the substance x (Cx) can be obtained by multiplying the urinary concentration of substance x (Ux) times the urinary flow rate in mL/min (V) divided by the plasma concentration of substance x (Px).

$$Cx = Ux * V / Px$$

Inulin

Determination of urinary inulin clearance during a continuous intravenous infusion is considered the "gold standard" method for measurement of GFR. Inulin has all the properties of an ideal marker. Inulin is inert and not synthesized or metabolized by the kidney. It is freely filtered by the glomerulus, and not secreted or reabsorbed in the tubules [32].

The measurement of urinary inulin clearance requires a constant intravenous infusion to maintain a constant level of inulin over a period of 3–4 h. After an equilibration period, timed urinary specimens and plasma are collected every 30 min and urinary and plasma inulin is measured to calculate urinary inulin clearance. The mean clearance of the 4–5 measurements determines the individual's GFR [33]. Urinary catheterization in young children is often required. To avoid this cumbersome procedure, two methods of plasma inulin clearance have been developed: the continuous infusion method and the single bolus method [34, 35]. The continuous infusion method is based on the concept that once a marker has reached steady state in the plasma and the volume of distribution is saturated, the rate of elimination of the marker will equal the rate of infusion (RI).

The clearance of the marker can then be measured [34]

$$Cx = RI\, x\, /\, Px$$

The equilibration period can take more than 12 h in certain situations. To avoid this long period, a bolus can be given prior to the infusion to reach steady state more rapidly.

After a single bolus injection, 10–12 blood samples are collected up to 240 min after injection and the inulin concentration measurements are used to construct a plasma concentration versus time curve (plasma disappearance curve). Plasma clearance of inulin can be calculated by dividing the dose by the area under the plasma concentration-time curve. This method has been shown to give accurate results in adults [36]. van Rossum et al. developed and validated sampling strategies to minimize the number of blood samples, making it more acceptable for children [37]. He concluded that two (at 90 and 240 min) to four samples (at 10, 30, 90, 240 min) allow accurate prediction of inulin clearance in pediatric patients with a non-significant bias and good imprecision (<15%) [37]. The single bolus injection method tends to overestimate GFR (average 9.7 mL/min 1.73 m^2), but the difference between the two methods becomes smaller at lower GFR (less than 50 mL/min/1.73 m^2) [37].

Although measurement of inulin clearance remains the gold standard for assessment of GFR, most laboratories cannot routinely measure inulin, which makes this test unpractical. Furthermore, simple, rapid determination of GFR is often needed in clinical practice.

The KDIGO 2012 Clinical Practice Guideline for the Evaluation and Management of Chronic Kidney Disease recommends the use of serum creatinine and a pediatric-specific GFR estimating equation which incorporates a height term in the initial assessment of pediatric renal function [38].

Serum Creatinine

Creatinine is an amino acid derivative produced in muscle cells. Its production increases in proportion to muscle mass, it is freely filtered, and about 10% of the creatinine found in urine is secreted by the proximal tubules. Tubular secretion varies between and within individuals [39]. Creatinine is used as a measure of renal function. In the past, laboratories used different measurement methods and the lack of standardization was clinically significant. In 2006, the National Kidney Disease Education Program published recommendations to improve creatinine measurement [40]. It is now recommended that creatinine measurements in all infants and children utilize methods that minimize confounders and that are calibrated against an international standard [38].

Creatinine Clearance (Ccr)

Creatinine clearance measurement has been widely used and correlates well with inulin clearance within the normal range of GFR [41]. Creatinine has the advantage of being an endogenous marker, which precludes the need to use an injection. However, as GFR declines the percentage of secreted creatinine increases; therefore, Ccr at low GFR will significantly overestimate true GFR [42]. In order to decrease tubular secretion of creatinine and obtain a creatinine clearance more reflective of the true GFR, cimetidine can be given in patients with renal disease since cimetidine decreases tubular secretion of creatinine [43, 44]. The cimetidine protocol involves the administration of cimetidine (20 mg/kg to a maximum of 1600 mg divided twice daily for a total of five doses) prior to assessment of urinary creatinine clearance. For the 24 h prior to the test, the patients were placed on a meat-free diet. Dose adjustments in cimetidine according to renal function are advised and the complete protocol is reported [45].

Equations to Predict GFR

Schwartz [46] and Counahan [47] first developed equations to predict GFR. In the clearance formula, the numerator UCr × V is the excretion rate of creatinine; in steady state this must equal the rate of production. Since the rate of production is a function of muscle mass, Schwartz tested different variables of body size to provide the best correlation with GFR measured by creatinine clearance. The body length had the best correlation. The GFR can be estimated using the equation known as the Schwartz formula:

$$GFR\left(mL/min/1.73\ m^2\right) = K*Ht/PCr$$

where K is a constant determined by regression analysis for different ages, Ht = height in cm and PCr = plasma creatinine.

Following the standardization of creatinine measurement, the pilot study for the Chronic Kidney Disease in Children (CKiD) study showed that the Schwartz formula overestimates GFR when compared to measured iohexol [48]. This was attributed to the fact that creatinine values determined by enzymatic creatinine assays are lower than those determined by the Jaffe method [49].

Subsequently, a number of new equations have been developed and validated. Many of these new equations were developed using a "gold standard" other than inulin and may overestimate GFR. Furthermore, the precision and accuracy of each equation may not be the same at all GFR levels, depending on which populations were used for validation. As per KDIGO, currently the most robust pediatric estimated GFR (eGFR) formula derived using iohexol disappearance and creatinine measurements, which were measured centrally and calibrated and traceable to international standards, is from the CKiD study [38, 50, 51].

The most common creatinine-based formulas recommended for use in clinical practice is the updated bedside Schwartz formula also known as the CKID 2009 equation [50]

$$eGFR\left(mL/min/1.73\ m^2\right) = 41.3 \times height\ \left(m\right)t/Scr\left(mg/dL\right)$$

or

$$eGFR\left(mL/min/1.73\ m^2\right) = 36.5 \times height\left(cm\right)/creatinine\left(\mu mol/L\right)$$

The CKID 2009 equation was validated in a population consisting primarily of children aged 8–15 years of age with reduced GFR and used creatinine as the marker.

Equations based on multivariate analyses are superior to those using univariate analysis. However, in some situations, a univariate equation might be preferred. For example, since creatinine is highly dependent on muscle mass, a cystatin C based equation may be preferable in patients with reduced muscle mass.

In 2012, the CKiD study group developed an improved equation to estimate GFR by adding cystatin c and urea as filtration markers and sex as additional variables [51].

$$eGFR\left(mL/min/1.73\ m^2\right) = 39.8 * \left[ht\left(m\right)/Scr\left(mg/dL\right)\right]^{0.456} \left[1.8/cystatin\,C\left(mg/L\right)\right]^{0.418}$$
$$\left[30/BUN\left(mg/dL\right)\right]^{0.079} \left[1.076^{male}\right]\left[ht\left(m\right)/1.4\right]^{0.179}$$

Cystatin C

Cystatin C is a low MW protein (MW = 13.36) member of the cystatin superfamily of cysteine protease inhibitors. It is produced at a stable rate by all nucleated cells. Cystatin C is freely filtered by the glomerulus and metabolized after tubular reabsorption [52]. Since it is not excreted in the urine, its clearance cannot be calculated.

Cystatin C is less influenced by age, gender and muscle mass than creatinine [53]. Levels decline from birth to one year of age then remain stable until about 50 years of age. However, cystatin C levels may be influenced by cigarette smoking, high c-reactive protein, steroid use and thyroid disorders [54–56]. One pediatric study showed that for children with CKD stage 3–5 the intrapatient coefficient of variation of cystatin C was significantly lower than serum creatinine and proposed that cystatin C is a better tool for longitudinally monitoring patients with advanced CKD [57]. Equations based on cystatin c and/or creatinine using different variables can be found in Table 4.

Some of the equations were developed using height as one of the variables whereas some are height independent to allow quick estimation of GFR when patient height is not available [58, 59]. These equations were externally validated against the gold standard single injection inulin clearance. The eGFR Pottell was superior to the eGFR-BCCH and comparable to the eGFR Schwartz [60]. Pottel developed an equation to be used in children, adolescents and young adults since none of the previous equations were validated for adolescent and young adults [61]. KDIGO suggest that measuring cystatin C based eGFR (not serum cystatin C) could be undertaken in adults with a creatinine-based eGFR of 45–59 mL/min/1.73 m² who do not have markers of kidney damage, such as proteinuria, in an attempt to confirm CKD. No specific recommendation for pediatrics or equation was made [38].

Since 2010, standards of measurement for cystatin C have been developed by the International Federation of Clinical Chemistry and Laboratory Medicine (IFCC) to reduce variability. The National Institute of Diabetes and Digestive and Kidney Diseases (NIDDK) recommends that eGFR based on cystatin C use an equation that was developed using data from measurement procedures that were standardized to the certified reference. This new IFCC-standardized assay increases measured cystatin C significantly and can thus affect the validity and reliability of GFR estimating equations [62]. The CKiD equation was one such equation initially affected by the change in standardization, but cystatin C values are now standardized to the appropriate IFCC reference. To correct older results to the new IFCC concentrations the value is multiplied by 1.17 [63].

Table 4 Equations to estimate GFR

Name	Equation to estimate GFR	Reference method used to derive
	Height dependent	
Updated Bedside Schwartz [50]	eGFR(mL/min/1.73 m²) = 41.3[Height (m)/Scr (mg/dL)] or eGFR(mL/min/1.73 m²) = 36.5[Height (cm)/Scr (µmol/L)]	Iohexol
Updated CKiD [51]	eGFR(mL/min/1.73 m²) = 39.8[ht (m)/Scr (mg/dL)]$^{0.456}$[1.8/CysC (mg/L)]$^{0.418}$[30/BUN (mg/dL)]$^{0.079}$[1.076^{male}][ht (m)/1.4]$^{0.179}$	Iohexol
	Height independent	
Pottel [59]	eGFR(mL/min/1.73 m²) = 107.3/[Scr (mg/dL)/Q] where Q is the median serum creatinine concentration for children based on age and sex Median serum creatinine (mg/dL) = 0.0270 × age + 0.2329 To express serum creatinine concentration in µmol/L, multiply by 88.4	Inulin
Modified BCCH equation [58]	eGFR(mL/min/1.73 m²) = Inverse ln of: 8.067 + (1.034 × ln[1/SCr (µmol/L)]) + (0.305 × ln[age (years)]) + 0.064 if male	Iothalamate
Filler [223]	eGFR(mL/min/1.73 m²) = 91.62[1/CysC]1.123	TcDTPA

Pediatric and adult equations for eGFR were developed using different datasets. The equations don't align at the transition from adolescent to adult. The CKiD equation generally underestimates GFR whereas the CKD-EPI equation, which is recommended for eGFR in adults, tends to overestimate GFR in young adults. Therefore, to improve the estimation of GFR in adolescent and younger adults, Pierce et al. modified the CKiD 2009 bedside estimation of GFR to include sex and age and used a dataset with patients 1–25 years old. The two equations, one for creatinine and one for cystatin C, are known as the CKiD U25 [64].

Bjork et al. also tried to improve the accuracy of eGFR in children and young adults [65]. They first established sex specific creatinine growth curves for children and young adults. These curves can be used to project childhood levels of serum creatinine to corresponding adult levels. Using the estimated adult creatinine, he then developed a modified CKD-EPI equation, the CKD-EPI 40, to improve precision and accuracy for both children and young adults at all measured GFR levels. This allows the use of the same equation for most patients without artificial change when transitioning from adolescent to adult care. However, the cohorts used for validation were from 4 European countries and may not be generalized to non-European populations or specific ethnic groups.

Other Methods

KDIGO suggests measuring GFR using an exogenous filtration marker when more accurate GFR will impact the treatment decisions. Since inulin is not widely available, other markers can be used.

Iohexol and Iothalamate
Iohexol is a safe nonionic low osmolar contrast agent (MW 821). It is eliminated exclusively by the kidneys, where it is filtered, but not secreted, metabolized, or reabsorbed. It has less than 2% binding to protein. Therefore, it makes it an ideal

marker of GFR and a good alternative to the use of radiotracers that are not suitable for some patients and require special handling, storage and disposal. Iohexol and iothalamate have similar kinetic profiles, but iohexol has a lower allergic potential [66].

Clearance of iohexol correlates well with measured inulin clearance [48, 66–68]. Gaspari et al. [69] showed a highly significant correlation between GFR measured by the plasma clearance of iohexol (using a two-compartment open–model) and the GFR measured by urinary inulin clearance.

EDTA, DTPA Nuclear GFR
GFR can be accurately measured using a radioactive tracer such as Chromium 51 (51Cr) EDTA or technetium 99m (^{99m}Tc) DTPA in children. The most accurate method is based on the plasma disappearance curve after a single bolus injection, fitted by a double exponential curve. The clearance of the radiotracer is calculated as the injected dose divided by the area under the curve [70]. The initial "fast curve" represents the diffusion of the radiotracer in its distribution volume whereas the late slow exponential curve represents its renal clearance. The two-compartment model requires serial blood sampling to obtain an accurate plasma disappearance curve. In general, the more numerous blood samples that are acquired over time, the more accurate the calculated GFR value will be. However, to avoid excessive blood sampling, two simplified methods have been proposed for routine clinical use in children [71].

The Slope-Intercept Method
The slope-intercept method requires two blood samples acquired 2 and 4 h post injection and is based on the determination of the late exponential curve. An algorithm must be used to correct for overestimation of the clearance because this method neglects the early exponential curve. Late blood sampling (between 5 and 24 h) is recommended to improve the accuracy in patients with renal clearance below 10–15 mL/min/1.73 m^2.

The Distribution Volume Method

This method only requires one blood sample acquired at 2 h post injection. It appears to be valid for children of any age except for those with very poor renal function (GFR < 30 mL/min/1.73 m²) [70].

One major limitation of these methods is decreased accuracy in the presence of significant edema. In such situations, the disappearance of the tracer will be influenced by its diffusion into an expanded extracellular volume, artifactually elevating the calculated GFR. Infiltration of the radiotracer at the injection site can also cause artifactual elevation of GFR.

The effective dose of radiation is approximately 0.011 mSv/examination regardless of the age of the child for Cr-EDTA and twice as high with low GFR (<10 min/1.73 m²). It is 0.1 mSV/examination for Tc-DTPA [70].

Assessment of Tubular Function

Fluid filtered by the glomerulus (plasma ultrafiltrate) enters the proximal tubule where 60–65% of the filtrate will be reabsorbed [72]. In disorders of the proximal tubule, excessive amount of the solutes will be found in the urine. The fractional excretion of sodium and tubular reabsorption of phosphate can be used to assess the integrity of the proximal tubules. Detection of glucosuria and aminoaciduria can also be indicative of a proximal tubular disorder in certain situations.

Fractional Excretion of Sodium (FeNa)

This is one of the most used tests of tubular integrity. There is no "normal" for fractional excretion of salt. It must be interpreted in the context of each patient's sodium and volume status.

In the face of hyponatremic dehydration the appropriate response will be conservation of sodium and water. Therefore, the fractional excretion of salt will be low, usually with a FeNa <1% in children and less than 2.5% in neonates. The urinary sodium concentration will be <20 mEq/L in children and <30 mEq/L in neonates. The FeNa can be useful in distinguishing prerenal, assumed reversible acute kidney injury (AKI) as first shown in a seminal paper in 1976 where patients who recovered from their acute oliguria had a FeNa <1%, and those that didn't recover after volume resuscitation had a FeNA >3% [73]. If tubular damage has occurred, such as in acute tubular necrosis, the fractional excretion of sodium will be inappropriately elevated. The FeNa will be >2% in children and >2.5% in neonates. Urinary sodium will generally be more than 30 mEq/L.

However, FeNa is unreliable in certain situations, such as when patients are on diuretic therapy, receiving intravenous saline or in patients with salt losing tubulopathies or CKD [74, 75]. The FeNa may be substituted by FeUrea, as urea is less influenced by diuretics, because urea reabsorption is mostly dependent on passive forces [76]. A FeUrea <35% implies prerenal AKI; it is >50% if there is intrinsic AKI. High FeNa combined with FeUrea >35% has a 95% negative predictive value for intrinsic AKI [77].

The FeNa can be calculated as below:

$$FeNa = \frac{U(Na) * PCr}{PNa * UCr} * 100$$

UNa = urinary concentration of sodium
PCr = plasma creatinine
PNa = plasma sodium
UCr = urinary creatinine

Tubular Reabsorption of Phosphate (TRP)

Eighty-five to ninety-five percent of phosphate is usually reabsorbed in the proximal tubule [72]. Phosphate transport is primarily regulated by the plasma phosphate concentration and parathyroid hormone, which alter the Na^+-phosphate carrier activity.

The normal tubular reabsorption of phosphate (TRP) is greater than 85% and can be calculated:

$$TRP\% = 1 - \frac{\left(UPO_4 * PCr\right)}{\left(PPO_4 * UCr\right)} * 100$$

UPO_4 = urinary concentration of phosphate
PCr = plasma creatinine
PPO_4 = plasma concentration of phosphate
UCr = urinary concentration of creatinine

The renal tubular maximum reabsorption rate of phosphate to glomerular filtration rate (TmP/GFR) was initially described by Bijvoet using phosphate infusion [78]. Its initial use was for diagnosis of hypercalcemia, parathyroid disorders and renal handling of phosphate. Although it is no longer used for evaluation of hypercalcemia, it can still be helpful for evaluation of hypophosphatemia. A nomogram [79] and algorithm [80] were derived from the initial infusion data of Bijvoet and can be used to calculate the TmP/GFR ratio from the TRP. The algorithm is less prone to error and therefore recommended instead of the nomogram [81]. Basically, if the TRP is ≤ 0.86 then TmP/GFR = TRP $\times P_p$ (where P_p = plasma phosphate) and if >0.86 then TmP/GFR = 0.3 $\times$ TRP/ $[1 - (0.8 \times TRP)] \times P_p$ [80, 81].

Glucosuria

Filtered glucose is usually almost completely reabsorbed in the three segments of the proximal tubule. Glucose is transported across the apical membrane by secondary active transport dependent on the sodium electrochemical gradient generated by the Na–K ATPase. Two sodium-glucose transporters are found in the proximal tubule. SGLT2, in the early proximal tubule, has high capacity and low affinity for glucose and SGLT1, found in segments 2 and 3, has high affinity and low capacity [82].

The plasma glucose at which glucose reabsorption is maximal is defined as the *threshold for glucose* and the transport capacity when the threshold is reached is called the maximal tubular glucose reabsorption (TmG).

In presence of glucosuria, it is important to determine the serum glucose concentration.

The presence of isolated glucosuria with normal serum glucose concentration is usually a result of familial renal glucosuria. Mutations of *SGLT2* were first described by Santer et al. [83]. Isolated glucosuria with elevated serum glucose is suggestive of diabetes.

The antidiabetic SGLT2 inhibitors enhance both urinary glucose and urate excretion, but the mechanism behind the uricosuric effect remains to be fully elucidated and is possibly related to an indirect effect of the glucosuria on the expression of the urate transporter, URAT1 [84].

Transtubular Potassium Gradient (TTKG)

Potassium is secreted in the late distal and cortical collecting tubules in response to aldosterone. The transtubular potassium gradient is an indirect measure of the activity of the potassium secretory process in the cortical distal nephron and reflects the action of aldosterone. It is an important component of the evaluation of hyperkalemia and hypokalemia.

It can be calculated using the formula proposed by West [85].

$$TTKG = \frac{UK \div \left(Uosm / Posm\right)}{Ppotassium}$$

UK = urinary potassium concentration
Uosm = urinary osmolality
Posm = plasma osmolality

The urinary sodium concentration should exceed 25 mmol/L. This ensures sodium reabsorption is not limiting potassium secretion, and urine osmolality should exceed plasma osmolality.

The luminal potassium of the terminal cortical collecting duct is estimated by dividing the urinary potassium by the urine/plasma osmolality since the luminal potassium concentration is influenced by removal of water in the medullary segments. The serum potassium is an estimate of the peritubular potassium concentration.

TTKG appears to be a good indicator of aldosterone activity in both normal children and in children with hypoaldosteronism and pseudohypoaldosteronism. A TTKG below 4.1 in children or 4.9 in infants is indicative of a state of hypoaldosteronism or pseudohypoaldosteronism [86]. Ethier et al. define expected values of TTKG under stimuli that are known to modulate excretion of potassium. The expected value during hypokalemia induced from a low potassium diet is less than 2.5 and during acute potassium loading is greater than 10.0 [87]. It may also be useful in distinguishing aldosterone deficiency from resistance by repeating the calculation after initiation of mineralocorticoid therapy [88]. Kamel and Halperin have recently questioned the validity of the TTKG because one of the principal assumptions involved in calculating the TTKG, that the majority of osmoles in the medullary collecting ducts are not reabsorbed, is incorrect, as this is where urea recycling occurs. If more urea is reabsorbed, then the TTKG may overestimate the potassium excretion. As the amount of urea being recycled and excreted in the cortical collecting duct cannot be measured to provide a correction for the formula, the TTKG is no longer considered a valid test [89]. Instead, the urinary potassium to creatinine ratio calculated on spot urine can be used. The expected urine potassium/urine creatinine (UK/UCr) ratio in a patient with hypokalemia should be less than <1.5 mmol K/mmol creatinine, whereas the appropriate renal response to hyperkalemia would be a UK/UCr ratio >20 mmol K/mmol creatinine [89].

Aminoaciduria

In the normal state, most of the amino acids are reabsorbed in the proximal tubule. Sodium dependent cotransporters are responsible for the transport of glycine and glutamine whereas sodium independents carriers are responsible for the transport of neutral amino acids (leucine, isoleucine and phenylalanine), cystine and dibasic amino acids (ornithine, arginine and lysine). Mutation in *SLC3A1*, which encodes a protein responsible for the transport of cystine and the dibasic amino acids, is the cause of cystinuria (type I/I) [90, 91].

The cyanide–nitroprusside test is an easy way to detect urinary amino acids which contain a free sulfhydryl group or disulfide bond such as cystine, cysteine, homocystine and homocysteine and can diagnose cystinuria in the evaluation of nephrolithiasis [3]. Generalized aminoaciduria is usually associated with Fanconi syndrome.

Assessment of Acid Base Status

Total Carbon Dioxide (Total CO_2) and Bicarbonate (HCO_3^-)

Total CO_2 content of blood, plasma or serum consists of an ionized (bicarbonate and carbonate) and a non-ionized (carbonic acid) fraction. The ionized fraction includes HCO_3^-, CO_3^{2-} and carbamino compounds. The non-ionized fraction contains H_2CO_3 and physically dissolved (anhydrous) carbon dioxide. Total CO_2 measurement typically includes both of these fractions.

HCO_3^- results obtained from a blood gas analyzer is a calculated parameter. First, pH and pCO_2 are measured and then HCO_3^- is calculated using the Henderson-Hasselbalch equation:

$$pH = pK1 + \log\left[\left(HCO_3^-\right) \div \left(0.03 * pCO_2\right)\right]$$

pK1 is usually equal to 6.1.

Discrepant values from calculated arterial bicarbonate and measured venous total CO_2 can be seen, especially in acutely ill pediatric patients who are prone to large fluctuations in pK1 [92].

Reference range for total CO_2 varies between 17 and 31 mEq/L depending on age.

Total CO_2 (tCO_2) and bicarbonate are reduced in the presence of acidosis. K/DOQI clinical practice guidelines for Bone metabolism and Disease in Children with CKD [93] recommends that serum level of tCO_2 be measured. Serum levels of tCO_2 should be maintained at ≥ 22 mmol/L in children over 2 years of age, and ≥ 20 mmol/L in neonates and young infants below age 2.

2 Laboratory Evaluation of Renal Disease in Childhood

Maintaining the serum tCO_2 in the normal range, as suggested by K/DOQI, may also be desirable for better growth in children with CKD [94].

Serum Anion Gap (SAG)

The serum anion gap (SAG) is used in the interpretation of metabolic acidosis to determine if there are additional unmeasured anions contributing to the acidosis. It is the difference between the most abundant cations and anions measured in the blood. The serum anion gap is calculated as follows.

$$SAG = Na^+ - \left[Cl^- + HCO3^- \right]$$

Potassium is generally not included in most references. However, if the serum K is significantly high or low, then it will alter the SAG. Reference values reported vary and depend on the method of quantification of the electrolytes by individual laboratories. A typical normal range is 8–16 with a mean of 12 ± 2 [95]. Correction for the serum albumin, a major anion, is advisable as the SAG changes by 2.5 mEq/L for every g/L change in serum albumin. Corrected SAG can be calculated by using the Figge equation as follows [96]:

$$Corrected\, SAG = SAG + 0.25 \times \left(normal\; albumin - measured\; albumin \left[g\,/\,L \right] \right)$$

or

$$Corrected\, SAG = SAG + 2.5 \times \left(normal\; albumin - measured\; albumin \left[g\,/\,dL \right] \right)$$

Not correcting for albumin, especially when it is low, may lead to an increased anion gap metabolic acidosis being missed in a significant number of cases [97].

Urine Anion Gap

The urine anion gap is normally positive (range 30–50 mmol/L) because there is excretion of unmeasured anions such as phosphate and sulfate. The urine anion gap can be used clinically as an indirect measurement of ammonium production by the distal nephron. Because ammonium is not routinely measured in most laboratories, clinicians need an index of ammonium secretion to use in the evaluation of normal anion gap metabolic acidosis. This was initially proposed by Goldstein et al. [98] and its clinical usefulness was also shown later by Batlle et al. [99]. In the setting of metabolic acidosis, ammonia production by the kidney is increased and ammonium is excreted into the urine with chloride.

If an excess of ammonium is present, the sum of sodium and potassium will be less than the chloride since ammonium is an unmeasured cation. This test presupposed that the chloride is the predominant anion in the urine balancing the positive charge in urine NH_4^+.

Therefore, the urine anion gap can be calculated by the equation:

$$Urine\; anion\; gap = \left(Na + K \right) - Cl$$

A negative urine anion gap suggests gastrointestinal loss of bicarbonate or renal bicarbonate loss whereas a positive urine anion gap suggests the presence of impaired distal urinary acidification [99].

The urine anion gap cannot be used in volume depletion with a urine sodium concentration of less than 25 mmol/L; when there is increased excretion of unmeasured anions such as ketoacid or hippurate; or in neonates.

Urine Osmolar Gap

Halperin et al. [100] proposed the urine osmolar gap in addition to urine anion gap to ascertain the etiology of normal or increased anion gap metabolic acidosis as well as mixed metabolic acidosis. The urine osmolar gap was defined as the difference between the measured urine osmolality and the sum of the concentration of sodium, potassium, chloride, bicarbonate, urea, and glucose. Normally this gap is 80–100 mOsmol/kg H_2O. Values >100 mOsmol/kg indicate increased urinary ammonium salts, the normal response to a metabolic acidosis [101]. A lower urine osmolar gap occurs in patients with dRTA.

Calculation of the urine osmolar gap is helpful in excluding glue sniffing, which causes a normal anion gap metabolic acidosis. A high urinary concentration of the unmeasured ions ammonium and benzoate will increase the osmolar gap, and can lead to a false exclusion of RTA as the cause of acidosis [102].

Urine-Blood pCO$_2$ (U-B pCO$_2$)

U-B pCO$_2$ can be used for the evaluation of normal anion gap metabolic acidosis with a positive urine net charge to differentiate between deficient ammonium production versus poor hydrogen secretion [103, 104]. The pCO$_2$ should be measured in alkaline urine. With adequate hydrogen secretion in the distal tubule, the hydrogen will couple with HCO_3 to form H_2CO_3 and then dissociate into CO_2 and H_2O.

Kim et al. [105] evaluated the diagnostic value of the U-B pCO$_2$ in patients diagnosed as having H^+-ATPase defect dRTA based on reduced urinary NH_4^+ and absolute decrease in H^+ ATPase immunostaining in intercalated cells. U-B pCO$_2$ during sodium bicarbonate loading was less than 30 mmHg in all patients with H^+ ATPase defect dRTA.

General Biochemistry

Serum Sodium

The reference range for plasma sodium varies with age and method of measurement used. The following reference range for serum sodium is rec-

ommended by the Canadian Laboratory Initiative in Pediatric Reference Intervals (CALIPER) database group and the Australasian Association of Clinical Biochemists (AACB); birth to <7 days 132–147 mmol/L, ≥7 days to <2 years 133–145 mmol/L, ≥2 to <12 years 134–145 mmol/L, and ≥12 to adult 135–145 mmol/L [106, 107]. Serum sodium outside that range can have serious consequences.

Hyponatremia is the result of excess free water or sodium loss. The former is usually associated with expended extracellular fluid, while the latter is often seen with volume contraction. Hyponatremia with normal serum osmolality is usually the result of hyperlipidemia, hyperproteinemia, or hyperglycemia. Most laboratories now measure serum sodium with ion-specific electrodes and the measurement will not be affected by hyperlipidemia and hyperproteinemia. In the presence of hyperglycemia every 3.4 mmol/L increment in glucose will reduce serum sodium by 1 mmol/L because of water shift from the intracellular space to the extracellular space.

Hypernatremia is usually secondary to water deficit, either because of poor intake or increased water loss such as in diabetes insipidus or mellitus. Salt intoxication is a less common cause of hypernatremia.

Serum Potassium

Approximately 98% of body potassium is located intracellularly. Cell potassium concentration is about 140 mmol/L, whereas normal range for serum potassium varies between 3.2 and 6.2 mmol/L, depending on age. Reference range varies with the method used and age of the child. In infants, the upper limit of normal can be as high as 6.2. The upper limit then progressively decreases to about 5.0 to reach the "adult" level. Reference ranges vary depending on the methodology [108].

Hyperkalemia can be the result of intracellular to extracellular shift in the presence of acidosis, beta blockers, or cellular breakdown; decreased excretion in renal failure, hypoaldosteronism or pseudohypoaldosteronism; and, less commonly, with increased potassium intake. Pseudohyperkalemia is defined as a serum K^+ that exceeds plasma K^+ by 0.4 mmol/L on a sample processed within 1 h of venipuncture (delay results in glucose depletion, and less ATP generation, which is the energy source of the sodium-potassium pump) and maintained at room temperature (lower temperatures inhibit the pump leading to potassium leak out of cells). It can occur with prolonged tourniquet use, mechanical factors, excessive crying and respiratory alkalosis, potassium EDTA contamination (associated also with hypocalcemia), leukocytosis, erythrocytosis and thrombocytosis. During the clotting process activated platelets degranulate and release potassium [109, 110]. The benign, dominantly inherited familial pseudohyperkalemia presents as hyperkalemia when the potassium is measured at or below room temperature, but no hyperkalemia when the potassium is measured at normal body temperature [111]. It has recently been linked to mutations in an erythrocyte porphyrin transporter, *ABCB6*, on chromosome 2 [112].

Hypokalemia not associated with diarrhea or emesis is mostly seen in renal tubular disorders such as Fanconi's syndrome, Bartter's syndrome, and Gitelman's syndrome and in hyperaldosteronism.

Serum Calcium, Phosphorus, and Calcium-Phosphorus Product

Evaluation of calcium, phosphorus and calcium phosphorus product is reviewed in detail in the guidelines published by K/DOQI [18, 93]. Representative normal values for serum phosphorus, ionized calcium and total calcium are in Table 5. Pseudohypocalcemia may be seen with gadolinium based contrast agents or in thrombocytosis [113]. The serum phosphate may appear falsely low after mannitol infusion and falsely elevated with hyperbilirubinemia, hyperlipidemia, amphotericin administration or if the sample is taken from a central line that has been treated with tissue plasminogen activator [113].

In CKD, serum levels of phosphorus should be maintained at or above the age-appropriate lower limits and no higher than the age–appropriate upper limits. For children with CKD stage 5, the serum level of phosphorus should be maintained between 3.5–5.5 mg/dL (1.13–1.78 mmol/L) during adolescence and between 4–6 mg/dL (1.29–1.94 mmol/L) for children between the ages of 1–12 years.

Calcium in blood exists in three fractions: protein-bound calcium, free (ionized) calcium and calcium complexes. Total measured calcium should be corrected if serum albumin is abnormal to better reflect the ionized calcium. The following formula can be used:

Table 5 Normal values for serum phosphorus, blood ionized calcium concentrations (adapted from [93])

Age	Serum phosphorus		Blood ionized calcium (mM)	Total calcium	
	mg/dL	mmol/L[a]		mg/dL	mmol/L[b]
0–3 months	4.8–7.4	1.55–2.39	1.22–1.40	8.8–11.3	2.20–2.83
1–5 years	4.5–6.5	1.45–2.10	1.22–1.32	9.4–10.8	2.35–2.70
6–12 years	3.6–5.8	1.16–1.87	1.15–1.32	9.4–10.3	2.35–2.57
13–20 years	2.3–4.5	0.74–1.45	1.12–1.30	8.8–10.2	2.20–2.55

[a] Serum phosphorus converted from mg/dL to mmol/L using a factor of 0.3229
[b] Serum calcium converted from mg/dL to mmol/L using a factor of 0.250

$$\text{Corrected calcium } (mg/dL) = \text{total calcium } (mg/dL) + 0.8 \times \left[4 - \text{serum albumin} (g/dL)\right]$$

Ionized calcium is affected by pH since hydrogen ion displaces calcium from albumin. A fall of 0.1 unit in pH will cause an approximately a 0.1 mEq/L rise in the concentration of ionized calcium. As serum ionized calcium is not routinely measured at most institutions, K/DOQI guidelines are based on corrected total calcium. Levels should be maintained within normal range for the laboratory and preferably toward the lower end in CKD stage 5. The serum calcium-phosphorus product should be maintained at <55 mg^2/dL^2 (4.4 mmol^2/L^2) in adolescents greater than 12 years and <65 mg^2/dL^2 (5.2 mmol^2/L^2) in younger children [93].

Serum Albumin

Serum albumin is used to assess the nutritional status in children with or without renal disease. Although it is used as a measure of the nutritional state of an individual, it can be affected by non-nutritional factors, especially in children with CKD, such as infection, inflammation, hydration status, peritoneal and urinary losses [114]. Children with low serum albumin should be assessed for protein-energy malnutrition if not losing protein.

Serum Uric Acid

Serum uric acid varies with both age and gender [115, 116]. An elevated serum uric acid is much less common in childhood as compared to adulthood, and in contrast to adults where gout is the primary cause, hereditary disorders of purine biosynthesis account for the majority of cases in children. These include a deficiency of the enzyme hypoxanthine-guanine phosphoribosyltransferase (Lesch-Nyhan syndrome) and hereditary xanthinuria [117]. Hyperuricemia is also found in familial juvenile hyperuricemic nephropathy in association with mutations in the uromodulin gene [118].

The combination of hyperuricemia, anemia, early onset kidney failure and hypotensive or presyncopal episodes should raise suspicion of the recently described disorder associated with a mutation in the renin gene [119]. The renal cysts and diabetes syndrome caused by mutations in the gene for hepatocyte nuclear factor 1β (*HNF1β*) is also associated with hyperuricemia [120]. Patients with *HNF1β* mutations may also present with hypomagnesemia [121].

The kidney is the primary site of excretion of uric acid. The fractional excretion of filtered urate is 15–30% in children compared to 10% adults [122]. Hyperuricemia can be seen in AKI, tumor lysis syndrome, and secondary to certain drugs such as thiazide diuretics, salicylates and cyclosporine [116]. In dehydration, serum uric acid correlates significantly with weight change, and increased significantly with dehydration severity in one study [123].

There is ongoing debate and uncertainty as to whether there is a causal link, or merely an association, between hyperuricemia and hypertension or CKD progression [124, 125]. Uric acid may be a clinically useful marker in the management of essential hypertension in adolescents and young children, where there is some evidence that even in preschool children those with higher serum uric acid have higher blood pressures [126–128]. A pediatric study of over 100 patients with CKD found that 70% of children with an eGFR <60 mL/min/1.73 m^2 had uric acid levels above the normal range [129]. A subsequent analysis including over 600 children and adolescents from North America found that those with hyperuricemia progressed faster to CKD [130].

Drugs that lower serum uric acid include allopurinol and rasburicase. In addition, the angiotensin receptor blocker losartan is uricosuric [131], and could be beneficial in hypertensive patients with hyperuricemia [125]. Allopurinol can increase xanthine and hypoxanthine levels, leading to xanthinuria and xanthine stones. It is also associated with severe dermatological reactions in children.

Urinary Calcium

Measurement of calcium excretion should be part of the evaluation of patients with hematuria, nephrocalcinosis and renal stones and can often be useful in the assessment of children with frequency, dysuria, urgency and recurrent UTI [132]. Urinary calcium excretion varies with age, being highest in infancy and reaching its nadir during puberty.

Hypercalciuria is usually defined as a urinary calcium excretion of more than 4 mg/kg/day based on the study of Ghazali and Barratt [133]. However, several authors have studied urinary calcium excretion and published reference ranges in their study population [134–138].

A spot urinary calcium/creatinine ratio (usually collected on the second morning fasting urine specimen) correlates well with 24-h calcium excretion, especially for children with normal muscle mass. They can be used clinically; however, they are more likely to be affected than a 24-h collection by factors such as recent dietary calcium intake [139]. Sodium, protein, phosphorus, potassium, and glucose intake can influence calcium excretion. There is no apparent seasonal variation of urinary calcium/creatinine ratio in children as seen in adults [140]. A 24-h urine collection for calcium assessment is typically stored in acidified bottles containing hydrochloric acid to prevent the crystallization of calcium oxalate although this may not be necessary [141]. For those who have reduced muscle mass, a urinary calcium/osmolality ratio predicts hypercalciuria with better sensitivity and specificity than a urine calcium/creatinine ratio [142, 143].

Urinary Sodium

Measurement of urinary sodium excretion should be assessed in children with hypercalciuria. Polito et al. found that urinary sodium excretion and 24-h urinary sodium/potassium ratio (U Na/K) was higher in children with hypercalciuria [144]. Twenty-four-hour urinary sodium can also be used to assess dietary sodium intake in adults on a low sodium diet for the treatment of hyperten-sion where a target 24 h intake of 50–100 mmol/day is recommended [145].

Urinary Magnesium

Magnesium is a known stone inhibitor as it forms complexes with oxalate and reduces supersaturation. Thirty-nine percent of children with calcium oxalate stones in one series had hypomagnesuria defined as magnesium excretion less than 1.2 mg/kg/24 h [146]. Urinary reference limits for Mg/Cr can be found in Table 6.

Urinary Citrate

Citrate inhibits calcium-oxalate and calcium-phosphate crystal nucleation, growth and aggregation. In normal circumstances, citrate is freely filtered at the glomerulus with a 65–90% reabsorption rate. Systemic acidosis, potassium depletion, starvation and acetazolamide therapy decrease urinary citrate. Citrate excretion is age and sex related. Mean molar excretion of citrate is higher in infants than in older children, and in infants is higher in females than males (Table 7) [147].

Table 6 Urinary reference limits for urinary magnesium/creatinine (adapted from [224])

Age in year	Urinary Mg/Cr mol/mol (mg/mg)	
	5th Percentile	95th Percentile
1/12–1	0.4 (0.10)	2.2 (0.48)
1–2	0.4 (0.09)	1.7 (0.37)
2–3	0.3 (0.07)	1.6 (0.34)
3–5	0.3 (0.07)	1.3 (0.29)
5–7	0.3 (0.06)	1.0 (0.21)
7–10	0.3 (0.05)	0.9 (0.18)
10–14	0.2 (0.05)	0.7 (0.15)
14–17	0.2 (0.05)	0.6 (0.13)

Table 7 Mean molar citrate/creatinine ratio based on [147]

Urinary citrate/creatinine	Girls	Boys
Infants	1.9	0.63
Childhood	0.27	0.33
Adolescence	0.32	0.28

Citrate excretion of more than 1.6 mmol/1.73 m^2 in girls and more than 1.9 mmol/1.73 m^2 in boys is considered normal [148].

Hypocitraturia, either alone or in association with hypercalciuria, is an important risk factor for nephrolithiasis in children [149, 150]. In one study, hypocitraturia defined as citrate excretion <320 mg/1.73 m^2/24 h [1.66 mmol/1.73 m^2/24 h] was observed in 60.6% of children with calcium oxalate stones [146]. A study in a stone-forming adult population suggests that urinary calcium to citrate ratio >0.25 mg/mg is predictive of litho-genesis [151].

Urinary calcium-to-citrate ratio >0.326 mg/mg has been found in children to predict stone form-ers in a random urine sample [152]. Furthermore, urinary calcium-to-citrate ratio calculated on 24-h collection can also distinguish between solitary and recurrent calcium stone forming children. The mean urinary calcium-to-citrate was 0.41 mg/mg in those with a single stone episode and 0.64 mg/mg in recurrent stone formers as compared to the mean of 0.33 mg/mg seen in normal children without stones [153]. Hypocitraturia is also rec-ognized as a major risk factor for nephrocalcino-sis in very low birth weight infants [154] and after kidney transplantation [155].

Urinary Oxalate

Urinary oxalate excretion is significantly increased in primary hyperoxaluria type I (PH I),

PH II and PH III and in secondary hyperoxaluria. In PH I, there is excessive endogenous production of oxalate caused by a deficiency of hepatic alanine:glyoxylate amino transferase (AGT), which catalyzes the peroxisomal conversion of glyoxylate to glycine and in PH II, a deficiency of cytosolic glyoxylate reductase/hydroxypyruvate reductase (GRHPR), an enzyme that catalyzes the reduction of glyoxylate and hydroxypyruvate as well as the dehydrogenation of glycerate [156, 157]. PH III is due to a defect in a hepatocyte specific mitochondrial enzyme, 4-hydroxy-2-oxoglutarate aldolase (HOGA) [158].

The secondary forms are due to increased intestinal absorption of oxalate due to malabsorp-tive states or impaired vitamin status. Reference values for oxalate/creatinine can be found in Table 8.

Patients suspected of having abnormalities in oxalate metabolism should have more extensive studies, including measurement of oxalate, gly-colate and L-glycerate and in some cases liver biopsy to assess the activity of AGT and GRHPR.

Elevated oxalate and glycolate is associated with PH1; however, normal glycolate is found in 25% of subject with PHI. Elevated urinary oxalate and L-glycerate is the typical finding of hyperox-aluria type II, but likewise elevated L-glycerate is not always present. Genetic analysis is now con-sidered the gold standard for diagnosis and liver biopsy, to measure intrahepatic enzyme levels, is generally reserved for patients in whom no muta-tion can be found [156, 157].

Table 8 Urinary reference limits for calcium/creatinine, oxalate/creatinine, urate/creatinine [224, 225]

	Urinary calcium/creatinine mol/mol (mg/mg)[a]		Urinary oxalate/creatinine mol/mol (mg/mg)[a]		Urinary urate/creatinine mol/mol (mg/mg)[a]	
Age	5th	95th	5th	95th	5th	95th
1–6 months	0.09 (0.03)	2.2 (0.81)	0.07 (0.0560)	0.22 (0.175)	0.80 (1/189)	1.60 (2.378)
6 months–1 year	0.09 (0.03)	2.2 (0.81)	0.06 (0.0480)	0.17 (0.139)	0.70 (1.040)	1.50 (2.299)
1–2	0.07 (0.03)	1.5 (0.500)	0.05 (0.04)	0.13 (0.103)	0.50 (0.743)	1.40 (2.080)
2–3	0.06 (0.02)	1.4 (0.41)	0.04 (0.032)	0.10 (0.080)	0.47 (0.698)	1.30 (1.932)
3–5	0.05 (0.02)	1.1 (0.30)	0.03 (0.024)	0.08 (0.064)	0/40 (0.594)	1.10 (1.635)
5–7	0.04 (0.01)	0.8 (0.25)	0.03 (0.024)	0.07 (0.056)	0.30 (0.446)	0.80 (1.189)
7–10	0.04 (0.01)	0.7 (0.24)	0.02 (0.016)	0.06 (0.048)	0.26 (0.386)	0.56 (0.832)
10–14	0.04 (0.01)	0.7 (0.24)	0.02 (0.016)	0.06 (0.048)	0.20 (0.297)	0.44 (0.654)
14–17	0.04 (0.01)	0.7 (0.24)	0.02 (0.016)	0.06 (0.048)	0.20 (0.297)	0.40 (0.594)

[a]Conversions have been performed with higher precision, then rounded for this presentation [224, 225]

Urinary Uric Acid

Increased urinary uric acid excretion can present with microscopic hematuria, abdominal and/or flank pain, dysuria, gravel and macroscopic hematuria. About half of patients with hyperuricosuria (HU) will have microlithiasis on ultrasonography [159]. HU may be defined by urine uric acid concentration corrected for creatinine clearance >0.53 mg/dL/GFR [160]. The excretion varies with age, being highest in infants. However, a simpler estimate of urinary urate excretion can be calculated from the urine urate/creatinine ratio. Reference values for urine urate/creatinine can be found in Table 8.

Assessment of the Renin-Angiotensin-Aldosterone System

Renin is a proteolytic enzyme predominantly formed and stored in the juxtaglomerular cells of the kidney. Renal hypoperfusion and increased sympathetic activity are the major physiologic stimuli to renin secretion [72]. When released in the circulation, renin cleaves angiotensinogen to produce a decapeptide angiotensin I. Angiotensin I is then converted to an octapeptide, angiotensin II, by the angiotensin I-converting enzyme. Angiotensin II is a potent vasoconstrictor and promotes salt and water retention. The converting enzyme is mainly located in the lung, but angiotensin II can be synthesized at a variety of sites, including the kidney, luminal membrane of vascular endothelial cells, adrenal gland and brain.

Angiotensin II promotes renal salt and water reabsorption by stimulation of sodium reabsorption in the early proximal tubule and by indirectly activating aldosterone biosynthesis in the zona glomerulosa of the adrenal cortex.

Measurement of plasma renin activity may not reflect the tissue activity of the local renin-angiotensin system.

Assessment of the renin-angiotensin-aldosterone system may be required in the evaluation of hypokalemia/hyperkalemia, adrenal insufficiency, and hypertension, see Table 9.

Renin

Renin release is dependent on renal tubular sodium concentration, renal perfusion pressure and beta-adrenergic vascular tone. The enzymatic activity of renin can be measured. It is expressed as the amount of angiotensin I generated per unit of time and is expressed in pmol or ng of generated angiotensin I per mL of plasma.

The "normal values" for plasma renin activity (PRA) are highly dependent on sodium intake, time of day, posture, age and methodology [161]. PRA varies inversely with age in infants and children. Reference values derived from measurement of PRA in 79 children age 1 month to 15 years in supine position were published in 1975 [162].

PRA can be useful in the management of hypertension to distinguish between a volume dependent hypertension, where renin is suppressed, and hypertension mediated by excess

Table 9 Assessment of the renin-angiotensin-aldosterone system

	PRA	PAC	PAC/PRA	BP	Potassium
Primary hyperaldosteronism	Decrease	Increase	Very high >20–50	High	Low
GRA	Decrease	Increase	High	High	Normal or low
Renin-secreting tumor	Increase	Increase		High	Low
Bartter' syndrome	Increased	Increased		Normal	Low
Renovascular disease	Increased	Increased	<10		
Apparent mineralocorticoid excess, Cushing, licorice ingestion	Low	Low		High	Low

PRA plasma renin activity, *PAC* plasma aldosterone concentration, *BP* blood pressure, *GRA* glucocorticoid remediable hypertension

renin secretion. A value less than 0.65 ng/mL/h suggests renin suppression, while a value above 6.5 ng/mL/h implies excess renin. This can help guide appropriate therapy [163].

During renal angiography, renal vein renin sampling may be done to predict feasibility of correcting hypertension or to identify which kidney contributes to the hypertension. A ratio of the renal vein renin from the diseased kidney (R) to the renal vein renin from the normal or less diseased contralateral kidney (RC) above 1.5 (R/RC >1.5) is considered significant, and there is greater probability that blood pressure will improve after surgery. A RC/infrarenal inferior vena cava ratio less than 1.3 further supports the presence of a lesion that may respond to repair. Segmental veins within a kidney may also be sampled [164–168].

Aldosterone

Aldosterone is synthesized in the zona glomerulosa of the adrenal gland. It regulates electrolyte excretion and intravascular volume, mainly through its effects on the distal tubules and cortical collecting ducts of the kidneys, where it acts to increase sodium reabsorption and potassium excretion [169].

Aldosterone is measured by radioimmunoassay. Like renin, it is dependent on sodium intake, posture and time of the day. Serum aldosterone concentration is highest at the time of awakening and lowest shortly after sleep onset. Hyperaldosteronism should be sought for in children with hypertension, hypokalemia and metabolic alkalosis [170].

Plasma Aldosterone Concentration (PAC) to Plasma Renin Activity Ratio

The PAC/PRA ratio is a screening test for hyperaldosteronism prior to confirmation with a suppression test. Patients should not be taking aldosterone receptor antagonists, ACE inhibitors and angiotensin receptor blockers for 3–6 weeks, and hypokalemia needs to be corrected prior to the test. Any medication that stimulates renin production, such as diuretics, may lead to a false negative result. False positives can be expected with the reduced renin and increased salt and water retention of renal impairment. The patient needs to be in the seated position for 10–15 min after ambulating for at least 2 h, and midmorning is considered the best time to perform the test [171]. The mean normal value is 4–10 compared to more than 30–50 in patients with primary hyperaldosteronism [172].

Endocrine Testing Relevant to Nephrology

ADH/Copeptin

Arginine vasopressin (AVP) or antidiuretic hormone (ADH) is one of the key hormones in the regulation of salt and water balance. The measurement of ADH can be helpful in the diagnosis and work-up of sodium disorders. However, due to its structural instability, very short plasma half-life, and long laboratory processing time, its use in clinical practice is limited. Copeptin is a well-established ADH surrogate. It is secreted in an equimolar amount to ADH and can be easily measured in plasma or serum. The distribution of copeptin levels in pediatric cohorts indicate a range between 2.4 and 8.6 pmol/L [173].

The distribution of plasma copeptin in percentiles in a population of children without disturbance of the AVP system can be found in a study published in 2021 [174]. Finally, measuring copeptin after infusion of 3% saline to induce hypernatremia of at least 150 mmol/L (hypertonic saline infusion test) may have greater diagnostic accuracy for diabetes insipidus (plasma copeptin <4.9 pmol/L) and primary polydipsia (plasma copeptin >4.9 pmol/L) than the indirect water-deprivation test [175].

Biochemical Testing for the Diagnosis of Pheochromocytoma

Typical testing of patients suspected of having pheochromocytoma includes measurement of catecholamines and metanephrines in the urine and plasma. Plasma and urinary metanephrines are recommended as they are more reliable, with the best negative predictive value. This is because metanephrines are produced continuously by the pheochromocytoma, whereas catecholamines are only intermittently secreted. Plasma metanephrines are most often measured using high-performance liquid chromatography coupled with either electrochemical detection or mass spectrometry. The sensitivity of plasma free metanephrines to diagnose pheochromocytoma is 97% and has a specificity of between 80 and 100%. Twenty-four-hour measurement of urinary fractionated metanephrines has similar sensitivities and specificities. Plasma metanephrines should ideally be obtained when the patient is fasting and has been in the supine position for at least 30 min to avoid sympathoadrenal activation. False positives due to interference with the analytical methods can be seen with acetaminophen, mesalamine and sulfasalazine. Alternatively, there may be false positives caused by drugs that affect metabolism or secretion, of catecholamines, such as caffeine, cocaine, amphetamines, ephedrine, venlafaxine (serotonin-noradrenaline reuptake inhibitor), tricyclic antidepressants, dihydropyridine calcium channel blockers, doxazocin and phenoxybenzamine [176].

Complement Pathway Assessment

The complement system consists of at least thirty plasma membrane proteins that provide an innate defense against microbes and an adjunct or complement to humoral immunity [177, 178]. The complement system is divided into three major pathways: classical, lectin and alternative. The lectin pathway is activated by the binding of lectin (which has a similar structure to C1q) to sugar residues on the surface of a pathogen and the alternative pathway which is an amplification loop for C3 activation is activated by polysaccharide antigens, aggregated IgA, injured cells or endotoxins. The classical pathway is activated by the binding of C1q to the Fc portion of antibody. The alternative pathway is a constitutively active and amplifiable system. Plasma factor H and factor I are important fluid phase complement regulators of the alternative pathway, while CD46 (membrane cofactor protein), CD55 (decay accelerating factor) and CD59 (protectin) are the principal surface bound regulators. Each of these three pathways lead to the deposition of an activated C3 fragment (C3b), inducing the final steps of the complement cascade, which include opsonisation, phagocytosis, induction of inflammation, and formation of the membrane attack complex (MAC) and cytolysis [179]. A fourth pathway by which thrombin can directly activate C5 and thus the terminal complement cascade was also identified and links the complement and coagulation cascades [180]. However, the significance of this pathway in the pathogenesis of disease is still unclear. There is an evolving spectrum of kidney diseases now recognized as being either complement-mediated or having complement dysregulation as part of their pathogenesis, and these will be discussed in a later chapter.

Evaluation of the complement system, or *complement analysis*, plays an integral part in the diagnosis of various infectious, inflammatory and autoimmune diseases as well as many glomerular diseases caused by either overactivity, or loss of regulation, of the complement system. Much progress has been made not just in the understanding of the role of complement in the pathogenesis of these diseases, but also in the quality and standardization of the methods of complement analysis [179, 181]. Concentrations of C3, C4 and C1q can be quantified by immunological methods. Glomerular disease associated with activation of the classical pathway will typically have a low C4 and C3, whereas disease associated with activation of the alternative pathway will have a low C3 and normal C4. Serial assessment of complement proteins can also be helpful in monitoring disease activity in immune complex mediated disease such as lupus. C4 is less likely to normalize because one or more C4 null genes are common in SLE; therefore, patients in remission can continue to have low C4. However, C3 is sensitive to change in disease activity [182]. The normal range for C3 varies considerably between laboratories [182]; therefore, no normal values are provided in this chapter.

There are functional assays that assess the total hemolytic activity of the entire classical (CH50) and alternative (AH50) pathways [181]. All nine components (C1–C9) are required to have a normal CH50, a test which in the past assessed the ability of the patient's serum to lyse sheep erythrocytes optimally sensitized with rabbit antibody, but now typically uses a synthetic liposome coated with antibody instead of erythrocytes [181]. A suppressed CH50 suggests a deficiency or consumption of one or more component, or complement activation and consumption of complement proteins. The CH50 is useful to diagnose hypocomplementemic states (for example congenital C2 deficiency) that would be missed if only C3 and C4 were measured.

AH50 is a functional assay of the alternative pathway. The assay typically used erythrocytes from rabbit, guinea pig or chicken, and the classical pathway is kept inactive by the addition of a calcium chelator (EGTA). Suppressed AH50 suggests a deficiency or consumption of one or more components of the alternative pathway. Depressed or absent AH50 activity, in the presence of a normal CH50, suggests a deficiency in an alternative pathway component (such as C3, C5, C6, C7, C8, C9, factor D, factor B, properdin or the regulators factor H or factor I). When the AH50 is normal, but the CH50 is absent, then there might be a classic pathway deficiency such as C1q, C2 or C4, or the presence of a C1 inhibitor. When both CH50 and AH50 are depressed this reflects either a late component deficiency or a setting of complement consumption and one should measure C3, C5–C9 as well as levels of factor H and I [183].

When a complement-mediated disease is suspected, more in-depth analysis of the complement system can be performed. The International Complement society provides guidelines for modern complement analysis [179]. There are a number of steps in order to complete a thorough analysis of the complement system including (1) functional assays of global complement pathway function, with the CH50, AH50 and lectin pathway (assessed by semiquantitative enzyme-linked immunosorbent assay [ELISA]), (2) analysis of individual complement components/proteins, such as C3, C4 and C1q, (3) analysis of key complement regulators such as CFH, CFI and C1-INH, (4) detection of complement activation or split products such as C3dg, C3a, Bb, sC5b-9, typically measured by ELISA in the serum, urine or tissues, (5) measuring auto-antibodies to various complement components, to the C3 convertase (C3 nephritic factor), or to the alternative pathway regulator CFH (anti-CFH) and (6) genetic analysis for mutations in C3, CFB, CFH, CFI, CD46/MCP, now linked to various diseases including atypical hemolytic uremic syndrome, membranoproliferative glomerulonephritis and antibody-mediated rejection.

The measurement of complement split products such as C3a, C3d, C4d or Bb and the soluble form of the membrane attack complex (sC5b-9) have allowed more sensitivity and accuracy in defining whether it is the classical, alternative, or terminal common pathway that is involved, and monitoring the degree of complement activation. Measuring these split products, and in particular sC5b-9, can be useful to ensure complete complement inactivation by complement inhibitors such as eculizumab [181].

Laboratory Assessment of Various Glomerulopathies

Antineutrophil Cytoplasmic Antibodies (ANCA)

Antineutrophil cytoplasmic antibodies (ANCA) are IgG autoantibodies directed against constituents of primary granules of neutrophil and monocyte lysosomes. They were first described in 1982 in patients with pauci-immune glomerulonephritis [184]. Indirect immunofluorescence (IIF) and ELISA are the most widely used techniques to detect ANCA. By IIF, two major immunostaining patterns can be seen: the diffuse granular cytoplasmic pattern with central accentuation known as C-ANCA and the perinuclear pattern which is defined as perinuclear fluorescence with nuclear extension known as P-ANCA. Diffuse flat cytoplasmic staining without interlobular accentuation can also be seen and is termed atypical C-ANCA. Atypical ANCA includes all other neutrophil-specific or monocyte-specific IIF reactivity, most commonly a combination of cytoplasmic and perinuclear fluorescence. Proteinase 3 and myeloperoxidase are two antigenic targets associated with vasculitis. The cytoplasmic pattern usually suggests the presence of serum proteinase 3 ANCA (PR3-ANCA), whereas the perinuclear pattern with nuclear extension is usually associated with myeloperoxidase ANCA (MPO-ANCA). Occasionally, antinuclear antibodies can give a false positive P-ANCA and this can be avoided by fixing the neutrophils with formalin rather than ethanol [185]. ELISA is used in addition to prove the presence of myeloperoxidase and proteinase 3 ANCA [186]. In order to enhance specificity, both IIF and ELISA have been recommended.

More novel assays for ANCA confirmation include capture ELISAs, high sensitivity or anchor ELISAs and automated immunoassays, the latter able to provide a result in under an hour, have become more widespread [187]. There are now several commercially available antigen-specific immunoassays that detect antibodies (IgG) to either MPO or PR3. These include first, second (monoclonal antibody capture-based) and third generation (peptide anchor-based) ELISA as well as fluorescent-enzyme immunoassays, chemiluminescent, or multiplex bead assays. These assays have excellent comparative performance with area under the curve (AUC) ranging from 0.92 to 0.98, better than those for IIF in recent studies [188, 189]. Current guidelines now recommend using a high-quality antigen-specific immunoassay to screen for MPO- or PR3-ANCA given that the turnaround time is faster and the cost is lower [190].

Antibodies to several azurophilic granule proteins (lactoferrin, elastase, cathepsin G, bactericidal permeability inhibitor, catalase, lysozyme and more) can cause a P-ANCA staining pattern.

The ELISA will determine the specific antibody responsible. Only anti-PR3 or anti-MPO antibodies, however, are clinically relevant [191].

ANCA measurement should only be done for patients who are strongly suspected of having vasculitis. Clinical indications for ANCA testing can be found in the International Consensus Statement on Testing and Reporting of Antineutrophil Cytoplasmic Antibodies [186]. Compliance with guidelines for ANCA testing would decrease the number of false positives, which may lead to misdiagnosis and potentially harmful treatments [192].

Granulomatosis with polyangiitis (GPA), microscopic polyangiitis, Churg-Strauss syndrome, renal limited vasculitis and drug induced ANCA-associated vasculitis are associated with positive ANCA. C-ANCA anti-PR3 ANCA suggests a diagnosis of GPA whereas P-ANCA anti-MPO associates more with MPA and Churg Strauss syndrome. ANCA are positive in 70–95% of patients with GPA and MPA, but only about 40% of patients with a diagnosis of Churg Strauss syndrome are positive [191].

ANCA can also be positive in non-vasculitic disease such as anti-glomerular basement membrane disease, inflammatory bowel disease, neoplasia, and other autoimmune disorders. Both PR3 and MPO ANCA may be found with infectious conditions such as tuberculosis, leprosy, HIV and subacute bacterial endocarditis. Various drugs can also be associated with ANCA positivity. These include propylthiouracil, hydralazine, penicillin, sulfonamides, quinolones, thiazides, and allopurinol [193].

Correlation with disease activity was first recognized by van der Woude et al. in 1985 [194]. Although the diagnostic value of ANCA is not disputed, the utility of measuring serial ANCA to monitor disease course, response to treatment or relapse prediction has overall been disappointing [191, 195]. A patient in clinical remission whose titers are rising, have returned to positivity or that remain persistently positive should be followed very closely as they may be at increased risk for relapse [190]. A rise in ANCA may be predictive of an imminent relapse, but this is not universal and may be limited to certain subgroups of patients, though this remains to be clarified. MPO-ANCA carries worse renal and adult patient survival [196, 197]. Relapse is more common with PR3-ANCA, especially if there is persistence of PR3 positivity after induction therapy [198–200].

Some progress in terms of the so called ANCA negative vasculitides has been made recently with the discovery of pathogenic versus naturally occurring MPO epitopes, previously undetectable by conventional testing [201]. In the future, epitope specificities may prove useful in distinguishing varying disease characteristics in ANCA-associated vasculitides [202].

Kain et al. detected antibodies against human lysosome-associated membrane protein-2 (LAMP-2), a protein localized to the same neutrophil granules as PR3 and MPO, in over 90% of patients with ANCA-associated vasculitis and glomerulonephritis [203]. These autoantibodies may only be present early post diagnosis and disappear with the initiation of immunosuppressive therapies and disease remission; however, their relevance as a pathological or serological marker is yet to be determined [204–206]. LAMP-2 ANCA titers have been detected by ELISA and typically coincide with MPO- or PR3-ANCA positivity in a cohort of children with systemic vasculitis, but this is just preliminary data that needs validation [207].

Antinuclear Antibodies (ANA) and Anti-doubled Stranded DNA (Anti-dsDNA)

ANAs are autoantibodies directed against chromatin and its individual components, including dsDNA, histones and some ribonucleoproteins [208]. Although ANAs are frequently found in children without a rheumatic disease [209], they have been associated with several systemic autoimmune diseases, including systemic lupus erythematosus (SLE), scleroderma, mixed connective tissue disease, polymyositis, dermatomyositis, rheumatoid arthritis, Sjögren's syndrome, drug induced lupus, discoid lupus, and pauciarticular juvenile chronic arthritis. They are also occasionally seen in autoimmune disease of the thyroid, liver and lungs as well as chronic infectious disease such as mononucleosis, hepatitis C infection, subacute bacterial endocarditis, tuberculosis and HIV, and some lymphoproliferative disorders. They do not always signify disease and 13.8% of the population over age 12 have detectable ANAs, with ANA positivity increasing with age and more common in females [210].

Different types of ANAs are known and classified based on their target antigens. Antibodies can be directed against dsDNA, individual nuclear histones, nuclear proteins, and RNA-protein complexes. As some of these antibodies are more specific for a particular disease, they are helpful tests for diagnosis. They are also used for monitoring disease activity. A positive ANA may also precede disease onset [211].

In most laboratories, ANAs are measured by an indirect immunofluorescence assay using a human epithelial cell tumor line (Hep2 cells) as the antigenic substrate. Different staining patterns can be seen, reflecting the presence of antibodies to one or a combination of nuclear antigens. The patterns are neither sensitive nor specific for a single disease. In general, a homogenous or chromosomal pattern is more likely in healthy individuals and in those with SLE, whereas a speckled or extrachromosomal pattern implies antibodies against extractable nuclear antigens (ENA) such as Smith antigen. A nucleolar pattern may suggest systemic sclerosis. It is important to emphasize that anti-dsDNA antibodies associated with SLE may also present a speckled or nucleolar pattern [212]. These different immunofluorescent staining patterns may correlate with disease manifestations in SLE. For instance, proliferative lupus nephritis is more commonly associated with a homogenous pattern and organ damage may be less likely with the speckled pattern in SLE [213]. A nuclear, coarse speckled, rather than a dense fine speckled pattern on immunofluorescence, may signify an autoimmune rheumatic disease [214]. This will need further validation before being employed in more widespread clinical practice [215].

The titer of ANAs can be helpful clinically. A negative ANA makes a diagnosis of SLE or mixed connective tissue disease very unlikely. ANAs in the sera of a normal healthy childhood population using Hep-2 cells as substrate is reported as 6% [216], and 16% at screening dilutions of 1:20 [217]. In healthy individuals, ANA titers above 1:40 are found in 32%, above 1:80 in 13% and above 1:320 in 3% [218].

The presence of a titer >1:640 should raise the suspicion of an autoimmune disease. If no diagnosis is made, the patient should be followed closely. Lower titers with no clinical sign or symptoms of disease are much less worrisome. In one study, no rheumatic disease was diagnosed in patients with ANA titers <1:160. Unless there is a high pretest likelihood of a rheumatic disease, a positive ANA has a very low positive predictive value [219].

Anti-dsDNA are relatively specific for SLE and fluctuate with disease activity [220].

Anti-nucleosome antibody is the earliest marker for the diagnosis of SLE. It is also a superior marker of lupus nephritis [208]. Among those with SLE, the prevalence of anti-nucleosome antibodies was higher in those with renal disease (58%) compared to those without nephritis (29%) [221]. Antibodies to the Smith antigen, which is a nuclear non-histone protein, are very specific for SLE but insensitive.

In SLE, autoantibodies to the complement component C1q are strongly associated with proliferative lupus nephritis, correlate with disease severity, can herald the onset of nephritis and be used to monitor response to therapy [220, 222]. Anti-dsDNA are also strongly associated with nephritis in SLE [220].

References

1. Sekhar DL, Wang L, Hollenbeak CS, Widome MD, Paul IM. A cost-effectiveness analysis of screening urine dipsticks in well-child care. Pediatrics. 2010;125(4):660–3.
2. Kavuru V, Vu T, Karageorge L, Choudhury D, Senger R, Robertson J. Dipstick analysis of urine chemistry: benefits and limitations of dry chemistry-based assays. Postgrad Med. 2020;132(3):225–33.
3. Graff SL. In: Biello LA, editor. A handbook of routine urinalysis. Philadelphia: Lippincott Williams & Wilkins; 1983.
4. Brodehl J, Franken A, Gellissen K. Maximal tubular reabsorption of glucose in infants and children. Acta Paediatr Scand. 1972;61(4):413–20.
5. Whiting P, Westwood M, Bojke L, Palmer S, Richardson G, Cooper J, et al. Clinical effectiveness and cost-effectiveness of tests for the diagnosis and investigation of urinary tract infection in children: a systematic review and economic model. Health Technol Assess. 2006;10(36):iii–iv, xi–xiii, 1–154.
6. Mori R, Yonemoto N, Fitzgerald A, Tullus K, Verrier-Jones K, Lakhanpaul M. Diagnostic performance of urine dipstick testing in children with suspected UTI: a systematic review of relationship with age and comparison with microscopy. Acta Paediatr. 2010;99(4):581–4.
7. Kazi BA, Buffone GJ, Revell PA, Chandramohan L, Dowlin MD, Cruz AT. Performance characteristics of urinalyses for the diagnosis of pediatric urinary tract infection. Am J Emerg Med. 2013;31(9):1405–7.
8. Coulthard MG. Using urine nitrite sticks to test for urinary tract infection in children aged <2 years: a meta-analysis. Pediatr Nephrol. 2019;34(7):1283–8.
9. Perazella MA, Coca SG. Traditional urinary biomarkers in the assessment of hospital-acquired AKI. Clin J Am Soc Nephrol (CJASN). 2012;7(1):167–74.
10. Cavanaugh C, Perazella MA. Urine sediment examination in the diagnosis and management of kidney disease: core curriculum 2019. Am J Kidney Dis. 2019;73(2):258–72.
11. Galpin JE, Shinaberger JH, Stanley TM, Blumenkrantz MJ, Bayer AS, Friedman GS, et al. Acute interstitial nephritis due to methicillin. Am J Med. 1978;65(5):756–65.
12. Muriithi AK, Nasr SH, Leung N. Utility of urine eosinophils in the diagnosis of acute interstitial nephritis. Clin J Am Soc Nephrol (CJASN). 2013;8(11):1857–62.
13. Oyaert M, Delanghe J. Progress in automated urinalysis. Ann Lab Med. 2019;39(1):15–22.
14. Trachtenberg F, Barregard L. The effect of age, sex, and race on urinary markers of kidney damage in children. Am J Kidney Dis. 2007;50(6):938–45.
15. Csernus K, Lanyi E, Erhardt E, Molnar D. Effect of childhood obesity and obesity-related cardiovascular risk factors on glomerular and tubular protein excretion. Eur J Pediatr. 2005;164(1):44–9.
16. Hjorth L, Helin I, Grubb A. Age-related reference limits for urine levels of albumin, orosomucoid, immunoglobulin G and protein HC in children. Scand J Clin Lab Invest. 2000;60(1):65–73.
17. Davies AG, Postlethwaite RJ, Price DA, Burn JL, Houlton CA, Fielding BA. Urinary albumin excretion in school children. Arch Dis Child. 1984;59(7):625–30.
18. Kidney Disease: Improving Global Outcomes CKDMBDWG. KDIGO clinical practice guideline for the diagnosis, evaluation, prevention, and treatment of Chronic Kidney Disease-Mineral and Bone Disorder (CKD-MBD). Kidney Int Suppl. 2009;113:S1–130.

19. Hogg RJ, Furth S, Lemley KV, Portman R, Schwartz GJ, Coresh J, et al. National Kidney Foundation's Kidney Disease Outcomes Quality Initiative clinical practice guidelines for chronic kidney disease in children and adolescents: evaluation, classification, and stratification. Pediatrics. 2003;111(6 Pt 1):1416–21.

20. Executive summary: standards of medical care in diabetes—2013. Diabetes Care. 2013;36(Suppl 1):S4–10.

21. Ettenger RB. The evaluation of the child with proteinuria. Pediatr Ann. 1994;23(9):486–94.

22. Hogg RJ, Portman RJ, Milliner D, Lemley KV, Eddy A, Ingelfinger J. Evaluation and management of proteinuria and nephrotic syndrome in children: recommendations from a pediatric nephrology panel established at the National Kidney Foundation conference on proteinuria, albuminuria, risk, assessment, detection, and elimination (PARADE). Pediatrics. 2000;105(6):1242–9.

23. Huang Y, Yang X, Zhang Y, Yue S, Mei X, Bi L, et al. Correlation of urine protein/creatinine ratios to 24-h urinary protein for quantitating proteinuria in children. Pediatr Nephrol. 2020;35(3):463–8.

24. Jones CA, Francis ME, Eberhardt MS, Chavers B, Coresh J, Engelgau M, et al. Microalbuminuria in the US population: third National Health and Nutrition Examination Survey. Am J Kidney Dis. 2002;39(3):445–59.

25. Brandt JR, Jacobs A, Raissy HH, Kelly FM, Staples AO, Kaufman E, et al. Orthostatic proteinuria and the spectrum of diurnal variability of urinary protein excretion in healthy children. Pediatr Nephrol. 2010;25(6):1131–7.

26. Park YH, Choi JY, Chung HS, Koo JW, Kim SY, Namgoong MK, et al. Hematuria and proteinuria in a mass school urine screening test. Pediatr Nephrol. 2005;20(8):1126–30.

27. Vehaskari VM, Rapola J. Isolated proteinuria: analysis of a school-age population. J Pediatr. 1982;101(5):661–8.

28. Mori Y, Hiraoka M, Suganuma N, Tsukahara H, Yoshida H, Mayumi M. Urinary creatinine excretion and protein/creatinine ratios vary by body size and gender in children. Pediatr Nephrol. 2006;21(5):683–7.

29. Kim HS, Cheon HW, Choe JH, Yoo KH, Hong YS, Lee JW, et al. Quantification of proteinuria in children using the urinary protein-osmolality ratio. Pediatr Nephrol. 2001;16(1):73–6.

30. Serdaroglu E, Mir S. Protein-osmolality ratio for quantification of proteinuria in children. Clin Exp Nephrol. 2008;12(5):354–7.

31. Hooman N, Otoukesh H, Safaii H, Mehrazma M, Shokrolah Y. Quantification of proteinuria with urinary protein to osmolality ratios in children with and without renal insufficiency. Ann Saudi Med. 2005;25(3):215–8.

32. Smith HS. The kidney structure and function in health and disease. New York: Oxford Univ. Press; 1951.

33. Arant BS Jr, Edelmann CM Jr, Spitzer A. The congruence of creatinine and inulin clearances in children: use of the Technicon AutoAnalyzer. J Pediatr. 1972;81(3):559–61.

34. Cole BR, Giangiacomo J, Ingelfinger JR, Robson AM. Measurement of renal function without urine collection. A critical evaluation of the constant-infusion technic for determination of inulin and para-aminohippurate. N Engl J Med. 1972;287(22):1109–14.

35. Swinkels DW, Hendriks JC, Nauta J, de Jong MC. Glomerular filtration rate by single-injection inulin clearance: definition of a workable protocol for children. Ann Clin Biochem. 2000;37(Pt 1): 60–6.

36. Florijn KW, Barendregt JN, Lentjes EG, van Dam W, Prodjosudjadi W, van Saase JL, et al. Glomerular filtration rate measurement by "single-shot" injection of inulin. Kidney Int. 1994;46(1):252–9.

37. van Rossum LK, Cransberg K, de Rijke YB, Zietse R, Lindemans J, Vulto AG. Determination of inulin clearance by single injection or infusion in children. Pediatr Nephrol. 2005;20(6):777–81.

38. Kidney Disease: Improving Global Outcomes (KDIGO) CKD Work Group. KDIGO 2012 clinical practice guideline for the evaluation and management of chronic kidney disease. Kidney Int Suppl. 2013(3):1–150.

39. Levey AS. Measurement of renal function in chronic renal disease. Kidney Int. 1990;38(1):167–84.

40. Myers GL, Miller WG, Coresh J, Fleming J, Greenberg N, Greene T, et al. Recommendations for improving serum creatinine measurement: a report from the Laboratory Working Group of the National Kidney Disease Education Program. Clin Chem. 2006;52(1):5–18.

41. Schwartz GJ, Brion LP, Spitzer A. The use of plasma creatinine concentration for estimating glomerular filtration rate in infants, children, and adolescents. Pediatr Clin N Am. 1987;34(3):571–90.

42. Atiyeh BA, Dabbagh SS, Gruskin AB. Evaluation of renal function during childhood. Pediatr Rev. 1996;17(5):175–80.

43. Hellerstein S, Berenbom M, Alon US, Warady BA. Creatinine clearance following cimetidine for estimation of glomerular filtration rate. Pediatr Nephrol. 1998;12(1):49–54.

44. van Acker BA, Koomen GC, Koopman MG, de Waart DR, Arisz L. Creatinine clearance during cimetidine administration for measurement of glomerular filtration rate. Lancet. 1992;340(8831):1326–9.

45. Hellerstein S, Berenbom M, DiMaggio S, Erwin P, Simon SD, Wilson N. Comparison of two formulae for estimation of glomerular filtration rate in children. Pediatr Nephrol. 2004;19(7):780–4.

46. Schwartz GJ, Haycock GB, Edelmann CM Jr, Spitzer A. A simple estimate of glomerular filtration rate in children derived from body length and plasma creatinine. Pediatrics. 1976;58(2):259–63.

47. Counahan R, Chantler C, Ghazali S, Kirkwood B, Rose F, Barratt TM. Estimation of glomerular filtra-

48. Schwartz GJ, Furth S, Cole SR, Warady B, Munoz A. Glomerular filtration rate via plasma iohexol disappearance: pilot study for chronic kidney disease in children. Kidney Int. 2006;69(11):2070–7.

49. Schwartz GJ, Work DF. Measurement and estimation of GFR in children and adolescents. Clin J Am Soc Nephrol (CJASN). 2009;4(11):1832–43.

50. Schwartz GJ, Munoz A, Schneider MF, Mak RH, Kaskel F, Warady BA, et al. New equations to estimate GFR in children with CKD. J Am Soc Nephrol (JASN). 2009;20(3):629–37.

51. Schwartz GJ, Schneider MF, Maier PS, Moxey-Mims M, Dharnidharka VR, Warady BA, et al. Improved equations estimating GFR in children with chronic kidney disease using an immunonephelometric determination of cystatin C. Kidney Int. 2012;82(4):445–53.

52. Rule AD, Bergstralh EJ, Slezak JM, Bergert J, Larson TS. Glomerular filtration rate estimated by cystatin C among different clinical presentations. Kidney Int. 2006;69(2):399–405.

53. Finney H, Newman DJ, Price CP. Adult reference ranges for serum cystatin C, creatinine and predicted creatinine clearance. Ann Clin Biochem. 2000;37(Pt 1):49–59.

54. Knight EL, Verhave JC, Spiegelman D, Hillege HL, de Zeeuw D, Curhan GC, et al. Factors influencing serum cystatin C levels other than renal function and the impact on renal function measurement. Kidney Int. 2004;65(4):1416–21.

55. Cimerman N, Brguljan PM, Krasovec M, Suskovic S, Kos J. Serum cystatin C, a potent inhibitor of cysteine proteinases, is elevated in asthmatic patients. Clin Chim Acta. 2000;300(1–2):83–95.

56. Wiesli P, Schwegler B, Spinas GA, Schmid C. Serum cystatin C is sensitive to small changes in thyroid function. Clin Chim Acta. 2003;338(1–2):87–90.

57. Sambasivan AS, Lepage N, Filler G. Cystatin C intrapatient variability in children with chronic kidney disease is less than serum creatinine. Clin Chem. 2005;51(11):2215–6.

58. Zappitelli M, Zhang X, Foster BJ. Estimating glomerular filtration rate in children at serial follow-up when height is unknown. Clin J Am Soc Nephrol (CJASN). 2010;5(10):1763–9.

59. Pottel H, Hoste L, Martens F. A simple height-independent equation for estimating glomerular filtration rate in children. Pediatr Nephrol. 2012;27(6):973–9.

60. Blufpand HN, Westland R, van Wijk JA, Roelandse-Koop EA, Kaspers GJ, Bokenkamp A. Height-independent estimation of glomerular filtration rate in children: an alternative to the Schwartz equation. J Pediatr. 2013;163(6):1722–7.

61. Hoste L, Dubourg L, Selistre L, De Souza VC, Ranchin B, Hadj-Aissa A, et al. A new equation to estimate the glomerular filtration rate in chil-dren, adolescents and young adults. Nephrol Dial Transplant. 2014;29(5):1082–91.

62. Benoit SW, Kathman T, Patel J, Stegman M, Cobb C, Hoehn J, et al. GFR estimation after cystatin C reference material change. Kidney Int Rep. 2021;6(2):429–36.

63. Schwartz GJ, Cox C, Seegmiller JC, Maier PS, DiManno D, Furth SL, et al. Recalibration of cystatin C using standardized material in Siemens nephelometers. Pediatr Nephrol. 2020;35(2):279–85.

64. Pierce CB, Munoz A, Ng DK, Warady BA, Furth SL, Schwartz GJ. Age- and sex-dependent clinical equations to estimate glomerular filtration rates in children and young adults with chronic kidney disease. Kidney Int. 2021;99(4):948–56.

65. Bjork J, Nyman U, Larsson A, Delanaye P, Pottel H. Estimation of the glomerular filtration rate in children and young adults by means of the CKD-EPI equation with age-adjusted creatinine values. Kidney Int. 2021;99(4):940–7.

66. Gaspari F, Perico N, Ruggenenti P, Mosconi L, Amuchastegui CS, Guerini E, et al. Plasma clearance of nonradioactive iohexol as a measure of glomerular filtration rate. J Am Soc Nephrol (JASN). 1995;6(2):257–63.

67. Stake G, Monn E, Rootwelt K, Monclair T. The clearance of iohexol as a measure of the glomerular filtration rate in children with chronic renal failure. Scand J Clin Lab Invest. 1991;51(8):729–34.

68. Berg UB, Back R, Celsi G, Halling SE, Homberg I, Krmar RT, et al. Comparison of plasma clearance of iohexol and urinary clearance of inulin for measurement of GFR in children. Am J Kidney Dis. 2011;57(1):55–61.

69. Gaspari F, Guerini E, Perico N, Mosconi L, Ruggenenti P, Remuzzi G. Glomerular filtration rate determined from a single plasma sample after intravenous iohexol injection: is it reliable? J Am Soc Nephrol (JASN). 1996;7(12):2689–93.

70. Piepsz A, Colarinha P, Gordon I, Hahn K, Olivier P, Sixt R, et al. Guidelines for glomerular filtration rate determination in children. Eur J Nucl Med. 2001;28(3):BP31–6.

71. Blaufox MD, Aurell M, Bubeck B, Fommei E, Piepsz A, Russell C, et al. Report of the radionuclides in nephrourology committee on renal clearance. J Nucl Med. 1996;37(11):1883–90.

72. Rose B. In: Dereck J, Muza N, editors. Clinical physiology of acid-base and electrolyte disorders. 4th ed. New York: McGraw-Hill Inc.; 1994. p. 66–103.

73. Espinel CH. The FENa test. Use in the differential diagnosis of acute renal failure. JAMA. 1976;236(6):579–81.

74. Perazella MA, Bomback AS. Urinary eosinophils in AIN: farewell to an old biomarker? Clin J Am Soc Nephrol (CJASN). 2013;8(11):1841–3.

75. Pepin MN, Bouchard J, Legault L, Ethier J. Diagnostic performance of fractional excretion of urea and fractional excretion of sodium in the

76. evaluations of patients with acute kidney injury with or without diuretic treatment. Am J Kidney Dis. 2007;50(4):566–73.

76. Carvounis CP, Nisar S, Guro-Razuman S. Significance of the fractional excretion of urea in the differential diagnosis of acute renal failure. Kidney Int. 2002;62(6):2223–9.

77. Vanmassenhove J, Glorieux G, Hoste E, Dhondt A, Vanholder R, Van Biesen W. Urinary output and fractional excretion of sodium and urea as indicators of transient versus intrinsic acute kidney injury during early sepsis. Crit Care. 2013;17(5):R234.

78. Bijvoet OL. Relation of plasma phosphate concentration to renal tubular reabsorption of phosphate. Clin Sci. 1969;37(1):23–36.

79. Walton RJ, Bijvoet OL. Nomogram for derivation of renal threshold phosphate concentration. Lancet. 1975;2(7929):309–10.

80. Kenny AP, Glen AC. Tests of phosphate reabsorption. Lancet. 1973;2(7821):158.

81. Barth JH, Jones RG, Payne RB. Calculation of renal tubular reabsorption of phosphate: the algorithm performs better than the nomogram. Ann Clin Biochem. 2000;37(Pt 1):79–81.

82. Hummel CS, Lu C, Loo DD, Hirayama BA, Voss AA, Wright EM. Glucose transport by human renal Na+/D-glucose cotransporters SGLT1 and SGLT2. Am J Physiol Cell Physiol. 2011;300(1):C14–21.

83. Santer R, Kinner M, Schneppenheim R, Hillebrand G, Kemper M, Ehrich J, et al. The molecular basis of renal glucosuria: mutations in the gene for a renal glucose transporter (SGLT2). J Inherit Metab Dis. 2000;23(Suppl 1):178.

84. Novikov A, Fu Y, Huang W, Freeman B, Patel R, van Ginkel C, et al. SGLT2 inhibition and renal urate excretion: role of luminal glucose, GLUT9, and URAT1. Am J Physiol Renal Physiol. 2019;316(1):F173–F85.

85. West ML, Bendz O, Chen CB, Singer GG, Richardson RM, Sonnenberg H, et al. Development of a test to evaluate the transtubular potassium concentration gradient in the cortical collecting duct in vivo. Miner Electrolyte Metab. 1986;12(4):226–33.

86. Rodriguez-Soriano J, Ubetagoyena M, Vallo A. Transtubular potassium concentration gradient: a useful test to estimate renal aldosterone bioactivity in infants and children. Pediatr Nephrol. 1990;4(2):105–10.

87. Ethier JH, Kamel KS, Magner PO, Lemann J Jr, Halperin ML. The transtubular potassium concentration in patients with hypokalemia and hyperkalemia. Am J Kidney Dis. 1990;15(4):309–15.

88. Choi MJ, Ziyadeh FN. The utility of the transtubular potassium gradient in the evaluation of hyperkalemia. J Am Soc Nephrol (JASN). 2008;19(3):424–6.

89. Kamel KS, Halperin ML. Intrarenal urea recycling leads to a higher rate of renal excretion of potassium: an hypothesis with clinical implications. Curr Opin Nephrol Hypertens. 2011;20(5):547–54.

90. Calonge MJ, Gasparini P, Chillaron J, Chillon M, Gallucci M, Rousaud F, et al. Cystinuria caused by mutations in rBAT, a gene involved in the transport of cystine. Nat Genet. 1994;6(4):420–5.

91. Saadi I, Chen XZ, Hediger M, Ong P, Pereira P, Goodyer P, et al. Molecular genetics of cystinuria: mutation analysis of SLC3A1 and evidence for another gene in type I (silent) phenotype. Kidney Int. 1998;54(1):48–55.

92. Kost GJ, Trent JK, Saeed D. Indications for measurement of total carbon dioxide in arterial blood. Clin Chem. 1988;34(8):1650–2.

93. K/DOQI Clinical practice guidelines for bone metabolism and disease in children with chronic kidney disease. Am J Kidney Dis. 2005;46(4). https://kidneyfoundation.cachefly.net/professionals/KDOQI/guidelines_pedbone/index.htm.

94. Rees L, Jones H. Nutritional management and growth in children with chronic kidney disease. Pediatr Nephrol. 2013;28(4):527–36.

95. Halperin ML, Kamel KS, Goldstein MB. Fluid, electrolyte, and acid-base physiology: a problem-based approach. 3rd ed. Philadelphia: W.B. Saunders; 2010.

96. Figge J, Jabor A, Kazda A, Fencl V. Anion gap and hypoalbuminemia. Crit Care Med. 1998;26(11):1807–10.

97. Srivastava T, Garg U, Chan YR, Alon US. Essentials of laboratory medicine for the nephrology clinician. Pediatr Nephrol. 2007;22(2):170–82.

98. Goldstein MB, Bear R, Richardson RM, Marsden PA, Halperin ML. The urine anion gap: a clinically useful index of ammonium excretion. Am J Med Sci. 1986;292(4):198–202.

99. Batlle DC, Hizon M, Cohen E, Gutterman C, Gupta R. The use of the urinary anion gap in the diagnosis of hyperchloremic metabolic acidosis. N Engl J Med. 1988;318(10):594–9.

100. Halperin ML, Margolis BL, Robinson LA, Halperin RM, West ML, Bear RA. The urine osmolal gap: a clue to estimate urine ammonium in "hybrid" types of metabolic acidosis. Clin Invest Med. 1988;11(3):198–202.

101. Palmer BF, Clegg DJ. The use of selected urine chemistries in the diagnosis of kidney disorders. Clin J Am Soc Nephrol (CJASN). 2019;14(2):306–16.

102. Carlisle EJ, Donnelly SM, Vasuvattakul S, Kamel KS, Tobe S, Halperin ML. Glue-sniffing and distal renal tubular acidosis: sticking to the facts. J Am Soc Nephrol (JASN). 1991;1(8):1019–27.

103. Halperin ML, Goldstein MB, Haig A, Johnson MD, Stinebaugh BJ. Studies on the pathogenesis of type I (distal) renal tubular acidosis as revealed by the urinary PCO2 tensions. J Clin Invest. 1974;53(3):669–77.

104. DuBose TD Jr, Caflisch CR. Validation of the difference in urine and blood carbon dioxide tension during bicarbonate loading as an index of distal nephron acidification in experimental models of dis-

tal renal tubular acidosis. J Clin Invest. 1985;75(4):1116–23.

105. Kim S, Lee JW, Park J, Na KY, Joo KW, Ahn C, et al. The urine-blood PCO gradient as a diagnostic index of H(+)-ATPase defect distal renal tubular acidosis. Kidney Int. 2004;66(2):761–7.

106. Southcott EK, Kerrigan JL, Potter JM, Telford RD, Waring P, Reynolds GJ, et al. Establishment of pediatric reference intervals on a large cohort of healthy children. Clin Chim Acta. 2010;411(19–20):1421–7.

107. Colantonio DA, Kyriakopoulou L, Chan MK, Daly CH, Brinc D, Venner AA, et al. Closing the gaps in pediatric laboratory reference intervals: a CALIPER database of 40 biochemical markers in a healthy and multiethnic population of children. Clin Chem. 2012;58(5):854–68.

108. Soldin SJ, Brugnara C, Wong EC, editors. Pediatric reference ranges. 4th ed. Washington: AACC Press; 2003.

109. Sevastos N, Theodossiades G, Archimandritis AJ. Pseudohyperkalemia in serum: a new insight into an old phenomenon. Clin Med Res. 2008;6(1):30–2.

110. Asirvatham JR, Moses V, Bjornson L. Errors in potassium measurement: a laboratory perspective for the clinician. N Am J Med Sci. 2013;5(4):255–9.

111. Stewart GW, Corrall RJ, Fyffe JA, Stockdill G, Strong JA. Familial pseudohyperkalaemia. A new syndrome. Lancet. 1979;2(8135):175–7.

112. Andolfo I, Alper SL, Delaunay J, Auriemma C, Russo R, Asci R, et al. Missense mutations in the ABCB6 transporter cause dominant familial pseudohyperkalemia. Am J Hematol. 2013;88(1):66–72.

113. Liamis G, Liberopoulos E, Barkas F, Elisaf M. Spurious electrolyte disorders: a diagnostic challenge for clinicians. Am J Nephrol. 2013;38(1):50–7.

114. Clinical practice guidelines for nutrition in chronic renal failure. K/DOQI, National Kidney Foundation. Am J Kidney Dis. 2000;35(6 Suppl 2):S1–140.

115. Clifford SM, Bunker AM, Jacobsen JR, Roberts WL. Age and gender specific pediatric reference intervals for aldolase, amylase, ceruloplasmin, creatine kinase, pancreatic amylase, prealbumin, and uric acid. Clin Chim Acta. 2011;412(9–10):788–90.

116. Fathallah-Shaykh SA, Cramer MT. Uric acid and the kidney. Pediatr Nephrol. 2014;29(6):999–1008.

117. Cameron JS, Moro F, Simmonds HA. Gout, uric acid and purine metabolism in paediatric nephrology. Pediatr Nephrol. 1993;7(1):105–18.

118. Dahan K, Devuyst O, Smaers M, Vertommen D, Loute G, Poux JM, et al. A cluster of mutations in the UMOD gene causes familial juvenile hyperuricemic nephropathy with abnormal expression of uromodulin. J Am Soc Nephrol (JASN). 2003;14(11):2883–93.

119. Zivna M, Hulkova H, Matignon M, Hodanova K, Vylet'al P, Kalbacova M, et al. Dominant renin gene mutations associated with early-onset hyperuricemia, anemia, and chronic kidney failure. Am J Hum Genet. 2009;85(2):204–13.

120. Bingham C, Ellard S, van't Hoff WG, Simmonds HA, Marinaki AM, Badman MK, et al. Atypical familial juvenile hyperuricemic nephropathy associated with a hepatocyte nuclear factor-1beta gene mutation. Kidney Int. 2003;63(5):1645–51.

121. Adalat S, Woolf AS, Johnstone KA, Wirsing A, Harries LW, Long DA, et al. HNF1B mutations associate with hypomagnesemia and renal magnesium wasting. J Am Soc Nephrol (JASN). 2009;20(5):1123–31.

122. Sanchez Bayle M, Vazquez Martul M, Ecija Peiro JL, Garcia Vao C, Ramo MC. Renal handling of uric acid in normal children by means of the pyrazinamide and sulfinpyrazone tests. Int J Pediatr Nephrol. 1987;8(1):5–8.

123. Kuge R, Morikawa Y, Hasegawa Y. Uric acid and dehydration in children with gastroenteritis. Pediatr Int. 2017;59(11):1151–6.

124. Johnson RJ, Bakris GL, Borghi C, Chonchol MB, Feldman D, Lanaspa MA, et al. Hyperuricemia, acute and chronic kidney disease, hypertension, and cardiovascular disease: report of a scientific workshop organized by the National Kidney Foundation. Am J Kidney Dis. 2018;71(6):851–65.

125. Stewart DJ, Langlois V, Noone D. Hyperuricemia and hypertension: links and risks. Integr Blood Press Control. 2019;12:43–62.

126. Yanik M, Feig DI. Serum urate: a biomarker or treatment target in pediatric hypertension? Curr Opin Cardiol. 2013;28(4):433–8.

127. Bharti S, Bharti B. Serum uric acid and childhood hypertension: association to causation to prevention. Am J Hypertens. 2017;30(7):658–60.

128. Park B, Lee HA, Lee SH, Park BM, Park EA, Kim HS, et al. Association between serum levels of uric acid and blood pressure tracking in childhood. Am J Hypertens. 2017;30(7):713–8.

129. Noone DG, Marks SD. Hyperuricemia is associated with hypertension, obesity, and albuminuria in children with chronic kidney disease. J Pediatr. 2013;162(1):128–32.

130. Rodenbach KE, Schneider MF, Furth SL, Moxey-Mims MM, Mitsnefes MM, Weaver DJ, et al. Hyperuricemia and progression of CKD in children and adolescents: the chronic kidney disease in children (CKiD) cohort study. Am J Kidney Dis. 2015;66(6):984–92.

131. Hamada T, Ichida K, Hosoyamada M, Mizuta E, Yanagihara K, Sonoyama K, et al. Uricosuric action of losartan via the inhibition of urate transporter 1 (URAT 1) in hypertensive patients. Am J Hypertens. 2008;21(10):1157–62.

132. Biyikli NK, Alpay H, Guran T. Hypercalciuria and recurrent urinary tract infections: incidence and symptoms in children over 5 years of age. Pediatr Nephrol. 2005;20(10):1435–8.

133. Ghazali S, Barratt TM. Urinary excretion of calcium and magnesium in children. Arch Dis Child. 1974;49(2):97–101.

134. Moore ES, Coe FL, McMann BJ, Favus MJ. Idiopathic hypercalciuria in children: prevalence and metabolic characteristics. J Pediatr. 1978;92(6):906–10.

135. Sorkhi H, Haji AM. Urinary calcium to creatinin ratio in children. Indian J Pediatr. 2005;72(12):1055–6.

136. De Santo NG, Di Iorio B, Capasso G, Paduano C, Stamler R, Langman CB, et al. Population based data on urinary excretion of calcium, magnesium, oxalate, phosphate and uric acid in children from Cimitile (southern Italy). Pediatr Nephrol. 1992;6(2):149–57.

137. So NP, Osorio AV, Simon SD, Alon US. Normal urinary calcium/creatinine ratios in African-American and Caucasian children. Pediatr Nephrol. 2001;16(2):133–9.

138. Vachvanichsanong P, Lebel L, Moore ES. Urinary calcium excretion in healthy Thai children. Pediatr Nephrol. 2000;14(8–9):847–50.

139. Butani L, Kalia A. Idiopathic hypercalciuria in children—how valid are the existing diagnostic criteria? Pediatr Nephrol. 2004;19(6):577–82.

140. Hilgenfeld MS, Simon S, Blowey D, Richmond W, Alon US. Lack of seasonal variations in urinary calcium/creatinine ratio in school-age children. Pediatr Nephrol. 2004;19(10):1153–5.

141. Chenevier-Gobeaux C, Rogier M, Dridi-Brahimi I, Koumakis E, Cormier C, Borderie D. Pre-, post- or no acidification of urine samples for calcium analysis: does it matter? Clin Chem Lab Med. 2019;58(1):33–9.

142. Richmond W, Colgan G, Simon S, Stuart-Hilgenfeld M, Wilson N, Alon US. Random urine calcium/osmolality in the assessment of calciuria in children with decreased muscle mass. Clin Nephrol. 2005;64(4):264–70.

143. Mir S, Serdaroglu E. Quantification of hypercalciuria with the urine calcium osmolality ratio in children. Pediatr Nephrol. 2005;20(11):1562–5.

144. Polito C, La Manna A, Maiello R, Nappi B, Siciliano MC, Di Domenico MR, et al. Urinary sodium and potassium excretion in idiopathic hypercalciuria of children. Nephron. 2002;91(1):7–12.

145. Bray GA, Vollmer WM, Sacks FM, Obarzanek E, Svetkey LP, Appel LJ, et al. A further subgroup analysis of the effects of the DASH diet and three dietary sodium levels on blood pressure: results of the DASH-Sodium Trial. Am J Cardiol. 2004;94(2):222–7.

146. Tefekli A, Esen T, Ziylan O, Erol B, Armagan A, Ander H, et al. Metabolic risk factors in pediatric and adult calcium oxalate urinary stone formers: is there any difference? Urol Int. 2003;70(4):273–7.

147. Hoppe B, Langman CB. Hypocitraturia in patients with urolithiasis. Arch Dis Child. 1997;76(2):174–5.

148. Hoppe B, Jahnen A, Bach D, Hesse A. Urinary calcium oxalate saturation in healthy infants and children. J Urol. 1997;158(2):557–9.

149. Karabacak OR, Ipek B, Ozturk U, Demirel F, Saltas H, Altug U. Metabolic evaluation in stone disease metabolic differences between the pediatric and adult patients with stone disease. Urology. 2010;76(1):238–41.

150. DeFoor WR, Jackson E, Minevich E, Caillat A, Reddy P, Sheldon C, et al. The risk of recurrent urolithiasis in children is dependent on urinary calcium and citrate. Urology. 2010;76(1):242–5.

151. Arrabal-Polo MA, Arrabal-Martin M, Arias-Santiago S, Garrido-Gomez J, Poyatos-Andujar A, Zuluaga-Gomez A. Importance of citrate and the calcium: citrate ratio in patients with calcium renal lithiasis and severe lithogenesis. BJU Int. 2013;111(4):622–7.

152. Srivastava T, Winston MJ, Auron A, Alon US. Urine calcium/citrate ratio in children with hypercalciuric stones. Pediatr Res. 2009;66(1):85–90.

153. DeFoor W, Jackson E, Schulte M, Alam Z, Asplin J. Calcium-to-citrate ratio distinguishes solitary and recurrent urinary stone forming children. J Urol. 2017;198(2):416–21.

154. Sikora P, Roth B, Kribs A, Michalk DV, Hesse A, Hoppe B. Hypocitraturia is one of the major risk factors for nephrocalcinosis in very low birth weight (VLBW) infants. Kidney Int. 2003;63(6):2194–9.

155. Stapenhorst L, Sassen R, Beck B, Laube N, Hesse A, Hoppe B. Hypocitraturia as a risk factor for nephrocalcinosis after kidney transplantation. Pediatr Nephrol. 2005;20(5):652–6.

156. Hoppe B. An update on primary hyperoxaluria. Nat Rev Nephrol. 2012;8(8):467–75.

157. Cochat P, Rumsby G. Primary hyperoxaluria. N Engl J Med. 2013;369(7):649–58.

158. Belostotsky R, Seboun E, Idelson GH, Milliner DS, Becker-Cohen R, Rinat C, et al. Mutations in DHDPSL are responsible for primary hyperoxaluria type III. Am J Hum Genet. 2010;87(3):392–9.

159. La Manna A, Polito C, Marte A, Iovene A, Di Toro R. Hyperuricosuria in children: clinical presentation and natural history. Pediatrics. 2001;107(1):86–90.

160. Stapleton FB, Nash DA. A screening test for hyperuricosuria. J Pediatr. 1983;102(1):88–90.

161. Azizi M, Menard J. Review: measurement of plasma renin: a critical review of methodology. J Renin Angiotensin Aldosterone Syst (JRAAS). 2010;11(2):89–90.

162. Dillon MJ, Ryness JM. Plasma renin activity and aldosterone concentration in children. Br Med J. 1975;4(5992):316–9.

163. Olson N, DeJongh B, Hough A, Parra D. Plasma renin activity-guided strategy for the management of hypertension. Pharmacotherapy. 2012;32(5):446–55.

164. Dillon MJ. The diagnosis of renovascular disease. Pediatr Nephrol. 1997;11(3):366–72.

165. Tash JA, Stock JA, Hanna MK. The role of partial nephrectomy in the treatment of pediatric renal hypertension. J Urol. 2003;169(2):625–8.

166. Goonasekera CD, Shah V, Wade AM, Dillon MJ. The usefulness of renal vein renin studies in hypertensive children: a 25-year experience. Pediatr Nephrol. 2002;17(11):943–9.

167. McLaren CA, Roebuck DJ. Interventional radiology for renovascular hypertension in children. Tech Vasc Interv Radiol. 2003;6(4):150–7.

168. Dillon MJ, Shah V, Barratt TM. Renal vein renin measurements in children with hypertension. Br Med J. 1978;2(6131):168–70.

169. White PC. Disorders of aldosterone biosynthesis and action. N Engl J Med. 1994;331(4):250–8.

170. Whitworth JA. Mechanisms of glucocorticoid-induced hypertension. Kidney Int. 1987;31(5):1213–24.

171. Stowasser M, Ahmed AH, Pimenta E, Taylor PJ, Gordon RD. Factors affecting the aldosterone/renin ratio. Horm Metab Res (Hormon-und Stoffwechselforschung = Hormones et metabolisme). 2012;44(3):170–6.

172. Blumenfeld JD, Sealey JE, Schlussel Y, Vaughan ED Jr, Sos TA, Atlas SA, et al. Diagnosis and treatment of primary hyperaldosteronism. Ann Intern Med. 1994;121(11):877–85.

173. Refardt J, Winzeler B, Christ-Crain M. Copeptin and its role in the diagnosis of diabetes insipidus and the syndrome of inappropriate antidiuresis. Clin Endocrinol (Oxford). 2019;91(1):22–32.

174. Tuli G, Munarin J, Tessaris D, Einaudi S, Matarazzo P, de Sanctis L. Distribution of plasma copeptin levels and influence of obesity in children and adolescents. Eur J Pediatr. 2021;180(1):119–26.

175. Fenske W, Refardt J, Chifu I, Schnyder I, Winzeler B, Drummond J, et al. A copeptin-based approach in the diagnosis of diabetes insipidus. N Engl J Med. 2018;379(5):428–39.

176. Sbardella E, Grossman AB. Pheochromocytoma: an approach to diagnosis. Best Pract Res Clin Endocrinol Metab. 2020;34(2):101346.

177. Walport MJ. Complement. First of two parts. N Engl J Med. 2001;344(14):1058–66.

178. Walport MJ. Complement. Second of two parts. N Engl J Med. 2001;344(15):1140–4.

179. Prohaszka Z, Nilsson B, Frazer-Abel A, Kirschfink M. Complement analysis 2016: clinical indications, laboratory diagnostics and quality control. Immunobiology. 2016;221(11):1247–58.

180. Huber-Lang M, Sarma JV, Zetoune FS, Rittirsch D, Neff TA, McGuire SR, et al. Generation of C5a in the absence of C3: a new complement activation pathway. Nat Med. 2006;12(6):682–7.

181. Prohaszka Z, Kirschfink M, Frazer-Abel A. Complement analysis in the era of targeted therapeutics. Mol Immunol. 2018;102:84–8.

182. Hebert LA, Cosio FG, Neff JC. Diagnostic significance of hypocomplementemia. Kidney Int. 1991;39(5):811–21.

183. Shih AR, Murali MR. Laboratory tests for disorders of complement and complement regulatory proteins. Am J Hematol. 2015;90(12):1180–6.

184. Davies DJ, Moran JE, Niall JF, Ryan GB. Segmental necrotising glomerulonephritis with antineutrophil antibody: possible arbovirus aetiology? Br Med J (Clin Res Ed). 1982;285(6342):606.

185. Elena C. L28. Relevance of detection techniques for ANCA testing. Presse Med. 2013;42(4 Pt 2):582–4.

186. Savige J, Gillis D, Benson E, Davies D, Esnault V, Falk RJ, et al. International consensus statement on testing and reporting of antineutrophil cytoplasmic antibodies (ANCA). Am J Clin Pathol. 1999;111(4):507–13.

187. Csernok E, Mahrhold J, Hellmich B. Anti-neutrophil cytoplasm antibodies (ANCA): Recent methodological advances-Lead to new consensus recommendations for ANCA detection. J Immunol Methods. 2018;456:1–6.

188. Damoiseaux J, Csernok E, Rasmussen N, Moosig F, van Paassen P, Baslund B, et al. Detection of anti-neutrophil cytoplasmic antibodies (ANCAs): a multicentre European Vasculitis Study Group (EUVAS) evaluation of the value of indirect immunofluorescence (IIF) versus antigen-specific immunoassays. Ann Rheum Dis. 2017;76(4):647–53.

189. Zhang W, Zheng Z, Jia R, Li X, Zuo X, Wu L, et al. Evaluation of 12 different assays for detecting ANCA in Chinese patients with GPA and MPA: a multicenter study in China. Clin Rheumatol. 2019;38(12):3477–83.

190. Mendel A, Ennis D, Go E, Bakowsky V, Baldwin C, Benseler SM, et al. CanVasc consensus recommendations for the management of antineutrophil cytoplasm antibody-associated vasculitis: 2020 update. J Rheumatol. 2020; https://doi.org/10.3899/jrheum.200721.

191. Radice A, Bianchi L, Sinico RA. Anti-neutrophil cytoplasmic autoantibodies: methodological aspects and clinical significance in systemic vasculitis. Autoimmun Rev. 2013;12(4):487–95.

192. Mandl LA, Solomon DH, Smith EL, Lew RA, Katz JN, Shmerling RH. Using antineutrophil cytoplasmic antibody testing to diagnose vasculitis: can test-ordering guidelines improve diagnostic accuracy? Arch Intern Med. 2002;162(13):1509–14.

193. Moiseev S, Cohen Tervaert JW, Arimura Y, Bogdanos DP, Csernok E, Damoiseaux J, et al. 2020 international consensus on ANCA testing beyond systemic vasculitis. Autoimmun Rev. 2020;19(9):102618.

194. van der Woude FJ, Rasmussen N, Lobatto S, Wiik A, Permin H, van Es LA, et al. Autoantibodies against neutrophils and monocytes: tool for diagnosis and marker of disease activity in Wegener's granulomatosis. Lancet. 1985;1(8426):425–9.

195. Sinclair D, Stevens JM. Role of antineutrophil cytoplasmic antibodies and glomerular basement membrane antibodies in the diagnosis and monitoring of systemic vasculitides. Ann Clin Biochem. 2007;44(Pt 5):432–42.

196. Flossmann O, Berden A, de Groot K, Hagen C, Harper L, Heijl C, et al. Long-term patient survival in ANCA-associated vasculitis. Ann Rheum Dis. 2011;70(3):488–94.

197. Sinico RA, Di Toma L, Radice A. Renal involvement in anti-neutrophil cytoplasmic autoanti-

198. body associated vasculitis. Autoimmun Rev. 2013;12(4):477–82.

198. Walsh M, Flossmann O, Berden A, Westman K, Hoglund P, Stegeman C, et al. Risk factors for relapse of antineutrophil cytoplasmic antibody-associated vasculitis. Arthritis Rheum. 2012;64(2):542–8.

199. Sanders JS, Stassen PM, van Rossum AP, Kallenberg CG, Stegeman CA. Risk factors for relapse in anti-neutrophil cytoplasmic antibody (ANCA)-associated vasculitis: tools for treatment decisions? Clin Exp Rheumatol. 2004;22(6 Suppl 36):S94–101.

200. Sanders JS, Huitma MG, Kallenberg CG, Stegeman CA. Prediction of relapses in PR3-ANCA-associated vasculitis by assessing responses of ANCA titres to treatment. Rheumatology (Oxford). 2006;45(6):724–9.

201. Roth AJ, Ooi JD, Hess JJ, van Timmeren MM, Berg EA, Poulton CE, et al. Epitope specificity determines pathogenicity and detectability in ANCA-associated vasculitis. J Clin Invest. 2013;123(4):1773–83.

202. Gou SJ, Xu PC, Chen M, Zhao MH. Epitope analysis of anti-myeloperoxidase antibodies in patients with ANCA-associated vasculitis. PLoS One. 2013;8(4):e60530.

203. Kain R, Exner M, Brandes R, Ziebermayr R, Cunningham D, Alderson CA, et al. Molecular mimicry in pauci-immune focal necrotizing glomerulonephritis. Nat Med. 2008;14(10):1088–96.

204. Kain R, Tadema H, McKinney EF, Benharkou A, Brandes R, Peschel A, et al. High prevalence of autoantibodies to hLAMP-2 in anti-neutrophil cytoplasmic antibody-associated vasculitis. J Am Soc Nephrol (JASN). 2012;23(3):556–66.

205. Roth AJ, Brown MC, Smith RN, Badhwar AK, Parente O, Chung H, et al. Anti-LAMP-2 antibodies are not prevalent in patients with antineutrophil cytoplasmic autoantibody glomerulonephritis. J Am Soc Nephrol (JASN). 2012;23(3):545–55.

206. Kain R. L29. Relevance of anti-LAMP-2 in vasculitis: why the controversy. Presse Med. 2013;42(4 Pt 2):584–8.

207. Gibson KM, Kain R, Luqmani RA, Ross CJ, Cabral DA, Brown KL. Autoantibodies against lysosome associated membrane protein-2 (LAMP-2) in pediatric chronic primary systemic vasculitis. Front Immunol. 2020;11:624758.

208. Saisoong S, Eiam-Ong S, Hanvivatvong O. Correlations between antinucleosome antibodies and anti-double-stranded DNA antibodies, C3, C4, and clinical activity in lupus patients. Clin Exp Rheumatol. 2006;24(1):51–8.

209. Malleson PN, Sailer M, Mackinnon MJ. Usefulness of antinuclear antibody testing to screen for rheumatic diseases. Arch Dis Child. 1997;77(4):299–304.

210. Satoh M, Chan EK, Ho LA, Rose KM, Parks CG, Cohn RD, et al. Prevalence and sociodemographic correlates of antinuclear antibodies in the United States. Arthritis Rheum. 2012;64(7):2319–27.

211. Pisetsky DS. Antinuclear antibodies in rheumatic disease: a proposal for a function-based classification. Scand J Immunol. 2012;76(3):223–8.

212. Servais G, Karmali R, Guillaume MP, Badot V, Duchateau J, Corazza F. Anti DNA antibodies are not restricted to a specific pattern of fluorescence on HEp2 cells. Clin Chem Lab Med. 2009;47(5):543–9.

213. Frodlund M, Dahlstrom O, Kastbom A, Skogh T, Sjowall C. Associations between antinuclear antibody staining patterns and clinical features of systemic lupus erythematosus: analysis of a regional Swedish register. BMJ Open. 2013;3(10):e003608.

214. Mariz HA, Sato EI, Barbosa SH, Rodrigues SH, Dellavance A, Andrade LE. Pattern on the antinuclear antibody-HEp-2 test is a critical parameter for discriminating antinuclear antibody-positive healthy individuals and patients with autoimmune rheumatic diseases. Arthritis Rheum. 2011;63(1):191–200.

215. Fritzler MJ. The antinuclear antibody test: last or lasting gasp? Arthritis Rheum. 2011;63(1):19–22.

216. Haynes DC, Gershwin ME, Robbins DL, Miller JJ 3rd, Cosca D. Autoantibody profiles in juvenile arthritis. J Rheumatol. 1986;13(2):358–63.

217. Cabral DA, Petty RE, Fung M, Malleson PN. Persistent antinuclear antibodies in children without identifiable inflammatory rheumatic or autoimmune disease. Pediatrics. 1992;89(3):441–4.

218. Tan EM, Feltkamp TE, Smolen JS, Butcher B, Dawkins R, Fritzler MJ, et al. Range of antinuclear antibodies in "healthy" individuals. Arthritis Rheum. 1997;40(9):1601–11.

219. Abeles AM, Abeles M. The clinical utility of a positive antinuclear antibody test result. Am J Med. 2013;126(4):342–8.

220. Marks SD, Tullus K. Autoantibodies in systemic lupus erythematosus. Pediatr Nephrol. 2012;27(10):1855–68.

221. Cervera R, Vinas O, Ramos-Casals M, Font J, Garcia-Carrasco M, Siso A, et al. Anti-chromatin antibodies in systemic lupus erythematosus: a useful marker for lupus nephropathy. Ann Rheum Dis. 2003;62(5):431–4.

222. Pickering MC, Botto M. Are anti-C1q antibodies different from other SLE autoantibodies? Nat Rev Rheumatol. 2010;6(8):490–3.

223. Filler G, Priem F, Vollmer I, Gellermann J, Jung K. Diagnostic sensitivity of serum cystatin for impaired glomerular filtration rate. Pediatr Nephrol. 1999;13(6):501–5.

224. Matos V, van Melle G, Boulat O, Markert M, Bachmann C, Guignard JP. Urinary phosphate/creatinine, calcium/creatinine, and magnesium/creatinine ratios in a healthy pediatric population. J Pediatr. 1997;131(2):252–7.

225. Matos V, Van Melle G, Werner D, Bardy D, Guignard JP. Urinary oxalate and urate to creatinine ratios in a healthy pediatric population. Am J Kidney Dis. 1999;34(2):e1.

Imaging and Radiological Interventions in the Pediatric Urinary Tract

3

Bernarda Viteri, Seth Vatsky, Amy Farkas, Mohamed Elsingergy, Richard D. Bellah, and Erum A. Hartung

Introduction

Imaging plays an important role in the diagnosis and monitoring of many diseases of the kidney and urinary tract in children [1–4]. Both congenital and acquired diseases of the urinary tract are imaged using a variety of modalities, and in many cases it is the imaging study that offers a diagnosis or at least narrows what may begin as a lengthy differential diagnosis. Radiography, excretory urography, contrast fluoroscopy, ultrasonography (US), computed tomography (CT), magnetic resonance imaging (MRI) and nuclear scintigraphy have all been used to assess the urinary tract, each

---

B. Viteri · E. A. Hartung (✉)
Division of Nephrology, Children's Hospital of Philadelphia, Philadelphia, PA, USA

Department of Pediatrics, Perelman School of Medicine at the University of Pennsylvania, Philadelphia, PA, USA
e-mail: viterib@chop.edu; hartunge@chop.edu

S. Vatsky · R. D. Bellah
Department of Radiology, Children's Hospital of Philadelphia, Philadelphia, PA, USA

Department of Radiology, Perelman School of Medicine at the University of Pennsylvania, Philadelphia, PA, USA
e-mail: vatskys@chop.edu; bellah@chop.edu

A. Farkas · M. Elsingergy
Department of Radiology, Children's Hospital of Philadelphia, Philadelphia, PA, USA
e-mail: farkasa1@chop.edu; elsingergm@chop.edu

with its own relative strengths and weaknesses. In some cases, two or more complementary modalities will be necessary to narrow the differential diagnosis. It is important not only to know the most appropriate modality for the investigation of a patient, but also to understand the risks and benefits associated with the various modalities. In this chapter, we provide an overview of these imaging modalities and their associated risks and benefits and present examples of their application in the evaluation of children with kidney and urinary tract abnormalities.

Imaging-Associated Risks

Ionizing Radiation

Several of the modalities used in urinary tract imaging employ ionizing radiation. It is well known that exposure to radiation has deleterious effects, including a strong association between exposure to radiation (particularly at doses reached in CT) and subsequent development of malignancies [5, 6].

The use of medical imaging that exposes patients to ionizing radiation has been increasing. Medical radiation, on average, accounts for the same radiation dose as background radiation in the United States [7]. The use of ionizing radiation is of particular concern in children due to their increased susceptibility to its negative effects. Compared to adult patients, pediatric

---

© The Author(s), under exclusive license to Springer Nature Switzerland AG 2023
F. Schaefer, L. A. Greenbaum (eds.), *Pediatric Kidney Disease*,
https://doi.org/10.1007/978-3-031-11665-0_3

patients have a higher lifetime radiation risk and higher relative dose for a given radiation exposure [5]. To decrease risks to children, it is important to minimize use of ionizing radiation when possible and employ radiation dose reduction strategies applicable to imaging modalities.

Fluoroscopy is an important imaging modality in the evaluation of pediatric genitourinary diseases, as voiding cystourethrography (VCUG) and retrograde urethrography provide necessary anatomic and functional information. A wide variation of radiation doses has been observed in pediatric fluoroscopy [8]. Technical considerations to reduce dose during imaging acquisition include proper collimation and position of patient close to the imaging receptor [9]. Further strategies include the removal of anti-scatter grids for smaller pediatric patients and use of grids for larger pediatric patients [10]. Fluoroscopy units can also be adjusted to optimize settings for pediatric patients, including the automatic brightness control [10]. A pulsed frame rate rather than continuous fluoroscopy can be used without sacrificing imaging quality with considerably less radiation exposure [11].

CT is used for the evaluation of pediatric stone disease and genitourinary trauma and is often the imaging modality of choice in the emergent setting. While CT represents 17% of radiologic procedures in the United States, it accounts for almost 50% of medical radiation [12], highlighting the importance of CT dose optimization. Dose mitigation strategies are of particular importance in the CT evaluation of genitourinary diseases, as the effective doses for pediatric CT of the abdomen and pelvis are the highest when compared to other scans such as head, chest, and spine [13]. Size-based protocols are essential for the reduction of pediatric radiation dose [14]. These protocols factor the patient size into the parameters used to acquire CT images, such as the tube voltage and tube current. Use of a lower tube voltage can cause a substantial dose reduction, and automated tube voltage selection systems can optimize the tube voltage and corresponding tube current based on the scout image [12]. Iterative reconstruction is a method of data processing that refines the raw data and reduces noise, allowing

decrease in the radiation dose necessary to acquire diagnostic quality images [12].

When available, dual energy CT (DECT) can also provide further dose reduction when multiphase contrast examinations are necessary. DECT is performed by scanning a patient with two x-ray tubes operating at different energies, one at a low energy and one at a high energy. DECT can be acquired with a dose comparable to conventional single source CT, but the image acquisition at different energies enables differentiation of structures based on atomic number rather than beam attenuation [15]. This data allows the virtual creation of an unenhanced phase, allowing a multiphasic examination without additional radiation dose. Applications of DECT for CT urography have been explored, demonstrating sufficient image quality with radiation dose reduction [16].

Intravenous Contrast Agents

Risks associated with the administration of intravenous (IV) contrast agents include contrast-induced nephropathy and adverse contrast reactions [17, 18]. The risk of post-contrast acute kidney injury (PC-AKI), defined as acute kidney injury (AKI) occurring within 48 h of IV administration of iodinated contrast media, has been controversial in recent decades. Observational studies designed to evaluate the association between iodinated CT contrast administration and PC-AKI have had conflicting results, likely due to differences in institutional contrast-enhanced CT protocols, variances in strategies for propensity matching, and discrepant subgroup sample sizes with different baseline kidney function [19–24]. Despite recent contributions to the pediatric literature by McDonald et al. [23] and Gilligan et al. [24], knowledge of the risk of PC-AKI in children remains limited.

Nephrotoxicity associated with gadolinium-based contrast agents for MRI has also been described, though the overall consensus is that the risk is low when used at approved doses, even in patients with kidney dysfunction [25, 26].

Another potential risk of IV contrast administration is nephrogenic systemic fibrosis (NSF) [27, 28], which has been described with the use of an older generation of gadolinium-based contrast agents in patients with kidney failure. This rare though significant side effect has limited gadolinium use in patients with advanced chronic kidney disease (CKD) [26]. Nevertheless, the risk of NSF is thought to be lower with newer macrocyclic gadolinium-based agents (e.g. gadobutrol, gadoteridol, gadoterate) [29]. There may also be a risk of gadolinium deposition throughout the body as studies have proven deposition in the bone, brain, and skin but further study is required to determine the clinical significance, if any [30–32]. Rarely, severe reactions to gadolinium-based contrast agents can occur [33].

Potential risks associated with US contrast agents are discussed in the subsequent section, "Contrast-Enhanced Ultrasonography."

Sedation and Anesthesia

Due to the scan times associated with some imaging modalities, some children will require sedation or general anesthesia, and these risks must also be considered when choosing an imaging modality [34, 35]. In some cases, techniques such as "feed and wrap" can be used to obtain high quality images in infants for specific studies such as functional MR urography [36].

Ultrasonography

US is arguably the most important part of the pediatric imaging armamentarium. Its main strengths are that it does not use ionizing radiation and sedation is very rarely required.

The most common indications for US of the kidneys and urinary tract include: urinary tract infection (UTI) [37–39], follow-up of antenatally diagnosed hydronephrosis, evaluation of a palpable mass, assessment for vascular abnormalities (including renal artery stenosis), assessment of medical kidney diseases, screening of patients at known risk to develop kidney neoplasms (for example Beckwith-Wiedemann syndrome and other cancer predisposition syndromes) [40], and assessment for possible urinary obstruction. US can also assess other findings noted on antenatal imaging such as kidney agenesis, ectopia, dysplasia or mass.

The US examination can be tailored in many ways to suit the patient and clinical situation. A patient who is upset or frightened can be scanned lying next to a parent or in the arms of a parent, which can alleviate some anxiety. Coupled with a calm and reassuring environment and various distractions (e.g. toys, music, videos, computer tablets), this setting often allows for the performance of a satisfactory diagnostic study. The need for sedation is extremely rare but may be considered on a case-by-case basis.

The patient can be scanned in various positions (supine, prone, decubitus) depending on the scenario. In fact, altering position can at times be helpful particularly in determining if a structure such as a calculus is mobile. In some situations, the US examination can be repeated after an intervention has been performed in order to determine whether it was successful or resulted in a complication. One can study the urinary tract before or after voiding, after placement of a bladder catheter, ureteral stent or nephrostomy catheter, and throughout a kidney biopsy procedure. These repeated examinations can be done without concern for the effects of radiation.

In general, the smaller body habitus of children allows for excellent US imaging of the kidneys and urinary tract. However, US of the urinary system can be suboptimal in some larger teenagers or obese children. Scanning of the kidneys is performed mainly with curved array transducers for assessment of kidney length and to examine the status of the kidney parenchyma, pelvicalyceal system, ureters, and bladder. These images can be supplemented with those obtained with a high-resolution linear transducer, which offers superior spatial resolution but is limited in penetration depth. For that reason, high-resolution US is particularly well suited to neonates, infants and younger children. In older children, the distance between the transducer and the kidneys may preclude this type of higher resolution examination.

The kidneys are ovoid organs that typically lie in the retroperitoneal renal fossae, although they can be ectopic. Their lengths can be measured and compared with published nomograms [41–43] (Fig. 3.1). Growth of the kidneys can be followed on serial examinations; however, it is important to keep in mind that kidney lengths can

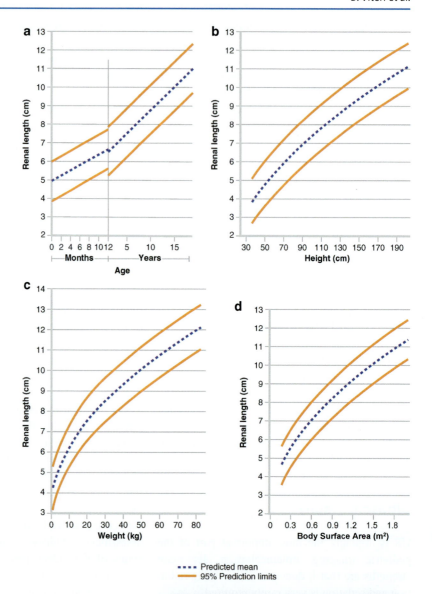

Fig. 3.1 Nomograms for kidney size. Nomograms delineate the predicted mean and 95% prediction limits of kidney length as a function of (**a**) age, (**b**) height, (**c**) weight, and (**d**) total body surface area

occasionally be over- or under-measured depending on the circumstances of the examination. Retardation in kidney growth can be a sign of ongoing insult such as vesicoureteral reflux [44].

Greyscale US

In healthy children there is a difference in echogenicity between normal kidney cortex and the medullary pyramids, with the former more echogenic and the latter more hypoechoic (Fig. 3.2). This difference is termed *corticomedullary differentiation*. The echogenicity of the kidney cortex can be compared to an internal and adjacent

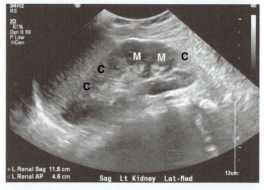

Fig. 3.2 US of normal kidney. Greyscale longitudinal US image of a 12-year-old child showing normal left kidney with relatively more echogenic cortex (C) and hypoechoic medulla (M)

standard—that is, the right kidney is compared to the liver, and the left kidney to the spleen. One must, however, ensure that this reference organ (the liver or spleen) is normal. The pattern of normal kidney echogenicity varies in childhood. In the neonate, the kidney cortex can be isoechoic or even hyperechoic compared to the liver and the renal pyramids are often profoundly hypoechoic, which can make corticomedullary differentiation quite marked [45] (Fig. 3.3a). By the time the child is several months of age the kidney cortex should be hypoechoic compared to the echogenicity of the liver [45, 46]. Any alteration in cortical echogenicity after that age suggests intrinsic kidney disease. The medullary pyramids, particularly in the neonate, can be so hypoechoic that they can be mistaken for a dilated collecting system. There are exceptions to the hypoechogenicity of the renal pyramids, the majority of which relate to disease states such as medullary nephrocalcinosis. The most common exception, however, seen in many neonates may be the transient increase in pyramidal echogenicity, which has been attributed to precipitation of Tamm Horsfall proteins [47]. In addition, there may be lobulation of the kidney outline, especially in neonates. This should not be confused with scarring. The notching of normal lobulation tends to be seen in the portion of the cortex between pyramids (Fig. 3.3b), whereas focal scarring tends to occur in portions of the cortex directly overlying the pyramid.

The degree of kidney collecting system dilation can be assessed both qualitatively and quantitatively. Measurement of pelvic dilation can be assessed at the level of the kidney hilum—or just beyond it in the case of an extrarenal pelvis. Classification of urinary tract dilation (UTD) is discussed in more detail later in this chapter in the section "Applications of Diagnostic and Interventional Radiology Techniques: Neonatal Diseases." A full bladder can exaggerate the degree of dilation. It is therefore prudent to assess the pelvic diameter after voiding if the bladder is overdistended. If the ureter is dilated, its diameter can be assessed along its course, although it can be visualized most reliably proximally and distally (Fig. 3.4). Overlying bowel gas often obscures the midportion of the ureter. The thickness of the wall of the intrarenal collecting system, ureter or bladder can also be assessed. Thickening of the urothelium anywhere along the urinary tract can be associated with, though is not pathognomonic for, infection or inflammation. Urolithiasis can be diagnosed as an echogenic focus with distal acoustic shadowing [48] and/or with twinkle artifact on color Doppler. The degree of obstruction caused by a calculus can also be assessed with US.

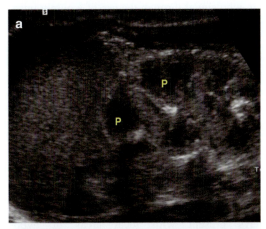

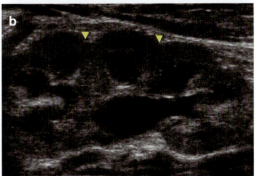

Fig. 3.3 US of normal neonatal kidney. (**a**) Greyscale longitudinal US image of a neonatal kidney showing hypoechoic pyramids (P) and hyperechoic cortex when compared to the liver with prominent corticomedullary differentiation. (**b**) Neonatal kidney showing "lobulations" (arrowheads) between pyramids

Color Doppler

Color Doppler and pulsed Doppler interrogation of the kidneys can be used to assess vascularity of the kidneys. The study can assess the

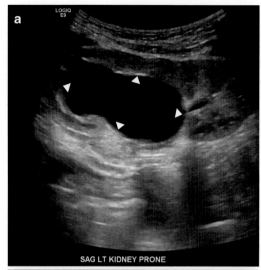

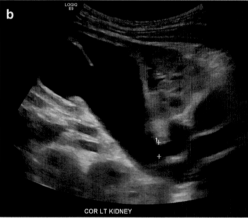

Fig. 3.4 US of urinary tract dilation and ureteral dilation. (**a**) Greyscale longitudinal US image of a 1-year-old child with congenital hydronephrosis of the left kidney showing marked dilatation of the upper pole collecting system (arrowheads) and thinning of the parenchyma with a relatively normal lower pole. The upper pole pelvis and calyces are markedly dilated. (**b**) The ureter is markedly dilated and tortuous with a proximal diameter of 0.53 cm (cross marks)

vessels from the ostia of the main renal arteries and veins through the arcuate vessels in the kidney parenchyma. Indications for Doppler evaluation include suspicion of renal arterial or venous thrombosis [49], arterial stenosis [50], trauma [51], infection [52], acute tubular necrosis, and transplant rejection [53]– though the role in the evaluation of rejection remains controversial [54].

Contrast-Enhanced Ultrasonography

Contrast-enhanced US (CEUS) is an innovative imaging modality that utilizes non-nephrotoxic microbubbles as an IV US contrast agent (UCA). UCAs consist of a gas core with lipid monolayer stabilizing shell no bigger than a red-blood cell. UCAs are currently approved by the United States Food and Drug Administration for IV use in cardiac and hepatic US, and for intravesical use in the evaluation of vesicoureteral reflux (VUR) in children. Despite being "off-label" in the United States, its kidney applications have grown in recent years, including evaluation of kidney trauma, masses and cysts, as well as to guide procedures [55–59]. CEUS is more sensitive in detecting perfusion abnormalities than Doppler (Fig. 3.5), as CEUS enhances the vascular echo signal through the use of a purely intravascular contrast agent, rather than detecting the Doppler shift, which is highly dependent on many technical factors such as speed of acquisition, angle of imaging, depth of imaging, and frequency [60]. CEUS in clinical practice provides dynamic information about an organ, such as microvascular perfusion, potential quantification of blood flow, and perfusion characteristics of masses and cystic lesions [61–63]. For example, inflammatory processes of the kidneys such as acute pyelonephritis and glomerulonephritis will show hyper-enhancement whereas scarred kidneys present with focal areas of hypo-enhancement. In the evaluation of lesions, cysts show no enhancement while solid lesions do. Moreover, malignant lesions usually enhance avidly and "wash out" because of their nearly complete arterial blood supply and abnormal arteriovenous shunts throughout. In kidney transplantation, CEUS has been able to detect early features of acute allograft dysfunction in the setting of acute tubular necrosis, rejection, cortical necrosis and other vascular complications such as local areas of hypoperfusion (Fig. 3.5) [64–66].

CEUS can also provide real-time images for guidance of interventional procedures, such as percutaneous drainage and biopsy, by providing

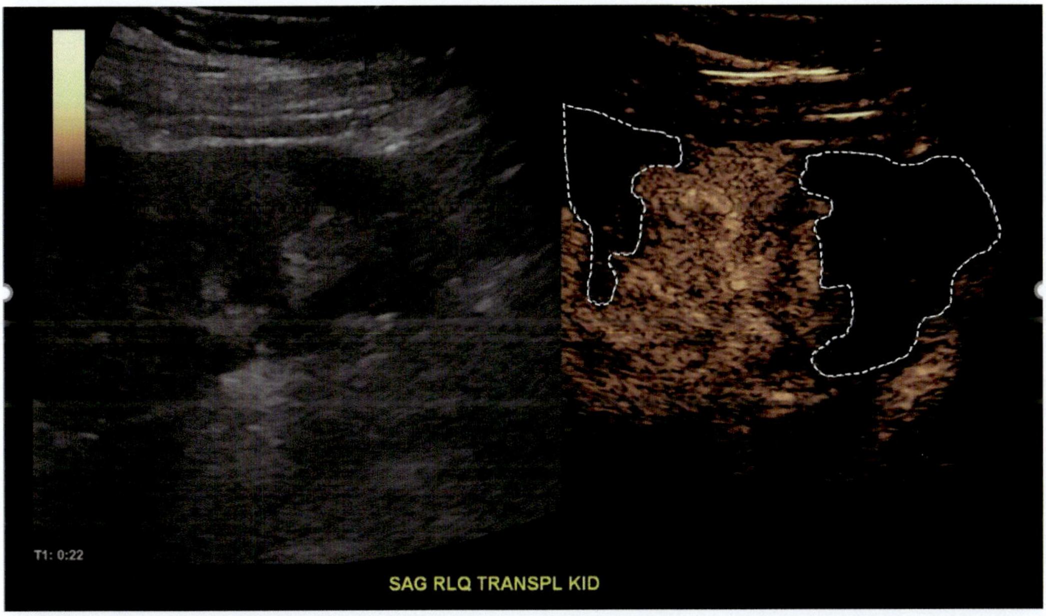

Fig. 3.5 Contrast enhanced US (CEUS) of kidney transplant. CEUS of a transplant kidney in an adolescent recipient showing lack of perfusion in the lower one third of the kidney along with a wedge-shaped perfusion defect in the anterior aspect of the upper-pole (dashed lines), highly suggestive of kidney infarction

evidence of communication between cavities or flow from the placed catheter into the region of interest. It can also be used during percutaneous nephrostomy and thermal ablation of tumors [56]. CEUS can also allow bedside evaluation of organ perfusion and lymphatic leakage without the need for ionizing radiation [67].

Post-acquisition quantification of perfusion or relative enhancement are, to date, a work in progress with no standardization but with promising preliminary results [68, 69]. Additionally, given that most US machines that have the capability to perform CEUS also perform conventional US, one can simultaneously evaluate images with both modalities.

Contrast-Enhanced Voiding Urosonography (ceVUS)

A special application of CEUS is contrast-enhanced voiding urosonography (ceVUS), an US-based alternative to evaluate for VUR or urethral pathology [70, 71]. CeVUS, like fluoroscopic VCUG, evaluates the urinary tract with contrast administration via a bladder catheter, but uses an US scanner for evaluation. Benefits of ceVUS include a more child-friendly imaging environment and lack of ionizing radiation. The detection of microbubbles within a ureter or kidney collecting system indicates VUR, which is graded similarly to VCUG [70, 72, 73]. ceVUS has been shown to be more sensitive in detecting VUR, with a higher grade of reflux in up to two thirds of patients, and as good for the evaluation of the urethra when compared to VCUG (Fig. 3.6) [74, 75]. CeVUS can also be used in the evaluation of posterior urethral valves (PUV) and urethral trauma [72, 76]. Moreover, in therapeutics, intraoperative applicability of ceVUS has improved the success rate of minimally invasive sub-trigonal injection procedure (Deflux®) for resolution of VUR by approximately 20% [77].

US Contrast Safety

US contrast agents have a good safety profile for intravesical use. The most common side effects relate to the urethral catheterization, with no known side effects from the actual US contrast agent [70].

Over two decades of experience with IV US contrast administration in thousands of pediatric

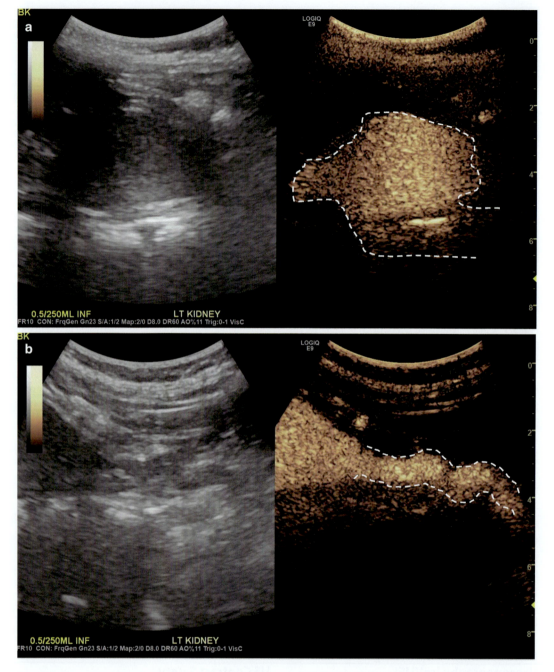

Fig. 3.6 Contrast enhanced voiding US (ceVUS). (**a**) CeVUS of a 4-year-old child shows grade 4 reflux to the left kidney. The renal pelvis and calyces are dilated (dashed lines). (**b**) The left ureter is moderately dilated and tortuous (dashed lines)

3 Imaging and Radiological Interventions in the Pediatric Urinary Tract

patients in Europe, Asia, and most recently in the United States, has shown a good track record of safety. Specifically, in over 1900 reported IV US contrast exams in children, two children had severe allergic reactions that were successfully treated [78–81]. Other reactions reported in children include tachypnea, unusual taste, mild itching and hives, and other minor reactions that did not require treatment [78–83]. Nausea and headache are the most common reactions associated with the administration of the commercially available US contrast agents Lumason® (approved in the United States) [84] and SonoVue (approved in Europe and Asia) [85].

Voiding Cystourethrography

VCUG has traditionally been the study of choice for diagnosing VUR and assessing the anatomy of the bladder and urethra. Indications include UTI [39], antenatally or postnatally diagnosed hydronephrosis, and suspected PUV, among others. At most institutions, sedation is not administered. In our experience, the examination can be performed without sedation in the vast majority of children, given proper explanation and reassurance.

A catheter is placed via the urethra into the bladder using aseptic technique; alternatively, a suprapubic catheter or appendicovesicostomy (Mitrofanoff) can be used if present. The bladder is filled with water soluble contrast under the pressure of gravity until pressure within the bladder induces micturition. The amount of contrast used will vary according to the patient's age and bladder capacity. If a child is unable to void on their own, the bladder can be drained via the catheter in situ. If the child is reticent or unable to void, warm water applied to the perineum can induce voiding. Some children will not void on the fluoroscopy table despite a variety of maneuvers. In these cases, the micturition phase of the study is not possible and the sensitivity of the study to detect reflux is diminished. In some institutions an image is taken after the child has been allowed to void in the toilet. At some institutions a single cycle of filling and voiding is performed. At others, two or three cycles are the routine [86]. This latter method, termed *cyclic VCUG*, has demonstrated greater sensitivity in detecting reflux, but results in a higher radiation dose compared to the single cycle method. In all cases, care is given to minimizing the dose of ionizing radiation [87].

Exact views obtained will vary between institutions, but all will include images of the bladder that will allow for assessment of its wall characteristics and detection of structural abnormalities such as diverticula, ureteroceles or urachal abnormalities. These images should demonstrate whether there is any reflux into the ureters. Images of the urethra will be obtained during voiding, either with the catheter in place or after its removal depending on the practice of the institution and the individual radiologist. At our institution an image of the urethra is obtained with the catheter in place as well as after its removal, thus ensuring an image of the urethra in cases in which the child stops voiding just as the catheter is removed. An image of the renal fossae will assess for any reflux to the level of the kidneys, characterize the collecting system anatomy (duplex or not) and assign a grade to that reflux [88]. The system of the International Reflux Study in Children classifies reflux into five grades. Reflux into the ureter alone is classified as Grade I. When contrast fills the intrarenal collecting system but without dilation, it is classified as Grade II. Grades III–V demonstrate progressive dilation of the ureter, pelvis and calyces [88] (Fig. 3.7).

Complications related to VCUG are similar to those encountered in any catheterization of the bladder, with infection and trauma being the most common. At our institution, we do not administer prophylactic antibiotics unless there is a clinical indication for procedure related prophylaxis. If the examination is positive and the patient is not on long-term antibiotic prophylaxis, a prompt communication of the results to the referring clinician is appropriate. One can also encounter urinary retention post-procedure.

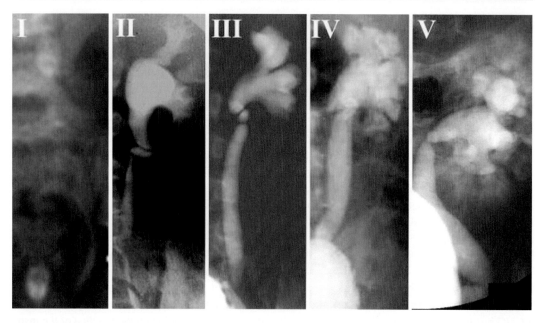

Fig. 3.7 Voiding cystourethrogram (VCUG). International Grading System of vesicoureteral reflux, illustrating VCUG grades I–V

Nuclear Medicine

Nuclear medicine is a modality that comprises a variety of examinations for evaluating the pediatric urinary tract. Nuclear medicine techniques differ from other imaging modalities in that they focus on function rather than detailed anatomic structure. As a result, nuclear imaging plays an important complementary role to other modalities, particularly to the structural evaluation obtained with US.

The physical principles of how scintigraphic images are generated also differ from those of other imaging modalities. Rather than transmitting x-rays through the patient as is done with fluoroscopy, radiography and CT, nuclear medicine introduces a radioactive tracer into the patient's body. An Anger camera is then positioned adjacent to the patient, and images are created by detecting the gamma-rays emitted from the patient's own body. In nuclear urinary tract imaging, depending on the specific examination being performed, the radiopharmaceutical can be injected IV to be extracted by the kidneys, or can be instilled via catheter into the bladder. Radiation doses in nuclear medicine examinations of the urinary tract are lower than those encountered in CT and lower or comparable to those in fluoroscopy.

Most pediatric patients do not require sedation, as they are either cooperative in lying still on the scintigraphy imaging table or are infants small enough to be safely restrained with swaddling. However, if a child is anticipated to have difficulty lying still for at least 30 min, sedation can be considered. Rarely, general anesthesia is necessary to perform a successful examination.

Urinary tract imaging comprises over half of the examinations performed in a typical pediatric nuclear medicine department. The most common clinical indications for performing nuclear kidney imaging examinations include UTI, ante- or post-natally detected hydronephrosis, vesicoureteral reflux, suspected urinary obstruction, and suspected impairment of kidney function.

Overview of Radiopharmaceuticals

Technetium-99m (99mTc) is the radionuclide (i.e. gamma-emitting isotope) that is used to label most radiopharmaceuticals in urinary tract imaging. It emits a 140 keV gamma-ray and has a physical half-life of 6 h.

Technetium-99m pertechnetate is the base form of 99mTc that is obtained from a portable generator unit found in any nuclear medicine radiopharmacy. 99mTc-pertechnetate can be used to radiolabel other pharmaceuticals using commercially available labeling kits. Other radiopharmaceuticals routinely used in nuclear urinary tract imaging are described in Table 3.1.

Table 3.1 Radiopharmaceuticals routinely used in nuclear urinary tract imaging

	Use	Mechanism of action	Imaging analysis
Glomerular filtration agents			
DTPA			
99mTc-diethylenetriaminepentaacetic acid	• Calculate GFR	Measuring the rate of DTPA extraction from plasma by serial blood sampling provides an accurate estimate of GFR. Approximately 90% of DTPA is filtered by the kidneys into the urine within 4 h after IV injection [126].	Kidney imaging can be performed using 99mTc-DTPA, providing additional information on excretion and drainage, as well as the ability to plot dynamic renogram time-activity curves.
EDTA			
51Cr-ethylenediaminetetraacetate	• Calculate GFR (standard GFR agent used in Europe)	Due to better radioisotope binding to the tracer, 51Cr-EDTA produces slightly higher values for GFR than 99mTc-DTPA. However, this difference is small (5% or less) and is not considered to be clinically relevant [284].	Kidney imaging is not performed with 51Cr-EDTA as it does not emit gamma-rays of suitable energy levels for imaging.
Tubular secretion agents			
MAG3			
99mTc-mercaptoacetyltriglycine	• Agent of choice for functional kidney imaging • Split kidney function • Detect obstruction • Evaluate kidney transplant allografts	MAG3 is cleared predominantly (95%) by the kidney tubules [126]. MAG3 clearance is proportional to effective kidney plasma flow.	Better image quality as the extraction fraction of MAG3 is more than twice that of DTPA, resulting in a much higher target-to-background ratio.
Kidney tubular fixation agents (cortical agents)			
DMSA			
99mTc-dimercaptosuccinic acid	• Agent of choice to detect cortical scarring	Binds to sulfhydryl groups of proximal kidney tubules after filtration [126]. Only 10% is excreted into the urine during the first several hours after IV injection.	Produces excellent high-resolution images of the kidney cortex without interference from urinary activity. Is the preferred cortical imaging agent.
GH			
99mTc-glucoheptonate	• Early imaging evaluates kidney perfusion, urinary excretion and drainage • Late imaging at 1–2 h visualizes kidney cortex	Cleared by the kidneys through both tubular secretion and glomerular filtration, with 10–15% remaining bound to the kidney tubules at 1 h after injection.	99mTc-GH has less cortical binding affinity than 99mTc-DMSA.

Direct Radionuclide Cystogram (DRC)

Direct radionuclide cystography (DRC) has good sensitivity to detect VUR, but provides very little anatomic detail for detecting bladder and urethral abnormalities [89, 90]. DRC is performed in a similar manner to VCUG, except the bladder is filled with a 99mTc-based radiopharmaceutical and an Anger camera is used for imaging, often for several cycles of filling and voiding. DRC can be used as a complementary modality to VCUG [89–91]. Typically, VCUG is the primary modality to evaluate for VUR in patients with febrile UTI or hydronephrosis [92]. Subsequently, DRC may be used as a follow-up examination to determine if VUR has resolved or is persistent, including post-operative evaluation after ureteral reimplantation surgery or minimally invasive sub-trigonal injection procedure (Deflux®). DRC can also be performed as a primary screening examination to detect reflux in asymptomatic patients with a small kidney or solitary kidney, or who have a family history of VUR (first degree relative, i.e. parent or sibling).

Indirect Radionuclide Cystogram

An alternative test for the detection of VUR reflux is the indirect radionuclide cystogram (IRC) [93–102]. This examination should be reserved for children >3 years of age [103] in whom bladder catheterization is impossible. IRC is performed by injecting 99mTc-mercaptuacetyltriglycine (MAG3) IV, then acquiring continuous dynamic images of the kidney and bladder during bladder filling and voiding. The patient must be able to remain still during imaging and to void on command after bladder filling. Regions of interest are drawn over the intrarenal collecting systems and the ureters, and time-activity curves are plotted. A sudden increase in activity in the renal pelvis and ureter indicates the presence of VUR.

Direct vs. Indirect Radionuclide Cystogram

There is ongoing debate regarding whether direct vs. indirect radionuclide cystography is preferable for detecting VUR. In theory, IRC is a better mimic of physiologic slow antegrade bladder filling, whereas DRC involves rapid retrograde bladder filling via a catheter, which some believe induces artificial reflux. Others assert that this higher sensitivity of DRC (up to 95%) [104] is an advantage, and may be a better comparator to prior VCUG results due to the same method of bladder filling. Patients with abnormal kidney function may have insufficient excretion of radiotracer during IRC, resulting in lower sensitivity ranging between 32% and 81% [94, 97, 104–106]. In practice, there is a high rate of failure of IRC due to the inability of children to remain still while voiding or the inability to void at all during image acquisition [107]. In the case of a negative IRC examination, a subsequent DRC or VCUG may be needed to confidently exclude vesicoureteral reflux [103].

Kidney Cortical Scan

Cortical scintigraphy with 99mTc-dimercaptosuccinic acid (DMSA) is a highly sensitive examination for the detection of both acute lesions (i.e. pyelonephritis) and late sequelae (i.e. permanent parenchymal scarring) in children with UTI. Acute lesions of pyelonephritis can take up to 6 months to resolve scintigraphically. Therefore, permanent scarring can only be reported when the DMSA scan is performed at least 6 months after the acute infection. If less than 6 months have elapsed since the acute infection, any cortical defects should be interpreted as either resolving pyelonephritis or potential scar. Therefore, kidney cortical scintigraphy should only be performed within 6 months of an acute infection if there is an acute need to document kidney involvement. Otherwise, a repeat scan will likely be needed later to exclude

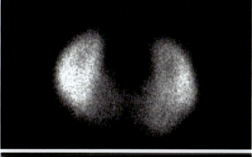

RELATIVE UPTAKE		
	Left	Right
Upper [%]		
Lower [%]		
% Diff/Total Vol	92	8
Counts/Total Vol	34212	2834
Counts/Unit Vol	22.8	2.8
% Diff/Unit Vol	89	11

Fig. 3.8 DMSA scan. DMSA scan in a 33-month-old boy with a history of posterior urethral valves and pyelonephritis showed small right kidney with significantly decreased uptake and irregular contour consistent with scarred right kidney and decreased activity in the lower pole of the left kidney suggestive of possible pyelonephritis vs. scar in the left lower pole

permanent scarring [39, 103, 108–110]. When requesting a DMSA scan, it is helpful for the referring physician to note the date of the most recent UTI.

Kidney scarring tends to occur at the upper and lower poles due to the round-shaped orifices of the compound papillae at these locations. The simple papillae at the mid-poles have slit-like orifices that are less prone to reflux of infected urine. Kidney cortical defects are reported as unilateral or bilateral, single or multiple, small or large, with or without loss of parenchymal volume. Permanent scarring tends to cause loss of parenchymal volume (Fig. 3.8), whereas acute infection does not. If present, a dilated renal pelvis can also be visualized. DMSA cortical scintigraphy is more sensitive than IV pyelography and US for the detection of both acute lesions and permanent scarring [52, 109, 111, 112].

Other causes of cortical defects on DMSA scan include kidney cysts and masses. Normal

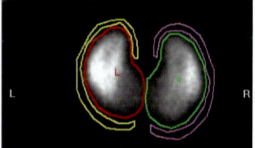

RELATIVE UPTAKE		
	Left	Right
Upper [%]		
Lower [%]		
% Diff/Total Vol	55	45
Counts/Total Vol	108964	89807
Counts/Unit Vol	30.6	24.0
% Diff/Unit Vol	56	44

Fig. 3.9 DMSA scan. DMSA scan in a patient with horseshoe kidney showing normal cortical activity in upper portions of both kidneys with relatively less activity in the lower portions and the isthmus. Differential function was 55% for the left moiety and 45% for the right

variations in appearance of the kidney cortex can include indentation by the adjacent spleen, fetal lobulation, columns of Bertin, duplex kidney, and malrotated kidney. Kidney cortical scans are often useful in confirming the diagnoses of horseshoe kidney, ectopic kidney, or cross-fused renal ectopia when US is equivocal (Fig. 3.9).

Images are acquired 2–3 h after injection of 99mTc-DMSA. Planar images are acquired in the posterior, and right and left posterior oblique positions. In infants, additional pinhole images may be acquired that offer higher spatial resolution. In older, sufficiently cooperative children, additional single photon emission computed tomography (SPECT) images may be acquired to improve spatial resolution [113–117]. SPECT iterative reconstruction algorithms can further improve spatial resolution, or maintain spatial resolution with a lower administered dose of radiopharmaceutical [118]. However, the clinical significance of any additional small cortical defects detected by these higher-resolution methods is unclear [119–125].

Functional Kidney Imaging and Renography

Functional kidney imaging uses dynamic image acquisition to evaluate kidney perfusion, uptake, excretion, and drainage of radiotracer by the urinary system. Renography refers to the process of plotting the radiotracer activity in the urinary system as a function of time, resulting in renogram (time-activity) curves. A large amount of information can be acquired with functional kidney imaging. For example, abnormal perfusion can suggest arterial stenosis or occlusion; delayed uptake and excretion of radiotracer suggest parenchymal disease; and poor drainage of radiotracer into the bladder can suggest obstructive uropathy or over-compliance of the collecting system. Functional kidney imaging can be custom-tailored for specific clinical problems. For example, a diuretic challenge can be administered to more sensitively evaluate for urinary obstruction (see below).

Although 99mTc-DTPA is widely used for functional kidney imaging, 99mTc-MAG3 is preferred due to its higher extraction fraction and better target-to-background ratio. This advantage is particularly important in patients with impaired kidney function or urinary obstruction, and in very young patients with immature kidney function.

Immediately after the injection of radiotracer, imaging of kidney perfusion can be performed. The patient lies supine with the camera positioned posteriorly. Radiotracer activity should reach the kidneys about 1 s after the tracer bolus in the abdominal aorta passes the renal arteries;

there should be symmetric perfusion of the kidneys [126]. Over the next 20–30 min, imaging of kidney function is performed. Maximal parenchymal activity is seen normally at 3–5 min after injection (T_{max}) [126]. Urinary activity in the renal pelvis is typically seen by 2–4 min after injection (calyceal transit time); however, there is no widespread consensus on what constitutes a normal calyceal transit time [127]. There should be prompt drainage of tracer into the bladder, with less than half of the activity at T_{max} remaining in the renal pelvis by 8–12 min after injection ($T_{1/2}$) [126].

Renogram curves are generated by plotting the activity within regions of interest drawn around each kidney. The renogram is a graphic representation of the uptake, excretion, and drainage phases of renal function, and the curves for each kidney should be reasonably symmetric. Patients should be well-hydrated, preferably with IV fluids, when functional kidney imaging is performed, as dehydration will result in an abnormal renogram with globally delayed function and slow drainage.

Diuretic Renogram

In the setting of urinary collecting system dilation not due to VUR, the possibility of urinary tract obstruction must be considered. Diuretic renography performed with furosemide is useful in determining the presence of a high-grade obstruction at the ureteropelvic junction (UPJ) or the ureterovesical junction (UVJ). Diuretic renography is commonly used to evaluate the results of surgery in patients who have undergone pyeloplasty for ureteropelvic junction obstruction.

Diuretic renography is performed as described above for dynamic kidney imaging, with the additional step of administering IV hydration and furosemide to cause maximal urine flow through the collecting system. The dose of furosemide is usually 1 mg/kg, with a maximum dose of 40 mg [128]. The timing of the furosemide administration varies among institutions, as several diuretic protocols have been described, validated, and debated in the literature [103, 129, 130]. The most commonly used protocols are: "F+20" (furosemide is given 20 min after radiotracer if normal spontaneous drainage has not occurred [131]; this protocol is endorsed by the American Society of Fetal Urology); "F−15" (furosemide is injected first, followed 15 min later by radiotracer; this protocol is the widely-used European standard) [128]; and "F0" (radiotracer and furosemide are injected immediately following one another) [132, 133]. Dynamic images are acquired from the time of radiotracer injection for approximately 20 min. In the case of the F+20 protocol, an additional 20 min of imaging is performed after injection of furosemide.

Bladder catheterization is not always necessary but should be performed in patients who are not toilet-trained, or who have known hydroureter, VUR, bladder dysfunction, or PUV. In this subset of patients, back pressure from urine in the bladder may cause a false-positive result.

In the absence of urinary obstruction, there is rapid drainage of radiotracer from the renal pelvis into the bladder to a minimal residual by 20 min. In quantitative terms, a drainage half-time, $T_{1/2}$, of less than 10 min usually means the absence of obstruction.

In an obstructed system, the drainage of radiotracer from the collecting system will be slow. In this case, a $T_{1/2}$ of greater than 20 min indicates obstruction (Fig. 3.10). When $T_{1/2}$ ranges between 10 and 20 min, this is usually considered an equivocal result, and a follow-up examination will typically be performed to see if the drainage remains unchanged, normalizes, or becomes frankly obstructed.

When UPJ obstruction is suspected, the above drainage parameters are used when analyzing a region of interest drawn around the renal pelvis. These values can also be applied to the ureter and to a region of interest combining the ureter and renal pelvis when UVJ obstruction is suspected.

If a large amount of radiotracer remains in the renal pelvis and/or ureter at the end of dynamic imaging, the patient can be positioned upright to void if possible. A final static image can then be acquired to see if the postural/gravitational effect caused additional drainage [103].

Pitfalls are common in the interpretation of diuretic renography. Poor kidney function from prolonged, severe obstruction can result in poor accumulation of radiotracer in the collecting system, making the renogram difficult or impossible to interpret. A very dilated, overly-compliant, but non-obstructed collecting system may have a prolonged $T_{1/2}$ because the capacious collecting system easily accommodates a large urine volume [128, 130]. This "reservoir effect" can be observed in the setting of primary megaureter, and in patients who have undergone successful pyeloplasty for UPJ obstruction.

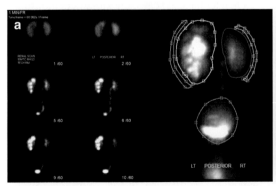
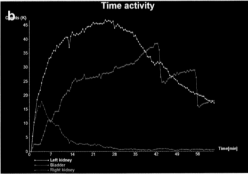
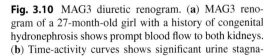

Fig. 3.10 MAG3 diuretic renogram. (**a**) MAG3 renogram of a 27-month-old girl with a history of congenital hydronephrosis shows prompt blood flow to both kidneys. (**b**) Time-activity curves shows significant urine stagnation on the left side at 25 min (white curve), which responds poorly to furosemide administration with a prolonged half-clearance time. Normal clearance of radiotracer of right kidney (blue curve)

Computed Tomography

CT is often the imaging modality of choice for evaluation of blunt or penetrating genitourinary trauma and may be used in the evaluation of stone disease or neoplasm. The indication for imaging determines the CT protocol and the need for the administration of IV contrast.

In the evaluation of trauma, IV contrast should be administered unless there is a contraindication. Obtaining a CT in the arterial phase, when contrast opacifies the arterial structures, can evaluate for arterial injury such as dissection or pseudoaneurysm, as well as active arterial hemorrhage. A delayed phase CT, obtained approximately 10 min after contrast administration when the contrast has been excreted into the collecting system, can be obtained if there is a suspicion for a collecting system injury, and will show extravasation from the collecting system when injured. A dedicated cystogram, or retrograde filling of the urinary bladder with contrast after placement of a catheter, can be performed if there is concern for bladder injury, as routine CT of the abdomen and pelvis is not sensitive for the detection of bladder injury [134].

Multiphasic CT evaluation with a single contrast bolus may offer increased clinical certainty to detect vascular extravasation (Fig. 3.11), devascularization and urinary leak, but results in increased radiation dose because multiple CT scans must be obtained at different time points corresponding with the structures that are opacified by the contrast [135, 136]. Double and triple split bolus techniques can opacify multiple structures during a single CT acquisition, reducing radiation dose [137–139].

Although rarely the initial imaging modality in the work-up of urinary tract disease, CT contributes significantly to the imaging of children with suspected urinary tract disorders. Indications include neoplasia [140], trauma [141, 142], severe infections [143] and occasionally complex questions regarding anatomy [144] (although MRI often would be the preferred modality). Though US is the mainstay of imaging urolithiasis in children, CT can be useful in cases that on US are equivocal or non-diagnostic.

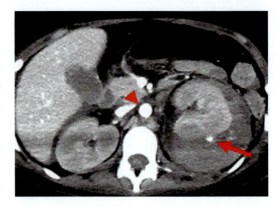

Fig. 3.11 Contrast enhanced CT of vascular extravasation. Arterial extravasation from the kidney on CT in a 14-year-old female following kidney biopsy. Contrast-enhanced axial CT image obtained in the arterial phase demonstrates opacification of the aorta (arrowhead) and remainder of the arterial system. There is arterial enhancement external to the left kidney (arrow) within a large perinephric hematoma, consistent with active arterial extravasation

CT allows for cross sectional imaging of the urinary tract and has the ability to reconstruct images in any plane for analysis. CT also provides excellent resolution of the urinary tract structures. The addition of IV contrast to the CT imaging allows for even greater accuracy in the detection of disease. Newer generations of CT technology provide higher spatial and temporal resolution and importantly can be done in many instances without sedation or general anesthesia, which may be required for MRI.

On unenhanced scans, the kidneys demonstrate similar attenuation to the normal liver or spleen. They are surrounded by a variable amount of retroperitoneal fat depending on the age and health status of the child. Administration of contrast results in a reliable pattern of enhancement beginning in the renal cortex, followed by enhancement of the renal pyramids, and later by opacification of the pelvicalyceal system, ureters and bladder.

The ability of CT to differentiate between tissues of various densities allows for the detection of hydronephrosis, calcifications (Fig. 3.12) and diseases extending into the perinephric fat even without the administration of IV contrast. With the addition of IV contrast, however, one can detect individual lesions of the kidney paren-

3 Imaging and Radiological Interventions in the Pediatric Urinary Tract

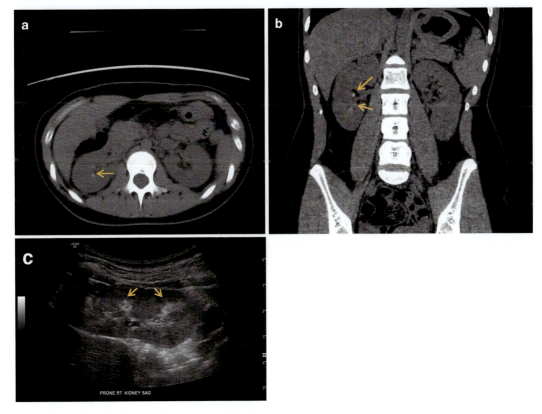

Fig. 3.12 Nephrocalcinosis. (**a**) Axial and (**b**) coronal planes of non-contrast CT of 17-year-old child showing variable hyperattenuation in multiple medullary papilla (arrows), which gradually decreases in density more proximally along the expected course of the medullary tubules. (**c**) Greyscale US shows diffuse increased echogenicity of the medullary pyramids. This is most suggestive of medullary calcifications (nephrocalcinosis)

chyma, such as cysts, tumors or nephroblastomatosis; focal areas of diminished enhancement, such as foci of pyelonephritis (Fig. 3.13) or contusion/laceration (Fig. 3.14); and global abnormalities of enhancement, such as is evident in renal artery stenosis (RAS) or thrombosis.

When ordering a CT examination, potential risks, including radiation exposure and possible contrast-induced nephropathy, must be considered and balanced with potential benefits such as avoidance of sedation or anesthesia.

Magnetic Resonance Imaging

MRI, like US, is uniquely suited to the imaging of children due to avoidance of ionizing radiation. Although radiofrequency energy is

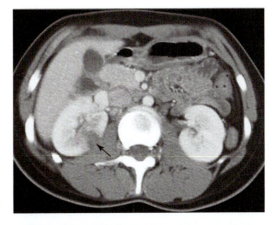

Fig. 3.13 Contrast enhanced CT for pyelonephritis. Contrast-enhanced CT at the level of the kidneys demonstrates an area in the posteromedial aspect of the right kidney with diminished enhancement (arrow), consistent with the clinical suspicion of pyelonephritis

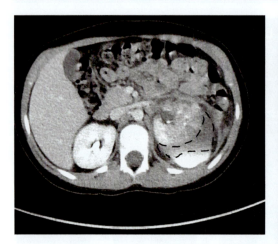

Fig. 3.14 Contrast enhanced CT of kidney laceration. Contrast-enhanced CT at the level of the kidneys demonstrates an area of diminished enhancement in the inferior aspect of the left kidney (dashed line), consistent with a laceration bisecting the lower pole of the kidney

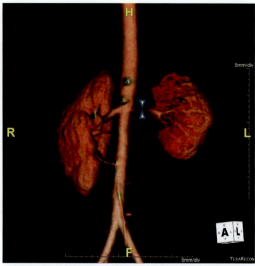

Fig. 3.15 MR angiography (MRA) of renal artery stenosis. MRA in a patient with hypertension showing stenosis in the left main renal artery (arrow heads)

imparted, MRI has not been shown to have the deleterious potential of CT. For that reason, MRI is often preferred over CT for children. However, longer scan times with MRI may necessitate sedation or general anesthesia in patients who are not able to lie still, such as children younger than 6 years and in those with development delay or claustrophobia [145]. In addition, access to an MR scanner remains limited in some regions of the world.

The superior tissue characterization of MRI makes it a powerful tool in assessing diseases of the urinary tract. Administration of gadolinium-based IV contrast can provide improved visualization but may be associated with risks such as NSF as discussed previously. For patients in whom gadolinium contrast is contraindicated, MRI without contrast can still provide detailed structural imaging of the urinary system.

MRI is particularly well suited in assessing neoplasms and tumor-like conditions of the kidneys [146, 147] including nephroblastomatosis [147]. MRI can help to characterize lesions, for example by demonstrating necrosis and hemorrhage in lesions such as Wilms tumor or renal cell carcinoma, or areas of fat in angiomyolipomas [148, 149]. Calcifications, however, are not as reliably seen with MRI as with CT.

As in adults, MRI can be used to assess the renal arteries and veins in children. Bland (non-tumor) thrombosis can readily be demonstrated, as can tumor extension into the vessels [150, 151]. MR angiography (MRA) can be used to assess for RAS in patients with hypertension [152–155] (Fig. 3.15). However, MRA may not be sensitive enough to definitively exclude RAS even in adults [156], and is additionally challenging in children due to their smaller vasculature. MRI can also be used in the assessment of infection [157–159] and trauma [160, 161]. Research is ongoing in adults and children into the application of additional advanced MR sequences in the kidney, such as diffusion-weighted MRI, diffusion tensor imaging, arterial spin labeling, and MR elastography [162–165].

Magnetic Resonance Urography

Magnetic resonance urography (MRU) is an advanced imaging technique that provides detailed anatomic information without ionizing radiation. The optimal visualization of the collecting system on MRU allows differentiation of complex genitourinary anatomy and evaluation

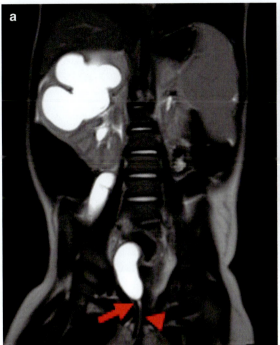 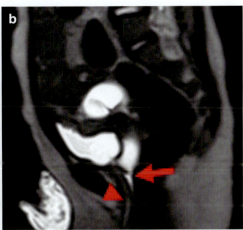

Fig. 3.16 MR urography (MRU) of ectopic ureter. Ectopic ureteral insertion on MRU in a 2-year-old with urinary tract infections. (**a**) Coronal and (**b**) sagittal T2-weighted images demonstrate a right-sided duplicated collecting system, with a markedly dilated upper pole system ectopically inserting into the urethra (arrows). A Foley catheter is in place (arrowheads), which demarcates the position of the urethra

of the course and insertion of the ureters (Fig. 3.16). This anatomic detail is provided by heavily T2-weighted, high spatial resolution two-dimensional and three-dimensional images [166]. With optimization of the imaging protocol, scan times with MRU can be reduced to 30 min [167].

Multiple technical factors of MRU must be considered and planned. Patients receive IV hydration and furosemide prior to imaging to distend the urinary tract and improve visualization [166]. A Foley catheter is often placed, allowing patients to tolerate the examination without the discomfort of needing to void. If evaluation of the bladder is necessary, the Foley catheter can be clamped during the examination to distend the bladder and allow better assessment. Patient positioning is also an important consideration, as patients with a dilated collecting system may need to be placed in a prone position to facilitate drainage of the system [167].

Functional information including differential kidney function, cortical transit time, calyceal transit time, and renal transit time can also be discerned with functional MRU (fMRU). Functional information coupled with delineation of anatomy is invaluable for treatment decisions and surgical planning [166]. If fMRU is desired, patients cannot have a contraindication to gadolinium contrast, as contrast enhancement and excretion provides the functional assessment.

MRU may require sedation in children younger than 6–10 years of age [166]. In infants, MRU without sedation is feasible using the "feed and wrap" technique [36]. In unsedated patients, motion robust sequences including radial volumetric interpolated breath-hold examination (VIBE) and periodically rotated overlapping parallel lines with enhanced reconstruction (PROPELLER) can be used. Respiratory or navigator gating can also be used to further improve image quality.

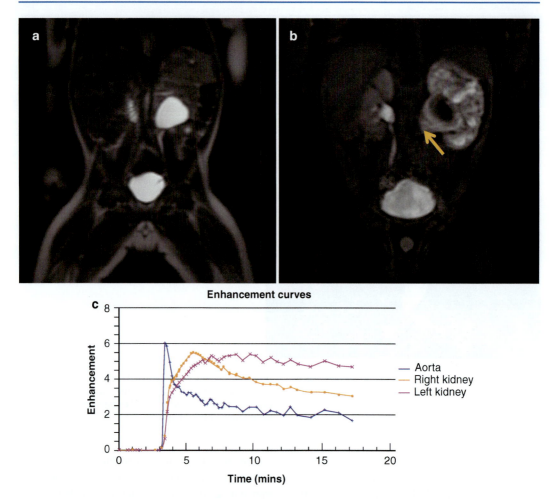

Fig. 3.17 Functional MR urography (fMRU). An 8-month-old boy with left ureteropelvic junction (UPJ) obstruction. (**a**) Coronal T2-weighted and (**b**) post-contrast VIBE images show left hydronephrosis with transition at the level of left UPJ (arrow). (**c**) Signal intensity versus time curves demonstrate asymmetric perfusion and excretion of contrast agent. The curve of the right kidney (blue line) is normal, and the left kidney (green line) reveals a dense delayed nephrogram and delayed excretion

MRU can be used to distinguish a capacious non-obstructed system from a UPJ obstruction. A UPJ obstruction should demonstrate delayed renal transit time correlating with the obstructed system (Fig. 3.17). MRU can confirm that the level of the obstruction is at the UPJ rather than at the level of the ureter, as seen with ureteral strictures. Additionally, arterial and venous phase postcontrast images can evaluate for crossing vessels as the etiology of the UPJ obstruction [166], a necessary step in surgical planning. MRU can also be used for postoperative reevaluation for UPJ obstruction following pyeloplasty or vessel reimplantation [168].

Radiography

Radiography is the oldest modality used in the evaluation of urinary tract disease, but its utility is limited. The normal urinary tract is not sufficiently different in tissue density compared to the surrounding abdominal and pelvic structures to be properly evaluated using radiography alone. There may, however, be cases in which there is sufficient retroperitoneal fat to outline the kidneys on plain radiographs and even assess their relative sizes. A kidney mass or severely hydronephrotic kidney might be detected by the presence of a soft tissue mass, calcification or fat, and

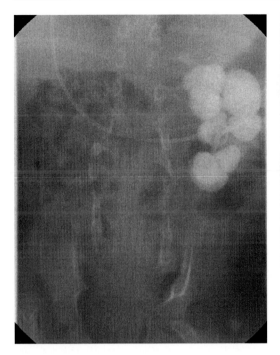

Fig. 3.18 Radiograph of staghorn calculus. Abdomen posteroanterior radiograph showing a radio-opaque staghorn calculus occupying the pelvis and collecting system of the left kidney

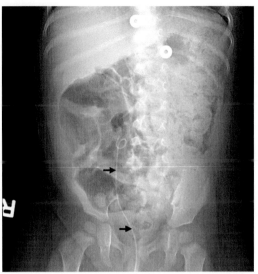

Fig. 3.19 Radiograph of ureteral stent. Abdomen posteroanterior radiograph showing right ureteral stent (arrows), which appears radiopaque

displacement of adjacent structures. A full bladder can also be seen as a midline structure in the pelvis, which will occasionally displace bowel loops out of the pelvis.

Calculi in the urinary collecting system can at times be seen on radiography depending on their composition [169–171] (Fig. 3.18). Nephrocalcinosis may also be detected depending on the degree of involvement [172]. Radiography is the mainstay of imaging for bone changes associated with advanced CKD, such as renal osteodystrophy [173].

Radiographs can also be beneficial in determining the correct positioning of various drainage catheters and stents. Most catheters and stents are sufficiently radio-opaque to be visible on radiographs (Fig. 3.19).

Overall, however, the role of radiography has largely been supplanted by the cross-sectional imaging modalities (US, CT and MRI) and by nuclear medicine.

Excretory Urography

Excretory urography (IV pyelography) relies on the administration of IV contrast to enhance the urinary tract relative to the remainder of the abdominal tissues [174–177]. Excretory urography was historically used to delineate and characterize the anatomy of the urinary tract, but has now largely been supplanted by other imaging modalities such as US, CT, MRI and nuclear medicine [178–181]. Current applications for excretory urography can include evaluation for ectopic ureters and diagnosis of urothelial disorders and papillary necrosis [182–184].

Retrograde Urethrography

Though retrograde urethrography is rarely performed, it remains useful in the evaluation of suspected acute trauma or stricture to the male urethra, [185] and both congenital and acquired urethral abnormalities [186–188] (Fig. 3.20). The examination involves placement of a balloon tipped catheter into the distal urethra and careful

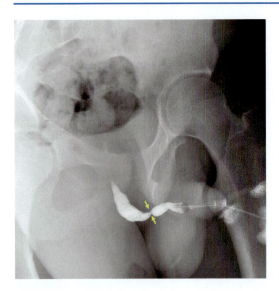

Fig. 3.20 Retrograde urethrogram. Retrograde urethrogram showing bulbar urethral stricture (arrows)

inflation of a balloon in the fossa navicularis. Images of the urethra are taken in an oblique projection during a hand injection of water-soluble contrast. Due to the presence of the external sphincter, the posterior urethra is usually not optimally assessed as part of this study but rather can be imaged during voiding after filling the bladder directly.

Interventional Radiology

Minimally invasive image-guided techniques are increasingly available and integrated into the diagnosis and treatment of pediatric kidney disease. Imaging innovations such as improved US imaging resolution and low radiation dose fluoroscopy and angiography allow for detailed evaluation and guidance in even the smallest patients. The development of pediatric interventional radiology (IR) as a subspecialty has resulted in innovative techniques specifically designed for application in children. Finally, innovative design has resulted in a greater selection of pediatric specific or applicable devices, allowing for application of adult techniques that were previously unavailable in children because of the technical limitations of devices designed for larger patients.

Patient Evaluation and Preparation

Pediatric patients frequently require deep procedural sedation or general anesthesia for minimally invasive image guided procedures, creating greater complexity for the performing proceduralist and health care system. Therefore, many pediatric institutions have adopted care teams with an additional care provider (critical care physician, nurse anesthetist, anesthesiologist) to monitor and manage the patient's sedation/anesthesia during genitourinary interventions, allowing the interventional radiologist to focus solely on the procedural goals. Patients must be screened for anesthetic risks and triaged appropriately to a team that can manage acute sedation or airway complications.

Procedure-specific evaluation includes review of the relevant presentation, medical history, goals of therapy, and allergies. Complete pediatric-specific guidelines for pre-procedure labs and anticoagulation protocols are not currently available from the Society of Pediatric Interventional Radiology, but pediatric literature increasingly incorporates guidelines published by the Society of Interventional Radiology (SIR). Pediatric interventional radiologists may use the SIR adult recommendations for procedural preparation or can develop institution-specific guidelines and protocols [189, 190]. Because of the robust blood supply of the kidneys, most interventions are considered at high risk for bleeding, and therefore anticipation of bleeding and/or the need for transfusion should be considered [189].

Facilities and Equipment

Proper equipment management and sterile technique are critical to reduce infectious complications. The portability of US, which has robust applications and favorable anatomic detail in the pediatric population, allows for the potential of bedside procedures. However, this increased portability should be used deliberately, as the IR suite frequently offers easier access and space to perform patient resuscitation in emergencies and adjunctive imaging modalities that can prevent complications and shorten procedures.

Types of Interventions

Pediatric renal interventions are often divided into two large subsets, vascular and non-vascular, and will be described in more detail in the next section, "Applications of Diagnostic and Interventional Radiology Techniques" Vascular interventions involve trans-arterial access to the renal arteries via the umbilical, femoral, brachial or radial artery. This technique can be utilized to treat renovascular hypertension, kidney hemorrhage in the setting of trauma, and benign kidney tumors using angioplasty, stenting or embolization. Non-vascular interventions frequently involve direct access to the collecting system of the kidney, ureter or bladder to address infection or obstruction. US guidance has become the standard of care for kidney biopsy and will be discussed specifically in a later chapter [191].

Applications of Diagnostic and Interventional Radiology Techniques

Neonatal Diseases

The increase in antenatal imaging (US and to a much lesser degree MRI) and prenatal detection of urinary tract abnormalities has resulted in a commensurate increase in postnatal imaging in the work-up of antenatal findings. The most common indications for postnatal imaging are follow-up of antenatally diagnosed UTD and renal ectopia, agenesis or dysplasia. US is the most common initial study to determine whether two kidneys are present, their location and the status of the parenchyma and collecting system. An increase in parenchymal echogenicity, loss of corticomedullary differentiation, parenchymal loss or scarring, and cyst formation can be signs of underlying kidney disease.

In many institutions, the initial postnatal US will be done after the first 48 h of life to avoid missing hydronephrosis during the relative dehydrated state of the newborn period and the non-distended state of the collecting system. The UTD classification system, described in further detail below, is used to quantify the degree of dilation. The region of dilatation helps to localize a urinary tract obstruction. Dilatation of only the pelvicalyceal system suggests UPJ obstruction [192] (Fig. 3.21); if the ureter is also dilated, UVJ obstruction may be present [193]; if the bladder is distended and perhaps trabeculated, the obstruction may involve the bladder outlet or urethra (Fig. 3.22) [194]. Any degree of pelvicalyceal and/or ureteral dilatation can also be due to VUR.

The work-up of a dilated collecting system may vary among institutions, but in general focuses on screening for VUR, obstruction, and other congenital anomalies of the kidneys and urinary tract (CAKUT). VCUG can be used to assess for VUR or urethral obstruction due to PUV or stenosis. If VCUG does not reveal VUR or PUV, nuclear medicine diuretic renography can assess for any degree and level of urinary obstruction.

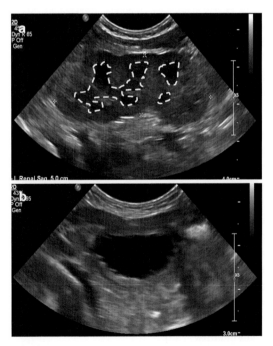

Fig. 3.21 US of urinary tract dilation (UTD) due to ureteropelvic junction (UPJ) obstruction. UTD due to UPJ obstruction in a 2-month-old male. (**a**) Longitudinal greyscale US image of the left kidney demonstrates central and peripheral calyceal dilation (dashed line). There was no abnormality of the kidney parenchyma or (**b**) the bladder

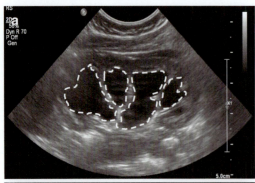
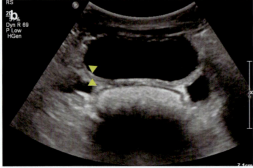

Fig. 3.22 US of urinary tract dilation (UTD) due to bladder outlet obstruction. UTD due to bladder outlet obstruction in a 2-month-old male. (**a**) Longitudinal greyscale US image of the left kidney demonstrates marked central and peripheral calyceal dilation (dashed line) with minimal renal parenchyma. (**b**) The urinary bladder is markedly distended with thickened bladder wall (arrow heads)

Urinary Tract Dilation Classification System

The UTD classification system is a multidisciplinary consensus intended to standardize the terminology used to describe and quantify the degree of pre- and postnatal UTD and to propose a management scheme based on risk stratification. The UTD classification system is based on the US findings of anterior-posterior renal pelvic diameter (APRPD), calyceal dilation, kidney parenchymal thickness, kidney parenchymal appearance, bladder abnormalities, and ureteral abnormalities [195].

Prenatally detected UTD is stratified into low risk (UTD A1) or increased risk (UTD A2–3) based on gestational age and US findings. Low risk patients have an APRPD of 4 to <7 mm at 16–27 weeks gestation and 7 to ≤10 mm at ≥28 weeks gestation, with central or no calyceal dilation. An increased APRPD of ≥7 mm at 16–27 weeks gestation or ≥10 mm at 28 weeks gestation is classified as increased risk. Additional findings such as peripheral calyceal dilation, parenchymal thinning, abnormalities of the parenchymal appearance, bladder abnormalities, ureteral abnormalities, and unexplained oligohydramnios classify patients as increased risk, with the classification based on the most concerning finding present.

As previously mentioned, initial postnatal US is typically performed greater than 48 h after birth to avoid underestimation of UTD due to dehydration. Patients that may require evaluation prior to 48 h after birth include those with oligohydramnios, urethral obstruction, bilateral high-grade dilation, or if there are concerns about patient compliance with postnatal evaluation. Low risk (UTD P1) patients have an APRPD of 10 to <15 mm and central calyceal dilation. APRPD of ≥15 mm, peripheral calyceal dilation, or ureteral abnormalities increase patient risk to the intermediate (UTD P2) category, whereas abnormal kidney parenchymal appearance or thickness and bladder abnormalities increase patient risk to the high (UTD P3) category.

The UTD classification system has been associated with clinical outcomes, with higher risk scores being associated with genitourinary diagnoses and need for surgical intervention [196].

Other Congenital Abnormalities of the Kidneys and Urinary Tract

Many other types of CAKUT can be diagnosed with antenatal or neonatal imaging. Multicystic dysplastic kidney (MCDK) is characterized by multiple non-communicating cysts with no identifiable normal kidney parenchyma [197, 198]. It is thought to arise either due to prenatal renal pelvic ureteral atresia or abnormal interaction between the ureteric bud and metanephric blastema [198]. Demonstration of the lack of communication between the cysts differentiates this process from pelvicalyceal dilation. Imaging can also demonstrate agenesis, ectopia, and horseshoe or cross-fused kidneys. Again, US is the preferred initial imaging modality, although in some cases the findings are discovered incidentally on other modalities (including DMSA renal cortical scintigraphy).

The presence of a duplicated collecting system can be inferred on US when the renal sinus echo complex is interrupted by a band of renal cortical tissue, though it can be difficult to distinguish this pattern from a prominent column of Bertin [199]. The presence of a duplex collecting system may be associated with obstruction (usually of the upper moiety) and/or reflux (usually of the lower moiety) according to the Weiger-Meyer rule [200]. This rule states that in a duplicated collecting system, the upper moiety is drained by a ureter, which inserts ectopically and the lower moiety is drained by a ureter that inserts orthotopically, with the former often obstructed by a ureterocele and the latter demonstrating VUR. These entities (obstruction and VUR) can coexist in the same patient.

Ureteroceles can be found using almost any modality but are most commonly diagnosed on US or VCUG [201]. Ureteroceles can occur with ectopic ureters or at the normal ureterovesical junction (termed orthotopic or simple ureteroceles), and like ectopic ureteroceles can be obstructive or non-obstructive [202].

Neonatal Renovascular Conditions

Conditions affecting the renal vasculature in the neonate, including thrombosis of the renal arteries or veins, can be assessed with Doppler US imaging of the vessels and kidneys. Associated thrombosis of the aorta and inferior vena cava (IVC) can also be assessed. If a central catheter is present, which can predispose a patient to thrombosis, its position can best be assessed with abdominal radiographs, although the catheters can also be seen with US. If a thrombus has occurred, recanalization can be assessed sonographically after anticoagulation or thrombolysis. Occasionally, residual thrombus can calcify and be visible as a linear hyperechoic structure, either along the vessel wall in major vessels or within the renal parenchyma in small vessels. Follow-up kidney US can also assess for any long-term sequelae of thrombosis, such as atrophy, abnormal parenchymal echogenicity or cyst formation.

Interventional Radiology in the Neonate

In most cases, neonatal UTD is managed surgically (ablation of PUV, ureteral reimplantation, pyeloplasty) or conservatively. Occasionally, urgent decompression of the upper urinary tract is necessary to prevent further injury to the kidney and allow postponement of definitive surgical intervention in the presence of significant comorbidities or prematurity [203].

Percutaneous nephrostomy (PCN) allows for rapid decompression of the upper urinary tract and is broadly used to treat urinary obstruction and infection in adults and children. The procedural success rate is consistently high (> 95%) in multiple case series in both neonates and larger children [203–207]. PCN is performed by placing the patient in the prone or semi-prone position and localizing the kidney using US. Periprocedural antibiotics are used routinely for infected systems and are recommended for all cases by SIR Quality Improvement Guidelines [190], although there is practice variation in antibiotic use for non-infected systems [206]. In cases with collecting system dilation, a "single stick" technique is employed to place a hollow tip or sheath needle into the collecting system via a peripheral calyx. Positioning within the collecting system is confirmed with a combination of US needle tip localization, return of urine via the needle hub, and injection of agitated saline, US contrast or iodinated contrast. Once peripheral access is confirmed, a guide wire is placed into the collecting system and coiled or advanced into the ureter or bladder. The tissues are then dilated over the wire and a pigtail drainage catheter is placed into the collecting system and secured (Fig. 3.23). In nondilated systems, a "two stick" technique may be used to access the central collecting system with a hollow tip needle to allow for distension and easier access to a peripheral calyx without endangering the central vasculature. An elegant modified technique for PCN in neonates has been described by Koral et al. that accommodates for their unique anatomy and tissue density [208]. Major complications are best avoided by using US guidance, avoiding central puncture of the renal collecting system, and using

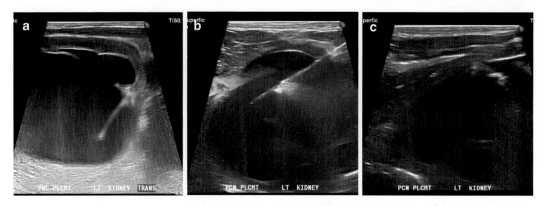

Fig. 3.23 Percutaneous nephrostomy (PCN). PCN placement in a 22-day old infant due to bilateral hydronephrosis and left sided urinoma with worsening abdominal distension despite bladder decompression. (**a**) Greyscale US showing a markedly dilated left kidney collecting system with parenchymal thinning. (**b**) The collecting system was accessed using a 21-gauge micro-puncture needle (**c**) Subsequently a 5 French Dawson-Mueller catheter was placed into the collecting system with US guidance

caution during tissue dilation with a supportive guide wire. In the immediate post-placement period, hemorrhage can occur due to central entry into the collecting system or inadvertent creation of an arterial fistula. Injury to the collecting system or ureter can occur due to needle or wire perforation during wire positioning or dilation, resulting in a urinoma. Sepsis is a feared complication in the setting of an infected collecting system. Appropriate antibiotic coverage and minimizing collecting system distension and manipulation during initial treatment of the infected system is recommended to reduce the risk of sepsis. Overall, the risk of major complication is the pediatric populations ranges from 0% to 9% [205, 209].

Retrograde placement of ureteral stents is less common in neonates than in older patients, as the size and rigidity of commercially available stents creates technical challenges.

Urinary Tract Infections and Vesicoureteral Reflux

The clinical management of UTI and VUR will be discussed more fully in later chapters. Multiple imaging modalities can contribute to the evaluation and management of UTI and VUR, including US, VCUG, ceVUS, and nuclear medicine. Imaging can help to identify urologic abnormalities such as obstruction or VUR, guide management strategies (e.g. need for antibiotic prophylaxis or surgical intervention such as ureteral reimplantation), and can aid in characterizing the extent of infection and potential complications (e.g. pyelonephritis, abscess, and kidney scarring). Clinical practice guidelines for imaging in pediatric UTI vary somewhat between international organizations [39, 210–212] but there are several unifying themes: (1) defining criteria for obtaining imaging based on risk factors for underlying urologic abnormalities (based on factors such as age, number of UTIs, and severity of symptoms); (2) using kidney and bladder US as the initial imaging method to assess for anatomic abnormalities; (3) evaluating for VUR in selected patients; and (4) using additional modalities such as DMSA based on various clinical criteria.

Kidney and bladder US can identify UTD that could suggest obstruction or reflux, evaluate bladder anatomy (e.g. wall thickness, bladder emptying [213]), and detect signs of either acute infection or sequelae of previous infection (e.g. scarring or global volume loss). Acute pyelonephritis can be associated with urothelial thickening [214], kidney enlargement [215], alterations in parenchymal echogenicity [216], or increased echogenicity of the renal sinus [217]. Focal bacterial nephritis (acute lobar nephronia) can resemble a kidney mass [218]. Echogenic debris in the collecting system can suggest, but is not pathognomonic for, infection. In patients with fungal UTI, particularly those who are immunosuppressed or have indwelling catheters, US can be used to assess for kidney parenchymal infection and the presence of fungal balls of the collecting systems.

Evaluation for VUR and urethral abnormalities such as PUV is most commonly performed using pulsed fluoroscopic VCUG. However, ceVUS is increasingly being used in some centers. Both VCUG and ceVUS can assess for the presence of VUR, whether it occurs during filling or voiding, and its severity in the five-grade system as described previously. Grading of VUR is similar between VCUG and ceVUS [73]. VCUG and ceVUS can also be used to assess for other anatomic abnormalities, including duplicated collected system, calyceal diverticula and PUV.

DMSA kidney cortical scintigraphy can be used to detect pyelonephritis and scars, both of which will appear as photopenic or "cold" areas. The distinction between acute pyelonephritis and scarring therefore depends on clinical signs and symptoms, as well as comparison with prior DMSA if available. If cortical defects persist beyond 6 months after clinical resolution of the acute infection, they are considered to be permanent scars that can predispose to CKD and hypertension [219].

Although contrast-enhanced CT (CECT) is the preferred imaging modality for acute pyelonephritis is adults [220], it is generally reserved for selected situations in children to minimize radiation exposure (for example, children with equivocal US findings at centers where MRI is unavailable, or when the risk of sedation for MRI is considered greater than that of radiation and IV contrast). CECT findings in acute pyelonephritis can include kidney enlargement and parenchymal hypodensities that can be wedge-shaped, linear, or patchy [220] (Fig. 3.13). The "striated nephrogram" is considered a classic finding of acute pyelonephritis, but can also be seen in other conditions such as renal vein thrombosis or ureteral obstruction [221].

MRI provides excellent anatomic definition of the kidneys without exposure to ionizing radiation. Contrast-enhanced MRI is generally considered to be the reference imaging technique for children with suspected acute pyelonephritis, but newer diffusion-weighted imaging sequences also appear to have comparable performance without the need for gadolinium contrast [222].

Interventional Radiology Techniques in UTI

Infection in the obstructed renal collecting system is considered a medical emergency and an indication for urgent decompression by stenting or percutaneous therapy. The need for minimally invasive decompression is less clear in infection occurring from ascending bacteria, direct spread from an adjacent source or hematogenous disseminated infection of the non-obstructed system.

Intraparenchymal kidney abscess and perinephric abscess are frequently grouped together in treatment algorithms. In general, collections smaller than 3 cm may be managed effectively with medical therapy alone, but percutaneous US-guided drainage may be advised in larger collections, immunocompromised or critically ill patients, or failure to improve despite appropriate antibiotics [223, 224] (Fig. 3.24).

Pyonephrosis refers to purulent material within the collecting system, and historically has been an indication for percutaneous drainage because of the risk of severe urosepsis with any extraneous manipulation. When collecting system decompression is indicated, US-drain placement, similar to PCN placement, is the technique of choice.

Neoplasm

Most kidney neoplasms in children present as a large palpable mass detected by the parent or physician. The initial imaging modality is most often US, which can suggest the renal origin of an abdominal mass by demonstrating extension of kidney tissue around the mass—the so-

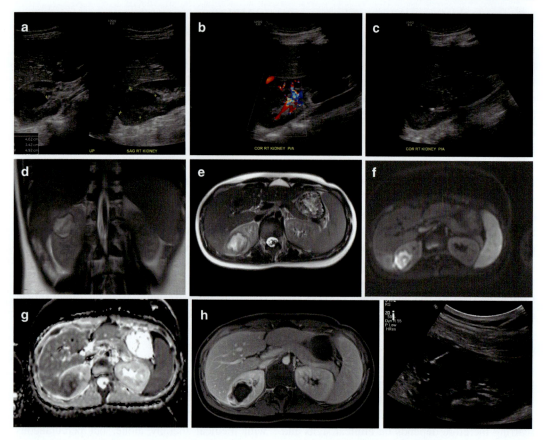

Fig. 3.24 Kidney abscess. 17-year-old female with acute pyelonephritis and increasing right flank pain despite appropriate antibiotic therapy. (**a–c**) US images with a heterogenous hypovascular expansile lesion of the right upper pole, with distortion of the adjacent vasculature and color Doppler signal. (**d, e**) MRI shows a T2 hyperintense collection with (**f**) restricted diffusion (**g**) confirmed with ADC map, with (**h**) no enhancement on post-contrast imaging (**h**). The collection was aspirated under US guidance (**i**)

called "claw sign" (Fig. 3.25). US can differentiate solid from cystic or necrotic areas, demonstrate if hemorrhage or calcification is present, and determine whether the tumor involves the renal vein or IVC or extends into the heart. Once an US confirms the presence of a tumor, CT or MRI can better assess the size, extent, involvement of adjacent structures, and spread, and are particularly useful for Wilms tumor staging [225–227]. Although CT and MRI are relatively equivalent in assessing the primary kidney mass, CT is the modality of choice to assess for lung metastases. If the tumor has a propensity to metastasize elsewhere, then appropriate imaging modalities (CT or MRI of the brain, bone scan, etc.) can be performed.

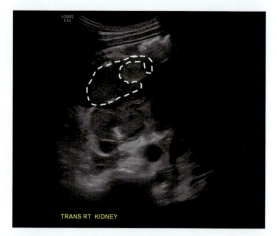

Fig. 3.25 US of kidney mass with "claw sign". Greyscale US showing transverse plane of right kidney with normal kidney tissue surrounding a mass ("claw sign," dashed outline)

Interventional Radiology in Pediatric Kidney Tumors

Interventional techniques can be applied in the management of pediatric kidney tumors in various situations. Percutaneous biopsy of Wilms tumor has been controversial since its use has been attributed to upstaging tumor classification in some staging systems [228] and it may not be necessary in patients with classical imaging presentation. Therefore, image guided diagnosis should be discussed with a pediatric oncologist before proceeding with a biopsy (Fig. 3.26). The technique for a targeted mass biopsy is similar to that of a non-targeted renal biopsy, although localization of a representative sample is critical. Adjunctive techniques, including image fusion and CEUS, can be helpful for targeting smaller lesions or obtaining viable tissue for pathologic analysis [229].

Rarely, a malignant kidney tumor can present with acute hemorrhage. Similar to kidney trauma, angiography and embolization can be useful either independently or in conjunction with surgery to stabilize patients and reduce blood loss [230].

Careful differentiation of kidney tumors from adrenal masses is critical prior to performing a biopsy. Tissue requirements for characterizing neuroblastoma are more extensive than other masses, necessitating larger coring needles and a greater number of samples for gene sequencing. Adrenal lesions, such as pheochromocytoma, can have catecholamine activity, and may result in hypertensive crisis if instrumented without alpha blockade [231].

The most common benign neoplasm of the kidney is angiomyolipoma (AML). In children, AML is seen almost exclusively in tuberous sclerosis complex (Fig. 3.27a, b), rather than as an independent lesion as seen in the middle-aged female population. These hamartomatous lesions are at risk for hemorrhage regardless of size, with increased risk in larger lesions or in the presence of intranidal aneurysm [232, 233]. Multiple lesions can be treated medically with mammalian target of rapamycin (mTOR) inhibitors, although embolization and partial nephrectomy have long been critical components of therapy. Embolization involves arterial access, renal angiography and microcatheter selection of the tumor vascularity of the AML (Fig. 3.27c, d) [233–235]. Liquid (dehydrated alcohol), glue (n-BCA) or particulates (PVA or Embospheres@) are administered until vascular stasis is achieved, resulting in tumor necrosis and lesion shrinkage over subsequent months [236].

Ablation therapy is a newer method of treating kidney tumors and has generally been accepted to treat small malignancies while preserving kidney parenchyma. In general, a probe is placed percutaneously into the target lesion and energy is imparted to the surrounding tissue to incur target

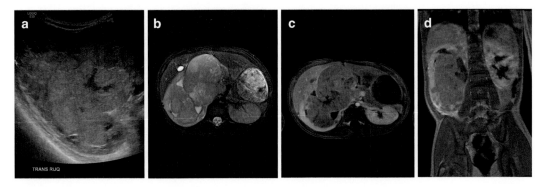

Fig. 3.26 Kidney mass. 6-year-old female with right abdominal mass. (**a**) Greyscale US demonstrates a heterogenous vascular mass expanding and distorting the contour of the right kidney. (**b**) T2, (**c**) post-contrast axial T1, (**d**) coronal MRI of the abdomen confirms a lesion arising from the right kidney. Staging evaluation confirmed metastatic spread to the lungs, therefore percutaneous biopsy was obtained for tissue diagnosis to guide presurgical chemotherapy

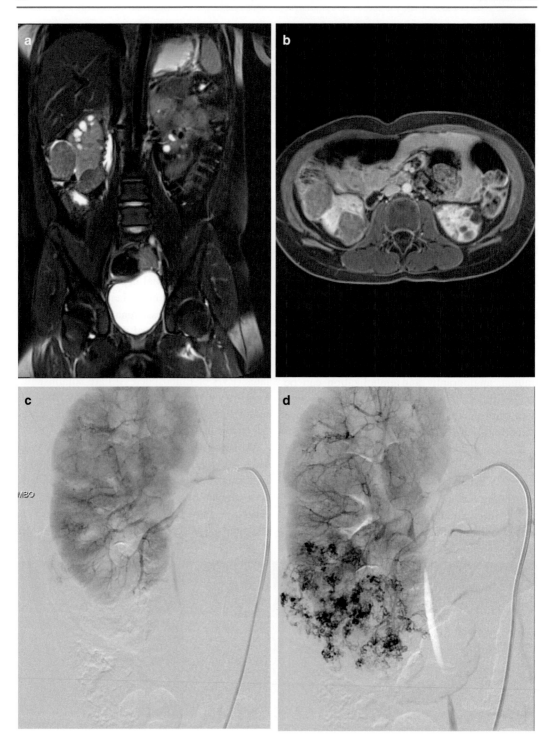

Fig. 3.27 Kidney angiomyolipoma. (**a**) Coronal T2 and (**b**) axial post contrast T1 abdominal MRI in a 12-year-old with tuberous sclerosis demonstrating interval growth of two pedunculated lesions from the lower pole of the right kidney. (**c**) Catheter directed angiography confirms angiomyolipoma with characteristic "cork-screw" vasculature. (**d**) Following particle embolization, the abnormal vasculature is no longer present and adjacent kidney parenchyma is preserved

cell injury and apoptosis. Currently, cryotherapy is commonly used in the GU system [237, 238], although radiofrequency ablation and microwave are also reported as effective for treatment of small kidney tumors. The primary limiting factors are proximity to critical structures or vascularity that can result in heat or cold sump, preventing target lesions reaching threshold damage.

Trauma

Due to the relatively large size of the kidneys compared to body size, decreased protection from the rib cage, and increased pliability of Gerota's fascia and capsule, there is increased frequency of kidney injury following blunt abdominal trauma in children and adolescents [239].

Imaging of trauma to the urinary tract has been studied extensively and remains a topic of debate [240]. In the acute setting, the imaging evaluation of the injured child is determined by the extent and type of injury as well as the practice of the particular institution [141, 241]. In some institutions, evaluation of trauma to the abdomen begins with abdominal US to assess for free fluid and obvious visceral injuries [242, 243]. At other institutions, CT is the modality of choice in the initial assessment [92, 142, 240]. The decision as to which modality is used will depend on the clinical situation. US has a high sensitivity in detecting intraperitoneal fluid; however, in the setting of trauma, the presence of fluid is not an absolute indication for surgery. Moreover, there can be injury to the urinary tract without the presence of free fluid [244]. CT, on the other hand, can accurately assess for the presence of free fluid and assess the solid and hollow abdominal viscera.

US imaging is effective for evaluating the kidneys and can be useful in triaging patients (FAST exam), in lower acuity patients, and to monitor patients following initial characterization of injuries [135]. US is not considered the primary study for trauma because of the lower sensitivity for kidney contusions and lacerations, operator dependence, length of the study, and patient dis-

comfort in the acutely injured patient. The adjunctive use of US contrast shows promise for increasing the sensitivity for parenchymal and vascular injury, but is not yet widely utilized and does not overcome the drawbacks of length of study and operator dependence [136].

US can depict a kidney laceration or contusion as a focal area of abnormal echotexture. The area can be hypoechoic, isoechoic or hyperechoic to the remainder of the kidney depending on the contents of the area and the stage of the evolution of the injury. US can also characterize the quality and amount of perinephric fluid (blood, urine or both) and follow the appearance to assess whether the collection is diminishing, remaining stable or increasing in size. Doppler US of the kidneys can assess both for areas of kidney parenchymal ischemia due to vascular interruption and for arterial or venous thrombosis and pseudoaneurysm formation. Renal vascular injury can also be visualized with nuclear medicine functional renal imaging, with non-perfused regions of the kidney appearing as cold defects.

CT is often the modality of choice in the evaluation of abdominal trauma, since most pediatric kidney injuries are related to blunt trauma and are associated with additional organ injuries [245]. Imaging is indicated in the setting of clinical suspicion based on mechanism or hematuria on presentation. As described previously in the section "Computed Tomography," IV contrast is generally used in the evaluation of trauma, and multiphase imaging can offer increased sensitivity to detect vascular disruptions or urinary leak. The appearance of the kidneys, particularly their patterns of enhancement on CT, can allow diagnosis of kidney contusions and lacerations. Areas devoid of enhancement, particularly if they are regional, suggest infarction. Perinephric and/or periureteral fluid can also be assessed. Delayed imaging may show disruption of the collecting system if dense contrast is seen outside of the collecting system (Fig. 3.28). CT cystography has also been used to assess for injuries to the urinary bladder and urethra.

In the past IV urography was used extensively in the evaluation of urinary tract trauma but is

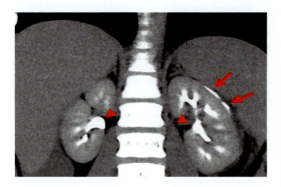

Fig. 3.28 Contrast enhanced CT (CECT) for trauma. CECT of collecting system injury in a 13-year-old following a snowboarding accident. CECT image obtained in the delayed phase shows opacification of the collecting system (arrowheads). There is contrast accumulation outside of the collecting system of the left kidney (arrows), compatible with collecting system injury

seldom used today. Fluoroscopic studies (retrograde urethrography and cystography) are, however, still used extensively in the imaging of bladder and urethral injury.

Interventional Radiology in Kidney Trauma

The American Association for the Surgery of Trauma (AAST) Organ Injury Scale (or the European Classification System) classifies kidney injury on a scale from grade I to V based on the depth and extent of injury, involvement of vascular structures, and urinary tract injury (Table 3.2). Most pediatric kidney injuries fall in grade I, II or III, and are frequently managed conservatively (Figs. 3.29 and 3.30) [246, 247]. Analysis of trauma registries and additional case series have described increased rates of surgical or interventional management within grades IV and V (Fig. 3.31) [246–248].

The goal of kidney trauma management is first to preserve life and second to preserve kidney integrity and function. The confined retroperitoneal space allows for tamponade of most hemorrhage when the facial plains remain intact. Initial patient instability frequently dictates the need for immediate operative intervention. However, delayed decompression of hemorrhage into the kidney collecting system or into the peritoneal space can result in refrac-

Table 3.2 American Association for the Surgery of Trauma (AAST) kidney injury scale (2018 revision)

AAST grade	Imaging criteria
I	Subcapsular hematoma and/or parenchymal contusion without laceration
II	Perirenal hematoma confined to Gerota's fascia Parenchymal laceration ≤1 cm in depth without urinary extravasation
III	Parenchymal laceration >1 cm without urinary extravasation or collecting system rupture Any injury in the presence of a kidney vascular injury or active bleeding contained within Gerota's fascia
IV	Parenchymal laceration extending into urinary collecting system with urinary extravasation Renal pelvis laceration and/or complete ureteropelvic disruption Segmental renal vein or artery injury Active bleeding beyond Gerota's fascia into the retroperitoneum or peritoneum Segmental or complete kidney infarction(s) due to vessel thrombosis without active bleeding
V	Main renal artery or vein laceration or avulsion of hilum Devascularized kidney with active bleeding Shattered kidney with loss of identifiable parenchymal renal anatomy

tory anemia and the need for persistent transfusion in the initially stable or stabilized patient. Patients requiring >3 transfusions in the initial 24–48 h should be deemed unstable, and angiographic intervention or surgery should be considered. Injury to the collecting system and ureter is a critical component of the trauma evaluation, as urine leak and urinoma can result in morbidity. Grade I–III injuries as well as most grade IV injuries can be successfully managed conservatively or with percutaneous or endoscopic therapy [249, 250].

When available, image guided intervention can successfully manage refractory hemorrhage while preserving kidney parenchyma. Trauma registries have demonstrated a high rate of nephrectomy when early surgery is performed for hemorrhage in the pediatric population [248]. Embolization can be performed rapidly and has been shown to be effective in salvaging

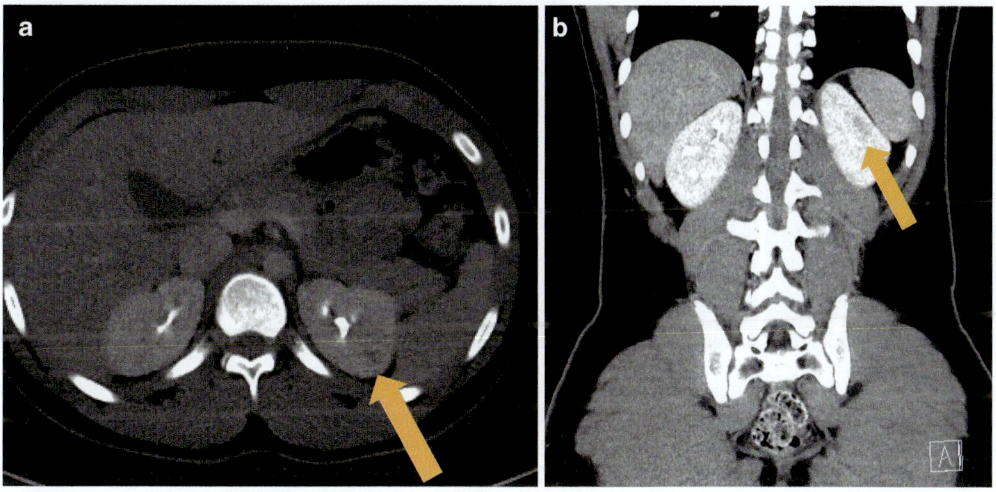

Fig. 3.29 Grade I left kidney parenchymal contusion on contrast enhanced CT. (**a**) Axial and (**b**) coronal contrast enhanced CT showing small focal hypoattenuating area (arrows) in the left interpolar region suggestive of grade I kidney contusion

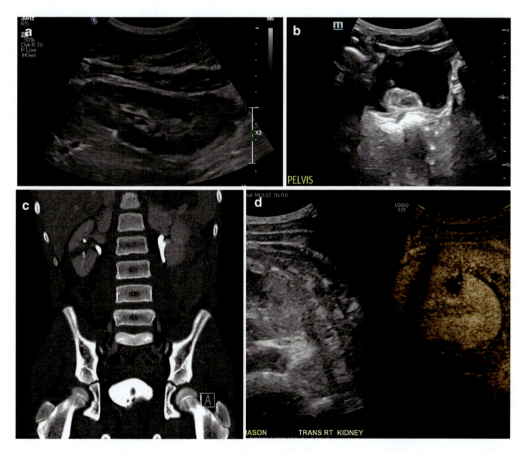

Fig. 3.30 Grade III right kidney injury. (**a**) Greyscale US of the right kidney shows increased lower pole echogenicity and a band of hypoechoic tissue at the juncture between the interpolar region and lower pole. (**b**) Bladder US provides visual confirmation of hematuria with a blood clot. (**c**, **d**) Contrast enhanced CT and US more accurately depict the extent of this Grade III right kidney injury

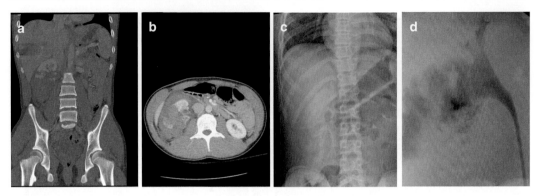

Fig. 3.31 Grade IV right kidney injury. Adolescent male following sports injury to the right flank. (**a**, **b**) Coronal and axial contrast enhanced CT angiography show a complex right kidney laceration involving the collecting system. Excretory phase imaging was not obtained. (**c**) Abdominal radiograph shows persistent contrast in the right kidney parenchyma with amorphous density in the perinephric tissues. (**d**) Retrograde ureterogram confirms urine leakage from the right kidney collecting system that was managed with placement of an endoscopic ureteral stent

the kidney without nephrectomy [245]. Embolization can be performed with a variety of agents, although temporary agents (such as Gelfoam®) and coils are the most common. A secondary procedure may be required if bleeding persists and has been shown to be beneficial for kidney salvage according to national trauma data bank [251].

Renovascular Hypertension

Imaging plays a critical role in identifying and managing renin-mediated renovascular hypertension. Renovascular hypertension can be described by stenosis location, extent and syndromic or non-syndromic association. Renovascular hypertension, once thought to be a rare cause of hypertension in children, has received growing attention in the past decade and is reported as a cause of hypertension in 10% of children with hypertension [252].

RAS can be unilateral or bilateral, involving the main, main branch or segmental renal arteries. Additionally, renal perfusion can be affected by upstream short or long segment stenosis of the lower thoracic or abdominal aorta. This distribution of disease, named middle aortic syndrome (MAS), can be isolated or can occur in combination with renal artery involvement.

Commonly identified causes for renovascular hypertension and MAS in children include fibromuscular dysplasia (FMD), vasculitis, neurofibromatosis type I, and Williams syndrome. However, the underlying cause is often difficult to confirm because of the overlapping imaging appearances, and the presumed diagnosis is made based on a combination of clinical and imaging features. For instance, "burned out" or senescent vasculitis can have imaging features identical to FMD. Additionally, the classically described "beaded string" appearance of FMD in adults is uncommon in children. In the young patient, the angiographic appearance of FMD is commonly a short segment uniform stenosis secondary to the involvement of both the intima and media within this age group.

Non-invasive imaging is critical for evaluating renovascular hypertension and determining the need for further intervention. US is the mainstay as it offers moderately high-resolution images with a combination of anatomic features and vascular flow assessment (Fig. 3.32) [253]. Differences in kidney lengths of >1 cm in the presence of hypertension may suggest main RAS and deserve additional evaluation. Established criteria for diagnosing RAS include direct visualization of stenosis, *parvus et tardus* wave form [acceleration time (time from onset of systole to peak systolic velocity) of >70 ms], main renal

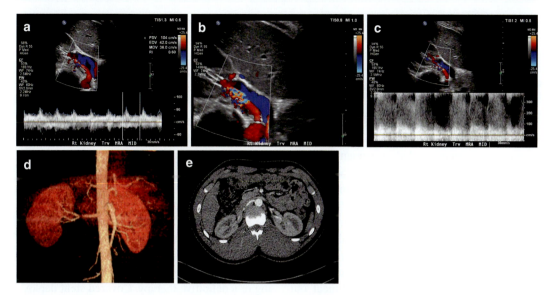

Fig. 3.32 Doppler US and CT angiography (CTA) of renal arteries. 16-year-old male with newly detected hypertension without hereditary risk factors. (**a–c**) Doppler US shows increased flow velocities in the mid- to distal right renal artery with aliasing on Doppler tracing and velocities in excess of 180 cm/s. (**d, e**) Contrast enhanced CTA confirms a short segment stenosis of the right renal artery, just proximal to a bifurcation into the upper and lower main branch renal arteries

Table 3.3 US criteria for renovascular hypertension (adapted from Dillman et al. [254])

US characteristic	Criteria suggesting renovascular hypertension
Kidney size	Asymmetric kidney lengths with difference of >1 cm
Doppler waveform	*Parvus et tardus* waveform Acceleration time of >70 ms
Main renal artery peak systolic velocity (PSV)	>180–200 cm/s
Renal-aortic (velocity) ratio (RAR)	>2.3–3.5
Renal-intrarenal (velocity) ratio (RIR)	>5

artery peak systolic velocity (PSV) of >180–200 m/s, main renal artery to aortic PSV ratio (RAR) of >2.3–3.5, or main renal artery to intrarenal artery PSV ratio (RIR) of >5 (Table 3.3) [254, 255]. Unfortunately, the sensitivity for RAS on Doppler US is low at 63–73% [256, 257].

CT angiography (CTA) (Fig. 3.32d) and MR angiography (MRA) (Fig. 3.15) have better sensitivity for detecting RAS, reported in the range of 93–94% and 77–93% respectively [256, 257]. Improved detection rates need to be balanced with the potential risks of ionizing radiation (for CTA) and sedation or anesthesia (for MRA). CTA image acquisition is much faster than MRA, and therefore conducive for non-sedated exams in the school-age child. Dose reduction, motion tolerant and image enhancement technology in newer MRI scanners will potentially offer no radiation exposure while maintaining image quality. However, currently MRA remains susceptible to even small amounts of motion that can occur in both sedated and non-sedated patients.

Catheter directed angiography remains the gold standard for the diagnosis of renovascular hypertension when there is a suggestive history and absence of non-invasive imaging findings [257]. In patients with appropriate histories as many as 40% of patients will have findings of clinically significant stenosis on angiography. Once identified, the lesion can be treated using angioplasty, stenting or ethanol ablation.

Angioplasty has, however, been the mainstay of endovascular therapy for renovascular hypertension and MAS. Lesions are confirmed with aortography or selective renal angiography, crossed using supportive wires and treated with balloon angioplasty following heparinization (Fig. 3.33). Adjunctive devices such as drug-eluting and cutting balloons have reportedly improved outcomes in small series [258–260]. Branch segmental artery stenoses may be difficult to traverse and current limitations of angioplasty devices may preclude treatment. In these cases, directed ethanol ablation may offer a mechanism to reduce renin secretion from the affected area of kidney parenchyma [261].

Angioplasty using a combination of traditional, high pressure and cutting balloons has high rates of technical angiographic success, up to 94% in reported series [262]. Features associated with favorable technical and clinical outcomes include short segment stenosis (<10 mm), and residual stenosis of <10% following angioplasty [259, 262]. Clinical responses vary among children and are lower than comparable disease in adults. This is most pronounced in FMD, where angioplasty alone has been reported to be beneficial in 93–98% of adult patients. In contrast, pediatric cases series have reported benefit in 56–72.8% of cases and cure in 23–39% of cases. Variability in the response rates may be due to regional variation and heterogenous disease etiology [259, 262, 263].

Renal artery angioplasty is well tolerated with infrequent life-threatening complications, even in the pediatric population. Potential complications include contrast toxicity (contrast-induced nephropathy), thrombosis, stent migration, vascular spasm, dissection, perforation and resulting hemorrhage with imminent threat to the kidney. Contrast toxicity is best managed by setting weight-based contrast notifications throughout the procedure and maintaining patient hydration. Hemorrhagic complications are more frequent when using cutting angioplasty balloon but can be treated with angioplasty as either a temporizing or a definitive therapy. Covered stent deployment is reserved for cases refractory to angioplasty and when appropriate sized devices are available but is associated with higher rates of re-stenosis [263]. If hemorrhage continues after a trial of balloon occlusion, then urgent engagement of the surgical team may be the only remaining option. Surgical interventions have been reported for primary or salvage therapy in the event of failed angioplasty or restenosis [264].

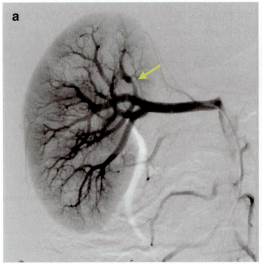

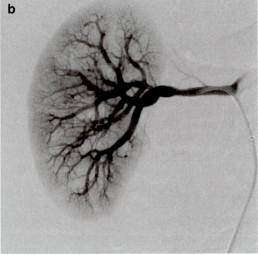

Fig. 3.33 Catheter directed angiography. Catheter directed angiography in a 9-year-old male with newly detected hypertension without hereditary risk factors. (**a**) Focal segmental branch stenosis in right upper pole with wedge-shaped parenchymal perfusion defect. (**b**) Repeat angiography following right upper pole segmental angioplasty showing improved lumen diameter and perfusion

Cystic Kidney Diseases

Kidney cysts can be seen at any age in the pediatric group. Cysts can be sporadic and unassociated with any systemic disease or may occur in a wide range of genetic and non-genetic diseases [265–267].

Kidney and bladder US is the primary imaging modality recommended for initial assessment of kidney cysts in children [267]. On US, a kidney macrocyst will appear anechoic with an imperceptible wall, whereas multiple microcysts may manifest as heterogeneous parenchymal echogenicity (e.g. "salt-and-pepper sign" in autosomal recessive polycystic kidney disease [ARPKD]) or just increased echogenicity without distinct cysts (Fig. 3.34) [267]. When distinct macrocysts are present, important characteristics to note include the number of cysts, location (e.g. cortical, medullary), sizes of larger cysts, and whether any complex features such as septations or debris are present [267]. The collecting system should be identified to ensure that a calyceal diverticulum or dilated calyces are not confused with cysts [267].

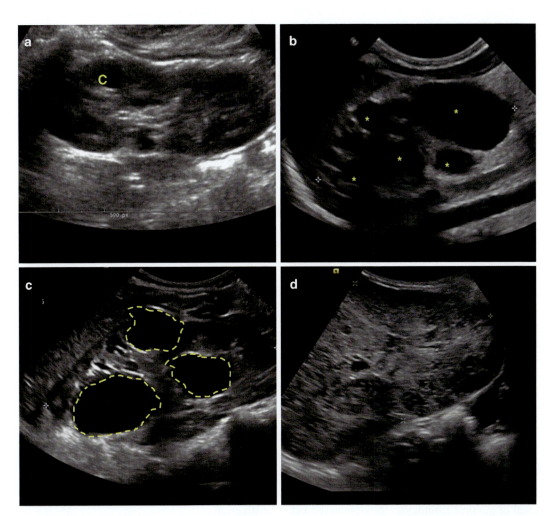

Fig. 3.34 US of cystic kidney diseases. US appearance of kidney cysts. (**a**) Simple cyst (c); (**b**) Multicystic dysplastic kidney, with numerous disorganized cysts (*) without intervening normal parenchyma; (**c**) ADPKD, with enlarged kidney with multiple macrocysts (dashed lines); (**d**) ARPKD, with numerous microcysts causing "salt-and-pepper" appearance of parenchyma and few resolvable cysts

Other imaging modalities such as CT or MRI are not routinely recommended for initial evaluation of kidney cysts in children due to cost and availability, as well as due to associated risks of ionization radiation (for CT) and need for sedation in younger children (for MRI). However, CT or MRI may be indicated in select circumstances, such as evaluation of complex cystic lesions with suspicion for malignancy or detection of angiomyolipomas in patients with tuberous sclerosis [267].

On CT, a cyst will have attenuation equal or near that of simple fluid and will have an imperceptible wall. There should be little to no change in the attenuation of the cyst after contrast administration. The Bosniak classification system was developed to assess the risk for malignancy based on cyst appearance on CT in adults, using factors such as cyst wall thickness, presence of septa, calcifications, or solid components, and degree of enhancement [268]. Studies in children suggest that modified versions of the Bosniak classification based on US appearance of cysts can adequately stratify malignancy risk [269–271]. CEUS also appears promising to classify kidney cystic lesions in native and transplant kidneys [57, 61, 62].

Non-genetic causes of kidney cysts in infants and children include cystic dysplasia, multicystic dysplastic kidney [272], medullary sponge kidney [273], cystic tumors or malformations, cystic nephroma, and solitary simple or acquired cysts [265, 267, 274]. Although simple cysts are common in adults, the reported incidence of simple cysts in children is as low as 0.2% [274]. Solitary cysts can also result from previous insult to the kidney, such as trauma or infection. In most cases of solitary cysts, the appearance of the remainder of the kidney is often normal.

Genetic causes of kidney cysts include autosomal dominant polycystic kidney disease (ADPKD), ARPKD, *HNF1B*-associated disease, nephronophthisis, and other genetic ciliopathies [267]. ADPKD is characterized by the development of multiple macrocysts throughout the kidney cortex and medulla (Fig. 3.34c), with progressive enlargement of the cysts and the kidneys throughout the lifetime [275, 276]. ARPKD

is typically characterized by enlarged, echogenic kidneys, sometimes with visible macroscopic cysts or dilated tubules predominantly in the medulla. Echogenic foci and the "twinkling sign" suggestive of calcifications can also be seen (Fig. 3.34d) [267, 277]. Juvenile nephronophthisis is characterized by relatively normal-sized or small kidneys with increased echogenicity and often cysts at the corticomedullary junction [267]. Imaging is also useful to assess for other complications or extra-renal manifestations of genetic cystic kidney diseases, such as angiomyolipomas in children with tuberous sclerosis, liver fibrosis in children with ARPKD, or liver cysts in children with ADPKD [278].

Kidney Stones and Nephrocalcinosis

Kidney Stone Imaging

US is typically the first-line modality in the evaluation of pediatric stone disease. Kidney stones can range from a few millimeters in size in a renal calyx to several centimeters in size filling the renal pelvis (staghorn calculus) (Fig. 3.35). They are most reliably detected by US when present in the kidney or bladder but may also be seen in the ureter when not obscured by overlying bowel gas. Kidney stones appear on greyscale US as echogenic foci, which may produce acoustic shadowing deep to the location of the stone. Small stones may be difficult to differentiate from vessels or portions of renal sinus fat, particularly if distal shadowing is not present. The twinkle artifact, or presence of alternating colors, is an imaging feature of kidney stones on color flow Doppler US (Fig. 3.35). Proper optimization of US settings is necessary to detect smaller stones, particularly in the selection of the focal zone and pulse repetition frequency. In addition to detecting stones, US may also assess for UTD suggestive of urinary obstruction due to stones. The bladder can also be evaluated for ureteral jets, the absence of which is suggestive of obstruction.

CT may also be indicated in the evaluation of stone disease if the US is equivocal or nondiagnostic. CT has a higher sensitivity than US

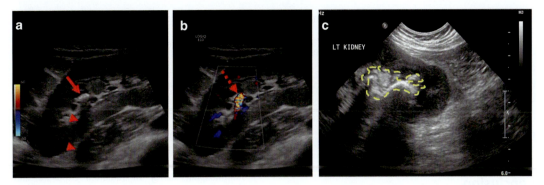

Fig. 3.35 US of kidney stones. (**a**) Greyscale longitudinal US of a non-obstructing stone, appearing as an echogenic focus (arrow) in the upper pole of the kidney with posterior acoustic shadowing (arrowheads). (**b**) Color Doppler longitudinal US demonstrates twinkle artifact (dashed arrow) associated with the echogenic focus, compatible with a kidney stone. There is no urinary tract dilation to suggest obstruction. (**c**) Obstructing staghorn calculus demonstrated by a large echogenic focus (dashed outline) occupying the collecting system of the left kidney

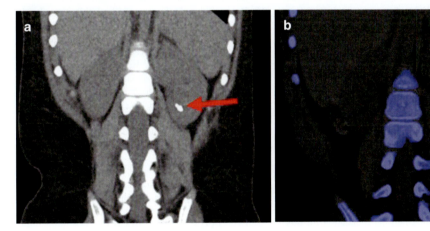

Fig. 3.36 Dual-energy CT (DECT) for detecting kidney stone composition. Non-obstructing kidney stone on DECT in an 8-year-old female. (**a**) Coronal DECT images demonstrate a dense focus in the left kidney lower pole (arrow), compatible with stone. (**b**) Color coding demonstrates that the stone is blue, correlating with non-uric acid/urate-composition, which is compatible with a cystine or calcium-based stone

for the detection of stones smaller than 3 mm [279], and can detect nearly all stones, except for matrix stones or medication stones, such as indinavir stones [280]. CT may also be necessary to evaluate for ureteral stones that may not be visualized on US, as well as complications of stone disease, including abscess and pyonephrosis. Stone evaluation is further enhanced by DECT, which can be used to determine stone composition based on the attenuation ratios (Fig. 3.36). Determining stone composition can help guide management, as certain compositions are less amenable to extracorporeal shock wave lithotripsy, and knowledge of the stone composition can help guide dietary recommendations and medical management [281]. In children, kidney stone size and Hounsfield attenuation values on CT have been shown to predict successful shock wave lithotripsy [282].

Nephrocalcinosis

US is often the modality of choice to assess nephrocalcinosis. While cortical nephrocalcinosis can be seen, it is a rare finding in children [283]. Medullary nephrocalcinosis is well described in children and can be accurately diagnosed and followed using US. Typically, medullary nephrocalcinosis appears as echogenic pyramids, often outlining the rim of the pyramid, with a normal appearing cortex (Fig. 3.12c). A pattern of peripheral increased echogenicity followed by progression toward the center of the pyramid has been described as the Anderson-Carr progression of nephrocalcinosis [172].

Conclusion

The role of radiologic imaging and interventions in the diagnosis and treatment of diseases of the kidneys and urinary tract continues to evolve. US, CT, MRI, and nuclear medicine remain the most common modalities for assessing the urinary tract, while new technologies such as CEUS, ceVUS, and MRU are starting to change practice patterns. Interventional radiology is playing an increasing role in the management of urinary tract and renovascular disease. Close collaboration between nephrologists, urologists, and radiologists will continue to allow optimal care for children with kidney and urinary tract abnormalities.

Acknowledgement The authors express their gratitude to Drs. Ruth Lim and Jeffrey Traubici, whose excellent work in the previous edition laid the foundation for this chapter.

References

1. Kuhn JP, Slovis TL, Haller JO, Caffey J. Caffey's pediatric diagnostic imaging. 10th ed. Philadelphia, PA: Mosby; 2004.
2. Thurman J, Gueler F. Recent advances in renal imaging. F1000Research. 2018;7 https://doi.org/10.12688/f1000research.16188.1.
3. Dillman JR, Trout AT, Smith EA, Towbin AJ. Hereditary renal cystic disorders: imaging of the kidneys and beyond. Radiographics. 2017;37:924–46. https://doi.org/10.1148/rg.2017160148.
4. Viteri B, Calle-Toro JS, Furth S, et al. State-of-the-art renal imaging in children. Pediatrics. 2020;145 https://doi.org/10.1542/peds.2019-0829.
5. Brenner D, Elliston C, Hall E, Berdon W. Estimated risks of radiation-induced fatal cancer from pediatric CT. AJR Am J Roentgenol. 2001;176:289–96. https://doi.org/10.2214/ajr.176.2.1760289.

6. Costello JE, Cecava ND, Tucker JE, Bau JL. CT radiation dose: current controversies and dose reduction strategies. AJR Am J Roentgenol. 2013;201:1283–90. https://doi.org/10.2214/AJR.12.9720.
7. Mettler FA, Bhargavan M, Faulkner K, et al. Radiologic and nuclear medicine studies in the United States and worldwide: frequency, radiation dose, and comparison with other radiation sources—1950-2007. Radiology. 2009;253:520–31. https://doi.org/10.1148/radiol.2532082010.
8. Brown PH, Silberberg PJ, Thomas RD, et al. A multihospital survey of radiation exposure and image quality in pediatric fluoroscopy. Pediatr Radiol. 2000;30:236–42. https://doi.org/10.1007/s002470050729.
9. Mahesh M. The AAPM/RSNA physics tutorial for residents. Fluoroscopy: patient radiation exposure issues. Radiographics. 2001;21:1033–45. https://doi.org/10.1148/radiographics.21.4.g01jl271033.
10. Brown Robert D, Thomas Phillip J, Silberberg Linda M, Johnson PH, Brown PH, Thomas RD, et al. Optimization of a fluoroscope to reduce radiation exposure in pediatric imaging. Springer; 2000.
11. Boland GWL, Murphy B, Arellano R, et al. Dose reduction in gastrointestinal and genitourinary fluoroscopy: use of grid-controlled pulsed fluoroscopy. AJR Am J Roentgenol. 2000;175:1453–7.
12. Nagayama Y, Oda S, Nakaura T, et al. Radiation dose reduction at pediatric CT: use of low tube voltage and iterative reconstruction. Radiographics. 2018;38:1421–40. https://doi.org/10.1148/rg.2018180041.
13. Miglioretti DL, Johnson E, Williams A, et al. The use of computed tomography in pediatrics and the associated radiation exposure and estimated cancer risk. JAMA Pediatr. 2013;167:700–7. https://doi.org/10.1001/jamapediatrics.2013.311.
14. Hollingsworth C, Frush DP, Cross M, Lucaya J. Helical CT of the body: a survey of techniques used for pediatric patients. Am J Roentgenol. 2003;180:401–6. https://doi.org/10.2214/ajr.180.2.1800401.
15. Siegel MJ, Schmidt B, Bradley D, et al. Radiation dose and image quality in pediatric CT: effect of technical factors and phantom size and shape. Radiology. 2004;233:515–22. https://doi.org/10.1148/radiol.2332032107.
16. Chen CY, Hsu JS, Jaw TS, et al. Split-Bolus portal venous phase dual-energy CT urography: protocol design, image quality, and dose reduction. Am J Roentgenol. 2015;205:W492–501. https://doi.org/10.2214/AJR.14.13687.
17. Morcos SK, Thomsen HS. Adverse reactions to iodinated contrast media. Eur Radiol. 2001;11:1267–75.
18. Lameier NH. Contrast-induced nephropathy—prevention and risk reduction. Nephrol Dial Transpl. 2006;21:i11–23.
19. Rao QA, Newhouse JH. Risk of nephropathy after intravenous administration of contrast material: a

critical literature analysis. Radiology. 2006;239:392–7. https://doi.org/10.1148/radiol.2392050413.

20. Aycock RD, Westafer LM, Boxen JL, et al. Acute kidney injury after computed tomography: a meta-analysis. Ann Emerg Med. 2018;71:44–53.e4. https://doi.org/10.1016/j.annemergmed.2017.06.041.

21. Sinert R, Brandler E, Subramanian RA, Miller AC. Does the current definition of contrast-induced acute kidney injury reflect a true clinical entity? Acad Emerg Med. 2012;19:1261–7. https://doi.org/10.1111/acem.12011.

22. Hinson JS, Ehmann MR, Fine DM, et al. Risk of acute kidney injury after intravenous contrast media administration. Ann Emerg Med. 2017;69:577–586.e4. https://doi.org/10.1016/j.annemergmed.2016.11.021.

23. McDonald JS, McDonald RJ, Tran CL, et al. Postcontrast acute kidney injury in pediatric patients: a cohort study. Am J Kidney Dis. 2018;72:811–8. https://doi.org/10.1053/j.ajkd.2018.05.014.

24. Gilligan LA, Davenport MS, Trout AT, et al. Risk of acute kidney injury following contrast-enhanced CT in hospitalized pediatric patients: a propensity score analysis. Radiology. 2020;294:548–56. https://doi.org/10.1148/radiol.2020191931.

25. Fujisaki K, Ono-Fujisaki A, Kura-Nakamura N, et al. Rapid deterioration of renal insufficiency after magnetic resonance imaging with gadolinium-based contrast agent. Clin Nephrol. 2011;75:251–4. https://doi.org/10.5414/cnp75251.

26. Rudnick MR, Wahba IM, Leonberg-Yoo AK, et al. Risks and options with gadolinium-based contrast agents in patients with CKD: a review. Am J Kidney Dis. 2021;77:517–28. https://doi.org/10.1053/j.ajkd.2020.07.012.

27. Thomsen HS, Morcos SK, Almen T, et al. Nephrogenic systemic fibrosis and gadolinium-based contrast media: updated ESUR Contrast Medium Safety Committee guidelines. Eur Radiol. 2013;23:307–18. https://doi.org/10.1007/s00330-012-2597-9.

28. Sadowski EA, Bennett LK, Chan MR, et al. Nephrogenic systemic fibrosis: risk factors and incidence estimation. Radiology. 2007;243(1):148–57.

29. Prybylski JP, Jay M. The impact of excess ligand on the retention of nonionic, linear gadolinium-based contrast agents in patients with various levels of renal dysfunction: a review and simulation analysis. Adv Chronic Kidney Dis. 2017;24:176–82. https://doi.org/10.1053/j.ackd.2017.03.002.

30. Holowka S, Shroff M, Chavhan GB. Use and safety of gadolinium based contrast agents in pediatric MR imaging. Indian J Pediatr. 2019; https://doi.org/10.1007/s12098-019-02891-x.

31. Gulani V, Calamante F, Shellock FG, et al. Gadolinium deposition in the brain: summary of evidence and recommendations. Lancet Neurol. 2017;16:564–70. https://doi.org/10.1016/S1474-4422(17)30158-8.

32. Akgun H, Gonlusen G, Cartwright J, et al. Are gadolinium-based contrast media nephrotoxic? A renal biopsy study. Arch Pathol Lab Med. 2006;130:1354–7. https://doi.org/10.1043/1543-2165(2006)130[1354:AGCMNA]2.0.CO;2.

33. Li A, Wong CS, Wong MK, et al. Acute adverse reactions to magnetic resonance contrast media—gadolinium chelates. Br J Radiol. 2006;79:368–71.

34. Malviya S, Voepel-Lewis T, Eldevik OP, et al. Sedation and general anaesthesia in children undergoing MRI and CT: adverse events and outcomes. Br J Anaesth. 2000;84:743–8.

35. Frush DP, Bisset GS, Hall SC. Pediatric sedation in radiology: the practice of safe sleep. AJR Am J Roentgenol. 1996;167:1381–7. https://doi.org/10.2214/ajr.167.6.8956563.

36. Kurugol S, Seager CM, Thaker H, et al. Feed and wrap magnetic resonance urography provides anatomic and functional imaging in infants without anesthesia. J Pediatr Urol. 2020;16:116–20. https://doi.org/10.1016/j.jpurol.2019.11.002.

37. Peratoner L, Pennesi M, Bordugo A, et al. Kidney length and scarring in children with urinary tract infection: importance of ultrasound scans. Abdom Imaging. 2005;30:780–5.

38. Dacher JN, Hitzel A, Avni FE, Vera P. Imaging strategies in pediatric urinary tract infection. Eur Radiol. 2005;15:1283–8.

39. Subcommittee on Urinary Tract Infection Steering Committee on Quality Improvement and Management, Roberts KB. Urinary tract infection: clinical practice guideline for the diagnosis and management of the initial UTI in febrile infants and children 2 to 24 months. Pediatrics. 2011;128:595–610. https://doi.org/10.1542/peds.2011-1330.

40. Monsalve J, Kapur J, Malkin D, Babyn PS. Imaging of cancer predisposition syndromes in children. Radiographics. 2011;31:263–80. https://doi.org/10.1148/rg.311105099.

41. Chen JJ, Pugach J, Patel M, et al. The renal length nomogram: multivariable approach. J Urol. 2002;168:2149–52. https://doi.org/10.1097/01.ju.0000033905.64110.91.

42. Blane CE, Bookstein FL, DiPietro MA, Kelsch RC. Sonographic standards for normal infant kidney length. AJR Am J Roentgenol. 1985;145:1289–91. https://doi.org/10.2214/ajr.145.6.1289.

43. Rosenbaum DM, Korngold E, Teele RL. Sonographic assessment of renal length in normal children. AJR Am J Roentgenol. 1984;142:467–9.

44. Ginalski JM, Michaud A, Genton N. Renal growth retardation in children: sign suggestive of vesicoureteral reflux? AJR Am J Roentgenol. 1985;145:617–9. https://doi.org/10.2214/ajr.145.3.617.

45. Hricak H, Slovis TL, Callen CW, et al. Neonatal kidneys: sonographic anatomic correlation. Radiology. 1983;147:699–702.

46. Haller JO, Berdon WE, Friedman AP. Increased renal cortical echogenicity: a normal finding in neonates and infants. Radiology. 1982;142:173–4.
47. Starinsky R, Vardi O, Batasch D, Goldberg M. Increased renal medullary echogenicity in neonates. Pediatr Radiol. 1995;25(Suppl 1):S43–5.
48. Nimkin K, Lebowitz RL, Share JC, Teele RL. Urolithiasis in a children's hospital: 1985-1990. Urol Radiol. 1992;14:139–43.
49. Ricci MA, Lloyd DA. Renal venous thrombosis in infants and children. Arch Surg. 1990;125:1195–9.
50. Brun P, Kchouk H, Mouchet B, et al. Value of Doppler ultrasound for the diagnosis of renal artery stenosis in children. Pediatr Nephrol. 1997;11:27–30. https://doi.org/10.1007/s004670050227.
51. Fang YC, Tiu CM, Chou YH, Chang T. A case of acute renal artery thrombosis caused by blunt trauma: computed tomographic and Doppler ultrasonic findings. J Formos Med Assoc. 1993;92:356–8.
52. Hitzel A, Liard A, Vera P, et al. Color and power Doppler sonography versus DMSA scintigraphy in acute pyelonephritis and in prediction of renal scarring. J Nucl Med. 2002;43:27–32.
53. Irshad A, Ackerman SJ, Campbell AS, Anis M. An overview of renal transplantation: current practice and use of ultrasound. Semin Ultrasound CT MR. 2009;30:298–314.
54. Sharma AK, Rustom R, Evans A, et al. Utility of serial Doppler ultrasound scans for the diagnosis of acute rejection in renal allografts. Transpl Int. 2004;17:138–44.
55. McArthur C, Baxter GM. Current and potential renal applications of contrast-enhanced ultrasound. Clin Radiol. 2012;67:909–22. https://doi.org/10.1016/j.crad.2012.01.017.
56. Huang DY, Yusuf GT, Daneshi M, et al. Contrast-enhanced ultrasound (CEUS) in abdominal intervention. Abdom Radiol. 2018;43:960–76. https://doi.org/10.1007/s00261-018-1473-8.
57. Bertolotto M, Bucci S, Valentino M, et al. Contrast-enhanced ultrasound for characterizing renal masses. Eur J Radiol. 2018;105:41–8. https://doi.org/10.1016/j.ejrad.2018.05.015.
58. Valentino M, Serra C, Zironi G, et al. Blunt abdominal trauma: emergency contrast-enhanced sonography for detection of solid organ injuries. AJR Am J Roentgenol. 2006;186:1361–7. https://doi.org/10.2214/AJR.05.0027.
59. Fetzer DT, Flanagan J, Nabhan A, et al. Impact of implementing contrast-enhanced ultrasound for antegrade nephrostogram after percutaneous nephrolithotomy. J Ultrasound Med. 2021;40:101–11. https://doi.org/10.1002/jum.15380.
60. Pan F-S, Liu M, Luo J, et al. Transplant renal artery stenosis: evaluation with contrast-enhanced ultrasound. Eur J Radiol. 2017;90:42–9. https://doi.org/10.1016/j.ejrad.2017.02.031.
61. Barr RG, Peterson C, Hindi A. Evaluation of indeterminate renal masses with contrast-enhanced US: a diagnostic performance study. Radiology. 2014;271:133–42. https://doi.org/10.1148/radiol.13130161.
62. Paudice N, Zanazzi M, Agostini S, et al. Contrast-enhanced ultrasound assessment of complex cystic lesions in renal transplant recipients with acquired cystic kidney disease: preliminary experience. Transplant Proc. 2012;44:1928–9. https://doi.org/10.1016/j.transproceed.2012.06.033.
63. Mueller-Peltzer K, Negrão de Figueiredo G, Fischereder M, et al. Vascular rejection in renal transplant: diagnostic value of contrast-enhanced ultrasound (CEUS) compared to biopsy. Clin Hemorheol Microcirc. 2018;69:77–82. https://doi.org/10.3233/CH-189115.
64. Benozzi L, Cappelli G, Granito M, et al. Contrast-enhanced sonography in early kidney graft dysfunction. Transplant Proc. 2009;41:1214–5. https://doi.org/10.1016/j.transproceed.2009.03.029.
65. Fernandez CP, Ripolles T, Martinez MJ, et al. Diagnosis of acute cortical necrosis in renal transplantation by contrast-enhanced ultrasound: a preliminary experience. Ultraschall Med. 2013;34:340–4. https://doi.org/10.1055/s-0032-1313007.
66. Mori G, Granito M, Favali D, Cappelli G. Long-term prognostic impact of contrast-enhanced ultrasound and power doppler in renal transplantation. Transplant Proc. 2015;47:2139–41. https://doi.org/10.1016/j.transproceed.2014.11.080.
67. Gokli A, Pinto E, Escobar FA, et al. Contrast-enhanced ultrasound: use in the management of lymphorrhea in generalized lymphatic anomaly. J Vasc Interv Radiol. 2020;31:1511–3. https://doi.org/10.1016/j.jvir.2020.05.001.
68. Yang WQ, Mou S, Xu Y, et al. Quantitative parameters of contrast-enhanced ultrasonography for assessment of renal pathology: a preliminary study in chronic kidney disease. Clin Hemorheol Microcirc. 2018;68:71–82. https://doi.org/10.3233/CH-170303.
69. Yang C, Wu S, Yang P, et al. Prediction of renal allograft chronic rejection using a model based on contrast-enhanced ultrasonography. Microcirculation. 2019;1–9 https://doi.org/10.1111/micc.12544.
70. Papadopoulou F, Ntoulia A, Siomou E, Darge K. Contrast-enhanced voiding urosonography with intravesical administration of a second-generation ultrasound contrast agent for diagnosis of vesicoureteral reflux: prospective evaluation of contrast safety in 1,010 children. Pediatr Radiol. 2014;44:719–28. https://doi.org/10.1007/s00247-013-2832-9.
71. Riccabona M, Vivier P-H, Ntoulia A, et al. ESPR uroradiology task force imaging recommendations in paediatric uroradiology, part VII: standardised terminology, impact of existing recommendations, and update on contrast-enhanced ultrasound of the paediatric urogenital tract. Pediatr Radiol. 2014;44:1478–84. https://doi.org/10.1007/s00247-014-3135-5.
72. Duran C, Beltrán VP, González A, et al. Contrast-enhanced voiding urosonography for vesicoure-

teral reflux diagnosis in children. Radiographics. 2017;37:1854–69. https://doi.org/10.1148/rg.2017170024.

73. Darge K, Troeger J. Vesicoureteral reflux grading in contrast-enhanced voiding urosonography. Eur J Radiol. 2002;43:122–8. https://doi.org/10.1016/S0720-048X(02)00114-6.

74. Papadopoulou F, Anthopoulou A, Siomou E, et al. Harmonic voiding urosonography with a second-generation contrast agent for the diagnosis of vesicoureteral reflux. Pediatr Radiol. 2009;39:239–44. https://doi.org/10.1007/s00247-008-1080-x.

75. Darge K. Voiding urosonography with US contrast agents for the diagnosis of vesicoureteric reflux in children. II. Comparison with radiological examinations. Pediatr Radiol. 2008;38:54–63; quiz 126–7. https://doi.org/10.1007/s00247-007-0528-8.

76. Grover S, Patra S, Grover H, Kumar A. Contrast-enhanced voiding urosonography (CEVUS) as a novel technique for evaluation in a case of male urethral diverticulum. Indian J Radiol Imaging. 2020;30:409. https://doi.org/10.4103/ijri.IJRI_50_20.

77. Woźniak MM, Osemlak P, Pawelec A, et al. Intraoperative contrast-enhanced urosonography during endoscopic treatment of vesicoureteral reflux in children. Pediatr Radiol. 2014;44:1093–100. https://doi.org/10.1007/s00247-014-2963-7.

78. Rosado E, Riccabona M. Off-label use of ultrasound contrast agents for intravenous applications in children: analysis of the existing literature. J Ultrasound Med. 2016;35:487–96. https://doi.org/10.7863/ultra.15.02030.

79. Yusuf GT, Sellars ME, Deganello A, et al. Retrospective analysis of the safety and cost implications of pediatric contrast-enhanced ultrasound at a single center. AJR Am J Roentgenol. 2017;208:446–52. https://doi.org/10.2214/AJR.16.16700.

80. Mao M, Xia B, Chen W, et al. The safety and effectiveness of intravenous contrast-enhanced sonography in Chinese children-a single center and prospective study in China. Front Pharmacol. 2019;10:1447. https://doi.org/10.3389/fphar.2019.01447.

81. Knieling F, Strobel D, Rompel O, et al. Spectrum, applicability and diagnostic capacity of contrast-enhanced ultrasound in pediatric patients and young adults after intravenous application—a retrospective trial. Ultraschall der Medizin—Eur J Ultrasound. 2016;37:619–26. https://doi.org/10.1055/s-0042-108429.

82. Torres A, Koskinen SK, Gjertsen H, Fischler B. Contrast-enhanced ultrasound using sulfur hexafluoride is safe in the pediatric setting. Acta Radiol. 2017;58:1395–9. https://doi.org/10.1177/0284185117690423.

83. Wang X, Yu Z, Guo R, et al. Assessment of postoperative perfusion with contrast-enhanced ultrasonography in kidney transplantation. Int J Clin Exp Med. 2015;8:18399–405.

84. Bracco Diagnostics Inc. LUMASON prescribing information (PDF). https://imaging.bracco.com/sites/braccoimaging.com/files/technica_sheet_pdf/us-en-2017-01-04-spc-lumason.pdf. Accessed 22 Jun 2021.

85. European Medicines Agency SonoVue. https://www.ema.europa.eu/en/medicines/human/EPAR/sonovue. Accessed 22 Jun 2021.

86. Fotter R. Pediatric uroradiology. New York: Springer; 2001.

87. Ward VL. Patient dose reduction during voiding cystourethrography. Pediatr Radiol. 2006;36(Suppl 2):168–72. https://doi.org/10.1007/s00247-006-0213-3.

88. Lebowitz RL, Olbing H, Parkkulainen KV, et al. International system of radiographic grading of vesicoureteric reflux. International Reflux Study in Children. Pediatr Radiol. 1985;15:105–9.

89. Unver T, Alpay H, Biyikli NK, Ones T. Comparison of direct radionuclide cystography and voiding cystourethrography in detecting vesicoureteral reflux. Pediatr Int. 2006;48:287–91. https://doi.org/10.1111/j.1442-200X.2006.02206.x.

90. Sükan A, Bayazit AK, Kibar M, et al. Comparison of direct radionuclide cystography and voiding direct cystography in the detection of vesicoureteral reflux. Ann Nucl Med. 2003;17:549–53. https://doi.org/10.1007/BF03006667.

91. Fettich J, Colarinha P, Fischer S, et al. Guidelines for direct radionuclide cystography in children. Eur J Nucl Med Mol Imaging. 2003;30:B39–44. https://doi.org/10.1007/s00259-003-1137-x.

92. Carpio F, Morey AF. Radiographic staging of renal injuries. World J Urol. 1999;17:66–70. https://doi.org/10.1007/s003450050108.

93. Peters AM, Morony S, Gordon I. Indirect radionuclide cystography demonstrates reflux under physiological conditions. Clin Radiol. 1990;41:44–7.

94. Gordon I, Peters AM, Morony S. Indirect radionuclide cystography: a sensitive technique for the detection of vesico-ureteral reflux. Pediatr Nephrol. 1990;4:604–6. https://doi.org/10.1007/BF00858633.

95. Gordon I. Indirect radionuclide cystography—the coming of age. Nucl Med Commun. 1989;10:457–8. https://doi.org/10.1097/00006231-198907000-00001.

96. Pollet JE, Sharp PF, Smith FW. Comparison of "direct" and "indirect" radionuclide cystography. J Nucl Med. 1985;26:1501–2.

97. Bower G, Lovegrove FT, Geijsel H, et al. Comparison of "direct" and "indirect" radionuclide cystography. J Nucl Med. 1985;26:465–8.

98. Pollet JE, Sharp PF, Smith FW, et al. Intravenous radionuclide cystography for the detection of vesicorenal reflux. J Urol. 1981;125:75–8.

99. Conway JJ, Kruglik GD. Effectiveness of direct and indirect radionuclide cystography in detecting vesicoureteral reflux. J Nucl Med. 1976;17:81–3.

100. Conway JJ, Belman AB, King LR, Filmer RB. Direct and indirect radionuclide cystography. J Urol. 1975;113:689–93. https://doi.org/10.1016/s0022-5347(17)59554-3.

101. Conway JJ, Belman AB, King LR. Direct and indirect radionuclide cystography. Semin Nucl Med. 1974;4:197–211. https://doi.org/10.1016/s0001-2998(74)80008-5.

102. Gordon I, Colarinha P, Fettich J, et al. Guidelines for indirect radionuclide cystography. Eur J Nucl Med. 2001;28:BP16–20.

103. Piepsz A, Ham HR. Pediatric applications of renal nuclear medicine. Semin Nucl Med. 2006;36:16–35.

104. De Sadeleer C, De Boe V, Keuppens F, et al. How good is technetium-99m mercaptoacetyltriglycine indirect cystography? Eur J Nucl Med. 1994;21:223–7. https://doi.org/10.1007/BF00188670.

105. Corso A, Ostinelli A, Trombetta MA. ["Indirect" radioisotope cystography after the furosemide test: its diagnostic efficacy compared to "direct" study]. Radiol Med. 1989;78:645–8.

106. Vlajković M, Ilić S, Bogićević M, et al. Radionuclide voiding patterns in children with vesicoureteral reflux. Eur J Nucl Med Mol Imaging. 2003;30:532–7. https://doi.org/10.1007/s00259-002-1077-x.

107. Mandell GA, Eggli DF, Gilday DL, et al. Procedure guideline for radionuclide cystography in children. Society of Nuclear Medicine. J Nucl Med. 1997;38:1650–4.

108. Hoberman A, Charron M, Hickey RW, et al. Imaging studies after a first febrile urinary tract infection in young children. N Engl J Med. 2003;348:195–202.

109. Stokland E, Hellstrom M, Jakobsson B, Sixt R. Imaging of renal scarring. Acta Paediatr Suppl. 1999;88:13–21.

110. Goldraich NP, Goldraich IH. Update on dimercaptosuccinic acid renal scanning in children with urinary tract infection. Pediatr Nephrol. 1995;9:221–6; discussion 227. https://doi.org/10.1007/BF00860755.

111. Mastin ST, Drane WE, Iravani A. Tc-99m DMSA SPECT imaging in patients with acute symptoms or history of UTI. Comparison with ultrasonography. Clin Nucl Med. 1995;20:407–12.

112. Majd M, Nussbaum Blask AR, Markle BM, et al. Acute pyelonephritis: comparison of diagnosis with 99mTc-DMSA, SPECT, spiral CT, MR imaging, and power Doppler US in an experimental pig model. Radiology. 2001;218:101–8.

113. Applegate KE, Connolly LP, Davis RT, et al. A prospective comparison of high-resolution planar, pinhole, and triple-detector SPECT for the detection of renal cortical defects. Clin Nucl Med. 1997;22:673–8. https://doi.org/10.1097/00003072-199710000-00002.

114. Cook GJ, Lewis MK, Clarke SE. An evaluation of 99Tcm-DMSA SPET with three-dimensional reconstruction in 68 patients with varied renal pathology. Nucl Med Commun. 1995;16:958–67. https://doi.org/10.1097/00006231-199511000-00012.

115. Yen TC, Chen WP, Chang SL, et al. A comparative study of evaluating renal scars by 99mTc-DMSA planar and SPECT renal scans, intravenous urography, and ultrasonography. Ann Nucl Med. 1994;8:147–52. https://doi.org/10.1007/BF03165020.

116. Takeda M, Katayama Y, Tsutsui T, et al. Value of dimercaptosuccinic acid single photon emission computed tomography and magnetic resonance imaging in detecting renal injury in pediatric patients with vesicoureteral reflux. Comparison with dimercaptosuccinic acid planar scintigraphy and intraven. Eur Urol. 1994;25:320–5.

117. Mouratidis B, Ash JM, Gilday DL. Comparison of planar and SPECT 99Tcm-DMSA scintigraphy for the detection of renal cortical defects in children. Nucl Med Commun. 1993;14:82–6.

118. Sheehy N, Tetrault TA, Zurakowski D, et al. Pediatric 99mTc-DMSA SPECT performed by using iterative reconstruction with isotropic resolution recovery: improved image quality and reduced radiopharmaceutical activity. Radiology. 2009;251:511–6. https://doi.org/10.1148/radiol.2512081440.

119. Piepsz A, Blaufox MD, Gordon I, et al. Consensus on renal cortical scintigraphy in children with urinary tract infection. Scientific Committee of Radionuclides in Nephrourology. Semin Nucl Med. 1999;29:160–74.

120. Itoh K, Yamashita T, Tsukamoto E, et al. Qualitative and quantitative evaluation of renal parenchymal damage by 99mTc-DMSA planar and SPECT scintigraphy. Ann Nucl Med. 1995;9:23–8.

121. Dhull RS, Joshi A, Saha A. Nuclear imaging in pediatric kidney diseases. Indian Pediatr. 2018;55:591–7.

122. Craig JC, Wheeler DM, Irwig L, Howman-Giles RB. How accurate is dimercaptosuccinic acid scintigraphy for the diagnosis of acute pyelonephritis? A meta-analysis of experimental studies. J Nucl Med. 2000;41:986–93.

123. Chiou YY, Wang ST, Tang MJ, et al. Renal fibrosis: prediction from acute pyelonephritis focus volume measured at 99mTc dimercaptosuccinic acid SPECT. Radiology. 2001;221:366–70. https://doi.org/10.1148/radiol.2212010146.

124. Yen TC, Tzen KY, Lin WY, et al. Identification of new renal scarring in repeated episodes of acute pyelonephritis using Tc-99m DMSA renal SPECT. Clin Nucl Med. 1998;23:828–31. https://doi.org/10.1097/00003072-199812000-00008.

125. Yen TC, Chen WP, Chang SL, et al. Technetium-99m-DMSA renal SPECT in diagnosing and monitoring pediatric acute pyelonephritis. J Nucl Med. 1996;37:1349–53.

126. Mettler FA, Guiberteau MJ. Essentials of nuclear medicine imaging. 5th ed. Philadelphia: Saunders Elsevier; 2006.

127. Ell PJ, Gambhir SS. Nuclear medicine in clinical diagnosis and treatment. 3rd ed. Edinburgh: Chuchill Livingstone; 2004.

128. Mandell GA, Cooper JA, Leonard JC, et al. Procedure guideline for diuretic renography in children. Society of Nuclear Medicine. J Nucl Med. 1997;38:1647–50.

129. Rossleigh MA. Renal cortical scintigraphy and diuresis renography in infants and children. J Nucl Med. 2001;42:91–5.

130. McCarthy CS, Sarkar SD, Izquierdo G, et al. Pitfalls and limitations of diuretic renography. Abdom Imaging. 1994;19:78–81.
131. Conway JJ, Maizels M. The "well tempered" diuretic renogram: a standard method to examine the asymptomatic neonate with hydronephrosis or hydroureteronephrosis. A report from combined meetings of The Society for Fetal Urology and members of The Pediatric Nuclear Medicine Counc. J Nucl Med. 1992;33:2047–51.
132. Donoso G, Kuyvenhoven JD, Ham H, Piepsz A. 99mTc-MAG3 diuretic renography in children: a comparison between F0 and F+20. Nucl Med Commun. 2003;24:1189–93. https://doi.org/10.1097/00006231-200311000-00010.
133. Wong DC, Rossleigh MA, Farnsworth RH. F+0 diuresis renography in infants and children. J Nucl Med. 1999;40:1805–11.
134. Ramchandani P, Buckler PM. Imaging of genitourinary trauma. Am J Roentgenol. 2009;192:1514–23.
135. Dane B, Baxter AB, Bernstein MP. Imaging genitourinary trauma. Radiol Clin N Am. 2017;55:321–35. https://doi.org/10.1016/j.rcl.2016.10.007.
136. Fernández-Ibieta M. Renal trauma in pediatrics: a current review. Urology. 2018;113:171–8.
137. Leung VJ, Grima M, Khan N, Jones HR. Early experience with a split-bolus single-pass CT protocol in paediatric trauma. Clin Radiol. 2017;72:497–501. https://doi.org/10.1016/j.crad.2017.01.004.
138. Jeavons C, Hacking C, Beenen LF, Gunn ML. A review of split-bolus single-pass CT in the assessment of trauma patients. Emerg Radiol. 2018;25:367–74. https://doi.org/10.1007/s10140-018-1591-1.
139. Godt JC, Eken T, Schulz A, et al. Triple-split-bolus versus single-bolus CT in abdominal trauma patients: a comparative study. Acta Radiol. 2018;59:1038–44. https://doi.org/10.1177/0284185117752522.
140. Lowe LH, Isuani BH, Heller RM, et al. Pediatric renal masses: Wilms tumor and beyond. Radiographics. 2000;20:1585–603. https://doi.org/10.1148/radiographics.20.6.g00nv051585.
141. Buckley JC, McAninch JW. The diagnosis, management, and outcomes of pediatric renal injuries. Urol Clin North Am. 2006;33(33–40):vi. https://doi.org/10.1016/j.ucl.2005.11.001.
142. McAleer IM, Kaplan GW. Pediatric genitourinary trauma. Urol Clin North Am. 1995;22:177–88.
143. Dacher JN, Boillot B, Eurin D, et al. Rational use of CT in acute pyelonephritis: findings and relationships with reflux. Pediatr Radiol. 1993;23:281–5. https://doi.org/10.1007/BF02010915.
144. Tunaci A, Yekeler E. Multidetector row CT of the kidneys. Eur J Radiol. 2004;52:56–66. https://doi.org/10.1016/j.ejrad.2004.03.033.
145. Volle E, Park W, Kaufmann HJ. MRI examination and monitoring of pediatric patients under sedation. Pediatr Radiol. 1996;26:280–1. https://doi.org/10.1007/BF01372113.
146. Hoffer FA. Magnetic resonance imaging of abdominal masses in the pediatric patient. Semin Ultrasound CT MR. 2005;26:212–23.
147. Rohrschneider WK, Weirich A, Rieden K, et al. US, CT and MR imaging characteristics of nephroblastomatosis. Pediatr Radiol. 1998;28:435–43.
148. Israel GM, Hindman N, Hecht E, Krinsky G. The use of opposed-phase chemical shift MRI in the diagnosis of renal angiomyolipomas. AJR Am J Roentgenol. 2005;184:1868–72.
149. Pretorius ES, Wickstrom ML, Siegelman ES. MR imaging of renal neoplasms. Magn Reson Imaging Clin N Am. 2000;8:813–36.
150. Ramchandani P, Soulen RL, Schnall RI, et al. Impact of magnetic resonance on staging of renal carcinoma. Urology. 1986;27:564–8.
151. Hallscheidt PJ, Fink C, Haferkamp A, et al. Preoperative staging of renal cell carcinoma with inferior vena cava thrombus using multidetector CT and MRI: prospective study with histopathological correlation. J Comput Assist Tomogr. 2005;29:64–8.
152. Kim D, Edelman RR, Kent KC, et al. Abdominal aorta and renal artery stenosis: evaluation with MR angiography. Radiology. 1990;174:727–31.
153. Zhang H, Prince MR. Renal MR angiography. Magn Reson Imaging Clin N Am. 2004;12:487–503, vi. https://doi.org/10.1016/j.mric.2004.03.002.
154. Schoenberg SO, Rieger J, Nittka M, et al. Renal MR angiography: current debates and developments in imaging of renal artery stenosis. Semin Ultrasound CT MR. 2003;24:255–67.
155. Marcos HB, Choyke PL. Magnetic resonance angiography of the kidney. Semin Nephrol. 2000;20:450–5.
156. Vasbinder GBC, Nelemans PJ, Kessels AGH, et al. Accuracy of computed tomographic angiography and magnetic resonance angiography for diagnosing renal artery stenosis. Ann Intern Med. 2004;141:674–82; discussion 682. https://doi.org/10.7326/0003-4819-141-9-200411020-00007.
157. Kovanlikaya A, Okkay N, Cakmakci H, et al. Comparison of MRI and renal cortical scintigraphy findings in childhood acute pyelonephritis: preliminary experience. Eur J Radiol. 2004;49:76–80.
158. Weiser AC, Amukele SA, Leonidas JC, Palmer LS. The role of gadolinium enhanced magnetic resonance imaging for children with suspected acute pyelonephritis. J Urol. 2003;169:2308–11. https://doi.org/10.1097/01.ju.0000068082.91869.29.
159. Leonidas JC, Berdon WE. MR imaging of urinary tract infections in children. Radiology. 1999;210:582–4.
160. Ku JH, Jeon YS, Kim ME, et al. Is there a role for magnetic resonance imaging in renal trauma? Int J Urol. 2001;8:261–7.
161. Marcos HB, Noone TC, Semelka RC. MRI evaluation of acute renal trauma. J Magn Reson Imaging. 1998;8:989–90.
162. Schmid-Tannwald C, Oto A, Reiser MF, Zech CJ. Diffusion-weighted MRI of the abdomen: cur-

rent value in clinical routine. J Magn Reson Imaging. 2013;37:35–47. https://doi.org/10.1002/jmri.23643.

163. Lee CU, Glockner JF, Glaser KJ, et al. MR elastography in renal transplant patients and correlation with renal allograft biopsy: a feasibility study. Acad Radiol. 2012;19:834–41. https://doi.org/10.1016/j.acra.2012.03.003.

164. Serai SD, Otero HJ, Calle-Toro JS, et al. Diffusion tensor imaging of the kidney in healthy controls and in children and young adults with autosomal recessive polycystic kidney disease. Abdom Radiol (New York). 2019; https://doi.org/10.1007/s00261-019-01933-4.

165. Wang Y-T, Li Y-C, Yin L-L, et al. Functional assessment of transplanted kidneys with magnetic resonance imaging. World J Radiol. 2015;7:343–9. https://doi.org/10.4329/wjr.v7.i10.343.

166. Dickerson EC, Dillman JR, Smith EA, et al. Pediatric MR urography: indications, techniques, and approach to review. Radiographics. 2015;35:1208–30. https://doi.org/10.1148/rg.2015140223.

167. Delgado J, Bedoya MA, Adeb M, et al. Optimizing functional MR urography: prime time for a 30-minutes-or-less fMRU. Pediatr Radiol. 2015;45:1333–43. https://doi.org/10.1007/s00247-015-3324-x.

168. Little SB, Jones RA, Grattan-Smith JD. Evaluation of UPJ obstruction before and after pyeloplasty using MR urography. Pediatr Radiol. 2008;38:S106–24.

169. Paulson DF, Glenn JF, Hughes J, et al. Pediatric urolithiasis. J Urol. 1972;108:811–4.

170. Breatnach E, Smith SE. The radiology of renal stones in children. Clin Radiol. 1983;34:59–64. https://doi.org/10.1016/s0009-9260(83)80384-5.

171. Day DL, Scheinman JI, Mahan J. Radiological aspects of primary hyperoxaluria. AJR Am J Roentgenol. 1986;146:395–401. https://doi.org/10.2214/ajr.146.2.395.

172. Patriquin H, Robitaille P. Renal calcium deposition in children: sonographic demonstration of the Anderson-Carr progression. AJR Am J Roentgenol. 1986;146:1253–6.

173. Jevtic V. Imaging of renal osteodystrophy. Eur J Radiol. 2003;46:85–95.

174. Lebowitz RL. Urography in children: when should it be done? 1. Infection. Postgr Med. 1978;64:63–72.

175. Lebowitz RL. Urography in children: when should it be done? 2. Conditions other than infection. Postgr Med. 1978;64:61–70.

176. American Academy of Pediatrics: Committee on Radiology. Excretory urography for evaluation of enuresis. Pediatrics. 1980;65:A49–50.

177. Lebowitz RL. Excretory urography in children. AJR Am J Roentgenol. 1994;163:990.

178. Sourtzis S, Thibeau JF, Damry N, et al. Radiologic investigation of renal colic: unenhanced helical CT compared with excretory urography. AJR Am J Roentgenol. 1999;172:1491–4.

179. McNicholas MM, Raptopoulos VD, Schwartz RK, et al. Excretory phase CT urography for opacification of the urinary collecting system. AJR Am J Roentgenol. 1998;170:1261–7.

180. O'Malley ME, Hahn PF, Yoder IC, et al. Comparison of excretory phase, helical computed tomography with intravenous urography in patients with painless haematuria. Clin Radiol. 2003;58:294–300.

181. Borthne AS, Pierre-Jerome C, Gjesdal KI, et al. Pediatric excretory MR urography: comparative study of enhanced and non-enhanced techniques. Eur Radiol. 2003;13:1423–7. https://doi.org/10.1007/s00330-002-1750-2.

182. Pollack HM, Banner MP. Current status of excretory urography. A premature epitaph? Urol Clin North Am. 1985;12:585–601.

183. Carrico C, Lebowitz RL. Incontinence due to an infrasphincteric ectopic ureter: why the delay in diagnosis and what the radiologist can do about it. Pediatr Radiol. 1998;28:942–9. https://doi.org/10.1007/s002470050506.

184. Smith H, Weaver D, Barjenbruch O, et al. Routine excretory urography in follow-up of superficial transitional cell carcinoma of bladder. Urology. 1989;34:193–6.

185. Kawashima A, Sandler CM, Wasserman NF, et al. Imaging of urethral disease: a pictorial review. Radiographics. 2004;24(Suppl 1):S195–216.

186. Yoder IC, Papanicolaou N. Imaging the urethra in men and women. Urol Radiol. 1992;14:24–8. https://doi.org/10.1007/BF02926897.

187. Pavlica P, Barozzi L, Menchi I. Imaging of male urethra. Eur Radiol. 2003;13:1583–96.

188. Sclafani SJ, Becker JA. Radiologic diagnosis of extrarenal genitourinary trauma. Urol Radiol. 1985;7:201–10.

189. Patel IJ, Rahim S, Davidson JC, et al. Society of Interventional Radiology Consensus Guidelines for the periprocedural management of thrombotic and bleeding risk in patients undergoing percutaneous image-guided interventions—part II : recommendations. J Vasc Interv Radiol. 2019;30:1168–1184.e1. https://doi.org/10.1016/j.jvir.2019.04.017.

190. Pabon-Ramos WM, Dariushnia SR, Walker TG, et al. Quality improvement guidelines for percutaneous nephrostomy. J Vasc Interv Radiol. 2016;27:410–4. https://doi.org/10.1016/j.jvir.2015.11.045.

191. Barnacle AM, Roebuck DJ, Racadio JM. Nephrourology interventions in children. Tech Vasc Interv Radiol. 2010;13:229–37. https://doi.org/10.1053/j.tvir.2010.04.005.

192. Grignon A, Filiatrault D, Homsy Y, et al. Ureteropelvic junction stenosis: antenatal ultrasonographic diagnosis, postnatal investigation, and follow-up. Radiology. 1986;160:649–51. https://doi.org/10.1148/radiology.160.3.3526403.

193. Wood BP, Ben-Ami T, Teele RL, Rabinowitz R. Ureterovesical obstruction and megaloureter: diagnosis by real-time US. Radiology. 1985;156:79–81. https://doi.org/10.1148/radiology.156.1.3890019.

194. Gilsanz V, Miller JH, Reid BS. Ultrasonic characteristics of posterior urethral valves. Radiology.

1982;145:143–5. https://doi.org/10.1148/radiology.145.1.7122871.

195. Nguyen HT, Benson CB, Bromley B, et al. Multidisciplinary consensus on the classification of prenatal and postnatal urinary tract dilation (UTD classification system). J Pediatr Urol. 2014; https://doi.org/10.1016/j.jpurol.2014.10.002.

196. Nelson CP, Lee RS, Trout AT, et al. The association of postnatal urinary tract dilation risk score with clinical outcomes. J Pediatr Urol. 2019;15:341.e1–6. https://doi.org/10.1016/j.jpurol.2019.05.001.

197. Hains DS, Bates CM, Ingraham S, Schwaderer AL. Management and etiology of the unilateral multicystic dysplastic kidney: a review. Pediatr Nephrol. 2009;24:233–41. https://doi.org/10.1007/s00467-008-0828-8.

198. Cardona-Grau D, Kogan BA. Update on multicystic dysplastic kidney. Curr Urol Rep. 2015;16:67. https://doi.org/10.1007/s11934-015-0541-7.

199. Mascatello VJ, Smith EH, Carrera GF, et al. Ultrasonic evaluation of the obstructed duplex kidney. AJR Am J Roentgenol. 1977;129:113–20.

200. El-Feky MM. Weigert-Meyer law. https://radiopaedia.org/articles/weigert-meyer-law. Accessed 25 Jun 2021.

201. Nussbaum AR, Dorst JP, Jeffs RD, et al. Ectopic ureter and ureterocele: their varied sonographic manifestations. Radiology. 1986;159:227–35.

202. Griffin J, Jennings C, MacErlean D. Ultrasonic evaluation of simple and ectopic ureteroceles. Clin Radiol. 1983;34:55–7. https://doi.org/10.1016/s0009-9260(83)80380-8.

203. Hwang JY, Shin JH, Lee YJ, et al. Percutaneous nephrostomy placement in infants and young children. Diagn Interv Imaging. 2018;99:157–62. https://doi.org/10.1016/j.diii.2017.07.002.

204. Laurin S, Sandström S, Ivarsson H. Percutaneous nephrostomy in infants and children. Acad Radiol. 2000;7:526–9. https://doi.org/10.1016/S1076-6332(00)80325-6.

205. Stanley P, Diament MJ. Pediatric percutaneous nephrostomy: experience with 50 patients. J Urol. 1986;135:1223–6. https://doi.org/10.1016/S0022-5347(17)46046-0.

206. Shellikeri S, Daulton R, Sertic M, et al. Pediatric percutaneous nephrostomy: a multicenter experience. J Vasc Interv Radiol. 2018;29 https://doi.org/10.1016/j.jvir.2017.09.017.

207. Irving HC, Arthur RJ, Thomas DFM. Percutaneous nephrostomy in paediatrics. Clin Radiol. 1987; https://doi.org/10.1016/S0009-9260(87)80057-0.

208. Koral K, Saker MC, Morello FP, et al. Conventional versus modified technique for percutaneous nephrostomy in newborns and young infants. J Vasc Interv Radiol. 2003;14:113–6. https://doi.org/10.1097/01.RVI.0000052301.26939.20.

209. Yavascan O, Aksu N, Erdogan H, et al. Original article: Percutaneous nephrostomy in children: diagnostic and therapeutic importance. Pediatr Nephrol. 2005;20:768–72. https://doi.org/10.1007/s00467-005-1845-5.

210. Back SJ, Hartung EA, Ntoulia A, Darge K. Imaging in pediatric urinary tract infections. J Pediatr Infect Dis. 2017;12:72–88. https://doi.org/10.1055/s-0037-1599121.

211. National Institute for Health and Care Excellence. Urinary tract infection in under 16s: diagnosis and management. 2007. https://www.nice.org.uk/guidance/cg54. Accessed 22 Sept 2016.

212. Stein R, Dogan HS, Hoebeke P, et al. Urinary tract infections in children: EAU/ESPU guidelines. Eur Urol. 2015;67:546–58. https://doi.org/10.1016/j.eururo.2014.11.007.

213. Tsai JD, Chang SJ, Lin CC, Yang SSD. Incomplete bladder emptying is associated with febrile urinary tract infections in infants. J Pediatr Urol. 2014;10:1222–6. https://doi.org/10.1016/j.jpurol.2014.06.013.

214. Gordon ZN, McLeod DJ, Becknell B, et al. Uroepithelial thickening on sonography improves detection of vesicoureteral reflux in children with first febrile urinary tract infection. J Urol. 2015;194:1074–9. https://doi.org/10.1016/j.juro.2015.05.001.

215. Pickworth FE, Carlin JB, Ditchfield MR, et al. Sonographic measurement of renal enlargement in children with acute pyelonephritis and time needed for resolution: implications for renal growth assessment. Am J Roentgenol. 1995;165:405–8. https://doi.org/10.2214/ajr.165.2.7618567.

216. Farmer KD, Gellett LR, Dubbins PA. The sonographic appearance of acute focal pyelonephritis 8 years experience. Clin Radiol. 2002;57:483–7. https://doi.org/10.1053/crad.2002.0935.

217. Dacher JN, Avni F, François A, et al. Renal sinus hyperechogenicity in acute pyelonephritis: description and pathological correlation. Pediatr Radiol. 1999;29:179–82. https://doi.org/10.1007/s002470050566.

218. Cheng CH, Tsau YK, Hsu SY, Lee TL. Effective ultrasonographic predictor for the diagnosis of acute lobar nephronia. Pediatr Infect Dis J. 2004;23:11–4. https://doi.org/10.1097/01.inf.0000105202.57991.3e.

219. Shaikh N, Craig JC, Rovers MM, et al. Identification of children and adolescents at risk for renal scarring after a first urinary tract infection: a meta-analysis with individual patient data. JAMA Pediatr. 2014;168:893–900. https://doi.org/10.1001/jamapediatrics.2014.637.

220. Zulfiqar M, Ubilla CV, Nicola R, Menias CO. Imaging of renal infections and inflammatory disease. Radiol Clin N Am. 2020;58:909–23.

221. Wolin EA, Hartman DS, Olson JR. Nephrographic and pyelographic analysis of CT urography: differential diagnosis. Am J Roentgenol. 2013;200:1197–203.

222. Vivier PH, Sallem A, Beurdeley M, et al. MRI and suspected acute pyelonephritis in children:

222. comparison of diffusion-weighted imaging with gadolinium-enhanced T1-weighted imaging. Eur Radiol. 2014;24:19–25. https://doi.org/10.1007/s00330-013-2971-2.

223. Linder BJ, Granberg CF. Pediatric renal abscesses: a contemporary series. J Pediatr Urol. 2016;12:99. e1–6. https://doi.org/10.1016/j.jpurol.2015.05.037.

224. Seguias L, Srinivasan K, Mehta A. Pediatric renal abscess: a 10-year single-center retrospective analysis. Hosp Pediatr. 2012;2:161–6. https://doi.org/10.1542/hpeds.2012-0010.

225. Khanna G, Naranjo A, Hoffer F, et al. Detection of preoperative wilms tumor rupture with CT: a report from the Children's Oncology Group. Radiology. 2013;266:610–7. https://doi.org/10.1148/radiol.12120670.

226. Khanna G, Rosen N, Anderson JR, et al. Evaluation of diagnostic performance of CT for detection of tumor thrombus in children with Wilms tumor: a report from the Children's Oncology Group. Pediatr Blood Cancer. 2012;58:551–5. https://doi.org/10.1002/pbc.23222.

227. McDonald K, Duffy P, Chowdhury T, McHugh K. Added value of abdominal cross-sectional imaging (CT or MRI) in staging of Wilms' tumours. Clin Radiol. 2013;68:16–20. https://doi.org/10.1016/j.crad.2012.05.006.

228. Metzger ML, Dome JS. Current therapy for Wilms' tumor. Oncologist. 2005;10:815–26. https://doi.org/10.1634/theoncologist.10-10-815.

229. Acord MR, Cahill AM, Durand R, et al. Contrast-enhanced ultrasound in pediatric interventional radiology. Pediatr Radiol. 2021; https://doi.org/10.1007/s00247-020-04853-4.

230. Ruff S, Bittman M, Lobko I, et al. Emergency embolization of a Wilms' tumor for life-threatening hemorrhage prior to nephrectomy. J Pediatr Surg Case Rep. 2014;2:280–3. https://doi.org/10.1016/j.epsc.2014.05.013.

231. Bholah R, Bunchman TE. Review of pediatric pheochromocytoma and paraganglioma. Front Pediatr. 2017;5:1–14. https://doi.org/10.3389/fped.2017.00155.

232. Yamakado K, Tanaka N, Nakagawa T, et al. Renal angiomyolipoma: relationship between tumor size, aneurysm formation, and rupture. Radiology. 2002;225:78–82.

233. Kiefer RM, Stavropoulos SW. The role of interventional radiology techniques in the management of renal angiomyolipomas. Curr Urol Rep. 2017;18 https://doi.org/10.1007/s11934-017-0687-6.

234. Warncke JC, Brodie KE, Grantham EC, et al. Pediatric renal angiomyolipomas in tuberous sclerosis complex. J Urol. 2017;197:500–6. https://doi.org/10.1016/j.juro.2016.09.082.

235. Williams JM, Racadio JM, Johnson ND, et al. Embolization of renal angiomyolipomata in patients with tuberous sclerosis complex. Am J Kidney Dis. 2005; https://doi.org/10.1053/j.ajkd.2005.09.028.

236. Ewalt DH, Diamond N, Rees C, et al. Long-term outcome of transcatheter embolization of renal angiomyolipomas due to tuberous sclerosis complex. J Urol. 2005;174:1764–6. https://doi.org/10.1097/01.ju.0000177497.31986.64.

237. Johnson SC, Graham S, D'Agostino H, et al. Percutaneous renal cryoablation of angiomyolipomas in patients with solitary kidneys. Urology. 2009;74:1246–9. https://doi.org/10.1016/j.urology.2008.09.005.

238. Shingleton WB, Sewell PE. Percutaneous renal tumor cryoablation with magnetic resonance imaging guidance. J Urol. 2001;165:773–6.

239. Brown SL, Elder JS, Spirnak JP. Are pediatric patients more susceptible to major renal injury from blunt trauma? A comparative study. J Urol. 1998;160:138–40. https://doi.org/10.1016/S0022-5347(01)63071-4.

240. Stein JP, Kaji DM, Eastham J, et al. Blunt renal trauma in the pediatric population: indications for radiographic evaluation. Urology. 1994;44:406–10.

241. John SD. Trends in pediatric emergency imaging. Radiol Clin N Am. 1999;37:995–1034, vi.

242. Rose JS. Ultrasound in abdominal trauma. Emerg Med Clin North Am. 2004;22:581–99, vii.

243. Soudack M, Epelman M, Maor R, et al. Experience with focused abdominal sonography for trauma (FAST) in 313 pediatric patients. J Clin Ultrasound. 2004;32:53–61.

244. Taylor GA, Sivit CJ. Posttraumatic peritoneal fluid: is it a reliable indicator of intraabdominal injury in children? J Pediatr Surg. 1995;30:1644–8.

245. Breyer BN, McAninch JW, Elliott SP, Master VA. Minimally invasive endovascular techniques to treat acute renal hemorrhage. J Urol. 2008;179:2248–53. https://doi.org/10.1016/j.juro.2008.01.104.

246. Lee JN, Lim JK, Woo MJ, et al. Predictive factors for conservative treatment failure in grade IV pediatric blunt renal trauma. J Pediatr Urol. 2016;12:93.e1–7. https://doi.org/10.1016/j.jpurol.2015.06.014.

247. McClung C, Hotaling JM, Wang J, et al. Contemporary trends in the immediate surgical management of renal trauma using a national database. J Trauma Acute Care Surg. 2013;75:1–10. https://doi.org/10.1097/TA.0b013e3182a53ac2.Contemporary.

248. Jacobs MA, Hotaling JM, Mueller BA, et al. Conservative management vs early surgery for high grade pediatric renal trauma—do nephrectomy rates differ? J Urol. 2012;187:1817–21. https://doi.org/10.1016/j.juro.2011.12.095.

249. Umbreit EC, Routh JC, Husmann DA. Nonoperative management of nonvascular grade IV blunt renal trauma in children: meta-analysis and systematic review. Urology. 2009;74:579–82. https://doi.org/10.1016/j.urology.2009.04.049.

250. Au JK, Tan X, Sidani M, et al. Imaging characteristics associated with failure of nonoperative management in high-grade pediatric blunt renal trauma. J Pediatr Urol. 2016;12:294.e1–6. https://doi.org/10.1016/j.jpurol.2016.02.021.

251. Hotaling JM, Sorensen MD, Smith TG, et al. Analysis of diagnostic angiography and angioembolization in the acute management of renal trauma using a national data set. J Urol. 2011;185:1316–20. https://doi.org/10.1016/j.juro.2010.12.003.

252. Wyszyńska T, Cichocka E, Wieteska-Klimczak A, et al. A single pediatric center experience with 1025 children with hypertension. Acta Paediatr. 1992;81:244–6. https://doi.org/10.1111/j.1651-2227.1992.tb12213.x.

253. Tullus K, Roebuck DJ, McLaren CA, Marks SD. Imaging in the evaluation of renovascular disease. Pediatr Nephrol. 2010;25:1049–56.

254. Dillman JR, Smith EA, Coley BD. Ultrasound imaging of renin-mediated hypertension. Pediatr Radiol. 2017;47:1116–24. https://doi.org/10.1007/s00247-017-3840-y.

255. Castelli PK, Dillman JR, Kershaw DB, et al. Renal sonography with Doppler for detecting suspected pediatric renin-mediated hypertension—is it adequate? Pediatr Radiol. 2014;44:42–9. https://doi.org/10.1007/s00247-013-2785-z.

256. Eklöf H, Ahlström H, Magnusson A, et al. A prospective comparison of duplex ultrasonography, captopril renography, MRA, and CTA in assessing renal artery stenosis. Acta Radiol. 2006;47:764–74. https://doi.org/10.1080/02841850600849092.

257. Trautmann A, Roebuck DJ, McLaren CA, et al. Non-invasive imaging cannot replace formal angiography in the diagnosis of renovascular hypertension. Pediatr Nephrol. 2017;32:495–502. https://doi.org/10.1007/s00467-016-3501-7.

258. Son JS. Successful cutting balloon angioplasty in a child with resistant renal artery stenosis. BMC Res Notes. 2015;8:670. https://doi.org/10.1186/s13104-015-1673-z.

259. Srinivasan A, Krishnamurthy G, Fontalvo-Herazo L, et al. Angioplasty for renal artery stenosis in pediatric patients: an 11-year retrospective experience. J Vasc Interv Radiol. 2010;21:1672–80. https://doi.org/10.1016/j.jvir.2010.07.012.

260. Morosetti D, Chiocchi M, De Crescenzo F, et al. Bilateral renal artery stenosis treated with drug-eluting balloon angioplasty in unique treatment. Radiol Case Rep. 2019;14:242–5. https://doi.org/10.1016/j.radcr.2018.10.033.

261. Teigen CL, Mitchell SE, Venbrux AC, et al. Segmental renal artery embolization for treatment of pediatric renovascular hypertension. J Vasc Interv Radiol. 1992;3:111–7. https://doi.org/10.1016/S1051-0443(92)72202-7.

262. Zhu G, He F, Gu Y, et al. Angioplasty for pediatric renovascular hypertension: a 13-year experience. Diagn Interv Radiol. 2014;20:285–92. https://doi.org/10.5152/dir.2014.13208.

263. Kari JA, Roebuck DJ, McLaren CA, et al. Angioplasty for renovascular hypertension in 78 children. Arch Dis Child. 2015;100:474–8. https://doi.org/10.1136/archdischild-2013-305886.

264. Eliason JL, Coleman DM, Criado E, et al. Remedial operations for failed endovascular therapy of 32 renal artery stenoses in 24 children. Pediatr Nephrol. 2016;31:809–17. https://doi.org/10.1007/s00467-015-3275-3.

265. Riccabona M, Avni FE, Damasio MB, et al. ESPR Uroradiology Task Force and ESUR Paediatric Working Group—Imaging recommendations in paediatric uroradiology, part V: childhood cystic kidney disease, childhood renal transplantation and contrast-enhanced ultrasonography in children. Pediatr Radiol. 2012;42:1275–83. https://doi.org/10.1007/s00247-012-2436-9.

266. Gimpel C, Avni FE, Bergmann C, et al. Perinatal diagnosis, management, and follow-up of cystic renal diseases. JAMA Pediatr. 2018;172:74. https://doi.org/10.1001/jamapediatrics.2017.3938.

267. Gimpel C, Avni EFF, Breysem L, et al. Imaging of kidney cysts and cystic kidney diseases in children: an International Working Group Consensus Statement. Radiology. 2019;290:181243. https://doi.org/10.1148/radiol.2018181243.

268. Bosniak MA. The Bosniak renal cyst classification: 25 years later. Radiology. 2012;262:781–5.

269. Karmazyn B, Tawadros A, Delaney LR, et al. Ultrasound classification of solitary renal cysts in children. J Pediatr Urol. 2015;11:149.e1–6. https://doi.org/10.1016/j.jpurol.2015.03.001.

270. Peng Y, Jia L, Sun N, et al. Assessment of cystic renal masses in children: comparison of multislice computed tomography and ultrasound imaging using the Bosniak classification system. Eur J Radiol. 2010;75:287–92. https://doi.org/10.1016/j.ejrad.2010.05.035.

271. Wallis MC, Lorenzo AJ, Farhat WA, et al. Risk assessment of incidentally detected complex renal cysts in children: potential role for a modification of the Bosniak classification. J Urol. 2008;180:317–21. https://doi.org/10.1016/j.juro.2008.03.063.

272. Stuck KJ, Koff SA, Silver TM. Ultrasonic features of multicystic dysplastic kidney: expanded diagnostic criteria. Radiology. 1982;143:217–21.

273. Patriquin HB, O'Regan S. Medullary sponge kidney in childhood. AJR Am J Roentgenol. 1985;145:315–9.

274. McHugh K, Stringer DA, Hebert D, Babiak CA. Simple renal cysts in children: diagnosis and follow-up with US. Radiology. 1991;178:383–5.

275. Cadnapaphornchai MA, McFann K, Strain JD, et al. Prospective change in renal volume and function in children with ADPKD. Clin J Am Soc Nephrol. 2009;4:820–9. https://doi.org/10.2215/CJN.02810608.

276. Irazabal MV, Rangel LJ, Bergstralh EJ, et al. Imaging classification of autosomal dominant polycystic kidney disease: a simple model for selecting patients for clinical trials. J Am Soc Nephrol. 2015;26:160–72. https://doi.org/10.1681/ASN.2013101138.

277. Traubici J, Daneman A. High-resolution renal sonography in children with autosomal recessive

polycystic kidney disease. AJR Am J Roentgenol. 2005;184:1630–3.

278. Srinath A, Shneider BL. Congenital hepatic fibrosis and autosomal recessive polycystic kidney disease. J Pediatr Gastroenterol Nutr. 2012;54:580–7. https://doi.org/10.1097/MPG.0b013e31824711b7.

279. Fowler KAB, Locken JA, Duchesne JH, Williamson MR. US for detecting renal calculi with nonenhanced CT as a reference standard. Radiology. 2002;222:109–13. https://doi.org/10.1148/radiol.2221010453.

280. Wu DSH, Stoller ML. Indinavir urolithiasis. Curr Opin Urol. 2000;10:557–61.

281. Hidas G, Eliahou R, Duvdevani M, et al. Determination of renal stone composition with dual-energy CT: in vivo analysis and comparison with X-ray diffraction. Radiology. 2010;257:394–401. https://doi.org/10.1148/radiol.10100249.

282. El-Assmy A, El-Nahas AR, Abou-El-Ghar ME, et al. Kidney stone size and Hounsfield units predict successful shockwave lithotripsy in children. Urology. 2013;81:880–4. https://doi.org/10.1016/j.urology.2012.12.012.

283. Wilson DA, Wenzl JE, Altshuler GP. Ultrasound demonstration of diffuse cortical nephrocalcinosis in a case of primary hyperoxaluria. AJR Am J Roentgenol. 1979;132:659–61. https://doi.org/10.2214/ajr.132.4.659.

284. Fleming JS, Zivanovic MA, Blake GM, et al. Guidelines for the measurement of glomerular filtration rate using plasma sampling. Nucl Med Commun. 2004;25:759–69. https://doi.org/10.1097/01.mnm.0000136715.71820.4a.

Molecular Diagnosis of Genetic Diseases of the Kidney: Primer for Pediatric Nephrologists

4

Aoife Waters and Mathieu Lemaire

Introduction

Over the past decade, remarkable advances have been made in our understanding of the human genome through the development of genotyping arrays and next-generation sequencing techniques. These technological advances have allowed us to examine the consequences of various types of genomic variations on the phenotype of patients in an unparalleled manner. Identification of mutations in novel genes associated with rare renal diseases has forced dramatic pathophysiological revisions owing to the discovery of links to unexpected biochemical pathways or structural scaffolds. These provide not only a firm molecular diagnosis for hitherto "idiopathic" conditions, but also offer hope for new therapeutic strategies for diseases that would otherwise have an unfavourable prognosis. The last few years have witnessed great improvements in our understanding of the role of common genetic variation in the pathogenesis of complex renal diseases, although the promises of clinical utility are far from reality. In this chapter, we will outline developments made in various fields related to genomic medicine, with a particular emphasis on how these will translate into the daily clinical practice of pediatric nephrologists.

General Genetic/Genomic Concepts

Deoxyribonucleic Acid (DNA)

In 1962, the Nobel Prize in Medicine was awarded to Watson and Crick together with Maurice Wilkins for their discovery of the structure of deoxyribonucleic acid (DNA). DNA is a critical participant in the execution and regulation of biological processes that are critical for living organisms to develop and survive. Constituting the double helix structure of DNA are two twisting, paired strands that are packed full of information via the systematic arrangement of four nucleotide bases—adenine (A), thymine (T), guanine (G), and cytosine (C)—the "genetic alphabet" [2]. Opposite strands anneal together specifically, via the pairing of bases: A binds to T, and C to G. If one strand's nucleotide sequence reads ATTCGG, the other strand will read TAAGCC; we refer to these as the positive and negative strands, respectively.

A. Waters
Paediatric Nephrology, Great Ormond Street Hospital, London, UK
e-mail: Aoife.Waters@gosh.nhs.uk

M. Lemaire (✉)
Nephrology, The Hospital for Sick Children, Toronto, ON, Canada
e-mail: mathieu.lemaire@sickkids.ca

© The Author(s), under exclusive license to Springer Nature Switzerland AG 2023
F. Schaefer, L. A. Greenbaum (eds.), *Pediatric Kidney Disease*,
https://doi.org/10.1007/978-3-031-11665-0_4

Gene

A gene refers to segments of DNA that carry the sequencing code for all building blocks necessary for cells to thrive. Two sequential processes are key: transcription and translation. Transcription is the process by which a ribonucleic acid (RNA) strand is made to match exactly the nucleotides that make up a particular gene. It is critical to preserve both nucleotide identity and order because it is a key determinant of the function of RNAs. The most well-known RNA molecule made this way is the messenger RNA (mRNA): it is the key player in the translation (or encoding) of proteins. During this process, which occurs in ribosomes, the sequence of mRNA molecules is read in triplets of nucleotides, known as codons, and this specifies which amino acid we add next during protein synthesis

(Fig. 4.1). The recent discovery of a dizzying array of noncoding RNA molecules has added an unexpected level of complexity: the RNA world is much more than mRNAs [3]. We are only starting to understand how these noncoding RNAs carry cellular functions by themselves, without requiring translation into proteins [4].

Genome

A genome represents an organism's complete DNA sequence. The Human Genome Project, an international effort to sequence the entire human genome (6 billion nucleotides), was completed in 2001 after more than 10 years of work and billions in research funding [5]. DNA from 13 anonymous individuals of European descent was used to build what is now referred to as the human ref-

1st base	2nd base								3rd base
	T		C		A		G		
T	TTT	(Phe/F) Phenylalanine	TCT	(Ser/S) Serine	TAT	(Tyr/Y) Tyrosine	TGT	(Cys/C) Cysteine	T
	TTC		TCC		TAC		TGC		C
	TTA		TCA		TAA	(X) STOP	TGA	(X) STOP	A
	TTG		TCG		TAG		TGG	(Trp/W) Tryptophan	G
C	CTT	(Leu/L) Leucine	CCT	(Pro/P) Proline	CAT	(His/H) Histidine	CGT	(Arg/R) Arginine	T
	CTC		CCC		CAC		CGC		C
	CTA		CCA		CAA	(Gln/Q) Glutamine	CGA		A
	CTG		CCG		CAG		CGG		G
A	ATT	(Ile/I) Isoleucine	ACT	(Thr/T) Threonine	AAT	(Asn/N) Asparagine	AGT	(Ser/S) Serine	T
	ATC		ACC		AAC		AGC		C
	ATA		ACA		AAA	(Lys/K) Lysine	AGA	(Arg/R) Arginine	A
	ATG	(Met/M) Methionine	ACG		AAG		AGG		G
G	GTT	(Val/V) Valine	GCT	(Ala/A) Alanine	GAT	(Asp/D) Aspartic Acid	GGT	(Gly/G) Glycine	T
	GTC		GCC		GAC		GGC		C
	GTA		GCA		GAA	(Glu/E) Glutamic Acid	GGA		A
	GTG		GCG		GAG		GGG		G

Amino acid properties: **Nonpolar** | **Polar** | **Basic** | **Acidic** | **Nonsense**

Fig. 4.1 DNA codons and associated amino acids. The three nucleotides (codons) that make up the 20 different amino acids (and stop signal) are presented, along with the single-letter database codes. To obtain the various codons, one simply needs to integrate the value of the first (left), second (top) and third (right) bases. To obtain the RNA codons, Key properties of amino acids are indicated in the color legend at the bottom. (Figure credits: Modified from Wikipedia, https://en.wikipedia.org/wiki/DNA_and_RNA_codon_tables#Translation_table_1)

erence genome. In principle, the human reference genome should be a repository containing a representative whole-genome sequence for a prototypical human. After the publication of the draft sequence in 2001 [6], a high-quality reference sequence followed in 2004 [7]; the Genome Reference Consortium continues to improve the quality and coverage of low-complexity, repetitive, and hard to resolve regions [8].

While the exact number of genes remains unknown, most experts estimate that there are ~20,000 protein-coding genes that occupy about 1% of the human genome. Other constituents of the genome include RNA genes, regulatory sequences, and repetitive DNA sequences. Ongoing research by the Encyclopedia of DNA Elements (ENCODE) project suggests that ~80% of the human genome is functionally active: non-protein-coding DNA must be implicated in a significant number of regulatory processes including gene-gene regulation, gene-protein interactions and the transcription of nontranslated RNA [9].

Genetic vs. Genomic

It is now common, but incorrect, to use the terms "Genetic" and "Genomic" as synonyms. The former refers to investigations restricted to a small number of genes at once, while the latter applies to tests that involve genome-wide interrogation.

Other Omics

Many other "-omics" sciences are actively developed in parallel to genomics, such as proteomics [10], transcriptomics [11], epigenomics [12], and metabolomics [13]. New forms of -omics are still emerging: for example, epitranscriptomics, which is the study of mechanisms that regulate RNA functions [14], is relevant to novel forms of nephrotic syndrome [15, 16]. The new frontier is to study one or more omics patterns at single-cell resolution [17]: it is widely anticipated that it is a key development to better understand the patho-

physiology of many kidney diseases [18]. Eventually, these methods will be combined to provide holistic insights into organ or cell functions [19]. It is, however, beyond the scope of this chapter to cover these methods in any detail.

Online Resources

Sources	URLs
MIT Pedigree	https://peds-renomics. clinic/MIT-pedigree
HapMap	http://hapmap.ncbi.nlm. nih.gov
Broad Institute's Primer on medical and population genetics	https://peds-renomics. clinic/ BI-Primer-Genetics

Variations in the Genome

Several different classes of DNA sequence variations are observed when comparing the genomes of different individuals. A variation may also be classified as a mutation, which is defined as a change of the nucleotide sequence when compared to the human reference genome; a mutation is not necessarily pathogenic. These alterations may be caused by a number of mechanisms, including unrepaired DNA damage (caused by mutagens such as radiation or chemicals), DNA polymerase errors during replication, or insertion or deletion of DNA segments by mobile genetic elements. Below, we will describe the different kinds of mutations after a short discussion on their key characteristics. Implicit to these discussions is that these mutations are all germline, which means that all cells of an individual carry the mutation, and this mutation is passed on to subsequent generations according to Mendel's law of allele segregation. This contrasts with somatic mutations that are only present in a restricted subset of cells. The concept of somatic mosaicism will not be covered further here: it has relevance well beyond that of cancer genetics [20], most notably in nephrology, for autosomal dominant polycystic kidney disease [21].

How to Assess Genomic Variations

One of the key features that will allow genomic medicine to flourish in the clinic is the ability to reliably assess whether a given mutation is likely to affect protein function or not. When appraising a particular mutation, there are a number of important characteristics to consider systematically before deciding on its pathogenic potential [22]. A recent review reveals that the nephrology literature is replete with spurious gene-disease associations, or "diagnoses of uncertain significance" [23]. Below, we will briefly describe four such characteristics, including frequency, location, mutation type, and conservation. This section introduces many key concepts that will be used frequently throughout this chapter. Please refer to Fig. 4.2 for an illustration of the various concepts.

Is the Allele Common or Rare?

The first consideration is to assess how frequently the mutation is observed in the general population. The minor allele frequency (MAF) is the most useful piece of information for this. It is calculated by dividing the number of mutant alleles in a sample by the number of wild-type alleles (each individual has two alleles since humans are diploid organisms). MAF data for common variants is easily retrieved from online databases, such as dbSNPs. The MAF for rare and common variants should be less than 1% and between 1% and 49%, respectively; the major allele frequency is usually more than 50%. This concept is important because common mutations are expected to have a low probability to cause rare conditions. The frequency of deleterious alleles is expected to remain low in the general population because of reduced reproductive fitness and natural selection.

Coding vs. Non-coding Variants

The second distinction relates to the location of the mutation in the genome: is it in a region that is involved in protein coding or not? Because we have rich knowledge about protein-coding DNA (exons) and their functions, most studies and clinical tests tend to focus on these regions of the genome, collectively known as the exome. "Non-coding" DNA, which is composed of intronic and intergenic segments, does not contain only "junk" DNA as this is where one finds a host of regula-

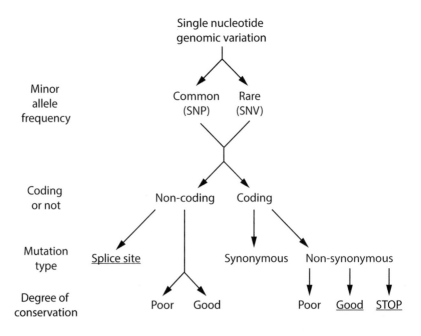

Fig. 4.2 An approach to assess a mutation. We present a simple workflow to assess mutations that include four steps. These are based on allele frequency, mutation location and type and degree of conservation. Underlined terminal nodes indicate the mutations most likely to cause human disease

tory elements such as promoters, enhancers, silencers and insulators, as well as microRNAs. There is mounting evidence that there is in fact no such thing as junk DNA as 80% of the entire genome plays an important role one way or another [24].

There is one type of intronic mutation that has a special status in clinical genetics: splice site mutations that change key nucleotides in one of the specific sites that are critical for splicing introns during the processing of precursor mRNA into mature mRNA. Abolishment of a splicing site results in the retention of introns in mature mRNA molecules and leads to the production of aberrant proteins (for an example relevant to nephrology, see Mele et al. [25]).

Mutation Types

Third, it is important to determine if an exonic mutation will result in the insertion of different amino acids in the encoded protein, in which case it is referred to as a nonsynonymous substitution (see Fig. 4.3). These changes are important in clinical genetics because they are most likely to alter the function of the encoded protein. To determine if a nonsynonymous mutation may be pathologic, one needs to assess if the physicochemical properties of the original amino acid are preserved (size, charge, and polarity) and the degree of amino acid conservation (see next section).

There are three instances where a substitution will be expected to be deleterious without requiring these analyses. First, changing any amino acid to a nonsense (or stop) codon will result in the production of a truncated protein. Second, substituting a start codon (which is always a methionine) for any other amino acid will cause problems because protein translation cannot be initiated properly: no protein is produced. Third, any mutations at a stop codon will also cause problems because the protein made will be longer than the wild type, and as a result, it will include extra amino acids that may interfere with the proper function of the protein.

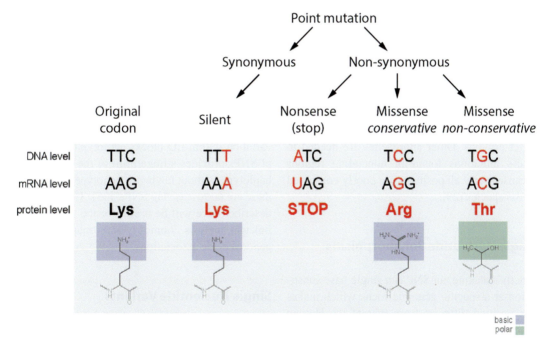

Fig. 4.3 Different types of point mutations. This figure illustrates how a single point mutation in a given codon can change the encoded amino acid in many ways. A conservative missense mutation is one that keeps some or all of the original amino acid properties intact. (Figure credits: Modified from Wikipedia, https://en.wikipedia.org/wiki/Synonymous_substitution)

Mutations that do not result in an amino acid change are referred to as synonymous variants (this is possible because many amino acids are generated from different codons; see Fig. 4.1). They are also known as silent mutations since in most instances (but not always [26]), they have little to no effect on the function of the encoded proteins.

Degree of Conservation

Finally, one needs to determine if the mutation occurs at a genomic position that is highly conserved when compared to the genomes of other species. It is possible to make this comparison rapidly since we have the entire genomic sequences of many different species (e.g., from humans to mice, frogs, and fruit flies). This analysis is most meaningful for coding segments because one can directly compare the amino acid sequences of the same protein in different organisms (orthologs) [27].

Such comparisons support the notion that the degree of interspecies amino acid variation is indirectly proportional to the functional importance of the amino acid. For example, key residues within the catalytic domain of protein kinases are conserved as a functional unit among all kinases of any species [28]. Kinases are enzymes that transfer a phosphate group from ATP to tyrosine, serine, or threonine residues on target proteins. Other approaches are needed to assess mutations found in noncoding regions because nearly all positions are poorly conserved across species [29].

Single Nucleotide Polymorphisms

Strictly speaking, an SNP is a single base substitution at a specific genomic locus which makes this position different from that of the Human Reference Genome [30]. However, common usage has SNPs also defined as a "common variant" on the basis of a population minor allele frequency of >1%. Single nucleotide mutations may occur anywhere in the genome. That the bulk of SNPs are located in noncoding segments is hardly surprising since they constitute ~99% of the genome. As discussed above, the vast majority of SNPs have long been thought to be benign because they are so common. However, the lack of clear clinical significance does not mean that SNPs are useless far from it.

Over the years, geneticists have long used a variety of genetic markers to study human genetic variation with greater depth and accuracy. SNPs emerged as the genetic marker of choice around 2000. It was preceded by three other "generations" of markers: restriction length fragment polymorphisms (~1980), variable number of tandem repeats (~1985), and short tandem repeat polymorphism (~1989) [31]. The rise of SNPs as markers is in large part due to the momentum created by the HapMap project [32], which aimed to catalogue millions of SNPs in hundreds of subjects from many ethnicities [33]. This resulted in marked improvements in the reliability, efficiency, and cost of high-throughput SNP genotyping (see the section below).

SNPs proved to be invaluable to study haplotype patterns in humans. Haplotypes are genomic segments on a chromosome that are defined by a combination of alleles that are consistently inherited together. This phenomenon is termed linkage disequilibrium (LD) [34] since these alleles are linked to each other more often than not because recombination events occur outside of the LD block. Because of the low diversity of genetic variation within LD blocks, genotyping a subset of SNPs provides a fingerprint of the underlying haplotype without having to genotype all alleles: these are known as "tag SNPs"[35]. The concepts described here will be useful for the sections on linkage analysis, homozygosity mapping, and genome-wide associations.

Single Nucleotide Variants

Single nucleotide variants (SNV) are often defined as alleles with a minor allele frequency of <1% in the general population. SNVs are found throughout the genome, both in noncoding (introns, intergenic segments) and coding (exons) regions. As described earlier, coding SNVs exist in two "flavours": synonymous and nonsynonymous variants. Since there is almost no selective pressure on synonymous variants, they are expected to be scattered anywhere in the genome. In contrast, nonsynonymous variants are often enriched in well-conserved amino acid positions owing to the strong selective pressure they sustain. As a result, it is not surprising that highly penetrant disease-causing variants in monogenic conditions are overwhelmingly nonsynonymous SNVs. It is commonplace to refer to disease-causing SNVs as pathogenic mutations [36]: this topic will be covered in the section on Mendelian conditions.

When dealing with a rare condition, one needs to determine whether the mutation is truly rare (or novel) by interrogating a variety of publicly available variant databases such as dbSNPs [37]. Most of these resources have been generated using samples from subjects of European descent. As a result, interpretation of variants from patients that are not "European" is problematic because usually, one does not have access to the optimal control group. This phenomenon, called population stratification, makes the search for pathogenic mutations more challenging because variants that are common in one population may be rare (or even absent) in another [38]. Hence, the validity of the interpretation of pathogenicity for a given variant is deeply impacted by the patient's ethnic background. The magnitude of this problem will be lessened as more non-European subjects are sequenced through various efforts worldwide [39].

An additional layer of complexity comes from the fact that reported ethnicity is notoriously unreliable [40]. This is particularly true in localities where multiethnic families are common: the genetic makeup of a patient may be much more complex than predicted based on recent family history [41]. For example, some self-identified "Europeans" have substantial genomic portions that are derived from African ancestors, whereas 99% of the genome of some self-identified "African Americans" is of European origin [42]. To circumvent this problem, researchers use unbiased measures of ethnicity that rely on the

SNPs genotyping data (such as principal component analysis) [43]. This approach is, however, not routinely used by clinical diagnostic laboratories to draw conclusions about the presence or absence of pathogenic mutations.

Structural Variations

We define structural variation as any genomic change that implicates more than a single base substitution at once. There are typically 5000–10,000 structural differences when comparing the genomes of two unrelated, apparently healthy individuals [44]. dbVar is a database equivalent to dbSNPs, but for variants >50 bp in length [45]. Below, we will briefly describe the most common types of structural variations while also providing, whenever possible, examples from the renal literature. We are only starting to grasp the magnitude, complexity, and ramifications of structural variations in human biology and diseases [46]. We still believe it is worthwhile for pediatric nephrologists to understand these topics since they will undoubtedly become "household" terminology in the clinic soon.

Insertions and Deletions (Indels)

There are two major types of structural variations that involve short genomic segments that are less than 1000 base pairs. These include situations where nucleotides are added or removed, which are respectively, known as insertions and deletions. Structural variants that affect more than 1000 base pairs are known as copy number variations (discussed in the next section).

Some events involve very short segments that are located within an exon. Whether such an alteration is deleterious for proteins depends largely on the number of nucleotides involved and the position of the alteration relative to the coding sequence. Any change that disrupts the normal sequence of bases is likely deleterious (it is key to remember that codons always include three bases) [47]. For example, any insertion that is not a multiple of three in terms of base number (for example, insertion of a single A) will dramatically change the interpretation of the mRNA sequence: its reading frame will be shifted, and the protein produced, truncated (Fig. 4.4a). In contrast, after insertion of three bases (for example, insertion of AGGACG), it simply adds a few extra amino acids to the protein (in this case, arginine "AGG" and threonine "ACG"). This type of alteration is usually benign because if it does not alter the way the mRNA sequence is "read" after the insertion (i.e., the amino acid sequence of the rest of the protein is unchanged).

Frameshift mutations are commonly found in genes known to cause Mendelian conditions affecting the kidney. Insertion of a single cystine residue in the gene mucin1 (*MUC1*) was recently found in multiple unrelated families with medullary cystic kidney disease type 1 using a unique combination of sequencing and bioinformatic techniques [48]. What is fascinating about this story is that while multiple linkage studies pointed to a small genomic segment on chromosome 1 (where *MUC1* is located) [50], the disease-causing mutations remained elusive even to next-generation sequencing approaches. Indeed, for all families, the C insertion lies in an exon that is enriched in C residues, thereby making it very difficult to distinguish *bone fide* mutations from sequencing errors [48] (see Fig. 4.4b).

For structural events involving slightly larger segments (for example, deletion of two exons), the functional consequences are related to either the absence of an important domain (e.g., these exons contain a kinase domain) or an aberrant

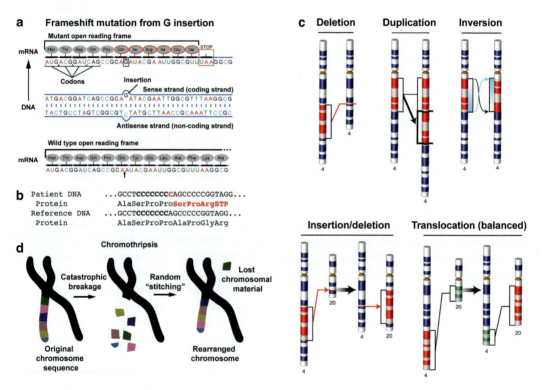

Fig. 4.4 Structural variations. Illustration of various types of structural variations. (**a**) Illustration of the impact of insertion of a single base in a coding exon. The shift in the reading frame causes a major change in the amino acid sequence. The encoded protein is truncated because a new stop codon is created by the frameshift. (**b**) Example of a C insertion (red) in a genomic segment that is highly enriched in cystine (bold). The impact on the amino acid sequence is presented below the DNA sequences. (**c**) Examples of large-scale structural changes. (**d**) This schematic presents the model by which the process of chromothripsis is explained. (Figure credits: Modified from (**a**, **c**) NHGRI digital image database. (**b**) Modified from Kirby et al. [48]. (**d**) Inspired from Fig. 1 in Tubio et al., 2011 [49])

tertiary protein structure (e.g., direct linking of the flanking exons results in a misfolded protein). These types of events are relevant to many conditions managed by nephrologists. For example, small deletions in *COL4A5* are described in patients with Alport syndrome [51], and a large duplication of the complement factor H-related protein 5 gene (*CFHR5*) gene is described in many patients with *C3* glomerulopathy [52].

Copy-Number Variations

Large-scale insertions or deletions are collectively referred to as copy-number variants (CNV; see Fig. 4.4c). They are detected using the same microarray-based technologies used for GWAS studies [53]. Most CNVs are predicted to be benign since the majority are common in the general population. Large hemizygous or homozygous deletions, especially when rare and leading to abrogation of a single gene, are the simplest CNVs to interpret phenotypically. Indeed, this copy number loss is equivalent to a gene knockout. Studies on patients with a large deletion of the X chromosome led to the discovery of *CLCN5* as the first molecular mechanism causing Dent's disease in an affected female with nonrandom X-inactivation [54]. Similar events were critical to the identification of *COL4A4* and *NPHP1* as the disease-causing genes for Alport syndrome [55] and nephronophthisis [56], respectively. Some syndromes associated with large chromosomal defects, such as Turner syndrome (loss of the X chromosome [57]) or Down syndrome (gain of chromosome 21 [58]), can also be associated with renal defects.

It is not straightforward to predict the functional impact of other types of CNVs, even those strongly associated with human diseases. In most instances, gene dosage is thought to be reflected proportionally in the levels of gene expression [59]. For example, mRNA and protein expression is higher when there is a copy number gain; important, the amino acid sequence of this protein is unchanged. The most prominent example of this in the renal literature comes from studies on the genetic basis of lupus nephritis: SLE patients with low copy numbers (0 or 1 per chromosome) of the gene encoding Fc receptor for IgG (*FCGR3B*) were more likely to develop kidney disease than those who had more than 1 [60]. It was recently shown that patients with congenital kidney malformations are much more likely to harbour large and rare heterozygous CNVs in any region of the genome when compared to unaffected controls [61]. Tumour-specific copy number gain and loss have been observed in clear cell renal cell carcinoma, particularly when there is no germline mutation in the gene VHL [62].

Copy-Neutral Variations

Copy-neutral variation, defined as genomic alterations that do not affect the overall number of copies of genes, includes inversion and translocation (see Fig. 4.4c). These may cause the disease in several ways. The function of genes may be abnormal if the inversion/translocation is accompanied by random loss of parts of the rearranged genomic segment that play an important role (i.e., it is "unbalanced"). Balanced copy-neutral variations can also be pathogenic. Indeed, if the boundaries of the structural change occur in the middle of a gene, it may disrupt the normal transcription of that gene (since contiguous exons are now far apart). Even if gene integrity is preserved, aberrant gene expression may be observed because of interference with the function of regulatory elements such as promoters, enhancers, silencers, insulators [63].

There are only a few examples of patients with renal conditions caused by balanced copy-neutral variations [64–66]. A unique type of disease-causing copy-neutral variation was also found by exome sequencing in a rare form of pheochromocytoma: the affected patient had homozygous *MAX* mutations because of uniparental disomy (a process by which two copies of a chromosome come from a single parent) [67]. One explanation for the apparent rarity of copy-neutral variants as the cause of disease is that commonly used genomic techniques are unable to detect these types of rearrangements. Thus, clinicians who have patients with a clear phenotype but without mutations in the known gene(s) should consider asking for copy-neutral variation testing.

Chromothripsis

Recent advances in DNA sequencing and bioinformatics now allow interrogation of genomes at an unprecedented resolution: it was instrumental in the discovery of yet another type of structural variation, namely, chromothripsis (which means chromosomes shattered to pieces). Chromothripsis is suspected when a chromosome is found to harbour two or more complex structural rearrangements (see Fig. 4.4d). This phenomenon was first described as a type of somatic structural variation present only in cancer cells [68]. Many similar reports followed shortly thereafter, suggesting that this mechanism is common in tumours [69]. The current working model states that chromothripsis arises from a single catastrophic event causing shattering of one or more chromosomes followed by the formation of a chromosome-like structure via random stitching of the fragments [70]. Chromothripsis was recently described in renal cell carcinomas [71].

Of utmost interest for pediatricians is the fact that a chromothripsis-like phenomenon has been reported as *a de novo* germline variation in patients with congenital diseases [72, 73]. Recent evidence suggests that the underlying mechanism is analogous to that described for cancer cells; the main difference being that the shattering process is much more circumscribed in so-called "constitutional chromothripsis"[74]. Chromothripsis was recently described as potentially causal in a child with multiple congenital anomalies, including vesicoureteral reflux [75]. However, there is still plenty to learn about the biological relevance of this process. Indeed, genetic investigations of a child with congenital anomalies ultimately uncovered parentally transmitted germline chromothripsis that was unlikely to be causal: besides his mother, 9 healthy carriers were found in this three-generation kindred [76].

Haploinsufficiency

Haploinsufficiency refers to a situation where adequate gene expression to preserve normal cell function requires the presence of two wild-type alleles being actively transcribed (diploid organisms have two copies of all autosomal genes) [77]. Disease occurs when one of the two alleles is absent or dysfunctional owing to a deletion event or a deleterious mutation, respectively [78]. Such conditions may arise *de novo* or via inheritance from an affected parent. Given their extreme dependence on gene dosage, it remains unclear why negative selection has not resulted in the disappearance of haploinsufficient genes [79].

There are several conditions that affect the kidneys that are driven by abnormalities in haploinsufficient genes. The most common is RCAD syndrome (renal cysts and diabetes) syndrome, a condition caused by either a heterozygous mutation in HNF1B or by the 17q12 microdeletion syndrome (this segment includes HNF1B) [80]. RCAD syndrome is characterized by its striking phenotypic variability among affected individuals (even between first-degree relatives with the same genotype) [81]. Recent data suggest that this phenomenon may be due to epigenetic modifications in many genes that occur in response to the haploinsufficiency state [82]. Other examples of haploinsufficient conditions that pediatric nephrologists should be aware of include SON deficiency syndrome [83] and various forms of CAKUT [84–86].

Online Resources

Sources	URLs
dbSNPs	http://www.ncbi.nlm.nih.gov/SNPs/
HapMap	http://hapmap.ncbi.nlm.nih.gov
dbVar	http://www.ncbi.nlm.nih.gov/dbvar/

Modes of Inheritance

An allele is one of a number of copies of the same gene or locus. Every person has two copies of every gene on autosomal chromosomes, one inherited from the mother and one inherited from the father. The occurrence of two copies of the same allele results in a homozygous genotype for that allele, whereas the presence of two different alleles results in a heterozygous genotype for each allele. How recessive or dominant genotype

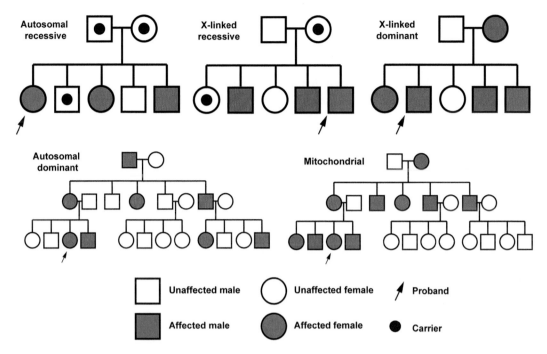

Fig. 4.5 Examples of pedigrees for most common types of inheritance. Examples of classic pedigrees for kindreds with patterns of inheritance consistent with autosomal recessive, autosomal dominant, X-linked recessive, X-linked dominant and mitochondrial

interactions can influence the expression of the characteristic traits of the underlying genetic variation are described in the following sections. Please see Fig. 4.5 for pedigrees displaying the typical inheritance patterns, and the sections below for clinical examples.

Dominant Genotypes

Dominant genotypes are seen when the heterozygous genotype is associated with phenotypic expression. Dominant genotypes arise when one allele dominates by masking the phenotypic expression of the other allele at the same genetic locus. For example, where a gene exists in two allelic forms (designated A and B), a combination of three different genotypes is possible: AA, AB, and BB. If AA and BB individuals (homozygotes) show different forms of some trait (phenotypes), and AB individuals (heterozygotes) show the same phenotype as AA individuals, then the allele A is said to dominate or be dominant to or show dominance to allele B, and B is said to be recessive to A. If instead, AB has the same phenotype as BB, B is said to be dominant to A. There are many autosomal dominant conditions that are relevant to pediatric nephrologists, such as autosomal dominant polycystic kidney disease (ADPKD) [87], tuberous sclerosis complex [88], or renal cyst and diabetes (RCAD) syndrome [80].

Recessive Genotypes

Recessive genotypes are seen when the homozygous genotype and not the heterozygous genotype are associated with phenotypic expression. Thus, both parents have to be carriers of a recessive trait in order for a child to express that trait. If both parents are carriers, there is a 25% chance for each child to show the recessive trait in the phenotype. Thus, if the parents are closely related (consanguineous), the probability of both having inherited the same allele is increased and as a result, the probability of children showing the recessive trait is increased as well. Most pediatric nephrologists will regularly manage patients with autosomal recessive conditions that affect the kidneys, including cystinosis [89], autosomal recessive polycystic kidney disease [90], Bartter syndrome [91], or pseudohypoaldosteronism type 1 [92].

X-Linked Inheritance

X-linked inheritance means that the gene causing the trait, or the disorder is located on the X chromosome. Females have two X chromosomes, while males have one X and one Y chromosome. X-linked recessive (XLR) inheritance is a mode of inheritance in which a mutation in a gene on the X chromosome causes the phenotype to be expressed (1) in males (who are necessarily hemizygous for the gene mutation because they have only one X chromosome) and (2) in females who are homozygous for the gene mutation (i.e., they have a copy of the gene mutation on each of their two X chromosomes). Carrier females who have only one copy of the mutation do not usually express the phenotype, although differences in X chromosome inactivation can lead to varying degrees of clinical expression in carrier females since some cells will express one X allele and some will express the other.

In contrast, X-linked dominant (XLD) conditions occur when a single mutated X-linked allele is responsible for the manifestations of the disorder: as such, both males and females are usually affected. The exact pattern of inheritance varies, depending on whether the father or the mother has the trait of interest. All daughters, but no son of an affected father, will have the same condition. In addition, the mother of an affected son would be expected to be affected. Examples of X-linked dominant conditions that primarily affect the kidneys include nephrogenic diabetes insipidus [93], and Dent Disease [94]. X-linked Alport syndrome can be either dominant or recessive [95]. X-linked hypophosphatemia is a rare X-linked recessive condition caused by mutations in *PHEX* [96].

Mitochondrial

Inheritance from a single parent can give rise to disease (uniparental isodisomy). Some renal phenotypes arise solely by maternal inheritance and are characterized by mitochondrial dysfunction. Mitochondrial DNA (mtDNA) is derived from the mother because it exists in much higher concentrations in ova compared to sperm. Furthermore, sperm mtDNA tends to get degraded in fertilized ova and sperm mtDNA fails to enter the ovum in several organisms. Most patients with mitochondrial cytopathies will present with evidence of proximal tubular dysfunction; it can also be associated with a distal tubulopathy, or even a glomerulopathy [97].

Genetic/Genomic Methods

SNPs Genotyping

Because of the unique properties of SNPs, there has been considerable interest in developing high-throughput technologies that would allow simultaneous testing of a large number of SNPs cheaply and reliably. The starting point is always a solution containing the patient's fragmented DNA. The two most successful approaches apply this solution to a microarray seeded with specific oligonucleotide probes directed against the sequence surrounding the target common variants (with minor allele frequencies of at least 1%).

The first method relies on non-enzymatic hybridization of single-stranded DNA with probes: a perfect match generates a light signal, but a fragment harbouring a variant does not. The second uses DNA polymerase to add one of four fluorescent-labelled nucleotides (A, C, T, or G), thus extending the probe by one base specifically at the SNPs locus. SNPs genotyping was rapidly adopted by investigators as the method of choice to investigate the links between common genetic variants and human disease [98].

Current estimates show that a typical human genome (3 billion base pairs in total) harbours 5 million SNPs: this corresponds to roughly 1 SNP every ~1000 bases. While early versions of these arrays contained <100,000 SNPs scattered throughout the genome, current platforms routinely interrogate 1–2 million SNPs at once (1 SNP every ~2000 bases). This means that we currently have unprecedented precision in our assessment of common genetic variation. As described below, SNPs genotyping has proved useful for many types of investigations, such as assessment of linkage, genome-wide association, ancestral heritage, and copy-number variations. The most recent application of this technology is the generation of polygenic risk scores to estimate the likelihood that a given individual will experience a specific clinical outcome based on genome-wide SNPs data [99]. The polygenic risk profiling tools developed to predict renal outcomes may soon be used in clinical practice [100].

Linkage Analysis

For decades, genetic linkage analysis has proved to be a powerful method to uncover short genomic segments that contain disease-causing genes for Mendelian conditions. The concepts of co-segregation, phase, linkage disequilibrium, and haplotype, which were described above, are central to this analysis (see Fig. 4.6). The goal is to identify nonrandom segregation of disease phenotypes with discrete chromosomal segments [101]. When performed with the current technology, the first step is to obtain dense SNPs geno-

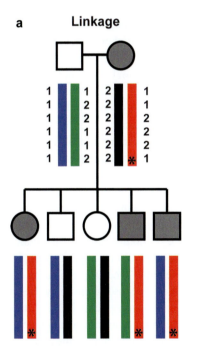
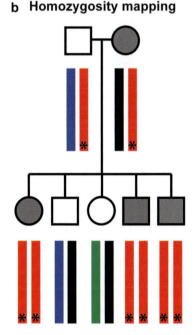
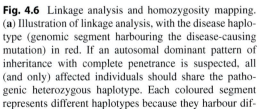

Fig. 4.6 Linkage analysis and homozygosity mapping. (**a**) Illustration of linkage analysis, with the disease haplotype (genomic segment harbouring the disease-causing mutation) in red. If an autosomal dominant pattern of inheritance with complete penetrance is suspected, all (and only) affected individuals should share the pathogenic heterozygous haplotype. Each coloured segment represents different haplotypes because they harbour different sequences of alleles at similar genomic positions (in this case, 6 loci are shown, each with 2 possible alleles, 1 or 2). (**b**) Homozygosity mapping seeks to identify homozygous segments that are present only in affected individuals (red). While a consanguineous union increases the probability of an autosomal recessive condition, outbred parents may share short genomic segments because of very distant common ancestors

typing data for all individuals in the family that provided a blood sample. Genotyping platforms typically record genotypes for millions of common variants (minor allele frequency >1% in the general population) that are scattered throughout the genome. On that basis, this approach is often referred to as a "genome-wide linkage scan."

Next is the identification of all series of contiguous SNPs that travel together (haplotypes) in all affected individuals, but not in healthy relatives (see Fig. 4.6). Using this approach, one can confidently exclude most of the genome and focus efforts on the incriminated genomic segments, which may contain any number of candidate genes (from zero to many). One key concept to understand is that the SNPs used for linkage analysis almost never turns out to be the disease-causing variant *per se* since the common variants on the SNPs genotyping platform cannot be the primary cause for a rare Mendelian condition. These SNPs are called tag SNPs because they effectively flag specific genomic segments (haplotypes) that contain the rare disease-causing variant.

The larger the number of samples from affected and unaffected individuals, the higher the precision of linkage analysis. This approach is thus most fruitful when dealing with a large kindred with multiple affected individuals, and it is not useful when dealing with families with a single affected individual. Obtaining a large number of blood samples from unaffected first-degree relatives is also key as one can exclude a larger number of "healthy" haplotypes. Combining linkage analysis performed on two or more unrelated kindreds with similar phenotypes allows for narrowing down the number and length of the target genomic segments since the disease-causing gene must lie within the segment that is shared between kindreds (if caused by mutations in the same gene).

Up until recently, most genes associated with Mendelian conditions were discovered using linkage analysis. This is true for renal conditions as well. Nowadays, gene discovery projects are done with whole-genome and whole-exome sequencing using analytical procedures that often include linkage analysis (see the section below)

[102]. Instead of using common variants as genomic markers for the disease locus, one can directly find the disease-causing mutation (which is expected to be rare or novel since the disease under scrutiny is rare).

Homozygosity Mapping

Genetic analysis of consanguineous families with multiple individuals exhibiting a similar disease phenotype is in theory simpler than for outbred kindreds because of a much higher prior probability that the disease follows an autosomal recessive pattern of inheritance (see Fig. 4.6) [103]. Homozygosity mapping [104], which is the method of choice in this context, is a version of linkage analysis that is streamlined by restricting the playing field to genomic segments that are homozygous only in affected individuals [105]. The entire set of homozygous segments has been termed the "autozygome" because autozygosity refers to homozygosity in the context of consanguinity [106]. This method relies on identity-by-descent because one would expect to find a single founder mutation that originated from a common ancestor. As in traditional linkage analyses, testing of unaffected parents and siblings is critical to make sure that only affected individuals carry recessive genotypes (monogenic disorders typically have complete penetrance).

Ideally, the homozygosity mapping points to a single homozygous genomic segment. Interestingly, homozygosity mapping is at times problematic when investigating highly inbred families because there may be many shared homozygous segments [107]. Alternatively, isolated communities can accumulate distinct pathogenic mutations in the same gene, resulting in the unexpected identification of affected individuals with compound heterozygous mutations despite being the product of a highly consanguineous union. The main example for this exceptional scenario is relevant to pediatric nephrologists since it stems from research on congenital nephrotic syndrome [108, 109]. There is evidence from the renal literature that homozygosity mapping may also be useful to investigate a subject from an outbred family for whom a recessive pattern of inheritance is suspected [110].

Since most of these conditions are first diagnosed clinically during childhood, pediatricians should know about this approach. The history of kidney disease genetics is replete with examples of successful applications of identity-by-descent methodology to identify novel disease-causing genes. While homozygosity mapping is better known as a research method for gene discovery, it is emerging as a critical tool for clinical genetics as well. It is particularly useful when dealing with patients from consanguineous unions that have a condition with many possible genetic causes [111]. For example, this approach reduced diagnostic costs and streamlined patient care when applied to a large number of patients with a clinical diagnosis of Bardet-Biedl syndrome [112].

Genome-Wide Association Studies

In many ways, a genome-wide association study (GWAS) is very similar to a linkage study. Indeed, both test to see if there is a statistical association between any of 1–2 million SNPs and a particular trait that may be recorded as a variable that is either continuous (systolic blood pressure, in mmHg) or dichotomous (hypertension: yes or no) [113]. There are two major differences between these study designs [114]. First, while the focus of linkage studies is on families with affected and unaffected individuals, GWAS methodology actively prohibits the inclusion of close relatives in the same study to avoid bias. Second, linkage and GWAS studies use the same set of tag SNPs to flag haplotypes harbouring rare disease-causing mutations or common risk alleles, respectively.

Anyone reading an article reporting on the results of a GWAS for the first time is usually struck by the extremely low p-values required to identify valid associations: the typical genome-wide significance threshold for GWAS studies is 5×10^{-8}. Such low p-values are necessary to minimize the chances of reporting false-positive associations, which become increasingly common as the number of tests performed increases

[115]. While on a different scale, this concept should be familiar to physicians ordering lab tests. The new p-value threshold is simple to calculate: 0.05 divided by the number of tests performed (in this case 1×10^{-6} SNPs). When reading an article, it is good practice for physicians to systematically calculate the number of tests performed and independently calculate the corrected p-value threshold, if applicable.

Flag SNPs with p values below the set threshold identify target haplotypes, each of which usually contains many genes. It is important to realize that a GWAS does not make it possible to pinpoint which of the genes contained in the haplotype is the culprit. This is critical because it influences the way GWAS results are reported in the literature. Early on, the tradition was to name a significant haplotype after one of the genes it contained, often based on the authors' best guess of pathogenic potential. This approach has backfired in the past because significant resources were allocated to the incorrect gene (see Box 4.1 for an exemplar taken from annals of Nephrology research history). Because of this problem, the authors now make it clear that the genes associated with haplotypes are merely signposts [116].

Box 4.1: The MYH9 vs. APOL1 Story
One of the best examples of an educated guess that misfired is from the nephrology literature. Simultaneous reports from two independent teams found a very strong genome-wide association between the haplotype containing the gene encoding myosin heavy chain 9 (*MYH9*) and glomerular disease in African-American adult patients [117, 118]. This was a reasonable guess given that many associated SNPs were clustered near or within *MYH9*, and given that autosomal dominant mutations in *MYH9* cause diseases with a complex, multisystemic phenotype that include an Alport-like glomerulonephritis that often leads to end-stage renal disease [119]. However, sequencing of all *MYH9* exons did not reveal the underlying risk allele(s).

Taking a deeper look at similar cohorts, a third team finally solved the riddle: the associated risk alleles were in a distinct gene named *APOL1*, located on the same haplotype [120]. These renal risk alleles are common in African Americans because they also confer a positive advantage via more efficient *APOL1*-dependent killing of trypanosome parasites. A prospective study later confirmed that African-American individuals harbouring the *APOL1* alleles do indeed have a higher risk of progression to ESKD or CKD over time [121]. Despite tremendous efforts to better understand the relationship between *APOL1* variants and kidney disease, the pathophysiology remains elusive [122, 123].

Polymerase Chain Reaction

Polymerase Chain Reaction (PCR) is the method of choice to amplify specific DNA segments. Most current DNA sequencing technologies depend on PCR amplification to generate a reliable signal that is translated into the DNA sequence itself through various ingenious means (see Fig. 4.7). PCR takes advantage of a DNA polymerase enzyme that is highly resistant to heat such that it is still functional following multiple rounds of heating/cooling. Heat is necessary to break the double-stranded DNA into single strands that can then be copied by the DNA polymerase using the supplied deoxynucleotide (dNTPs). The reaction also requires primer pairs that are synthesized in the laboratory: these are made out of a series of ~20 nucleotides that

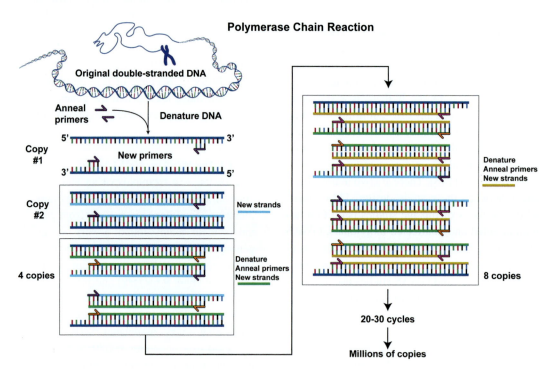

Fig. 4.7 Polymerase chain reaction. Illustration of the amplification process that occurs when DNA is subjected to PCR. Specific oligonucleotide primers, heat-resistant DNA polymerase and unlabelled nucleotides are added to the solution containing the starting DNA. The mix is subjected to heat to denature DNA. Once the temperature is reduced, the primers anneal to single-stranded DNA segments and new strands are synthesized by DNA polymerase enzyme. The first cycle generates two new strands, the second cycle four new strands. Ultimately, millions of copies of this segment are generated after 20–30 cycles. (Figure credits: Modified from NHGRI Image Gallery, https://www.genome.gov/genetics-glossary/Polymerase-Chain-Reaction)

match a very specific region of the genome. Now that the human reference genome is well established, it is simple to design primer pairs located around the target genomic segment of interest that is no more than 1000 base pairs in length.

The main drawback of PCR-based methods is that the DNA polymerase sometimes inserts the wrong nucleotide at a given position during the copying process. When one such amplified segment is subjected to DNA sequencing, one could be mistaken to think that it is a mutation when in fact there is none in the original DNA. It is thus important to validate all mutations deemed "pathologic" via PCR reamplification of a fresh sample of DNA followed by Sanger sequencing (method discussed below). The reason this step is useful is that most of these errors occur at random, which means that the same mistake is very unlikely to be observed at the same locus in a separate experiment.

DNA Sequencing Technologies

DNA sequencing determines the precise order of the four bases adenine, guanine, cytosine, and thymidine in a single strand of DNA. Sequences of individual genes or clusters of genes, full chromosomes, or the whole genome have greatly facilitated our understanding of the basic biological mechanisms of human disease. DNA sequencing was first developed in the 1970s [124] and a rapid sequencing method using the 'chain termination Method' was developed by Sanger in 1977 [125].

Sanger Method

DNA replication requires the presence of a single strand of DNA template, dNTPs, DNA polymerase, and DNA primers. Under normal conditions, the 3′-OH terminus of the dNTPs facilitates the formation of a phosphodiesterase bond between two nucleotides catalysed by the enzyme, DNA polymerase. The 'chain termination method' relies on the incorporation of dideoxy NTPs (ddNTPs) lacking a 3′-OH terminus such that the extension of DNA thereby ceases during the replication process (Fig. 4.8). Fluorescent-labelled ddNTPs are employed in automated sequencing methods which rely on wavelength determination to identify the different ddNTPs in a given sequence [126].

Next-Generation Sequencing Methods

Sanger sequencing can be laborious and expensive. A number of new sequencing technologies called next-generation sequencing (NGS) technologies have been developed that have significantly reduced the cost and time required for sequencing [127]. Unlike the Sanger method where a single predefined target is required for each sequencing reaction, NGS platforms allow for the sequencing of many millions of target molecules in parallel (Fig. 4.9). DNA molecules are immobilized on a solid surface and are sequenced in situ by stepwise incorporation of fluorescent-labelled nucleotides or oligonucleotides. "Clusters" of identical DNA are generated by the clonal amplification of template DNA, hence the term 'massive parallel deep sequencing' used to describe NGS. Platforms vary, with some covering fewer genomic regions than others, some are able to detect a greater total number of variants with additional sequencing, while others capture untranslated regions, which are not targeted by other platforms [128].

Massive parallel sequencing has greatly facilitated investigations of variations within the human genome. In January 2008, the 1000-Genome Project was launched with the objective of establishing a detailed catalogue of human genetic variation [129]. Utilizing the genomic sequences of 2500 anonymous participants from a number of different ethnic groups worldwide and using a combination of methods including low-coverage genome sequencing and targeted resequencing of coding regions, the primary goals of this project were to discover SNPs at frequencies of 1% or higher in diverse populations; to uncover rare SNPs with frequencies of 0.1–0.5% in functional gene regions; and to reveal structural variants, such as copy number variants, insertions, and

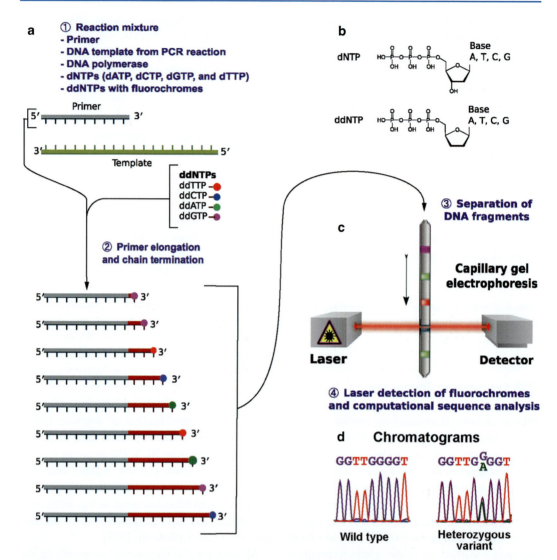

Fig. 4.8 Sanger sequencing with fluorescent-labelled ddNTPs. (**a**) Reagents necessary for Sanger sequencing. (**b**) Illustration of the structural difference between dNTP and ddNTP. (**c**) Capillary gel electrophoresis of elongated fragments and detection of the added fluorochrome-labelled base with laser detection. (**d**) Example of the output in the form of a chromatogram; the same sequence is presented from a subject that is wild-type and another that harbours a heterozygous G to A substitution. (Figure credits: Modified from a file that is licensed under the Creative Commons Attribution Share Alike 3.0 Unported license. The author of the original figure is Wikipedia user "Estevezj". It is available: https://en.wikipedia.org/wiki/Sanger_sequencing)

deletions. The pilot project involving more than 1000 genomes was completed in May 2011 [130]. This resource is publicly available and can be used by researchers to identify variants in regions that are suspected of being associated with the disease. By identifying and cataloguing most of the common genetic variants in the populations studied, this project has generated data that will serve as an invaluable reference for clinical interpretation of genomic variation.

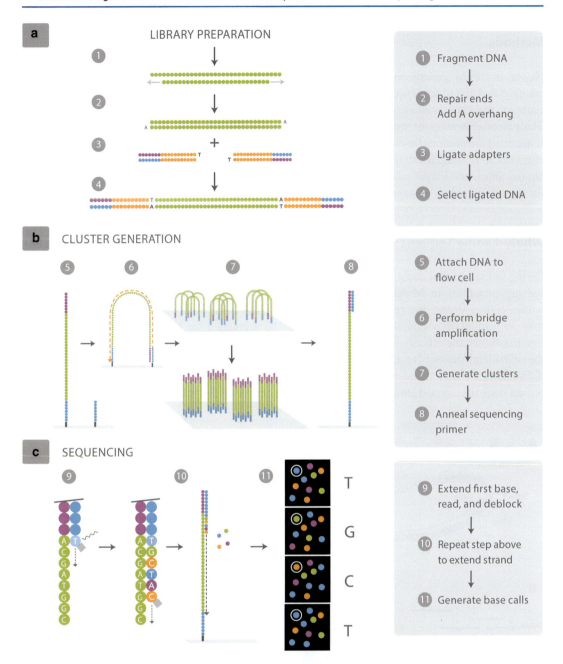

Fig. 4.9 Illumina® sequencing technology overview. This figure illustrates the steps necessary to sequence genomic DNA fragments using the Illumina® sequencing technology. These include (**a**) library preparation, (**b**) cluster generation and (**c**) sequencing. Additional details are provided in the gray boxes. (Figure credits: Image courtesy of Illumina, Inc. All rights reserved)

Third Generation Sequencing Methods

Newer or 'third generation' approaches have emerged that aim to sequence a single DNA molecule in real-time without prior amplification. The potential benefits of using single-molecule sequencing are minimal input DNA requirements, elimination of amplification bias, faster turn-around times, and longer read lengths that allow for some haplotyping of sequence information.

Whole-Exome Sequencing

Owing to the fact that about 85% of all disease-causing mutations in Mendelian disorders are within coding exons, the recent application of massive parallel deep sequencing with exon capture has shown the efficacy of this technique for the rapid identification of mutations in single-gene disorders [131, 132]. Almost 15 years have now passed since the targeted enrichment of an exome by hybridization of shotgun libraries was first described [133]. Two years later, the targeted capture and massively parallel sequencing of the exomes of 12 humans was published [134]. The following year, the first reports emerged on the use of whole-exome sequencing in gene identification [135]. Since then, investigators have discovered the genetic etiology of hundreds of Mendelian diseases.

Exome sequencing involves the targeted resequencing of all protein-coding sequences, which requires 5% as much sequencing as the whole human genome (Fig. 4.10) [134]. As the majority of Mendelian disorders are due to mutations that disrupt protein-coding sequences, the use of exome capture to identify allelic variants in rare monogenic disorders is well justified. Furthermore, highly functional variation can also be accounted for by changes in splice acceptor and donor sites, the sequences of which will also be targeted by exome capture.

The major advantage of whole-exome sequencing is that virtually all variants within

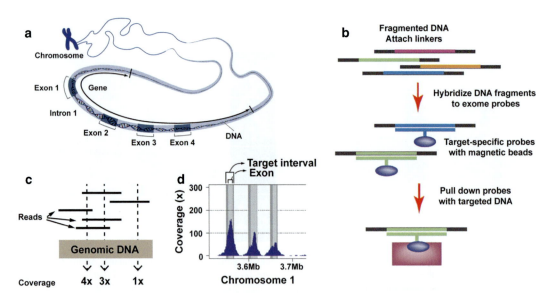

Fig. 4.10 Whole-exome capture and sequencing. (**a**) Representation of a gene and its exons and introns. (**b**) Illustration of the exome capture process. In this case, the oligonucleotide probes designed to specifically anneal to all exons in the genomes are in solution. They are easily pulled out from the solution, the probes are linked to magnetic beads. Another exome capture system has probes attached to a microarray. (**c**) Illustration of the concept of reads and coverage for a small genomic segment. These are key concepts in genomics. (**d**) Illustration of the skewed distribution of read coverage with exome capture to the exonic segments. (Figure credits: Modified from (**a**) NHGRI Image Gallery, https://peds-renomics.clinic/NHGRI-images. (**b**) Wikipedia, author SarahKusala, https://peds-renomics.clinic/Capture. (**d**) Dr. Murim Choi, Seoul National University)

an individual's genome are uncovered simultaneously. This allows for direct examination of the list of variants and candidate gene selection in the presence or absence of mapping studies. Variant listing depends on several factors that depend on the technology used. For example, the type of capture kit, the sequencing platform, and sequencing depth can influence the variant listing. Additionally, the lists produced will depend on the alignment algorithms and the stringency settings of the bioinformatics tools employed for identifying variants. Capture kits are continuously improving, initially covering 27 Mb and 180,000 coding exons to now up to 62 Mb of the human genome and over 201,121 coding exons. Each platform uses biotinylated oligonucleotide baits complementary to the exome targets to hybridize sequencing libraries prepared from fragmented genomic DNA. These bound libraries are enriched for targeted regions by pulldown with magnetic streptavidin beads and then sequenced.

Whole-Genome Sequencing

Whole-genome sequencing (WGS) involves sequencing the complete DNA sequence encompassing all 6 billion nucleotide bases in 23 chromosome pairs of a diploid human genome [136]. The main difference between WGS and WES is that WGS covers the entire genome, including all exons [137]. As a result, it includes the exome and allows the detection of mutations in noncoding DNA elements that are missed by WES. While we cannot efficiently analyse such mutations right now, it is fair to assume that we will be in a good position to do so in a few years. Once the tools exist to assess noncoding variants, re-analysis of "negative" WGS datasets would be very simple. On the other hand, patients who underwent WES studies that proved uninformative (i.e., no causative coding variant was identified) would have to be studied again with WGS.

Yet another significant advantage over WES is the much improved ability to uncover various types of CNVs, such as insertions, duplications, and deletions [138]. This is possible because of the introduction of paired-end mapping of sequence reads: a CNV is flagged when the 75 bp reads generated from both ends of genomic fragments of known length (~300 bp) are aligned farther (or closer) than anticipated (Fig. 4.11) [139]. The earliest example of genome-wide CNV interrogation using WGS data revealed 1000 large structural variations per genome, which is much more than anticipated [140]. However, the gold standard for a thorough investigation of structural variations remains comparative genomic hybridization (CGH) microarray techniques.

We will use one of the first published WGS studies (based on James Watson's DNA) to illustrate how comprehensive is the dataset created [141]. More than 100 million high-quality short-read sequences were produced, containing a total of 24.5 billion DNA bases. This allowed the investigators to "read" every base of Watson's genome on average seven-times—this is referred to as the "coverage", and the higher it is, the more confident you are that the mutations identified are true. After processing the data with various bioinformatics tools, a total of 3 million high-quality variants were ultimately identified, of which ~10,000 were nonsynonymous mutations (0.3%). More than 65,000 insertions and twice as many deletions were also found in these data.

When compared to WES, one of the biggest challenges of WGS is the substantially larger volume of data generated (estimated to be over 1 TB per genome). This has significant implications because the raw aligned data will typically be stored long-term. The issue is that sequencing costs have decreased much more rapidly than the costs associated with the infrastructure necessary to store and process these data [142]. For example, even when Watson's team was done processing his data back in 2008 [141], they would have to keep the data indefinitely in case reanalysis was deemed necessary. Consequently, teams interested in implementing WGS as opposed to WES have to be ready to face significant challenges with regards to storing data.

Another big challenge is the much higher number of variants identified in a WGS dataset. Indeed, it is not easy to pinpoint the disease-causing variant from the many hundreds of variants that remain after various bioinformatics

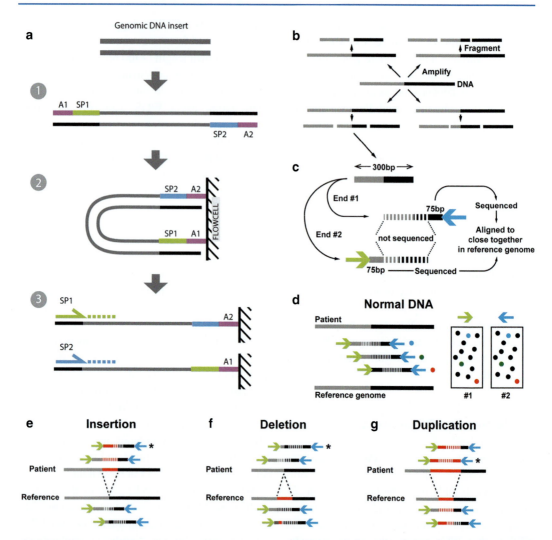

Fig. 4.11 Paired-end sequencing to detect structural variations. (**a**) Preparation DNA sample for standard next-generation sequencing using paired-end. Genomic DNA from the patient were amplified and then fragmented into small pieces. Only fragments with lengths ~200–250 base pairs are selected for sequencing (genomic DNA inserts). The steps described are as follows: (1) Adapter (A1 and A2) with sequencing primer sites (SP1 and SP2) are ligated onto DNA fragments; (2) Template clusters are formed on the flow cell by bridge amplification; (3) Clusters are then sequenced by synthesis from the paired primers sequentially. (**b**) Illustration of amplification of DNA, random fragmentation of amplified segments; in this case, fragments of similar sizes are illustrated. (**c**) Illustration of the two-step process leading to paired-end sequencing. The fragment size selected for is 300 base pairs, and 75 base pairs are sequenced at each end. The dotted lines represent segments that are not directly sequenced in that fragment. (**d**) Schematic showing how paired-end reads from a small genomic region from a patient with normal DNA align to the reference genome. The right-hand side shows the position of the clusters from which the data for each read come from. Each DNA fragment is linked to a specific cluster on the flow cell, thus linking the first and second sequencing data. Also shown are examples of how paired-end sequencing is useful to identify for insertions (**e**), deletion (**f**) or duplications (**g**). (Figure credits: Panel **a**: Figure modified from the original Illumina® paired-end sequencing workflow. All rights reserved)

filters. In comparison, one has to investigate ~50–100 coding variants after filtering WES data.

Furthermore, it will be essential for accurate and comprehensive characterization of disease phenotypes to greatly assist the analysis of an individual's phenotype. It has been shown that the presence of bi-allelic variants can greatly influence a disease phenotype and the data generated by WGS will likely increase our understanding of the molecular intersection of biologically relevant pathways.

As whole-genome is still expensive, currently over £2000 per genome, whole-exome sequencing remains the preferred strategy for molecular genetic diagnosis as this remains a more cost-effective strategy than Sanger sequencing in genetically heterogeneous conditions. However, limitations exist with both technologies and the major challenges posed by both strategies will involve the logistics of delivering genome sequence information to clinicians and how we as clinicians use the data, and how patients and their families deal with the incidental findings.

Online Resources

Topics	URLs
PCR	https://peds-renomics.clinic/PCR
Single base primer extension genotyping	https://peds-renomics.clinic/Genotyping
Linkage	https://peds-renomics.clinic/Linkage
Sanger sequencing	https://peds-renomics.clinic/Sanger-seq
Exome sequencing	https://peds-renomics.clinic/Exome
Illumina on YouTube	https://peds-renomics.clinic/YouTube-Illumina
NHGRI on YouTube	https://peds-renomics.clinic/YouTube-NHGRI

Clinical Implementation in Nephrology

Finding Pathogenic Mutations for Mendelian Disease

Nowadays, most pediatric nephrologists will send blood samples for genetic testing a few times a year for patients with a wide range of conditions. This may be done to establish a firm molecular diagnosis for a patient, to verify if the relatives are carriers. Non-invasive techniques are also emerging to obtain an antenatal molecular diagnosis from maternal blood [143]. The interested reader is directed to a recent review on the topic of genetic testing applied to nephrology [144].

The first set of investigations is usually to sequence genes known to cause a particular condition to uncover possible pathogenic mutations. Until recently, this was done using PCR amplification and Sanger sequencing of all exons of these genes. However, when the number of genes under investigation is less than 50, the same diagnostic procedure is usually now done using targeted exome sequencing because it is fast, cheap, customisable, widely available, and reliable [145]. The difference between the targeted exome and the whole exome lies in the number of genes investigated at once: all known genes known to cause disease X vs. all genes of the genome. This approach has been applied to various groups of kidney diseases with great success [146]. A gene panel was designed to allow for the rapid discovery of pathogenic mutations in ~4500 genes relevant to genetic conditions with neonatal or infantile onset: "RapSeq" includes many genes that cause renal diseases [147].

Whole-exome sequencing is usually reserved for conditions caused by >50 genes, cases that remain undiagnosed using targeted sequencing panels, or for patients with atypical phenotypes. Recent data suggest, however, that the added benefits of whole-genome sequencing may result in this approach soon becoming the standard test [148]. A clear advantage and yet another challenge of this approach is the ability to interrogate all genes and all noncoding regions at once, and the improved yields for structural variations.

The simplest scenario is when a mutation identified in your patient is described in other patients with the same phenotype. Unfortunately, the alternative scenario is much more common: the report states that there is a variant of "uncertain significance" in one of the genes tested. This means that the genetic testing company, using a systematic approach to evaluate novel variants, cannot determine with high certainty that your patient's mutation is causal [149]. With a little extra work, it is however possible to provide families with more information about the pathogenic potential of the variant. We provide a case that illustrates what a pediatric nephrologist can do to evaluate such a report (see clinical vignette). It emphasizes the usefulness of simple concepts that were discussed earlier in this chapter, such as co-segregation, allele frequency, and amino acid conservation.

Physicians need to be prepared to revisit the diagnosis since databases are evolving and should make this clear to the patient and his/her parents. Current protocols used by leaders in the field stipulate systematic rechecks of all datasets every 6 months, with automatic reporting to the ordering physician if new findings emerge [150, 151]. This is critical because as public databases are populated with an increasing number of pathogenic variants over time, the output of bioinformatic analyses performed changes. Table 4.1 shows the significant increase in the number of pathogenic genotypes in HGMD between 2012 and 2020 for congenital nephrotic syndrome caused by *NPHS1* mutations. Thus, an initial negative report from next-generation sequencing testing may yield a firm molecular diagnosis later on. A recent study on millions of genetic tests done for hereditary forms of cancer found that ~25% of variants of uncertain significance were later confidently labelled as pathogenic or benign [152].

Since the criteria for a mutation to be deemed pathogenic are very stringent, one may assume that the interpretation of such a mutation is unlikely to be overturned. However, the curation of mutation databases is surprisingly unreliable: sequencing of ~438 target genes in 52 parent-child trios revealed that ~25% of mutations flagged as "likely pathogenic" (on the basis of being already described as such) were likely to be benign since they were found in healthy, asymptomatic parents [153]. To address this issue (and many others in the field), the NIH created the Clinical Genome Resource, or ClinGen [154]. This group devised a comprehensive and systematic approach to evaluate the robustness of all gene-disease and mutation-disease causal links [155]. The assessment of renal genetic conditions will soon improve as ClinGen recently established a Clinical Domain Working Group on tubulopathies, and another one focused on kidney cystic and ciliopathy disorders (https://peds--renomics.clinic/ClinGen-kidney).

Clinical Vignette

A young patient with a clinical diagnosis of congenital nephrotic syndrome spent many months as an inpatient. Since the parents are first cousins, an autosomal recessive form of CNS was expected; the patient has a 2-year-old female sibling that is apparently healthy (Fig. 4.12). There is no prior family history of CNS. A few months back, your colleagues made sure to send blood samples from all first-degree relatives for genetic testing of the usual CNS gene panel, which includes Sanger sequencing of the genes *NPHS1* and *NPHS2*. You are seeing the patient and his parents today in the clinic to discuss the report issued by the diagnostic laboratory.

Table 4.1 Change in the number of pathogenic *NPHS1* mutations in HGMD between 2012 and 2020

Mutation types	Yearly data for *NPHS1* in HGMD database								
	2012	2013	2014	2015	2016	2017	2018	2019	2020
Missense/nonsense	87	97	113	125	145	152	152	163	180
Splicing	14	16	20	22	25	28	28	33	39
Regulatory	0	0	0	0	0	0	0	1	1
Small deletions	20	24	25	28	33	35	36	38	40
Small insertions	10	10	10	10	13	14	14	14	16
Small indels	2	2	2	2	3	3	3	3	4
Gross deletions	0	0	1	1	3	3	3	3	3
All mutations	133	149	171	188	222	235	236	255	283
% Freely available	62	66	72	67	79	76	75	78	79

Note: These data were compiled yearly by the author (ML) directly from the HGMD website

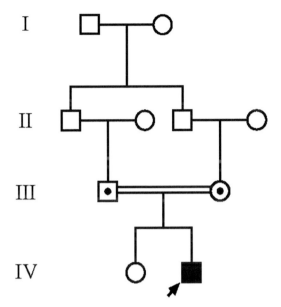

Fig. 4.12 Pedigree for a patient with Congenital Nephrotic Syndrome. Black and white symbols represent affected and unaffected subjects, respectively. Black dots and double lines denote heterozygous carriers and consanguineous unions, respectively. Black arrowhead identifies the proband

The report highlights potentially relevant alterations. The homozygous mutation in *NPHS1* (c.2276 T>C; p.I759T) is considered a "variant of uncertain significance" (VUS) because it has not been described before in other patients with CNS. It is important to note that mutations should always be described with "c." and "p.", which are the base change relative to the cDNA (mRNA) and the resulting amino acid change in the encoded protein, respectively. Not surprisingly, for a novel variant, there are no *in vitro* studies that have tested its functional impact experimentally. We confirmed that the two healthy parents and the unaffected sibling were heterozygous carriers: thus, the pattern of cosegregation is consistent with this mutation being potentially pathogenic. In preparation for our meeting with the family, we decided to investigate further to see if this mutation could be pathogenic. Indeed, finding a convincing mutation in a gene known to be associated with CNS would help our team provide a more accurate prognosis while also providing some closure for the family [156].

First, we visited the public version of the Human Gene Mutation Database (HGMD [157]) to make sure that this mutation remained novel (free registration required for access; Fig. 4.13a). We then confirmed that conclusion using ClinVar (Fig. 4.13b) [158]. These two resources present comprehensive lists of mutations causing Mendelian conditions curated by experts. A major advantage of ClinVar is that it also provides information on the variant of interest if it was reported as VUS by any genetic testing facility or if there are any data in control databases, such as the gnomAD browser (see the bottom of Fig. 4.13b) [159] or dbSNPs [37]. As shown in Fig. 4.13b (bottom panel), ClinVar also reported that the Broad Institute Rare Disease Group reported an unrelated case of congenital nephrotic syndrome with *NPHS1* p.I759T in compound heterozygosity.

To get a better understanding of the pathogenic potential of this variant, we also consulted gnomAD [159]: it was observed in the heterozygous state in 4 out of >125,000 individuals that were all of South Asian descent (like our patient; Fig. 4.13c). This database includes whole-exome and whole-genome data from adults that are unlikely to have a severe pediatric syndrome [159]. Another port of entry to access all this information is dbSNPs [37], particularly if the report includes the rs# associated with the variant (in our case, rs775313529; Fig. 4.13d).

The gnomAD page for the variant includes a wealth of information [159], including the likelihood of it being pathogenic based on two of the most widely used prediction tools, Polyphen [160] and SIFT [161]. There are now dozens of such bioinformatic tools, all claiming to be better than the others. All evaluate the pathogenic potential of missense mutations by using information about the degree of amino acid conservation between various species, the predicted impact of the specific amino acid change (based on physicochemical properties of amino acids, such as size, charge, and polarity) compounded by some advanced computing methodologies (machine learning). An alternative approach is to use software like Condel [162] because it inte-

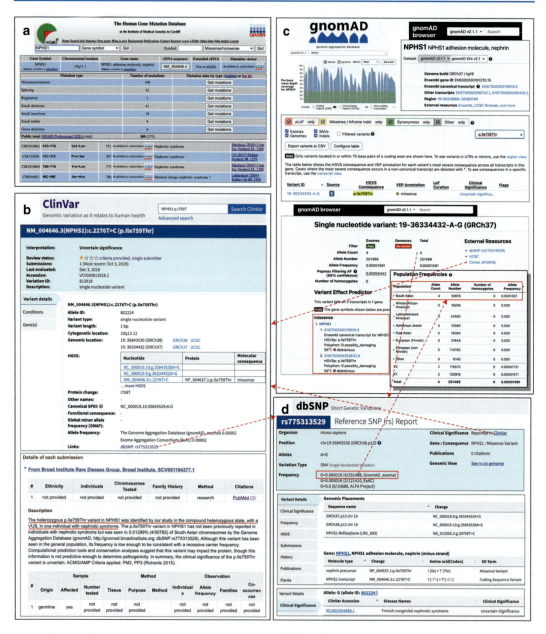

Fig. 4.13 Assessing a variant of uncertain significance in *NPHS1*. (**a**) A visit to the HGMD website suggest that the variant *NPHS1* p.I759T has yet to be reported in a patient. (**b**) While the ClinVar website corroborates this finding, it also suggest that there is one report of a patient with the same variant in the context of compound heterozygosity. (**c**) Data from gnomAD suggest that variant is rare and is only described in South Asian individuals. (**d**) dbSNP is the simplest point of entry to all these data if the genetic test report include the rs#. Note that most of these resources are densely linked to each other (red arrows)

4 Molecular Diagnosis of Genetic Diseases of the Kidney: Primer for Pediatric Nephrologists

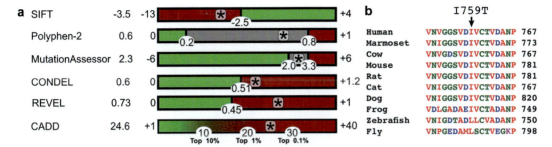

Fig. 4.14 Assessing mutations for pathogenicity with various prediction softwares. (**a**) The ranges of scores for SIFT, Polyphen2, MutationAssessor, Condel, REVEL and CADD. For a mutation to be considered as pathogenic, its score should lie in the red zone of the score gradients. Because all softwares use slightly different inputs and analytical methods, it is not unusual to generate contradictory predictions for the same mutation. (**b**) Multiple species protein sequence alignment was done using BLAST shows that position I759 is well conserved down to the fruit fly (note: leucine and isoleucine are interchangeable). Each letter represents an amino acid; the number on the right-hand side indicates the position of the last amino acid of the series presented in a given ortholog

grates the outputs of Polyphen [160], SIFT [161] and MutationAssessor [163] (Fig. 4.14a). Newer tools that attempt to further refine the output include CADD [164] and REVEL [165] (Fig. 4.14a). Interestingly, the isoleucine at position 759 is well conserved across orthologs, down to the fruit fly (Fig. 4.14b).

Overall, it is likely that this VUS will soon be upgraded to "pathogenic" on the basis that it was found in two unrelated patients with congenital nephrotic syndrome, familial cosegregation analysis was consistent with a recessive mode of inheritance (as expected), the mutated amino acid is well conserved, the mutation is only observed in the heterozygous states with very low MAF in South Asians (0.01%), and most prediction softwares predict that p.I759T should be deleterious.

Genetic Heterogeneity

Genetic (or locus) heterogeneity is recognized when a particular phenotype may be caused by mutations in different genes. Nephronophthisis is one of the best examples of locus heterogeneity in the renal literature, with disease-causing mutations reported in ~30 genes (Table 4.2). Functional studies have shown that the majority of the proteins encoded by these genes are localized and play important roles at the centrosome, basal body, and cilia. This led to the proposition that these structures are central in the pathogenesis of nephronophthisis [166]. It is important to note that locus heterogeneity is common among many monogenic renal conditions, such as atypical hemolytic-uremic syndrome [167], nephrotic syndrome [168], distal renal tubular acidosis [169], Dent's disease [170], or primary hyperoxaluria [171].

Pleiotropy is the mirror image of genetic heterogeneity: mutations in the same gene cause different phenotypes. Incidentally, nephronophthisis also provides many well-documented cases of pleiotropy (Table 4.1). For example, the study of patients with unique phenotypes within the nephronophthisis spectrum using whole-exome sequencing led to the identification of novel candidate genes that were previously associated with completely distinct disorders, such as *SLC4A1* or *AGXT* [172]. The first gene, which encodes the anion exchanger 1 protein, was previously associated with hereditary spherocytosis [173] or distal tubular renal acidosis [169], while the second one is a well-established cause for primary hyperoxaluria (it encodes an enzyme involved in glyoxylate metabolism) [171].

Interestingly, a substantial number of patients with nephronophthisis (~40%) remain genetically undefined. The same is true for many other renal conditions. This will prove to be a fertile

Table 4.2 Genetic heterogeneity among nephronophthisis-associated ciliopathies

Genes	Nephronophthisis syndromes											OMIM #
	BBS	CED	COACH	JATD	JBTS	LCA	MKS	MSS	MORM	NPHP	SLS	
AGXT										■		604285
AH1					■							608894
ANKS6										■		615370
ARL13B					■							608922
CC2D2A			■		■		■					612013
CEP164						■				■		614848
CEP290	■				■		■			■		610142
CEP41					■							610523
GLIS2										■		608539
IFT122		■										606045
IFT140				■				■				614620
IFT43		■										614068
INPP5E					■				■			613037
INVS										■		243305
IQCB1										■		609237
MRE11										■		600814
NEK8										■		609799
NPHP1					■					■	■	607100
NPHP3							■			■		608002
NPHP4										■	■	607215
RPGRIPL1			■		■							610937
SDCCAG8	■										■	613524
SLC4A1										■		109270
SLC41A1										■		610801
TMEM138					■							614459
TMEM216					■							613277
TMEM67	■											609884
TTC21B				■						■		612014
WDR19			■	■								608151
XPNPEP3										■		613553
ZNF423										■		604557

BBS Bardet-Biedl Syndrome, CED Cranioectodermal dysplasia, COACH syndrome characterized by cerebellar vermis hypo/aplasia, oligophrenia, congenital ataxia, ocular coloboma, and hepatic fibrosis, JATD Jeune asphyxiating thoracic dystrophy, JBTS Joubert Syndrome, LCA Leber's Congenital Amaurosis, MKS Meckel-Gruber Syndrome, MMS Mainzer-Saldino syndrome, MORM syndrome characterized by mental retardation, truncal obesity, retinal dystrophy, and micropenis, NPHP nephronopthisis, SLS Senior Loken Syndrome

ground to display the utility of whole-exome and/or whole-genome sequencing and will undoubtedly lead to the identification of many other unexpected candidate genes [174, 175].

Finding Risk Alleles for Complex Diseases

One of the promises of genomic medicine is for knowledge about a patient's genome to play a central role in the management of complex medical conditions. Classic examples of complex diseases include essential hypertension, diabetes mellitus type 2, steroid-sensitive nephrotic syndrome, and congenital malformations of the kidney and/or urinary tract. For example, pediatric nephrologists could optimize the prevention and/or treatment of steroid-sensitive nephrotic syndrome, thus realizing the guiding principles of personalized medicine. While this will undoubtedly change the face of clinical medicine, as described below, we are unfortunately years away from enacting this scenario.

In contrast to Mendelian conditions that are caused by highly penetrant mutations in a single gene, complex diseases are not rare and are caused by multiple factors. Detailed epidemiological studies have shown that for many of these conditions, environmental and genetic factors are the major determinants of trait expression. Current models implicate the interaction of multiple low penetrance variants in many genes. These are based on studies of heritability, defined as the fraction of phenotypic variation that is likely explained by genetic variation [176]. Heritability is estimated from the phenotypic correlations among related individuals, using families with multiple affected individuals as well as twin studies. A prime example of a complex trait with high heritability is adult essential hypertension [177].

Finding the genetic basis for complex traits could have significant public health implications. First, it may help identify at-risk individuals early on, thereby perhaps allowing for the prevention of long-term, largely preventable health consequences. Second, it may be an important tool to decide the type and dose of medication that is best suited for a given patient, which would be a major advance towards the realization of personalized medicine. Below, we will discuss the two competing theories of complex trait genetics and the methodologies employed to find associations, while providing examples from the renal literature.

Complex Diseases: Associated with Common and/or Rare Variants?

There are two predominant explanatory models of complex disease genetic causation: the complex disease, common variants (CDCV) and the complex disease, rare variants (CDRV) hypotheses (see Fig. 4.15) [178]. Both assume that multiple genes are implicated in the pathophysiology of common traits. The first hypothesis states that the genetic landscape of common traits mostly comprises common variants (minor allele frequency >1%), each with a very small contribution to the overall phenotype. The alternative hypothesis suggests that rare variants (minor allele frequency <1%) with larger effects are largely responsible. Up until recently, the technology to perform the comprehensive genomic analyses required to unravel the genetic architecture of complex diseases did not exist: the predominant working model was CDRV.

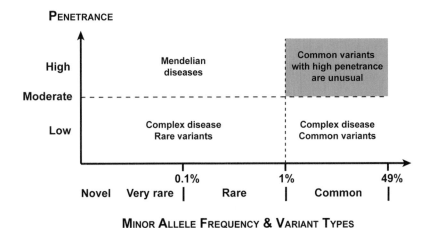

Fig. 4.15 The relationship between minor allele frequency and penetrance to explain the genetic basis of complex diseases. This graph illustrates the relationship between minor allele frequency and penetrance of phenotype. Typically, common variants that have a phenotypic effect have low penetrance. On the other hand, rare variants are expected to result in a much higher penetrance. This is due to the fact that penetrance is one of the main factors driving the selective pressure for/against a particular phenotype. Most variants identified thus far for Mendelian conditions are in the left upper quadrant, while those associated with complex diseases fit in the right lower quadrant

The CDCV hypothesis was the first to be tested rigorously owing to technological and methodological developments related to SNPs genotyping. This opened the gates for a flurry of genome-wide association scans (GWAS) performed on common SNPs. Reliable investigations of the CDRV hypothesis were beyond reach until the emergence of cheap high-throughput sequencing and the development of exome capture.

Clinical Implications of Genome-Wide Association Studies

Most of the GWAS studies focused on renal conditions include only adult subjects [113]. Some studies were focused on dichotomous disease outcomes, such as hypertension, diabetic nephropathy, IgA nephropathy, CKD, ESKD/FSGS and kidney stones [113]. Others tested the association with relevant continuous variables like blood pressure, eGFR, serum creatinine, creatinine clearance, albumin-to-creatinine ratio, or serum cystatin C [113]. Unfortunately, there are few variants showing robust association with a given trait that is replicated across distinct studies. These SNPs typically explain very little of the phenotypic variability observed in patients: this phenomenon, which is not unique to nephrology studies, has been termed "missing heritability" [179]. Many of these studies have, however, provided unique insights into the biological pathways that cause disease that were hitherto immune to detection [180].

There are now a few published GWAS that enrolled children with kidney disease [181]. As a result of this research lag, children may not benefit from the realization of genomic medicine as rapidly as adult patients [182]. Indeed, it is likely that advances percolating from adult studies will not translate into concrete measures for children for two main reasons. First, the important pediatric public health problems that could be addressed "genomically" are not on the adult medicine "radar" (e.g., nephrotic syndrome). Second, even when diagnoses are congruent (e.g., hypertension), it is unclear how useful results from large adult studies will apply to pediatric care since the underlying pathophysiology is often distinct (due to growth and development) [183, 184].

Thankfully, this state of affair is changing. The first GWAS, which included more than one thousand children with CKD, was inconclusive because of low power [185]. A number of small GWAS (sample sizes <500) focused on nephrotic syndrome yielded statistically significant SNPs, particularly in the HLA genes [186–189]. The largest GWAS published in 2020, which included many of the subjects from earlier cohorts, confirmed this association and also uncovered new loci of interest in the regions of *NEPHS1-KIRREL2* and *TNFS15* [190].

Source of Missing Heritability: Rare Variants?

A substantial proportion of the genetic contribution to complex traits thus remains unexplained. The next logical step is to determine the impact of rare variants on such phenotypes using whole-genome or -exome sequencing [191]. Unfortunately, because the variants are rare, the sample sizes required to draw conclusions are prohibitively large (10,000–100,000 subjects at a minimum) [192, 193]. As a result, few studies testing the CDRV hypothesis have been published [194]. Other aspects that could also play a role in the pathophysiology of complex traits include epigenetic factors [195], gene-gene interactions (epistasis) [196], and/or gene-environment interactions [197]. An alternative explanation recently put forward is that heritability may have been overestimated all along [198]. Finally, the complexity of the underlying genetic architecture of these diseases may be such that it is not possible to unravel with our current experimental tools [199].

Pharmacogenetics/Pharmacogenomics

Most current studies attempt to link genetic polymorphisms in a small number of genes with known functions in drug metabolism. As such, they establish the pharmacogenetic profiles for patients. Very few studies, particularly when enrolling pediatric subjects, perform pharmacogenomic profiling, which involves genome-wide interrogation. One of the major promises of personalized medicine is that drug prescriptions will be tailored based on a patient's pharmacogenetic profile. This promise is within reach because of the extensive knowledge accumulated about two of the key determinants of drugs' pharmacokinetic and pharmacodynamics properties.

First, a group of enzymes add specific chemical groups to the parent compound: this way, drugs are metabolized to their active form, or they are modified to enhance excretion. Cytochrome P-450 oxidases (CYP) and uridine diphosphate-glucuronosyltransferase (UGT) are two of the most prominent families of enzymes of this class. The second class are transporters that mediate the efflux of drugs outside of cells, thereby limiting their therapeutic benefits. Many great examples are provided by transporter proteins that are part of the ATP-binding Cassette (ABC) superfamily. The other key development is the increasing knowledge about the physiological impact of SNPs in genes encoding proteins that play important roles in both of these processes. Below, we will describe issues that relate specifically to the realization of pharmacogenetics for pediatric nephrology patients, while also providing concrete examples from the literature.

Four main issues plague the field of pediatric pharmacogenetics in general. First, the vast majority of pharmacogenetics studies are done exclusively on adult subjects. Unfortunately, these findings cannot be directly extrapolated to children because of the impact that growth and development have on pharmacologic parameters. Second, there are currently very few studies reporting specifically on the association of genetic polymorphisms with pharmacologic parameters in pediatric subjects. Third, the predictive power of most pediatric studies is effectively limited by small sample sizes (typically less than 100). Finally, all studies conducted thus far are retrospective and have not been able to test if the inclusion of pharmacogenetic data influences outcomes. It is therefore not surprising that there are currently very few tests that are ready for prime time for pediatric patients.

In both adult [200] and pediatric nephrology [201], the most active research in pharmacogenetics relates to key agents used in current renal transplantation cocktails. Calcineurin inhibitors were logical candidates for such studies since they have proved to be valuable as steroid-sparing agents but are known to cause significant level-dependent nephrotoxicity. A single study with 104 pediatric kidney transplant recipients treated with cyclosporin showed no evidence that genotyping for polymorphisms in genes from the CYP and ABC families helped optimize patient care [202]; these results largely echo the consensus opinion derived from similar adult studies [200]. In contrast, the implementation of pharmacogenetic profiling is probably closer to reality for tacrolimus: testing for polymorphisms in *CYP3A5* identified in adult studies [200] were found to be predictive when tested in 30 teenage kidney transplant recipients [203]. There are also data from two small studies on pediatric kidney transplant recipients treated with MMF that report promising associations with UGT polymorphisms that require corroboration [204, 205].

Two additional hurdles will complicate the implementation of pharmacogenetics specifically in renal transplant protocols. First, the benefits of genotyping above and beyond the current gold standard will have to be demonstrated. This may prove a difficult task since therapeutic drug monitoring (TDM) of various immunosuppressive medications allows personalization of doses within days to weeks [200]. There is evidence that at least in adult patients, pharmacogenetics leads to more rapid optimization of drug dosage, but it does not appear to translate into better outcomes [206]. Second, the ability of any predictive indices, including pharmacogenetics, to impact clinical outcomes will always be hampered by the polypharmacy that is inherent to most renal transplant drug cocktails because of complex drug-drug interactions [200].

Warfarin is yet another medication relevant to pediatric nephrologists that has been extensively studied for pharmacogenetic applications.

Studies in adult subjects have shown that polymorphisms in the genes encoding the target of warfarin, *VKORC1* (vitamin K epoxide reductase complex subunit 1) or its main metabolizing CYP (*CYP2C9*) are helpful to predict warfarin disposition [207]. Data emerging from pediatric studies testing the same polymorphism are unfortunately not as clear [208].

While pharmacogenetics offers the potential of individualized treatment strategies, it is critical to obtain solid evidence of clinical utility before widespread clinical implementation. A great source of information for interested physicians is the Clinical Pharmacogenetics Implementation Consortium (CPIC), a project aimed at addressing "some of the barriers to the implementation of pharmacogenetic tests into clinical practice".

Online Resources

Sources	URLs
Clinical Pharmacogenetics Implementation Consortium	https://cpicpgx.org/
Renal genes	http://www.renalgenes.org/
HGMD	http://www.hgmd.cf.ac.uk/
ClinVar	http://www.ncbi.nlm.nih.gov/clinvar/
The gnomAD browser	https://gnomad.broadinstitute.org/
SIFT	http://provean.jcvi.org/index.php
Polyphen2	http://genetics.bwh.harvard.edu/pph2/
MutationAssessor	http://mutationassessor.org/
BLAST	http://blast.ncbi.nlm.nih.gov/

Barriers to Implementation in the Clinic

There is a lot of hype and high expectations that remain largely unrealistic. Apart from the diagnosis of rare diseases and some rare applications in pharmacogenomics, the real-world impact of genomics has yet to be shown in the clinic. Notwithstanding the knowledge limitations that are inherent in the implementation delays, there are a number of other issues that will hamper this process, some of which are discussed below.

Patients' Health Literacy and Numeracy

Adequate health literacy skills are necessary for patients to understand a discussion about genomic issues and to appropriately consent for testing. Health literacy is defined as "the degree to which individuals can obtain, process, and understand the basic health information and services needed to make appropriate health decisions" [209]. A survey of general US adults demonstrated poor health literacy in ~30–40% [210]. Not surprisingly, the situation is even worse when these skills are assessed in the context of genomics issues [211]. Apparent familiarity with genetic concepts is common in adults, but physicians should be alert to the fact that understanding of basic genetic concepts is often limited [212].

Health numeracy skills are also critical for patients to grasp the predictive nature of most discussions that relate to genomic health decisions. Indeed, statistics and probabilities are an integral part of these discussions. Health numeracy is defined as "the degree to which individuals have the capacity to access, process, interpret, communicate, and act on numerical, quantitative, graphical, biostatistical, probabilistic health information needed to make effective health decisions" [213]. A recent survey revealed that ~50% of adult subjects have basic or minimal numeracy skills [210]. In contrast to health literacy, this subject has been little studied [211].

While these issues cannot be ignored, they should not jeopardize patient care. Given that time is limited in the clinic, it may not be possible for the treating physician to spend time explaining basic concepts. The critical point is to rapidly assess if the patient (or their caretaker) has at least a basic understanding of the issues at stake and take measures to try to address perceived inadequacies. If the family has access to the Internet and is motivated to learn independently, the physician may provide the address of reputa-

4 Molecular Diagnosis of Genetic Diseases of the Kidney: Primer for Pediatric Nephrologists

ble websites focused on teaching basic genetic concepts to a general audience (see the list below).

Online Resources for Patients

Sources	URLs
Genetic Science Learning Centre	http://learn.genetics.utah.edu/
NHGRI educational material	https://www.genome.gov/about-genomics
MedLine Plus—Genetics	https://medlineplus.gov/genetics/
All about genetics (Kids Health)	http://bit.ly/all-about-genetics
CDC Family health history	http://bit.ly/CDC-family-health-history

Physicians' Health Literacy and Numeracy

Another important issue that is emerging is the gap between what physicians will need to know to implement genomic science in clinical practice, and what they actually know [1, 214]. Given the scarcity of healthcare professionals with expertise in genetics and genomics [215], which is unlikely to change in the next few years, it is possible that these inadequacies may hamper the deployment of genomic medicine when it is ready for widespread implementation. There are many resources in the literature [1], in print and online (see the list below) that may help bridge that gap for practicing physicians.

While most physicians agree that a good understanding of basic statistical concepts is necessary in contemporary medicine, very few feel confident of their own skills [216]. This is a long-standing problem that has been repeatedly documented in Europe and North America [217–219]. Up until recently, these skills were deemed important by physicians espousing the principles of evidence-based medicine. The advent of genomic medicine will hopefully trigger a renewed interest for physicians to acquire basic quantitative skills. Medical schools have adapted their curricula to reflect these changes such that

current physicians-in-training will be better prepared [220–222].

Online Resources for Physicians

Book from AAP: Robert A Saul, Medical Genetics in Pediatric Practice, 2013, 503 p., American Academy of Pediatrics. ISBN: 978-1-58110-496-7.

Mobile Apps:

Human Genome; iPhone
GeneticCode; iPhone
Gene Screen (CSHL); iPhone
Gene tutor; iPhone & Android
Genetics 4 Medics; iPhone ($5), Android (free)

Type	Sources	URLs
Genetic testing	Gene Reviews	http://Genetests.org
	NCI—Gene testing	https://peds-renomics.clinic/NCI-genetic-testing
	Lab tests Online	https://peds-renomics.clinic/lab-test-genetics
	NIH Genetic Testing Registry	http://www.ncbi.nlm.nih.gov/gtr/
Online tutorials	Open Helix	http://openhelix.eu/
	OMIM	https://www.omim.org/
	Medline Plus—Genetics	https://medlineplus.gov/genetics/
	Genetics in Primary Care (AAP)	https://peds-renomics.clinic/AAP-Genetics
Free resources	European Rare Disease	http://www.orpha.net/
	CDC—Public Health Genomics	http://www.cdc.gov/genomics/
	Human Gene Mutation Database	http://www.hgmd.cf.ac.uk/
	Gene Forum	http://www.geneforum.org/

Test Costs and Gene Patents

Both governmental programs and insurance companies will usually agree to defray the costs of tests that are ordered by physicians, are relevant to the patient's condition, and may lead to a concrete change in the plan of care. Ideally, the cost of tests would not play a major role in this decision, but up until recently, it did for a few genetic tests that were prohibitively expensive (thousands of dollars). These high prices were driven in large part by the strict enforcement of gene patents held by a few companies. For example, the price of BRCA1 and 2 tripled once the company Myriad Genetics decided to exercise a strict monopoly on its gene patents [223].

Since ~40% of the human genes have been patented [224], this has the potential to be a major hurdle in the development of personalized medicine based on genomic testing [225]. This situation changed dramatically following the US Supreme Court judgment that invalidated the gene patents held by Myriad Genetics [226].

Demonstration of Efficacy and Cost-Effectiveness

With the gene patent barriers now down and cheap sequencing being available, the next big obstacle to the promised widespread clinical implementation of genomic tests [227] will be the demonstration of efficacy and cost-effectiveness for common conditions [228]. At the request of the CDC, a committee of experts proposed to use a specific set of criteria to assess whether a particular genetic test ought to be implemented in the clinic. It is referred to as ACCE, an acronym that reflects the four criteria that need to be fulfilled: Analytical validity, Clinical validity, Clinical utility, and associated ethical, legal, and social implications.

As seen in Fig. 4.16, this is an ambitious task that requires the integration of data from many different spheres of expertise. Genomic tests will also need to be analysed using the ACCE multifaceted approach: this will likely prove to be a lengthier process since, in theory, each gene-disease combination will undergo a similar in-depth examination. The CDC also formed another committee, named Evaluation of Genomic Applications in Practice and Prevention (EGAPP), that is aimed at the prospective integration of published data within the ACCE framework [229].

It is sobering to review the most up-to-date EGAPP recommendations, which are focused only on common diseases with a significant public health burden: there is "insufficient evidence to recommend for or against the use" of well-studied genetic tests for breast cancer, cardiovascular disease, depression, diabetes, and prostate cancer [230]. In fact, only genetic testing for KRAS mutations in colorectal cancer fulfils all requirements. Children are typically not mentioned in articles on this topic; if they are mentioned, it is as part of the subjects that are excluded [231].

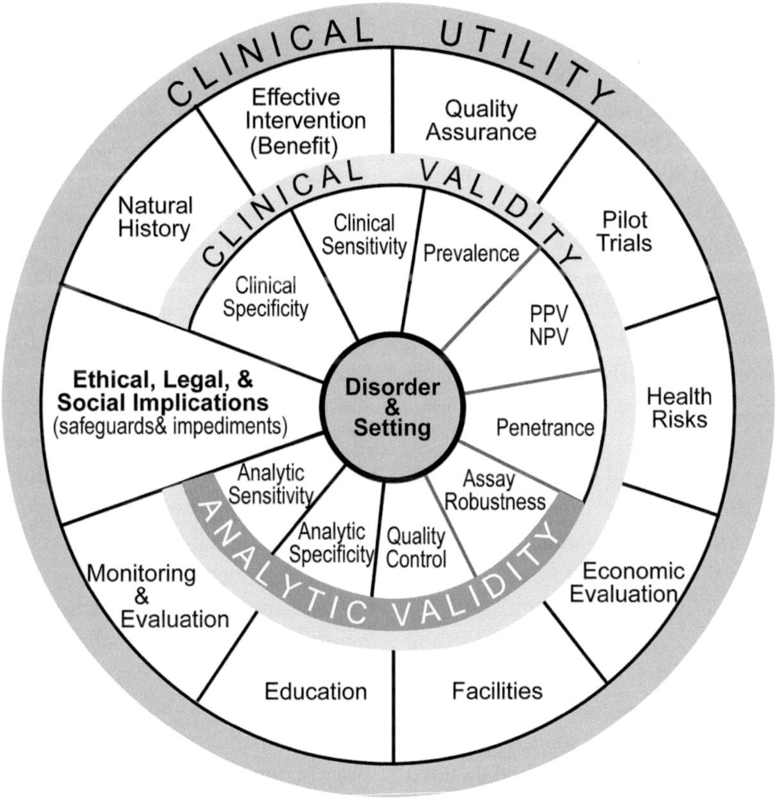

Fig. 4.16 Illustration of the ACCE framework used to evaluate genetic tests. Evaluation of genetic tests with ACCE is based on four criteria: analytic validity, clinical validity, clinical utility and associated ethical, legal and social implications (ELSI). It is meant to be an up-to-date source of information for policymakers to allow informed decision-making. This figure illustrates the various components that are studied for each category. Analytical validity is defined as how accurately and reliably the test measures the genotype of interest. Clinical validity is defined as how consistently and accurately the test detects or predicts the intermediate or final outcomes of interest. Clinical utility is defined as how likely the test is to significantly improve patient outcomes. ELSI is defined as the ethical, legal, and social implications that may arise in the context of using the test. (Figure credits: CDC, https://www.cdc.gov/genomics/gtesting/acce/index.htm)

Ethical and Legal Issues

As the clinical use of sequencing technologies becomes increasingly widespread, practicing nephrologists should expect to have to deal with a new set of issues when discussing results with their patients. With the price of whole-exome and/or exome sequencing decreasing over time, these technologies have now supplanted current approaches that are more targeted, such as Sanger sequencing. This is a dramatic change in practice since clinicians will now have to deal with genome-wide data that are not restricted to genes known to be associated with a given condition. With these changes comes a complex set of issues that every physician is likely to encounter in the near future. These include dealing with mis-attributed paternity and handling incidental genetic findings. Physicians should also be able to discuss how genomic medicine may affect patient privacy and how these results may lead to genetic discrimination. Below, we provide a brief introduction to these concepts that will provide interested physicians with a good starting point or springboard to learn more about these topics. The interested readers are directed to more in-depth reviews on these topics [232, 233].

Mis-attributed Paternity

One important consideration when performing genetic testing is to be cognizant of the fact that misattributed paternity, also referred to as non-paternity, is observed in ~10% of tested individuals (range 1–30%) [234]. In the clinical arena, this problem will be encountered in two main scenarios. First, in the context of HLA testing when assessing parents as potential organ donors [235]. The other situation is when diagnosing a genetic condition, particularly if it is a recessive disease and the father does not harbour the mutation [236].

The treating team should strongly consider consulting a medical geneticist or a genetic counsellor since they are trained to handle these situations. In addition, they can help to calculate and interpret the paternity index, the most useful measure of paternity testing [237]. This method relies on genotyping of 10–15 additional loci for each member of the trio, the assumption being that: each parent shares ~50% of the variants with their child. Rarely, a paternally inherited de novo mutation may explain these findings when paternity testing confirms that the father is indeed genetically related to the patient.

In most jurisdictions, there are no guidelines, rules, or laws that dictate what a clinical team should do in these circumstances. Proponents of nondisclosure emphasize the importance of non-maleficence, while those that advocate for disclosure invoke respect for patient autonomy and truth telling [238]. Treating physicians should be aware that nearly all genetic specialists in the US [239] or abroad [240] have consistently favoured disclosure, but only to the mother. This was also the recommendation from a report published by the Institute of Medicine in 1994 [241].

Medically Actionable Variants

Another dilemma that stems from the introduction of genome sequencing in the clinic is how incidental genomic findings, also known as "incidentalomas", should be handled. This dilemma is particularly acute when dealing with so-called "medically actionable pathologic mutations". These are defined as variants in genes known to be associated with severe Mendelian diseases for which there is good evidence of benefit from specific preventive measures or therapies. A debate on whether one has a duty to report such findings has been raging for a few years in the genetic research community: a recent consensus opinion states that such findings should be reported to subjects who have a priori consented to receive information about incidental findings [242]. The debate is now overflowing to the clinical world.

Recently published policy guidelines put forth by the American College of Medical Genetics recommend mandatory reporting of variants found via clinical sequencing and deemed to be likely pathogenic in 57 genes associated with 24 monogenic conditions [243]. In stark contrast to the research guidelines mentioned above, these incidental findings would have to be reported to patients even if they did not consent to receive this information. While providing valuable information to patients and their families, the enactment of these guidelines would add extra work that may not be accommodated easily by the current clinical workforce. Interrogation of whole-genome sequencing data from 500 Caucasians and 500 African-American "healthy" adults revealed that ~1–3% of subjects tested harbour at least 1 mutation in one of these genes [244]. Adjudication of which incidental findings are actionable is not straightforward [245].

Importantly for pediatricians, these recommendations make no exception regarding children, even for genes that cause adult-onset conditions [243]. This suggestion is based on the fact that it may be critical for the parents themselves to know about these incidental findings. It is predicted that more restricted reporting of such variants will be recommended for children once clinical sequencing becomes more widespread: indeed, this argument will be moot when the parents also have their own sequencing data [243]. Table 4.3 provides a list of genes that are relevant to the practice of pediatric nephrologists: all follow an autosomal dominant pattern of inheritance and are the primary cause for a variety of cancers [243]. A recent study on more than 2000 adults

4 Molecular Diagnosis of Genetic Diseases of the Kidney: Primer for Pediatric Nephrologists

Table 4.3 Conditions and/or syndromes with clinically actionable mutations that are relevant to pediatric nephrologists

Conditions	Gene	OMIM #	Patients affected	Mode of inheritance	Clinical impact
VHLS	VHL	193300	Child/adult	AD	Known and expected
MEN type 1	MEN1	131100	Child/adult	AD	Known and expected
MEN type 2	RET	171400, 162300	Child/adult	AD	Known
HPPS type 1	SDHD	168000	Child/adult	AD	Known and expected
HPPS type 2	SDHAF2	601650	Child/adult	AD	Known
HPPS type 3	SDHC	605373	Child/adult	AD	Known and expected
HPPS type 4	SDHB	115310	Child/adult	AD	Unknown
TSC type 1	TSC1	191100	Child	AD	Known and expected
TSC type 2	TSC2	613254	Child	AD	Known and expected
Wilms tumour	WT1	194070	Child	AD	Known and expected
NF type 2	NF2	101100	Child/adult	AD	Known and expected

HPPS hereditary paraganglioma-pheochromocytoma syndrome, *MEN* multiple endocrine neoplasia, *NF* neurofibromatosis, *TSC* tuberous sclerosis complex, *VHLS* von Hippel-Lindau syndrome

with CKD who underwent exome sequencing revealed that 1.6% had a medically actionable variant [144].

Privacy

All physicians are keenly aware that patient privacy is paramount. Most are also cognizant of data that could be used as unique identifiers: name, birth date, home address, social security number, etc. When stripped of these data, samples or datasets are deemed deidentified. Like most pediatric subspecialists, pediatric nephrologists routinely take care of patients with very rare conditions. For such patients, it is unclear how "deidentified" the information really is if the diagnosis is part of the data that may be shared. For example, the inclusion of this information in public databases could lead to the de facto identification of a specific patient, particularly if the condition is associated with a visible phenotype. For this reason, some jurisdictions have added rare (UK) or unique (USA) characteristics of patients to the list of unique identifiers [246].

One recent challenge to the privacy of patients stems from the emergence of genomic medicine because genomic data is not considered as a unique identifier per se. This is likely to become even more challenging as the pressures from the research community grow to have as many genomes available publicly as possible [247].

Given the fact that humans differ at ~0.1% of the 3.2 billion bases of the genome, and given a world population of 6 billion, current estimates show that genotyping data from 30 to 80 alleles would be sufficient to provide unique genomic fingerprinting for every individual [248]. This number is amazingly small when compared to the datasets from whole-exome and whole-genome sequencing, which provide thousands of such alleles. Thus, reidentification of a deidentified dataset is simple if one can genotype a sample obtained from an individual that may then be used to find a perfect match against all available genomic datasets (or near-perfect match for close relatives).

In a recent tour-de-force, it was shown that it is possible to trace the original subject linked to a particular genomic dataset by combining the analysis with data from publicly available genealogical databases [249]. The "investigator hackers" were able to do this with the following publicly available information in hand: whole-genome sequencing data, gender (males), age when the samples were provided, and state where the men lived at the time (Utah).

As front-line responders deal with keen parents who are very likely to use the internet to find health information [250], pediatricians should be prepared to answer questions about the impact of genomic medicine on the privacy of their patients. The current status is that there is still considerable uncertainty in the field, but the consensus appears to be that complete deidentification of genomic datasets is far more complex than expected [251].

Genetic Discrimination

The rapid developments in the sequencing and analysis of genomic information have forced a debate about the potential real-life consequences for patients when it is used in the clinic [252]. The reporting of diagnostic and/or incidental findings opens the door to genetic discrimination, which is defined as an "adverse treatment that is based solely on the genotype of asymptomatic individuals" [253].

Knowledge about genetic or familial risks for a variety of diseases has been used to justify health insurers' refusal of at-risk patients [254] or employers' dismissal of potential or current employees [255]. Most European countries have enacted legislation against this type of discrimination since the 1990s [256]. The US congress followed suit in 2008 with the passage of the Genetic Information Nondiscrimination Act (GINA) [257]. Canada remains the only G8 country without such legislation, and Canadians are routinely refused life and/or disability insurance because of genetic risk factors [258]. Similar problems also occur in other developed nations with national health care systems, such as Japan [259] or Australia [260].

All pediatricians ordering genetic tests for their patients should seek information about the current legal framework in their country as these may have immediate implications for the family as a whole. These issues should ideally be discussed with the family before ordering the tests.

Direct-to-Consumer Testing of Presymptomatic Minors

The first direct-to-consumer (DTC) genetic testing companies started to operate more than 10 years ago. Up until recently, they existed in a legislative void: because the tests used were developed internally (known as "home brews"), they are exempt from the tight regulations that apply to most diagnostic tests [261]. As a result of this, they were able to offer tests of questionable value, without oversight and without interaction with a healthcare professional before or after testing [262]. Once it became clear that thousands of people were paying for these services, regulatory bodies in many countries started to pay closer attention to the products offered by these companies [263], but changes in regulation have been slow to come [264]. The interested reader is directed to recent exhaustive reviews for more details on this complex topic [265, 266]. In this discussion, we will focus on issues that relate to DTC testing when applied specifically to children.

Many direct-to-consumer (DTC) genetic testing companies, most notably 23andMe, agree to perform pre-symptomatic or predictive genetic testing on children [267]. This is in direct contradiction with the professional guidelines promulgated by most professional organizations, which state that such tests should only be performed once the child can provide informed consent for themselves [268]. Additional concerns raised by the behaviour of DTC companies are that there is no requirement for these findings to be medically actionable (i.e., at a minimum, a way to prevent or treat the condition must exist to offer such tests to minors) [267]. The FDA has been investigating to determine whether tighter regulations are necessary for these companies.

A pediatrician should expect to be asked for advice regarding performing DTC genetic testing on their patients, or they may be asked to help interpret the results of such tests [269]. It may also lead to new consultations for asymptomatic children because a number of renal conditions are included in mainstream DTC reports (for example, carrier status for ARPKD, primary hyperoxaluria type 2, and tyrosinemia type 1). Since DTC companies do not spend time explaining the ethical and legal issues that stem from such testing (discussed above), the onus will be on the treating physician to do so. Unless clinically indicated, pediatricians should strongly consider refraining from ordering additional diagnostic tests triggered solely from the results of DTC genetic testing as the clinical validity of many of the findings has yet to be established [270]. In a significant turn of events, the US Federal Drug Administration (FDA) asked 23andme to stop marketing these tests to consumers starting in November 2013; the FDA will now require DTC genomic companies to undergo regulatory clearances that are typical for genetic tests used in the clinic.

Online Resources

Sources	URLs
FDA letter to 23andme	https://peds-renomics.clinic/FDA-vs-23andme
23andme website	https://www.23andme.com/health/

Glossary

Alleles Alternative forms of a gene at the same locus.

Alternative splicing Formation of diverse mRNAs through differential splicing of an mRNA precursor.

Autosome Any chromosome (1–22) other than the sex chromosomes X and Y.

cDNA, complementary DNA DNA sequence that contains only exonic sequences and was made from an mRNA molecule.

Centimorgan Length of DNA that on average has 1 crossover per 100 gametes.

Cis Location of two genes/changes on the same chromosome.

Codon Three consecutive bases/nucleotides in DNA/RNA that specifies an amino acid.

Compound heterozygote Individual with two different mutant alleles at a locus.

Consanguineous Mating between individuals who share at least one common ancestor.

Conservation Sequence similarity for genes present in two distinct organisms or for gene families; can be detected by measuring the sequence similarity at the nucleotide (DNA or RNA) or amino acid (protein) level.

Crossover Exchange of genetic material between homologous chromosomes during meiosis.

Digenic inheritance Two genes interacting to produce a disease phenotype.

Diploid Chromosome number of somatic cells.

Domain Segment of a protein associated with a specialized structure or function.

Dominant Trait expressed in the heterozygote.

Downstream Sequence that is distal or 3′ from the reference point.

Empiric risk Recurrence risk based on experience rather than calculation.

Epigenetics Term describing non-mutational phenomena (e.g., methylation and acetylation) that modify the expression of a gene.

Euchromatin Majority of nuclear DNA that remains relatively unfolded during most of the cell cycle and is therefore accessible to transcriptional machinery.

Exon Segment of a gene (usually protein-coding) that remains after splicing of the primary RNA transcript.

Expressivity Variation in the severity of a genetic trait.

Genotype Genetic constitution of the organism; usually refers to a particular pair of alleles the individual carries at a given locus of the genome.

Germline Cell lineage resulting in eggs or sperm.

Germline mutation Any detectable, heritable variation in the lineage of germ cells transmitted to offspring while those in somatic cells are not.

Gonadal (germline) mosaicism Occurrence of more than one genetic constitution in the precursor cells of eggs or sperm.

Haplotype Group of nearby, closely linked alleles inherited together as a unit.

Heterozygote Person with one normal and one mutant allele at a given locus on a pair of homologous chromosomes.

Homozygote Person with identical alleles at a given locus on a pair of homologous chromosomes.

Imprinting Parent-specific expression or repression of genes or chromosomes in offspring.

Intron Segment of a gene transcribed into the primary RNA transcript but excised during exon splicing, thus does not code for a protein.

Isodisomy, uniparental Inheritance of two copies of one homologue of a chromosome from one parent, with loss of the corresponding homologue from the other parent.

Karyotype Classified chromosome complement of an individual or a cell.

Lyon hypothesis (X inactivation) Principle of inactivation of one of the two X chromosomes in normal female cells (first proposed by Dr. Mary Lyon).

Mendelian Following patterns of inheritance originally proposed by Gregor Mendel.

Monogenic disorder Caused by mutations in a single gene.

Mosaicism Occurrence of more than one genetic constitution arising in an individual after fertilization.

Multifactorial disorder Caused by the interaction of multiple genetic and environmental factors.

Mutation Change from the normal to an altered form of a particular gene that has harmful; pathogenic effects.

Oligogenic inheritance Character that is determined by a small number of genes acting together.

Penetrance Frequency with which a genotype manifests itself in a given phenotype.

Phenotype Visible expression of the action of a particular gene; the clinical picture resulting from a genetic disorder.

Pleiotropy Multiple effects of a single gene.

Polymerase chain reaction (PCR) Amplification of DNA using a specific technique that allows analysis of minute original amounts of DNA.

Polymorphism Usually used for any sequence variant present at a frequency greater than 1% in a population.

Recessive A trait expressed only when both alleles at a given genetic locus are altered.

Recombination Separation of alleles that are close together on the same chromosome by crossing over of homologous chromosomes at meiosis.

SNPs (single nucleotide polymorphism) Usually used for any sequence variant present at a frequency greater than 1% in a population.

Somatic Involving the body cells rather than the germline.

Syndrome, genetic Nonrandom combination of features.

Teratogen Any agent causing congenital malformations.

Trans Location of two genes/changes on opposite chromosomes of a pair.

Transcription Production of mRNA from the DNA template.

Translation The process by which a protein is synthesized from an mRNA sequence.

References

1. Guttmacher AE, Porteous ME, McInerney JD. Educating health-care professionals about genetics and genomics. Nat Rev Genet. 2007;8:151–7. https://doi.org/10.1038/nrg2007.
2. Watson JD, Crick FH. Molecular structure of nucleic acids; a structure for deoxyribose nucleic acid. Nature. 1953;171:737–8. https://doi.org/10.1038/171737a0.
3. Wei L-H, Guo JU. Coding functions of "noncoding" RNAs. Science. 2020:1074–5. https://doi.org/10.1126/science.aba6117.
4. Statello L, Guo C-J, Chen L-L, Huarte M. Gene regulation by long non-coding RNAs and its biological functions. Nat Rev Mol Cell Biol. 2021;22:96–118. https://doi.org/10.1038/s41580-020-00315-9.
5. Hood L, Rowen L. The Human Genome Project: big science transforms biology and medicine. Genome Med. 2013;5:79. https://doi.org/10.1186/gm483.
6. Lander ES, Linton LM, Birren B, Nusbaum C, Zody MC, Baldwin J, et al. Initial sequencing and analysis of the human genome. Nature. 2001;409:860–921. https://doi.org/10.1038/35057062.
7. International Human Genome Sequencing Consortium. Finishing the euchromatic sequence of the human genome. Nature. 2004;431:931–45. https://doi.org/10.1038/nature03001.
8. Eisenstein M. Closing in on a complete human genome. Nature. 2021;590:679–81. https://doi.org/10.1038/d41586-021-00462-9.
9. Kellis M, Wold B, Snyder MP, Bernstein BE, Kundaje A, Marinov GK, et al. Defining functional DNA elements in the human genome. Proc Natl Acad Sci U S A. 2014;111:6131–8. https://doi.org/10.1073/pnas.1318948111.
10. Gregorich ZR, Ge Y. Top-down proteomics in health and disease: challenges and opportunities. Proteomics. 2014;14:1195–210. https://doi.org/10.1002/pmic.201300432.
11. Oliverio AL, Bellomo T, Mariani LH. Evolving clinical applications of tissue transcriptomics in kidney disease. Front Pediatr. 2019;7:306. https://doi.org/10.3389/fped.2019.00306.

12. Zhang L, Lu Q, Chang C. Epigenetics in health and disease. Adv Exp Med Biol. 2020;1253:3–55. https://doi.org/10.1007/978-981-15-3449-2_1.
13. Wishart DS. Metabolomics for investigating physiological and pathophysiological processes. Physiol Rev. 2019;99:1819–75. https://doi.org/10.1152/physrev.00035.2018.
14. Peer E, Rechavi G, Dominissini D. Epitranscriptomics: regulation of mRNA metabolism through modifications. Curr Opin Chem Biol. 2017;41:93–8. https://doi.org/10.1016/j.cbpa.2017.10.008.
15. Braun DA, Rao J, Mollet G, Schapiro D, Daugeron M-C, Tan W, et al. Mutations in KEOPS-complex genes cause nephrotic syndrome with primary microcephaly. Nat Genet. 2017;49:1529–38. https://doi.org/10.1038/ng.3933.
16. Balogh E, Chandler JC, Varga M, Tahoun M, Menyhárd DK, Schay G, et al. Pseudouridylation defect due to DKC1 and NOP10 mutations causes nephrotic syndrome with cataracts, hearing impairment, and enterocolitis. Proc Natl Acad Sci U S A. 2020;117:15137–47. https://doi.org/10.1073/pnas.2002328117.
17. Potter SS. Single-cell RNA sequencing for the study of development, physiology and disease. Nat Rev Nephrol. 2018;14:479–92. https://doi.org/10.1038/s41581-018-0021-7.
18. Wu H, Humphreys BD. The promise of single-cell RNA sequencing for kidney disease investigation. Kidney Int. 2017;92:1334–42. https://doi.org/10.1016/j.kint.2017.06.033.
19. Karczewski KJ, Snyder MP. Integrative omics for health and disease. Nat Rev Genet. 2018;19:299–310. https://doi.org/10.1038/nrg.2018.4.
20. Erickson RP. Somatic gene mutation and human disease other than cancer: an update. Mutat Res. 2010;705:96–106. https://doi.org/10.1016/j.mrrev.2010.04.002.
21. Tan AY, Zhang T, Michaeel A, Blumenfeld J, Liu G, Zhang W, et al. Somatic mutations in renal cyst epithelium in autosomal dominant polycystic kidney disease. J Am Soc Nephrol. 2018;29:2139–56. https://doi.org/10.1681/ASN.2017080878.
22. MacArthur DG, Manolio TA, Dimmock DP, Rehm HL, Shendure J, Abecasis GR, et al. Guidelines for investigating causality of sequence variants in human disease. Nature. 2014;508:469–76. https://doi.org/10.1038/nature13127.
23. Gale DP, Mallett A, Patel C, Sneddon TP, Rehm HL, Sampson MG, et al. Diagnoses of uncertain significance: kidney genetics in the 21st century. Nat Rev Nephrol. 2020;16:616–8. https://doi.org/10.1038/s41581-020-0277-6.
24. Ko Y-A, Susztak K. Epigenomics: the science of no-longer-junk DNA. Why study it in chronic kidney disease? Semin Nephrol. 2013;33:354–62. https://doi.org/10.1016/j.semnephrol.2013.05.007.
25. Mele C, Lemaire M, Iatropoulos P, Piras R, Bresin E, Bettoni S, et al. Characterization of a new DGKE intronic mutation in genetically unsolved cases of familial atypical hemolytic uremic syndrome. Clin J Am Soc Nephrol. 2015;10:1011–9. https://doi.org/10.2215/CJN.08520814.
26. Hunt RC, Simhadri VL, Iandoli M, Sauna ZE, Kimchi-Sarfaty C. Exposing synonymous mutations. Trends Genet. 2014;30:308–21. https://doi.org/10.1016/j.tig.2014.04.006.
27. Camps M, Herman A, Loh E, Loeb LA. Genetic constraints on protein evolution. Crit Rev Biochem Mol Biol. 2007;42:313–26. https://doi.org/10.1080/10409230701597642.
28. Hanks SK, Quinn AM, Hunter T. The protein kinase family: conserved features and deduced phylogeny of the catalytic domains. Science. 1988;241:42–52. https://doi.org/10.1126/science.3291115.
29. Gloss BS, Dinger ME. Realizing the significance of noncoding functionality in clinical genomics. Exp Mol Med. 2018;50:1–8. https://doi.org/10.1038/s12276-018-0087-0.
30. Landegren U, Nilsson M, Kwok PY. Reading bits of genetic information: methods for single-nucleotide polymorphism analysis. Genome Res. 1998;8:769–76. https://doi.org/10.1101/gr.8.8.769.
31. Nakamura Y. DNA variations in human and medical genetics: 25 years of my experience. J Hum Genet. 2009;54:1–8. https://doi.org/10.1038/jhg.2008.6.
32. International HapMap Consortium, Frazer KA, Ballinger DG, Cox DR, Hinds DA, Stuve LL, et al. A second generation human haplotype map of over 3.1 million SNPs. Nature. 2007;449:851–61. https://doi.org/10.1038/nature06258.
33. Bustamante CD, Burchard EG, De la Vega FM. Genomics for the world. Nature. 2011;475:163–5. https://doi.org/10.1038/475163a.
34. Neale BM. Introduction to linkage disequilibrium, the HapMap, and imputation. Cold Spring Harb Protoc. 2010;2010:db.top74. https://doi.org/10.1101/pdb.top74.
35. Stram DO. Tag SNP selection for association studies. Genet Epidemiol. 2004;27:365–74. https://doi.org/10.1002/gepi.20028.
36. Karki R, Pandya D, Elston RC, Ferlini C. Defining "mutation" and "polymorphism" in the era of personal genomics. BMC Med Genet. 2015;8:37. https://doi.org/10.1186/s12920-015-0115-z.
37. Sherry ST, Ward MH, Kholodov M, Baker J, Phan L, Smigielski EM, et al. dbSNP: the NCBI database of genetic variation. Nucleic Acids Res. 2001;29:308–11. https://doi.org/10.1093/nar/29.1.308.
38. Jiang Y, Epstein MP, Conneely KN. Assessing the impact of population stratification on association studies of rare variation. Hum Hered. 2013;76:28–35. https://doi.org/10.1159/000353270.
39. Sirugo G, Williams SM, Tishkoff SA. The missing diversity in human genetic studies. Cell. 2019;177:26–31. https://doi.org/10.1016/j.cell.2019.02.048.
40. Shraga R, Yarnall S, Elango S, Manoharan A, Rodriguez SA, Bristow SL, et al. Evaluating genetic

40. ancestry and self-reported ethnicity in the context of carrier screening. BMC Genet. 2017;18:99. https://doi.org/10.1186/s12863-017-0570-y.

41. Alves I, Srámková Hanulová A, Foll M, Excoffier L. Genomic data reveal a complex making of humans. PLoS Genet. 2012;8:e1002837. https://doi.org/10.1371/journal.pgen.1002837.

42. Mersha TB, Abebe T. Self-reported race/ethnicity in the age of genomic research: its potential impact on understanding health disparities. Hum Genomics. 2015;9:1. https://doi.org/10.1186/s40246-014-0023-x.

43. Reich D, Price AL, Patterson N. Principal component analysis of genetic data. Nat Genet. 2008:491–2. https://doi.org/10.1038/ng0508-491.

44. Mills RE, Walter K, Stewart C, Handsaker RE, Chen K, Alkan C, et al. Mapping copy number variation by population-scale genome sequencing. Nature. 2011;470:59–65. https://doi.org/10.1038/nature09708.

45. Church DM, Lappalainen I, Sneddon TP, Hinton J, Maguire M, Lopez J, et al. Public data archives for genomic structural variation. Nat Genet. 2010;42:813–4. https://doi.org/10.1038/ng1010-813.

46. Nowakowska B. Clinical interpretation of copy number variants in the human genome. J Appl Genet. 2017;58:449–57. https://doi.org/10.1007/s13353-017-0407-4.

47. Roth JR. Frameshift mutations. Annu Rev Genet. 1974;8:319–46. https://doi.org/10.1146/annurev.ge.08.120174.001535.

48. Kirby A, Gnirke A, Jaffe DB, Barešová V, Pochet N, Blumenstiel B, et al. Mutations causing medullary cystic kidney disease type 1 lie in a large VNTR in MUC1 missed by massively parallel sequencing. Nat Genet. 2013;45:299–303. https://doi.org/10.1038/ng.2543.

49. Tubio JMC, Estivill X. Cancer: when catastrophe strikes a cell. Nature. 2011;470:476–7. https://doi.org/10.1038/470476a.

50. Christodoulou K, Tsingis M, Stavrou C, Eleftheriou A, Papapavlou P, Patsalis PC, et al. Chromosome 1 localization of a gene for autosomal dominant medullary cystic kidney disease (ADMCKD). Hum Mol Genet. 1998;7:905–11.

51. Antignac C, Knebelmann B, Drouot L, Gros F, Deschênes G, Hors-Cayla MC, et al. Deletions in the COL4A5 collagen gene in X-linked Alport syndrome. Characterization of the pathological transcripts in nonrenal cells and correlation with disease expression. J Clin Invest. 1994;93:1195–207. https://doi.org/10.1172/JCI117073.

52. Gale DP, de Jorge EG, Cook HT, Martinez-Barricarte R, Hadjisavvas A, McLean AG, et al. Identification of a mutation in complement factor H-related protein 5 in patients of Cypriot origin with glomerulonephritis. Lancet. 2010;376:794–801. https://doi.org/10.1016/S0140-6736(10)60670-8.

53. Barnes MR, Breen G. A short primer on the functional analysis of copy number variation for biomedical scientists. Methods Mol Biol. 2010;628:119–35. https://doi.org/10.1007/978-1-60327-367-1_7.

54. Pook MA, Wrong O, Wooding C, Norden AGW, Feest TG, Thakker RV. Dent's disease, a renal Fanconi syndrome with nephrocalcinosis and kidney stones, is associated with a microdeletion involving DXS25 and maps to Xp11.22. Hum Mol Genet. 1993;2:2129–34.

55. Barker DF, Hostikka SL, Zhou J, Chow LT, Oliphant AR, Gerken SC, et al. Identification of mutations in the COL4A5 collagen gene in Alport syndrome. Science. 1990;248:1224–7. https://doi.org/10.1126/science.2349482.

56. Hildebrandt F, Otto E, Rensing C, Nothwang HG, Vollmer M, Adolphs J, et al. A novel gene encoding an SH3 domain protein is mutated in nephronophthisis type 1. Nat Genet. 1997;17:149–53. https://doi.org/10.1038/ng1097-149.

57. Lippe B, Geffner ME, Dietrich RB, Boechat MI, Kangarloo H. Renal malformations in patients with Turner syndrome: imaging in 141 patients. Pediatrics. 1988;82:852–6. Available from: https://www.ncbi.nlm.nih.gov/pubmed/3054787.

58. Málaga S, Pardo R, Málaga I, Orejas G, Fernández-Toral J. Renal involvement in Down syndrome. Pediatr Nephrol. 2005;20:614–7. https://doi.org/10.1007/s00467-005-1825-9.

59. Henrichsen CN, Chaignat E, Reymond A. Copy number variants, diseases and gene expression. Hum Mol Genet. 2009;18:R1–8. https://doi.org/10.1093/hmg/ddp011.

60. Aitman TJ, Dong R, Vyse TJ, Norsworthy PJ, Johnson MD, Smith J, et al. Copy number polymorphism in Fcgr3 predisposes to glomerulonephritis in rats and humans. Nature. 2006;439:851–5. https://doi.org/10.1038/nature04489.

61. Sanna-Cherchi S, Kiryluk K, Burgess KE, Bodria M, Sampson MG, Hadley D, et al. Copy-number disorders are a common cause of congenital kidney malformations. Am J Hum Genet. 2012;91:987–97. https://doi.org/10.1016/j.ajhg.2012.10.007.

62. Girgis AH, Iakovlev VV, Beheshti B, Bayani J, Squire JA, Bui A, et al. Multilevel whole-genome analysis reveals candidate biomarkers in clear cell renal cell carcinoma. Cancer Res. 2012;72:5273–84. https://doi.org/10.1158/0008-5472.CAN-12-0656.

63. Riethoven J-JM. Regulatory regions in DNA: promoters, enhancers, silencers, and insulators. Methods Mol Biol. 2010;674:33–42. https://doi.org/10.1007/978-1-60761-854-6_3.

64. Vervoort VS, Smith RJH, O'Brien J, Schroer R, Abbott A, Stevenson RE, et al. Genomic rearrangements of EYA1 account for a large fraction of families with BOR syndrome. Eur J Hum Genet. 2002;10:757–66. https://doi.org/10.1038/sj.ejhg.5200877.

65. Hertz JM, Persson U, Juncker I, Segelmark M. Alport syndrome caused by inversion of a 21 Mb fragment

of the long arm of the X-chromosome comprising exon 9 through 51 of the COL4A5 gene. Hum Genet. 2005;118:23–8. https://doi.org/10.1007/s00439-005-0013-0.

66. Reilly DS, Lewis RA, Ledbetter DH, Nussbaum RL. Oculocerebrorenal syndrome, with application to carrier assessment. Am J Hum Genet. 1988;42:748–55.

67. Comino-Méndez I, Gracia-Aznárez FJ, Schiavi F, Landa I, Leandro-García LJ, Letón R, et al. Exome sequencing identifies MAX mutations as a cause of hereditary pheochromocytoma. Nat Genet. 2011;43:663–7. https://doi.org/10.1038/ng.861.

68. Stephens PJ, Greenman CD, Fu B, Yang F, Bignell GR, Mudie LJ, et al. Massive genomic rearrangement acquired in a single catastrophic event during cancer development. Cell. 2011;144:27–40. https://doi.org/10.1016/j.cell.2010.11.055.

69. Forment JV, Kaidi A, Jackson SP. Chromothripsis and cancer: causes and consequences of chromosome shattering. Nat Rev Cancer. 2012;12:663–70. https://doi.org/10.1038/nrc3352.

70. Maher CA, Wilson RK. Chromothripsis and human disease: piecing together the shattering process. Cell. 2012;148:29–32. https://doi.org/10.1016/j.cell.2012.01.006.

71. Mitchell TJ, Turajlic S, Rowan A, Nicol D, Farmery JHR, O'Brien T, et al. Timing the landmark events in the evolution of clear cell renal cell cancer: TRACERx renal. Cell. 2018;173:611–623.e17. https://doi.org/10.1016/j.cell.2018.02.020.

72. Kloosterman WP, Guryev V, van Roosmalen M, Duran KJ, de Bruijn E, Bakker SCM, et al. Chromothripsis as a mechanism driving complex de novo structural rearrangements in the germline. Hum Mol Genet. 2011;20:1916–24. https://doi.org/10.1093/hmg/ddr073.

73. Chiang C, Jacobsen JC, Ernst C, Hanscom C, Heilbut A, Blumenthal I, et al. Complex reorganization and predominant non-homologous repair following chromosomal breakage in karyotypically balanced germline rearrangements and transgenic integration. Nat Genet. 2012;44(390–7):S1. https://doi.org/10.1038/ng.2202.

74. Kloosterman WP, Tavakoli-Yaraki M, van Roosmalen MJ, van Binsbergen E, Renkens I, Duran K, et al. Constitutional chromothripsis rearrangements involve clustered double-stranded DNA breaks and nonhomologous repair mechanisms. Cell Rep. 2012;1:648–55. https://doi.org/10.1016/j.celrep.2012.05.009.

75. de Pagter MS, van Roosmalen MJ, Baas AF, Renkens I, Duran KJ, van Binsbergen E, et al. Chromothripsis in healthy individuals affects multiple protein-coding genes and can result in severe congenital abnormalities in offspring. Am J Hum Genet. 2015;96:651–6. https://doi.org/10.1016/j.ajhg.2015.02.005.

76. Bertelsen B, Nazaryan-Petersen L, Sun W, Mehrjouy MM, Xie G, Chen W, et al. A germline chromothripsis event stably segregating in 11 individuals through three generations. Genet Med. 2016;18:494–500. https://doi.org/10.1038/gim.2015.112.

77. Veitia RA, Birchler JA. Dominance and gene dosage balance in health and disease: why levels matter! J Pathol. 2010;220:174–85. https://doi.org/10.1002/path.2623.

78. Johnson AF, Nguyen HT, Veitia RA. Causes and effects of haploinsufficiency. Biol Rev Camb Philos Soc. 2019;94:1774–85. https://doi.org/10.1111/brv.12527.

79. Morrill SA, Amon A. Why haploinsufficiency persists. Proc Natl Acad Sci U S A. 2019;116:11866–71. https://doi.org/10.1073/pnas.1900437116.

80. Clissold RL, Hamilton AJ, Hattersley AT, Ellard S, Bingham C. HNF1B-associated renal and extra-renal disease-an expanding clinical spectrum. Nat Rev Nephrol. 2015;11:102–12. https://doi.org/10.1038/nrneph.2014.232.

81. Bockenhauer D, Jaureguiberry G. HNF1B-associated clinical phenotypes: the kidney and beyond. Pediatr Nephrol. 2016;31:707–14. https://doi.org/10.1007/s00467-015-3142-2.

82. Clissold RL, Ashfield B, Burrage J, Hannon E, Bingham C, Mill J, et al. Genome-wide methylomic analysis in individuals with HNF1B intragenic mutation and 17q12 microdeletion. Clin Epigenetics. 2018;10:97. https://doi.org/10.1186/s13148-018-0530-z.

83. Kim J-H, Park EY, Chitayat D, Stachura DL, Schaper J, Lindstrom K, et al. SON haploinsufficiency causes impaired pre-mRNA splicing of CAKUT genes and heterogeneous renal phenotypes. Kidney Int. 2019;95:1494–504. https://doi.org/10.1016/j.kint.2019.01.025.

84. Lopez-Rivera E, Liu YP, Verbitsky M, Anderson BR, Capone VP, Otto EA, et al. Genetic drivers of kidney defects in the DiGeorge syndrome. N Engl J Med. 2017;376:742–54. https://doi.org/10.1056/NEJMoa1609009.

85. Le Tanno P, Breton J, Bidart M, Satre V, Harbuz R, Ray PF, et al. PBX1 haploinsufficiency leads to syndromic congenital anomalies of the kidney and urinary tract (CAKUT) in humans. J Med Genet. 2017;54:502–10. https://doi.org/10.1136/jmedgenet-2016-104435.

86. Yang N, Wu N, Dong S, Zhang L, Zhao Y, Chen W, et al. Human and mouse studies establish TBX6 in Mendelian CAKUT and as a potential driver of kidney defects associated with the 16p11.2 microdeletion syndrome. Kidney Int. 2020;98:1020–30. https://doi.org/10.1016/j.kint.2020.04.045.

87. Cordido A, Besada-Cerecedo L, García-González MA. The genetic and cellular basis of autosomal dominant polycystic kidney disease-a primer for clinicians. Front Pediatr. 2017;5:279. https://doi.org/10.3389/fped.2017.00279.

88. Henske EP, Jóźwiak S, Kingswood JC, Sampson JR, Thiele EA. Tuberous sclerosis complex. Nat Rev Dis Primers. 2016;2:16035. https://doi.org/10.1038/nrdp.2016.35.

89. Veys KR, Elmonem MA, Arcolino FO, van den Heuvel L, Levtchenko E. Nephropathic cystinosis: an update. Curr Opin Pediatr. 2017;29:168–78. https://doi.org/10.1097/MOP.0000000000000462.

90. Bergmann C. Genetics of autosomal recessive polycystic kidney disease and its differential diagnoses. Front Pediatr. 2017;5:221. https://doi.org/10.3389/fped.2017.00221.

91. Besouw MTP, Kleta R, Bockenhauer D. Bartter and Gitelman syndromes: questions of class. Pediatr Nephrol. 2020;35:1815–24. https://doi.org/10.1007/s00467-019-04371-y.

92. Furgeson SB, Linas S. Mechanisms of type I and type II pseudohypoaldosteronism. J Am Soc Nephrol. 2010;21:1842–5. https://doi.org/10.1681/ASN.2010050457.

93. Bockenhauer D, Bichet DG. Nephrogenic diabetes insipidus. Curr Opin Pediatr. 2017;29:199–205. https://doi.org/10.1097/MOP.0000000000000473.

94. Ehlayel AM, Copelovitch L. Update on dent disease. Pediatr Clin N Am. 2019;66:169–78. https://doi.org/10.1016/j.pcl.2018.09.003.

95. Zhang X, Zhang Y, Zhang Y, Gu H, Chen Z, Ren L, et al. X-linked Alport syndrome: pathogenic variant features and further auditory genotype-phenotype correlations in males. Orphanet J Rare Dis. 2018;13:229. https://doi.org/10.1186/s13023-018-0974-4.

96. Haffner D, Emma F, Eastwood DM, Duplan MB, Bacchetta J, Schnabel D, et al. Clinical practice recommendations for the diagnosis and management of X-linked hypophosphataemia. Nat Rev Nephrol. 2019;15:435–55. https://doi.org/10.1038/s41581-019-0152-5.

97. Govers LP, Toka HR, Hariri A, Walsh SB, Bockenhauer D. Mitochondrial DNA mutations in renal disease: an overview. Pediatr Nephrol. 2021;36:9–17. https://doi.org/10.1007/s00467-019-04404-6.

98. Ragoussis J. Genotyping technologies for genetic research. Annu Rev Genomics Hum Genet. 2009;10:117–33. https://doi.org/10.1146/annurev-genom-082908-150116.

99. Torkamani A, Wineinger NE, Topol EJ. The personal and clinical utility of polygenic risk scores. Nat Rev Genet. 2018;19:581–90. https://doi.org/10.1038/s41576-018-0018-x.

100. Liu L, Kiryluk K. Genome-wide polygenic risk predictors for kidney disease. Nat Rev Nephrol. 2018:723–4. https://doi.org/10.1038/s41581-018-0067-6.

101. Lander ES, Schork NJ. Genetic dissection of complex traits. Science. 1994;265:2037–48. https://doi.org/10.1126/science.8091226.

102. Ott J, Wang J, Leal SM. Genetic linkage analysis in the age of whole-genome sequencing. Nat Rev Genet. 2015;16:275–84. https://doi.org/10.1038/nrg3908.

103. Hamamy H, Antonarakis SE, Cavalli-Sforza LL, Temtamy S, Romeo G, Kate LPT, et al. Consanguineous marriages, pearls and perils: Geneva International Consanguinity Workshop Report. Genet Med. 2011;13:841–7. https://doi.org/10.1097/GIM.0b013e318217477f.

104. Lander ES, Botstein D. Homozygosity mapping: a way to map human recessive traits with the DNA of inbred children. Science. 1987;236:1567–70. https://doi.org/10.1126/science.2884728.

105. Alkuraya FS. Discovery of rare homozygous mutations from studies of consanguineous pedigrees. Curr Protoc Hum Genet. 2012;Chapter 6:Unit6.12. https://doi.org/10.1002/0471142905.hg0612s75.

106. Alkuraya FS. Autozygome decoded. Genet Med. 2010;12:765–71. https://doi.org/10.1097/GIM.0b013e3181fbfcc4.

107. Miano MG, Jacobson SG, Carothers A, Hanson I, Teague P, Lovell J, et al. Pitfalls in homozygosity mapping. Am J Hum Genet. 2000;67:1348–51. Available from: https://linkinghub.elsevier.com/retrieve/pii/S0002929707629668.

108. Bolk S, Puffenberger EG, Hudson J, Morton DH, Chakravarti A. Elevated frequency and allelic heterogeneity of congenital nephrotic syndrome, Finnish type, in the old order Mennonites. Am J Hum Genet. 1999;65:1785–90. https://doi.org/10.1086/302687.

109. Frishberg Y, Ben-Neriah Z, Suvanto M, Rinat C, Männikkö M, Feinstein S, et al. Misleading findings of homozygosity mapping resulting from three novel mutations in NPHS1 encoding nephrin in a highly inbred community. Genet Med. 2007;9:180–4. https://doi.org/10.1097/gim.0b013e318031c7de.

110. Hildebrandt F, Heeringa SF, Rüschendorf F, Attanasio M, Nürnberg G, Becker C, et al. A systematic approach to mapping recessive disease genes in individuals from outbred populations. PLoS Genet. 2009;5:e1000353. https://doi.org/10.1371/journal.pgen.1000353.

111. Alkuraya FS. Homozygosity mapping: one more tool in the clinical geneticist's toolbox. Genet Med. 2010;12:236–9. https://doi.org/10.1097/GIM.0b013e3181ceb95d.

112. Abu Safieh L, Aldahmesh MA, Shamseldin H, Hashem M, Shaheen R, Alkuraya H, et al. Clinical and molecular characterisation of Bardet-Biedl syndrome in consanguineous populations: the power of homozygosity mapping. J Med Genet. 2010;47:236–41. https://doi.org/10.1136/jmg.2009.070755.

113. Köttgen A. Genome-wide association studies in nephrology research. Am J Kidney Dis. 2010;56:743–58. https://doi.org/10.1053/j.ajkd.2010.05.018.

114. Borecki IB, Province MA. Linkage and association: basic concepts. Adv Genet. 2008;60:51–74. https://doi.org/10.1016/S0065-2660(07)00403-8.

115. Pan Q. Multiple hypotheses testing procedures in clinical trials and genomic studies. Front Public Health. 2013;1:63. https://doi.org/10.3389/fpubh.2013.00063.

116. Visscher PM, Brown MA, McCarthy MI, Yang J. Five years of GWAS discovery. Am J Hum Genet. 2012;90:7–24. https://doi.org/10.1016/j.ajhg.2011.11.029.

117. Kao WHL, Klag MJ, Meoni LA, Reich D, Berthier-Schaad Y, Li M, et al. MYH9 is associated with nondiabetic end-stage renal disease in African Americans. Nat Genet. 2008;40:1185–92. https://doi.org/10.1038/ng.232.

118. Kopp JB, Smith MW, Nelson GW, Johnson RC, Freedman BI, Bowden DW, et al. MYH9 is a major-effect risk gene for focal segmental glomerulosclerosis. Nat Genet. 2008;40:1175–84. https://doi.org/10.1038/ng.226.

119. Seri M, Pecci A, Di Bari F, Cusano R, Savino M, Panza E, et al. MYH9-related disease: may-Hegglin anomaly, Sebastian syndrome, Fechtner syndrome, and Epstein syndrome are not distinct entities but represent a variable expression of a single illness. Medicine. 2003;82:203–15. https://doi.org/10.1097/01.md.0000076006.64510.5c.

120. Genovese G, Friedman DJ, Ross MD, Lecordier L, Uzureau P, Freedman BI, et al. Association of trypanolytic ApoL1 variants with kidney disease in African Americans. Science. 2010;329:841–5. https://doi.org/10.1126/science.1193032.

121. Parsa A, Kao WHL, Xie D, Astor BC, Li M, Hsu C-Y, et al. APOL1 risk variants, race, and progression of chronic kidney disease. N Engl J Med. 2013;369:2183–96. https://doi.org/10.1056/NEJMoa1310345.

122. Friedman DJ, Pollak MR. APOL1 and kidney disease: from genetics to biology. Annu Rev Physiol. 2020;82:323–42. https://doi.org/10.1146/annurev-physiol-021119-034345.

123. Bruggeman LA, O'Toole JF, Sedor JR. APOL1 polymorphisms and kidney disease: loss-of-function or gain-of-function? Am J Physiol Renal Physiol. 2019;316:F1–8. https://doi.org/10.1152/ajprenal.00426.2018.

124. Min Jou W, Haegeman G, Ysebaert M, Fiers W. Nucleotide sequence of the gene coding for the bacteriophage MS2 coat protein. Nature. 1972;237:82–8. https://doi.org/10.1038/237082a0.

125. Sanger F, Nicklen S, Coulson AR. DNA sequencing with chain-terminating inhibitors. Biotechnology. 1992;24:104–8. Available from: https://www.ncbi.nlm.nih.gov/pubmed/1422003.

126. Smith LM, Sanders JZ, Kaiser RJ, Hughes P, Dodd C, Connell CR, et al. Fluorescence detection in automated DNA sequence analysis. Nature. 1986;321:674–9. https://doi.org/10.1038/321674a0.

127. Metzker ML. Sequencing technologies—the next generation. Nat Rev Genet. 2010;11:31–46. https://doi.org/10.1038/nrg2626.

128. Loman NJ, Misra RV, Dallman TJ, Constantinidou C, Gharbia SE, Wain J, et al. Performance comparison of benchtop high-throughput sequencing platforms. Nat Biotechnol. 2012;30:434–9. https://doi.org/10.1038/nbt.2198.

129. Abecasis GR, Altshuler D, Auton A, Brooks LD, Durbin RM, Gibbs RA, et al. A map of human genome variation from population-scale sequencing. Nature. 2010;467:1061–73. https://doi.org/10.1038/nature09534.

130. Buchanan CC, Torstenson ES, Bush WS, Ritchie MD. A comparison of cataloged variation between International HapMap Consortium and 1000 Genomes Project data. J Am Med Inform Assoc. 2012;19:289–94. https://doi.org/10.1136/amiajnl-2011-000652.

131. Ng PC, Levy S, Huang J, Stockwell TB, Walenz BP, Li K, et al. Genetic variation in an individual human exome. PLoS Genet. 2008;4:e1000160. https://doi.org/10.1371/journal.pgen.1000160.

132. Choi M, Scholl UI, Ji W, Liu T, Tikhonova IR, Zumbo P, et al. Genetic diagnosis by whole exome capture and massively parallel DNA sequencing. Proc Natl Acad Sci U S A. 2009;106:19096–101. https://doi.org/10.1073/pnas.0910672106.

133. Hodges E, Xuan Z, Balija V, Kramer M, Molla MN, Smith SW, et al. Genome-wide in situ exon capture for selective resequencing. Nat Genet. 2007;39:1522–7. https://doi.org/10.1038/ng.2007.42.

134. Ng SB, Turner EH, Robertson PD, Flygare SD, Bigham AW, Lee C, et al. Targeted capture and massively parallel sequencing of 12 human exomes. Nature. 2009;461:272–6. https://doi.org/10.1038/nature08250.

135. Ng SB, Bigham AW, Buckingham KJ, Hannibal MC, McMillin MJ, Gildersleeve HI, et al. Exome sequencing identifies MLL2 mutations as a cause of Kabuki syndrome. Nat Genet. 2010;42:790–3. https://doi.org/10.1038/ng.646.

136. Levy S, Sutton G, Ng PC, Feuk L, Halpern AL, Walenz BP, et al. The diploid genome sequence of an individual human. PLoS Biol. 2007;5:e254. https://doi.org/10.1371/journal.pbio.0050254.

137. Bick D, Dimmock D. Whole exome and whole genome sequencing. Curr Opin Pediatr. 2011;23:594–600. https://doi.org/10.1097/MOP.0b013e32834b20ec.

138. Stankiewicz P, Lupski JR. Structural variation in the human genome and its role in disease. Annu Rev Med. 2010;61:437–55. https://doi.org/10.1146/annurev-med-100708-204735.

139. Medvedev P, Stanciu M, Brudno M. Computational methods for discovering structural variation with next-generation sequencing. Nat Methods. 2009;6:S13–20. https://doi.org/10.1038/nmeth.1374.

140. Korbel JO, Urban AE, Affourtit JP, Godwin B, Grubert F, Simons JF, et al. Paired-end mapping reveals extensive structural variation in the human genome. Science. 2007;318:420–6. https://doi.org/10.1126/science.1149504.

141. Wheeler DA, Srinivasan M, Egholm M, Shen Y, Chen L, McGuire A, et al. The complete genome of an individual by massively parallel DNA sequencing. Nature. 2008;452:872–6. https://doi.org/10.1038/nature06884.

142. Sboner A, Mu XJ, Greenbaum D, Auerbach RK, Gerstein MB. The real cost of sequencing: higher

143. Sabbagh R, Van den Veyver IB. The current and future impact of genome-wide sequencing on fetal precision medicine. Hum Genet. 2020;139:1121–30. https://doi.org/10.1007/s00439-019-02088-4.

144. Groopman EE, Marasa M, Cameron-Christie S, Petrovski S, Aggarwal VS, Milo-Rasouly H, et al. Diagnostic utility of exome sequencing for kidney disease. N Engl J Med. 2019;380:142–51. https://doi.org/10.1056/NEJMoa1806891.

145. Sun Y, Ruivenkamp CAL, Hoffer MJV, Vrijenhoek T, Kriek M, van Asperen CJ, et al. Next-generation diagnostics: gene panel, exome, or whole genome? Hum Mutat. 2015;36:648–55. https://doi.org/10.1002/humu.22783.

146. Connaughton DM, Hildebrandt F. Personalized medicine in chronic kidney disease by detection of monogenic mutations. Nephrol Dial Transplant. 2020;35:390–7. https://doi.org/10.1093/ndt/gfz028.

147. Brunelli L, Jenkins SM, Gudgeon JM, Bleyl SB, Miller CE, Tvrdik T, et al. Targeted gene panel sequencing for the rapid diagnosis of acutely ill infants. Mol Genet Genomic Med. 2019;7:e00796. https://doi.org/10.1002/mgg3.796.

148. Lionel AC, Costain G, Monfared N, Walker S, Reuter MS, Hosseini SM, et al. Improved diagnostic yield compared with targeted gene sequencing panels suggests a role for whole-genome sequencing as a first-tier genetic test. Genet Med. 2017; https://doi.org/10.1038/gim.2017.119.

149. Richards S, Aziz N, Bale S, Bick D, Das S, Gastier-Foster J, et al. Standards and guidelines for the interpretation of sequence variants: a joint consensus recommendation of the American College of Medical Genetics and Genomics and the Association for Molecular Pathology. Genet Med. 2015;17:405. https://doi.org/10.1038/gim.2015.30.

150. Jacob HJ, Abrams K, Bick DP, Brodie K, Dimmock DP, Farrell M, et al. Genomics in clinical practice: lessons from the front lines. Sci Transl Med. 2013;5:194cm5. https://doi.org/10.1126/scitranslmed.3006468.

151. Yang Y, Muzny DM, Reid JG, Bainbridge MN, Willis A, Ward PA, et al. Clinical whole-exome sequencing for the diagnosis of mendelian disorders. N Engl J Med. 2013;369:1502–11. https://doi.org/10.1056/NEJMoa1306555.

152. Mersch J, Brown N, Pirzadeh-Miller S, Mundt E, Cox HC, Brown K, et al. Prevalence of variant reclassification following hereditary cancer genetic testing. JAMA. 2018;320:1266–74. https://doi.org/10.1001/jama.2018.13152.

153. Bell CJ, Dinwiddie DL, Miller NA, Hateley SL, Ganusova EE, Mudge J, et al. Carrier testing for severe childhood recessive diseases by next-generation sequencing. Sci Transl Med. 2011;3:65ra4. https://doi.org/10.1126/scitranslmed.3001756.

154. Rehm HL, Berg JS, Brooks LD, Bustamante CD, Evans JP, Landrum MJ, et al. ClinGen—the clinical genome resource. N Engl J Med. 2015;372:2235–42. https://doi.org/10.1056/NEJMsr1406261.

155. Patel RY, Shah N, Jackson AR, Ghosh R, Pawliczek P, Paithankar S, et al. ClinGen pathogenicity calculator: a configurable system for assessing pathogenicity of genetic variants. Genome Med. 2017;9:3. https://doi.org/10.1186/s13073-016-0391-z.

156. Krabbenborg L, Vissers LELM, Schieving J, Kleefstra T, Kamsteeg EJ, Veltman JA, et al. Understanding the psychosocial effects of WES test results on parents of children with rare diseases. J Genet Couns. 2016;25:1207–14. https://doi.org/10.1007/s10897-016-9958-5.

157. Stenson PD, Mort M, Ball EV, Evans K, Hayden M, Heywood S, et al. The human gene mutation database: towards a comprehensive repository of inherited mutation data for medical research, genetic diagnosis and next-generation sequencing studies. Hum Genet. 2017;136:665–77. https://doi.org/10.1007/s00439-017-1779-6.

158. Landrum MJ, Kattman BL. ClinVar at five years: delivering on the promise. Hum Mutat. 2018;39:1623–30. https://doi.org/10.1002/humu.23641.

159. Koch L. Exploring human genomic diversity with gnomAD. Nat Rev Genet. 2020:448. https://doi.org/10.1038/s41576-020-0255-7.

160. Adzhubei I, Jordan DM, Sunyaev SR. Predicting functional effect of human missense mutations using PolyPhen-2. Curr Protoc Hum Genet. 2013;Chapter 7:Unit7.20. https://doi.org/10.1002/0471142905.hg0720s76.

161. Kumar P, Henikoff S, Ng PC. Predicting the effects of coding non-synonymous variants on protein function using the SIFT algorithm. Nat Protoc. 2009;4:1073–81. https://doi.org/10.1038/nprot.2009.86.

162. González-Pérez A, López-Bigas N. Improving the assessment of the outcome of nonsynonymous SNVs with a consensus deleteriousness score, Condel. Am J Hum Genet. 2011;88:440–9. https://doi.org/10.1016/j.ajhg.2011.03.004.

163. Reva B, Antipin Y, Sander C. Predicting the functional impact of protein mutations: application to cancer genomics. Nucleic Acids Res. 2011;39:e118 [cited 2021 Apr 15]. Available from: https://academic.oup.com/nar/article-pdf/39/17/e118/16776369/gkr407.pdf.

164. Rentzsch P, Witten D, Cooper GM, Shendure J, Kircher M. CADD: predicting the deleteriousness of variants throughout the human genome. Nucleic Acids Res. 2019;47:D886–94 [cited 2021 Apr 15]. Available from: https://academic-oup-com.myaccess.library.utoronto.ca/nar/article-pdf/47/D1/D886/27436395/gky1016.pdf.

165. Ioannidis NM, Rothstein JH, Pejaver V, Middha S, McDonnell SK, Baheti S, et al. REVEL: an ensemble method for predicting the pathogenicity of rare missense variants. Am J Hum Genet. 2016;99:877–85. https://doi.org/10.1016/j.ajhg.2016.08.016.

166. Bettencourt-Dias M, Hildebrandt F, Pellman D, Woods G, Godinho SA. Centrosomes and cilia in

of the long arm of the X-chromosome comprising exon 9 through 51 of the COL4A5 gene. Hum Genet. 2005;118:23–8. https://doi.org/10.1007/s00439-005-0013-0.

66. Reilly DS, Lewis RA, Ledbetter DH, Nussbaum RL. Oculocerebrorenal syndrome, with application to carrier assessment. Am J Hum Genet. 1988;42:748–55.

67. Comino-Méndez I, Gracia-Aznárez FJ, Schiavi F, Landa I, Leandro-García LJ, Letón R, et al. Exome sequencing identifies MAX mutations as a cause of hereditary pheochromocytoma. Nat Genet. 2011;43:663–7. https://doi.org/10.1038/ng.861.

68. Stephens PJ, Greenman CD, Fu B, Yang F, Bignell GR, Mudie LJ, et al. Massive genomic rearrangement acquired in a single catastrophic event during cancer development. Cell. 2011;144:27–40. https://doi.org/10.1016/j.cell.2010.11.055.

69. Forment JV, Kaidi A, Jackson SP. Chromothripsis and cancer: causes and consequences of chromosome shattering. Nat Rev Cancer. 2012;12:663–70. https://doi.org/10.1038/nrc3352.

70. Maher CA, Wilson RK. Chromothripsis and human disease: piecing together the shattering process. Cell. 2012;148:29–32. https://doi.org/10.1016/j.cell.2012.01.006.

71. Mitchell TJ, Turajlic S, Rowan A, Nicol D, Farmery JHR, O'Brien T, et al. Timing the landmark events in the evolution of clear cell renal cell cancer: TRACERx renal. Cell. 2018;173:611–623.e17. https://doi.org/10.1016/j.cell.2018.02.020.

72. Kloosterman WP, Guryev V, van Roosmalen M, Duran KJ, de Bruijn E, Bakker SCM, et al. Chromothripsis as a mechanism driving complex de novo structural rearrangements in the germline. Hum Mol Genet. 2011;20:1916–24. https://doi.org/10.1093/hmg/ddr073.

73. Chiang C, Jacobsen JC, Ernst C, Hanscom C, Heilbut A, Blumenthal I, et al. Complex reorganization and predominant non-homologous repair following chromosomal breakage in karyotypically balanced germline rearrangements and transgenic integration. Nat Genet. 2012;44(390–7):S1. https://doi.org/10.1038/ng.2202.

74. Kloosterman WP, Tavakoli-Yaraki M, van Roosmalen MJ, van Binsbergen E, Renkens I, Duran K, et al. Constitutional chromothripsis rearrangements involve clustered double-stranded DNA breaks and nonhomologous repair mechanisms. Cell Rep. 2012;1:648–55. https://doi.org/10.1016/j.celrep.2012.05.009.

75. de Pagter MS, van Roosmalen MJ, Baas AF, Renkens I, Duran KJ, van Binsbergen E, et al. Chromothripsis in healthy individuals affects multiple protein-coding genes and can result in severe congenital abnormalities in offspring. Am J Hum Genet. 2015;96:651–6. https://doi.org/10.1016/j.ajhg.2015.02.005.

76. Bertelsen B, Nazaryan-Petersen L, Sun W, Mehrjouy MM, Xie G, Chen W, et al. A germline chromothripsis event stably segregating in 11 individuals through three generations. Genet Med. 2016;18:494–500. https://doi.org/10.1038/gim.2015.112.

77. Veitia RA, Birchler JA. Dominance and gene dosage balance in health and disease: why levels matter! J Pathol. 2010;220:174–85. https://doi.org/10.1002/path.2623.

78. Johnson AF, Nguyen HT, Veitia RA. Causes and effects of haploinsufficiency. Biol Rev Camb Philos Soc. 2019;94:1774–85. https://doi.org/10.1111/brv.12527.

79. Morrill SA, Amon A. Why haploinsufficiency persists. Proc Natl Acad Sci U S A. 2019;116:11866–71. https://doi.org/10.1073/pnas.1900437116.

80. Clissold RL, Hamilton AJ, Hattersley AT, Ellard S, Bingham C. HNF1B-associated renal and extra-renal disease-an expanding clinical spectrum. Nat Rev Nephrol. 2015;11:102–12. https://doi.org/10.1038/nrneph.2014.232.

81. Bockenhauer D, Jaureguiberry G. HNF1B-associated clinical phenotypes: the kidney and beyond. Pediatr Nephrol. 2016;31:707–14. https://doi.org/10.1007/s00467-015-3142-2.

82. Clissold RL, Ashfield B, Burrage J, Hannon E, Bingham C, Mill J, et al. Genome-wide methylomic analysis in individuals with HNF1B intragenic mutation and 17q12 microdeletion. Clin Epigenetics. 2018;10:97. https://doi.org/10.1186/s13148-018-0530-z.

83. Kim J-H, Park EY, Chitayat D, Stachura DL, Schaper J, Lindstrom K, et al. SON haploinsufficiency causes impaired pre-mRNA splicing of CAKUT genes and heterogeneous renal phenotypes. Kidney Int. 2019;95:1494–504. https://doi.org/10.1016/j.kint.2019.01.025.

84. Lopez-Rivera E, Liu YP, Verbitsky M, Anderson BR, Capone VP, Otto EA, et al. Genetic drivers of kidney defects in the DiGeorge syndrome. N Engl J Med. 2017;376:742–54. https://doi.org/10.1056/NEJMoa1609009.

85. Le Tanno P, Breton J, Bidart M, Satre V, Harbuz R, Ray PF, et al. PBX1 haploinsufficiency leads to syndromic congenital anomalies of the kidney and urinary tract (CAKUT) in humans. J Med Genet. 2017;54:502–10. https://doi.org/10.1136/jmedgenet-2016-104435.

86. Yang N, Wu N, Dong S, Zhang L, Zhao Y, Chen W, et al. Human and mouse studies establish TBX6 in Mendelian CAKUT and as a potential driver of kidney defects associated with the 16p11.2 microdeletion syndrome. Kidney Int. 2020;98:1020–30. https://doi.org/10.1016/j.kint.2020.04.045.

87. Cordido A, Besada-Cerecedo L, García-González MA. The genetic and cellular basis of autosomal dominant polycystic kidney disease-a primer for clinicians. Front Pediatr. 2017;5:279. https://doi.org/10.3389/fped.2017.00279.

88. Henske EP, Jóźwiak S, Kingswood JC, Sampson JR, Thiele EA. Tuberous sclerosis complex. Nat Rev Dis Primers. 2016;2:16035. https://doi.org/10.1038/nrdp.2016.35.

89. Veys KR, Elmonem MA, Arcolino FO, van den Heuvel L, Levtchenko E. Nephropathic cystinosis: an update. Curr Opin Pediatr. 2017;29:168–78. https://doi.org/10.1097/MOP.0000000000000462.

90. Bergmann C. Genetics of autosomal recessive polycystic kidney disease and its differential diagnoses. Front Pediatr. 2017;5:221. https://doi.org/10.3389/fped.2017.00221.

91. Besouw MTP, Kleta R, Bockenhauer D. Bartter and Gitelman syndromes: questions of class. Pediatr Nephrol. 2020;35:1815–24. https://doi.org/10.1007/s00467-019-04371-y.

92. Furgeson SB, Linas S. Mechanisms of type I and type II pseudohypoaldosteronism. J Am Soc Nephrol. 2010;21:1842–5. https://doi.org/10.1681/ASN.2010050457.

93. Bockenhauer D, Bichet DG. Nephrogenic diabetes insipidus. Curr Opin Pediatr. 2017;29:199–205. https://doi.org/10.1097/MOP.0000000000000473.

94. Ehlayel AM, Copelovitch L. Update on dent disease. Pediatr Clin N Am. 2019;66:169–78. https://doi.org/10.1016/j.pcl.2018.09.003.

95. Zhang X, Zhang Y, Zhang Y, Gu H, Chen Z, Ren L, et al. X-linked Alport syndrome: pathogenic variant features and further auditory genotype-phenotype correlations in males. Orphanet J Rare Dis. 2018;13:229. https://doi.org/10.1186/s13023-018-0974-4.

96. Haffner D, Emma F, Eastwood DM, Duplan MB, Bacchetta J, Schnabel D, et al. Clinical practice recommendations for the diagnosis and management of X-linked hypophosphataemia. Nat Rev Nephrol. 2019;15:435–55. https://doi.org/10.1038/s41581-019-0152-5.

97. Govers LP, Toka HR, Hariri A, Walsh SB, Bockenhauer D. Mitochondrial DNA mutations in renal disease: an overview. Pediatr Nephrol. 2021;36:9–17. https://doi.org/10.1007/s00467-019-04404-6.

98. Ragoussis J. Genotyping technologies for genetic research. Annu Rev Genomics Hum Genet. 2009;10:117–33. https://doi.org/10.1146/annurev-genom-082908-150116.

99. Torkamani A, Wineinger NE, Topol EJ. The personal and clinical utility of polygenic risk scores. Nat Rev Genet. 2018;19:581–90. https://doi.org/10.1038/s41576-018-0018-x.

100. Liu L, Kiryluk K. Genome-wide polygenic risk predictors for kidney disease. Nat Rev Nephrol. 2018:723–4. https://doi.org/10.1038/s41581-018-0067-6.

101. Lander ES, Schork NJ. Genetic dissection of complex traits. Science. 1994;265:2037–48. https://doi.org/10.1126/science.8091226.

102. Ott J, Wang J, Leal SM. Genetic linkage analysis in the age of whole-genome sequencing. Nat Rev Genet. 2015;16:275–84. https://doi.org/10.1038/nrg3908.

103. Hamamy H, Antonarakis SE, Cavalli-Sforza LL, Temtamy S, Romeo G, Kate LPT, et al. Consanguineous marriages, pearls and perils: Geneva International Consanguinity Workshop Report. Genet Med. 2011;13:841–7. https://doi.org/10.1097/GIM.0b013e318217477f.

104. Lander ES, Botstein D. Homozygosity mapping: a way to map human recessive traits with the DNA of inbred children. Science. 1987;236:1567–70. https://doi.org/10.1126/science.2884728.

105. Alkuraya FS. Discovery of rare homozygous mutations from studies of consanguineous pedigrees. Curr Protoc Hum Genet. 2012;Chapter 6:Unit6.12. https://doi.org/10.1002/0471142905.hg0612s75.

106. Alkuraya FS. Autozygome decoded. Genet Med. 2010;12:765–71. https://doi.org/10.1097/GIM.0b013e3181fbfcc4.

107. Miano MG, Jacobson SG, Carothers A, Hanson I, Teague P, Lovell J, et al. Pitfalls in homozygosity mapping. Am J Hum Genet. 2000;67:1348–51. Available from: https://linkinghub.elsevier.com/retrieve/pii/S0002929707629668.

108. Bolk S, Puffenberger EG, Hudson J, Morton DH, Chakravarti A. Elevated frequency and allelic heterogeneity of congenital nephrotic syndrome, Finnish type, in the old order Mennonites. Am J Hum Genet. 1999;65:1785–90. https://doi.org/10.1086/302687.

109. Frishberg Y, Ben-Neriah Z, Suvanto M, Rinat C, Männikkö M, Feinstein S, et al. Misleading findings of homozygosity mapping resulting from three novel mutations in NPHS1 encoding nephrin in a highly inbred community. Genet Med. 2007;9:180–4. https://doi.org/10.1097/gim.0b013e318031c7de.

110. Hildebrandt F, Heeringa SF, Rüschendorf F, Attanasio M, Nürnberg G, Becker C, et al. A systematic approach to mapping recessive disease genes in individuals from outbred populations. PLoS Genet. 2009;5:e1000353. https://doi.org/10.1371/journal.pgen.1000353.

111. Alkuraya FS. Homozygosity mapping: one more tool in the clinical geneticist's toolbox. Genet Med. 2010;12:236–9. https://doi.org/10.1097/GIM.0b013e3181ceb95d.

112. Abu Safieh L, Aldahmesh MA, Shamseldin H, Hashem M, Shaheen R, Alkuraya H, et al. Clinical and molecular characterisation of Bardet-Biedl syndrome in consanguineous populations: the power of homozygosity mapping. J Med Genet. 2010;47:236–41. https://doi.org/10.1136/jmg.2009.070755.

113. Köttgen A. Genome-wide association studies in nephrology research. Am J Kidney Dis. 2010;56:743–58. https://doi.org/10.1053/j.ajkd.2010.05.018.

114. Borecki IB, Province MA. Linkage and association: basic concepts. Adv Genet. 2008;60:51–74. https://doi.org/10.1016/S0065-2660(07)00403-8.

115. Pan Q. Multiple hypotheses testing procedures in clinical trials and genomic studies. Front Public Health. 2013;1:63. https://doi.org/10.3389/fpubh.2013.00063.

116. Visscher PM, Brown MA, McCarthy MI, Yang J. Five years of GWAS discovery. Am J Hum Genet. 2012;90:7–24. https://doi.org/10.1016/j.ajhg.2011.11.029.

117. Kao WHL, Klag MJ, Meoni LA, Reich D, Berthier-Schaad Y, Li M, et al. MYH9 is associated with nondiabetic end-stage renal disease in African Americans. Nat Genet. 2008;40:1185–92. https://doi.org/10.1038/ng.232.

118. Kopp JB, Smith MW, Nelson GW, Johnson RC, Freedman BI, Bowden DW, et al. MYH9 is a major-effect risk gene for focal segmental glomerulosclerosis. Nat Genet. 2008;40:1175–84. https://doi.org/10.1038/ng.226.

119. Seri M, Pecci A, Di Bari F, Cusano R, Savino M, Panza E, et al. MYH9-related disease: may-Hegglin anomaly, Sebastian syndrome, Fechtner syndrome, and Epstein syndrome are not distinct entities but represent a variable expression of a single illness. Medicine. 2003;82:203–15. https://doi.org/10.1097/01.md.0000076006.64510.5c.

120. Genovese G, Friedman DJ, Ross MD, Lecordier L, Uzureau P, Freedman BI, et al. Association of trypanolytic ApoL1 variants with kidney disease in African Americans. Science. 2010;329:841–5. https://doi.org/10.1126/science.1193032.

121. Parsa A, Kao WHL, Xie D, Astor BC, Li M, Hsu C-Y, et al. APOL1 risk variants, race, and progression of chronic kidney disease. N Engl J Med. 2013;369:2183–96. https://doi.org/10.1056/NEJMoa1310345.

122. Friedman DJ, Pollak MR. APOL1 and kidney disease: from genetics to biology. Annu Rev Physiol. 2020;82:323–42. https://doi.org/10.1146/annurev-physiol-021119-034345.

123. Bruggeman LA, O'Toole JF, Sedor JR. APOL1 polymorphisms and kidney disease: loss-of-function or gain-of-function? Am J Physiol Renal Physiol. 2019;316:F1–8. https://doi.org/10.1152/ajprenal.00426.2018.

124. Min Jou W, Haegeman G, Ysebaert M, Fiers W. Nucleotide sequence of the gene coding for the bacteriophage MS2 coat protein. Nature. 1972;237:82–8. https://doi.org/10.1038/237082a0.

125. Sanger F, Nicklen S, Coulson AR. DNA sequencing with chain-terminating inhibitors. Biotechnology. 1992;24:104–8. Available from: https://www.ncbi.nlm.nih.gov/pubmed/1422003.

126. Smith LM, Sanders JZ, Kaiser RJ, Hughes P, Dodd C, Connell CR, et al. Fluorescence detection in automated DNA sequence analysis. Nature. 1986;321:674–9. https://doi.org/10.1038/321674a0.

127. Metzker ML. Sequencing technologies—the next generation. Nat Rev Genet. 2010;11:31–46. https://doi.org/10.1038/nrg2626.

128. Loman NJ, Misra RV, Dallman TJ, Constantinidou C, Gharbia SE, Wain J, et al. Performance comparison of benchtop high-throughput sequencing platforms. Nat Biotechnol. 2012;30:434–9. https://doi.org/10.1038/nbt.2198.

129. Abecasis GR, Altshuler D, Auton A, Brooks LD, Durbin RM, Gibbs RA, et al. A map of human genome variation from population-scale sequencing. Nature. 2010;467:1061–73. https://doi.org/10.1038/nature09534.

130. Buchanan CC, Torstenson ES, Bush WS, Ritchie MD. A comparison of cataloged variation between International HapMap Consortium and 1000 Genomes Project data. J Am Med Inform Assoc. 2012;19:289–94. https://doi.org/10.1136/amiajnl-2011-000652.

131. Ng PC, Levy S, Huang J, Stockwell TB, Walenz BP, Li K, et al. Genetic variation in an individual human exome. PLoS Genet. 2008;4:e1000160. https://doi.org/10.1371/journal.pgen.1000160.

132. Choi M, Scholl UI, Ji W, Liu T, Tikhonova IR, Zumbo P, et al. Genetic diagnosis by whole exome capture and massively parallel DNA sequencing. Proc Natl Acad Sci U S A. 2009;106:19096–101. https://doi.org/10.1073/pnas.0910672106.

133. Hodges E, Xuan Z, Balija V, Kramer M, Molla MN, Smith SW, et al. Genome-wide in situ exon capture for selective resequencing. Nat Genet. 2007;39:1522–7. https://doi.org/10.1038/ng.2007.42.

134. Ng SB, Turner EH, Robertson PD, Flygare SD, Bigham AW, Lee C, et al. Targeted capture and massively parallel sequencing of 12 human exomes. Nature. 2009;461:272–6. https://doi.org/10.1038/nature08250.

135. Ng SB, Bigham AW, Buckingham KJ, Hannibal MC, McMillin MJ, Gildersleeve HI, et al. Exome sequencing identifies MLL2 mutations as a cause of Kabuki syndrome. Nat Genet. 2010;42:790–3. https://doi.org/10.1038/ng.646.

136. Levy S, Sutton G, Ng PC, Feuk L, Halpern AL, Walenz BP, et al. The diploid genome sequence of an individual human. PLoS Biol. 2007;5:e254. https://doi.org/10.1371/journal.pbio.0050254.

137. Bick D, Dimmock D. Whole exome and whole genome sequencing. Curr Opin Pediatr. 2011;23:594–600. https://doi.org/10.1097/MOP.0b013e32834b20ec.

138. Stankiewicz P, Lupski JR. Structural variation in the human genome and its role in disease. Annu Rev Med. 2010;61:437–55. https://doi.org/10.1146/annurev-med-100708-204735.

139. Medvedev P, Stanciu M, Brudno M. Computational methods for discovering structural variation with next-generation sequencing. Nat Methods. 2009;6:S13–20. https://doi.org/10.1038/nmeth.1374.

140. Korbel JO, Urban AE, Affourtit JP, Godwin B, Grubert F, Simons JF, et al. Paired-end mapping reveals extensive structural variation in the human genome. Science. 2007;318:420–6. https://doi.org/10.1126/science.1149504.

141. Wheeler DA, Srinivasan M, Egholm M, Shen Y, Chen L, McGuire A, et al. The complete genome of an individual by massively parallel DNA sequencing. Nature. 2008;452:872–6. https://doi.org/10.1038/nature06884.

142. Sboner A, Mu XJ, Greenbaum D, Auerbach RK, Gerstein MB. The real cost of sequencing: higher

than you think! Genome Biol. 2011;12:125. https://doi.org/10.1186/gb-2011-12-8-125.

143. Sabbagh R, Van den Veyver IB. The current and future impact of genome-wide sequencing on fetal precision medicine. Hum Genet. 2020;139:1121–30. https://doi.org/10.1007/s00439-019-02088-4.

144. Groopman EE, Marasa M, Cameron-Christie S, Petrovski S, Aggarwal VS, Milo-Rasouly H, et al. Diagnostic utility of exome sequencing for kidney disease. N Engl J Med. 2019;380:142–51. https://doi.org/10.1056/NEJMoa1806891.

145. Sun Y, Ruivenkamp CAL, Hoffer MJV, Vrijenhoek T, Kriek M, van Asperen CJ, et al. Next-generation diagnostics: gene panel, exome, or whole genome? Hum Mutat. 2015;36:648–55. https://doi.org/10.1002/humu.22783.

146. Connaughton DM, Hildebrandt F. Personalized medicine in chronic kidney disease by detection of monogenic mutations. Nephrol Dial Transplant. 2020;35:390–7. https://doi.org/10.1093/ndt/gfz028.

147. Brunelli L, Jenkins SM, Gudgeon JM, Bleyl SB, Miller CE, Tvrdik T, et al. Targeted gene panel sequencing for the rapid diagnosis of acutely ill infants. Mol Genet Genomic Med. 2019;7:e00796. https://doi.org/10.1002/mgg3.796.

148. Lionel AC, Costain G, Monfared N, Walker S, Reuter MS, Hosseini SM, et al. Improved diagnostic yield compared with targeted gene sequencing panels suggests a role for whole-genome sequencing as a first-tier genetic test. Genet Med. 2017; https://doi.org/10.1038/gim.2017.119.

149. Richards S, Aziz N, Bale S, Bick D, Das S, Gastier-Foster J, et al. Standards and guidelines for the interpretation of sequence variants: a joint consensus recommendation of the American College of Medical Genetics and Genomics and the Association for Molecular Pathology. Genet Med. 2015;17:405. https://doi.org/10.1038/gim.2015.30.

150. Jacob HJ, Abrams K, Bick DP, Brodie K, Dimmock DP, Farrell M, et al. Genomics in clinical practice: lessons from the front lines. Sci Transl Med. 2013;5:194cm5. https://doi.org/10.1126/scitranslmed.3006468.

151. Yang Y, Muzny DM, Reid JG, Bainbridge MN, Willis A, Ward PA, et al. Clinical whole-exome sequencing for the diagnosis of mendelian disorders. N Engl J Med. 2013;369:1502–11. https://doi.org/10.1056/NEJMoa1306555.

152. Mersch J, Brown N, Pirzadeh-Miller S, Mundt E, Cox HC, Brown K, et al. Prevalence of variant reclassification following hereditary cancer genetic testing. JAMA. 2018;320:1266–74. https://doi.org/10.1001/jama.2018.13152.

153. Bell CJ, Dinwiddie DL, Miller NA, Hateley SL, Ganusova EE, Mudge J, et al. Carrier testing for severe childhood recessive diseases by next-generation sequencing. Sci Transl Med. 2011;3:65ra4. https://doi.org/10.1126/scitranslmed.3001756.

154. Rehm HL, Berg JS, Brooks LD, Bustamante CD, Evans JP, Landrum MJ, et al. ClinGen—the clinical genome resource. N Engl J Med. 2015;372:2235–42. https://doi.org/10.1056/NEJMsr1406261.

155. Patel RY, Shah N, Jackson AR, Ghosh R, Pawliczek P, Paithankar S, et al. ClinGen pathogenicity calculator: a configurable system for assessing pathogenicity of genetic variants. Genome Med. 2017;9:3. https://doi.org/10.1186/s13073-016-0391-z.

156. Krabbenborg L, Vissers LELM, Schieving J, Kleefstra T, Kamsteeg EJ, Veltman JA, et al. Understanding the psychosocial effects of WES test results on parents of children with rare diseases. J Genet Couns. 2016;25:1207–14. https://doi.org/10.1007/s10897-016-9958-5.

157. Stenson PD, Mort M, Ball EV, Evans K, Hayden M, Heywood S, et al. The human gene mutation database: towards a comprehensive repository of inherited mutation data for medical research, genetic diagnosis and next-generation sequencing studies. Hum Genet. 2017;136:665–77. https://doi.org/10.1007/s00439-017-1779-6.

158. Landrum MJ, Kattman BL. ClinVar at five years: delivering on the promise. Hum Mutat. 2018;39:1623–30. https://doi.org/10.1002/humu.23641.

159. Koch L. Exploring human genomic diversity with gnomAD. Nat Rev Genet. 2020:448. https://doi.org/10.1038/s41576-020-0255-7.

160. Adzhubei I, Jordan DM, Sunyaev SR. Predicting functional effect of human missense mutations using PolyPhen-2. Curr Protoc Hum Genet. 2013;Chapter 7:Unit7.20. https://doi.org/10.1002/0471142905.hg0720s76.

161. Kumar P, Henikoff S, Ng PC. Predicting the effects of coding non-synonymous variants on protein function using the SIFT algorithm. Nat Protoc. 2009;4:1073–81. https://doi.org/10.1038/nprot.2009.86.

162. González-Pérez A, López-Bigas N. Improving the assessment of the outcome of nonsynonymous SNVs with a consensus deleteriousness score, Condel. Am J Hum Genet. 2011;88:440–9. https://doi.org/10.1016/j.ajhg.2011.03.004.

163. Reva B, Antipin Y, Sander C. Predicting the functional impact of protein mutations: application to cancer genomics. Nucleic Acids Res. 2011;39:e118 [cited 2021 Apr 15]. Available from: https://academic.oup.com/nar/article-pdf/39/17/e118/16776369/gkr407.pdf.

164. Rentzsch P, Witten D, Cooper GM, Shendure J, Kircher M. CADD: predicting the deleteriousness of variants throughout the human genome. Nucleic Acids Res. 2019;47:D886–94 [cited 2021 Apr 15]. Available from: https://academic-oup-com.myaccess.library.utoronto.ca/nar/article-pdf/47/D1/D886/27436395/gky1016.pdf.

165. Ioannidis NM, Rothstein JH, Pejaver V, Middha S, McDonnell SK, Baheti S, et al. REVEL: an ensemble method for predicting the pathogenicity of rare missense variants. Am J Hum Genet. 2016;99:877–85. https://doi.org/10.1016/j.ajhg.2016.08.016.

166. Bettencourt-Dias M, Hildebrandt F, Pellman D, Woods G, Godinho SA. Centrosomes and cilia in

human disease. Trends Genet. 2011;27:307–15. https://doi.org/10.1016/j.tig.2011.05.004.

167. Kavanagh D, Goodship TH, Richards A. Atypical hemolytic uremic syndrome. Semin Nephrol. 2013;33:508–30. https://doi.org/10.1016/j.semnephrol.2013.08.003.

168. Joshi S, Andersen R, Jespersen B, Rittig S. Genetics of steroid-resistant nephrotic syndrome: a review of mutation spectrum and suggested approach for genetic testing. Acta Paediatr. 2013;102:844–56. https://doi.org/10.1111/apa.12317.

169. Batlle D, Haque SK. Genetic causes and mechanisms of distal renal tubular acidosis. Nephrol Dial Transplant. 2012;27:3691–704. Available from: https://academic.oup.com/ndt/article-lookup/doi/10.1093/ndt/gfs442.

170. Devuyst O, Thakker RV. Dent's disease. Orphanet J Rare Dis. 2010;5:28. https://doi.org/10.1186/1750-1172-5-28.

171. Hoppe B. An update on primary hyperoxaluria. Nat Rev Nephrol. 2012;8:467–75. https://doi.org/10.1038/nrneph.2012.113.

172. Gee HY, Otto EA, Hurd TW, Ashraf S, Chaki M, Cluckey A, et al. Whole-exome resequencing distinguishes cystic kidney diseases from phenocopies in renal ciliopathies. Kidney Int. 2014;85:880–7. https://doi.org/10.1038/ki.2013.450.

173. Gallagher PG. Disorders of red cell volume regulation. Curr Opin Hematol. 2013;20:201–7. https://doi.org/10.1097/MOH.0b013e32835f6870.

174. Chaki M, Airik R, Ghosh AK, Giles RH, Chen R, Slaats GG, et al. Exome capture reveals ZNF423 and CEP164 mutations, linking renal ciliopathies to DNA damage response signaling. Cell. 2012;150:533–48. https://doi.org/10.1016/j.cell.2012.06.028.

175. Hurd TW, Otto EA, Mishima E, Gee HY, Inoue H, Inazu M, et al. Mutation of the Mg2+ transporter SLC41A1 results in a nephronophthisis-like phenotype. J Am Soc Nephrol. 2013;24:967–77. https://doi.org/10.1681/ASN.2012101034.

176. Zaitlen N, Kraft P. Heritability in the genome-wide association era. Hum Genet. 2012;131:1655–64. https://doi.org/10.1007/s00439-012-1199-6.

177. Ehret GB. Genome-wide association studies: contribution of genomics to understanding blood pressure and essential hypertension. Curr Hypertens Rep. 2010;12:17–25. https://doi.org/10.1007/s11906-009-0086-6.

178. Schork NJ, Murray SS, Frazer KA, Topol EJ. Common vs. rare allele hypotheses for complex diseases. Curr Opin Genet Dev. 2009;19:212–9. https://doi.org/10.1016/j.gde.2009.04.010.

179. Eichler EE, Flint J, Gibson G, Kong A, Leal SM, Moore JH, et al. Missing heritability and strategies for finding the underlying causes of complex disease. Nat Rev Genet. 2010;11:446–50. https://doi.org/10.1038/nrg2809.

180. Hirschhorn JN. Genomewide association studies—illuminating biologic pathways. N Engl J Med. 2009:1699–701. https://doi.org/10.1056/NEJMp0808934.

181. Gupta J, Kanetsky PA, Wuttke M, Köttgen A, Schaefer F, Wong CS. Genome-wide association studies in pediatric chronic kidney disease. Pediatr Nephrol. 2016;31:1241–52 [cited 2021 Apr 16]. https://doi.org/10.1007/s00467-015-3235-y.

182. Arnold D, Jones BL. Personalized medicine: a pediatric perspective. Curr Allergy Asthma Rep. 2009;9:426–32. Available from: http://link.springer.com/10.1007/s11882-009-0063-9.

183. Kearns GL, Abdel-Rahman SM, Alander SW, Blowey DL, Leeder JS, Kauffman RE. Developmental pharmacology—drug disposition, action, and therapy in infants and children. N Engl J Med. 2003;349:1157–67. https://doi.org/10.1056/NEJMra035092.

184. Leeder JS. Translating pharmacogenetics and pharmacogenomics into drug development for clinical pediatrics and beyond. Drug Discov Today. 2004;9:567–73. https://doi.org/10.1016/S1359-6446(04)03129-0.

185. Wuttke M, Wong CS, Wühl E, Epting D, Luo L, Hoppmann A, et al. Genetic loci associated with renal function measures and chronic kidney disease in children: the Pediatric Investigation for Genetic Factors Linked with Renal Progression Consortium. Nephrol Dial Transplant. 2016;31:262–9. https://doi.org/10.1093/ndt/gfv342.

186. Debiec H, Dossier C, Letouzé E, Gillies CE, Vivarelli M, Putler RK, et al. Transethnic, genome-wide analysis reveals immune-related risk alleles and phenotypic correlates in pediatric steroid-sensitive nephrotic syndrome. J Am Soc Nephrol. 2018;29:2000–13. https://doi.org/10.1681/ASN.2017111185.

187. Dufek S, Cheshire C, Levine AP, Trompeter RS, Issler N, Stubbs M, et al. Genetic identification of two novel loci associated with steroid-sensitive nephrotic syndrome. J Am Soc Nephrol. 2019;30:1375–84. https://doi.org/10.1681/ASN.2018101054.

188. Gbadegesin RA, Adeyemo A, Webb NJA, Greenbaum LA, Abeyagunawardena A, Thalgahagoda S, et al. HLA-DQA1 and PLCG2 are candidate risk loci for childhood-onset steroid-sensitive nephrotic syndrome. J Am Soc Nephrol. 2015;26:1701–10. https://doi.org/10.1681/ASN.2014030247.

189. Jia X, Horinouchi T, Hitomi Y, Shono A, Khor S-S, Omae Y, et al. Strong association of the HLA-DR/DQ locus with childhood steroid-sensitive nephrotic syndrome in the Japanese population. J Am Soc Nephrol. 2018;29:2189–99. https://doi.org/10.1681/ASN.2017080859.

190. Jia X, Yamamura T, Gbadegesin R, McNulty MT, Song K, Nagano C, et al. Common risk variants in NPHS1 and TNFSF15 are associated with childhood steroid-sensitive nephrotic syndrome. Kidney Int. 2020;98:1308–22. https://doi.org/10.1016/j.kint.2020.05.029.

191. Goldstein DB. Common genetic variation and human traits. N Engl J Med. 2009;360:1696–8. https://doi.org/10.1056/NEJMp0806284.

192. Kryukov GV, Shpunt A, Stamatoyannopoulos JA, Sunyaev SR. Power of deep, all-exon resequencing for discovery of human trait genes. Proc Natl Acad Sci U S A. 2009;106:3871–6. https://doi.org/10.1073/pnas.0812824106.

193. Tennessen JA, Bigham AW, O'Connor TD, Fu W, Kenny EE, Gravel S, et al. Evolution and functional impact of rare coding variation from deep sequencing of human exomes. Science. 2012;337:64–9. https://doi.org/10.1126/science.1219240.

194. Panoutsopoulou K, Tachmazidou I, Zeggini E. In search of low-frequency and rare variants affecting complex traits. Hum Mol Genet. 2013;22:R16–21. https://doi.org/10.1093/hmg/ddt376.

195. Slatkin M. Epigenetic inheritance and the missing heritability problem. Genetics. 2009;182:845–50. https://doi.org/10.1534/genetics.109.102798.

196. Hemani G, Knott S, Haley C. An evolutionary perspective on epistasis and the missing heritability. PLoS Genet. 2013;9:e1003295. https://doi.org/10.1371/journal.pgen.1003295.

197. Kaprio J. Twins and the mystery of missing heritability: the contribution of gene-environment interactions. J Intern Med. 2012;272:440–8. https://doi.org/10.1111/j.1365-2796.2012.02587.x.

198. Zuk O, Hechter E, Sunyaev SR, Lander ES. The mystery of missing heritability: genetic interactions create phantom heritability. Proc Natl Acad Sci U S A. 2012;109:1193–8. https://doi.org/10.1073/pnas.1119675109.

199. Janssens ACJW, van Duijn CM. Genome-based prediction of common diseases: advances and prospects. Hum Mol Genet. 2008;17:R166–73. https://doi.org/10.1093/hmg/ddn250.

200. Elens L, Bouamar R, Shuker N, Hesselink DA, van Gelder T, van Schaik RHN. Clinical implementation of pharmacogenetics in kidney transplantation: calcineurin inhibitors in the starting blocks. Br J Clin Pharmacol. 2014;77:715–28. https://doi.org/10.1111/bcp.12253.

201. Zhao W, Fakhoury M, Jacqz-Aigrain E. Developmental pharmacogenetics of immunosuppressants in pediatric organ transplantation. Ther Drug Monit. 2010;32:688–99. https://doi.org/10.1097/FTD.0b013e3181f6502d.

202. Fanta S, Niemi M, Jönsson S, Karlsson MO, Holmberg C, Neuvonen PJ, et al. Pharmacogenetics of cyclosporine in children suggests an age-dependent influence of ABCB1 polymorphisms. Pharmacogenet Genomics. 2008;18:77–90. https://doi.org/10.1097/FPC.0b013e3282f3ef72.

203. Ferraresso M, Tirelli A, Ghio L, Grillo P, Martina V, Torresani E, et al. Influence of the CYP3A5 genotype on tacrolimus pharmacokinetics and pharmacodynamics in young kidney transplant recipients. Pediatr Transplant. 2007;11:296–300. https://doi.org/10.1111/j.1399-3046.2006.00662.x.

204. Prausa SE, Fukuda T, Maseck D, Curtsinger KL, Liu C, Zhang K, et al. UGT genotype may contribute to adverse events following medication with myco-phenolate mofetil in pediatric kidney transplant recipients. Clin Pharmacol Ther. 2009;85:495–500. https://doi.org/10.1038/clpt.2009.3.

205. Zhao W, Fakhoury M, Deschênes G, Roussey G, Brochard K, Niaudet P, et al. Population pharmacokinetics and pharmacogenetics of mycophenolic acid following administration of mycophenolate mofetil in de novo pediatric renal-transplant patients. J Clin Pharmacol. 2010;50:1280–91. https://doi.org/10.1177/0091270009357429.

206. Thervet E, Loriot MA, Barbier S, Buchler M, Ficheux M, Choukroun G, et al. Optimization of initial tacrolimus dose using pharmacogenetic testing. Clin Pharmacol Ther. 2010;87:721–6. https://doi.org/10.1038/clpt.2010.17.

207. Eby C. Warfarin pharmacogenetics: does more accurate dosing benefit patients? Semin Thromb Hemost. 2012;38:661–6. https://doi.org/10.1055/s-0032-1326789.

208. Vear SI, Stein CM, Ho RH. Warfarin pharmacogenomics in children. Pediatr Blood Cancer. 2013;60:1402–7. https://doi.org/10.1002/pbc.24592.

209. Institute of Medicine. In: Nielsen-Bohlman L, Panzer AM, Kindig DA, editors. Health literacy: a prescription to end confusion. Washington, DC: The National Academies Press; 2004. Available from: https://www.nap.edu/catalog/10883/health-literacy-a-prescription-to-end-confusion.

210. Kutner M, Greenberg E, Jin Y, Paulsen C. The Health Literacy of America's Adults: results from the 2003 National Assessment of Adult Literacy (NCES 2006-483). Washington, DC: U.S. Department of Education, National Center for Education Statistics; 2006. Available from: https://nces.ed.gov/pubs2006/2006483.pdf.

211. Lea DH, Kaphingst KA, Bowen D, Lipkus I, Hadley DW. Communicating genetic and genomic information: health literacy and numeracy considerations. Public Health Genomics. 2011;14:279–89. https://doi.org/10.1159/000294191.

212. Lanie AD, Jayaratne TE, Sheldon JP, Kardia SLR, Anderson ES, Feldbaum M, et al. Exploring the public understanding of basic genetic concepts. J Genet Couns. 2004;13:305–20. Available from: https://www.ncbi.nlm.nih.gov/pubmed/19736696.

213. Golbeck AL, Ahlers-Schmidt CR, Paschal AM, Dismuke SE. A definition and operational framework for health numeracy. Am J Prev Med. 2005;29:375–6. https://doi.org/10.1016/j.amepre.2005.06.012.

214. Selkirk CG, Weissman SM, Anderson A, Hulick PJ. Physicians' preparedness for integration of genomic and pharmacogenetic testing into practice within a major healthcare system. Genet Test Mol Biomarkers. 2013;17:219–25. https://doi.org/10.1089/gtmb.2012.0165.

215. Cooksey JA, Forte G, Benkendorf J, Blitzer MG. The state of the medical geneticist workforce: findings of the 2003 survey of American Board of Medical Genetics certified geneticists. Genet Med.

215. 2005;7:439–43 [cited 2015 Dec 3]. https://doi.org/10.1097/01.GIM.0000172416.35285.9F.

216. West CP, Ficalora RD. Clinician attitudes toward biostatistics. Mayo Clin Proc. 2007;82:939–43. https://doi.org/10.4065/82.8.939.

217. Weiss ST, Samet JM. An assessment of physician knowledge of epidemiology and biostatistics. J Med Educ. 1980;55:692–7. Available from: https://www.ncbi.nlm.nih.gov/pubmed/7401147.

218. Rao G. Physician numeracy: essential skills for practicing evidence-based medicine. Fam Med. 2008;40:354–8. Available from: http://www.stfm.org/fmhub/fm2008/May/Goutham354.pdf.

219. Wulff HR, Andersen B, Brandenhoff P, Guttler F. What do doctors know about statistics? Stat Med. 1987;6:3–10. https://doi.org/10.1002/sim.4780060103.

220. Rao G, Kanter SL. Physician numeracy as the basis for an evidence-based medicine curriculum. Acad Med. 2010;85:1794–9. https://doi.org/10.1097/ACM.0b013e3181e7218c.

221. Patay BA, Topol EJ. The unmet need of education in genomic medicine. Am J Med. 2012;125:5–6. https://doi.org/10.1016/j.amjmed.2011.05.005.

222. Dhar SU, Alford RL, Nelson EA, Potocki L. Enhancing exposure to genetics and genomics through an innovative medical school curriculum. Genet Med. 2012;14:163–7. https://doi.org/10.1038/gim.0b013e31822dd7d4.

223. Matloff E, Caplan A. Direct to confusion: lessons learned from marketing BRCA testing. Am J Bioeth. 2008;8:5–8. https://doi.org/10.1080/15265160802248179.

224. Rosenfeld JA, Mason CE. Pervasive sequence patents cover the entire human genome. Genome Med. 2013;5:27. https://doi.org/10.1186/gm431.

225. Klein RD. AMP v myriad: the supreme court gives a win to personalized medicine. J Mol Diagn. 2013;15:731–2. Available from: https://linkinghub.elsevier.com/retrieve/pii/S1525157813001530.

226. Graff GD, Phillips D, Lei Z, Oh S, Nottenburg C, Pardey PG. Not quite a myriad of gene patents. Nat Biotechnol. 2013;31:404–10. https://doi.org/10.1038/nbt.2568.

227. Guttmacher AE, Collins FS. Realizing the promise of genomics in biomedical research. JAMA. 2005;294:1399–402. https://doi.org/10.1001/jama.294.11.1399.

228. Janssens ACJW. Is the time right for translation research in genomics? Eur J Epidemiol. 2008;23:707–10. https://doi.org/10.1007/s10654-008-9293-8.

229. Veenstra DL, Piper M, Haddow JE, Pauker SG, Klein R, Richards CS, et al. Improving the efficiency and relevance of evidence-based recommendations in the era of whole-genome sequencing: an EGAPP methods update. Genet Med. 2013;15:14–24. https://doi.org/10.1038/gim.2012.106.

230. Evaluation of Genomic Applications in Practice and Prevention (EGAPP) Working Group. The EGAPP initiative: lessons learned. Genet Med. 2014;16:217–24. https://doi.org/10.1038/gim.2013.110.

231. Wade CH, McBride CM, Kardia SLR, Brody LC. Considerations for designing a prototype genetic test for use in translational research. Public Health Genomics. 2010;13:155–65. Available from: https://www.karger.com/DOI/10.1159/000236061.

232. Botkin JR. Ethical issues in pediatric genetic testing and screening. Curr Opin Pediatr. 2016;28:700–4. https://doi.org/10.1097/MOP.0000000000000418.

233. Botkin JR, Belmont JW, Berg JS, Berkman BE, Bombard Y, Holm IA, et al. Points to consider: ethical, legal, and psychosocial implications of genetic testing in children and adolescents. Am J Hum Genet. 2015;97:6–21. https://doi.org/10.1016/j.ajhg.2015.05.022.

234. Lucassen A, Parker M. Revealing false paternity: some ethical considerations. Lancet. 2001;357:1033–5. https://doi.org/10.1016/S0140-6736(00)04240-9.

235. Schroder NM. The dilemma of unintentional discovery of misattributed paternity in living kidney donors and recipients. Curr Opin Organ Transplant. 2009;14:196–200. https://doi.org/10.1097/mot.0b013e328327b21f.

236. Macintyre S, Sooman A. Non-paternity and prenatal genetic screening. Lancet. 1991;338:869–71. https://doi.org/10.1016/0140-6736(91)91513-t.

237. Gjertson DW, Brenner CH, Baur MP, Carracedo A, Guidet F, Luque JA, et al. ISFG: recommendations on biostatistics in paternity testing. Forensic Sci Int Genet. 2007;1:223–31. https://doi.org/10.1016/j.fsigen.2007.06.006.

238. Ross LF. Disclosing misattributed paternity. Bioethics. 1996;10:114–30. https://doi.org/10.1111/j.1467-8519.1996.tb00111.x.

239. Wertz DC, Fletcher JC. Ethics and medical genetics in the United States: a national survey. Am J Med Genet. 1988;29:815–27. https://doi.org/10.1002/ajmg.1320290411.

240. Wertz DC, Fletcher JC, Mulvihillt JJ. Medical geneticists confront ethical dilemmas: cross-cultural comparisons among nations. Am Hum Genet. 1990;46:1200–13.

241. Institute of Medicine (US) Committee on Assessing Genetic Risks. In: Andrews LB, Fullarton JE, Holtzman NA, Motulsky AG, editors. Assessing genetic risks: implications for health and social policy. Washington, DC: National Academies Press (US); 2014. https://doi.org/10.17226/2057.

242. Wolf SM, Crock BN, Van Ness B, Lawrenz F, Kahn JP, Beskow LM, et al. Managing incidental findings and research results in genomic research involving biobanks and archived data sets. Genet Med. 2012;14:361–84. https://doi.org/10.1038/gim.2012.23.

243. Green RC, Berg JS, Grody WW, Kalia SS, Korf BR, Martin CL, et al. ACMG recommendations for reporting of incidental findings in clinical exome and genome sequencing. Genet Med. 2013;15:565–74. https://doi.org/10.1038/gim.2013.73.

244. Dorschner MO, Amendola LM, Turner EH, Robertson PD, Shirts BH, Gallego CJ, et al. Actionable, pathogenic incidental findings in 1,000 participants' exomes. Am J Hum Genet. 2013;93:631–40. https://doi.org/10.1016/j.ajhg.2013.08.006.

245. Hayeems RZ, Miller FA, Li L, Bytautas JP. Not so simple: a quasi-experimental study of how researchers adjudicate genetic research results. Eur J Hum Genet. 2011;19:740–7. https://doi.org/10.1038/ejhg.2011.34.

246. Eguale T, Bartlett G, Tamblyn R. Rare visible disorders/diseases as individually identifiable health information. AMIA Annu Symp Proc. 2005;947. Available from: https://www.ncbi.nlm.nih.gov/pubmed/16779234.

247. Kaye J. The tension between data sharing and the protection of privacy in genomics research. Annu Rev Genomics Hum Genet. 2012;13:415–31. https://doi.org/10.1146/annurev-genom-082410-101454.

248. Lin Z, Owen AB, Altman RB. Genetics. Genomic research and human subject privacy. Science. 2004;305:183. https://doi.org/10.1126/science.1095019.

249. Gymrek M, McGuire AL, Golan D, Halperin E, Erlich Y. Identifying personal genomes by surname inference. Science. 2013;339:321–4. https://doi.org/10.1126/science.1229566.

250. Fox S. After Dr Google: peer-to-peer health care. Pediatrics. 2013;131(Suppl 4):S224–5. https://doi.org/10.1542/peds.2012-3786K.

251. Rodriguez LL, Brooks LD, Greenberg JH, Green ED. The complexities of genomic identifiability. Science. 2013;339:275.

252. Collins FS, McKusick VA. Implications of the Human Genome Project for medical science. JAMA. 2001;285:540–4. https://doi.org/10.1001/jama.285.5.540.

253. Rothstein MA, Anderlik MR. What is genetic discrimination, and when and how can it be prevented? Genet Med. 2001;3:354–8.

254. Hudson KL, Rothenberg KH, Andrews LB, Kahn MJ, Collins FS. Genetic discrimination and health insurance: an urgent need for reform. Science. 1995;270:391–3. Available from: https://www.ncbi.nlm.nih.gov/pubmed/7569991.

255. Rothenberg K, Fuller B, Rothstein M, Duster T, Ellis Kahn MJ, Cunningham R, et al. Genetic information and the workplace: legislative approaches and policy changes. Science. 1997;275:1755–7. Available from: https://www.ncbi.nlm.nih.gov/pubmed/9122681.

256. Van Hoyweghen I, Horstman K. European practices of genetic information and insurance: lessons for the Genetic Information Nondiscrimination Act.

JAMA. 2008;300:326–7. https://doi.org/10.1001/jama.2008.62.

257. Hudson KL, Holohan MK, Collins FS. Keeping pace with the times—the Genetic Information Nondiscrimination Act of 2008. N Engl J Med. 2008;358:2661–3. https://doi.org/10.1056/NEJMp0803964.

258. Bombard Y, Veenstra G, Friedman JM, Creighton S, Currie L, Paulsen JS, et al. Perceptions of genetic discrimination among people at risk for Huntington's disease: a cross sectional survey. BMJ. 2009;338:b2175. https://doi.org/10.1136/bmj.b2175.

259. Murashige N, Tanimoto T, Kusumi E. Fear of genetic discrimination in Japan. Lancet. 2012;380:730. https://doi.org/10.1016/S0140-6736(12)61407-X.

260. Taylor S, Treloar S, Barlow-Stewart K, Stranger M, Otlowski M. Investigating genetic discrimination in Australia: a large-scale survey of clinical genetics clients. Clin Genet. 2008;74:20–30. https://doi.org/10.1111/j.1399-0004.2008.01016.x.

261. Anon. What's brewing in genetic testing. Nat Genet. 2002;32:553–4. https://doi.org/10.1038/ng1202-553.

262. Hudson K, Javitt G, Burke W, Byers P, American Society of Human Genetics Social Issues Committee. ASHG statement* on direct-to-consumer genetic testing in the United States. Obstet Gynecol. 2007;110:1392–5. https://doi.org/10.1097/01.AOG.0000292086.98514.8b.

263. McCarthy M. FDA halts sale of genetic test sold to consumers. BMJ. 2013;347:f7126. https://doi.org/10.1136/bmj.f7126.

264. Borry P, van Hellemondt RE, Sprumont D, Jales CFD, Rial-Sebbag E, Spranger TM, et al. Legislation on direct-to-consumer genetic testing in seven European countries. Eur J Hum Genet. 2012;20:715–21. https://doi.org/10.1038/ejhg.2011.278.

265. Bloss CS, Darst BF, Topol EJ, Schork NJ. Direct-to-consumer personalized genomic testing. Hum Mol Genet. 2011;20:R132–41. https://doi.org/10.1093/hmg/ddr349.

266. Caulfield T, McGuire AL. Direct-to-consumer genetic testing: perceptions, problems, and policy responses. Annu Rev Med. 2012;63:23–33. https://doi.org/10.1146/annurev-med-062110-123753.

267. Howard HC, Avard D, Borry P. Are the kids really all right? Eur J Hum Genet. 2011;19:1122–6. https://doi.org/10.1038/ejhg.2011.94.

268. Borry P, Fryns J-P, Schotsmans P, Dierickx K. Carrier testing in minors: a systematic review of guidelines and position papers. Eur J Hum Genet. 2006;14:133–8. https://doi.org/10.1038/sj.ejhg.5201509.

269. Tracy EE. Are doctors prepared for direct-to-consumer advertising of genetics tests? Obstet Gynecol. 2007:1389–91. https://doi.org/10.1097/01.AOG.0000295601.75089.6f.

270. McGuire AL, Burke W. An unwelcome side effect of direct-to-consumer personal genome testing: raiding the medical commons. JAMA. 2008;300:2669–71. https://doi.org/10.1001/jama.2008.803.

271. Reed FA, Aquadro CF. Mutation, selection and the future of human evolution. Trends Genet. 2006;22:479–84. https://doi.org/10.1016/j.tig.2006.07.005.

272. MacArthur DG, Balasubramanian S, Frankish A, Huang N, Morris J, Walter K, et al. A systematic survey of loss-of-function variants in human protein-coding genes. Science. 2012;335:823–8. https://doi.org/10.1126/science.1215040.

Tools for Kidney Tissue Analysis

5

Anette Melk

Introduction

The gold standard for renal tissue analysis is the kidney biopsy. It is routinely performed to allow histological diagnoses of kidney diseases and determine the extent of damage in native and allograft kidneys. However, there has been controversy over the use and interpretation of kidney biopsies. Issues include sampling errors and reproducibility between different observers. More importantly, histopathological assessment has failed to predict progression or regression of kidney diseases reducing the value of kidney biopsies as a guide for clinical therapeutic approaches. Because of this, researchers have always tried to use new methods in order to add more validity and prognostication. Needle biopsies were performed already in the 1930s, but kidney biopsies as clinical diagnostic tool were introduced in the 1960s when Jones silver stain and the new techniques of electron microscopy (EM) and immunofluorescence (IF) became available. In the 1970s, immunohistological methods were applied to identify, localize and semi-quantify immune deposits, extracellular matrix proteins and cellular infiltrates. The developments in the late 1980s and 1990s have been focused on methods to measure RNA and DNA. With the ongoing advances in kidney imaging this non-invasive, indirect technique may become the ultimate way of analyzing kidney tissue in the future.

Kidney Biopsy

Indication

There are multiple indications to perform a kidney biopsy. The most frequent indications for native kidney biopsies in the pediatric population are nephrotic syndrome, non-nephrotic range proteinuria, asymptomatic hematuria and acute kidney injury [1, 2]. Other indications are unexplained kidney failure, nephritic syndrome, and potential kidney involvement in case of systemic diseases. Kidney transplant biopsies are performed in case of allograft dysfunction, suspected rejection, virus-associated nephropathy, and suspected *de novo* or recurrent kidney diseases. Some transplant centers advocate for the use of protocol biopsies in pediatric kidney transplantation [3, 4].

Absolute contraindications to kidney biopsy include uncorrected severe coagulopathy, uncontrolled severe hypertension, active renal or perirenal infection, or a skin infection at biopsy site. The following conditions represent relative contraindications to kidney biopsy: complex anat-

A. Melk (✉)
Childrens' Hospital, Hannover Medical School, Hannover, Germany
e-mail: melk.anette@mh-hannover.de

© The Author(s), under exclusive license to Springer Nature Switzerland AG 2023
F. Schaefer, L. A. Greenbaum (eds.), *Pediatric Kidney Disease*,
https://doi.org/10.1007/978-3-031-11665-0_5

omy of the kidney that may increase the risk of the biopsy (e.g. multiple cysts, anatomical abnormalities as in horseshoe kidneys), small kidneys or the presence of a solitary native kidney.

Procedure

In children, kidney biopsies were done using open exposure of the kidney until 1962 when White in England and in 1970 Metcoff in the United States described a modified needle biopsy procedure for children including infants [5–7]. Today percutaneous kidney biopsies in children are done under ultrasound guidance and have become a routine procedure. A report on the 22-year experience on 9288 native kidneys biopsies (715 from children) from the Norwegian Kidney Biopsy Registry came to the conclusion that the percutaneous kidney biopsy is a low-risk procedure at all ages [8]. However, in case of contraindications or after failed attempts at percutaneous kidney biopsy, open (surgical), laparoscopic or transvascular biopsies may be performed.

Despite differences in details, the procedures for a kidney biopsy are relatively standardized. In preparation for the biopsy the patient and the parents have to be informed about the possible risks of the biopsy and the potential therapeutic consequences. For safety, laboratory values that should be obtained include hemoglobin, platelet count, prothrombin time, partial thromboplastin time and bleeding time if uremic. In addition, serum creatinine, electrolytes and a urine dip stick analysis are useful as baseline parameters in case of occurring complications. Prior to performing the biopsy the nephrologist should be aware of the patient's kidney anatomy. Ultrasound examination is used to exclude contraindications.

Small children will receive general anesthesia. In larger children the procedure can safely be performed with mild sedation allowing for cooperation of the patient, but many centers use general anesthesia even in larger children. Briefly, the patient is placed in prone position with a foam roll under the upper part of the abdomen. The kidneys are localized by ultrasound from the back. The kidney, of which the lower pole is easiest to reach, is chosen for biopsy. In most cases, this will be the right kidney. The exact position of the kidney during inspiration is determined and after marking the intended entry position of the needle on the skin, the skin is cleaned with an antiseptic solution. If the patient is only sedated, the skin, the subcutaneous tissue and the muscle are infiltrated with a local anesthetic. After a small incision, the needle mounted on the semi-automated spring loaded biopsy gun is carefully introduced under ultrasound guidance until the kidney is almost reached. Manually operated needles have been widely replaced by biopsy guns because of the easier use and lower complication rates. The patient is then advised to take a breath and hold the air. In case of general anesthesia, the anesthetist will hold the patient in deep inspiration. The needle is quickly advanced to the capsule of the kidney and the biopsy is taken (Fig. 5.1). Ideally, the whole procedure is followed on the ultrasound screen to visualize the path of the biopsy needle.

After the procedure, the patient usually stays in bed for 24 h with compression of the puncture site. However, during the past several years, kidney biopsies have been performed on an outpatient basis, where stable patients are discharged after about 8 h [9]. To assure brisk diuresis the patient receives either a glucose/sodium chloride solution intravenously and/or is asked to drink a lot. Urine is collected in single portions and is examined with urine dip sticks. Hemoglobin levels and ultrasound controls are performed in most centers after 4–6 h and after 24 h. Hourly controls of blood pressure and heart rate have to be done.

The primary major complication remains macroscopic hematuria that occurs in 0.8–12% of biopsies performed in pediatric patients. Other complications may include subcapsular or perirenal hematoma, possible need for transfusion, infection, and pain requiring medication. Arteriovenous fistulas are diagnosed more often in recent years because of the improvement in Doppler ultrasound technique. Table 5.1 provides on overview of the efficacy and most frequent complications with regard to different biopsy techniques over a period of three decades [10].

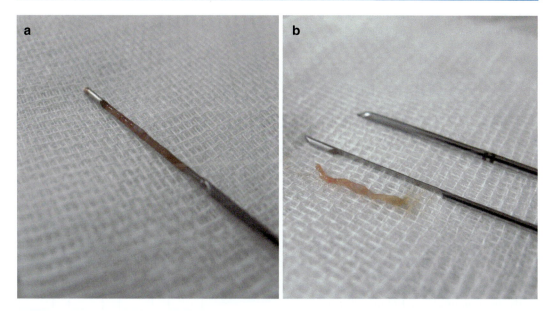

Fig. 5.1 Kidney biopsy needle and biopsy specimen. (**a**) Biopsy specimen still captured in the notch of the stylet. (**b**) Biopsy specimen sitting next to the inner needle and outer trocar

Table 5.1 Historical evolution of percutaneous biopsy technology in children (modified after [10]). While the efficacy significantly improved over time, the rate of complications did not change

Periods	1969–1974	1974–1985	1985–1990	1990–1992	1992–1996
Needle	Silverman	TrueCut	TrueCut	Biopsy	Biopsy
Localization of kidney	Radiocontrast imaging	Radiocontrast imaging	Pre-biopsy ultrasound	Pre-biopsy ultrasound	Ultrasound guidance
Efficacy					
No. of passes per session, %	3.04	2.98	2.86	2.60	2.45
Tissue-yielding punctures, %	78	87	90	87	94
No. of glomeruli per session	22.3	24.3	26.4	28.4	33.7
Complications					
Microhematuria, %	21.7	32.5	26.3	47.0	40.3
Macrohematuria, %	2.7	16.7	15.8	8.3	4.4
Perirenal hematoma, %			32.3	46.7	55.8

Processing of Biopsy Specimens

As important as accurate performance of the biopsy is adequate processing and interpretation of the specimen [11, 12]. The Renal Pathology Society has published practice guidelines that address specimen handling and processing [13].

Prior to fixation, each core should be examined for the presence and number of glomeruli by light microscopy with tenfold magnification. Based on sample size and location this examination should lead to a decision on whether more kidney tissue is needed. One should take into account the number of glomeruli as well as the suspected diseases process. It cannot be emphasized enough that adequacy of sample size is crucial for the validity of a biopsy specimen. In order to diagnose a focal disease process such as focal segmental glomerulosclerosis (FSGS) recognition of a single abnormal glomerulus is required.

Table 5.2 Minimum number of harvested glomeruli required to allow concluding a minimal fractional involvement (e.g. % sclerotic glomeruli in FSGS, % crescents in extracapillary GN) (from [100])

Number of harvested glomeruli	Minimal number of abnormal glomeruli (absolute and %) required to reliably estimate extent of involvement		
	≥80%	≥50%	≥20%
8	8 (100)	7 (88)	3 (38)
10	10 (100)	8 (80)	4 (40)
12	12 (100)	9 (75)	5 (42)
15	14 (93)	11 (73)	6 (40)
20	19 (95)	14 (70)	7 (35)
25	23 (92)	17 (68)	9 (36)
30	28 (93)	20 (66)	10 (33)
35	32 (91)	23 (66)	11 (31)
40	36 (90)	26 (65)	12 (30)

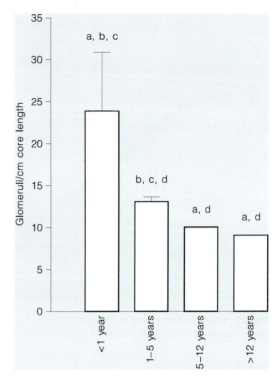

Fig. 5.2 Number of glomeruli per centimeter core length derived from native kidneys shown for different age groups. (From [10])

The probability to make this diagnosis depends on the fraction of affected glomeruli per kidney as well as on the glomeruli present in a given biopsy specimen. The same holds true for the assessment of the extent of a disease with variable pathologic involvement among glomeruli. Corwin and colleagues have published estimates on the minimum number of abnormal glomeruli that have to be present in a biopsy core that contains a certain number of glomeruli to infer with 95% confidence that a disease process involves 20%, 50% or 80% of the kidney (Table 5.2). Glomeruli within the juxtamedullary region are the ones to be involved first with FSGS, highlighting the importance that this area is represented in the sample. Overrepresentation of global sclerosis, however, may result from subcapsular cortical specimens and needs to be considered when dealing with wedge biopsy taken during an open biopsy of the native kidney or at implantation of a kidney transplant. It is also of note that the number of glomeruli that are retrieved per centimeter core length decreases with age (Fig. 5.2) [10].

Appropriate processing and potentially fixation of the biopsy should be done as soon as possible because small cores can dry out fast. The choice of fixatives should be discussed with the local nephropathologist. In pediatric kidney diseases, light microscopy (LM) alone can be insufficient to make a diagnosis. Therefore, specimens for IF and EM should be obtained. Because of the superior morphology, some nephropathologists prefer fixation with Bouin's alcohol picrate solution. This, however, may lead to problems if immunohistochemistry (IHC) staining needs to be performed. Fixation with paraformaldehyde or buffered formalin (4%, pH 7.2–7.4) followed by paraffin embedding is therefore common practice in most pathology departments. For IF, kidney tissue should be "snap-frozen" in liquid nitrogen or can be placed in tissue transport media or isotonic sodium chloride solution if transported to the laboratory immediately. Specimens for EM are usually fixed in a solution containing 0.1–3% glutaraldehyde.

LM specimens should be sectioned at a thickness of 2 μm or less by an experienced technician. Subtle pathologic changes are more easily detected in thinner sections and section thickness is an important issue for glomerular pathology, especially when assessing for cellularity.

A number of histochemical stains are used to evaluate kidney biopsies (Fig. 5.3). Typically,

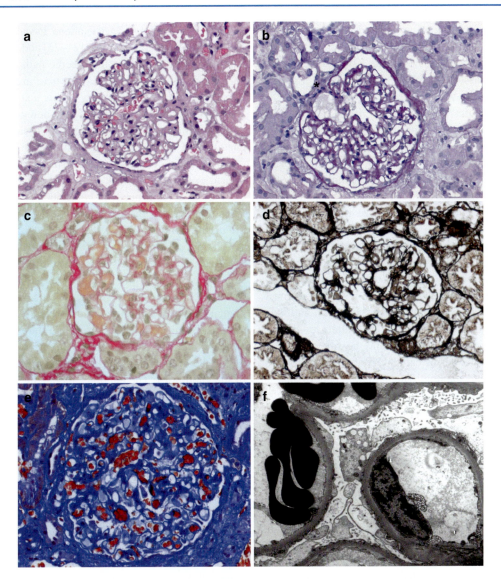

Fig. 5.3 Overview of the different stainings that are used to evaluate a kidney biopsy. Representative light (**a–e**) and electron microscopy (**f**) of minimal change glomerulopathy (MCGN) with mild hypercellularity. (**a**) Hematoxylin eosin stain (HE): the HE stain is the work horse of pathology; it is useful to get a first idea about glomerular changes such as proliferation and matrix deposition. In the case of MCGN the glomerulus shows a slightly increased number of mesangial cells, open capillaries, no evidence of intra- or extracapillary proliferation and normal thickness of glomerular basement membrane (GBM). (**b**) Periodic acid-Schiffs (PAS) stain: PAS staining is helpful to analyze changes in glomerular cell number and GBM in more detail. In the case of MCGN mild segmental hypercellularity (*) and normal thickness of GBM without any irregularities is seen. Some podocytes (arrows) are slightly enlarged and appear detached from the GBM. (**c**) Sirius red stain (fibrous tissue stain): this fibrous tissue stain is helpful to analyze the amount of fibrous tissue (fibrosis) of glomeruli and most importantly the interstitial tissue (interstitial fibrosis). In the case of MCGN a normal amount of fibrous tissue is found in Bowmans capsule and no increase in mesangial matrix is visible. (**d**) Silver stain: the silver stain is most useful to detect thickening and irregularities of the GBM. In the case of MCGN no thickening and spike formation is seen. (**e**) Acid fuchsin-Orange G stain (SFOG): this stain is helpful to detect protein deposition, i.e. immune complex formation, which appear in bright red within the mesangial matrix or the GBM. In the case of MCGN no immune deposits are present. (**f**) Electron microscopy of a capillary loop shows typical changes in MCGN, i.e. normal thickness of GBM with no evidence immune complex deposition, but with effacement of podocyte foot processes and loss of endothelial fenestration. (Pictures are courtesy of Dr. Amann, Erlangen)

biopsy specimens are stained with hematoxylin and eosin (H+E), periodic acid-Schiff (PAS) or periodic acid-methenamine silver (Jones silver) and Masson's trichrome. H+E is used for general morphology and reference, whereas the other three stains provide a clear distinction of extracellular matrix from cytoplasm. Depending on indication Congo red stain (amyloid), Kossa stain (calcifications), elastic tissue stain (loss of elasticity in arteries, arterial thickening) and other stains are used. IF uses fluorophore-labelled antibodies to detect and localize immunoglobulins (IgA, IgG, IgM) and their light chains (κ, λ), components of the classical or alternative complement pathways (C1q, C3c, C4), albumin and fibrinogen. In transplant biopsies, staining for C4d, a fragment within the complement pathway, has become a major diagnostic tool in antibody-mediated rejection [14]. The pattern of fluorescence positive stain should be noted, such as mesangial versus capillary staining and linear or granular staining. The granular pattern has an EM counterpart and corresponds to extracellular, electron dense masses.

EM studies do not need to be part of the routine work up of every kidney biopsy. However, EM plays an important diagnostic role in almost 50% of cases and is essential for a correct diagnosis in up to 21% [15, 16]. Even though it is sometimes possible to omit EM after evaluation of LM and IF, specimens for EM studies should always be procured. EM can localize deposits (mesangial, subendothelial, or subepithelial). EM is able to detect changes in cell structure (e.g. fusion of podocyte foot process, podocyte vacuolization) and alterations of the basement membrane (thickening, thinning, splicing, duplication and other irregularities). The definite diagnosis of e.g. minimal change nephropathy, Alport's disease or thin basement membrane disease requires EM [17, 18].

Histopathological Assessment

Abnormalities in kidney structures can occur in all four compartments of the kidney: glomeruli, tubules, interstitium and vasculature [19, 20].

Numerous consensus classifications have been developed for specific diseases [21–25] and those classifications, as well as the specific pathological changes seen with certain diseases, are discussed in the relevant chapters of this textbook. This chapter provides a general overview on the various histopathological features that can be encountered while reading a biopsy [12, 26, 27].

Glomerular changes are the primary pathological event in many kidney diseases. If glomeruli are affected it needs to be decided whether these changes are diffuse (defined as ≥50% of glomeruli involved) or whether the disease process is focal (defined as <50% of glomeruli involved). By assessing single glomeruli a decision has to be made whether the disease process involves only part of the glomerulus, i.e. is segmental, or the whole glomerulus, which is considered global. Glomerular sclerosis refers to an increase in extracellular material (e.g. hyaline) within the mesangium that leads to compression of the capillaries. The capillary basement membrane has a wrinkled appearance and adhesions to Bowman's capsule are found. Depending on the expansion of the sclerotic lesion, it can be either segmental or global. Hypercellularity is a descriptive term reflecting an increased number of cells (e.g. mesangial cells, endothelial cells, inflammatory cells) in the mesangial space, internal to the glomerular basement membrane or in the Bowman's space, which is called mesangial, endocapillary or extracapillary hypercellularity respectively. Glomerular diseases involving hypercellularity are often called "proliferative". Changes of the basement membrane that can be seen by light microscopy involve thickening of the basement membrane and basement membrane double layering. Whereas the first is caused by the accumulation of basement membrane material, the latter is meant to be caused by peripheral interposition of mesangial material. Severe glomerular diseases show the formation of crescents. Crescents are located in the urinary space of the glomerulus and consist of cells and extracellular material. The proportion of glomeruli affected by crescents is of enormous prognostic importance in acute glomerulonephritis/ vasculitis. The most subtle glomerular damage is

5 Tools for Kidney Tissue Analysis

effacement of foot process and refers to the loss of normal podocyte morphology with an undivided cytoplasmic mass covering the basement membrane. Effacement of foot processes cannot be seen by light microscopy, but is easily found by electron microscopy.

Tubular cells can show various signs of damage. This includes loss of brush border (in proximal tubules), flattening of the tubular epithelium, and detachment of tubular cells from the basement membrane, necrosis and apoptosis. Mitosis of tubular cells is often found after an episode of acute tubular necrosis as a sign of repair. Tubulitis, an important feature in acute allograft rejection, refers to the presence of inflammatory cells that have crossed the tubular basement membrane and infiltrate the tubular epithelium. Tubular changes when chronic occur as tubular atrophy. Atrophic tubules have a reduced diameter and a thickened basement membrane. Tubular atrophy is often accompanied by interstitial fibrosis. Another type of tubular pathology is the accumulation of droplets containing various substances. This for example can occur in patients with heavy proteinuria or with various storage diseases. A foamy appearance of the tubular epithelium is called vacuolization and can occur with several conditions. Intranuclear inclusions can indicate viral infection (see below), can occur non-specifically with different nephropathies, and can also reflect regeneration after acute tubular necrosis. The occurrence of coagulated proteins or formed elements in the tubular lumen is described as tubular casts (e.g. RBC casts).

Interstitial changes are edema, fibrosis and infiltration by inflammatory cells. Edema indicates acute diseases whereas fibrosis is the sequelae of chronic kidney damage. In both cases, tubules are no longer "sitting back to back" but are separated by interstitial material. The degree of interstitial fibrosis is of prognostic importance in chronic kidney diseases. In many instances, the degree of interstitial fibrosis found in a primary glomerular disease is a more powerful predictor of outcome than the glomerular changes itself. Infiltration of inflammatory cells can be the cause of kidney disease such as acute interstitial nephritis or acute transplant rejection, but an interstitial infiltrate can also be a mere accompanying phenomenon, e.g. in fibrosis.

The kidney vasculature can also show a range of pathological changes. Inflammation (vasculitis) may affect any vessel. If only the arterial subendothelial space is affected, this subtype is called endothelialitis, a finding peculiar to vascular rejection. Direct damage of endothelial cells, e.g. through *E. coli* toxins in hemolytic uremic syndrome (see Chap. 24), leads to thrombotic microangiopathy with endothelial cell swelling and intimal edema that is followed by platelet fibrin thrombi. Hypertension can lead to vascular changes affecting all parts of the arterial wall. This includes fibrous intimal thickening and medial hypertrophy. Overall, the vessel walls can be thickened and hyalinized, in extreme cases leading to complete obstruction of the vessel lumen. Very high blood pressure can result in fibrinoid necrosis, an endpoint also seen in other thrombotic microangiopathies.

Pathologists summarize the findings seen in the different kidney compartments based on their assessment using LM, IF, IHC and EM. Recently, a minimum reporting standard for nonneoplastic biopsies has been proposed to facilitate optimal communication between pathologists and nephrologists and eventually to optimize patient care [28].

Protein Analysis

Proteins in kidney tissue are classically analyzed by immunostaining, using either IF or IHC for visualization. Both techniques use antibodies or antisera directed against the protein of interest. They can be performed both in native and formalin-fixed tissues. As fixatives can mask protein epitopes, antigen retrieval steps become necessary, particularly for nuclear antigens. Detection and visualization of unlabeled primary antibody that specifically binds the target epitope is achieved by a secondary antibody, which for IF carries a fluorophore or for IHC either peroxidase or alkaline phosphatase. In order to further enhance the signal, especially if the target antigen is rarely expressed, amplification systems such as the streptavidin-biotin-peroxidase system are used for IHC. Direct IF or IHC, for which the primary antibody is linked to a fluorophore or peroxidase, is also possible.

Both IF and IHC have advantages and disadvantages. IF is most often performed on frozen sections. It is a technically easy and fast procedure. Processing, sectioning and staining can be performed within 1–2 h. Even though the cost of the procedure itself is low, storage is difficult as the fluorophores fade over time. A broad range of suitable antibodies is available and background staining is usually not a problem. However, in case of frozen sections an additional sample for assessment of histopathological details may be required to provide good morphology. IHC can be done using the same tissue as for LM. It provides much better morphological details and causes permanent staining, in contrast to IF. IHC is highly sensitive because of the possibility to enhance the signal by certain amplifiers, but can be technically challenging (e.g. due to higher background staining) and expensive.

Some of the applications of IF and IHC in non-neoplastic kidney biopsies have already been described above as they are part of the standard work-up of biopsy specimens. Some pathology centers prefer to use IHC even for the standard workup because of the possibility to store and archive the slides for future comparisons. In addition, IHC is used to detect subtypes of type IV collagen (see Chap. 16) and viral antigens, especially in allograft biopsies, although PCR techniques are currently taking over because of their higher sensitivity. A practical example for virus detection with IHC is BK polyoma virus. Demonstration of typical smudgy tubular cells with enlarged nuclei gives direct evidence for viral tissue invasiveness [29]. A pleomorphic infiltrate with lymphocytes, plasma cells and PMNs is highly suspicious of BK virus nephropathy. Diagnostic confirmation can be achieved by IHC using a monoclonal antibody directed against simian virus 40 (SV-40) large T antigen, which is common to all known polyoma viruses [19]. In case expansile/dysplastic plasma cells are found in the interstitium of an allograft biopsy specimen, staining for Epstein-Barr virus (EBV) may be useful to make the diagnosis of post-transplant lymphoproliferative disorder (PTLD) as most but not all PTLDs are EBV positive [30].

While proteomic tools represent a major technological advancement in protein analysis, they have not been included in the routine work-up of kidney biopsies to date. Proteomics has been coined the "non-invasive kidney biopsy", reflecting that most proteomics approaches nowadays are performed in urine. Proteomic analysis in kidney tissue has been used to identify biomarkers enabling diagnosis, disease monitoring, and treatment of kidney malignancies, especially renal cell carcinoma [31–33]. Proteomic tools may become increasingly interesting to study microdissected structures from biopsies [34, 35] as demonstrated for different glomerular diseases [34–37] and amyloidosis [38–41]. For example, mass spectrometry, by providing the molecular composition of micro-dissected deposits, is a sensitive and specific technique accurately diagnosing kidney amyloidosis [39, 40, 42]. The fact that formalin-fixed tissue even from archived tissue blocks can be used for such analyses will support future use of this approach [43, 44]. The Kidney Precision Medicine Project has recently proposed to combine traditional and digital pathology with transcriptomic, proteomic, and metabolomic analysis of the kidney tissue not only to create a reference kidney atlas, but also to characterize disease subgroups [37].

RNA Analysis

Transcriptomic analysis allows to gain insight in physiologic and pathologic processes within the kidney. RNA expression can be evaluated from as little as 10% of a biopsy core [45]. The use of RNase inhibitors stabilizes and protects the integrity of RNA in unfrozen tissue samples. Importantly, kidney tissue can be stored in these agents allowing for later micro-dissection and immunohistochemical analysis [45]. Hence, RNA expression can be evaluated from fixed and processed kidney biopsy samples, allowing for molecular analysis in combination with routine histology assessments. RNA can be isolated from frozen sections, but also from formaldehyde-fixed, paraffin-embedded tissues [46]. This methodology enables RNA analysis even after years of storage, allowing for a correlation of expression profiles from archived materials with the subsequent clinical disease course.

Even with these sensitive methods of RNA detection, the different compartments of the kidney contribute or respond differently to diseases or injury and signals may be underestimated or even missed. Manual dissection or sieving allows to compare glomeruli with tubulointerstitium [47]. Laser-assisted microdissection allows to select a defined histological structure from a given biopsy slide, allowing direct correlation of information from histology and gene expression for the same nephron segments. While the technique has been used successfully in fixed kidney tissue [48, 49], the challenge is to retrieve sufficient high-quality material. Several technical reports have been published [46, 50–52]. Laser-assisted microdissection is often used in combination with RNA amplification protocols with 1000-fold linear amplification efficiency to generate gene profiles that are specific for a certain nephron segment. This approach has been used to generate expression profiles of single glomeruli derived from biopsies of lupus nephritis [53]. The study revealed considerable kidney-to-kidney heterogeneity, whereas glomerulus-to-glomerulus variation within a kidney was less marked.

High throughput gene expression technologies emerged in the mid 1990s and a number of different microarray platforms became available. A microarray chip assembles a number of gene-specific probes (clones or oligonucleotides) spotted on a small surface area with high density. The underlying principle of microarray is that after labeling transcripts from a specific sample and hybridizing them to an array, the amount of sample material bound to the specific complementary probe set is measured. As variation across the different platforms is an important issue, a number of studies have compared different platforms. Some claimed significant divergence across technologies, whereas others found an acceptable level of concordance [54, 55]. Nowadays chips are commercially available from different suppliers and the method is highly standardized, which allows for comparison and exchange of data between different laboratories as long as the same chips are utilized. In contrast to those high density arrays, low density arrays allow for the simultaneous evaluation of a few hundred genes and are based on a reverse transcriptase-polymerase chain reaction (RT-PCR) technique.

Gene expression profiling has been performed investigating large cohorts of patients with native kidney diseases or after transplantation [56, 57]. The major challenge of any of those expression analyses remains the extraction of biological insight from such information. Ideally, one would like to recognize specific patterns or pathways involved in certain diseases (Fig. 5.4). Approaches combining conventional histological assessment with molecular analysis for transplant biopsies, called the molecular microscope [58], have created a new understanding of transplant disease states and their outcomes [59–61]. Despite strong associations described for certain genes with specific diseases, none of those genes have made it into routine diagnostics to date.

The introduction of single cell RNA sequencing has revolutionized the field of tissue transcriptomics [62] (Fig. 5.5). While methods that measure RNA in small biopsy samples had previously been applied to analyze diseased native kidneys as well as allografts, single cell RNA sequencing allows to monitor gene expression in thousands of individual cells in a single experiment. Importantly, a combination with other Omics approaches in single-cell multi-omics analyses (mRNA plus genome, mRNA plus DNA methylation, mRNA plus chromatin accessibility, and mRNA plus protein) is often applied to gain a comprehensive understanding of cellular pathways [63–67]. The single-cell transcriptomic landscape of certain kidney structures (e.g. glomeruli [68]) or diseases [69, 70] have been described. A pre-requisite for an accurate assessment of gene expression on a single cell level is, however, the creation of a single cell suspension that preserves the viability of cells and mirrors the cellular composition in the kidney, which can be a challenge. Data from such experiments is generally made available to the public, e.g. as

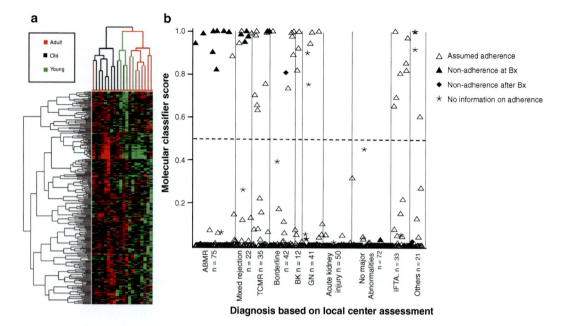

Fig. 5.4 (**a**) Dendrogram used in gene array analysis. Hierarchical cluster of genes that are differentially expressed based on kidney age (Y, young kidneys, A, adult kidneys, O, old kidneys). The color from green to red reflects increasing gene expression. Based on such gene array analysis in large cohorts, researchers have described molecular classifiers shown in (**b**) relationship between a molecular classifier score and diagnoses based on local center assessment. Molecular classifiers are able to distinguish antibody- and T-cell-mediated rejection. The order within each diagnostic category is random. Horizontal line represents arbitrary threshold of 0.5 for defining high versus low scores. Symbols indicate information about medication adherence. (Figure kindly provided by Dr. Einecke, Hannover)

single cell data sets or atlases, allowing exploration and comparison of own data against these existing data sets.

New technologies usually come along with some challenges. An important limitation of single cell RNA sequencing is the low coverage. Compared to traditional experiments using bulk RNA, the number of reads per sample is considerably lower for single cell experiments. This is especially important for genes with low expression levels, e.g. the senescence gene $p16^{INK4a}$, for which rarely any or only few corresponding reads are captured. Considerable variation in gene expression between two cells of the same type may occur as a result of the stochasticity in capturing and therefore require appropriate statistical modelling. Filtering of low-quality cells and especially of so-called doublets (libraries representing more than one cell captured in a single bead) are important quality control steps. Another important limitation is the loss of spatial information caused by the dissociation of the tissue. While techniques to overcome these limitations have been described [71–73], the need to work with fresh materials remains a major pre-analytical challenge and prevents large scale collection and analysis of human samples. Isolation protocols for archived tissues have been published; these also promise less bias between cell types [74]. Other approaches propose the use of nuclei, so-called single nucleus RNA-sequencing allowing the use of frozen tissue [75]. As further techniques are being developed, bioinformatic integration of multi-omics datasets from single-cell analyses represents a major challenge [76]. Innovative computational tools will be required that will accommodate the current limitations [77].

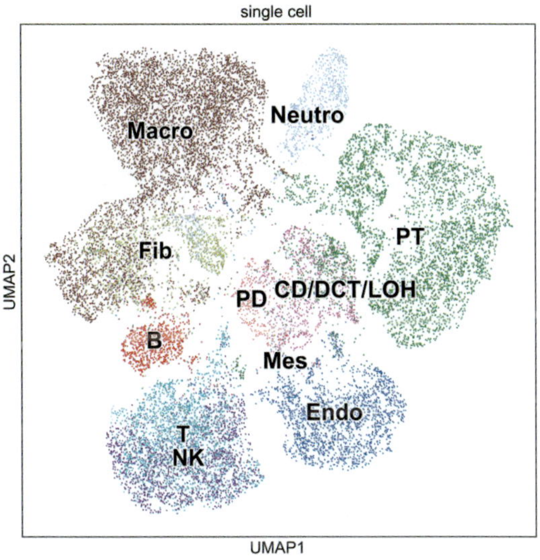

Fig. 5.5 Visualization of data from a single cell RNA-sequencing experiment using mouse kidney tissue. The high-dimensional data from such experiments is typically presented as so-called t-SNE (t-Distributed Stochastic Neighbor Embedding) plot. This technique assembles cell populations based on their expression profile. *B* B cells, *CD* collecting duct cells, *DCT* distal tubular cells, *Endo* endothelial cells, *Fib* fibroblasts, *LOH* loop of henle cells, *Macro* macrophages, *Mes* mesenchymal cells, *Neutro* neutrophils, *NK* natural killer cells, *PT* proximal tubular cells, *Podo* poocytes, *T* T cells. (Figure is retrieved from unpublished data, Drs. Melk and Schmitt)

DNA Analysis

Detection of viral DNA by PCR using sequence specific primers for a large panel of viruses such as BK virus, CMV, EBV, other herpes viruses, and hepatitis B virus is possible [78–81], but rarely used in clinical practice. Measurements of viral load to diagnose and monitor affected patients, especially after transplantation (see also Chap. 69), are preferentially performed in blood and urine [82–84]. Pathologists typically combine this information, the histopathological features and the available immunostaining methods to make the diagnosis of a virus-associated process in the kidney.

Molecular cytogenetic techniques such as chromosomal comparative genomic hybridization (CGH) are performed on tumor tissue. These techniques have improved the diagnosis of chro-

mosomal aberrations e.g. in Wilms' tumor, but have only a limited resolution across the whole genome. The development of genomic arrays allows the assessment of the whole genome at a much higher resolution at a sub-microscopic or sub-band level [85, 86].

Indirect Measurements

Even though the complication rate with kidney biopsies is low, taking a biopsy is still an invasive procedure. Therefore, methodological progress should aim for indirect and non-invasive methods to assess the status of a kidney *in vivo* in order to minimize the need for biopsies. The kidney is well suited for such indirect measurements, as urine represents an easily accessible direct read-out of the organ of interest. Indeed, proteinuria has been used for decades as a biomarker of disease activity, however it lacks disease specificity. Ideally, one would like to use urinary markers that are highly sensitive and specific for individual disease entities to screen and diagnose a kidney disease.

Urinary extracellular vesicles have become such attractive tools in biomarker development. These vesicles are secreted membrane-coated structures that allow conclusions on the cells of their origin through extraction of protein, mRNA, miRNA and lipid [87]. Urinary exosome signatures have been proposed to diagnose kidney transplant rejection [88], but also for autosomal dominant polycystic kidney disease [89]. In addition, some of the technologies discussed above have been applied to cells derived from urine. Recently single cell profiling was applied to human urine samples and shows that almost all cell types from the kidney and urinary tract can be detected and quantified in urine [90].

Transcriptome studies of urine cell extracts have identified a number of candidate biomarkers; e.g., CD3ε mRNA, IP-10 mRNA, and 18S rRNA levels in urinary cells have been postulated to detect or predict the outcome of acute rejection in kidney allograft recipients [91]. However, such measurements have not entered routine diagnostic practice to date, highlighting the challenges in biomarker development. More advances have been made for the use of the urinary proteome [92].

Imaging methods as indirect tools to evaluate kidney tissue are also discussed elsewhere (see Chap. 3), Novel functional magnetic resonance imaging (MRI) techniques allow for detailed assessments of both kidney structure and function. While arterial spin labeling measures perfusion [93], diffusion-weighted MRI enables the assessment of fibrosis and microstructure and blood oxygen level dependent imaging detects hypoxia [94, 95]. A high cortical relaxation rate, which indicates lesser oxygenation, has been associated with faster eGFR decline [96, 97]. A longitudinal study on patients with CKD could not confirm an association between a low apparent diffusion coefficient (ADC), used as a an indicator of tissue fibrosis, and changes in eGFR over a period of 12 months after adjustment for albuminuria [98]. A much smaller study in transplant patients suggested that ADC may detect fibrotic changes and thereby disease progression earlier than through eGFR decline [99]. While it is not predictable when MRI biomarkers become available for clinical use, it is conceivable that with further technological progress applications assessing indicating oxygenation and fibrosis could replace the need for histopathological assessment in certain clinical settings.

References

1. Paripovic D, Kostic M, Kruscic D, Spasojevic B, Lomic G, Markovic-Lipkovski J, et al. Indications and results of renal biopsy in children: a 10-year review from a single center in Serbia. J Nephrol. 2012;25(6):1054–9.
2. Santangelo L, Netti GS, Giordano P, Carbone V, Martino M, Torres DD, et al. Indications and results of renal biopsy in children: a 36-year experience. World J Pediatr. 2018;14(2):127–33.
3. Zotta F, Guzzo I, Morolli F, Diomedi-Camassei F, Dello Strologo L. Protocol biopsies in pediatric renal transplantation: a precious tool for clinical management. Pediatr Nephrol. 2018;33(11):2167–75.
4. Gordillo R, Munshi R, Monroe EJ, Shivaram GM, Smith JM. Benefits and risks of protocol biopsies

in pediatric renal transplantation. Pediatr Nephrol. 2019;34(4):593–8.
5. Morales P, Hamilton K, Brown J, Hotchkiss RS. Open renal biopsy. J Urol. 1961;86:501–3.
6. White RH. Observations on percutaneous renal biopsy in children. Arch Dis Child. 1963;38:260–6.
7. Metcoff J. Needles for percutaneous renal biopsy in infants and children. Pediatrics. 1970;46(5):788–9.
8. Tondel C, Vikse BE, Bostad L, Svarstad E. Safety and complications of percutaneous kidney biopsies in 715 children and 8573 adults in Norway 1988-2010. Clin J Am Soc Nephrol. 2012;7(10):1591–7.
9. Sweeney C, Geary DF, Hebert D, Robinson L, Langlois V. Outpatient pediatric renal transplant biopsy—is it safe? Pediatr Transplant. 2006;10(2):159–61.
10. Feneberg R, Schaefer F, Zieger B, Waldherr R, Mehls O, Scharer K. Percutaneous renal biopsy in children: a 27-year experience. Nephron. 1998;79(4):438–46.
11. Amann K, Haas CS. What you should know about the work-up of a renal biopsy. Nephrol Dial Transplant. 2006;21(5):1157–61.
12. Fogo AB. Approach to renal biopsy. Am J Kidney Dis. 2003;42(4):826–36.
13. Walker PD, Cavallo T, Bonsib SM. Practice guidelines for the renal biopsy. Mod Pathol. 2004;17(12):1555–63.
14. Racusen LC, Colvin RB, Solez K, Mihatsch MJ, Halloran PF, Campbell PM, et al. Antibody-mediated rejection criteria—an addition to the Banff'97 classification of renal allograft rejection. Am J Transplant. 2003;3:708–14.
15. Haas M. A reevaluation of routine electron microscopy in the examination of native renal biopsies. J Am Soc Nephrol. 1997;8(1):70–6.
16. Siegel NJ, Spargo BH, Kashgarian M, Hayslett JP. An evaluation of routine electron microscopy in the examination of renal biopsies. Nephron. 1973;10(4):209–15.
17. Pirson Y. Making the diagnosis of Alport's syndrome. Kidney Int. 1999;56(2):760–75.
18. Morita M, White RH, Raafat F, Barnes JM, Standring DM. Glomerular basement membrane thickness in children. A morphometric study. Pediatr Nephrol. 1988;2(2):190–5.
19. Liptak P, Kemeny E, Ivanyi B. Primer: histopathology of polyomavirus-associated nephropathy in renal allografts. Nat Clin Pract Nephrol. 2006;2(11):631–6.
20. Jennette JC, Olson JL, Schwartz MM, Silva FG. Primer on the pathologic diagnosis of renal disease. In: Jennette JC, Olson JL, Schwartz MM, Silva FG, editors. Heptinstall's pathology of the kidney. 6th ed. Philadelphia: Lippincott Williams & Wilkins; 2007. p. 97–123.
21. D'Agati VD, Fogo AB, Bruijn JA, Jennette JC. Pathologic classification of focal segmental glomerulosclerosis: a working proposal. Am J Kidney Dis. 2004;43(2):368–82.

22. Weening JJ, D'Agati VD, Schwartz MM, Seshan SV, Alpers CE, Appel GB, et al. The classification of glomerulonephritis in systemic lupus erythematosus revisited. Kidney Int. 2004;65(2):521–30.
23. Coppo R, Troyanov S, Camilla R, Hogg RJ, Cattran DC, Cook HT, et al. The Oxford IgA nephropathy clinicopathological classification is valid for children as well as adults. Kidney Int. 2010;77(10):921–7.
24. Cattran DC, Coppo R, Cook HT, Feehally J, Roberts IS, Troyanov S, et al. The Oxford classification of IgA nephropathy: rationale, clinicopathological correlations, and classification. Kidney Int. 2009;76(5):534–45.
25. Roberts IS, Cook HT, Troyanov S, Alpers CE, Amore A, Barratt J, et al. The Oxford classification of IgA nephropathy: pathology definitions, correlations, and reproducibility. Kidney Int. 2009;76(5):546–56.
26. Camous X, Pera A, Solana R, Larbi A. NK cells in healthy aging and age-associated diseases. J Biomed Biotechnol. 2012;2012:195956.
27. Racusen LC, Solez K, Colvin RB, Bonsib SM, Castro MC, Cavallo T, et al. The Banff 97 working classification of renal allograft pathology. Kidney Int. 1999;55(2):713–23.
28. Chang A, Gibson IW, Cohen AH, Weening JJ, Jennette JC, Fogo AB. A position paper on standardizing the nonneoplastic kidney biopsy report. Clin J Am Soc Nephrol. 2012;7(8):1365–8.
29. Drachenberg CB, Papadimitriou JC. Polyomavirus-associated nephropathy: update in diagnosis. Transpl Infect Dis. 2006;8(2):68–75.
30. Meehan SM, Domer P, Josephson M, Donoghue M, Sadhu A, Ho LT, et al. The clinical and pathologic implications of plasmacytic infiltrates in percutaneous renal allograft biopsies. Hum Pathol. 2001;32(2):205–15.
31. Boysen G, Bausch-Fluck D, Thoma CR, Nowicka AM, Stiehl DP, Cima I, et al. Identification and functional characterization of pVHL-dependent cell surface proteins in renal cell carcinoma. Neoplasia. 2012;14(6):535–46.
32. Kurban G, Gallie BL, Leveridge M, Evans A, Rushlow D, Matevski D, et al. Needle core biopsies provide ample material for genomic and proteomic studies of kidney cancer: observations on DNA, RNA, protein extractions and VHL mutation detection. Pathol Res Pract. 2012;208(1):22–31.
33. Zacchia M, Vilasi A, Capasso A, Morelli F, De VF, Capasso G. Genomic and proteomic approaches to renal cell carcinoma. J Nephrol. 2011;24(2):155–64.
34. Sethi S, Theis JD, Vrana JA, Fervenza FC, Sethi A, Qian Q, et al. Laser microdissection and proteomic analysis of amyloidosis, cryoglobulinemic GN, fibrillary GN, and immunotactoid glomerulopathy. Clin J Am Soc Nephrol. 2013;8(6):915–21.
35. Satoskar AA, Shapiro JP, Bott CN, Song H, Nadasdy GM, Brodsky SV, et al. Characterization of glomerular diseases using proteomic analysis of laser capture microdissected glomeruli. Mod Pathol. 2012;25(5):709–21.
36. Nakatani S, Wei M, Ishimura E, Kakehashi A, Mori K, Nishizawa Y, et al. Proteome analysis of laser microdissected glomeruli from formalin-fixed paraffin-embedded kidneys of autopsies of diabetic patients: nephronectin is associated with the development of diabetic glomerulosclerosis. Nephrol Dial Transplant. 2012;27(5):1889–97.
37. Sethi S, Madden B, Debiec H, Morelle J, Charlesworth MC, Gross L, et al. Protocadherin 7-associated membranous nephropathy. J Am Soc Nephrol. 2021;32(5):1249–61.
38. Brambilla F, Lavatelli F, Merlini G, Mauri P. Clinical proteomics for diagnosis and typing of systemic amyloidoses. Proteomics Clin Appl. 2013;7(1-2):136–43.
39. Sethi S, Vrana JA, Theis JD, Leung N, Sethi A, Nasr SH, et al. Laser microdissection and mass spectrometry-based proteomics aids the diagnosis and typing of renal amyloidosis. Kidney Int. 2012;82(2):226–34.
40. Sethi S, Theis JD, Leung N, Dispenzieri A, Nasr SH, Fidler ME, et al. Mass spectrometry-based proteomic diagnosis of renal immunoglobulin heavy chain amyloidosis. Clin J Am Soc Nephrol. 2010;5(12):2180–7.
41. Klein CJ, Vrana JA, Theis JD, Dyck PJ, Dyck PJ, Spinner RJ, et al. Mass spectrometric-based proteomic analysis of amyloid neuropathy type in nerve tissue. Arch Neurol. 2011;68(2):195–9.
42. Nasr SH, Said SM, Valeri AM, Sethi S, Fidler ME, Cornell LD, et al. The diagnosis and characteristics of renal heavy-chain and heavy/light-chain amyloidosis and their comparison with renal light-chain amyloidosis. Kidney Int. 2013;83(3):463–70.
43. Nasr SH, Fidler ME, Cornell LD, Leung N, Cosio FG, Sheikh SS, et al. Immunotactoid glomerulopathy: clinicopathologic and proteomic study. Nephrol Dial Transplant. 2012;27(11):4137–46.
44. Maes E, Broeckx V, Mertens I, Sagaert X, Prenen H, Landuyt B, et al. Analysis of the formalin-fixed paraffin-embedded tissue proteome: pitfalls, challenges, and future prospectives. Amino Acids. 2013;45(2):205–18.
45. Cohen CD, Frach K, Schlondorff D, Kretzler M. Quantitative gene expression analysis in renal biopsies: a novel protocol for a high-throughput multicenter application. Kidney Int. 2002;61(1):133–40.
46. Jonigk D, Modde F, Bockmeyer CL, Becker JU, Lehmann U. Optimized RNA extraction from non-deparaffinized, laser-microdissected material. Methods Mol Biol. 2011;755:67–75.
47. Emmert-Buck MR, Bonner RF, Smith PD, Chuaqui RF, Zhuang Z, Goldstein SR, et al. Laser capture microdissection. Science. 1996;274:998–1001.
48. Jiang R, Scott RS, Hutt-Fletcher LM. Laser capture microdissection for analysis of gene expression in formalin-fixed paraffin-embedded tissue. Methods Mol Biol. 2011;755:77–84.
49. Cohen CD, Grone HJ, Grone EF, Nelson PJ, Schlondorff D, Kretzler M. Laser microdissection

and gene expression analysis on formaldehyde-fixed archival tissue. Kidney Int. 2002;61(1):125–32.

50. Woroniecki RP, Bottinger EP. Laser capture microdissection of kidney tissue. Methods Mol Biol. 2009;466:73–82.

51. Noppert SJ, Eder S, Rudnicki M. Laser-capture microdissection of renal tubule cells and linear amplification of RNA for microarray profiling and real-time PCR. Methods Mol Biol. 2011;755:257–66.

52. De SW, Cornillie P, Van PM, Peelman L, Burvenich C, Van den Broeck W. Quantitative mRNA expression analysis in kidney glomeruli using microdissection techniques. Histol Histopathol. 2011;26(2):267–75.

53. Peterson KS, Huang JF, Zhu J, D'Agati V, Liu X, Miller N, et al. Characterization of heterogeneity in the molecular pathogenesis of lupus nephritis from transcriptional profiles of laser-captured glomeruli. J Clin Invest. 2004;113(12):1722–33.

54. Sarmah CK, Samarasinghe S. Microarray gene expression: a study of between-platform association of Affymetrix and cDNA arrays. Comput Biol Med. 2011;41(10):980–6.

55. Carter SL, Eklund AC, Mecham BH, Kohane IS, Szallasi Z. Redefinition of Affymetrix probe sets by sequence overlap with cDNA microarray probes reduces cross-platform inconsistencies in cancer-associated gene expression measurements. BMC Bioinformatics. 2005;6:107.

56. Halloran PF, Pereira AB, Chang J, Matas A, Picton M, De FD, et al. Microarray diagnosis of antibody-mediated rejection in kidney transplant biopsies: an international prospective study (INTERCOM). Am J Transplant. 2013;13(11):2865–74.

57. Halloran PF, Reeve JP, Pereira AB, Hidalgo LG, Famulski KS. Antibody-mediated rejection, T cell-mediated rejection, and the injury-repair response: new insights from the Genome Canada studies of kidney transplant biopsies. Kidney Int. 2014;85(2):258–64.

58. Halloran PF, Madill-Thomsen KS, group Is. The molecular microscope((R)) diagnostic system meets eminence-based medicine: a clinician's perspective. Am J Transplant. 2020;20(10):2964–5.

59. Mengel M, Campbell P, Gebel H, Randhawa P, Rodriguez ER, Colvin R, et al. Precision diagnostics in transplantation: from bench to bedside. Am J Transplant. 2013;13(3):562–8.

60. Ozluk Y, Blanco PL, Mengel M, Solez K, Halloran PF, Sis B. Superiority of virtual microscopy versus light microscopy in transplantation pathology. Clin Transpl. 2012;26(2):336–44.

61. Einecke G, Reeve J, Sis B, Mengel M, Hidalgo L, Famulski KS, et al. A molecular classifier for predicting future graft loss in late kidney transplant biopsies. J Clin Invest. 2010;120(6):1862–72.

62. Park J, Shrestha R, Qiu C, Kondo A, Huang S, Werth M, et al. Single-cell transcriptomics of the mouse kidney reveals potential cellular targets of kidney disease. Science. 2018;360(6390):758–63.

63. Cao J, Cusanovich DA, Ramani V, Aghamirzaie D, Pliner HA, Hill AJ, et al. Joint profiling of chromatin accessibility and gene expression in thousands of single cells. Science. 2018;361(6409):1380–5.

64. Cusanovich DA, Daza R, Adey A, Pliner HA, Christiansen L, Gunderson KL, et al. Multiplex single cell profiling of chromatin accessibility by combinatorial cellular indexing. Science. 2015;348(6237):910–4.

65. Gerlach JP, van Buggenum JAG, Tanis SEJ, Hogeweg M, Heuts BMH, Muraro MJ, et al. Combined quantification of intracellular (phospho-)proteins and transcriptomics from fixed single cells. Sci Rep. 2019;9(1):1469.

66. Stoeckius M, Hafemeister C, Stephenson W, Houck-Loomis B, Chattopadhyay PK, Swerdlow H, et al. Simultaneous epitope and transcriptome measurement in single cells. Nat Methods. 2017;14(9):865–8.

67. Stuart T, Butler A, Hoffman P, Hafemeister C, Papalexi E, Mauck WM, et al. Comprehensive integration of single-cell data. Cell. 2019;177(7):1888–902.e21.

68. Chung JJ, Goldstein L, Chen YJ, Lee J, Webster JD, Roose-Girma M, et al. Single-cell transcriptome profiling of the kidney glomerulus identifies key cell types and reactions to injury. J Am Soc Nephrol. 2020;31(10):2341–54.

69. Wilson PC, Wu H, Kirita Y, Uchimura K, Ledru N, Rennke HG, et al. The single-cell transcriptomic landscape of early human diabetic nephropathy. Proc Natl Acad Sci. 2019;116(39):19619–25.

70. Menon R, Otto EA, Hoover P, Eddy S, Mariani L, Godfrey B, et al. Single cell transcriptomics identifies focal segmental glomerulosclerosis remission endothelial biomarker. JCI Insight. 2020;5(6):e133267.

71. Chen KH, Boettiger AN, Moffitt JR, Wang S, Zhuang X. RNA imaging. Spatially resolved, highly multiplexed RNA profiling in single cells. Science. 2015;348(6233):aaa6090.

72. Codeluppi S, Borm LE, Zeisel A, La Manno G, van Lunteren JA, Svensson CI, et al. Spatial organization of the somatosensory cortex revealed by osmFISH. Nat Methods. 2018;15(11):932–5.

73. Halpern KB, Shenhav R, Matcovitch-Natan O, Toth B, Lemze D, Golan M, et al. Single-cell spatial reconstruction reveals global division of labour in the mammalian liver. Nature. 2017;542(7641):352–6.

74. Habib N, Avraham-Davidi I, Basu A, Burks T, Shekhar K, Hofree M, et al. Massively parallel single-nucleus RNA-seq with DroNc-seq. Nat Methods. 2017;14(10):955–8.

75. Slyper M, Porter CBM, Ashenberg O, Waldman J, Drokhlyansky E, Wakiro I, et al. A single-cell and single-nucleus RNA-Seq toolbox for fresh and frozen human tumors. Nat Med. 2020;26(5):792–802.

76. Barkas N, Petukhov V, Nikolaeva D, Lozinsky Y, Demharter S, Khodosevich K, et al. Wiring together large single-cell RNA-seq sample collections. bioRxiv. 2018; https://doi.org/10.1101/460246.

77. Kuppe C, Perales-Paton J, Saez-Rodriguez J, Kramann R. Experimental and computational technologies to dissect the kidney at the single-cell level. Nephrol Dial Transplant. 2020; https://doi.org/10.1093/ndt/gfaa233.

78. Liapis H, Storch GA, Hill DA, Rueda J, Brennan DC. CMV infection of the renal allograft is much more common than the pathology indicates: a retrospective analysis of qualitative and quantitative buffy coat CMV-PCR, renal biopsy pathology and tissue CMV-PCR. Nephrol Dial Transplant. 2003;18(2):397–402.

79. Gupta M, Filler G, Kovesi T, Shaw L, Forget C, Carpenter B, et al. Quantitative tissue polymerase chain reaction for Epstein-Barr virus in pediatric solid organ recipients. Am J Kidney Dis. 2003;41(1):212–9.

80. Randhawa P, Shapiro R, Vats A. Quantitation of DNA of polyomaviruses BK and JC in human kidneys. J Infect Dis. 2005;192(3):504–9.

81. Gupta M, Diaz-Mitoma F, Feber J, Shaw L, Forget C, Filler G. Tissue HHV6 and 7 determination in pediatric solid organ recipients—a pilot study. Pediatr Transplant. 2003;7(6):458–63.

82. Bechert CJ, Schnadig VJ, Payne DA, Dong J. Monitoring of BK viral load in renal allograft recipients by real-time PCR assays. Am J Clin Pathol. 2010;133(2):242–50.

83. Kotton CN, Kumar D, Caliendo AM, Asberg A, Chou S, Danziger-Isakov L, et al. Updated international consensus guidelines on the management of cytomegalovirus in solid-organ transplantation. Transplantation. 2013;96(4):333–60.

84. Lautenschlager I, Razonable RR. Human herpesvirus-6 infections in kidney, liver, lung, and heart transplantation: review. Transpl Int. 2012;25(5):493–502.

85. Rassekh SR, Chan S, Harvard C, Dix D, Qiao Y, Rajcan-Separovic E. Screening for submicroscopic chromosomal rearrangements in Wilms tumor using whole-genome microarrays. Cancer Genet Cytogenet. 2008;182(2):84–94.

86. Gambin T, Stankiewicz P, Sykulski M, Gambin A. Functional performance of aCGH design for clinical cytogenetics. Comput Biol Med. 2013;43(6):775–85.

87. Blijdorp CJ, Tutakhel OAZ, Hartjes TA, van den Bosch TPP, van Heugten MH, Rigalli JP, et al. Comparing approaches to normalize, quantify, and characterize urinary extracellular vesicles. J Am Soc Nephrol. 2021;32(5):1210–26.

88. El Fekih R, Hurley J, Tadigotla V, Alghamdi A, Srivastava A, Coticchia C, et al. Discovery and validation of a urinary exosome mRNA signature for the diagnosis of human kidney transplant rejection. J Am Soc Nephrol. 2021;32:994–1004.

89. Magayr TA, Song X, Streets AJ, Vergoz L, Chang L, Valluru MK, et al. Global microRNA profiling in human urinary exosomes reveals novel disease biomarkers and cellular pathways for autosomal dominant polycystic kidney disease. Kidney Int. 2020;98(2):420–35.

90. Abedini A, Zhu YO, Chatterjee S, Halasz G, Devalaraja-Narashimha K, Shrestha R, et al. Urinary single-cell profiling captures the cellular diversity of the kidney. J Am Soc Nephrol. 2021;32(3):614–27.

91. Suthanthiran M, Schwartz JE, Ding R, Abecassis M, Dadhania D, Samstein B, et al. Urinary-cell mRNA profile and acute cellular rejection in kidney allografts. N Engl J Med. 2013;369(1):20–31.

92. Decramer S, Wittke S, Mischak H, Zurbig P, Walden M, Bouissou F, et al. Predicting the clinical outcome of congenital unilateral ureteropelvic junction obstruction in newborn by urinary proteome analysis. Nat Med. 2006;12(4):398–400.

93. Hueper K, Gutberlet M, Rong S, Hartung D, Mengel M, Lu X, et al. Acute kidney injury: arterial spin labeling to monitor renal perfusion impairment in mice-comparison with histopathologic results and renal function. Radiology. 2014;270(1):117–24.

94. Inoue T, Kozawa E, Okada H, Inukai K, Watanabe S, Kikuta T, et al. Noninvasive evaluation of kidney hypoxia and fibrosis using magnetic resonance imaging. J Am Soc Nephrol. 2011;22(8):1429–34.

95. Gloviczki ML, Glockner JF, Crane JA, McKusick MA, Misra S, Grande JP, et al. Blood oxygen level-dependent magnetic resonance imaging identifies cortical hypoxia in severe renovascular disease. Hypertension. 2011;58(6):1066–72.

96. Sugiyama K, Inoue T, Kozawa E, Ishikawa M, Shimada A, Kobayashi N, et al. Reduced oxygenation but not fibrosis defined by functional magnetic resonance imaging predicts the long-term progression of chronic kidney disease. Nephrol Dial Transplant. 2020;35(6):964–70.

97. Pruijm M, Milani B, Pivin E, Podhajska A, Vogt B, Stuber M, et al. Reduced cortical oxygenation predicts a progressive decline of renal function in patients with chronic kidney disease. Kidney Int. 2018;93(4):932–40.

98. Srivastava A, Cai X, Lee J, Li W, Larive B, Kendrick C, et al. Kidney functional magnetic resonance imaging and change in eGFR in individuals with CKD. Clin J Am Soc Nephrol. 2020;15(6):776–83.

99. Berchtold L, Crowe LA, Friedli I, Legouis D, Moll S, de Perrot T, et al. Diffusion magnetic resonance imaging detects an increase in interstitial fibrosis earlier than the decline of renal function. Nephrol Dial Transplant. 2020;35(7):1274–6.

100. Corwin HL, Schwartz MM, Lewis EJ. The importance of sample size in the interpretation of the renal biopsy. Am J Nephrol. 1988;8(2):85–9.

Part II

Disorders of Kidney Development

Functional Development of the Nephron

6

Aoife Waters

Abbreviations

ACE	Angiotensin converting enzyme
ACEI	Angiotensin converting enzyme inhibitors
ADH	Antidiuretic hormone
ANP	Atrial natriuretic peptide
AQ2	Aquaporin-2
AT1	Angiotensin type 1 receptors
BK	Bradykinin
CA	Carbonic anhydrase
cAMP	Cyclic adenosine monophosphate
CCD	Cortical collecting duct
CD	Collecting duct
cGMP	Cyclic guanosine monophosphate
COX-2	Cyclooxygenase type-2
ENaC	Epithelial sodium channel
ET	Endothelin
FGF-23	Fibroblast growth factor 23
GA	Gestational age
GFB	Glomerular filtration barrier
GFR	Glomerular filtration rate
GH	Growth hormone
IGF-1	Insulin growth factor-1
KK	Kallikrein
NaCl	Sodium chloride
NAG	N-acetyl-β-D-glucosaminidase
NCC	Sodium chloride co-transporter
NHE3	Sodium-hydrogen antiporter 3
NKCC$_2$	Sodium-potassium-chloride cotransporter
NO	Nitric oxide
PGs	Prostaglandins
PTH	Parathyroid hormone
RAS	Renin–angiotensin–aldosterone system
ROMK	Renal outer medullary potassium channel
RVR	Renal vascular resistance
TALH	Thick ascending limb of loop of Henle
TRPV5	Transient receptor potential cation channel subfamily V member 5
TTKG	Transtubular potassium gradient
VMNP	Vasomotor nephropathy

A. Waters (✉)
Department of Nephrology, Great Ormond Street Hospital NHS Foundation Trust, London, UK
e-mail: aoife.waters@gosh.nhs.uk

General Overview of Antenatal, Perinatal, and Postnatal Fluid and Electrolyte Homeostasis

Fluid and electrolyte homeostasis in the fetus is controlled by the placenta. As a result, the placenta receives a significant proportion of the fetal cardiac output (33%), whereas the fetal kidneys receive only 2.5% even in late gestation [1]. The low fetal renal blood flow (RBF) results in a low creatinine clearance which correlates well with gestational age (GA) (Fig. 6.1a, b). Urine pro-

© The Author(s), under exclusive license to Springer Nature Switzerland AG 2023
F. Schaefer, L. A. Greenbaum (eds.), *Pediatric Kidney Disease*,
https://doi.org/10.1007/978-3-031-11665-0_6

Fig. 6.1 (a) Creatinine clearance for human fetuses from 20 weeks. (■) and corresponding preterm neonates (●). Creatinine clearance increases with increasing gestational age (used with permission of John Wiley and Sons from Haycock [2]). (b) GFR doubles over the first 2 weeks of life in term infants and reaches almost 50 mL/min/1.73 m² between 2 and 4 weeks after birth and adult values by 2 years of age. (Used with permission of Vieux et al. [3])

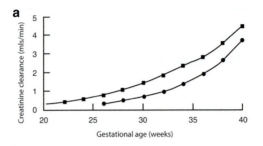

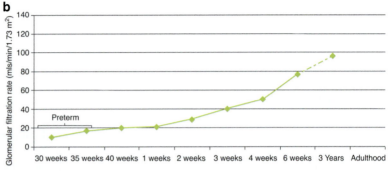

duction begins at approximately 10 weeks of gestation in the human kidney. This coincides with the acquisition of the first capillary loops by the inner medullary metanephric nephrons. Subsequently, hourly fetal urine production increases from 5 mL at 20 weeks to approximately 50 mL at 40 weeks [4]. After 20 weeks, the kidneys provide over 90% of the amniotic fluid volume [5]. Severe oligohydramnios due to abnormal fetal renal function in the second trimester can result in pulmonary hypoplasia and in severe cases, Potter's syndrome [6].

At birth, the newborn consists largely of water, with total body water comprising 75% of body weight at full term and about 80–85% in preterm infants [7]. Adaptation to the extrauterine environment involves an increase in glomerular filtration with an immediate postnatal natriuresis. High circulating levels of atrial natriuretic peptide (ANP) in the newborn are responsible for the postnatal physiological natriuresis [8]. In addition, maturation of tubular function occurs postnatally [9]. Changes include an increase in resorptive surface area, transporter number and function, together with further modification of paracrine regulatory mechanisms [9]. In the following section, we will discuss the developmental changes in the neonatal kidney that are necessary for extrauterine adaptation. Regulatory mechanisms of the mature kidney will be discussed elsewhere.

Glomerular Function in the Fetal, Perinatal, and Postnatal Period

Glomerular filtration is the transudation of plasma across the glomerular filtration barrier (GFB) and is the first step in the formation of urine (Fig. 6.2). Filtration depends both on Starling's forces and an adequate RBF [10]. The total glomerular filtration rate (GFR) is the sum of the GFR of each single functioning nephron, SNGFR [where SNGFR = $(k \times S) \times (\Delta P - \Delta \pi)$]. ΔP, is the hydrostatic pressure difference between the glomerular capillary pressure (P_{GC}) and the hydrostatic pressure in Bowman's space (P_{BS}). $\Delta \pi$ is the oncotic pressure difference between the glomerular capillary pressure (π_{GC}) and the oncotic pressure in Bowman's space (π_{BS}). K_f is the product of the hydraulic permeability of glomerular capillary walls (k) and the surface area available for filtration, (S), ($K_f = k \times S$). In an adult, the rate of glomerular filtration is about 100–120 mL/min/1.73 m². Even though the term neonate has the full number of glomeruli, its

6 Functional Development of the Nephron

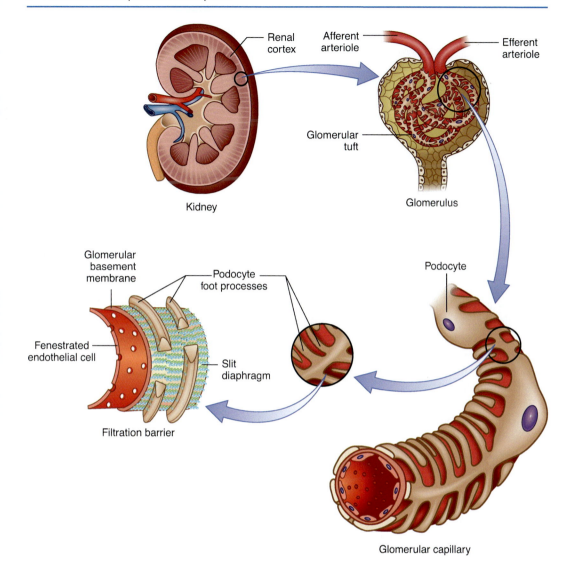

Fig. 6.2 Schematic of the structure and function of the glomerular filtration barrier. It consists of layers that block the passage of plasma macromolecules and also maintain plasma oncotic pressure. A fenestrated capillary endothelium lines each capillary loop. A porous glomerular basement membrane attached to highly dynamic epithelial cells (podocytes) is on the other side of this lining. The slit diaphragm is the prime barrier to filtration of plasma macromolecules. This slit diaphragm consists of podocytes that have interdigitating foot processes with neighbor podocytes and are connected to each other by a platform of signaling molecules

GFR is about 30 mL/min/1.73 m². In this section, we will discuss the functional development of glomerular filtration in the perinatal period.

Fetal GFR

During nephrogenesis, the increase in renal mass parallels an increase in fetal GFR [11]. Indeed, fetal GFR correlates well with both GA and body weight [11]. Preterm infants of 30 week GA have a creatinine clearance of less than 10 mL/min/1.73 m² within the first 24–40 h of birth [12], whereas creatinine clearance in term infants is higher and ranges between 10 and 40 mL/min/1.73 m² [13]. A study involving 275 neonates between 27 and 31 weeks GA reported GFR reference values as 3rd, 10th, 50th, 90th,

Table 6.1 Glomerular filtration rate reference values in premature infants

| Gestational age at birth | Glomerular filtration rate, mL/min/1.73 m^2 | | | | | | | | |
| | Day 7 | | | Day 14 | | | Day 21 | | |
	10th	Median	90th	10th	Median	90th	10th	Median	90th
27 weeks	8.7	13.4	18.1	11.5	16.2	20.9	13.3	18	22.7
28 weeks	11.5	16.2	20.9	14.4	19.1	23.8	16.1	20.8	25.5
29 weeks	14.4	19.1	23.8	17.2	21.9	26.6	19	23.7	28.4
30 weeks	17.2	21.9	26.6	20.1	24.8	29.4	21.8	26.5	31.2
31 weeks	20.1	24.8	29.5	22.9	27.6	32.3	24.7	29.4	34.1

Used with permission from Vieux et al. [3]

and 97th percentiles and provide useful reference ranges of the various GAs (Table 6.1) [3].

All four determinants of SNGFR contribute to the maturational increase in GFR to varying degrees [14]. Mean arterial pressure increases during fetal development and an increase in P_{GC} occurs as a result [15]. An increase in renal plasma flow leads to a further increase in SNGFR [16]. In addition, the oncotic pressure also rises with advancing GA [17]. However, the increase in P_{GC} is greater than that observed for π_{GC}, favoring ultrafiltration.

Fetal RBF can be measured by Doppler ultrasound techniques and increases from 20 mL/min at 25 weeks of gestation to more than 60 mL/min at 40 weeks [12]. Fetal RBF is low due to the high renal vascular resistance (RVR) [1, 18]. RVR depends on arteriolar tone and on the number of resistance vessels. As nephrogenesis proceeds, there is an increase in the number of glomerular vessels and in preterm infants born before 36 weeks gestation, the postnatal fall in RVR can, in part be attributable to new nephron formation [18]. Concomitantly, a re-distribution of RBF occurs from the inner medullary nephrons to the more superficial cortical nephrons. The superficial cortex is the site of more recent glomerulogenesis and the increase in SNGFR of the superficial nephrons significantly contributes to the increase in total GFR [14, 19].

Assessment of fetal glomerular function is possible by measurement of fetal serum cystatin C, α1-microglobulin and β2-microglobulin [20]. Cystatin C is a proteinase inhibitor involved in intracellular catabolism of proteins, produced by all nucleated cells, freely filtered across glomeruli and completely catabolized and reabsorbed in the proximal tubule. Fetal serum cystatin C is independent of GA and has been shown to have a high specificity (92%) for the prediction of postnatal kidney dysfunction. Reference intervals were calculated in a study of 129 cordocentesis involving 54 fetuses without renal disease [21]. Mean serum cystatin C levels were 1.6 mg/L with 2.0 mg/L being the upper limit of normal. In the same study, the authors showed that fetal serum β2-microglobulin decreased significantly with GA. In the same study, serum β2-microglobulin was demonstrated to have a higher sensitivity (87%) than cystatin C in predicting postnatal renal dysfunction. Both tests, therefore, may be used to assess fetal glomerular function in antenatally diagnosed renal malformations.

Neonatal GFR

A rapid rise in GFR occurs in term infants over the first 4 days of life. Preterm infants also experience a rise in GFR, but the rise occurs more slowly than that in term neonates [22]. Overall, a doubling of GFR is seen over the first 2 weeks of life in term infants and reaches almost 50 mL/min/1.73 m^2 between 2 and 4 weeks after birth and adult values by 2 years of age (Fig. 6.1b) [23, 24]. Postnatally, the mean arterial pressure increases and consequently an increase in glomerular hydraulic pressure occurs, resulting in an increase in GFR. A dramatic postnatal fall in RVR with redistribution of intrarenal blood flow from the juxtamedullary nephrons to the superficial cortical nephrons also contributes to the increased GFR. The fraction of cardiac output supplying the neonatal kidneys increases to

15–18% over the first 6 weeks of life [25]. In addition, an increase in the area available for glomerular filtration also contributes to the increase in GFR seen postnatally [14]. Glomerular size, glomerular basement membrane surface area and capillary permeability to macromolecules all contribute to the increase in GFR seen from the neonatal period to adulthood [26]. Maturation of glomerular filtration also occurs, as result of changes in both afferent and efferent arteriolar tone. A decrease in renal vasoconstrictors and activation of renal vasodilators occurs over the first 2 weeks of life and will be discussed in the following section.

Neonatal renal function is often assessed by measurement of serum creatinine, which is derived from creatinine and phosphocreatine of muscles and therefore reflects muscle mass. The serum creatinine concentration in the neonate is determined by maturation of the renal tubules, the total muscle mass of the body, GFR and tubular secretion. Several studies have now shown that the plasma creatinine in most infants actually increases after birth (Table 6.2) [27–30]. This is consistent with the idea that the tubules in the neonate are reabsorbing creatinine and not secreting it. Clearly, this has important implications for misinterpreting a rising creatinine in many neonatal ICU (NICU) patients as renal impairment.

Emerging evidence suggests that cystatin C is a more reliable marker of GFR in the neonatal period. A recent report involving 60 preterm (<37 weeks' GA) and 40 term infants studied from birth demonstrated that creatinine-based equations consistently underestimated GFR, whereas cystatin C and combined equations were more consistent with referenced inulin clearance studies [31].

Table 6.2 Reference values for serum creatinine levels in term neonates

Age	Serum creatinine, mg/dL		
	10th	Median	90th
Day 1	0.49	0.62	0.79
Day 3	0.37	0.48	0.61
Week 1	0.31	0.38	0.50
Week 2	0.27	0.35	0.45
Week 4	0.23	0.28	0.36

Used with permission of Springer Science + Business Media from Boer et al. [27]

Vasoregulatory Mechanisms of the Neonatal Kidney

Renal Vasoconstrictors in the Developing Nephron

The Renin-Angiotensin System (RAS)

The renin-angiotensin system (RAS) plays an important role in the regulation of RBF and glomerular filtration. Angiotensin II is a potent vasoconstrictor of the efferent arteriole, causing a resultant increase in P_{GC} and, therefore, GFR. Both plasma renin activity and angiotensin II levels are high in the neonate. Renal angiotensin converting enzyme (ACE) levels are higher than adult levels during first 2 weeks of life and expression is localized to the proximal tubules and capillaries in the developing human kidney [32, 33]. Expression of angiotensinogen and ACE increases during late gestation and peaks after birth [34, 35]. In addition, the number of angiotensin type 1 receptors (AT1) are also twice that of adult levels at 2 weeks of age [35, 36]. Angiotensin II receptors, on the other hand, are more abundant in the fetal kidney with progressive downregulation during fetal maturation. In contrast, AT1 receptors undergo upregulation as the fetal kidney matures [36, 37].

Animal studies have shown that angiotensin II constricts the fetal renal arteries via the AT1 receptor and during fetal life plays an important role in controlling the resistance of the umbilical arteries and, therefore, the total fetal peripheral vascular resistance [38]. Maintenance of arterial pressure and baroreceptor control of heart rate and renal sympathetic nerve activity is controlled by circulating and endogenous angiotensin II in newborn lambs [39]. Therefore, the RAS plays a significant role in maintaining blood pressure as well as vascular resistance in the developing fetus.

Indeed, the importance of the fetal RAS is highlighted by studies reporting cases of ACE fetopathy with the use of ACE inhibitors (ACEI) in pregnancy. Maternal ACEI use can result in decreased placental perfusion, fetal hypotension, oligohydramnios and neonatal renal failure [40]. Recently, mutations in genes coding for renin, angiotensinogen, ACE and AT1 have been described in association with autosomal recessive renal tubular dysgenesis with fetal hypotension [41]. Both inherited and acquired defects of the RAS, therefore, can alter fetal renal haemodynamics, with deleterious effects on renal development.

Renal Nerves and Catecholamines

The high RVR in the perinatal period can in part be due to increased renal sympathetic nerve activity (through α1 receptor stimulation) and rising circulating catecholamine levels [42]. The renal sympathetic nerves cause renal vasoconstriction, primarily of the afferent arteriole, which results in a decrease in P_{GC} and GFR (Fig. 6.3)

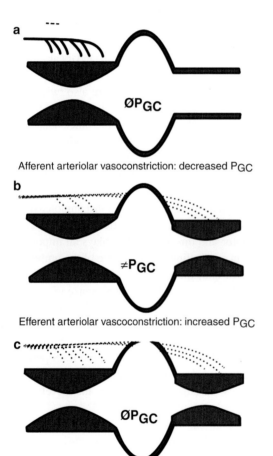

Fig. 6.3 (a–c) The renal nerves constrict the renal vasculature, causing decreases in renal blood flow and glomerular filtration. (Used with permission of John Wiley and Sons from Denton et al. [43])

[44]. Renal sympathetic nerve activity increases immediately after birth in sheep and plasma epinephrine and norepinephrine increase several fold immediately following birth [45, 46]. A fall in catecholamine levels subsequently occurs over the first few days of life [47]. Renal denervation in maturing piglets has been shown to increase RBF, demonstrating the role of renal nerves in maintaining high RVR. The sympathetic nervous system also has an important secondary role by stimulating the release of renin. Rodent studies have shown that renin-containing cells and nerve fibers are detected at 17 days of gestation, in close spatial relationship along the main branches of the renal artery [48]. Innervation of renin-containing cells follows the centrifugal pattern of renin distribution and nephrovascular development. The density and organization of nerve fibers increases with age along the arterial vascular tree [48]. Therefore, an interplay between increased sympathetic nerve activity and high plasma renin is likely necessary for the high RVR during the perinatal period.

Endothelin

Endothelin (ET) is a potent vasoconstrictor secreted by the endothelial cells of renal vessels, mesangial cells, and distal tubular cells in response to angiotensin II, bradykinin, epinephrine and shear stress [48]. Renal vasomotor tone is exquisitely sensitive to ET. An increase in RVR occurs following ET-induced contraction of glomerular arterioles (afferent > efferent) with a subsequent reduction in GFR [49]. In the first days of life, ET is elevated both in term and preterm neonates. A subsequent reduction in ET levels occur after the first week of life [50]. Newborn rat kidneys have a higher number of ET receptors than adult rat kidneys. A comparable binding affinity for ET has also been shown [51]. In addition, ET can also cause vasodilatation. Activation of ET_B receptors on the vascular endothelium evokes the release of vasodilators. The renal vasculature of fetal renal lambs reacts with vasodilatation to low doses of ET which may be due to the secondary release of nitric oxide (NO) which blunts the vasoconstrictor effects of ET [52, 53]. ET, therefore, may have both vasoconstrictor effects and vasodilatory effects on the neonatal kidney.

Renal Vasodilators in the Developing Nephron

Prostaglandins

The major prostaglandins (PGs), PGE_2, PGD_2, and PGI_2, increase RBF by stimulating afferent arteriolar vasodilatation, free water clearance, urine flow, and natriuresis. PGs are synthesized by the fetal and neonatal kidney [54]. Alterations in the synthetic and catabolic activity of renal prostaglandins occur with advancing gestational and postnatal age. Concomitant alterations in RBF, GFR, water and electrolyte excretion occur, suggesting an important role for PGs in renal functional development.

Newborns have high circulating levels of PGs that counteract the highly activated vasoconstrictor state of the neonatal microcirculation [55]. The deleterious renal vasoconstrictor effect of PG synthesis inhibitors illustrates the protective role of PGs in the immature kidney. Long-term maternal indomethacin treatment may decrease fetal urine output enough to alter amniotic fluid volume [56]. Severe renal impairment leading to fetal or neonatal death has been reported with the use of PG synthesis inhibitors which include indomethacin [57]. Neonatal indomethacin therapy may cause transient dose-related renal dysfunction characterized by a decrease in urine output. Renal dysfunction depends in part, on dosage, timing of therapy, and the cardiovascular and renal status of the infant prior to treatment [58]. In addition, recent data from studies in rodents with targeted gene disruption have shown that cyclooxygenase type-2 (COX-2) are necessary for late stages of kidney development and lack of COX-2 activity leads to pathological change in cortical architecture and eventually to renal failure [59]. Therefore, both the RAS and PGs are not only important for renal hemodynamics but are also necessary for kidney development.

Nitric Oxide

Nitric oxide (NO) plays a major role in maintaining basal renal vascular tone in the mature kidney. Through activation of its second messenger, cGMP, NO results in vasodilatation, modification of renin release and change in GFR [60]. Nitric oxide plays an important role in the maintenance of glomerular filtration in the developing kidney. Animal studies have shown that inhibition of NO synthesis by infusion with L-arginine analogues significantly decreases GFR in the developing kidney but not in the adult [61–63]. Treatment with angiotensin receptor blockers abolishes the decrease in GFR observed in the developing kidneys treated with L-arginine analogues [63]. Therefore, NO plays a critical role in the developing kidney by counter-regulating the vasoconstricting effects of angiotensin II and protecting the immature kidney.

The Kallikrein-Kinin System

Bradykinin (BK) is a vasodilator and diuretic peptide, produced by the action of kallikrein (KK), an enzyme produced by the collecting duct (CD) epithelial cells. Activation of the BK-2 receptor by BK stimulates NO and PG production, resulting in vasodilation and natriuresis. An endogenous kallikrein-kinin system is expressed in the developing kidney with higher neonatal expression than that found in adult kidneys [64, 65]. Renal expression and urinary excretion of KK rapidly rises in the postnatal period with excretion of KK correlating well with the rise in RBF [66, 67]. Blockade of the BK-2 receptor results in renal vasoconstriction in newborn rabbits, demonstrating the renal vasodilatory action of BK in the neonatal kidney [68].

Disordered Vasoregulatory Mechanisms

Vasomotor Nephropathy (VMNP)

Vasomotor nephropathy (VMNP) is defined as renal dysfunction due to reduced renal perfusion, and the preterm infant is particularly vulnerable to VMNP [69]. The main causes of neonatal acute renal failure are prerenal mechanisms and include hypotension, hypovolemia, hypoxemia and neonatal septicemia. Hypotension can stimulate vasoconstrictive mediators such as angiotensin II, causing renal vasoconstriction and hypoperfusion and thus further reduce the GFR in the newborn. The treatment of neonatal hypotension can involve inotropic support and dopamine is usually considered as the first line agent. Dopamine has a direct effect on renal function via renal dopaminergic receptors located in the renal arteries, glomeruli, and proximal and distal tubules [70]. At low doses (0.5–2 μg/kg/min), dopamine causes renal vasodilatation and increases GFR and electrolyte excretion. In neonatal intensive care units, higher doses of dopamine (6–10 μg/kg/min) are needed to achieve systemic cardiovascular effects. Such doses have an opposite effect on renal function, causing renal vasoconstriction and reduction in sodium and water excretion [71]. Hypoxemia reduces RBF and GFR. In a study of severely asphyxiated neonates, 61% developed acute renal failure [72]. Hypoxemia stimulates ET, ANP and PG release. In addition, mechanical ventilation can reduce venous return and cardiac output and can thus cause renal hypoperfusion and impair renal function [69]. Therefore, in the neonate, VMNP can result from disturbances of glomerular hemodynamics through complex interplay of the renal vasoregulatory mechanisms.

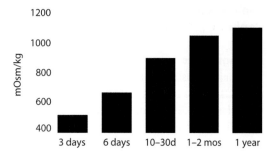

Fig. 6.4 Renal concentrating capacity increases in the postnatal period in the term infant, reaching adult values by the first month of life. (Used with permission of BMJ Publishing Group from Polacek et al. [75])

sick premature infant at greater risk for serious disturbances in water and electrolyte homeostasis [77]. The reasons for the limited concentrating capacity include diminished responsiveness of the CDs to antidiuretic hormone (ADH), anatomical immaturity of the renal medulla and decreased medullary concentration of sodium chloride (NaCl) and urea [78, 79]. In the following section, we will discuss each of these components in detail.

Water Transport in the Developing Kidney

Term neonates can dilute their urine to an osmolality as low 50 mOsm/L which is similar to adults [73]. However, the ability to excrete a water load is limited by the neonate's low GFR. As a result, the newborn infant is largely water, with total body water comprising 75% of body weight at full term and about 80–85% in babies between 26 and 31 weeks gestation [7]. Under normal physiological conditions, the kidneys have to excrete this water load during the first week of life [74]. Therefore, maximal concentrating abilities are not necessary at birth and, in fact, are low in the neonatal period. A progressive increase in concentrating capacity occurs postnatally and in term infants reaches adult levels by the first month of life (Fig. 6.4) [75]. In the premature neonate, maximal concentrating capacity is about 500 mOsm/L for a more prolonged period [76], which places the

Antidiuretic Hormone in the Development of Water Transport

Normal ADH Physiology

ADH exerts its antidiuretic effect in the CD via the V_2 receptor on the basolateral membrane of the principal and inner medullary CD cells [80, 81]. Binding of ADH to the V_2 receptor results in activation of adenyl cyclase, increased cAMP and activation of protein kinase A. Subsequent phosphorylation of the cytoplasmic COOH terminus at serine 256 of the aquaporin-2 water channel (AQ2) occurs and results in the insertion of AQ2 into the apical membrane of the CD cells [82–84]. Water enters the cells via AQ2 and exits the cell via the AQ3 and AQ4 water channels located on the basolateral membrane of the CD cells [85]. Water reabsorption depends on a hypertonic medullary interstitium, which drives water from the luminal fluid across the tubular epithelium [86].

Development of Water Transport in the Collecting Duct

Neonatal low urine concentrating capacity is not attributable to low ADH levels. During labour, ADH levels are elevated, which is consistent with the raised intracranial pressure and hypoxemia acting as stimuli for ADH release [87]. Despite adequate ability to secrete ADH, no correlation exists between ADH levels and urine osmolality in the first 3 weeks of life [88]. ADH stimulation of the neonatal cortical CD (CCD) results in a lower permeability response to water than that seen in the adult [89, 90]. The response to ADH does, however, improve with age [91]. Similarly, studies have shown that the concentrating capacity is even lower in infants who have sustained neonatal asphyxia [92]. V_2 receptor mRNA expression is observed in rodents as early as day 16 of gestation in cells of the developing medullary and cortical CD [93]. During the first 2 weeks of life in rats, the number of receptors does not change. By the fifth week of life, the number of receptors reaches adult levels [94]. However, the low response of the immature kidney to ADH is more likely due to immaturity of the intracellular second messenger systems rather than inadequate receptor number. ADH binding sites precede the onset of adenyl cyclase responsiveness [95]. In addition, ADH stimulation of adenyl cyclase generation is markedly lower in the neonatal period and is only about one-third that of the cAMP response seen in the adult CCD [96]. However, even when cAMP generation is rescued using cAMP analogs, the hydraulic permeability of isolated, microperfused rabbit CCD remains low [97]. Intracellular phosphodiesterases degrade cAMP. Indeed, an increase in phosphodiesterase IV and inhibition of the production of cAMP by PGE2 acting through EP3 receptors has been shown to inhibit adenyl cyclase generation on ADH stimulation. Therefore, cAMP inhibition likely accounts for the immature kidney's reduced response to ADH [98, 99].

AQ-2 levels (mRNA and protein) are lower in early postnatal life and reach maximal expression at 10 weeks of age (Fig. 6.5) [100]. AQ2 trafficking can be appropriately stimulated by dehydration and vasopressin in the immature kidney but

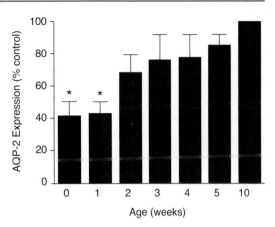

Fig. 6.5 Aquaporin-2 (AQ2) expression between 0 and 10 weeks of age. An increase in protein expression occurs in the postnatal period. (Used with permission from Bonilla-Felix [78])

the urine osmolality remains low [100]. Glucocorticoids regulate the AQ2 expression in the infant and not in the adult by increasing expression of both AQ2 protein and mRNA [101]. The expression of AQ3 and AQ4 does not change significantly after birth and they do not seem to play a role in the maturation of water transport in the CD [102].

Tonicity of the Developing Medullary Interstitium

In addition to low CD responsiveness to ADH, two other factors are responsible for the low concentrating capacity of the neonatal nephron. The medullary interstitium of the neonate has a low tonicity due to a low concentration of NaCl and urea [103]. Factors such as low protein intake, low sodium transport by the thick ascending limb of loop of Henle (TALH) [104], immaturity of the medullary architecture with shorter loops of Henle [105, 106] and alterations in urea transport [107] all contribute to the lower tonicity of the medullary interstitium. The activity of the Na-K-ATPase in the TALH increases after birth, with the most pronounced increase in activity between the second and third week of life, correlating well with the increase in urine concentrating capacity [108]. The loops of Henle elongate and penetrate the medulla, forming tubulovascular units that are completed by the fourth postnatal week in rodents [109].

The medulla/cortex urea ratio increases over the first 3 weeks of life in newborn rabbits [103]. Rodent studies have shown that there is a striking increase in the number of urea transporters during the first 2 weeks of life [107]. The urea transporters prevent the loss of urea from the medulla into the circulation thereby ensuring a high concentration of urea in the medullary interstitium. Renal concentrating capacity is dependent on dietary protein intake [103] and infants fed high protein diets show a significant improvement in urinary concentrating capacity [92, 110].

In summary, the neonatal kidney's ability to concentrate urine is dependent on a number of steps involving the ADH-signal transduction pathway (Fig. 6.6), the maturation of Henle's loop and tonicity of the medullary interstitium.

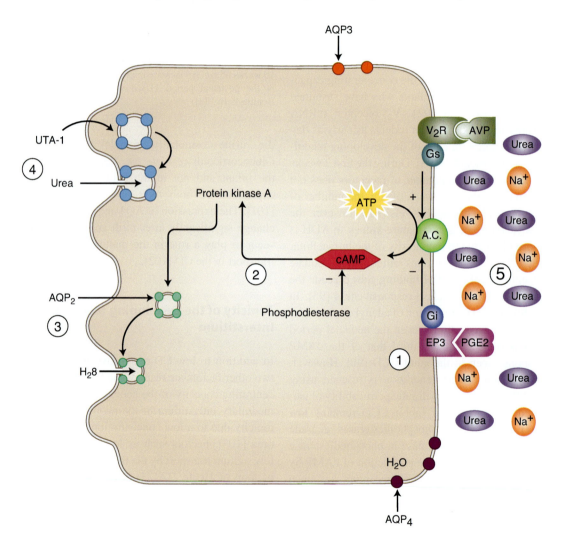

Fig. 6.6 The immature kidney's response to ADH: Responsible mechanisms are illustrated as follows: (1) Inhibition of cAMP generation by PGE$_2$ through EP3 receptor, (2) rapid degradation of formed cAMP resulting from increased phosphodiesterase activity, (3) low expression of AQP2 during early postnatal life, (4) low expression of UTA-1 during early postnatal life, (5) low concentration of urea and sodium in the medullary interstitium resulting from low rates of sodium transport, low dietary protein intake, and low expression of urea transporters

Postnatal Urine Flow

Oliguria is the most helpful sign of renal impairment in the neonate and a delay in the first void in a newborn may signal a renal disorder. Preterm neonates void earlier than term or post-term neonates [111] and the majority of normal newborns void within the first 24 h of life regardless of GA. Therefore, any neonate who remains anuric beyond the first day of life should be evaluated for renal insufficiency. The factors determining urine output include water balance, solute load and renal concentrating ability.

Minimum urine volume (L) = Urine solutes to be excreted/urine osmolality (max). As a result, a neonate receiving the usual renal solute load (7–15 mOsm/kg daily) with a maximal renal concentrating capacity of 500 mOsm/kg would require a minimal urine output of approximately 1 mL/kg/h to remain in solute balance. Since acute renal failure results in progressively positive solute balance, a urine flow rate less than 1 mL/kg/h has become an accepted criterion for the definition of oliguria in the neonate.

Sodium Transport in the Developing Kidney

Adaptation to the extrauterine environment involves a physiological natriuresis in the immediate postnatal period with preterm infants losing up to 16% of their birth weight in the first 3 days of life and term infants losing slightly less [112]. Human neonates remain in negative sodium balance for the first 4 days of life and then shift to a positive sodium balance by the second and third weeks of life (Fig. 6.7) [113]. Sodium conservation occurs because sodium is essential for growth in the neonate. In contrast to term neonates, preterm infants less than 35 weeks of gestation do not tolerate sodium deprivation, and hyponatremia may develop due to tubular immaturity and sodium wasting [114]. For this reason, sodium supplementation is important. Thus, the sodium requirements for a term newborn range from 1 to 1.5 mEq/kg daily, whereas the requirements for a preterm neonate range from 3 to 5 mEq/kg daily. Sodium supplementation in the

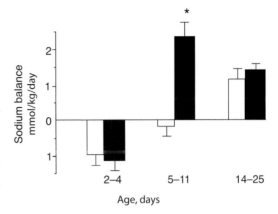

Fig. 6.7 Net external sodium balance for preterm infants in the first 3 weeks of life. Symbols are: (□) control infants; (■) sodium-supplemented infants, 4–5 mEq/kg/day; *$P < 0.0005$ vs. controls. In the first 2–4 days after birth, infants undergo natriuresis regardless of sodium intake, whereas by 1 week, supplemented infants achieve positive sodium balance sooner than controls. (Used with permission of BMJ Publishing Group from Al-Dahhan et al. [113])

preterm infant enhances the cumulative weight gain following the initial postnatal diuresis [113]. In the following section, we will discuss the mechanisms involved in the postnatal natriuresis and then the factors involved in the neonatal transition from negative to positive sodium balance.

Early Postnatal Natriuresis

High perinatal circulating levels of ANP have been implicated in the immediate postnatal natriuresis seen in both term and preterm infants [8]. ANP is a natriuretic hormone produced within the cardiac myocytes and released by stretch of the atrial wall. At birth, pulmonary vascular resistance falls and left atrial venous return increases, stimulating the release of ANP. ANP exerts a number of physiological effects, including an increase in GFR, natriuresis, diuresis, inhibition of renin and aldosterone release, vasorelaxation and an increase in vascular permeability [115].

ANP modulates sodium homeostasis by binding to physiologically active receptors, increasing intracellular cGMP [116]. Inhibition of sodium transport occurs through inhibition of apical sodium channels in renal tubular epithelial cells, leading to natriuresis. Plasma ANP concentration decreases with maturation [117, 118]. A fall in right atrial volume occurs over the first 4 days of fetal life with parallel reductions in ANP concentration and urinary cGMP excretion [119]. In addition, a decrease in cGMP production per ANP binding site has been shown to occur rapidly in the suckling period in neonatal rats [120]. Therefore, sodium excretion is reduced after the first few postnatal days and the neonatal kidney subsequently aims to conserve sodium.

Neonatal Transition to Positive Sodium Balance

A reduction in the fractional excretion of sodium occurs after the first week of life, with fractions <1% in the majority of infants (Fig. 6.8) [122]. Factors contributing to the decrease in the fractional excretion of sodium include maturation of the sodium transport mechanisms in the postnatal nephron, in addition to high circulating levels of angiotensin II, catecholamines, glucocorticoids and a reduction in ANP. Each of these factors will be discussed in the following section.

Maturation of Sodium Transport Mechanisms in the Developing Nephron

A progressive maturation of each tubular segment occurs in the postnatal kidney [123]. Each tubular segment will be discussed separately in the following section.

Proximal Tubule

Solute transport in the neonatal proximal tubule is similar to that in the adult and follows both chloride and bicarbonate reabsorption. Several animal studies have shown an increase in the activity of the Na^+/H^+ exchanger as the neonate matures [124, 125]. In addition, an increase in activity of the chloride/formate exchanger has also been shown to occur [126]. The Na-K-ATPase transporter plays a key role in sodium reabsorption in the proximal tubule and slower transport has been shown in neonates compared to adults, with a progressive maturation occurring from birth (Fig. 6.9) [127, 128]. In guinea pigs, posttranslational increase in the $\alpha 1$ and $\beta 1$ subunits of the Na-K-ATPase transporter occurs immediately after birth [129].

Loop of Henle

NaCl transport in the TALH occurs by paracellular and transcellular pathways via the apical

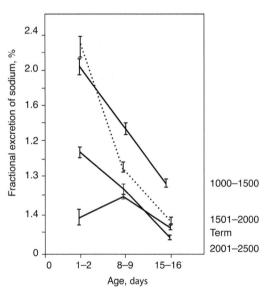

Fig. 6.8 Fractional excretion of sodium during the first 2 weeks of life in preterm and term infants. Sodium is conserved despite an increase in GFR. (Used with permission of Elsevier from Chevalier [121])

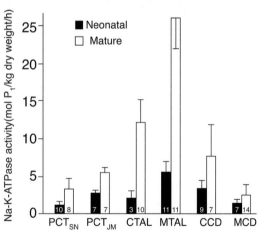

Fig. 6.9 Na^+/K^+ ATPase activity in the neonatal and adult nephron. The Na^+/K^+/ATPase activity is lower in the neonate compared to the adult. (Used with permission of Schmidt and Horster [127])

sodium-potassium-chloride cotransporter (NKCC2) and sodium-hydrogen antiporter 3 (NHE3) exchangers. The basolateral cell membrane utilizes the Na-K-ATPase to extrude sodium. Transcription of NKCC2 is observed early in development, prior to the onset of filtration in the descending loop of Henle. Physiological studies show, however, that the NKCC2 is unlikely to be functional until postnatally, as a low reabsorptive capacity has been shown for this segment in early postnatal life [109]. Compared to the adult, the expression of all of these transporters is lower in the neonate [130–133]. A postnatal five to tenfold increase in activity of the Na-K-ATPase co-transporter occurs and is greater than that seen in other tubular segments (Fig. 6.9) [127, 134]. Na-K-ATPase consists of a catalytic (α subunit) and a regulatory (β subunit). Both the α1 and β1 isoforms are present in the mature kidney. On the other hand, the α1 subunit is detected early in fetal life whereas the β1 subunit is detected only after birth. Interestingly, the β2 isoform is expressed in the fetal kidney and, in contrast to the adult, Na-K-ATPase is expressed on both the apical and basolateral cell membranes. After birth, the β2 isoform is downregulated and the α1 and β1 isoforms are upregulated [135]. Heterodimerization of the α1 and β1 isoforms is essential for the function of the Na-K-ATPase. Of note, treatment with glucocorticoids increases the synthesis of mRNA for both the catalytic and regulatory subunits of the Na-K-ATPase. During postnatal life, there is a 20% increase in the amount of sodium reabsorbed along this segment, which reflects functional maturation of transporters, an increase in the resorptive surface area and maturation mechanisms of hormonal control.

Distal Tubule
The Na$^+$–Cl$^-$ co-transporter (NCC) is the major sodium influx co-transporter in the distal tubule. In the mature nephron, NCC is expressed along the entire distal tubule, starting beyond the NKCC2-expressing post-macular segment and ending at the transition into the collecting tubules [136]. During development, NCC mRNA is detected in distal tubule segments before the expression of NKCC2 mRNA and sodium-phosphate type 2 co-transporter mRNA. Later in development, NCC expression proceeds gradually into the post-macula segment of the TALH [132].

Cortical Collecting Duct
Fine-tuning of sodium reabsorption occurs in the CCD where the amiloride-sensitive epithelial sodium channel (ENaC) plays an important role. ENaC is located on the apical membrane of distal tubular, cortical and outer medullary CD cells [137]. ENaC is comprised of three subunits, α,β and γ. Rodent studies show that the amount of total renal embryonic rat ENaC subunit mRNA is low but increases from murine gestational day 16–19 [138]. A sharp rise to almost adult levels occurs in the first three postnatal days [139]. After birth, the mRNA for α ENaC increases, whereas that for β- and γ-decreases. In the immature kidney, the greatest expression is seen in the terminal CD for all three subunits. As the kidney matures, the expression in the cortical distal nephron increases and in rodents is complete by the ninth postnatal day [140]. Endogenous glucocorticoids do not appear to have any effect on the prenatal maturation of ENaC in the kidney [141]. Although this response has long been assumed to be solely the result of liganded nuclear hormone receptors transactivating αENaC, epigenetic controls of basal and aldosterone-induced transcription of αENaC in the CD were recently described [142].

The Na-K-ATPase is also present in the CCD on the basolateral cell membrane. Tracer uptake assays of individual CCDs have shown that the activity of the Na-K-ATPase increases within the same time interval as it takes for maturation of the net transepithelial reabsorption of sodium and potassium [143]. The capacity of the CCD to reabsorb sodium increases immediately after birth [144] and reflects the increase in expression of the aforementioned sodium channels.

Developmental Paracrine Regulation of Renal Sodium Excretion

Renin: Angiotensin: Aldosterone System (RAS)

Studies have shown that the RAS is involved in renal tubular sodium reabsorption in the neonate. Acute volume expansion in neonatal rat pups results in natriuresis and AT1 blockade attenuates the natriuretic response, demonstrating that angiotensin II mediates sodium reabsorption via the ATI receptor [145]. The proximal tubule is the likely site of sodium reabsorption because angiotensin II augments sodium reabsorption in the proximal tubule in adult rats during volume contraction [146]. In addition, angiotensin II stimulates aldosterone, which stimulates sodium reabsorption in the TALH as well as the distal tubule and the CD. Preterm neonates without sodium supplementation demonstrate markedly increased plasma renin and aldosterone activity compared to their sodium supplemented counterparts, indicating that the neonatal RAS is involved in sodium homeostatic mechanisms [147].

Catecholamines

Catecholamines stimulate NaCl and water reabsorption by the proximal tubule, ascending limb of Henle's loop, distal tubule and CD. Circulating plasma catecholamines are high in the neonatal period and then fall over the first few days of life as discussed earlier (see section on "Glomerular Function in the Fetal, Perinatal, and Postnatal Period"). Catecholamines stimulate an increase in renin release, which promotes sodium reabsorption. In addition, dopamine acting via the D2 receptor in preterm neonates enhances sodium reabsorption in the proximal tubule [148].

Glucocorticoids and Thyroid Hormone

Plasma cortisol levels increase markedly after birth [149]. Maturation of the Na^+/H^+ exchanger occurs under the influence of glucocorticoids, as demonstrated by the attenuated postnatal increase of Na^+/H^+ exchanger activity and protein and mRNA abundance in the brush border of proximal tubular cells of adrenalectomized newborn rodents [150]. Glucocorticoids also play a role in the maturation of transporters along the entire nephron [151, 152]. Thyroid hormone plays a role in the maturation of the paracellular pathways of sodium reabsorption [153] and in the regulation of the Na^+/K^+ ATPase activity [154].

Fractional Excretion of Sodium

In the oliguric term neonate (urine flow less than 1 mL/kg/h), fractional excretion of sodium of less than 2.5% suggests a pre-renal cause, such as volume depletion, hypoalbuminemia or reduced cardiac output [155]. The criterion of 2.5% is valid after the first 10 days of life in the low birth weight newborn after the period of postnatal natriuresis [122]. In addition, very low birth weight infants have greater fractional sodium excretion due to immaturity of the sodium reabsorptive capacity [156].

Potassium Transport in the Developing Kidney

Like sodium, potassium is critical for somatic growth and an increase in total body potassium content is associated with growth [157]. In contrast to the adult, neonates greater than 30 weeks GA must maintain a positive potassium balance [157, 158]. Premature newborns, as a result, tend to have higher plasma potassium concentrations than children [158]. In utero, the placenta transports potassium from the mother to the fetus [159]. Interestingly, potassium levels >6.5 mmol/L are observed in 30–50% of very low birth weight infants in the first 48 h in the absence of potassium intake and not after 72 h [160]. A shift from the intracellular to the extracellular fluid compartment, as a result of either Na/K ATPase pump failure and/or a limited renal potassium excretory capacity have been postulated to account for this increase [161, 162].

Renal potassium excretion is determined by the rate of potassium excretion by the principal cells of the distal tubule and CD. Net potassium secretion cannot be detected in microperfused CCD of newborn rabbits until after the third week of life (Fig. 6.10) [164] and flow-stimulated transport is not detected until after the first postnatal month [165].

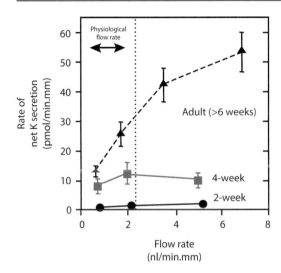

Fig. 6.10 Net potassium secretion in maturing rabbits. (Used with permission of Elsevier from Zhou and Satlin [163])

Maturation of Potassium Transport Mechanisms in the Developing Nephron

Maturation of tubular transport mechanisms will be discussed for each tubular segment in this section.

Proximal Tubule and Loop of Henle

In the mature nephron, 65% of the filtered potassium load is reabsorbed passively in the proximal tubule [166] and only 10% reaches the early distal tubule. In contrast, 35% of the filtered potassium load reaches the distal tubule of the newborn rat [167]. Therefore, postnatal maturation of the TALH is required for further potassium reabsorption. Indeed, both the diluting capacity and Na-K-ATPase activity increase after birth [108, 127]. As discussed earlier, transcription of NKCC2 is observed early in development, prior to the onset of filtration in the descending loop of Henle, but is unlikely to be functional until postnatally in view of the low reabsorptive capacity shown for this segment in early postnatal life [104]. Apical renal outer medullary potassium channel (ROMK) has been detected in the TALH at an earlier developmental stage compared to the CCD. Functional analyses on ROMK in the developing TALH have not been performed.

Cortical Collecting Duct

In the fully differentiated CCD, two types of potassium channels are involved in potassium secretion: (1) the ROMK channel mediates potassium secretion under baseline conditions [168, 169] and (2) the maxi-K^+ channel, which mediates flow-stimulated potassium secretion [170]. ROMK has only been shown in principal cells of the CCD. Maxi-K^+ exists in both the principal and intercalated cells of the CCD [170]. In isolated CCDs of neonatal rabbits, apical ROMK channels are not detected in the first 7 days of life and, subsequently, a threefold increase in the number of ROMK channels is seen in the principal cells of CCD between the third and fifth week of life [171]. The initial increase in expression follows 1 week after an increase in ENaC activity is detected [172]. Also, expression of the ROMK protein on apical cell membranes of the TALH and occasional CCD in the inner cortex and outer medulla is detected in 1-week old animals by indirect immunofluorescence studies [173]. By 3 weeks of age, expression has increased to involve the mid and outer CCDs [173]. Maxi-K^+ channels mediate flow stimulated K^+ secretion and do not appear to be functional in 4-week old rabbits subjected to a sixfold increase in tubular flow rate [165]. However, a small but significant increase in net potassium secretion after 5 weeks of age is observed. An associated increase in the mRNA and protein expression of the α subunit of the maxi-K^+ channel is seen on the apical surface of the intercalated cells of the CCD [165]. In addition to potassium excretion, potassium reabsorption also occurs in the distal nephron via the apical H^+/K^+ ATPase. Fluorescent functional assays identify significant H^+/K^+ ATPase activity on the apical cell membranes of neonatal intercalated cells [174], which suggests that neonatal CDs have a capacity to retain potassium. Indeed, a longitudinal prospective study of fractional potassium excretion in 23–31 week GA infants demonstrated that despite a threefold increase of filtered potassium, the renal excretion fell by half between 26 and 30 weeks [157]. This study supports the idea that the developing kidney has the capacity for potassium reabsorption.

Regulation of Potassium Balance in the Neonate

Table 6.3 illustrates the factors which acutely regulate plasma potassium in the neonate. The immature kidney displays an insensitivity to aldosterone despite high circulating levels of aldosterone [158]. The number of mineralocorticoid receptors, the receptor affinity and degree of nuclear binding of hormone-receptor is similar in adult and neonatal rats [175]. Aldosterone insensitivity may result from immature intracellular signal transduction mechanisms. Aldosterone insensitivity in the immature kidney is supported by the low transtubular potassium gradients (TTKG) reported in 27 week GA infants compared to 30-week infants followed over the first 5 days of postnatal life [176]. However, the low TTKG may also reflect a low secretory ability. Glucocorticoids have a significant effect on potassium balance in extremely low birth weight infants during the first week of life. Infants whose mothers received a full course of prenatal steroids had no hyperkalemia (>6.5 mmol/L) and a less negative potassium balance at the end of the first week of life [177]. Several studies have shown that glucocorticoids upregulate the expression of the Na^+/K^+ ATPase [178], resulting in a decrease of the intracellular to extracellular potassium shift.

Acid-Base Regulation in the Developing Kidney

The term neonate has a lower bicarbonate concentration than the adult (Fig. 6.11) [179, 180]. In the low birth weight newborn, total bicarbonate may be as low as 15 mmol/L during the early postnatal period and is within normal limits [179]. Bicarbonate gradually increases with increasing GFR. Misdiagnosis of renal tubular acidosis may occur if one does not take into account the physiologically low plasma bicarbonate in neonates. In addition, neonates need to excrete 2–3 mEq/kg/day of acid due to their high protein intake and formation of new bone. The neonate has a reduced ability to respond to an acid load while ammoniagenesis and titratable acidity mature after 4–6 weeks in the low birth weight newborn [181]. Renal regulation of acid-base balance undergoes complex changes during development and will be discussed in detail.

Table 6.3 Neonatal potassium regulation

	Effect on cell uptake of K^+
Physiologic	
Plasma K concentration	
↑	↑
↓	↓
Insulin	↑
Catecholamines	
α-Agonists	↓
β-Agonists	↑
Pathologic	
Acid-base balance	
Acidosis	↓
Alkalosis	↑
Hyperosmolality	↑ cell efflux
Cell breakdown	↑ cell efflux

Used with permission of Elsevier from Zhou and Satlin [163]

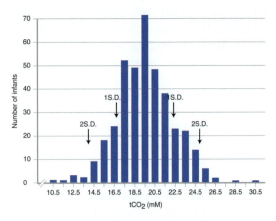

Fig. 6.11 Frequency distribution of serum total bicarbonate (tCO_2) in low birth weight neonates during first month of life. Mean is approximately 20 mM and normal range ±2 standard deviations (S.D.) is 14.5–24.5 mM. (Used with permission of Elsevier from Schwartz et al. [179])

Proximal Tubule Handling of Bicarbonate in the Neonate

Neonatal bicarbonate reabsorption in the proximal tubule is one third that of the adult [182] and is due to lower activity of the transporters present in the adult [183]. The number of apical NHE3 antiporters is lower than that in the mature nephron and has about one-third the activity [124]. The H^+/ATPase does not appear to be active in the neonate while the basolateral Na-K-ATPase has about one-half of activity compared to the adult [184]. The carbonic anhydrase (CA) type IV isoform which is expressed on the brush border of proximal tubular epithelial cells has a lower activity in the developing nephron of rabbits, but activity does increase during maturation and parallels the increase in bicarbonate reabsorption occurring in the proximal tubule [185]. Ammoniagenesis does occur in the neonatal kidney, but at a much lower rate compared to the adult [186, 187]. Glutamine and activity of the deaminating enzyme, glutaminase, is lower in the neonatal kidney while glutaminate, an inhibitor of glutaminase, is higher. Neonates, as a result, cannot generate the same amount of ammonia during an acid load and take a longer time to recover their acid-base balance.

Thick Ascending Limb of Henle's Loop

While transcription of NKCC2 is observed early in development, NKCC2 is unlikely to be functional until postnatally as a low reabsorptive capacity has been shown for this segment in early postnatal life [104]. As discussed earlier, the expression of all of the TALH transporters is lower in the neonate [130–133]. As a result, bicarbonate and ammonium reabsorption occur at a lower rate compared to the adult. A postnatal five to tenfold increase in activity of the Na-K-ATPase co-transporter has been shown and is greater than that seen in other tubular segments (Fig. 6.9) [127, 134].

Cortical Collecting Duct

Microperfusion studies of neonatal rabbit kidneys demonstrate a lower capacity to secrete acid compared to adult controls [188]. The neonatal number of intercalated cells is half that of the adult [189–191]. In addition, lower levels of the CA II isoform have been shown in neonatal rat kidneys [191, 192]. The CA II isoform is important for the function of the α-intercalated cell and may be indicative of the increase in acid secreting capability of the developing CCD.

Regulation of Maturational Acid-Base Homeostatic Mechanisms

Glucocorticoids

Glucocorticoids can stimulate bicarbonate reabsorption and a developmental increase in circulating cortisol levels precedes the increase in bicarbonate reabsorption [193]. Pregnant rabbits injected with glucocorticoids give birth to neonatal rabbits with proximal tubular bicarbonate reabsorption rates similar to that of adults [193]. An increase in NHE3 antiporters occurs with prenatal glucocorticoids [194]. Adrenalectomy prevents this maturational increase in NHE3 antiporter expression at both the level of protein and mRNA. Therefore, the maturational increase in glucocorticoids is responsible for the postnatal increase seen in proximal tubule acidification.

Renal Calcium Handling in the Developing Kidney

Higher calcium and phosphate levels are required for the growing skeleton in the fetus to ensure a positive calcium balance when bone calcium deposition rate is at its highest [195, 196]. A high geomaterial calcium ratio is maintained during pregnancy and is mediated by active transport in the placenta [197]. The elevated fetal calcium suppresses PTH release [198]. PTH is the main regulator of calcium metabolism after birth.

Circulating fetal calcium levels increase with advancing GA and at term the fetus is hypercalcemic relative to the maternal levels [199]. Serum calcium levels fall over the first 24 h in the absence of the placenta. As a result, PTH secretion is stimulated [200], but the response to the falling calcium is not sufficient such that a physiological nadir of serum calcium occurs in the first 2 days of life. This nadir is still within the adult range but represents a significant decrease compared to fetal levels [198]. Term infants typically achieve normal serum calcium levels by the second week of life, with typical circulating concentrations of ionized calcium in neonates being in the range of 1–1.5 mmol/L (2–3 mEq/L) [201].

After birth, the kidney plays an important role in calcium and phosphate homeostasis (Table 6.4). Calcium filtered by the kidney is reabsorbed along the nephron to maintain the serum concentration [202]. Only 1–2% of filtered calcium is excreted in urine by the mature nephron [203]. Most reabsorption of filtered calcium, about 70% in the proximal tubule and 20% in the thick ascending limb, is paracellular, a passive process occurring down an electrochemical gradient. Calcium diffuses across the apical cell membrane into the cell. Sodium-driven water absorption plays a significant role in this process

Table 6.4 Summarises the developmental expression of the proteins involved in renal handling of calcium

Age	<3 weeks	3–8 weeks	>8 weeks
Paracellular			
Cldn 2	Yes	Yes	Yes
Cldn 6	Yes	NK	No
Cldn 9	Yes	NK	No
Cldn 14	NK	Yes	Yes
Cldn 16	Yes	Yes	Yes
Cldn 19	NK	Yes	Yes
Transcellular			
TRPV5	Yes	Yes	Yes
TRPV6	Yes	NK	Yes
CaBP9K	Yes	Yes	Yes
CaBP28K	Yes	Yes	Yes
Pmca1	NK	Yes	Yes
Pmca4	NK	Yes	Yes
Ncx1	NK	NK	Yes

NK not known
Modified from Beggs and Alexander [202]

as highlighted by a two-fold increase in the fractional excretion of calcium (FECa) in mice null for the *Nhe3* transporter, which mediates the majority of sodium reabsorption from the proximal tubule [204]. Paracellular movement of calcium is mediated by tight junction proteins called claudins (Cldn) [205]. Claudin-2 is responsible for calcium permeability in the proximal tubule. *Cldn2* deficient mice have a three-fold increase in the fractional excretion of calcium (FECa) associated with decreased proximal tubular monovalent cation permeability [206]. Little is known about the role of other claudins in paracellular calcium permeability across the proximal tubule.

Claudins 16 and 19, in the TALH, form a cation permeable pore [207]. Upregulation of Claudin-14 occurs in hypercalcaemia and is associated with increased transepithelial resistance (TER) and decreased absolute calcium permeability, similar to the effect of pharmacological inhibition of Claudin-14. Activating mutations in the calcium sensing receptor (CaSR) mediate downregulation of Claudin-14 transcript, supporting the role of claudin-14 as an important negative regulator of calcium reabsorption in the TALH [202]. The regulatory role of the CaSR during postnatal development has yet to be determined. Autosomal dominant hypocalcaemia is associated with gain of function mutations, whilst loss of function mutations cause hypercalcemia, ranging from benign familial hypocalciuric hypercalcemia (autosomal dominant) to potentially fatal neonatal severe hyperparathyroidism (autosomal recessive).

Eighty percent of filtered calcium is reabsorbed by the proximal tubule whilst the remainder of calcium is reabsorbed in the distal nephron and, in particular, the distal convoluted tubule and connecting tubule via an active transcellular process. Active calcium reabsorption occurs through the highly Ca^{2+}-selective TRPV5 channel and binds to calbindin/D28K. The calbindin/D28K ferries Ca^{2+} to the basolateral $3Na^+/Ca^{2+}$ exchanger (NCX1) and the plasma membrane calcium ATPase 1b which extrude calcium into the blood compartment. Animal studies have shown that TRPV6, calbindin/

D9K, TRPV5 and calbindin/D28K are expressed in the kidneys of fetal mice at GA 18 days [208]. TRPV6 reaches a maximum level at 1 week of age and then decreases to <10% of TRPV5 expression, suggesting a possible role for TRPV6 during developmental regulation of calcium homeostasis. The expression of TRPV5 and calbindin/D28K peaks at the third postnatal week and then falls [208].

Renal Calcium Handling in Postnatal Period

The amount of calcium excreted increases over the first 2 weeks of life [209], and normal calcium:creatinine ratios are accordingly higher in infants. Premature and low birth weight infants have a high incidence of nephrocalcinosis on ultrasound that is most likely secondary to a three-fold higher urine calcium excretion than the upper limit of normal for term infants.

During childhood, urine calcium excretion declines by 50% between 1 month and 2 years of age. By 10 years of age, a further reduction of 30% occurs [210].

Renal Phosphate Handling in the Developing Kidney

Phosphate is of critical importance to body functions, particularly during periods of growth. Neonates excrete only 60% of intestinally absorbed phosphate and have a higher phosphate concentration than adults [211]. In neonates, the transtubular reabsorption of phosphate is high. Neonates reabsorb 99% of the filtered load of phosphate on the first day of life and 90% by the end of the first week [212]. Micropuncture studies performed on guinea pig neonatal proximal tubules demonstrated a higher phosphate reabsorption rate than adult guinea pigs [213]. Reabsorption does not occur through the $2Na^+/Pi$ IIa antiporter but rather through its developmental isoform, the $2Na^+/Pi$ IIc antiporter, the expression of which is higher in weaning animals and has a reduced function in adults [214].

Regulation of Renal Phosphate Handling in the Developing Kidney

The increased phosphate reabsorption in the early postnatal period is thought to be multifactorial. Parathyroidectomy in immature rats results in a greater increase in the maximal tubular phosphate reabsorption than in mature rats, suggesting a role for PTH in neonatal phosphaturia [215]. However, a decline in resorptive capacity is also observed with age in the presence of parathyroid glands, suggesting that there is an enhanced capacity of the immature tubule to reabsorb phosphate. In addition, responsiveness to PTH increases threefold during the first few weeks of life, suggesting a maturation of second messenger systems [216]. In the mature nephron, Klotho and PTH both increase the expression and activity of the $2Na^+/Pi$ symporter [217] resulting in phosphaturia. Future research will provide interesting insights into the ontogeny of Klotho and fibroblast growth factor 23 (FGF-23), a phosphaturic hormone, during maturation of the renal phosphate transport systems.

Growth hormone (GH) has also been shown to upregulate $2Na^+/Pi$ symporter in micropuncture studies performed on 4 week old rat proximal tubules, an effect that is independent of PTH [218, 219]. As GH levels in rodents peak in the first week of life, high serum GH in the neonate may contribute to the elevated phosphate reabsorption observed in the kidneys of neonates [220].

The mechanism enhancing the GH effect is unknown as developmental differences in the expression of GH receptors have not been shown. Both GH and IGF-1 mRNA have been localized to the apical membrane of proximal tubular epithelial cells suggesting a role of the GH/IGF-1 axis in phosphate reabsorption [221].

Magnesium Handling in the Developing Kidney

In the adult kidney, 80% of total serum magnesium is filtered and >95% is reabsorbed along the nephron [222]. The proximal tubule reabsorbs 15–20% in the adult kidney but interestingly 70%

in the developing proximal tubule [222]. A maturational decrease in the paracellular permeability at the level of the tight junction has been suggested as a reason for the decline in proximal magnesium reabsorption. From early childhood on, the majority of magnesium transport (70% of the filtered load) occurs in the loop of Henle. The distal convoluted tubule reabsorbs 5–10%. Transport in the TALH is passive and paracellular, driven by the lumen positive transepithelial voltage and involves paracellin-1, a member of the claudin family involved in tight junction formation [223]. Active and transcellular reabsorption of magnesium occurs in the distal convoluted tubule and probably through the apical TRPM6 channel [224]. Ontogeny of the TRPM6 channel and its family members and paracellin-1 requires further research.

Renal Glucose Handling in the Developing Kidney

In the mature nephron, more than 99% of the filtered glucose is reabsorbed [225]. Glucosuria is more common among neonates, with the highest levels in preterm infants [226]. The maximum tubular reabsorption of glucose is lower in preterm and term infants than in adults [227]. Age-related differences in glucose transport activity correlate with differences in sodium conductance. Changes in membrane permeability to sodium affect membrane potential, a factor which modifies glucose reabsorption. Therefore, factors such as an increase in cell membrane surface area and in basolateral Na^+/K^+-ATPase, increased density of transporter proteins and the development of new nephrons are implicated in the increase in glucose resorptive capacity observed as the fetus matures [228–230].

Renal Amino Acid Handling in the Developing Kidney

Amino acids are reabsorbed in the proximal one third of the proximal tubule in an active, sodium-dependent process [231]. Specific amino acid transport systems on the luminal cell membrane reabsorb the amino acids by secondary active transport against an uphill concentration gradient along with sodium. Aminoaciduria is frequently observed in the neonate. Factors include decreased activity of the amino acid-sodium cotransporter, increased Na^+/H^+ exchange at the luminal membrane and decreased activity of the $Na^+/K^+/ATPase$ at the basolateral membrane [232]. Of note, not all of the amino acids are wasted to the same degree [233]. Developmental differences have been shown for the amino acid system and the glycine transporter systems [234, 235].

Assessment of Renal Functional Maturation

Renal functional maturation can be measured by either glomerular or tubular indicators. Glomerular function is assessed by serum creatinine and cystatin C levels, urinary microalbumin and immunoglobulin G and GFR. Tubular function can be assessed by the fractional excretion of sodium or urinary α1-microglobulin and urinary levels of other tubular proteins normally reabsorbed by the proximal tubule such as N-acetyl-β-D-glucosaminidase or β2-microglobulin [236]. All markers have been closely associated with GA. A decrease in urinary tubular proteins occurs with increasing GA [237].

References

1. Rudolph AM. Distribution and regulation of blood flow in the fetal and neonatal lamb. Circ Res. 1985;57:811–21.
2. Haycock GB. Development of glomerular filtration and tubular sodium reabsorption in the human fetus and newborn. Br J Urol. 1998;81(Suppl 2):33–8.
3. Vieux R, Hascoet JM, Merdariu D, et al. Glomerular filtration rate reference values in very preterm infants. Pediatrics. 2010;125:e1186–92.
4. Rabinowitz R, Peters MT, Vyas S, Campbell S, Nicolaides KH. Measurement of fetal urine production in normal pregnancy by real-time ultrasonography. Am J Obstet Gynecol. 1989;161:1264–6.
5. Vanderheyden T, Kumar S, Fisk NM. Fetal renal impairment. Semin Neonatol. 2003;8:279–89.

6. Potter EL. Bilateral renal agenesis. J Pediatr. 1946;29:68–76.
7. Friis-Hansen B. Water distribution in the foetus and newborn infant. Acta Paediatr Scand Suppl. 1983;305:7–11.
8. Tulassay T, Seri I, Rascher W. Atrial natriuretic peptide and extracellular volume contraction after birth. Acta Paediatr Scand. 1987;76:444–6.
9. Baum M, Quigley R, Satlin L. Maturational changes in renal tubular transport. Curr Opin Nephrol Hypertens. 2003;12:521–6.
10. Pappenheimer JR. Permeability of glomerulomembranes in the kidney. Klin Wochenschr. 1955;33:362–5.
11. Kleinman LI, Lubbe RJ. Factors affecting the maturation of renal PAH extraction in the new-born dog. J Physiol. 1972;223:411–8.
12. Veille JC, Hanson RA, Tatum K, Kelley K. Quantitative assessment of human fetal renal blood flow. Am J Obstet Gynecol. 1993;169:1399–402.
13. Chevalier RL. Developmental renal physiology of the low birth weight pre-term newborn. J Urol. 1996;156:714–9.
14. Spitzer A, Edelmann CM Jr. Maturational changes in pressure gradients for glomerular filtration. Am J Phys. 1971;221:1431–5.
15. Ichikawa I, Maddox DA, Brenner BM. Maturational development of glomerular ultrafiltration in the rat. Am J Phys. 1979;236:F465–71.
16. Aperia A, Herin P. Development of glomerular perfusion rate and nephron filtration rate in rats 17–60 days old. Am J Phys. 1975;228:1319–25.
17. Allison ME, Lipham EM, Gottschalk CW. Hydrostatic pressure in the rat kidney. Am J Phys. 1972;223:975–83.
18. Gruskin AB, Edelmann CM Jr, Yuan S. Maturational changes in renal blood flow in piglets. Pediatr Res. 1970;4:7–13.
19. Aperia A, Broberger O, Herin P, Joelsson I. Renal hemodynamics in the perinatal period. A study in lambs. Acta Physiol Scand. 1977;99:261–9.
20. Nguyen C, Dreux S, Heidet L, Czerkiewicz I, Salomon LJ, Guimiot F, Schmitz T, Tsatsaris V, Boulot P, Rousseau T, Muller F. Fetal serum α-1 microglobulin for renal function assessment: comparison with β2-microglobulin and cystatin C. Prenat Diagn. 2013;33(8):775–81.
21. Bokenkamp A, Dieterich C, Dressler F, Muhlhaus K, Gembruch U, Bald R, Kirschstein M. Fetal serum concentrations of cystatin C and beta2-microglobulin as predictors of postnatal kidney function. Am J Obstet Gynecol. 2001;185:468–75.
22. Aperia A, Broberger O, Elinder G, Herin P, Zetterstrom R. Postnatal development of renal function in pre-term and full-term infants. Acta Paediatr Scand. 1981;70:183–7.
23. Bueva A, Guignard JP. Renal function in preterm neonates. Pediatr Res. 1994;36:572–7.
24. Guignard JP, Torrado A, Da Cunha O, Gautier E. Glomerular filtration rate in the first three weeks of life. J Pediatr. 1975;87:268–72.
25. Paton JB, Fisher DE, DeLannoy CW, Behrman RE. Umbilical blood flow, cardiac output, and organ blood flow in the immature baboon fetus. Am J Obstet Gynecol. 1973;117:560–6.
26. Fetterman GH, Shuplock NA, Philipp FJ, Gregg HS. The growth and maturation of human glomeruli and proximal convolutions from term to adulthood: studies by microdissection. Pediatrics. 1965;35:601–19.
27. Boer DP, de Rijke YB, Hop WC, Cransberg K, Dorresteijn EM. Reference values for serum creatinine in children younger than 1 year of age. Pediatr Nephrol. 2010;25:2107–13.
28. Miall LS, Henderson MJ, Turner AJ, et al. Plasma creatinine rises dramatically in the first 48 h of life in preterm infants. Pediatrics. 1999;104:e76.
29. Auron A, Mhanna MJ. Serum creatinine in very low birth weight infants during their first days of life. J Perinatol. 2006;26:755–60.
30. Jacobelli S, Bonsante F, Ferdinus C, et al. Factors affecting postnatal changes in serum creatinine in preterm infants with gestational age <32 weeks. J Perinatol. 2009;29:232–6.
31. Abitbol CL, Seeherunvong W, Galarza MG, Katsoufis C, Francoeur D, Defreitas M, Edwards-Richards A, Master Sankar Raj V, Chandar J, Duara S, Yasin S, Zilleruelo G. Neonatal kidney size and function in preterm infants: what is a true estimate of glomerular filtration rate? J Pediatr. 2014;164:1026–31.
32. Kotchen TA, Strickland AL, Rice TW, Walters DR. A study of the renin-angiotensin system in newborn infants. J Pediatr. 1972;80:938–46.
33. Wolf G. Angiotensin II and tubular development. Nephrol Dial Transplant. 2002;17(Suppl 9):48–51.
34. Niimura F, Okubo S, Fogo A, Ichikawa I. Temporal and spatial expression pattern of the angiotensinogen gene in mice and rats. Am J Phys. 1997;272:R142–7.
35. Yosipiv IV, El-Dahr SS. Developmental biology of angiotensin-converting enzyme. Pediatr Nephrol. 1998;12:72–9.
36. Tufro-McReddie A, Harrison JK, Everett AD, Gomez RA. Ontogeny of type 1 angiotensin II receptor gene expression in the rat. J Clin Invest. 1993;91:530–7.
37. Kakuchi J, Ichiki T, Kiyama S, Hogan BL, Fogo A, Inagami T, Ichikawa I. Developmental expression of renal angiotensin II receptor genes in the mouse. Kidney Int. 1995;47:140–7.
38. Segar JL, Barna TJ, Acarregui MJ, Lamb FS. Responses of fetal ovine systemic and umbilical arteries to angiotensin II. Pediatr Res. 2001;49:826–33.
39. Segar JL, Minnick A, Nuyt AM, Robillard JE. Role of endogenous ANG II and AT1 receptors in regulating arterial baroreflex responses in newborn lambs. Am J Phys. 1997;272:R1862–73.

40. Robillard JE, Weismann DN, Gomez RA, Ayres NA, Lawton WJ, VanOrden DE. Renal and adrenal responses to converting-enzyme inhibition in fetal and newborn life. Am J Phys. 1983;244:R249–56.
41. Lacoste M, Cai Y, Guicharnaud L, Mounier F, Dumez Y, Bouvier R, Dijoud F, Gonzales M, Chatten J, Delezoide AL, et al. Renal tubular dysgenesis, a not uncommon autosomal recessive disorder leading to oligohydramnios: role of the renin-angiotensin system. J Am Soc Nephrol. 2006;17:2253–63.
42. Nakamura KT, Matherne GP, McWeeny OJ, Smith BA, Robillard JE. Renal hemodynamics and functional changes during the transition from fetal to newborn life in sheep. Pediatr Res. 1987;21:229–34.
43. Denton KM, Luff SE, Shweta A, Anderson WP. Differential neural control of glomerular ultrafiltration. Clin Exp Pharmacol Physiol. 2004;31:380–6.
44. DiBona GF, Kopp UC. Neural control of renal function. Physiol Rev. 1997;77:75–197.
45. Buckley NM, Brazeau P, Gootman PM, Frasier ID. Renal circulatory effects of adrenergic stimuli in anesthetized piglets and mature swine. Am J Phys. 1979;237:H690–5.
46. Smith FG, Smith BA, Guillery EN, Robillard JE. Role of renal sympathetic nerves in lambs during the transition from fetal to newborn life. J Clin Invest. 1991;88:1988–94.
47. Segar JL, Mazursky JE, Robillard JE. Changes in ovine renal sympathetic nerve activity and baroreflex function at birth. Am J Phys. 1994;267:H1824–32.
48. Pupilli C, Gomez RA, Tuttle JB, Peach MJ, Carey RM. Spatial association of renin-containing cells and nerve fibers in developing rat kidney. Pediatr Nephrol. 1991;5:690–5.
49. Naicker S, Bhoola KD. Endothelins: vasoactive modulators of renal function in health and disease. Pharmacol Ther. 2001;90:61–88.
50. Mattyus I, Zimmerhackl LB, Schwarz A, Brandis M, Miltenyi M, Tulassay T. Renal excretion of endothelin in children. Pediatr Nephrol. 1997;11:513–21.
51. Abadie L, Blazy I, Roubert P, Plas P, Charbit M, Chabrier PE, Dechaux M. Decrease in endothelin-1 renal receptors during the 1st month of life in the rat. Pediatr Nephrol. 1996;10:185–9.
52. Bogaert GA, Kogan BA, Mevorach RA, Wong J, Gluckman GR, Fineman JR, Heymann MA. Exogenous endothelin-1 causes renal vasodilation in the fetal lamb. J Urol. 1996;156:847–53.
53. Semama DS, Thonney M, Guignard JP. Role of endogenous endothelin in renal haemodynamics of newborn rabbits. Pediatr Nephrol. 1993;7:886–90.
54. Gleason CA. Prostaglandins and the developing kidney. Semin Perinatol. 1987;11:12–21.
55. Guignard JP, Gouyon JB, John EG. Vasoactive factors in the immature kidney. Pediatr Nephrol. 1991;5:443–6.
56. Cantor B, Tyler T, Nelson RM, Stein GH. Oligohydramnios and transient neonatal anuria: a possible association with the maternal use of prostaglandin synthetase inhibitors. J Reprod Med. 1980;24:220–3.
57. Simeoni U, Messer J, Weisburd P, Haddad J, Willard D. Neonatal renal dysfunction and intrauterine exposure to prostaglandin synthesis inhibitors. Eur J Pediatr. 1989;148:371–3.
58. Marpeau L, Bouillie J, Barrat J, Milliez J. Obstetrical advantages and perinatal risks of indomethacin: a report of 818 cases. Fetal Diagn Ther. 1994;9:110–5.
59. Jensen BL, Stubbe J, Madsen K, Nielsen FT, Skott O. The renin-angiotensin system in kidney development: role of COX-2 and adrenal steroids. Acta Physiol Scand. 2004;181:549–59.
60. Bachmann S, Mundel P. Nitric oxide in the kidney: synthesis, localization, and function. Am J Kidney Dis. 1994;24:112–29.
61. Ballevre L, Solhaug MJ, Guignard JP. Nitric oxide and the immature kidney. Biol Neonate. 1996;70:1–14.
62. Bogaert GA, Kogan BA, Mevorach RA. Effects of endothelium-derived nitric oxide on renal hemodynamics and function in the sheep fetus. Pediatr Res. 1993;34:755–61.
63. Solhaug MJ, Wallace MR, Granger JP. Nitric oxide and angiotensin II regulation of renal hemodynamics in the developing piglet. Pediatr Res. 1996;39:527–33.
64. El-Dahr SS, Figueroa CD, Gonzalez CB, Muller-Esterl W. Ontogeny of bradykinin B2 receptors in the rat kidney: implications for segmental nephron maturation. Kidney Int. 1997;51:739–49.
65. El-Dahr SS. Spatial expression of the kallikrein-kinin system during nephrogenesis. Histol Histopathol. 2004;19:1301–10.
66. El-Dahr SS, Chao J. Spatial and temporal expression of kallikrein and its mRNA during nephron maturation. Am J Phys. 1992;262:F705–11.
67. Robillard JE, Lawton WJ, Weismann DN, Sessions C. Developmental aspects of the renal kallikrein-like activity in fetal and newborn lambs. Kidney Int. 1982;22:594–601.
68. Toth-Heyn P, Guignard JP. Endogenous bradykinin regulates renal function in the newborn rabbit. Biol Neonate. 1998;73:330–6.
69. Toth-Heyn P, Drukker A, Guignard JP. The stressed neonatal kidney: from pathophysiology to clinical management of neonatal vasomotor nephropathy. Pediatr Nephrol. 2000;14:227–39.
70. Felder RA, Felder CC, Eisner GM, Jose PA. The dopamine receptor in adult and maturing kidney. Am J Phys. 1989;257:F315–27.
71. Seri I. Cardiovascular, renal, and endocrine actions of dopamine in neonates and children. J Pediatr. 1995;126:333–44.
72. Karlowicz MG, Adelman RD. Nonoliguric and oliguric acute renal failure in asphyxiated term neonates. Pediatr Nephrol. 1995;9:718–22.
73. Rodriguez-Soriano J, Vallo A, Castillo G, Oliveros R. Renal handling of water and sodium in infancy and childhood: a study using clearance methods

during hypotonic saline diuresis. Kidney Int. 1981;20:700–4.

74. Rodriguez G, Ventura P, Samper MP, Moreno L, Sarria A, Perez-Gonzalez JM. Changes in body composition during the initial hours of life in breast-fed healthy term newborns. Biol Neonate. 2000;77:12–6.

75. Polacek E, Vocel J, Neugebauerova L, Sebkova M, Vechetova E. The osmotic concentrating ability in healthy infants and children. Arch Dis Child. 1965;40:291–5.

76. Sujov P, Kellerman L, Zeltzer M, Hochberg Z. Plasma and urine osmolality in full-term and pre-term infants. Acta Paediatr Scand. 1984;73:722–6.

77. Day GM, Radde IC, Balfe JW, Chance GW. Electrolyte abnormalities in very low birth-weight infants. Pediatr Res. 1976;10:522–6.

78. Bonilla-Felix M. Development of water transport in the collecting duct. Am J Physiol Renal Physiol. 2004;287:F1093–101.

79. Edelmann CM, Barnett HL, Troupkou V. Renal concentrating mechanisms in newborn infants. Effect of dietary protein and water content, role of urea, and responsiveness to antidiuretic hormone. J Clin Invest. 1960;39:1062–9.

80. Grantham JJ, Burg MB. Effect of vasopressin and cyclic AMP on permeability of isolated collecting tubules. Am J Phys. 1996;211:255–9.

81. Sands JM, Nonoguchi H, Knepper MA. Vasopressin effects on urea and H2O transport in inner medullary collecting duct subsegments. Am J Phys. 1987;253:F823–32.

82. Fushimi K, Sasaki S, Marumo F. Phosphorylation of serine 256 is required for cAMP-dependent regulatory exocytosis of the aquaporin-2 water channel. J Biol Chem. 1997;272:14800–4.

83. Fushimi K, Uchida S, Hara Y, Hirata Y, Marumo F, Sasaki S. Cloning and expression of apical membrane water channel of rat kidney collecting tubule. Nature. 1993;361:549–52.

84. Nielsen S, Chou CL, Marples D, Christensen EI, Kishore BK, Knepper MA. Vasopressin increases water permeability of kidney collecting duct by inducing translocation of aquaporin-CD water channels to plasma membrane. Proc Natl Acad Sci U S A. 1995;92:1013–7.

85. Liu H, Wintour EM. Aquaporins in development—a review. Reprod Biol Endocrinol. 2005;3:18.

86. Knepper MA, Nielsen S, Chou CL, DiGiovanni SR. Mechanism of vasopressin action in the renal collecting duct. Semin Nephrol. 1994;14:302–21.

87. Hadeed AJ, Leake RD, Weitzman RE, Fisher DA. Possible mechanisms of high blood levels of vasopressin during the neonatal period. J Pediatr. 1979;94:805–8.

88. Rees L, Forsling ML, Brook CG. Vasopressin concentrations in the neonatal period. Clin Endocrinol (Oxf). 1980;12:357–62.

89. Horster MF, Zink H. Functional differentiation of the medullary collecting tubule: influence of vasopressin. Kidney Int. 1982;22:360–5.

90. Siga E, Horster MF. Regulation of osmotic water permeability during differentiation of inner medullary collecting duct. Am J Phys. 1991;260:F710–6.

91. Ivanova LN, Zelenina MN, Melidi NN, Solenov EI, Khegaĭ II. Vasopressin: the ontogeny of antidiuretic action at the cellular level. Fiziol Zh SSSR Im I M Sechenova. 1989;7:970–9.

92. Svenningsen NW, Aronson AS. Postnatal development of renal concentration capacity as estimated by DDAVP-test in normal and asphyxiated neonates. Biol Neonate. 1974;25:230–41.

93. Ostrowski NL, Young WS 3rd, Knepper MA, Lolait SJ. Expression of vasopressin V1a and V2 receptor messenger ribonucleic acid in the liver and kidney of embryonic, developing, and adult rats. Endocrinology. 1993;133:1849–59.

94. Ammar A, Roseau S, Butlen D. Postnatal ontogenesis of vasopressin receptors in the rat collecting duct. Mol Cell Endocrinol. 1992;86:193–203.

95. Rajerison RM, Butlen D, Jard S. Ontogenic development of antidiuretic hormone receptors in rat kidney: comparison of hormonal binding and adenylate cyclase activation. Mol Cell Endocrinol. 1976;4:271–85.

96. Bonilla-Felix M, John-Phillip C. Prostaglandins mediate the defect in AVP-stimulated cAMP generation in immature collecting duct. Am J Phys. 1994;267:F44–8.

97. Bonilla-Felix M, Vehaskari VM, Hamm LL. Water transport in the immature rabbit collecting duct. Pediatr Nephrol. 1999;13:103–7.

98. Quigley R, Chakravarty S, Baum M. Antidiuretic hormone resistance in the neonatal cortical collecting tubule is mediated in part by elevated phosphodiesterase activity. Am J Physiol Renal Physiol. 2004;286:F317–22.

99. Negishi M, Sugimoto Y, Hayashi Y, Namba T, Honda A, Watabe A, Narumiya S, Ichikawa A. Functional interaction of prostaglandin E receptor EP3 subtype with guanine nucleotide-binding proteins, showing low-affinity ligand binding. Biochim Biophys Acta. 1993;1175:343–50.

100. Bonilla-Felix M, Jiang W. Aquaporin-2 in the immature rat: expression, regulation, and trafficking. J Am Soc Nephrol. 1997;8:1502–9.

101. Yasui M, Marples D, Belusa R, Eklof AC, Celsi G, Nielsen S, Aperia A. Development of urinary concentrating capacity: role of aquaporin-2. Am J Phys. 1996;271:F461–8.

102. Yamamoto T, Sasaki S, Fushimi K, Ishibashi K, Yaoita E, Kawasaki K, Fujinaka H, Marumo F, Kihara I. Expression of AQP family in rat kidneys during development and maturation. Am J Phys. 1997;272:F198–204.

103. Forrest JN Jr, Stanier MW. Kidney composition and renal concentration ability in young rabbits. J Physiol. 1996;187:1–4.

104. Horster M. Loop of Henle functional differentiation: in vitro perfusion of the isolated thick ascending segment. Pflugers Arch. 1978;78:15–24.

105. Cha JH, Kim YH, Jung JY, Han KH, Madsen KM, Kim J. Cell proliferation in the loop of henle in the developing rat kidney. J Am Soc Nephrol. 2001;12:1410–21.

106. Liu W, Morimoto T, Kondo Y, Iinuma K, Uchida S, Imai M. "Avian-type" renal medullary tubule organization causes immaturity of urine-concentrating ability in neonates. Kidney Int. 2001;60:680–93.

107. Kim YH, Kim DU, Han KH, Jung JY, Sands JM, Knepper MA, Madsen KM, Kim J. Expression of urea transporters in the developing rat kidney. Am J Physiol Renal Physiol. 2002;282:F530–40.

108. Zink H, Horster M. Maturation of diluting capacity in loop of Henle of rat superficial nephrons. Am J Phys. 1977;233:F519–24.

109. Speller AM, Moffat DB. Tubulo-vascular relationships in the developing kidney. J Anat. 1977;123:487–500.

110. Edelmann CM Jr, Barnett HL, Stark H. Effect of urea on concentration of urinary nonurea solute in premature infants. J Appl Physiol. 1966;21:1021–5.

111. Clark DA. Times of first void and first stool in 500 newborns. Pediatrics. 1977;60:457–9.

112. Hansen JD, Smith CA. Effects of withholding fluid in the immediate postnatal period. Pediatrics. 1953;12:99–113.

113. Al-Dahhan J, Haycock GB, Nichol B, Chantler C, Stimmler L. Sodium homeostasis in term and preterm neonates. III. Effect of salt supplementation. Arch Dis Child. 1984;59:945–50.

114. Engelke SC, Shah BL, Vasan U, Raye JR. Sodium balance in very low-birth-weight infants. J Pediatr. 1978;93:837–41.

115. Goetz KL. Physiology and pathophysiology of atrial peptides. Am J Phys. 1988;254:E1–15.

116. Chevalier RL. Atrial natriuretic peptide in renal development. Pediatr Nephrol. 1993;7:652–6.

117. Kikuchi K, Shiomi M, Horie K, Ohie T, Nakao K, Imura H, Mikawa H. Plasma atrial natriuretic polypeptide concentration in healthy children from birth to adolescence. Acta Paediatr Scand. 1988;77:380–4.

118. Weil J, Bidlingmaier F, Dohlemann C, Kuhnle U, Strom T, Lang RE. Comparison of plasma atrial natriuretic peptide levels in healthy children from birth to adolescence and in children with cardiac diseases. Pediatr Res. 1986;20:1328–31.

119. Bierd TM, Kattwinkel J, Chevalier RL, Rheuban KS, Smith DJ, Teague WG, Carey RM, Linden J. Interrelationship of atrial natriuretic peptide, atrial volume, and renal function in premature infants. J Pediatr. 1990;116:753–9.

120. Semmekrot B, Chabardes D, Roseau S, Siaume-Perez S, Butlen D. Developmental pattern of cyclic guanosine monophosphate production stimulated by atrial natriuretic peptide in glomeruli microdissected from kidneys of young rats. Pflugers Arch. 1990;416:519–25.

121. Chevalier RL. The moth and the aspen tree: sodium in early postnatal development. Kidney Int. 2001;59(5):1617–25.

122. Ross B, Cowett RM, Oh W. Renal functions of low birth weight infants during the first two months of life. Pediatr Res. 1977;11:1162–4.

123. Spitzer A. The role of the kidney in sodium homeostasis during maturation. Kidney Int. 1982;21:539–45.

124. Baum M. Neonatal rabbit juxtamedullary proximal convoluted tubule acidification. J Clin Invest. 1990;85:499–506.

125. Guillery EN, Karniski LP, Mathews MS, Robillard JE. Maturation of proximal tubule Na+/H+ antiporter activity in sheep during transition from fetus to newborn. Am J Phys. 1994;267:F537–45.

126. Guillery EN, Huss DJ. Developmental regulation of chloride/formate exchange in guinea pig proximal tubules. Am J Phys. 1995;269:F686–95.

127. Schmidt U, Horster M. Na-K-activated ATPase: activity maturation in rabbit nephron segments dissected in vitro. Am J Phys. 1977;233:F55–60.

128. Fukuda Y, Bertorello A, Aperia A. Ontogeny of the regulation of Na+, K(+)-ATPase activity in the renal proximal tubule cell. Pediatr Res. 1991;30:131–4.

129. Guillery EN, Huss DJ, McDonough AA, Klein LC. Posttranscriptional upregulation of Na(+)-K(+)-ATPase activity in newborn guinea pig renal cortex. Am J Phys. 1997;273:F254–63.

130. Biemesderfer D, Rutherford PA, Nagy T, Pizzonia JH, Abu-Alfa AK, Aronson PS. Monoclonal antibodies for high-resolution localization of NHE3 in adult and neonatal rat kidney. Am J Phys. 1997;273:F289–99.

131. Igarashi P, Vanden Heuvel GB, Payne JA, Forbush B 3rd. Cloning, embryonic expression, and alternative splicing of a murine kidney-specific Na-K-Cl cotransporter. Am J Phys. 1995;269:F405–18.

132. Schmitt R, Ellison DH, Farman N, Rossier BC, Reilly RF, Reeves WB, Oberbaumer I, Tapp R, Bachmann S. Developmental expression of sodium entry pathways in rat nephron. Am J Phys. 1999;276:F367–81.

133. Bachmann S, Bostanjoglo M, Schmitt R, Ellison DH. Sodium transport-related proteins in the mammalian distal nephron—distribution, ontogeny and functional aspects. Anat Embryol (Berl). 1999;200:447–68.

134. Rane S, Aperia A. Ontogeny of Na-K-ATPase activity in thick ascending limb and of concentrating capacity. Am J Phys. 1985;249:F723–8.

135. Burrow CR, Devuyst O, Li X, Gatti L, Wilson PD. Expression of the beta2-subunit and apical localization of Na+-K+-ATPase in metanephric kidney. Am J Phys. 1999;277:F391–403.

136. Obermuller N, Bernstein P, Velazquez H, Reilly R, Moser D, Ellison DH, Bachmann S. Expression of the thiazide-sensitive Na-Cl cotransporter in rat and human kidney. Am J Phys. 1995;269:F900–10.

137. Duc C, Farman N, Canessa CM, Bonvalet JP, Rossier BC. Cell-specific expression of epithelial sodium channel alpha, beta, and gamma subunits in aldosterone-responsive epithelia from the rat: localization by in situ hybridization and immuno cytochemistry. J Cell Biol. 1994;127:1907–21.

138. Vehaskari VM, Hempe JM, Manning J, Aviles DH, Carmichael MC. Developmental regulation of ENaC subunit mRNA levels in rat kidney. Am J Phys. 1998;274:C1661–6.
139. Horster M. Embryonic epithelial membrane transporters. Am J Physiol Renal Physiol. 2000;279:F982–96.
140. Watanabe S, Matsushita K, McCray PB Jr, Stokes JB. Developmental expression of the epithelial Na+ channel in kidney and uroepithelia. Am J Phys. 1999;276:F304–14.
141. Nakamura K, Stokes JB, McCray PB Jr. Endogenous and exogenous glucocorticoid regulation of ENaC mRNA expression in developing kidney and lung. Am J Physiol Cell Physiol. 2002;283:C762–72.
142. Kone BC. Epigenetics and the control of the collecting duct epithelial sodium channel. Semin Nephrol. 2013;33(4):383–91.
143. Constantinescu AR, Lane JC, Mak J, Zavilowitz B, Satlin LM. Na(+)-K(+)-ATPase-mediated basolateral rubidium uptake in the maturing rabbit cortical collecting duct. Am J Physiol Renal Physiol. 2000;279:F1161–8.
144. Vehaskari VM. Ontogeny of cortical collecting duct sodium transport. Am J Phys. 1994;267:F49–54.
145. Chevalier RL, Thornhill BA, Belmonte DC, Baertschi AJ. Endogenous angiotensin II inhibits natriuresis after acute volume expansion in the neonatal rat. Am J Phys. 1996;270:R393–7.
146. Quan A, Baum M. Endogenous angiotensin II modulates rat proximal tubule transport with acute changes in extracellular volume. Am J Phys. 1998;275:F74–8.
147. Sulyok E. In: Spitzer A, editor. The kidney during development: morphogenesis and function. New York: Masson; 1982. p. 273.
148. Sulyok E. Dopaminergic control of neonatal salt and water metabolism. Pediatr Nephrol. 1988;2:163–5.
149. Magyar DM, Fridshal D, Elsner CW, Glatz T, Eliot J, Klein AH, Lowe KC, Buster JE, Nathanielsz PW. Time-trend analysis of plasma cortisol concentrations in the fetal sheep in relation to parturition. Endocrinology. 1980;107:155–9.
150. Gupta N, Tarif SR, Seikaly M, Baum M. Role of glucocorticoids in the maturation of the rat renal Na+/H+ antiporter (NHE3). Kidney Int. 2001;60:173–81.
151. Guillery EN, Karniski LP, Mathews MS, Page WV, Orlowski J, Jose PA, Robillard JE. Role of glucocorticoids in the maturation of renal cortical Na+/H+ exchanger activity during fetal life in sheep. Am J Phys. 1995;268:F710–7.
152. Celsi G, Nishi A, Akusjarvi G, Aperia A. Abundance of Na(+)-K(+)-ATPase mRNA is regulated by glucocorticoid hormones in infant rat kidneys. Am J Phys. 1991;260:F192–7.
153. Shah M, Quigley R, Baum M. Maturation of proximal straight tubule NaCl transport: role of thyroid hormone. Am J Physiol Renal Physiol. 2000;278:F596–602.
154. McDonough AA, Brown TA, Horowitz B, Chiu R, Schlotterbeck J, Bowen J, Schmitt CA. Thyroid hormone coordinately regulates Na+-K+-ATPase alpha- and beta-subunit mRNA levels in kidney. Am J Phys. 1988;254:C323–9.
155. Mathew OP, Jones AS, James E, Bland H, Groshong T. Neonatal renal failure: usefulness of diagnostic indices. Pediatrics. 1980;65:57–60.
156. Siegel SR, Oh W. Renal function as a marker of human fetal maturation. Acta Paediatr Scand. 1976;65:481–5.
157. Delgado MM, Rohatgi R, Khan S, Holzman IR, Satlin LM. Sodium and potassium clearances by the maturing kidney: clinical-molecular correlates. Pediatr Nephrol. 2003;18:759–67.
158. Sulyok E, Nemeth M, Tenyi I, Csaba IF, Varga F, Gyory E, Thurzo V. Relationship between maturity, electrolyte balance and the function of the renin-angiotensin-aldosterone system in newborn infants. Biol Neonate. 1979;35:60–5.
159. Serrano CV, Talbert LM, Welt LG. Potassium deficiency in the pregnant dog. J Clin Invest. 1964;43:27–31.
160. Lorenz JM, Kleinman LI, Markarian K. Potassium metabolism in extremely low birth weight infants in the first week of life. J Pediatr. 1997;131:81–6.
161. Sato K, Kondo T, Iwao H, Honda S, Ueda K. Internal potassium shift in premature infants: cause of nonoliguric hyperkalemia. J Pediatr. 1995;126:109–13.
162. Stefano JL, Norman ME, Morales MC, Goplerud JM, Mishra OP, Delivoria-Papadopoulos M. Decreased erythrocyte Na+, K(+)-ATPase activity associated with cellular potassium loss in extremely low birth weight infants with non oliguric hyperkalemia. J Pediatr. 1993;122:276–84.
163. Zhou H, Satlin LM. Renal potassium handling in healthy and sick newborns. Semin Perinatol. 2004;28(2):103–11.
164. Satlin LM. Postnatal maturation of potassium transport in rabbit cortical collecting duct. Am J Phys. 1994;266:F57–65.
165. Woda CB, Miyawaki N, Ramalakshmi S, Ramkumar M, Rojas R, Zavilowitz B, Kleyman TR, Satlin LM. Ontogeny of flow-stimulated potassium secretion in rabbit cortical collecting duct: functional and molecular aspects. Am J Physiol Renal Physiol. 2003;285:F629–39.
166. Giebisch G. Renal potassium transport: mechanisms and regulation. Am J Phys. 1998;274:F817–33.
167. Lelievre-Pegorier M, Merlet-Benichou C, Roinel N, de Rouffignac C. Developmental pattern of water and electrolyte transport in rat superficial nephrons. Am J Phys. 1983;245:F15–21.
168. Frindt G, Palmer LG. Low-conductance K channels in apical membrane of rat cortical collecting tubule. Am J Phys. 1989;256:F143–51.
169. Wang WH, Schwab A, Giebisch G. Regulation of small-conductance K+ channel in apical membrane of rat cortical collecting tubule. Am J Phys. 1990;259:F494–502.

170. Pacha J, Frindt G, Sackin H, Palmer LG. Apical maxi K channels in intercalated cells of CCT. Am J Phys. 1991;261:F696–705.

171. Satlin LM, Palmer LG. Apical K+ conductance in maturing rabbit principal cell. Am J Phys. 1997;272:F397–404.

172. Satlin LM, Palmer LG. Apical Na+ conductance in maturing rabbit principal cell. Am J Phys. 1996;270:F391–7.

173. Zolotnitskaya A, Satlin LM. Developmental expression of ROMK in rat kidney. Am J Phys. 1999;276:F825–36.

174. Hunter M, Lopes AG, Boulpaep EL, Giebisch GH. Single channel recordings of calcium-activated potassium channels in the apical membrane of rabbit cortical collecting tubules. Proc Natl Acad Sci U S A. 1984;81:4237–9.

175. Stephenson G, Hammet M, Hadaway G, Funder JW. Ontogeny of renal mineralocorticoid receptors and urinary electrolyte responses in the rat. Am J Phys. 1984;247:F665–71.

176. Rodriguez-Soriano J, Ubetagoyena M, Vallo A. Transtubular potassium concentration gradient: a useful test to estimate renal aldosterone bioactivity in infants and children. Pediatr Nephrol. 1990;4:105–10.

177. Omar SA, DeCristofaro JD, Agarwal BI, LaGamma EF. Effect of prenatal steroids on potassium balance in extremely low birth weight neonates. Pediatrics. 2000;106:561–7.

178. Celsi G, Wang ZM, Akusjarvi G, Aperia A. Sensitive periods for glucocorticoids' regulation of Na+, K(+)-ATPase mRNA in the developing lung and kidney. Pediatr Res. 1993;33:5–9.

179. Schwartz GJ, Haycock GB, Edelmann CM Jr, Spitzer A. Late metabolic acidosis: a reassessment of the definition. J Pediatr. 1979;95:102–7.

180. Edelmann CM, Soriano JR, Boichis H, Gruskin AB, Acosta MI. Renal bicarbonate reabsorption and hydrogen ion excretion in normal infants. J Clin Invest. 1967;46:1309–17.

181. Kerpel-Fronius E, Heim T, Sulyok E. The development of the renal acidifying processes and their relation to acidosis in low-birth-weight infants. Biol Neonate. 1970;15:156–68.

182. Schwartz GJ, Evan AP. Development of solute transport in rabbit proximal tubule. I. HCO-3 and glucose absorption. Am J Phys. 1983;245:F382–90.

183. Baum M, Quigley R. Ontogeny of proximal tubule acidification. Kidney Int. 1995;48:1697–704.

184. Schwartz GJ, Brown D, Mankus R, Alexander EA, Schwartz JH. Low pH enhances expression of carbonic anhydrase II by cultured rat inner medullary collecting duct cells. Am J Phys. 1994;266:C508–14.

185. Winkler CA, Kittelberger AM, Watkins RH, Maniscalco WM, Schwartz GJ. Maturation of carbonic anhydrase IV expression in rabbit kidney. Am J Physiol Renal Physiol. 2001;280:F895–903.

186. Goldstein L. Renal ammonia and acid excretion in infant rats. Am J Phys. 1970;218:1394–8.

187. Goldstein L. Ammonia metabolism in kidneys of suckling rats. Am J Phys. 1971;220:213–7.

188. Mehrgut FM, Satlin LM, Schwartz GJ. Maturation of HCO3− transport in rabbit collecting duct. Am J Phys. 1990;259:F801–8.

189. Kim J, Tisher CC, Madsen KM. Differentiation of intercalated cells in developing rat kidney: an immunohistochemical study. Am J Phys. 1994;266:F977–90.

190. Satlin LM, Matsumoto T, Schwartz GJ. Postnatal maturation of rabbit renal collecting duct. III. Peanut lectin-binding intercalated cells. Am J Phys. 1992;262:F199–208.

191. Satlin LM, Schwartz GJ. Postnatal maturation of rabbit renal collecting duct: intercalated cell function. Am J Phys. 1987;253:F622–35.

192. Karashima S, Hattori S, Ushijima T, Furuse A, Nakazato H, Matsuda I. Developmental changes in carbonic anhydrase II in the rat kidney. Pediatr Nephrol. 1998;12:263–8.

193. Baum M, Quigley R. Prenatal glucocorticoids stimulate neonatal juxtamedullary proximal convoluted tubule acidification. Am J Phys. 1991;261:F746–52.

194. Baum M, Moe OW, Gentry DL, Alpern RJ. Effect of glucocorticoids on renal cortical NHE-3 and NHE-1 mRNA. Am J Phys. 1994;267:F437–42.

195. David L, Anast CS. Calcium metabolism in newborn infants. The interrelationship of parathyroid function and calcium, magnesium, and phosphorus metabolism in normal, "sick," and hypocalcemic newborns. J Clin Invest. 1974;54:287–96.

196. Moniz CF, Nicolaides KH, Tzannatos C, Rodeck CH. Calcium homeostasis in second trimester fetuses. J Clin Pathol. 1986;39:838–41.

197. Care AD. The placental transfer of calcium. J Dev Physiol. 1991;15:253–7.

198. Kovacs CS, Kronenberg HM. Maternal-fetal calcium and bone metabolism during pregnancy, puerperium, and lactation. Endocr Rev. 1997;18:832–72.

199. Hsu SC, Levine MA. Perinatal calcium metabolism: physiology and pathophysiology. Semin Neonatol. 2004;9:23–36.

200. Saggese G, Baroncelli GI, Bertelloni S, Cipolloni C. Intact parathyroid hormone levels during pregnancy, in healthy term neonates and in hypocalcemic preterm infants. Acta Paediatr Scand. 1991;80:36–41.

201. Wandrup J, Kroner J, Pryds O, Kastrup KW. Age-related reference values for ionized calcium in the first week of life in premature and full-term neonates. Scand J Clin Lab Invest. 1988;48:255–60.

202. Beggs M, Alexander RT. Intestinal absorption and renal reabsorption of calcium throughout postnatal development. Exp Biol Med. 2017;242:840–49.

203. Dimke H, Hoenderop JGJ, Bindels RJM. Molecular basis of epithelial Ca2þ and Mg2þ transport: insights from the TRP channel family. J Physiol. 2011;589:1535–42.

204. Woudenberg-Vrenken TE, Lameris AL, Weissgerber P, Olausson J, Flockerzi V, Bindels RJ, Freichel

M, Hoenderop JG. Functional TRPV6 channels are crucial for transepithelial Ca2þ absorption. Am J Physiol Gastrointest Liver Physiol. 2012;303:G879–85.

205. Alexander RT, Rievaj J, Dimke H. Paracellular calcium transport across renal and intestinal epithelia. Biochem Cell Biol. 2014;92:467–80.

206. Schnermann J, Huang Y, Mizel D. Fluid reabsorption in proximal convoluted tubules of mice with gene deletions of claudin-2 and/or aquaporin1. Am J Physiol Renal Physiol. 2013;305:F1352–64.

207. Hou J, Renigunta A, Gomes AS, Hou M, Paul DL, Waldegger S, Goodenough DA. Claudin-16 and claudin-19 interaction is required for their assembly into tight junctions and for renal reabsorption of magnesium. Proc Natl Acad Sci U S A. 2009;106:15350–5.

208. Song Y, Peng X, Porta A, Takanaga H, Peng JB, Hediger MA, Fleet JC, Christakos S. Calcium transporter 1 and epithelial calcium channel messenger ribonucleic acid are differentially regulated by 1,25 dihydroxyvitamin D3 in the intestine and kidney of mice. Endocrinology. 2003;144:3885–94.

209. Karlen J, Aperia A, Zetterstrom R. Renal excretion of calcium and phosphate in preterm and term infants. J Pediatr. 1985;106:814–9.

210. Esbjorner E, Jones I. Urinary calcium excretion in Swedish children. Acta Paediatr. 1995;84:156–9.

211. Brodehl J, Gellissen K, Weber HP. Postnatal development of tubular phosphate reabsorption. Clin Nephrol. 1982;17:163–71.

212. Hohenauer L, Rosenberg TF, Oh W. Calcium and phosphorus homeostasis on the first day of life. Biol Neonate. 1970;15:49–56.

213. Kaskel FJ, Kumar AM, Feld LG, Spitzer A. Renal reabsorption of phosphate during development: tubular events. Pediatr Nephrol. 1988;2:129–34.

214. Segawa H, Kaneko I, Takahashi A, Kuwahata M, Ito M, Ohkido I, Tatsumi S, Miyamoto K. Growth-related renal type II Na/Pi cotransporter. J Biol Chem. 2002;277:19665–72.

215. Haramati A, Mulroney SE, Webster SK. Developmental changes in the tubular capacity for phosphate reabsorption in the rat. Am J Phys. 1988;255:F287–91.

216. Imbert-Teboul M, Chabardes D, Clique A, Montegut M, Morel F. Ontogenesis of hormone-dependent adenylate cyclase in isolated rat nephron segments. Am J Phys. 1984;247:F316–25.

217. Hu MC, Shi M, Zhang J, Pastor J, Nakatani T, Lanske B, Razzaque MS, Rosenblatt KP, Baum MG, Kuro-o M, Moe OW. Klotho: a novel phosphaturic substance acting as an autocrine enzyme in the renal proximal tubule. FASEB J. 2010;24:3438–50.

218. Mulroney SE, Lumpkin MD, Haramati A. Antagonist to GH-releasing factor inhibits growth and renal Pi reabsorption in immature rats. Am J Phys. 1989;257:F29–34.

219. Woda CB, Halaihel N, Wilson PV, Haramati A, Levi M, Mulroney SE. Regulation of renal NaPi-2 expression and tubular phosphate reabsorption by growth hormone in the juvenile rat. Am J Physiol Renal Physiol. 2004;287:F117–23.

220. Toriz CG, Melo AI, Solano-Agama C, Gómez-Domínguez EG, Martínez-Muñoz MDLA, Castañeda-Obeso J, Vera-Aguilar E, Aguirre-Benítez EL, Romero-Aguilar L, González-del Pliego M, Jiménez-Estrada I, Luna M, Pardo JP, Camacho J, Mendoza-Garrido ME. Physiological changes of growth hormone during lactation in pup rats artificially reared. PLoS One. 2019;14:8.

221. Hammerman MR, Karl IE, Hruska KA. Regulation of canine renal vesicle Pi transport by growth hormone and parathyroid hormone. Biochim Biophys Acta. 1980;603:322–35.

222. de Rouffignac C, Quamme G. Renal magnesium handling and its hormonal control. Physiol Rev. 1994;74:305–22.

223. Simon DB, Lu Y, Choate KA, Velazquez H, Al-Sabban E, Praga M, Casari G, Bettinelli A, Colussi G, Rodriguez-Soriano J, et al. Paracellin-1, a renal tight junction protein required for paracellular Mg2+ resorption. Science. 1999;285:103–6.

224. Voets T, Nilius B, Hoefs S, van der Kemp AW, Droogmans G, Bindels RJ, Hoenderop JG. TRPM6 forms the Mg2+ influx channel involved in intestinal and renal Mg2+ absorption. J Biol Chem. 2004;279:19–25.

225. Rossi R, Danzebrink S, Linnenburger K, Hillebrand D, Gruneberg M, Sablitzky V, Deufel T, Ullrich K, Harms E. Assessment of tubular reabsorption of sodium, glucose, phosphate and amino acids based on spot urine samples. Acta Paediatr. 1994;83:1282–6.

226. Arant BS Jr. Developmental patterns of renal functional maturation compared in the human neonate. J Pediatr. 1978;92:705–12.

227. Brodehl J, Franken A, Gellissen K. Maximal tubular reabsorption of glucose in infants and children. Acta Paediatr Scand. 1972;61:413–20.

228. Beck JC, Lipkowitz MS, Abramson RG. Characterization of the fetal glucose transporter in rabbit kidney. Comparison with the adult brush border electrogenic Na+-glucose symporter. J Clin Invest. 1988;82:379–87.

229. LeLievre-Pegorier M, Geloso JP. Ontogeny of sugar transport in fetal rat kidney. Biol Neonate. 1980;38:16–24.

230. Robillard JE, Sessions C, Kennedy RL, Smith FG Jr. Maturation of the glucose transport process by the fetal kidney. Pediatr Res. 1978;12:680–4.

231. Silbernagl S. The renal handling of amino acids and oligopeptides. Physiol Rev. 1988;68:911–1007.

232. Zelikovic I, Chesney RW. Development of renal amino acid transport systems. Semin Nephrol. 1989;9:49–55.

233. Baerlocher KE, Scriver CR, Mohyuddin F. The ontogeny of amino acid transport in rat kidney. I. Effect on distribution ratios and intracellular metabolism of proline and glycine. Biochim Biophys Acta. 1971;249:353–63.

234. Baerlocher KE, Scriver CR, Mohyuddin F. The ontogeny of amino acid transport in rat kidney. II. Kinetics of uptake and effect of anoxia. Biochim Biophys Acta. 1971;249:364–72.

235. Muller F, Dommergues M, Bussieres L, Lortat-Jacob S, Loirat C, Oury JF, Aigrain Y, Niaudet P, Aegerter P, Dumez Y. Development of human renal function: reference intervals for 10 biochemical markers in fetal urine. Clin Chem. 1996;42:1855–60.

236. Ojala R, Ala-Houhala M, Harmoinen AP, Luukkaala T, Uotila J, Tammela O. Tubular proteinuria in pre-term and full-term infants. Pediatr Nephrol. 2006;21:68–73.

237. Awad H, el-Safty I, el-Barbary M, Imam S. Evaluation of renal glomerular and tubular functional and structural integrity in neonates. Am J Med Sci. 2002;324:261–6.

Structural Development of the Kidney

7

Melissa Anslow and Jacqueline Ho

Abbreviations

Agt	Angiotensinogen
Agtr1	Angiotensinogen receptor 1
Agtr2	Angiotensinogen receptor 2
Alk3	Bone morphogenetic protein receptor, type 1A
Alk6	Bone morphogenetic protein receptor, type 1B
Ang1	Angiopoietin-1
Ap-2	Transcription factor AP-2
Bcl2	B-cell lymphoma 2
Bmp4	Bone morphogenetic protein 4
Bmp5	Bone morphogenetic protein 5
Bmp7	Bone morphogenetic protein 7
Brn1	Brain specific homeobox 1
Cited1	Cbp/p300-interacting transactivator, with Glu/Asp-rich carboxy-terminal domain, 1
Ctnnb1	β-Catenin
Cxcr4	Chemokine (C-X-C motif) receptor 4
Dsch1/2	Dachsous ½
Ecm1	Extracellular matrix protein 1
Egf	Epidermal growth factor
Emx2	Empty spiracles homolog 2
Etv4	ETS transcription factor 4
Etv5	ETS transcription factor 5
Eya1	Eyes absent homolog 1
Fat4	Fat atypical cadherin 4
Fgf20	Fibroblast growth factor 20
Fgf8	Fibroblast growth factor 8
Fgf9	Fibroblast growth factor 9
Fgfr1	Fibroblast growth factor receptor 1
Fgfr2	Fibroblast growth factor receptor 2
Foxc1	Forkhead box C1
Foxc2	Forkhead box C2
Foxd1	Forkhead box D1
FoxF1	Forkhead box F1
Frs2α	Fibroblast growth factor receptor substrate 2α
Gata3	Gata binding protein 3
Gdf11	Growth/differentiation factor-11
Gdnf	Glial-derived neurotrophic factor
Gfrα-1	Glial-derived neurotrophic factor receptor alpha-1
Gli3	Gli family zinc finger 3
Gpc3	Glypican 3
Grem1	Gremlin 1
Hgf	Hepatocyte growth factor
Hnf1β	Hepatic nuclear factor 1β
Hnf4a	Hepatic nuclear factor 4a
Hoxa11	Homeobox A11
Hoxc11	Homeobox C11
Hoxd11	Homeobox D11
Hs2st	Heparan sulfate 2-sulfotransferase
Igf2	Insulin-like growth factor 2
Lhx1	Lim homeobox 1
Lmx1b	Lim homeobox 1b

M. Anslow · J. Ho (✉)
Division of Pediatric Nephrology, UPMC Children's Hospital of Pittsburgh, University of Pittsburgh School of Medicine, Pittsburgh, PA, USA
e-mail: melissa.anslow@chp.edu;
jacqueline.ho2@chp.edu

© The Author(s), under exclusive license to Springer Nature Switzerland AG 2023
F. Schaefer, L. A. Greenbaum (eds.), *Pediatric Kidney Disease*,
https://doi.org/10.1007/978-3-031-11665-0_7

Met	Met proto-oncogene
Mmp14	Matrix metallopeptidase 14
mTor	Mechanistic target of rapamycin
Myb	Myb proto-oncogene
Osr1	Odd-skipped related1
Pax2	Paired box gene 2
Pax8	Paired box gene 8
Pdgfβ	Platelet derived growth factor beta
Pod1	Podocyte expressed 1
Psen1	Presenilin 1
Psen2	Presenilin 2
Ptch1	Patched1
Raldh2	Aldehyde dehydrogenase 1 family, member A2
Rarα	Retinoic acid receptor α
Rarβ2	Retinoic acid receptor β2
Rbpsuh	Recombining binding protein suppressor of hairless
Ret	Ret proto-oncogene
Robo2	Roundabout, axon guidance receptor, homolog 2
Ror1	Receptor tyrosine kinase like orphan receptor 1
Ror2	Receptor tyrosine kinase like orphan receptor 2
Sall1	Sal-like 1
sFrp	secreted Frizzled-related protein
Shh	Sonic hedgehog
Six1	Sine oculis homeobox homolog 1
Six2	Sine oculis homeobox homolog 2
Slit2	Slit homolog 2
Spry1	Sprouty1
Tak1	TGF-β-activated kinase
Tbx18	T box transcription factor 18
Tbx2	T box transcription factor 2
Tbx3	T box transcription factor 3
TGFα	Transforming growth factor alpha
TGFβ2	Transforming growth factor beta2
Tie2	Angiopoietin-1 receptor
Timp	Tissue inhibitor of metalloproteinase
Tsc1	Hamartin
Tshz3	Teashirt zinc finger homeobox 3
Vegf	Vascular endothelial growth factor
Vegfr2	Vascular endothelial growth factor receptor 2
Wnt11	Wingless-type MMTV integration site family 11
Wnt4	Wingless-type MMTV integration site family 4
Wnt5a	Wingless-type MMTV integration site family 5a
Wnt7b	Wingless-type MMTV integration site family 7b
Wnt9b	Wingless-type MMTV integration site family 9b
Wt1	Wilms tumour 1

Overview of Human Kidney Development

Human kidney development begins in the fifth week of gestation, with the first functioning nephrons making urine by the ninth week [1]. The formation of new nephrons continues until approximately 32–34 weeks gestation [2, 3]. Further renal growth is the result of growth and maturation of already formed nephrons, rather than the generation of new nephrons. Remarkably, there exists wide variability in the number of nephrons that occur naturally in humans, from 200,000 to 1.8 million per person [4]. In humans that suffer fetal or perinatal renal injury, the developing kidney is incapable of compensating for irreversible nephron loss by either accelerating the rate of nephron formation *ex utero* in infants born prematurely, or by *de novo* generation of nephrons once nephrogenesis is completed [2, 5]. Thus, the number of nephrons formed at birth is thought to be an important determinant of renal function later in life.

This concept is supported by the association of renal failure in humans with oligomeganephronia [6, 7], and by the demonstration of reduced glomerular number in humans with primary hypertension and chronic kidney disease [8, 9]. Quantitative analyses in humans and rodents using stereological methods of glomerular counting in renal autopsy specimens have revealed a relationship between birth weight and glomerular number [4, 10]. The latter data are consistent with the "Barker Hypothesis", which proposes that adult disease has fetal origins and is based on epidemiological studies showing a correlation between birth weight and the incidence of cardiovascular disease [11, 12]. Equally important is the normal structural development of each nephron (or, nephron pattern), which is critical for nephron function. Abnormal nephron pattern results in renal dysplasia. Consequently, mechanisms that control congenital nephron endowment and nephron pattern are likely to be crucial factors in determining long-term as well as short-term renal function.

Our understanding of human kidney development historically began with histological descriptions of microdissected human fetal kidney autopsy specimens performed by Edith Potter and Vitoon Osathanondh [1, 13, 14]. Their seminal work was complemented by analyses of mouse kidney development performed by Lauri Saxen [15]. The mammalian kidney derives from two parts of the metanephros, its embryonic precursor. The first part is the ureteric bud, which gives rise to the collecting duct system, including the cortical and medullary collecting ducts, the renal calyces, the renal pelvis, the ureter, and the trigone of the bladder [2, 15]. The second part is the metanephric mesenchyme, which differentiates into all the epithelial cell types comprising the mature nephron, including the visceral and parietal epithelium of the glomerulus, the proximal convoluted tubule, the ascending and descending limbs of the Loops of Henle, and the distal convoluted tubule [2, 15]. Reciprocal signals between these two tissues are critical for normal kidney development.

The molecular and genetic control of kidney morphogenesis is the subject of several comprehensive reviews [16–20]. Mutational analyses in mice have yielded important insights into the molecular pathways that regulate key events during the formation of nephrons, including the specification and differentiation of the metanephric mesenchyme, ureteric bud induction, renal branching morphogenesis, nephron segmentation and glomerulogenesis. The phenotypes resulting from murine gene mutations also serve as paradigms for renal malformations (*viz.* renal agenesis, duplex kidney) that predict roles for corresponding human gene mutations in the

pathogenesis of these conditions. Thus, advances in human genomics and mammalian developmental genetics have accelerated the tempo of discovery in the field of developmental nephrology, providing novel insights into the genetic, epigenetic and environmental factors that impact nephron number and pattern. In the following sections, the morphologic events and molecular underpinnings of these developmental processes will be described.

Origin of the Mammalian Kidney

The mammalian kidney is derived from the intermediate mesoderm of the urogenital ridge, which develops along the posterior abdominal wall of the developing fetus between the dorsal somites and the lateral plate mesoderm. The Wolffian (also known as the mesonephric or nephric duct) is a paired embryonic epithelial tubule extending in an anterior-posterior orientation on either side of the midline, which arises from the intermediate mesoderm. The Wolffian duct is divided into three segments—the pronephros, mesonephros, and metanephros (Fig. 7.1). At its anterior end, the pronephros forms the renal anlage in fish [21] and frogs [22], but degenerates in mammals. The mid-portion of the Wolffian duct, the mesonephros, gives rise to male reproductive organs including the rete testis, efferent ducts, epididymis, vas deferens, seminal vesicle, and prostate [23]. In females, the mesonephric portion of the Wolffian duct degenerates. The caudal portion of the Wolffian duct, the metanephros, becomes the mature mammalian kidney. The posterior segment of the Wolffian duct ultimately communicates with the cloaca to form the trigone of the bladder [23].

Several molecules have been identified as necessary in establishing the immediate precursors to the ureteric bud and metanephric mesenchyme of the developing metanephros in the intermediate mesoderm. The regional specification of metanephric mesenchyme at the posterior intermediate mesoderm next to the Wolffian duct requires the transcription factor, *Odd-skipped related 1 (Osr1)* [24]. Cell-fate tracing studies

tors, *Paired box gene 2* (*Pax2*) [26], *Pax8* [27], *Lim homeobox 1* (*Lhx1*) [28] and *Gata binding protein 3* (*Gata3*) [29], along with signaling through the tyrosine kinase receptor, *Ret* [30], and *β-catenin* (*Ctnnb1*) [31].

The ureteric bud forms as an outgrowth of the Wolffian duct in response to external cues provided by the surrounding metanephric mesenchyme. Signals that promote and direct ureteric bud branching morphogenesis originate from all derivative cell types of the metanephric mesenchyme, including induced and uninduced mesenchyme [32–34], stromal cells [35–39], and angioblasts [40, 41], as well as the ureteric bud itself [42]. The metanephric mesenchyme, in turn, originates from undifferentiated cells in the intermediate mesoderm adjacent to the Wolffian duct, to form nephrons and the renal stroma [25]. Similarly, the metanephric mesenchyme responds to inductive cues supplied by the ureteric bud and renal stroma to initiate nephron formation [43–47]. Subsequent patterning and differentiation of the cell types of the nephron is highly dependent on factors secreted by developing epithelial and stromal cells [38, 48, 49].

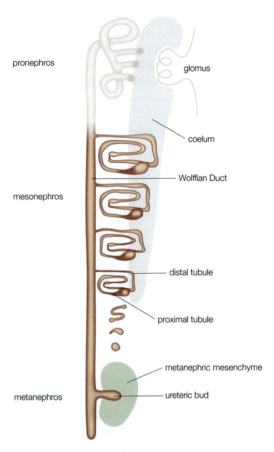

Fig. 7.1 Schematic overview of kidney development. Mammalian kidney development begins with the formation of the Wolffian duct, which is divided into three segments: pronephros, mesonephros and metanephros. The pronephros degenerates in mammals, whereas the mesonephros forms the male reproductive organs (rete testis, efferent ducts, epididymis, vas deferens, seminal vesicles and prostate). The metanephros becomes the mature mammalian kidney, and forms via inductive interactions between the metanephric mesenchyme and the ureteric bud. (Reproduced with kind permission from Springer Science+Business Media: Factors Influencing Mammalian Kidney Development: Implications for Health in Adult Life, Morphological Development of the Kidney, Advances in Anatomy and Cell Biology, Volume 196, 2008, pp. 9–16, Moritz K, et al., Figure 1)

have identified *Osr1*-expressing cells of the intermediate mesoderm as the origin of the principal cellular components of the metanephric kidney: the main body of the nephron, vascular and interstitial cell types, and the Wolffian duct [25]. The establishment and development of the Wolffian duct requires the function of the transcription fac-

Induction of Nephrons from the Metanephric Mesenchyme

Once induced by the ureteric bud, the metanephric mesenchyme condenses around the ureteric bud tip, resulting in formation of the cap mesenchyme (Fig. 7.2). The cap mesenchyme is thought to represent a population of nephron progenitors, as these cells have the capacity to self-renew to generate an appropriate number of nephrons at the end of kidney development, and to differentiate into the multiple cell types required to form a mature nephron [50, 51]. The molecules that regulate the specification, proliferation, survival and differentiation of nephron progenitors are a focus of many studies, because an improved understanding of these processes may guide the development of novel cell-based therapies for chronic kidney disease [52].

The differentiation of the cap mesenchyme involves a process termed mesenchymal-

7 Structural Development of the Kidney

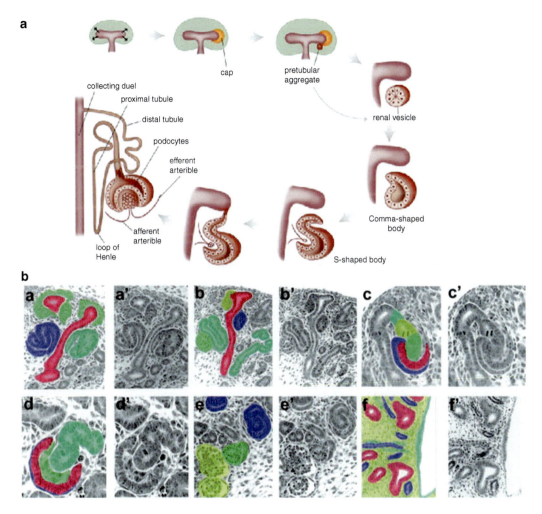

Fig. 7.2 Stages of nephrogenesis. (**A**) Induction of the metanephric mesenchyme by the ureteric bud promotes aggregation of the cap mesenchyme around the tip of the ureteric bud. The cap mesenchyme subsequently undergoes a mesenchymal to epithelial transition to form the pre-tubular aggregate, followed by a polarized renal vesicle. A cleft forms in the renal vesicle giving rise to the comma-shaped body. The development of the S-shaped body involves the formation of a proximal cleft which is subsequently invaded by angioblasts and starts the process of glomerulogenesis. Fusion of S-shaped body occurs with the collecting ducts (reproduced with kind permission from Springer Science+Business Media: Factors Influencing Mammalian Kidney Development: Implications for Health in Adult Life, Morphological Development of the Kidney, Advances in Anatomy and Cell Biology, Volume 196, 2008, pp. 9–16, Moritz, K., et al.). (**B**) Series of matched-pair histological images from a developing metanephric kidney with coloring for specific developmental stages. (a, a′) The ureteric tip and renal cortical collecting duct are in red, with the cap mesenchyme in green. Derivatives of the cap mesenchyme include the comma-shaped body in light blue and S-shaped body in dark blue. (b, b′) Next to the ureteric bud and renal cortical collecting duct (red) is a pre-tubular aggregate (yellow), a renal vesicle (dark blue), capillary loop stage developing glomerulus (green) and renal tubules (light blue). (c, c′) Segments of the S-shaped body include the visceral epithelium (red), parietal epithelium (dark blue), medial segment (green), distal segment (yellow) and renal junctional tubule (light blue). (d, d′) Segments of the capillary loop stage developing glomerulus include the visceral epithelium (red), parietal epithelium (dark blue), presumptive mesangium (green) and renal tubule (light blue). (e, e′) Image of the cortex of the metanephros showing different stages of glomerular development: an S-shaped body (dark blue), capillary loop stage (green) and maturing glomeruli (yellow). (f, f′) Image of the renal medulla and pelvis of the metanephros showing the renal medullary interstitium (yellow), medullary collecting ducts (red), immature loop of Henle (dark blue), renal medullary vasculature (green) and renal pelvic urothelial lining (blue) (reprinted from Gene Expression Patterns, Vol. 7(6), Little MH et al., A high-resolution anatomical ontology of the developing murine genitourinary tract, p. 688, 2007, Figure 3C, with permission from Elsevier)

epithelial transformation (MET). A localized cluster of cells separates from the cap mesenchyme under the ureteric bud tip, and acquires epithelial characteristics, becoming a "pre-tubular aggregate" (Fig. 7.2) [53]. Simultaneous with epithelialization, an internal cavity forms within the pre-tubular aggregate, at which point the structure is termed a renal vesicle. The renal vesicle subsequently forms a connection with its neighboring ureteric bud ampulla, permitting the ureteric bud lumen to communicate with the internal cavity of the renal vesicle. Further differentiation of the renal vesicle in a spatially organized proximal-distal pattern results in formation of the glomerular and tubular segments of the mature nephron (discussed in section "Formation of Nephrons").

Specification of the Metanephric Mesenchyme

The formation of the metanephric mesenchyme is molecularly marked by expression of the transcription factors *Wilms tumour 1 (Wt1)* [54], *Cbp/p300-interacting transactivator, with Glu/Asp-rich carboxy-terminal domain, 1 (Cited1)* [55], *Eyes absent homolog 1 (Eya1)* [56, 57], *sine oculis homeobox homolog 1 (Six1)* [58], *Six2* [59], *Sal-like 1 (Sall1)* [60], *Pax2* [26], and *Lhx1* [61], as well as by expression of transmembrane molecules *cadherin-11 (Cdh11)* [62] and *α8 integrin* (Fig. 7.3A, B) [63]. *Sall1* [60], *Six1* [58], *Eya1* [56, 57] and the secreted peptide growth factor, *Glial-derived neurotrophic factor (Gdnf)* [64], are expressed in intermediate mesoderm in the presumptive metanephric mesenchyme. Indeed, the cap mesenchyme is now understood to represent a heterologous population of nephron progenitors, which differ in their relative response to cues for self-renewal and differentiation. Molecular evidence of this is the differing expression patterns of key transcription factors. Thus, *Wt1, Cited1* and *Six2* expression is induced in the cap mesenchyme at the onset of ureteric bud outgrowth [54, 55, 59]. *Pax2* [65] and *Lhx1* [61] are also expressed in cap mesenchyme and its early epithelial derivatives. Recent single cell

RNA-sequencing studies in developing mouse [66–71] and human kidneys [72–74] have contributed to our understanding of these subpopulations of nephron progenitors as well as the differences between mouse and human kidney development (Table 7.1).

Phenotypic analyses of mice with targeted gene deletions or tissue-specific inactivation of conditional alleles for these transcription factors have been informative regarding their role in specification of the cap mesenchyme, and subsequent induction of ureteric bud outgrowth. Homozygous deletion in many of these genes (including: *Eya1* [57], *Six1* [58], *Pax2* [75, 76], *Wt1* [54], *Sall1* [60], *Six2* [59] and *Lhx1* [61, 77]) causes ureteric bud outgrowth failure, and results in bilateral renal agenesis or severe renal dysgenesis with variable penetrance depending on the gene involved (Fig. 7.3E, F). However, the underlying molecular mechanism responsible for renal agenesis/severe dysgenesis in each of these mutants varies. For example, *Pax2* mutants fail to form the posterior Wolffian duct from which derives the ureteric bud [76]. In contrast, *Lhx1* [61, 78] and *Sall1* [60] mutants initiate, but do not complete, ureteric bud induction. *Wt1* mutants also exhibit failed ureteric bud induction and show apoptosis of the metanephric mesenchyme [54] (Fig. 7.3E, F). Tissue recombination experiments show that isolated metanephric mesenchyme explants from *Wt1* knock-out mice are neither competent to respond to signals from wild-type ureteric buds, nor able to induce growth and branching of isolated wild-type ureteric bud explants [54, 79]. In contrast, *Sall1*-deficient mesenchyme, which expresses *Wt1*, responds to a heterologous inducer in *ex vivo* tissue recombination experiments [60], suggesting that *Sall1* functions downstream of *Wt1* in a genetic regulatory cascade. Taken together, these data present an emerging image of intricate interplay between transcription factors that are required for the establishment of the nephric duct, subsequent specification of the cap mesenchyme, induction of *Gdnf* expression, and regulation of the differentiation capacity of the cap mesenchyme in response to inductive cues.

Indeed, insights into this interplay come from recent genome-wide studies of transcription fac-

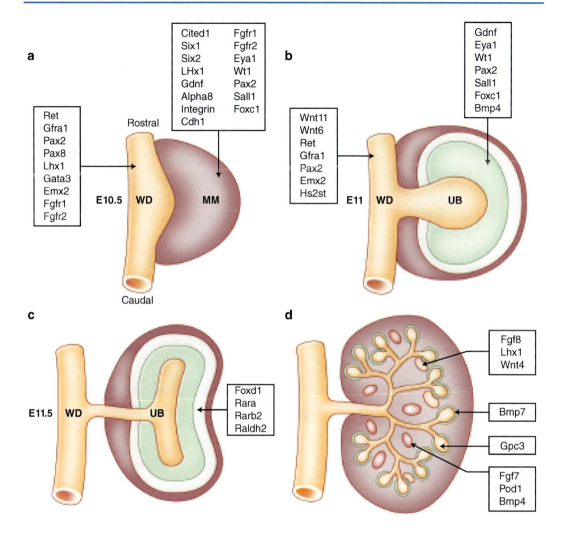

Fig. 7.3 Molecules involved in specification of the metanephric mesenchyme and nephron induction. (**A**) The mammalian kidney starts to develop when the ureteric bud forms at the caudal end of the Wolffian duct (WD) at about embryonic day (E)10.5 in mice. The ureteric bud grows into the metanephric mesenchyme (MM) and (**B**) induces the mesenchyme that is adjacent to the tips of the ureteric bud (UB) to condense to form the cap mesenchyme, as well as the stromal cells that are peripheral to the cap. (**C**) The cap mesenchyme induces the ureteric bud to branch from E11.5 onwards. (**D**) In association with ureteric branching morphogenesis, mesenchymal cells are induced at each ureteric bud tip to undergo a mesenchymal-to-epithelial transformation to form the nephron. *Bmp7* bone morphogenetic protein 7, *Emx2* empty spiracles 2, *Eya1* Eya1, eyes absent 1, *Fgf7* fibroblast growth factor 7, *Foxc1* forkhead box C1, *Foxd1* forkhead box D1, *Gdnf1* glial cell-line-derived neurotrophic factor 1, *Gfra1* glial cell-line derived neurotrophic factor receptor-α1, *Gpc3* glypican-3, *Hs2st* heparan sulfate 2-*O*-sulphotransferase 1, *Pax1* paired-box gene 1, *Rara* retinoic acid receptor-α, *Ret* Ret proto-oncogene, *Sall1* sal-like 1, *Wnt* Wingless-related, *Wt1* Wilms tumour 1 (adapted with permission from Macmillan Publishers Ltd.: Nature Reviews Genetics, Coordinating early kidney development: lessons from gene targeting, Vol. 4(7), p. 535, 2002, Vainio S and Lin Y, Figure 1). Representative kidney phenotypes of mice with targeted deletions affecting nephron progenitors and nephron induction. (**E–F′**) Histological transverse sections from E11.5 embryos showing a wild-type (**E**) and *Wt1* mutant embryo (**F**) with the ureteric bud (U), Wolffian duct (W) and metanephric mesenchyme (M) labeled. (**E′–F′**) At higher magnification, a cluster of apoptotic cells with dark nuclear fragments is visualized in the Wt1 mutant kidney, resulting in loss of nephron progenitors (arrow) (reprinted from Cell, Vol. 74(4), Kreidberg et al., WT-1 is required for early kidney development, p. 682, 1993, with permission from Elsevier). (**G–H′**) Loss of *Wnt4* results in renal hypoplasia and failure of nephron induction, with no epithelial to mesenchymal transition when comparing control (**G–G′**) to control kidneys (**H–H′**) (reprinted with permission from Macmillan Publishers Ltd.: Nature, Epithelial transformation of metanephric mesenchyme in the developing kidney regulated by Wnt-4, 372(6507), p. 682, 1994, Stark et al., Figure 3)

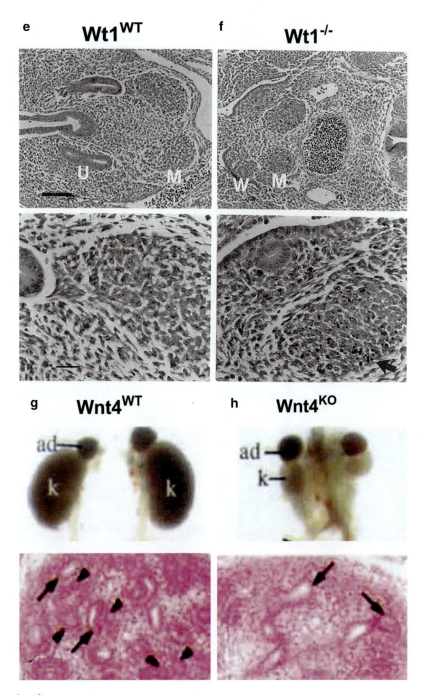

Fig. 7.3 (continued)

tor binding using chromatin immunoprecipitation followed by sequencing (ChIP-seq). The transcription factors Six2, Hoxd11, Osr1, and Wt1 have been shown to bind enhancer sequences located in "regulatory hot-spots" in the genome in nephron progenitors [80]. In addition, Six2 co-binds enhancers with β-catenin to drive expression of genes associated with nephron progenitor self-renewal and differentiation [81]. These studies have also identified differences in the transcriptional regulation of mouse and human nephron progenitors mediated by Six1 and Six2 [82].

There is a growing body of work defining the signals required to induce and regulate nephron progenitors, to enable the generation of induced pluripotent stem cell (iPSC)-derived nephron progenitors and optimize the culture of kidney organoids (reviewed in [83]). Of these, the growth factor, *Wingless-type MMTV integration site family 9b (Wnt9b)*, is required in the ureteric bud for induction of the cap mesenchyme (Fig. 7.3B). The loss of *Wnt9b* activity results in failure of the cap mesenchyme to undergo MET [84]. Moreover, *Wnt9b* plays an important role in regulating the balance between nephron progenitor differentiation and self-renewal, in cooperation with signals mediated by stromal cells [47, 85].

Fibroblast growth factor (FGF) signaling has also been shown to be critical in regulating nephron progenitors. The FGF ligands belong to a large family of secreted peptides that signal

Table 7.1 Mouse mutations exhibiting defects in kidney morphogenesis and predominant accompanying renal phenotypes

Mutant gene	Morphogenetic defect	Predominant mutant renal malformation phenotype
Failed ureteric bud outgrowth		
Metanephric mesenchyme-derived		Renal aplasia
Eya1		
Fgf9/20		
Fgfr1/2		
Frs2α		
Gdnf		
Grem1		
Lhx1		
Osr1		
Pax2		
Sall1		
Six1		
Wt1		
Ureteric bud-derived		
Emx2		
Etv4/5		
Gata3		
Gfrα1		
Hoxa11/Hoxd11/Hoxc11		
Hs2st		
Itgα8		
Lhx1		
Pax2/8		
Ret		
Wnt9b		
Ectopic ureteric bud outgrowth		
Bmp4		Duplex collecting system
Foxc1/c2		
Robo2		
Slit2		
Spry1		
Decreased ureteric bud branching		

Table 7.1 (continued)

Mutant gene	Morphogenetic defect	Predominant mutant renal malformation phenotype
Alk3		Renal hypoplasia, renal dysplasia
Alk6		
Dsch1/2		
Ecm1		
Fat4		
Fgfr2		
Foxd1		
Hnf1β		
Pod1		
Raldh2		
Rarα/Rarβ2		
Spry2		
Wnt11		
Defective renal medulla formation		
Fgf7		Medullary dysplasia
Fgf10		
Gpc3		
Hnf1β		
p57^{KIP2}		
Agt		Hydronephrosis
Agtr1		
Agtr2		
Bmp4		
Bmp5		
Defective tubulogenesis		
Bmp7		Renal hypoplasia, renal dysplasia
Brn1		
Fgf8		
Hnf4a		
Lhx1		
Notch1		
Notch2		
Pod1		
Psen1/Psen2		
Rbpsuh		
Six2		
Wnt4		
Wnt9b		
Defective glomerulogenesis		
Jag1		Glomerular malformation
Notch2		
Pdgfβ		
Pdgfrβ		
Pod1		
Vegf		
Col4α3/Col4α4/Col4α5		Loss of glomerular filtration selectivity
Lamb		
Lmx1β		
Mafβ		
Wt1		

Adapted with permission from Comprehensive Pediatric Nephrology, Structural and Functional Development of the Kidney, 1st edition, p. 98, 2008, Tino Piscione

through their cognate receptor tyrosine kinases, FGF receptors (FGFRs). Several FGFs are expressed in the developing kidney, including FGF2, FGF7, FGF8, and FGF10 [39, 86, 87] (Fig. 7.3). Two FGF ligands, *Fgf9* and *Fgf20*, have been shown to be critical in regulating nephron progenitor survival, proliferation and competence to respond to inductive signals in mice and humans, with loss of these signals resulting in renal agenesis [88]. These *in vivo* findings were supported by *in vitro* studies showing that the addition of FGF1, 2, 9 and 20 protein results in the ability to maintain early nephron progenitor cells in culture [89]. In addition, *in vivo* data is consistent with a functionally important role for *Fgfr1* and *Fgfr2* in the metanephric mesenchyme during kidney development, with loss of *Fgr1* and *Fgfr2* function in the metanephric mesenchyme resulting in renal agenesis [90–92].

Bone morphogenetic protein (BMP) signaling interacts with FGF signaling to balance the self-renewal and differentiation of nephron progenitors. Bmp7 induces the initial exit of nephron progenitors into a state "primed" for differentiation by ureteric bud-derived Wnt 9/β-catenin signaling (Fig. 7.3). Conversely, remaining nephron progenitors are kept in an undifferentiated and self-renewing state in response to FGF9, Wnt and BMP7 signals [81, 85, 88, 89, 93–97]. Mice deficient for *Bmp7* demonstrate developmental arrest and rudimentary kidneys without the inhibition of differentiation of already induced cells, which is likely to due to failure to expand and renew the epithelial precursor population [98, 99]. Together, these data have now informed several *in vitro* protocols to propagate nephron progenitors that rely on a combination of FGF ligands and manipulation of BMP signaling, amongst other growth factors in the culture media [100–103].

The regulation of nephron progenitor survival also contributes to determining nephron number. Archetypal organ culture experiments have demonstrated that isolated metanephric mesenchyme undergoes apoptosis unless induced by co-culture with ureteric buds or a heterologous inducer (e.g. spinal cord) [15, 33]. Several soluble factors have been described to be essential to prevent mesenchymal apoptosis, e.g. epidermal growth factor (EGF), FGF2, and BMP7 [43, 104, 105]. In addition, microRNAs (miRNAs) have been implicated in regulating nephron progenitor survival [106, 107]. However, inhibition of apoptosis by pharmacologic or genetic manipulation causes defects in ureteric bud branching and nephrogen-

esis [108, 109], suggesting that alterations in cell survival disrupt important functional interactions between mesenchymal and epithelial cells. Possible roles for apoptosis in the metanephric mesenchyme include regulation of nephron number or establishment of tissue boundaries between cells destined to become epithelial or stromal [110, 111].

Recent studies have also shed light on the molecular mechanisms that regulate the cessation of nephrogenesis. Transcriptional changes in nephron progenitors occur as kidney development proceeds, and they are associated with genes and pathways that influence stem cell aging, in particular *Mechanistic target of rapamycin (mTor)* and its repressor *Hamartin (Tsc1)* [112, 113]. These changes are thought to desensitize nephron progenitors to signals for self-renewal, contributing to the cessation of nephrogenesis [113]. Furthermore, miRNA in the *let-7* family are thought to play an important role in the timing of cessation of nephrogenesis. Ectopic expression of *Lin28b*, a known let-7 family repressor, is sufficient to prolong nephrogenesis [114].

Nephron Induction

Seminal experiments involving isolated kidney rudiments cultured *ex vivo* established the role of ureteric bud-derived secreted factors in providing inductive cues for cap mesenchyme to undergo epithelial differentiation to initiate tubulogenesis [33]. The isolation of ureteric bud cell lines has subsequently facilitated the identification of several secreted factors that function individually or in combination to cause mesenchymal-epithelial conversion and tubulogenesis, including FGF2 [115], leukemia inhibitory factor (LIF) [44, 116, 117], transforming growth factor-β2 (TGFβ2) [117, 118], and growth/differentiation factor-11 (GDF-11) [117, 119].

Wnt genes also play a key role in epithelial conversion, as suggested by the observation that cells expressing WNT proteins are potent inducers of tubulogenesis in isolated metanephric mesenchyme [120, 121]. A genetic requirement for *Wnt4* in MET is revealed by the demonstration of the arrest of the cap mesenchyme, and the inability to form pre-tubular aggregates in *Wnt4* mutant mice [84] (Fig. 7.3D, G, H). The effects of Wnt signals are modulated by mesenchymal-derived secreted Wnt binding proteins, including secreted Frizzled-related protein (sFrp). sFrp antagonizes the actions of Wnt4 and Wnt9b by binding secreted Wnt proteins *in vitro* and preventing them from activating membrane-bound Wnt receptors [122]. Similar to the induction of nephron progenitors, FGF signaling is also critical for MET. Mice with deletions in *Fgf8* fail to undergo tubulogenesis, and the data suggests that *Wnt4* and *Fgf8* cooperate in the conversion of mesenchymal to epithelial cells, possibly by up-regulating *Lhx1* expression [123, 124]. The transcription factor, *Lhx1*, is uniformly expressed in renal vesicles [61], and conditional knockout of *Lhx1* in metanephric mesenchyme causes developmental arrest at the renal vesicle stage [61].

Ureteric Bud Induction and Branching

Ureteric bud formation begins at week 5 of human fetal gestation and at embryonic day 10.5 (E10.5) in mice. Signaling from the metanephric mesenchyme induces the ureteric bud from the Wolffian duct (Fig. 7.4A). The ureteric bud then elongates and branches into the surrounding mesenchyme, a process termed *branching morphogenesis*, to ultimately pattern the collecting ducts and pelvicaliceal system [125, 126]. Renal branching morphogenesis occurs as a sequence of tightly regulated events: (1) ureteric bud outgrowth; (2) ureteric bud branching and derivation of collecting ducts; (3) cortical and medullary patterning of the collect ducts; and (4) formation of the renal pelvises and calyces.

Ureteric Bud Induction and Outgrowth

Genes encoding *Gdnf* [127], its tyrosine kinase receptor *Ret* [128], and its co-receptor *Gfra1* [129] are crucial regulators of ureteric bud outgrowth. Targeted *Gdnf* mutations in mice cause

failure of ureteric bud induction and bilateral renal aplasia [130, 131] (Fig. 7.4B). Homozygous deletion of *Ret* or *Gfra1* cause the same defect [128, 132–135] (Fig. 7.4C). However, initial ureteric bud outgrowth was evident in 20–40% of *Gdnf*$^{-/-}$ or *Ret*$^{-/-}$ mutants [128, 130], indicating that GDNF-RET signaling is not the only molecular pathway involved in ureteric bud induction and outgrowth. Mice with homozygous null mutations in *heparan sulfate 2-sulfotransferase* (*Hs2st*), which is involved in proteoglycan synthesis, show bilateral renal agenesis and induction of the ureteric bud, but no further outgrowth [136]. Mice with a mutation in integrin $\alpha 8$ show a similar phenotype in 50% of the mutant mouse embryos [137], implicating integrin signaling as an important molecular pathway for ureteric bud outgrowth.

The downstream effect of GDNF-RET signaling is ureteric bud proliferation, cell survival, and epithelial branching. Downstream genes of GDNF-RET signaling include *ETS transcription factor 4* (*Etv4*) and *Etv5*, which are upregulated in response to RET signaling, and loss of both transcription factors results in bilateral renal agenesis due to ureteric bud formation defects [138]. Expression of several genes in the ureteric bud tip depend on *Etv4* and *Etv5*, including *Chemokine (C-X-C motif) receptor 4* (*Cxcr4*), *matrix metallopeptidase 14* (*Mmp14*), *Myb proto-oncogene* (*Myb*), *Met proto-oncogene* (*Met*), and *Wnt11* [138]. Loss of *Wnt11* in mice leads to abnormal ureteric branching with resultant renal hypoplasia and decreased levels of GDNF in the metanephric mesenchyme; conversely, *Wnt11* expression is reduced in the absence of GDNF, suggesting a feedback loop that coordinates ureteric branching [97]. Furthermore, *hepatocyte nuclear factor-1 beta* (*Hnf1β*) has been implicated as a transcriptional regulator of *Etv5*, and mice lacking *Hnf1β* also show abnormal ureteric bud outgrowth and branching [139, 140]. Thus, these studies highlight that improper ureteric bud induction and outgrowth lead to renal agenesis or renal hypoplasia.

GDNF in organ cultures induce ectopic ureteric buds along the Wolffian duct [127, 141], indicating that additional signals are required to

7 Structural Development of the Kidney

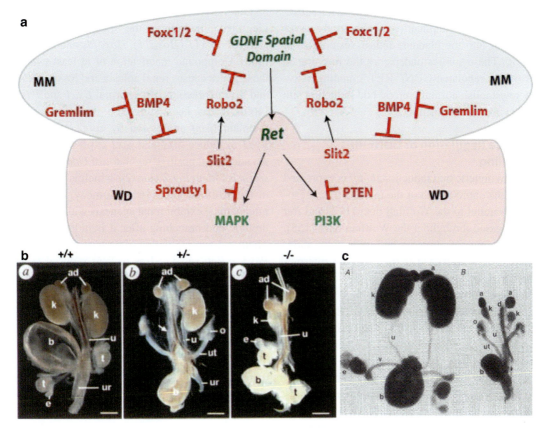

Fig. 7.4 Schematic demonstrating the molecular control of ureteric bud branching. (**A**) Glial cell-line derived neurotrophic factor (GDNF) is secreted from the mesenchyme (grey) and binds to the Ret receptor to induce a thickening of the WD (pink); the WD will then elongate to form the UB. Binding of GDNF to RET leads to activation of the MAPK and PI3K signal transduction pathways. These pathways are negatively regulated by SPROUTY1 and PTEN, respectively. SLIT2/ROBO2, FOXC1 and FOXC2 inhibit the spatial GDNF expression domain and limit UB outpouching to a single site. BMP4 inhibits branching, in a manner that is opposed by Gremlin. RED Inhibitory, Green stimulatory, Grey MM and GDNF spatial domain, Pink WD (with kind permission from Springer Science+Business Media: Pediatric Nephrology, Stimulatory and inhibitory signaling molecules that regulate renal branching morphogenesis, Vol. 24, p. 1616, 2009, Bridgewater D and Rosenblum ND, Figure 4). Representative kidney phenotypes of mice having targeted mutations affecting branching morphogenesis. (**B**) Bilateral renal agenesis in *GDNF* mutant mice (reprinted with permission from Macmillan Publishers Ltd.: Nature, Defects in enteric innervation and kidney development in mice lacking GDNF, 382(6586), p. 74, 1996, Pichel et al., Figure 2). (**C**) Severe bilateral renal hypoplasia in *Ret* null mutants. A, adrenal; K, kidney; U, ureter; B, bladder (reprinted with permission from Macmillan Publishers Ltd.: Nature, Defects in the kidney and enteric nervous system of mice lacking the tyrosine kinase receptor Ret, 367(6461), p. 382, 1994, Schuchardt et al., Figure 2)

restrict the number of ureteric buds induced, as well as the position of ureteric bud induction. When multiple ureteric buds form from a single Wolffian duct, renal and urogenital malformations occur (e.g. duplex kidney) [142]. The position of ureteric bud outgrowth from the Wolffian duct is also critical for the formation of a single ureter and competent vesicoureteral junction. Outgrowth of the ureteric bud at an ectopic site leads to ectopic insertion of the ureter into the bladder [143]. Mice with mutations in *Bmp4* [144], *Slit homologue 2* (*Slit2*) or its receptor *Roundabout guidance receptor 2* (*Robo2*) [145], components of the renin-angiotensin cascade [109], *Forkhead box C1* (*Foxc1*), *Foxc2* [146], *Fgfr2* [147, 148], *FGF receptor substrate 2α* (*Frs2α*) [149], *Dicer1* [150–152], *Ret* [153], and *Pax2* [154] exhibit abnormal ureteric bud induction sites and/or ureteric branching with subsequent ureteral duplications, abnormal ureter insertion into the bladder, and/or vesicoureteral reflux. These studies underscore the importance of tightly regulated GDNF-RET signaling activity to establish normal ureteric bud induction site and subsequent branching.

Positive Regulation of GDNF-RET Signaling

Prior to ureteric bud induction, *Gdnf* is expressed along the entire length of the intermediate mesoderm parallel to the Wolffian duct [127] and *Ret* is expressed throughout the Wolffian duct [155]. By the time of ureteric bud induction, *Gdnf* expression is restricted to the posterior intermediate mesoderm, marking the location of the presumptive metanephric mesenchyme close to the site of ureteric bud outgrowth. Once the ureteric bud enters the metanephric mesenchyme, *Ret* expression becomes restricted to the epithelial cells of the branching ureteric bud [155]. As noted above, mice that ectopically express *Gdnf* or *Ret* during ureteric bud induction and branching have renal malformations, which underscores the importance of regulation of the spatial activity of GDNF-RET signaling [156, 157].

Three transcription factor genes expressed in the intermediate mesoderm—*Eya1*, *Six1*, and *Pax2*—promote *Gdnf* expression during kidney development (Fig. 7.3A). Genetic mutations in *Eya1* or *Pax2* in mouse models both result in no *Gdnf* expression [57, 158]. *Eya1* knock-out mice fail to undergo ureteric bud induction due to loss of *Gdnf* expression and the result is renal agenesis [57]. *Eya1* mutant mice also show a loss of *Six1* expression, suggesting an Eya-Six-Gdnf signaling cascade [57, 159]. *Six1* null mice fail ureteric bud induction into the mesenchyme, which subsequently undergoes apoptosis [58]. *Eya1* expression in the *Six1* null mice is normal, further supporting that it is upstream of *Six1* [58]. *Pax2* is expressed in the intermediate mesoderm and homozygous null mice do not undergo ureteric bud outgrowth and *Gdnf* expression is absent [158]. *Gdnf* transcription is directly activated by *Pax2* [158].

Other activators of *Gdnf* expression have been identified, including the paralogous genes *Homeobox A11* (*Hoxa11*), *Hoxc11*, and *Hoxd11* [160]. Compound inactivation of at least two of these genes causes renal aplasia and loss of *Gdnf* and *Six2* expression, with normal *Eya1* and *Pax2* [160]. It has been suggested that Hox genes maintain *Gdnf* expression by cooperating with *Eya1* to induce *Six1* and *Six2* expression [159]. An additional positive regulator of *Gdnf* is *Empty spiracles homolog 2* (*Emx2*), which is expressed in the Wolffian duct [161]. Homozygous *Emx2* mutant mice exhibit renal agenesis with failure of ureteric bud branching after it is induced [161]. There is down-regulation of ureteric bud markers *Pax2*, *c-Ret*, and *Lim1* as well as reduced *Gdnf* expression in the metanephric mesenchyme [161]. In explant culture experiments, branching of the *Emx2* mutant ureteric bud was not induced by wild-type mesenchyme; whereas, mutant mesenchyme was able to induce wild-type ureteric bud branching [161]. These data suggest that *Emx2* may be important in the ureteric bud to provide cues to maintain *Gdnf* expression in the mesenchyme and sustain ureteric bud branching.

Negative Regulation of GDNF-RET Signaling

Negative regulation of Gdnf expression is equally important to control the location and number of ureteric buds induced. *Foxc1*, *Slit2*, and *Robo2* are involved in restricting *Gdnf* expression to the posterior intermediate mesoderm (Fig. 7.4A). Mice lacking either *Slit2* or its receptor *Robo2* develop supernumerary ureteric buds and multiple ureters, with *Gdnf* expression inappropriately maintained in the anterior metanephric mesenchyme [145]. The anterior expansion of *Gdnf* occurs without alterations in expression of *Foxc1*, *Eya1*, or *Pax2* [145], suggesting that SLIT2 and ROBO2 function in a parallel pathway to restrict GDNF-RET activity during ureteric bud outgrowth. The secreted protein SLIT2 and its receptor ROBO2 are encoded by genes best known for their role in axon guidance, functioning as chemorepellents that cause axons or migrating cells to move away from the source of SLIT2 [162], which may be the mechanism by which they regulate *Gdnf* expression domain. Their expression pattern supports this: *Slit2* is primary expressed at the tips of the branching ureteric buds and *Robo2* is expressed in a complementary pattern in the metanephric mesenchyme [163]. More recently, further evaluation of *Robo2* null mice shows failure of the nephrogenic cord to separate from the Wolffian duct, leading to increased proliferation signals, which suggests a possible second mechanism by which *Gdnf* domain expands and aberrant ureteric buds form [164]. *Foxc1* homozygous null mutant mice have anterior expansion of *Gdnf* and *Eya1*, leading to ectopic anterior ureteric buds that result in ureter and renal abnormalities [146]. *Foxc1* encodes a transcription factor that overlaps in domain with *Gdnf* in the intermediate mesoderm and these data suggest that *Foxc1* regulates either *Eya1* or its upstream genes [146].

The gene *Sprouty1* (*Spry1*), a receptor tyrosine kinase agonist, is implicated in a regulatory feedback loop involving GDNF-RET signaling and downstream effector, *Wnt11*. *Spry1* is expressed along the Wolffian duct, with highest levels of expression in the posterior aspect [165] (Fig. 7.4A). Loss of *Spry1* function in mice results in ectopic ureteric bud induction and urogenital malformations such as multiple ureters and kidneys [165, 166]. Recently, tyrosine 53 of *Spry1* is implicated as essential for *Spry1* function, showing the same phenotype as *Spry1* null mice [167]. *Gdnf* and *Wnt11* expression extends more anteriorly in *Spry1* null mice [165, 166]. Metanephric cultures showed more sensitivity to GDNF in *Spry1* null mutants, inducing supernumerary ureteric buds at low concentrations compared to wildtype [165]. Further, *Ret* is required to maintain *Spry1* expression in the Wolffian duct [165]. Ectopic expression of human *SPRY2*, a related homologue to *Spry1*, in the ureteric bud in transgenic mice leads to decreased ureteric branching [168]. Together, these data suggest that *Spry1* acts as a negative regulator of a GDNF/RET/*Wnt11* feedback loop to prevent supernumerary ureteric budding and guide branching.

Another example of negative feedback in GDNF-RET signaling and branching morphogenesis involves secreted growth factors belonging to the Bone Morphogenetic Protein (BMP) family. Kidney organ culture studies reveal inhibitory roles for BMP-2, -4, and -7 in ureteric bud branching morphogenesis [169–172]. However, only *Bmp4* shows convincing evidence *in vivo* for modulating ureteric bud outgrowth [144] (Fig. 7.4A). *Bmp4* is expressed in stromal cells adjacent to the Wolffian duct and the early ureteric bud and its receptors are expressed in the Wolffian duct [144, 173]. Mice heterozygous for *Bmp4* exhibit ectopic or multiple ureteric buds, shortened ureteric trunk and first branch stem, and a spectrum of urinary tract and renal malformations [144]. The abnormal sites of ureteric bud outgrowth in *Bmp4* heterozygous mice suggests that BMP4 inhibits the local effect of GDNF-RET signaling to constrain ureteric bud induction at the appropriate site and promotes elongation at the stalk of the branching ureteric bud [144]. BMP4 can block the ability of GDNF to induce ureteric bud outgrowth from the Wolffian duct *in vitro* [158], and also inhibits further ureteric bud branching *in vitro* in an asymmetric manner [169, 170]. *Gremlin1* (*Grem1*) inhibits BMP4 activity, enabling ureteric bud outgrowth [174].

Other signaling factors have been implicated in regulating the appropriate position of the ureteric bud. For example, *Receptor tyrosine kinase like orphan receptor-1* (*Ror1*) and *-2* (*Ror2*) bind Wnt5a, and have recently been implicated in ureteric bud formation. *Ror2* and *Wnt5a* deficient mice exhibit ectopic rostral ureteric buds and abnormal *Gdnf* expression domain [175, 176].

Renal Branching Morphogenesis

Renal branching morphogenesis begins between the fifth and sixth week of gestation in humans [2], and at E11.5 in mice [177] when the ureteric bud invades the metanephric mesenchyme and forms a T-shaped, branched structure (Fig. 7.3C). The T-shaped structure then undergoes further iterative branching events to generate approximately 15 generations of branches. In human kidney development, the first 9 generations of branching are complete by approximately

15 weeks gestation [2]. During this time, new nephrons are induced through reciprocal inductive interactions between the newly formed tips of the ureteric bud and the surrounding metanephric mesenchyme. By the 20th–22nd week of gestation, ureteric bud branching is completed, and the remainder of collecting duct development occurs by extension of peripheral (or cortical) segments and remodeling of central (or medullary) segments [2]. During these final stages, new nephrons form predominantly through the induction of approximately four to seven nephrons around the tips of terminal collecting duct branches that have completed their branching program, while retaining the capacity to induce new nephron formation [2, 177].

Analysis of renal branching morphogenesis in organ culture systems employing kidneys of transgenic mice expressing the fluorescent reporter, enhanced green fluorescent protein (EGFP), in the ureteric bud lineage have been informative regarding the sequence and pattern of branching events that occur following the formation of the initial T structure [178, 179]. Throughout renal branching morphogenesis, the branching ureteric bud recapitulates a patterned, morphogenetic sequence. This sequence includes: (1) expansion of the advancing ureteric bud branch at its leading tip (called the ampulla); (2) division of the ampulla causing the formation of new ureteric bud branches; and (3) elongation of the newly formed branch segment.

Proliferation and Apoptosis in Branching Morphogenesis

During branching morphogenesis, there is a zone of high proliferation at the site of ureteric bud and then at the tips of the branching ureteric buds/collecting ducts [180]. Proliferation rates are highest at and localized to sites undergoing active branching morphogenesis [180] and as new branches form, proliferation rates are higher in branch tips than trunks [42, 180, 181], which suggests that localized cell proliferation contributes to evagination of the ureteric bud from the Wolffian duct and formation of ampullae. A time-lapse imaging study traced individual ureteric bud tip cells to find that most tip cells are self-renewing progenitors whose progeny either populate the growing ureteric bud trunk or remain at the tips [182].

Apoptotic cells are rarely seen in the ureteric branches [183], and cultured ureteric bud cells do not demonstrate apoptosis *ex vivo* [184]. This suggests that ureteric bud-derived cells may have an intrinsic survival tendency. Further evidence that cell survival is tightly regulated during branching morphogenesis is provided by several studies in which dysregulated apoptosis and cell proliferation are associated with defective collecting duct development. *Glypican-3-(Gpc3)* deficient mice exhibit increased cell proliferation with increased ureteric bud branching, increased cortical collecting duct proliferation, and increased medullary collecting duct system apoptosis leading to cystic and dysplastic kidneys [185, 186]. Additionally, increased apoptosis was associated with collecting duct cyst formation in mice with mutated genes associated with cell survival including *B-cell lymphoma 2 (bcl2)* [187] and *transcription factor AP2 (AP-2)* [188]. Also, apoptosis is prominent in dilated collecting ducts in experimental models of fetal and neonatal urinary tract obstruction [189, 190]. These data suggest a relationship between collecting duct apoptosis and two frequent features of renal dysplasia—cystogenesis and urinary tract dilation.

Signaling Molecules in Branching Morphogenesis

In addition to stimulating ureteric bud induction, GDNF is also a stimulus for subsequent ureteric bud branching [157, 191]. Transgenic mice that express *Gdnf* ectopically in the Wolffian duct and ureteric buds develop multiple, ectopic ureteric buds that branch independently of the metanephric mesenchyme [157]. However, *in vitro* studies demonstrate that GDNF is not sufficient to induce robust branching in isolated ureteric bud culture [127, 192], which suggests that other factors cooperate with GDNF-RET to control ureteric branching.

Retinoic acid (RA) signaling is also essential for ureteric bud induction and branching. Inactivation of retinoic acid receptors RARα and RARβ2 leads to decreased ureteric bud branch-

ing and downregulation of *Ret* in the ureteric bud [36]. Forced expression of *Ret* in the ureteric bud lineage in *Rarα* and *Rarβ2* double mutant mice is sufficient to restore ureteric bud outgrowth [37]. Retinoic acid activates RA-receptor signaling in the ureteric bud and regulates *Ret* expression in the ureteric bud tips and subsequent proper branching morphogenesis [37, 193]. More recently, *in vitro* studies suggest that retinoic acid-regulated *Extracellular matrix 1 (Ecm1)* restricts *Ret* expression to the ureteric bud tip for proper branching morphogenesis [194].

WNT signaling acts in concert with GDNF-RET signaling to regulate branching morphogenesis. *Wnt11* is expressed at the tips of the ureteric bud and mice that are deficient in *Wnt11* have defects in branching morphogenesis [97, 195] (Fig. 7.3B). This data suggests that *Wnt11* functions at least in part to maintain GDNF expression; conversely, *Wnt11* expression is reduced in the absence of GDNF-RET signaling [97]. β-catenin is an effector that regulates downstream transcriptional targets of the canonical WNT pathway. Mice with β-Catenin deficiency in the ureteric bud cell lineage [196] and the Wolffian duct epithelium [31] display abnormal ureteric branching, loss of gene expression in the ureteric bud tip, and premature expression of differentiated collecting duct epithelial genes. However, β-Catenin overexpression in the metanephric mesenchyme also leads to ectopic and abnormal branching as well as overexpression of *Gdnf* [197], which highlights the complex nature of interacting compartmental signals that coordinate for proper branching. The Prorenin receptor also appears to control branching morphogenesis via the Wnt/β-Catenin pathway [198]. Together, these data suggest that WNT/β-catenin and GDNF-RET signaling pathways act to regulate branching morphogenesis.

The FGF family is also involved in growth and cell proliferation of the ureteric bud [86]. FGF family members exert unique spatial effects on ureteric bud cell proliferation *in vitro*, suggesting that they may coordinate control of three-dimensional growth. For example, FGF10 preferentially simulates cell proliferation at the ureteric bud tips, whereas FGF7 induces prolif-

eration in a non-selective manner throughout the developing collecting duct system [86]. Displaced ureteric buds and aberrant ureteric branching occur in mice with conditional inactivation of the FGF receptor gene, *Fgfr2*, or the docking protein, fibroblast receptor substrate 2α *(Frs2α)* [91, 147, 149, 199, 200]. Increased ureteric bud apoptosis and reduced proliferation are present when *Fgfr2* is conditionally inactivated in the ureteric bud tissue or metanephric mesenchyme [91, 200]. *Fgfr2* appears to function downstream of *Eya1* and *Six1*, but upstream of *Six2*, *Sall1*, and *Pax2* [91]. FGF7 induces expression of the Sprouty gene, *Spry2*, *in vitro,* so FGF7 may also participate with *Spry2* in the feedback loop that controls ureteric bud branching by regulating *Gdnf* and *Wnt11* expression [168]. Further, *Fgf-7* null mice had smaller developing ureteric bud and collecting systems than wild-type [201].

Hepatocyte nuclear factor-1 beta (Hnf1β) inactivation in the ureteric bud cell lineage leads to decreased ureteric branching morphogenesis and defective collecting duct differentiation, with subsequent collecting duct system cystic dilations, renal dysplasia, hypoplasia, or agenesis [139]. Importantly, *HNF1β* mutations in humans present with various renal (and extra-renal) manifestations [202]. *Ex vivo* kidney culture studies in the *Hnf1β* null mice suggest a role in both the ureteric bud tip domain and ureteric bud stalks to organize the epithelium and cell polarity of the ureteric bud branches [139]. HNF1β is believed to directly regulate *Gfrα1* and *Etv5*, so may be involved in regulation both upstream and downstream of GDNF-RET pathway to regulate ureteric bud branching [139].

GDNF, FGF7, and TGF-β also promote expression of *Tissue inhibitors of metalloproteinases (TIMPs)* from cultured ureteric bud cells [203, 204]. TIMPS regulate the local activity of extracellular matrix metalloproteases (MMPs), which are implicated in altering the composition of the extracellular matrix to facilitate branch initiation. This concept is supported by demonstration that TIMPs block ureteric bud branching *in vitro* [203, 205]. Consequently, growth factors may play an important role in regulating the local activity of matrix-degrading proteases by controlling TIMP expression.

Various other signaling factors also stimulate ureteric branching, including *Vascular endothelial growth factor (VEGF)* [206]. *VEGF receptor 2 (VEGFR2)* (critical for endothelial cell development) blockade or deletion both *in vitro* and *in vivo* leads to reduced ureteric branching [40, 207], which further highlights a role for endothelial cell involvement in renal branching morphogenesis. Finally, components of the tight junction such as claudin proteins have also been implicated in branching morphogenesis [208].

Formation of Nephrons

Proximal-distal patterning of nephron epithelial cell fate, as reflected by the formation of tubular and glomerular cell fate domains, is a crucial step in nephron segmentation. Nephron segmentation begins with the sequential formation of two clefts in the renal vesicle, the earliest epithelial derivative of nephron progenitors [2] (Fig. 7.2). Creation of a lower cleft, termed the vascular cleft, heralds formation of the comma-shaped body. The comma-shaped body is a transient structure that rapidly undergoes morphogenetic conversion into an S-shaped structure (termed S-shaped body) upon generation of an upper cleft. The S-shaped body is characterized by three segments or limbs. The middle and upper limbs give rise to the tubular segments of the mature nephron. While the middle limb of the S-shaped body gives rise to the proximal convoluted tubule [2], the descending and ascending limbs of the loops of Henle and the distal convoluted tubule originate from the upper limb of the S-shaped body [2, 15] (Fig. 7.5A). As the vascular cleft broadens and deepens, the lower limb of the S-shaped body forms a cup-shaped unit (Fig. 7.5B). Epithelial cells lining the inner wall of this cup will comprise the visceral glomerular epithelium, or podocytes. Cells lining the outer wall of the cup will form parietal glomerular epithelium, or Bowman's capsule.

All parts of the developing nephron increase in size as they become mature. However, the most striking changes consist of increased tortuosity of the proximal convoluted tubule, and elongation of the loop of Henle [2]. Cellular maturation of the proximal tubule involves transition from columnar to cuboidal epithelium, elaboration of apical and basal microvilli, and gradual increase in tubular diameter and length [209]. The human kidney at birth shows marked heterogeneity in proximal tubule length as one progresses from the outer cortex to the inner cortex [210]. Uniformity in proximal tubule length is achieved by 1 month of life, and the proximal tubule subsequently lengthens at a uniform rate. Prospective cells of the loop of Henle are thought to be first positioned at the junctional region of the middle and upper limbs of the S-shaped body near the vascular pole of the glomerulus, where it will form the macula densa [211]. The descending and ascending limbs of the presumptive loop of Henle are first recognizable as a U-shaped structure in the periphery of the developing renal cortex, termed the nephrogenic zone [211, 212]. Maturation of the primitive loop involves elongation of both ascending and descending limbs through the corticomedullary boundary. Continued maturation involves differentiation of descending and ascending limb epithelia [213]. Development of the presumptive distal tubule involves elongation of the connecting segment, which joins with the ureteric bud/collecting duct.

Longitudinal growth of the medulla contributes to lengthening of the loops of Henle such that all but a small percentage of the loops of Henle extend below the corticomedullary junction in full term newborn infants [2]. As the kidney increases in size postnatally, the loops of Henle further elongate and reach the inner two-thirds of the renal medulla in the mature kidney. Functional development of the kidney's urine concentrating mechanism is dependent on elongation of the loops of Henle during nephrogenesis since longer loops favor urine concentrating capacity. In the extremely premature fetus, the loops of Henle are short owing to the relative distance between the renal capsule and the renal papilla. Consequently, the urine concentrating capacity of the premature kidney is limited by generation of a shallow medullary tonicity gradient.

7 Structural Development of the Kidney

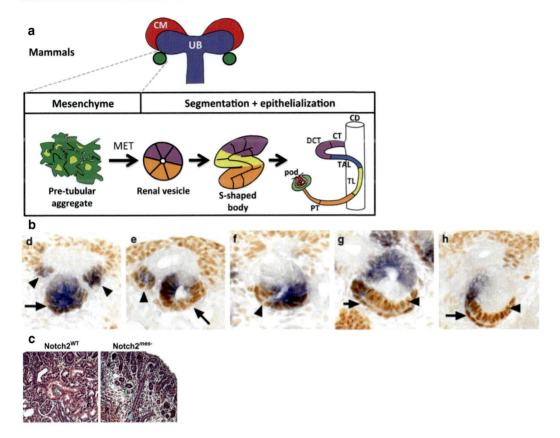

Fig. 7.5 Schematic of nephron segmentation. (**A**) The stages of mammalian metanephric nephron developed are shown, with colors denoting the segmentation of the renal vesicle, S-shaped body and mature nephron (with kind permission from Springer Science+Business Media: Pediatric Nephrology, Hnf1beta and nephron segmentation, published online Nov 5, 2013, Naylor RW and Davidson AJ, Figure 1). (**B**) Dual section in situ hybridization and immunohistochemistry for Wt1 (brown) and Wnt4 (purple) in the mouse kidney at embryonic day 15.5. (d) Wt1 and Wnt4 expression in a pre-tubular aggregate. (e) Wt1 in a pre-tubular aggregate (arrowhead) and the proximal portion of the renal vesicle (arrow). (f) Wt1 expression in the lower limb of the comma-shaped body. (g) Wt1 in the podocytes and parietal epithelium of the proximal segment of an early S-shape body. (h) Wt1 in podocyte and parietal epithelium of the proximal segment of an S-shape body (with kind permission from Springer Science+Business Media: Histochemistry and Cell Biology, Use of dual section mRNA in situ hybridization/immunohistochemistry to clarify gene expression patterns during the early stages of nephron development in the embryo and in the mature nephron of the adult mouse kidney, Vol. 130, p. 937, 2008, Georgas et al., Figure 5). (**C**) Representative kidney phenotype of mice with a conditional mutation affecting nephron segmentation. Loss of Notch2 in the metanephric mesenchyme results in loss of proximal nephron elements (glomeruli, proximal tubules and S-shaped bodies). Red arrows, glomeruli; green, proximal tubule; yellow, S-shaped bodies; turquoise, collecting duct (reprinted with permission from: Company of Biologists: Development, Notch2, but not Notch1, is required for proximal cell fate acquisition in the mammalian nephron, 134(4), p. 803, 2007, Cheng et al., Figure 1)

Nephron Segmentation

Proximal-distal patterning of nephron epithelial cell fate, as reflected by the formation of glomerular and tubular cell fate domains, is a crucial step in nephron segmentation. Recently, elegant studies have provided a high resolution view of comparative histology, RNA expression and protein localization of mouse and human developing kidneys throughout nephrogenesis [214, 215]. These studies offer insights into when proximal-distal patterning is established in renal vesicles, along with differences in marker genes in the mouse and human.

One mechanism for patterning glomerular and tubular cell fates in the S-shaped body appears to be dependent on negative feedback between *Wt1* and *Pax2* [216–218] (Fig. 7.5B). During early kidney development, the expression patterns of *Pax2* and *Wt1* become restricted in S-shaped bodies such that the expression domain of *Pax2* is complementary to the corresponding domain for *Wt1*. *Wt1* expression is restricted to glomerular epithelial precursors, which give rise to podocytes later in glomerular development [219]. In contrast, *Pax2* expression is restricted to that portion which gives rise to tubular epithelial precursors of the proximal and distal nephron segments and is later repressed in differentiated tubular epithelium [123, 220]. The precise roles for *Wt1* or *Pax2* in nephron differentiation is not evident from the analyses of renal phenotypes in mice with targeted *Wt1* or *Pax2* mutations since these mutants fail to form kidneys [54, 76]. However, evidence from transgenic mice that over-express PAX2 in all nephrogenic cell types illustrates the importance of spatially restricting *Pax2* expression during early nephrogenesis since these mice exhibit dysplastic kidneys with defective differentiation of both tubular and glomerular epithelia [221].

Two other transcription factors expressed at the renal vesicle stage, *Lhx1* and *Brn1*, also appear to be involved in initiating proximal-distal nephron epithelial cell fate patterning. While *Lhx1* is uniformly expressed in renal vesicles [61], *Brain specific homeobox 1* (*Brn1*) expression occurs in a more spatially restricted pattern in renal vesicles [212]. Conditional knockout of *Lhx1* in the metanephric mesenchyme causes developmental arrest at the renal vesicle stage, and results in loss of *Brn1* expression [61]. In contrast, targeted deletion of *Brn1* in the metanephric mesenchyme does not prevent the early stages of nephron morphogenesis, but blocks formation of the loop of Henle, and suppresses terminal differentiation of distal nephron epithelia [212]. Taken together, these data suggest that *Brn1* functions downstream of *Lhx1* in a genetic hierarchy which establishes distal cell fates. An additional role for *Lhx1* in specifying podocyte cell fate is revealed by the analysis of *Lhx1* chimeric mutant mice [61].

Genetic evidence in mice suggests that the process for selecting which nephrogenic progenitors will comprise the proximal portion of the developing nephron (i.e. the podocytes and proximal convoluted tubule) is dependent on Notch signaling [222–224]. Conditional knock-out of *Notch2* and *Recombining binding protein suppressor of hairless* (*Rbpsuh*), but not *Notch1*, in metanephric mesenchyme prior to nephron segmentation results in complete lack of both proximal tubule and glomerular epithelia [223] (Fig. 7.5C). Similar effects were observed in mutant mice when presenilin-mediated Notch activation was abrogated by mutagenesis of *Psen1* and *Psen2* [224]. Moreover, ectopic Notch activation in nephron progenitors results in premature differentiation and MET, with a preference towards proximal tubule cell fate [225].

There is limited information regarding the subsequent specification of cell types in the proximal tubule, loop of Henle and distal tubule. Mutations in the transcription factor, *Hepatic nuclear factor 4a* (*Hnf4a*), are associated with Fanconi syndrome, and *Hnf4a* has been shown to be required for the formation of differentiated proximal tubules [226].

Glomerulogenesis

During embryonic development, formation of the lower limb of the S-shaped body heralds the onset of glomerulogenesis [2, 227] (Fig. 7.6A). The vascular cleft provides an entry point to which progenitor endothelial and mesangial cells are recruited [228]. Cells residing along the inner surface of the lower S-shaped body limb represent nascent podocytes. At this stage, immature podocytes are proliferative and exhibit a columnar shape, apical cell attachments and a single-layer basement membrane [227]. Development of the glomerular capillary tuft is a dynamic process involving recruitment and proliferation of endothelial and mesangial cell precursors, formation of a capillary plexus, and concomitant assembly of podocytes and mesangial cells distributed around the newly formed capillary loops [227].

Recruitment of angioblasts and mesangial precursors into the vascular cleft results in formation of the lower S-shaped body limb into a cup-like structure [2] (Fig. 7.6A). Formation of a primitive vascular plexus occurs at this so-called capillary loop stage. Podocytes of capillary loop stage glomeruli lose mitotic capacity [229] and begin to demonstrate complex cellular architecture, including the formation of actin-based cytoplasmic extensions, or foot processes, and the formation of specialized intercellular junctions, termed slit diaphragms [230, 231] (Fig. 7.6B). Subsequent development of the glomerular capillary tuft involves extensive branching of capillaries and formation of endothelial fenestrae [2]. Mesangial cells, in turn, populate the core of the tuft and provide structural support to capillary loops through the deposition of extracellular matrix [232, 233]. The full complement of glomeruli in the fetal human kidney is attained by 32–34 weeks when nephrogenesis ceases [2]. At birth, superficial glomeruli, which are chronologically the last to be formed, are significantly smaller than juxtamedullary glomeruli, which are the earliest formed glomeruli [210]. Subsequent glomerular development involves hypertrophy, and glomeruli reach adult size by 3½ years of age [210].

Podocyte Terminal Differentiation

Functional and genetic evidence support the role of Notch signaling in the determination of podocyte cell fate early in nephron development [222, 224]. Additional roles for the Notch receptor gene, *Notch2*, and its ligand, *Jagged1*, at later stages of glomerular capillary tuft assembly are revealed by the analysis of compound mutant mice which show avascular glomeruli or aneurysmal defects and absent mesangial cells in glomerular capillary tuft formation [234].

Following podocyte cell fate determination, the transcription factors *Wt1*, *podocyte expressed 1* (*Pod1*), *Lim homeobox 1b* (*Lmx1b*), *Foxc2*, *Mafb*, and *Osr1* [235, 236] have been shown to have important roles in podocyte terminal differentiation. Loss of function mutations in *Foxc2*, *Pod1*, *Lmx1b*, and *Mafb* cause podocyte defects in mice which become evident at the capillary loop stage (in the case of *Pod1*) or later (in the case of *Foxc2*,

Lmx1b, *Mafb*) [237–240]. Analysis of chimeric mice reveal that normal glomerular epithelial differentiation requires the function of *Pod1* in neighboring stromal cells, suggesting that *Pod1* regulates stromal factors that act to promote podocyte cell fate [49]. In humans, *LMX1b* mutations are identified in patients with Nail-Patella Syndrome, which is associated with focal segmental glomerulosclerosis [241]. A role for *Wt1* in podocyte differentiation is suggested by the identification of *WT1* mutations in humans with Denys-Drash and Frasier syndromes [242–244], which are inherited disorders associated with mesangial sclerosis, a form of glomerular disease characterized by defects in podocyte differentiation [245]. The demonstration of an identical glomerular phenotype in mice with targeted *Wt1* mutations, genetically similar to the *WT1* mutation in humans with Denys-Drash and Frasier syndromes, [246–249] serves as additional support that *Wt1* has important roles in podocyte differentiation. *TGF-β-activated kinase* (*Tak1*) targeted deletion in podocytes results in disrupted podocyte architecture associated with decreased *Wt1* expression [250].

Podocyte maturation coincides with a loss of mitotic activity and cell cycle blockade [229]. The limited capacity of mature podocytes to undergo cell proliferation has important implications on the glomerular response to injury since damaged podocytes are not capable of compensating for their loss of function by way of regeneration. Moreover, escape from cell cycle blockade in mature podocytes has been associated with severe changes in glomerular cytoarchitecture and a rapidly progressive decline in renal function, as demonstrated by the deleterious course of idiopathic collapsing and human immunodeficiency virus (HIV) nephropathies [251].

Glomerular Capillary Tuft Development

Lineage tracing studies show that the precursors of most glomerular endothelial cells (angioblasts) are Foxd1-positive stromal cells [252, 253]. Studies of autologous transplantation of embryonic kidney rudiments into adult renal cortex suggests that angioblasts originate from a unique subpopulation of induced metanephric mesenchyme that do not differentiate along epithelial lineages (vasculogenesis) [228, 254, 255]. An alternate theory is provided by evidence that glomerular capillaries originate from ingrowth of primitive sprouts from external vessels through experiments involving engraftment of rodent fetal kidneys onto avian chorioallantoic membrane [256], suggesting that angiogenesis also plays a role in glomerular endothelial development.

Several signaling systems are involved in the recruitment of endothelial and mesangial precursors during the formation and assembly of the glomerular capillary tuft. Vascular endothelial growth factor (VEGF) is secreted by podocyte precursors of early S-shaped bodies [257]. VEGF promotes recruitment of VEGFR2-expressing angioblasts into the vascular cleft to initiate glomerular vasculogenesis [258] and is required to induce apoptosis for lumen capillary formation [259, 260]. This process is under tight regulatory control, as suggested by the demonstration of severe glomerular defects in mice when the gene dosage of *Vegf* is genetically manipulated [261, 262] (Fig. 7.6C). Appropriate development of the glomerular mesangial cells is also important to provide structural and functional support to the glomerular capillary network. Recruitment of mesangial cells is under the guidance of platelet-derived growth factor (PDGF)–β, expressed by endothelial cells, which binds to its receptor, PDGF receptor-β (PDGFRβ) [263]. This axis is required for proliferation and assembly of glomerular capillaries and mesangium as revealed by the absence of glomerular capillary tufts in mice deficient for either *Pdgfβ* or *Pdgfrβ* [264, 265]. Other regulators required for normal renal vasculogenesis include the renin angiotensin system genes [266–270], *Angiopoietin1* and its tyrosine receptor *Angiopoietin-1 receptor* (*Tie2*) [271–273], *Dicer* [274, 275], Notch signaling [276, 277] and TGFβ signaling [278–280]. Other

---

Fig. 7.6 Development of the glomerulus. (**A**) Immunohistochemical staining for Wt1 (brown) in the developing glomerulus. (i) Wt1 in podocytes and parietal epithelium in a late S-shaped body. Endothelial cells are recruited into the cup-shaped glomerular precursor region of the S-shaped body forming a primitive vascular tuft. (j, k) Wt1 in podocytes and parietal epithelium in a capillary loop stage glomerulus. Podocyte precursors contact invading endothelial cells and begin to differentiate. In turn, endothelial cells form a primitive capillary plexus (capillary loop stage). (l, m) Wt1 is strongly expressed in podocytes in maturing glomeruli. Parietal epithelial cells encapsulate the developing glomerulus. (**B**) (a) Immunohistochemistry of maturing glomeruli using antibodies to Tjp1, Wt1, Des and Aqp1. Tjp1 expression in the glomerular basement membrane (gbm) and parietal epithelium (pe); Wt1 in podocytes or visceral epithelium (ve); Desmin in the extraglomerular mesangium (egm), glomerular mesangium of Bowman's capsule (gmbc) and the glomerular mesangium (gm); and Aqp1 in endothelial cells of the glomerular capillary system (gcs) and red blood cells (rbc). (b) Schematic of a developing glomerulus showing the structures present in both the adult and embryonic kidney. The developing glomerulus is composed of a central glomerular tuft, which contains a capillary loop network arising from the afferent arteriole termed the glomerular capillary system. Forming a tight association with the endothelial cells of the capillaries is the visceral epithelium (or podocytes), a layer of highly specialized epithelial cells specific to the nephron. The fused basal lamina of the endothelial and visceral epithelial cells forms the glomerular basement membrane, an extracellular component of the renal corpuscle. In the interstitial spaces between the capillaries is the glomerular mesangium, a complex of mesangial cells and extracellular matrix. The glomerular tuft is surrounded by the Bowman's capsule, which is composed of the parietal epithelium, mesangium and the urinary space of the renal corpuscle. Extraglomerular mesangium located outside the renal corpuscle is a component of the juxtaglomerular complex and is associated with the afferent arteriole. The antibodies used to identify each of the structures are shown; Aqp1 (orange), Wt1 (red), Tjp1 (green) and Des (blue) (with kind permission from Springer Science+Business Media: Histochemistry and Cell Biology, Use of dual section mRNA in situ hybridization/immunohistochemistry to clarify gene expression patterns during the early stages of nephron development in the embryo and in the mature nephron of the adult mouse kidney, Vol. 130, p. 932 and 937, 2008, Georgas et al., Figure 2 and 5). (**C**) Representative kidney phenotype of mice with a conditional deletion affecting glomerulogenesis. Loss of VEGFA in the podocyte results in a failure of the glomerular endothelial cells to undergo fenestration and progressive loss of endothelial cells. +/+, wild-type glomerulus; −/−, VEGF-null glomerulus; green, Wt1 staining; red PECAM staining (reprinted with permission from: American Society for Clinical Investigation: Journal of Clinical Investigation, Glomerular-specific alterations of VEGF-A lead to distinct congenital and acquired renal diseases, 111(5), p. 712, 2003, Eremina et al., Figure 5)

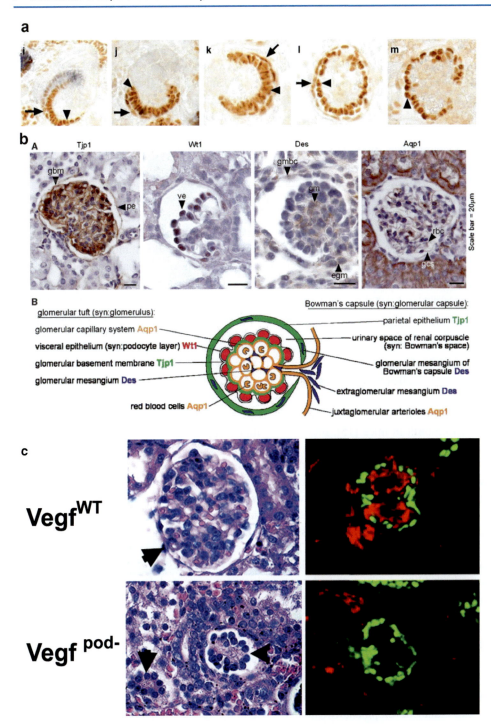

molecules implicated in exerting attraction and repulsion guidance for glomerular capillary formation include the chemokine Stromal cell derived factor 1 (SDF1) [281], which acts on CXCR3 and CXCR7, the transmembrane protein EphrinB2 [282–284] and chemorepellent glycoprotein Semaphorin 3a [285].

During the S-shaped stage, podocyte progenitors express a primitive glomerular basement membrane which is composed predominantly of laminin-1, and α-1 and α-2 subchains of type IV collagen [286]. During glomerular development, composition of the glomerular basement membrane undergoes transition as laminin-1 is replaced by laminin-11, and α-1 and α-2 type IV collagen chains are replaced by α-3, α-4, and α-5 subchains [286]. As demonstrated in several mouse models, failure of these changes result in severe structural and functional defects [287–289].

Formation of the Collecting System

Between the 22nd–34th week of human fetal gestation [2], or E15.5-birth in mice [15], morphologic changes result in the establishment of peripheral (i.e. cortical) and central (i.e. medullary) domains in the developing kidney. The renal cortex, which represents 70% of total kidney volume at birth [290], becomes organized as a relatively compact, circumferential rim of tissue surrounding the periphery of the kidney. The renal medulla, which represents 30% of total kidney volume at birth [290], has a modified cone shape with a broad base contiguous with cortical tissue. The apex of the cone is formed by convergence of collecting ducts in the inner medulla and is termed the papilla.

Distinct morphologic differences emerge between collecting ducts located in the medulla compared to those located in the renal cortex during this stage of kidney development. Medullary collecting ducts are organized into elongated, relatively unbranched linear arrays which converge centrally in a region devoid of glomeruli. In contrast, collecting ducts located in the renal cortex continue to induce metanephric mesenchyme. The specification of cortical and medullary

domains is essential to the eventual function of the mature collecting duct system. The most central segments of the collecting duct system formed from the first five generations of ureteric bud branching undergo remodeling by increased growth and dilatation of these tubules to form the pelvis and calyces (reviewed in [291]).

The developing renal cortex and medulla exhibit distinct axes of growth. The renal cortex grows along a circumferential axis, resulting in a ten-fold increase in volume while preserving compact organization of cortical tissue around the developing kidney [290]. In this manner, differentiating glomeruli and tubules maintain their relative position in the renal cortex with respect to the external surface of the kidney, or renal capsule. In contrast to the circumferential pattern of growth exhibited by the developing renal cortex, the developing renal medulla expands 4.5-fold in thickness along a longitudinal axis perpendicular to the axis of cortical growth [290]. This pattern of renal medulla growth is largely due to elongation of outer medullary collecting ducts [290]. The development of a medullary zone coincides with the appearance of stromal cells between the seventh and eighth generations of ureteric bud branches [290]. It has been suggested that stromal cells provide stimulatory cues to promote the growth of medullary collecting ducts [290]. Additional support for this hypothesis is provided by analyses of mutant mice lacking functional expression of the stromal transcription factors *Pod1* and *Forkhead box d1* (*Foxd1*) [35, 49, 292], which demonstrate defects in medullary collecting duct patterning.

In the developing collecting system, apoptosis is infrequently detected in the tips and trunks of the branching ureteric bud [110]. At later stages of embryonic and post-natal kidney development, apoptosis is prominent in the medullary regions of the rat collecting duct system that give rise to the calyces, renal pelvis and renal papilla [110]. The prominence of apoptosis in these regions suggests a potential role for apoptosis in remodeling the first 3–5 generations of the branched ureteric bud/developing collecting duct system. The extent to which apoptosis contributes to this morphogenetic process is, however, unknown. Other suggested roles for medullary apoptosis include elimination of medullary interstitial cells as a mechanism for making room for new blood vessel ingrowth [293].

Medullary Patterning and Formation of the Pelvicaliceal System

Regional specification of cortical and medullary domains of the renal collecting duct system is a relatively late event in kidney development. At least five soluble growth factor genes (*Fgf7*, *Fgf10*, *Bmp4*, *Bmp5* and *Wnt7b*), one proteoglycan gene (*Gpc3*), one cell cycle regulatory gene (*p57^{KIP2}*), and molecular components of the renin-angiotensin axis (*Angiotensinogen* (*Agt*), *Angiotensinogen receptor* 1 and 2 (*Agtr1*, *Agtr2*)) are implicated in medullary collecting duct morphogenesis as revealed by the demonstration of defects in renal medulla development in mutant mice.

The kidneys of *Fgf7* null mice are characterized by marked underdevelopment of the papilla [39]. Similarly, *Fgf10* null kidneys exhibit modest medullary dysplasia with reduced numbers of loops of Henle and medullary collecting ducts, increased medullary stromal cells, and enlargement of the renal calyx [294]. Cellular responses to FGFs are modulated through interactions with cell surface proteoglycans [295]. Syndecans and glypicans are heparan sulfate proteoglycans expressed in developing collecting ducts [186, 296], and their expression is required for normal collecting duct growth and branching [136, 297]. Moreover, treatment of embryonic kidney explants with pharmacologic inhibitors of sulfated proteoglycan synthesis leads to loss of *Wnt11* expression at the ureteric bud branch tips [298], suggesting that sulfated proteoglycans interact with multiple mechanisms that control ureteric bud branching.

Functional and genetic evidence in humans and mice demonstrate that GPC3, a glycosylphosphatidylinositol (GPI)-linked cell surface heparan sulfate proteoglycan, is required for normal patterning of the medulla [186, 299]. Medullary dysplasia in the *Gpc3* deficient mouse arises from overgrowth of the ureteric bud and collecting ducts due to increased cell proliferation in the ureteric bud lineage [299], with subsequent destruction of these elements due to apoptosis [186]. The defect is thought to be caused by an altered cellular response of GPC3-deficient collecting duct cells to growth factors such as FGFs [186, 300, 301]. The defective renal medulla formation in *Gpc3* null mutant mice illustrates the importance of tightly regulated cell proliferation and apoptosis in this process. Other signals that promote collecting duct cell survival include Wnt7b and Egf [302, 303].

Additional support for this concept is provided by the phenotypic analysis of mice carrying a null mutation for *p57^{KIP2}*, a cell cycle regulatory gene. *p57^{KIP2}* knock-out mice show medullary dysplasia characterized by a decreased number of inner medullary collecting ducts, in addition to abdominal, skeletal, and adrenal defects [304]. Genetic studies in humans and mice suggest a potential functional interaction between *p57^{KIP2}* and the *Insulin-like growth factor-2* (*Igf2*) gene in the formation of the renal medulla. For example, phenotypic features of mice with *p57^{KIP2}* null mutations are exhibited by approximately 15% of individuals with Beckwith-Wiedemann Syndrome, a heterogeneous disorder characterized by somatic overgrowth and renal dysplasia [305]. Genetic linkage studies in humans with this syndrome have mapped the disease to chromosome 11p15.5, which harbors loci for *p57^{KIP2}* as well as for *IGF2* and *H19*. Murine *H19* mutations result in enhanced *Igf2* expression, but do not cause renal dysplasia [306]. However, *H19^{-/-}*; *p57^{KIP2-/-}* double knock-out mice exhibit elevated serum levels of IGF2, and more severe renal dysplasia than that observed in *p57^{KIP2}* single knock-out mice [307]. These findings support an additional mechanism for the cause of renal medullary dysplasia resulting from dysregulated stimulation of cell proliferation through the inactivation of p57^{KIP2} and overexpression of IGF2.

Elaboration of the medullary collecting duct network is thought to require oriented cell divisions that permit elongation of the medullary collecting ducts through proliferation during development. One means by which this occurs is through the activity of the secreted factor, WNT7b, in up-regulating canonical Wnt signaling in medullary collecting ducts to promote oriented cell division and cell survival [302, 308]. α3β1 integrin and the receptor tyrosine kinase c-Met (receptor for hepatocyte growth factor) appear to coordinately regulate *Wnt7b* expression in the medullary collecting duct [308]. Another member of the Wnt family, *Wnt9b*, also plays a role in elongation and appears to regulate planar cell polarity [309]. Post-transcriptional regulation by miRNAs also drives collecting duct elongation and differentiation [310, 311].

Development of the Ureteral Smooth Muscle

Urinary filtrate removal also requires coordinated ureteric contractions, which in turn is the result of development of a "pacemaker" at the base of the renal papilla and smooth muscle around the ureter. *Bmp4* heterozygous mutant mice develop both hydronephrosis and hydroureter [144], suggesting that *Bmp4* may play additional roles that involve formation of the ureter and renal pelvis. Support for this concept is provided by the finding in kidney explants that recombinant BMP4 induces smooth muscle actin, an early marker for smooth muscle differentiation, in peri-ureteric mesenchymal cells [312]. Both *Bmp4* and *Bmp5* are expressed in mesenchymal cells lining the ureter and the developing renal pelvis [144, 173, 313], and BMP receptors *Bone morphogenetic protein receptor, type 1A (Alk3)* and *Bone morphogenetic protein receptor, type 1B (Alk6)* are expressed in neighboring collecting ducts [144]. Moreover, mice mutant for *Bmp4* in the ureteric mesenchyme show similar defects in renal pelvis and ureter development with reduced ureter smooth muscle [314]. This study suggested SMAD as a downstream effector of BMP4. Indeed, mice with inactivation of *Smad4* show a similar phenotype with decreased ureteral smooth muscle and abnormal function [315, 316].

In addition to BMP signaling, the Sonic hedgehog (SHH) pathway plays a critical role in regulating ureteral mesenchymal development. SHH is secreted from the medullary collecting duct and ureteric stalk, and signals to the surrounding interstitium through its receptor, Patched1 (Ptch1) [317]. BMP4, together with SHH, induces the expression of the transcription factor, *Teashirt zinc finger homeobox 3 (Tshz3)*, which regulates the development of smooth muscle [318]. Interestingly, loss of the *Gli family zinc finger 3 (Gli3)* repressor (resulting in inappropriate Hedgehog pathway activation) results in hydronephrosis due to ureteric dyskinesis and reduced numbers of pacemaker cells [319]. Mutations in *GLI3* are associated with Pallister-Hall syndrome in humans [320]. Loss of another zinc factor transcription factor gene, *Gata2*, in the ureteric mesenchyme also leads to abnormal smooth muscle differentiation and dilated ureters [321]. More recently, SHH was shown to use FOXF1-BMP4 signaling to program ureter elongation and differentiation [322].

Mutations in genes encoding components of the renin-angiotensin axis also cause abnormalities in the development of the renal calyces, pelvis and ureter. Mice homozygous for a null mutation in the *Agt* gene demonstrate progressive widening of the calyx and atrophy of the papillae and underlying medulla [323]. Identical defects occur in homozygous mutants for the *Agtr1* gene [324]. The underlying defect in these mutants appears to be decreased cell proliferation of the smooth muscle cell layer lining the renal pelvis, resulting in decreased thickness of this layer in the proximal ureter. Mutational inactivation of *Agtr2* results in a range of anomalies, including vesicoureteral reflux, duplex kidney, renal ectopia, uretero-pelvic or ureterovesical junction stenoses, renal dysplasia or hypoplasia, multicystic dysplastic kidney, or renal agenesis [109]. Null mice demonstrate a decreased rate of apoptosis of the cells around the ureter, suggesting that *Agtr2* also plays a role in morphogenetic remodeling of the ureter.

Other regulators of ureteral smooth muscle differentiation include *Tbx18* [325], *Tbx2* and *Tbx3 (Tbx2 and Tbx3)* [326], *Robo2* [327] and retinoic acid signaling [328]. Deletion of *Dicer* also led to impaired ureter morphology and function with ureteral smooth muscle abnormalities [329], suggesting that miRNAs are important in regulating ureter smooth muscle differentiation.

Renal Stroma

Stromal cells are comprised of interstitial cells that secrete extracellular matrix and growth factors that provide a supportive framework and developmental patterning signals around the developing nephrons, collecting system and vasculature. In keeping with this idea, stromal cells are found in close proximity to developing nephrons, ureteric bud branches and blood vessels (Fig. 7.3C). Developmentally, stromal cells are derived from a population of *Foxd1*-expressing stromal progenitors [330]. As the renal cortex and medulla become morphologically distinct regions, stromal cells become defined geographically into two separate populations—cortical stroma, which form interstitium between induced nephrons and express *Foxd1*, *Aldehyde dehydrogenase 1 family, member A2 (Raldh2)*, *Retinoic acid receptor α (Rarα)* and *Rarβ2*; and medullary stroma, which form interstitium between medullary collecting ducts and express *Fgf7*, *Pod1*, and *Bmp4*. Many of these stromal genes have been shown to be critical for nephrogenesis and ureteric branching morphogenesis in transgenic mouse studies [35, 36, 38, 39, 144, 239]. Further evidence of the importance of the renal stroma for kidney development comes from transgenic animal studies which result in ablation of the renal stroma with diphtheria toxin, causing an abnormally thickened cap mesenchyme and decreased ability of progenitors to differentiate [47, 331]. scRNA-seq studies have recently identified 17 molecularly distinct cell clusters of renal interstitium in the developing kidney [71]. Once nephrogenesis is complete, stromal cells differentiate into a diverse population which includes fibroblasts, lymphocyte-like cells, glomerular mesangial cells, renin-expressing cells and pericytes [330, 332, 333].

One important role for the renal stroma is regulation of *Ret* expression, and hence branching morphogenesis. RARα and RARβ2, members of the retinoic acid receptor (RAR) and retinoid X receptor (RXR) families of transcription factors, are both expressed in stromal cells and *Ret*-expressing ureteric bud branch tips [36]. *Rarα*$^{-/-}$; *Rarβ2*$^{-/-}$ double mutant mice have small kidneys characterized by a decreased number of ureteric bud branches and loss of normal cortical stromal patterning between induced nephrons [36]. In the collecting ducts of *Rarα*$^{-/-}$; *Rarβ2*$^{-/-}$ double mutant mice, *Ret* expression is down-regulated whereas *Gdnf* expression in the metanephric mesenchyme is maintained. The renal defect in these mice can be rescued by overexpressing a *Ret* transgene in the ureteric bud lineage [37]. Recent data suggests that retinoic acid derived from the renal stroma via the enzyme Raldh2 signals to the ureteric bud to up-regulate expression of *Rarα* and *Rarβ2* to induce *Ret* expression in the ureteric bud [193].

The transcription factors *Foxd1* and *Pod1* have roles in regulating the spatially restricted pattern of *Ret* expression during collecting duct development. *Foxd1* is most strongly expressed in the developing kidney in the cortical, or subcapsular, stroma [35, 38] (Fig. 7.3C). In contrast, *Pod1* is most abundant in medullary stromal cells [239, 334]. Homozygous deletion of either *Foxd1* or *Pod1* results in decreased renal branching morphogenesis and misexpression of *Ret* throughout the developing collecting system [35, 239]. These data suggest that stromal cues expressed under the control of *Foxd1* and *Pod1* are involved in inhibiting *Ret* expression in the truncal segments of the developing ureteric bud. It is not clear from the analyses of these mutants whether secreted stromal factors directly block *Ret* expression in collecting ducts. Since *Foxd1* and *Pod1* mutants show additional defects in nephron morphogenesis [35, 239], these stromal genes may indirectly control *Ret* expression through the production of nephron-derived factors that secondarily act on collecting duct cells to inhibit *Ret* expression.

Although the mechanisms by which the renal stroma regulates nephron differentiation are not entirely clear, Wnt and Hippo signaling have been implicated. With regards to Hippo signaling, loss of the protocadherin *Fat atypical cadherin 4 (Fat4)* in the stroma results in expansion of the cap mesenchyme, and this appears to be due to binding to *Dachsous 1/2 (Dsch1/2)* on the cap mesenchyme [47, 335]. Interestingly, activation of β-catenin in the renal stroma prevents the differentiation of nephron progenitors and results in histological and molecular features similar to Wilm's tumour [336].

Acknowledgments The authors would like to express their gratitude to Tino Piscione for his contributions to the second edition of this chapter.

References

1. Osathanondh V, Potter EL. Development of human kidney as shown by microdissection. Arch Pathol. 1966;82:391–402.
2. Potter EL. Normal and abnormal development of the kidney. Chicago: Year Book Medical Publishers Inc.; 1972. p. 305.
3. Hinchliffe SA, Sargent PH, Howard CV, Chan YF, van Velzen D. Human intrauterine renal growth expressed in absolute number of glomeruli assessed by the disector method and Cavalieri principle. Lab Invest. 1991;64(6):777–84.
4. Hughson M, Farris AB 3rd, Douglas-Denton R, Hoy WE, Bertram JF. Glomerular number and size in autopsy kidneys: the relationship to birth weight. Kidney Int. 2003;63(6):2113–22.
5. Rodriguez MM, Gomez AH, Abitbol CL, Chandar JJ, Duara S, Zilleruelo GE. Histomorphometric analysis of postnatal glomerulogenesis in extremely preterm infants. Pediatr Dev Pathol. 2004;7(1):17–25.
6. Brenner BM, Chertow GM. Congenital oligonephropathy and the etiology of adult hypertension and progressive renal injury. Am J Kidney Dis. 1994;23(2):171–5.
7. Brenner BM, Mackenzie HS. Nephron mass as a risk factor for progression of renal disease. Kidney Int Suppl. 1997;63:S124–7.
8. Keller G, Zimmer G, Mall G, Ritz E, Amann K. Nephron number in patients with primary hypertension. N Engl J Med. 2003;348(2):101–8.
9. Hoy WE, Hughson MD, Singh GR, Douglas-Denton R, Bertram JF. Reduced nephron number and glomerulomegaly in Australian aborigines: a group at high risk for renal disease and hypertension. Kidney Int. 2006;70(1):104–10.
10. Manalich R, Reyes L, Herrera M, Melendi C, Fundora I. Relationship between weight at birth and the number and size of renal glomeruli in humans: a histomorphometric study. Kidney Int. 2000;58(2):770–3.
11. Barker DJ, Osmond C, Golding J, Kuh D, Wadsworth ME. Growth in utero, blood pressure in childhood and adult life, and mortality from cardiovascular disease. BMJ (Clin Res Ed). 1989;298(6673):564–7.
12. Barker DJ, Eriksson JG, Forsen T, Osmond C. Fetal origins of adult disease: strength of effects and biological basis. Int J Epidemiol. 2002;31(6):1235–9.
13. Osathanondh V, Potter EL. Development of human kidney as shown by microdissection. II. Renal pelvis, calyces, and papillae. Arch Pathol. 1963;76:277–89.
14. Osathanondh V, Potter EL. Development of human kidney as shown by microdissection. III. Formation and interrelationship of collecting tubules and nephrons. Arch Pathol. 1963;76:66–78.
15. Saxen L. Organogenesis of the kidney. Cambridge: Cambridge University Press; 1987.
16. Short KM, Smyth IM. The contribution of branching morphogenesis to kidney development and disease. Nat Rev Nephrol. 2016;12(12):754–67.
17. Costantini F, Kopan R. Patterning a complex organ: branching morphogenesis and nephron segmentation in kidney development. Dev Cell. 2010;18(5):698–712.
18. Little MH, McMahon AP. Mammalian kidney development: principles, progress, and projections. Cold Spring Harb Perspect Biol. 2012;4(5):a008300.
19. Dressler GR. The cellular basis of kidney development. Annu Rev Cell Dev Biol. 2006;22:509–29.
20. Takasato M, Little MH. The origin of the mammalian kidney: implications for recreating the kidney in vitro. Development (Cambridge, England). 2015;142(11):1937–47.
21. Drummond IA, Majumdar A, Hentschel H, Elger M, Solnica-Krezel L, Schier AF, et al. Early development of the zebrafish pronephros and analysis of mutations affecting pronephric function. Development (Cambridge, England). 1998;125:4655–67.
22. Vize PD, Seufert DW, Carroll TJ, Wallingford JB. Model systems for the study of kidney development: use of the pronephros in the analysis of organ induction and patterning. Dev Biol. 1997;188:189–204.
23. Staack A, Donjacour AA, Brody J, Cunha GR, Carroll P. Mouse urogenital development: a practical approach. Differentiation. 2003;71(7):402–13.
24. James RG, Kamei CN, Wang Q, Jiang R, Schultheiss TM. Odd-skipped related 1 is required for development of the metanephric kidney and regulates formation and differentiation of kidney precursor cells. Development (Cambridge, England). 2006;133(15):2995–3004.
25. Mugford JW, Sipila P, McMahon JA, McMahon AP. Osr1 expression demarcates a multi-potent population of intermediate mesoderm that undergoes progressive restriction to an Osr1-dependent nephron progenitor compartment within the mammalian kidney. Dev Biol. 2008;324(1):88–98.
26. Dressler GR, Deutsch U, Chowdhury K, Nornes HO, Gruss P. Pax-2, a new murine paired-box-containing gene and its expression in the developing excretory system. Development (Cambridge, England). 1990;109:787–95.
27. Bouchard M, Souabni A, Mandler M, Neubuser A, Busslinger M. Nephric lineage specification by Pax2 and Pax8. Genes Dev. 2002;16(22):2958–70.
28. Fujii T, Pichel JG, Taira M, Toyama R, Dawid IB, Westphal H. Expression patterns of the murine LIM class homeobox gene lim1 in the developing brain and excretory system. Dev Dyn. 1994;1:73–83.
29. Grote D, Souabni A, Busslinger M, Bouchard M. Pax 2/8-regulated Gata 3 expression is necessary for morphogenesis and guidance of the nephric duct

in the developing kidney. Development (Cambridge, England). 2006;133(1):53–61.

30. Pachnis V, Mankoo B, Costantini F. Expression of the *c-ret* proto-oncogene during mouse embryogenesis. Development. 1993;119:1005–17.

31. Marose TD, Merkel CE, McMahon AP, Carroll TJ. Beta-catenin is necessary to keep cells of ureteric bud/Wolffian duct epithelium in a precursor state. Dev Biol. 2008;314(1):112–26.

32. Erickson RA. Inductive interactions in the development of the mouse metanephros. J Exp Zool. 1968;169(1):33–42.

33. Grobstein C. Morphogenetic interaction between embryonic mouse tissues separated by a membrane filter. Nature. 1953;172:869–71.

34. Grobstein C. Inductive interaction in the development of the mouse metanephros. J Exp Zool. 1955;130:319–40.

35. Hatini V, Huh SO, Herzlinger D, Soares VC, Lai E. Essential role of stromal mesenchyme in kidney morphogenesis revealed by targeted disruption of Winged Helix transcription factor *BF-2*. Genes Dev. 1996;10:1467–78.

36. Mendelsohn C, Batourina E, Fung S, Gilbert T, Dodd J. Stromal cells mediate retinoid-dependent functions essential for renal development. Development (Cambridge, England). 1999;126:1139–48.

37. Batourina E, Gim S, Bello N, Shy M, Clagett-Dame M, Srinivas S, et al. Vitamin A controls epithelial/mesenchymal interactions through Ret expression. Nat Genet. 2001;27:74–8.

38. Levinson RS, Batourina E, Choi C, Vorontchikhina M, Kitajewski J, Mendelsohn CL. Foxd1-dependent signals control cellularity in the renal capsule, a structure required for normal renal development. Development (Cambridge, England). 2005;132(3):529–39.

39. Qiao J, Uzzo R, Obara-Ishihara T, Degenstein L, Fuchs E, Herzlinger D. FGF-7 modulates ureteric bud growth and nephron number in the developing kidney. Development. 1999;126:547–54.

40. Gao X, Chen X, Taglienti M, Rumballe B, Little MH, Kreidberg JA. Angioblast-mesenchyme induction of early kidney development is mediated by Wt1 and Vegfa. Development (Cambridge, England). 2005;132(24):5437–49.

41. Tufro-McReddie A, Norwood VF, Aylor KW, Botkin SJ, Carey RM, Gomez RA. Oxygen regulates vascular endothelial growth factor-mediated vasculogenesis and tubulogenesis. Dev Biol. 1997;183(2):139–49.

42. Meyer TN, Schwesinger C, Bush KT, Stuart RO, Rose DW, Shah MM, et al. Spatiotemporal regulation of morphogenetic molecules during in vitro branching of the isolated ureteric bud: toward a model of branching through budding in the developing kidney. Dev Biol. 2004;275(1):44–67.

43. Barasch J, Qiao J, McWilliams G, Chen D, Oliver JA, Herzlinger D. Ureteric bud cells secrete multiple factors, including bFGF, which rescue renal progenitors from apoptosis. Am J Phys. 1997;273:F757–67.

44. Barasch J, Yang J, Ware CB, Taga T, Yoshida K, Erdjument-Bromage H, et al. Mesenchymal to epithelial conversion in rat metanephros is induced by LIF. Cell. 1999;99(4):377–86.

45. Shah MM, Sampogna RV, Sakurai H, Bush KT, Nigam SK. Branching morphogenesis and kidney disease. Development (Cambridge, England). 2004;131(7):1449–62.

46. Piscione TD, Rosenblum ND. The molecular control of renal branching morphogenesis: current knowledge and emerging insights. Differentiation. 2002;70(6):227–46.

47. Das A, Tanigawa S, Karner CM, Xin M, Lum L, Chen C, et al. Stromal-epithelial crosstalk regulates kidney progenitor cell differentiation. Nat Cell Biol. 2013;15(9):1035–44.

48. Yang J, Blum A, Novak T, Levinson R, Lai E, Barasch J. An epithelial precursor is regulated by the ureteric bud and by the renal stroma. Dev Biol. 2002;246(2):296–310.

49. Cui S, Schwartz L, Quaggin SE. Pod1 is required in stromal cells for glomerulogenesis. Dev Dyn. 2003;226(3):512–22.

50. Boyle S, Misfeldt A, Chandler KJ, Deal KK, Southard-Smith EM, Mortlock DP, et al. Fate mapping using Cited1-CreERT2 mice demonstrates that the cap mesenchyme contains self-renewing progenitor cells and gives rise exclusively to nephronic epithelia. Dev Biol. 2008;313(1):234–45.

51. Kobayashi A, Valerius MT, Mugford JW, Carroll TJ, Self M, Oliver G, et al. Six2 defines and regulates a multipotent self-renewing nephron progenitor population throughout mammalian kidney development. Cell Stem Cell. 2008;3(2):169–81.

52. Little MH. Returning to kidney development to deliver synthetic kidneys. Dev Biol. 2021;474:22–36.

53. Bard JB. Growth and death in the developing mammalian kidney: signals, receptors and conversations. BioEssays. 2002;24(1):72–82.

54. Kreidberg JA, Sariola H, Loring JM, Maeda M, Pelletier J, Housman D, et al. WT-1 is required for early kidney development. Cell. 1993;74:679–91.

55. Boyle S, Shioda T, Perantoni AO, de Caestecker M. Cited1 and Cited2 are differentially expressed in the developing kidney but are not required for nephrogenesis. Dev Dyn. 2007;236(8):2321–30.

56. Kalatzis V, Sahly I, El-Amraoui A, Petit C. Eya1 expression in the developing ear and kidney: towards the understanding of the pathogenesis of Branchio-Oto-Renal (BOR) syndrome. Dev Dyn. 1998;213:486–99.

57. Xu P-X, Adams J, Peters H, Brown MC, Heaney S, Maas R. Eya1-deficient mice lack ears and kidneys and show abnormal apoptosis of organ primordia. Nat Genet. 1999;23:113–7.

58. Xu PX, Zheng W, Huang L, Maire P, Laclef C, Silvius D. Six1 is required for the early organogenesis of mammalian kidney. Development (Cambridge, England). 2003;130(14):3085–94.

59. Self M, Lagutin OV, Bowling B, Hendrix J, Cai Y, Dressler GR, et al. Six2 is required for suppression of nephrogenesis and progenitor renewal in the developing kidney. EMBO J. 2006;25(21):5214–28.

60. Nishinakamura R, Matsumoto Y, Nakao K, Nakamura K, Sato A, Copeland NG, et al. Murine homolog of SALL1 is essential for ureteric bud invasion in kidney development. Development (Cambridge, England). 2001;128:3105–15.

61. Kobayashi A, Kwan KM, Carroll TJ, McMahon AP, Mendelsohn CL, Behringer RR. Distinct and sequential tissue-specific activities of the LIM-class homeobox gene Lim1 for tubular morphogenesis during kidney development. Development (Cambridge, England). 2005;132(12):2809–23.

62. Cho EA, Patterson LT, Brookhiser WT, Mah S, Kintner C, Dressler GR. Differential expression and function of cadherin-6 during renal epithelium development. Development (Cambridge, England). 1998;125(5):803–12.

63. Müller U, Wang D, Denda S, Meneses JJ, Pedersen RA, Reichardt LF. Integrin a8b1 is critically important for epithelial-mesenchymal interactions during kidney morphogenesis. Cell. 1997;88:603–13.

64. Hellmich HL, Kos L, Cho ES, Mahon KA, Zimmer A. Embryonic expression of glial cell-line derived neurotrophic factor (GDNF) suggests multiple developmental roles in neural differentiation and epithelial-mesenchymal interactions. Mech Dev. 1996;54:95–105.

65. Brophy PD, Ostrom L, Lang KM, Dressler GR. Regulation of ureteric bud outgrowth by Pax2-dependent activation of the glial derived neurotrophic factor gene. Development. 2001;128:4747–56.

66. Adam M, Potter AS, Potter SS. Psychrophilic proteases dramatically reduce single-cell RNA-seq artifacts: a molecular atlas of kidney development. Development (Cambridge, England). 2017;144(19):3625–32.

67. Brunskill EW, Park JS, Chung E, Chen F, Magella B, Potter SS. Single cell dissection of early kidney development: multilineage priming. Development (Cambridge, England). 2014;141(15):3093–101.

68. Magella B, Adam M, Potter AS, Venkatasubramanian M, Chetal K, Hay SB, et al. Cross-platform single cell analysis of kidney development shows stromal cells express Gdnf. Dev Biol. 2018;434(1):36–47.

69. Combes AN, Phipson B, Lawlor KT, Dorison A, Patrick R, Zappia L, et al. Single cell analysis of the developing mouse kidney provides deeper insight into marker gene expression and ligand-receptor crosstalk. Development (Cambridge, England). 2019;146(12) https://doi.org/10.1242/dev.178673.

70. Combes AN, Phipson B, Lawlor KT, Dorison A, Patrick R, Zappia L, et al. Correction: single cell analysis of the developing mouse kidney provides deeper insight into marker gene expression and ligand-receptor crosstalk. Development (Cambridge, England). 2019;146(13) https://doi.org/10.1242/dev.178673.

71. England AR, Chaney CP, Das A, Patel M, Malewska A, Armendariz D, et al. Identification and characterization of cellular heterogeneity within the developing renal interstitium. Development (Cambridge, England). 2020;147(15) https://doi.org/10.1242/dev.190108.

72. Menon R, Otto EA, Kokoruda A, Zhou J, Zhang Z, Yoon E, et al. Single-cell analysis of progenitor cell dynamics and lineage specification in the human fetal kidney. Development (Cambridge, England). 2018;145(16) https://doi.org/10.1242/dev.164038.

73. Wang P, Chen Y, Yong J, Cui Y, Wang R, Wen L, et al. Dissecting the global dynamic molecular profiles of human fetal kidney development by single-cell RNA sequencing. Cell Rep. 2018;24(13):3554–67.e3.

74. Lindstrom NO, Guo J, Kim AD, Tran T, Guo Q, De Sena Brandine G, et al. Conserved and divergent features of mesenchymal progenitor cell types within the cortical nephrogenic niche of the human and mouse kidney. J Am Soc Nephrol (JASN). 2018;29:806–24.

75. Rothenpieler UW, Dressler GR. Pax-2 is required for mesenchyme-to-epithelium conversion during kidney development. Development (Cambridge, England). 1993;119:711–20.

76. Torres M, Gomez-Pardo E, Dressler GR, Gruss P. *Pax-2* controls multiple steps of urogenital development. Development (Cambridge, England). 1995;121:4057–65.

77. Tsang TE, Shawlot W, Kinder SJ, Kobayashi A, Kwan KM, Schughart K, et al. Lim1 activity is required for intermediate mesoderm differentiation in the mouse embryo. Dev Biol. 2000;223(1):77–90.

78. Shawlot W, Behringer RR. Requirement for *Lim1* in head-organizer function. Nature. 1995;374:425–30.

79. Donovan MJ, Natoli TA, Sainio K, Amstutz A, Jaenisch R, Sariola H, et al. Initial differentiation of the metanephric mesenchyme is independent of WT1 and the ureteric bud. Dev Genet. 1999;24:252–62.

80. O'Brien LL, Guo Q, Bahrami-Samani E, Park JS, Hasso SM, Lee YJ, et al. Transcriptional regulatory control of mammalian nephron progenitors revealed by multi-factor cistromic analysis and genetic studies. PLoS Genet. 2018;14(1):e1007181.

81. Park JS, Ma W, O'Brien LL, Chung E, Guo JJ, Cheng JG, et al. Six2 and Wnt regulate self-renewal and commitment of nephron progenitors through shared gene regulatory networks. Dev Cell. 2012;23(3):637–51.

82. O'Brien LL, Guo Q, Lee Y, Tran T, Benazet JD, Whitney PH, et al. Differential regulation of mouse and human nephron progenitors by the Six family of transcriptional regulators. Development (Cambridge, England). 2016;143(4):595–608.

83. Little MH, Lawlor KT. Recreating, expanding and using nephron progenitor populations. Nat Rev Nephrol. 2020;16(2):75–6.

84. Carroll TJ, Park JS, Hayashi S, Majumdar A, McMahon AP. Wnt9b plays a central role in the regulation of mesenchymal to epithelial transitions

underlying organogenesis of the mammalian urogenital system. Dev Cell. 2005;9(2):283–92.

85. Karner CM, Das A, Ma Z, Self M, Chen C, Lum L, et al. Canonical Wnt9b signaling balances progenitor cell expansion and differentiation during kidney development. Development (Cambridge, England). 2011;138(7):1247–57.

86. Qiao J, Bush KT, Steer DL, Stuart RO, Sakurai H, Wachsman W, et al. Multiple fibroblast growth factors support growth of the ureteric bud but have different effects on branching morphogenesis. Mech Dev. 2001;109(2):123–35.

87. Cancilla B, Davies A, Cauchi JA, Risbridger GP, Bertram JF. Fibroblast growth factor receptors and their ligands in the adult rat kidney. Kidney Int. 2001;60(1):147–55.

88. Barak H, Huh SH, Chen S, Jeanpierre C, Martinovic J, Parisot M, et al. FGF9 and FGF20 maintain the stemness of nephron progenitors in mice and man. Dev Cell. 2012;22(6):1191–207.

89. Brown AC, Adams D, de Caestecker M, Yang X, Friesel R, Oxburgh L. FGF/EGF signaling regulates the renewal of early nephron progenitors during embryonic development. Development (Cambridge, England). 2011;138(23):5099–112.

90. Hains D, Sims-Lucas S, Kish K, Saha M, McHugh K, Bates CM. Role of fibroblast growth factor receptor 2 in kidney mesenchyme. Pediatr Res. 2008;64(6):592–8.

91. Poladia DP, Kish K, Kutay B, Hains D, Kegg H, Zhao H, et al. Role of fibroblast growth factor receptors 1 and 2 in the metanephric mesenchyme. Dev Biol. 2006;291(2):325–39.

92. Sims-Lucas S, Cusack B, Baust J, Eswarakumar VP, Masatoshi H, Takeuchi A, et al. Fgfr1 and the IIIc isoform of Fgfr2 play critical roles in the metanephric mesenchyme mediating early inductive events in kidney development. Dev Dyn. 2011;240(1):240–9.

93. Muthukrishnan SD, Yang X, Friesel R, Oxburgh L. Concurrent BMP7 and FGF9 signalling governs AP-1 function to promote self-renewal of nephron progenitor cells. Nat Commun. 2015;6:10027.

94. Di Giovanni V, Walker KA, Bushnell D, Schaefer C, Sims-Lucas S, Puri P, et al. Fibroblast growth factor receptor-Frs2alpha signaling is critical for nephron progenitors. Dev Biol. 2015;400(1):82–93.

95. Blank U, Brown A, Adams DC, Karolak MJ, Oxburgh L. BMP7 promotes proliferation of nephron progenitor cells via a JNK-dependent mechanism. Development (Cambridge, England). 2009;136(21):3557–66.

96. Brown AC, Muthukrishnan SD, Guay JA, Adams DC, Schafer DA, Fetting JL, et al. Role for compartmentalization in nephron progenitor differentiation. Proc Natl Acad Sci U S A. 2013;110(12):4640–5.

97. Majumdar A, Vainio S, Kispert A, McMahon J, McMahon AP. Wnt11 and Ret/Gdnf pathways cooperate in regulating ureteric branching during metanephric kidney development. Development (Cambridge, England). 2003;130(14):3175–85.

98. Dudley AT, Lyons KM, Robertson EJ. A requirement for bone morphogenetic protein-7 during development of the mammalian kidney and eye. Genes Dev. 1995;9:2795–807.

99. Luo G, Hofmann C, Bronckers ALJJ, Sohocki M, Bradley A, Karsenty G. BMP-7 is an inducer of nephrogenesis, and is also required for eye development and skeletal patterning. Genes Dev. 1995;9:2808–20.

100. Brown AC, Muthukrishnan SD, Oxburgh L. A synthetic niche for nephron progenitor cells. Dev Cell. 2015;34(2):229–41.

101. Li Z, Araoka T, Wu J, Liao HK, Li M, Lazo M, et al. 3D culture supports long-term expansion of mouse and human nephrogenic progenitors. Cell Stem Cell. 2016;19(4):516–29.

102. Tanigawa S, Taguchi A, Sharma N, Perantoni AO, Nishinakamura R. Selective in vitro propagation of nephron progenitors derived from embryos and pluripotent stem cells. Cell Rep. 2016;15(4):801–13.

103. Tanigawa S, Naganuma H, Kaku Y, Era T, Sakuma T, Yamamoto T, et al. Activin is superior to BMP7 for efficient maintenance of human iPSC-derived nephron progenitors. Stem Cell Rep. 2019;13(2):322–37.

104. Dudley AT, Godin RE, Robertson EJ. Interaction between FGF and BMP signaling pathways regulates development of metanephric mesenchyme. Genes Dev. 1999;13:1601–13.

105. Koseki C, Herzlinger D, Al-Awqati Q. Apoptosis in metanephric development. J Cell Biol. 1992;119(5):1327–33.

106. Cerqueira DM, Bodnar AJ, Phua YL, Freer R, Hemker SL, Walensky LD, et al. Bim gene dosage is critical in modulating nephron progenitor survival in the absence of microRNAs during kidney development. FASEB J. 2017;31(8):3540–54.

107. Ho J, Pandey P, Schatton T, Sims-Lucas S, Khalid M, Frank MH, et al. The pro-apoptotic protein Bim is a microRNA target in kidney progenitors. J Am Soc Nephrol (JASN). 2011;22(6):1053–63.

108. Araki T, Saruta T, Okano H, Miura M. Caspase activity is required for nephrogenesis in the developing mouse metanephros. Exp Cell Res. 1999;248(2):423–9.

109. Nishimura H, Yerkes E, Hohenfellner K, Miyazaki Y, Ma J, Hunley TE, et al. Role of the angiotensin type 2 receptor gene in congenital anomalies of the kidney and urinary tract, CAKUT, of mice and men. Mol Cell. 1999;3:1–10.

110. Coles HSR, Burne JF, Raff MC. Large-scale normal cell death in the developing rat kidney and its reduction by epidermal growth factor. Development (Cambridge, England). 1993;117:777–84.

111. Winyard PJD, Nauta J, Lirenman DS, Hardman P, Sams VR, Risdon RA, et al. Deregulation of cell survival in cystic and dysplastic renal development. Kidney Int. 1996;49:135–46.

112. Volovelsky O, Nguyen T, Jarmas AE, Combes AN, Wilson SB, Little MH, et al. Hamartin regulates cessation of mouse nephrogenesis inde-

pendently of Mtor. Proc Natl Acad Sci U S A. 2018;115(23):5998–6003.

113. Chen S, Brunskill EW, Potter SS, Dexheimer PJ, Salomonis N, Aronow BJ, et al. Intrinsic age-dependent changes and cell-cell contacts regulate nephron progenitor lifespan. Dev Cell. 2015;35(1):49–62.

114. Yermalovich AV, Osborne JK, Sousa P, Han A, Kinney MA, Chen MJ, et al. Lin28 and let-7 regulate the timing of cessation of murine nephrogenesis. Nat Commun. 2019;10(1):168.

115. Karavanov AA, Karavanova I, Perantoni A, Dawid IB. Expression pattern of the rat Lim-1 homeobox gene suggests a dual role during kidney development. Int J Dev Biol. 1998;42:61–6.

116. Stewart CL, Kaspar P, Brunet LJ, Bhatt H, Gadi I, Kontgen F, et al. Blastocyst implantation depends on maternal expression of leukaemia inhibitory factor. Nature. 1992;359(6390):76–9.

117. Plisov SY, Yoshino K, Dove LF, Higinbotham KG, Rubin JS, Perantoni AO. TGF beta 2, LIF and FGF2 cooperate to induce nephrogenesis. Development (Cambridge, England). 2001;128(7):1045–57.

118. Sanford LP, Ormsby I, Gittenberger-de Groot AC, Sariola H, Friedman R, Boivin GP, et al. TGFb2 knockout mice have multiple developmental defects that are non-overlapping with other TGFb knockout phenotypes. Development (Cambridge, England). 1997;124:2659–70.

119. McPherron AC, Lawler AM, Lee SJ. Regulation of anterior/posterior patterning of the axial skeleton by growth/differentiation factor 11. Nat Genet. 1999;22(3):260–4.

120. Herzlinger D, Qiao J, Cohen D, Ramakrishna N, Brown AMC. Induction of kidney epithelial morphogenesis by cells expressing wnt-1. Dev Biol. 1994;166:815–8.

121. Kispert A, Vainio S, McMahon AP. Wnt-4 is a mesenchymal signal for epithelial transformation of metanephric mesenchyme in the developing kidney. Development (Cambridge, England). 1998;125:4225–34.

122. Yoshino K, Rubin JS, Higinbotham KG, Uren A, Anest V, Plisov SY, et al. Secreted Frizzled-related proteins can regulate metanephric development. Mech Dev. 2001;102(1–2):45–55.

123. Grieshammer U, Cebrian C, Ilagan R, Meyers E, Herzlinger D, Martin GR. FGF8 is required for cell survival at distinct stages of nephrogenesis and for regulation of gene expression in nascent nephrons. Development (Cambridge, England). 2005;132(17):3847–57.

124. Perantoni AO, Timofeeva O, Naillat F, Richman C, Pajni-Underwood S, Wilson C, et al. Inactivation of FGF8 in early mesoderm reveals an essential role in kidney development. Development (Cambridge, England). 2005;132(17):3859–71.

125. Goodwin K, Nelson CM. Branching morphogenesis. Development (Cambridge, England). 2020;147(10):dev184499.

126. Hu MC, Rosenblum ND. Genetic regulation of branching morphogenesis: lessons learned from loss-of-function phenotypes. Pediatr Res. 2003;54(4):433–8.

127. Sainio K, Suvanto P, Davies J, Wartiovaara J, Wartiovaara K, Saarma M, et al. Glial-cell-line-derived neurotrophic factor is required for bud initiation from ureteric epithelium. Development (Cambridge, England). 1997;124(20):4077–87.

128. Schuchardt A, D'Agati V, Larsson-Blomberg L, Costantini F, Pachnis V. Defects in the kidney and enteric nervous system of mice lacking the tyrosine kinase receptor Ret. Nature. 1994;367(6461):380–3.

129. Enomoto H, Araki T, Jackman A, Heuckeroth RO, Snider WD, Johnson EM Jr, et al. GFR alpha1-deficient mice have deficits in the enteric nervous system and kidneys. Neuron. 1998;21(2):317–24.

130. Pichel JG, Shen L, Sheng HZ, Granholm AC, Drago J, Grinberg A, et al. Defects in enteric innervation and kidney development in mice lacking GDNF. Nature. 1996;382(6586):73–6.

131. Sánchez MP, Silos-Santiago I, Frisén J, He B, Lira SA, Barbacid M. Renal agenesis and the absence of enteric neurons in mice lacking GDNF. Nature. 1996;382(6586):70–3.

132. Schuchardt A, D'Agati V, Pachnis V, Costantini F. Renal agenesis and hypodysplasia in ret-k-mutant mice result from defects in ureteric bud development. Development (Cambridge, England). 1996;122(6):1919–29.

133. Cacalano G, Fariñas I, Wang LC, Hagler K, Forgie A, Moore M, et al. GFRalpha1 is an essential receptor component for GDNF in the developing nervous system and kidney. Neuron. 1998;21(1):53–62.

134. Jain S, Encinas M, Johnson EM Jr, Milbrandt J. Critical and distinct roles for key RET tyrosine docking sites in renal development. Genes Dev. 2006;20(3):321–33.

135. Jain S, Knoten A, Hoshi M, Wang H, Vohra B, Heuckeroth RO, et al. Organotypic specificity of key RET adaptor-docking sites in the pathogenesis of neurocristopathies and renal malformations in mice. J Clin Invest. 2010;120(3):778–90.

136. Bullock SL, Fletcher JM, Beddington RS, Wilson VA. Renal agenesis in mice homozygous for a gene trap mutation in the gene encoding heparan sulfate 2-sulfotransferase. Genes Dev. 1998;12(12):1894–906.

137. Müller U, Wang D, Denda S, Meneses JJ, Pedersen RA, Reichardt LF. Integrin alpha8beta1 is critically important for epithelial-mesenchymal interactions during kidney morphogenesis. Cell. 1997;88(5):603–13.

138. Lu BC, Cebrian C, Chi X, Kuure S, Kuo R, Bates CM, et al. Etv4 and Etv5 are required downstream of GDNF and Ret for kidney branching morphogenesis. Nat Genet. 2009;41(12):1295–302.

139. Desgrange A, Heliot C, Skovorodkin I, Akram SU, Heikkilä J, Ronkainen V-P, et al. HNF1B controls epithelial organization and cell polarity during

140. Lokmane L, Heliot C, Garcia-Villalba P, Fabre M, Cereghini S. vHNF1 functions in distinct regulatory circuits to control ureteric bud branching and early nephrogenesis. Development (Cambridge, England). 2010;137(2):347–57.

ureteric bud branching and collecting duct morphogenesis. Development (Cambridge, England). 2017;144(24):4704–19.

141. Towers PR, Woolf AS, Hardman P. Glial cell line-derived neurotrophic factor stimulates ureteric bud outgrowth and enhances survival of ureteric bud cells in vitro. Exp Nephrol. 1998;6(4):337–51.

142. Woolf AS, Winyard PJ. Molecular mechanisms of human embryogenesis: developmental pathogenesis of renal tract malformations. Pediatr Dev Pathol. 2002;5(2):108–29.

143. Mackie GG, Stephens FD. Duplex kidneys: a correlation of renal dysplasia with position of the ureteral orifice. J Urol. 1975;114(2):274–80.

144. Miyazaki Y, Oshima K, Fogo A, Hogan BL, Ichikawa I. Bone morphogenetic protein 4 regulates the budding site and elongation of the mouse ureter. J Clin Invest. 2000;105(7):863–73.

145. Grieshammer U, Le M, Plump AS, Wang F, Tessier-Lavigne M, Martin GR. SLIT2-mediated ROBO2 signaling restricts kidney induction to a single site. Dev Cell. 2004;6(5):709–17.

146. Kume T, Deng K, Hogan BL. Murine forkhead/winged helix genes Foxc1 (Mf1) and Foxc2 (Mfh1) are required for the early organogenesis of the kidney and urinary tract. Development (Cambridge, England). 2000;127(7):1387–95.

147. Walker KA, Sims-Lucas S, Di Giovanni VE, Schaefer C, Sunseri WM, Novitskaya T, et al. Correction: deletion of fibroblast growth factor receptor 2 from the Peri-Wolffian duct stroma leads to ureteric induction abnormalities and vesicoureteral reflux. PLoS One. 2016;11(11):e0167191.

148. Hains DS, Sims-Lucas S, Carpenter A, Saha M, Murawski I, Kish K, et al. High incidence of vesicoureteral reflux in mice with Fgfr2 deletion in kidney mesenchyma. J Urol. 2010;183(5):2077–84.

149. Narla D, Slagle SB, Schaefer CM, Bushnell DS, Puri P, Bates CM. Loss of peri-Wolffian duct stromal Frs2alpha expression in mice leads to abnormal ureteric bud induction and vesicoureteral reflux. Pediatr Res. 2017;82(6):1022–9.

150. Anslow MJ, Bodnar AJ, Cerqueira DM, Bushnell D, Shrom BE, Sims-Lucas S, et al. Increased rates of vesicoureteral reflux in mice from deletion of Dicer in the peri-Wolffian duct stroma. Pediatr Res. 2020;88:382–90.

151. Yu J. miRNAs in mammalian ureteric bud development. Pediatr Nephrol (Berlin, Germany). 2014;29(4):745–9.

152. Chu JY, Sims-Lucas S, Bushnell DS, Bodnar AJ, Kreidberg JA, Ho J. Dicer function is required in the metanephric mesenchyme for early kidney development. Am J Physiol Renal Physiol. 2014;306(7):F764–72.

153. Yu OH, Murawski IJ, Myburgh DB, Gupta IR. Overexpression of RET leads to vesicoureteric reflux in mice. Am J Physiol Renal Physiol. 2004;287(6):F1123–30.

154. Murawski IJ, Myburgh DB, Favor J, Gupta IR. Vesico-ureteric reflux and urinary tract development in the Pax2 1Neu+/− mouse. Am J Physiol Renal Physiol. 2007;293(5):F1736–45.

155. Pachnis V, Mankoo B, Costantini F. Expression of the c-ret proto-oncogene during mouse embryogenesis. Development (Cambridge, England). 1993;119(4):1005–17.

156. Srinivas S, Wu Z, Chen CM, D'Agati V, Costantini F. Dominant effects of RET receptor misexpression and ligand-independent RET signaling on ureteric bud development. Development (Cambridge, England). 1999;126(7):1375–86.

157. Shakya R, Jho E-h, Kotka P, Wu Z, Kholodilov N, Burke R, et al. The role of GDNF in patterning the excretory system. Dev Biol. 2005;283(1):70–84.

158. Brophy PD, Ostrom L, Lang KM, Dressler GR. Regulation of ureteric bud outgrowth by Pax2-dependent activation of the glial derived neurotrophic factor gene. Development (Cambridge, England). 2001;128(23):4747–56.

159. Brodbeck S, Englert C. Genetic determination of nephrogenesis: the Pax/Eya/Six gene network. Pediatr Nephrol (Berlin, Germany). 2004;19(3):249–55.

160. Wellik DM, Hawkes PJ, Capecchi MR. Hox11 paralogous genes are essential for metanephric kidney induction. Genes Dev. 2002;16(11):1423–32.

161. Miyamoto N, Yoshida M, Kuratani S, Matsuo I, Aizawa S. Defects of urogenital development in mice lacking Emx2. Development (Cambridge, England). 1997;124(9):1653–64.

162. Brose K, Bland KS, Wang KH, Arnott D, Henzel W, Goodman CS, et al. Slit proteins bind Robo receptors and have an evolutionarily conserved role in repulsive axon guidance. Cell. 1999;96(6):795–806.

163. Piper M, Georgas K, Yamada T, Little M. Expression of the vertebrate Slit gene family and their putative receptors, the Robo genes, in the developing murine kidney. Mech Dev. 2000;94(1–2):213–7.

164. Wainwright EN, Wilhelm D, Combes AN, Little MH, Koopman P. ROBO2 restricts the nephrogenic field and regulates Wolffian duct-nephrogenic cord separation. Dev Biol. 2015;404(2):88–102.

165. Basson MA, Akbulut S, Watson-Johnson J, Simon R, Carroll TJ, Shakya R, et al. Sprouty1 is a critical regulator of GDNF/RET-mediated kidney induction. Dev Cell. 2005;8(2):229–39.

166. Basson MA, Watson-Johnson J, Shakya R, Akbulut S, Hyink D, Costantini FD, et al. Branching morphogenesis of the ureteric epithelium during kidney development is coordinated by the opposing functions of GDNF and Sprouty1. Dev Biol. 2006;299(2):466–77.

167. Vaquero M, Cuesta S, Anerillas C, Altés G, Ribera J, Basson MA, et al. Sprouty1 controls genitourinary

223. the mammalian nephron. Development (Cambridge, England). 2007;134:801–11.

224. Wang P, Pereira FA, Beasley D, Zheng H. Presenilins are required for the formation of comma- and S-shaped bodies during nephrogenesis. Development (Cambridge, England). 2003;130(20):5019–29.

225. Boyle SC, Kim M, Valerius MT, McMahon AP, Kopan R. Notch pathway activation can replace the requirement for Wnt4 and Wnt9b in mesenchymal-to-epithelial transition of nephron stem cells. Development (Cambridge, England). 2011;138(19):4245–54.

226. Marable SS, Chung E, Adam M, Potter SS, Park JS. Hnf4a deletion in the mouse kidney phenocopies Fanconi renotubular syndrome. JCI Insight. 2018;3(14):e97497.

227. Kreidberg JA. Podocyte differentiation and glomerulogenesis. J Am Soc Nephrol. 2003;14(3):806–14.

228. Robert B, St John PL, Hyink DP, Abrahamson DR. Evidence that embryonic kidney cells expressing flk-1 are intrinsic, vasculogenic angioblasts. Am J Phys. 1996;271(3 Pt 2):F744–53.

229. Nagata M, Nakayama K, Terada Y, Hoshi S, Watanabe T. Cell cycle regulation and differentiation in the human podocyte lineage. Am J Pathol. 1998;153(5):1511–20.

230. Garrod DR, Fleming S. Early expression of desmosomal components during kidney tubule morphogenesis in human and murine embryos. Development (Cambridge, England). 1990;108(2):313–21.

231. Pavenstadt H, Kriz W, Kretzler M. Cell biology of the glomerular podocyte. Physiol Rev. 2003;83(1):253–307.

232. Ekblom P. Formation of basement membranes in embryonic kidney: an immunohistological study. J Cell Biol. 1981;91:1–10.

233. Sariola H, Timpl R, von der Mark K, Mayne R, Fitch JM, Linsenmayer TF, et al. Dual origin of glomerular basement membrane. Dev Biol. 1984;101:86–96.

234. McCright B, Gao X, Shen L, Lozier J, Lan Y, Maguire M, et al. Defects in development of the kidney, heart and eye vasculature in mice homozygous for a hypomorphic Notch2 mutation. Development (Cambridge, England). 2001;128:491–502.

235. Tomar R, Mudumana SP, Pathak N, Hukriede NA, Drummond IA. osr1 is required for podocyte development downstream of wt1a. J Am Soc Nephrol (JASN). 2014;25(11):2539–45.

236. Drummond BE, Chambers BE, Wesselman HM, Ulrich MN, Gerlach GF, Kroeger PT, et al. *osr1* maintains renal progenitors and regulates podocyte development by promoting *wnt2ba* through antagonism of *hand2*. bioRxiv. 2020; https://doi.org/10.1101/2020.12.21.423845.

237. Sadl V, Jin F, Yu J, Cui S, Holmyard D, Quaggin S, et al. The mouse Kreisler (Krml1/MafB) segmentation gene is required for differentiation of glomerular visceral epithelial cells. Dev Biol. 2002;249(1):16–29.

238. Miner JH, Morello R, Andrews KL, Li C, Antignac C, Shaw AS, et al. Transcriptional induction of slit diaphragm genes by Lmx1b is required in podocyte differentiation. J Clin Invest. 2002;109(8):1065–72.

239. Quaggin SE, Schwartz L, Cui S, Igarashi P, Deimling J, Post M, et al. The basic-helix-loop-helix protein pod1 is critically important for kidney and lung organogenesis. Development (Cambridge, England). 1999;126:5771–83.

240. Nilsson D, Heglind M, Arani Z, Enerbäck S. Foxc2 is essential for podocyte function. Physiol Rep. 2019;7(9):e14083.

241. Dreyer SD, Zhou G, Baldini A, Winterpacht A, Zabel B, Cole W, et al. Mutations in LMX1B cause abnormal skeletal patterning and renal dysplasia in nail patella syndrome. Nat Genet. 1998;19:47–50.

242. Barbaux S, Niaudet P, Gubler M-C, Grünfeld J-P, Jaubert F, Kuttenn F, et al. Donor splice-site mutations in WT1 are responsible for Frasier syndrome. Nat Genet. 1997;17:467–70.

243. Klamt B, Koziell A, Poulat F, Wieacker P, Scambler P, Berta P, et al. Frasier syndrome is caused by defective alternative splicing of WT1 leading to an altered ratio of WT1+/-KTS splice isoforms. Hum Mol Genet. 1998;7:709–14.

244. Coppes MJ, Liefers GJ, Higuchi M, Zinn AB, Balfe JW, Williams BR. Inherited WT1 mutation in Denys-Drash syndrome. Cancer Res. 1992;52(21):6125–8.

245. Yang Y, Jeanpierre C, Dressler GR, Lacoste M, Niaudet P, Gubler MC. WT1 and PAX-2 podocyte expression in Denys-Drash syndrome and isolated diffuse mesangial sclerosis. Am J Pathol. 1999;154(1):181–92.

246. Gao F, Maiti S, Sun G, Ordonez NG, Udtha M, Deng JM, et al. The Wt1+/R394W mouse displays glomerulosclerosis and early-onset renal failure characteristic of human Denys-Drash syndrome. Mol Cell Biol. 2004;24(22):9899–910.

247. Patek CE, Little MH, Fleming S, Miles C, Charlieu JP, Clarke AR, et al. A zinc finger truncation of murine WT1 results in the characteristic urogenital abnormalities of Denys-Drash syndrome. Proc Natl Acad Sci U S A. 1999;96(6):2931–6.

248. Hammes A, Guo JK, Lutsch G, Leheste JR, Landrock D, Ziegler U, et al. Two splice variants of the Wilms' tumor 1 gene have distinct functions during sex determination and nephron formation. Cell. 2001;106(3):319–29.

249. Guo JK, Menke AL, Gubler MC, Clarke AR, Harrison D, Hammes A, et al. WT1 is a key regulator of podocyte function: reduced expression levels cause crescentic glomerulonephritis and mesangial sclerosis. Hum Mol Genet. 2002;11(6):651–9.

250. Kim SI, Lee S-Y, Wang Z, Ding Y, Haque N, Zhang J, et al. TGF-β-activated kinase 1 is crucial in podocyte differentiation and glomerular capillary formation. J Am Soc Nephrol (JASN). 2014;25(9):1966–78.

251. Barisoni L, Kriz W, Mundel P, D'Agati V. The dysregulated podocyte phenotype: a novel concept in the pathogenesis of collapsing idiopathic focal segmen-

251. tal glomerulosclerosis and HIV-associated nephropathy. J Am Soc Nephrol (JASN). 1999;10(1):51–61.

252. Sims-Lucas S, Schaefer C, Bushnell D, Ho J, Logar A, Prochownik E, et al. Endothelial progenitors exist within the kidney and lung mesenchyme. PLoS One. 2013;8(6):e65993.

253. Sequeira-Lopez MLS, Lin EE, Li M, Hu Y, Sigmund CD, Gomez RA. The earliest metanephric arteriolar progenitors and their role in kidney vascular development. Am J Phys Regul Integr Comp Phys. 2014;308(2):R138–R49.

254. Hyink DP, Tucker DC, St John PL, Leardkamolkarn V, Accavitti MA, Abrass CK, et al. Endogenous origin of glomerular endothelial and mesangial cells in grafts of embryonic kidneys. Am J Phys. 1996;270(5 Pt 2):F886–99.

255. Ricono JM, Xu YC, Arar M, Jin DC, Barnes JL, Abboud HE. Morphological insights into the origin of glomerular endothelial and mesangial cells and their precursors. J Histochem Cytochem. 2003;51(2):141–50.

256. Sariola H, Ekblom P, Lehtonen E, Saxen L. Differentiation and vascularization of the metanephric kidney grafted on the chorioallantoic membrane. Dev Biol. 1983;96(2):427–35.

257. Kitamoto Y, Tokunaga H, Tomita K. Vascular endothelial growth factor is an essential molecule for mouse kidney development: glomerulogenesis and nephrogenesis. J Clin Invest. 1997;99(10):2351–7.

258. Tufro A, Norwood VF, Carey RM, Gomez RA. Vascular endothelial growth factor induces nephrogenesis and vasculogenesis. J Am Soc Nephrol (JASN). 1999;10(10):2125–34.

259. Ferrari G, Cook BD, Terushkin V, Pintucci G, Mignatti P. Transforming growth factor-beta 1 (TGF-beta1) induces angiogenesis through vascular endothelial growth factor (VEGF)-mediated apoptosis. J Cell Physiol. 2009;219(2):449–58.

260. Choi ME, Ballermann BJ. Inhibition of capillary morphogenesis and associated apoptosis by dominant negative mutant transforming growth factor-beta receptors. J Biol Chem. 1995;270(36):21144–50.

261. Eremina V, Cui S, Gerber H, Ferrara N, Haigh J, Nagy A, et al. Vascular endothelial growth factor a signaling in the podocyte-endothelial compartment is required for mesangial cell migration and survival. J Am Soc Nephrol (JASN). 2006;17(3):724–35.

262. Eremina V, Sood M, Haigh J, Nagy A, Lajoie G, Ferrara N, et al. Glomerular-specific alterations of VEGF-A expression lead to distinct congenital and acquired renal diseases. J Clin Invest. 2003;111(5):707–16.

263. Lindahl P, Hellström M, Kalén M, Karlsson L, Pekny M, Pekna M, et al. Paracrine PDGF-B/PDGF-Rß signaling controls mesangial cell development in kidney glomeruli. Development (Cambridge, England). 1998;125:3313–22.

264. Leveen P, Pekny M, Gebre-Medhin S, Swolin B, Larsson E, Betsholtz C. Mice deficient for PDGF B show renal, cardiovascular, and hematological abnormalities. Genes Dev. 1994;8:1875–87.

265. Soriano P. Abnormal kidney development and hematological disorders in PDGF ß-receptor mutant mice. Genes Dev. 1994;8:1888–96.

266. Oka M, Medrano S, Sequeira-López MLS, Gómez RA. Chronic stimulation of renin cells leads to vascular pathology. Hypertension. 2017;70(1):119–28.

267. Takahashi N, Lopez ML, Cowhig JE Jr, Taylor MA, Hatada T, Riggs E, et al. Ren1c homozygous null mice are hypotensive and polyuric, but heterozygotes are indistinguishable from wild-type. J Am Soc Nephrol (JASN). 2005;16(1):125–32.

268. Gomez RA, Belyea B, Medrano S, Pentz ES, Sequeira-Lopez ML. Fate and plasticity of renin precursors in development and disease. Pediatr Nephrol (Berlin, Germany). 2014;29(4):721–6.

269. Makhanova N, Lee G, Takahashi N, Sequeira Lopez ML, Gomez RA, Kim HS, et al. Kidney function in mice lacking aldosterone. Am J Physiol Renal Physiol. 2006;290(1):F61–9.

270. Yosypiv IV, Sequeira-Lopez MLS, Song R, De Goes MA. Stromal prorenin receptor is critical for normal kidney development. Am J Physiol Regul Integr Comp Physiol. 2019;316(5):R640–r50.

271. Satchell SC, Harper SJ, Tooke JE, Kerjaschki D, Saleem MA, Mathieson PW. Human podocytes express angiopoietin 1, a potential regulator of glomerular vascular endothelial growth factor. J Am Soc Nephrol (JASN). 2002;13(2):544–50.

272. Kolatsi-Joannou M, Li XZ, Suda T, Yuan HT, Woolf AS. Expression and potential role of angiopoietins and Tie-2 in early development of the mouse metanephros. Dev Dyn. 2001;222(1):120–6.

273. Woolf AS, Yuan HT. Angiopoietin growth factors and Tie receptor tyrosine kinases in renal vascular development. Pediatr Nephrol (Berlin, Germany). 2001;16(2):177–84.

274. Phua YL, Chu JY, Marrone AK, Bodnar AJ, Sims-Lucas S, Ho J. Renal stromal miRNAs are required for normal nephrogenesis and glomerular mesangial survival. Physiol Rep. 2015;3(10):e12537.

275. Sequeira-Lopez ML, Weatherford ET, Borges GR, Monteagudo MC, Pentz ES, Harfe BD, et al. The microRNA-processing enzyme dicer maintains juxtaglomerular cells. J Am Soc Nephrol (JASN). 2010;21(3):460–7.

276. Lin EE, Sequeira-Lopez ML, Gomez RA. RBP-J in FOXD1+ renal stromal progenitors is crucial for the proper development and assembly of the kidney vasculature and glomerular mesangial cells. Am J Physiol Renal Physiol. 2014;306(2):F249–58.

277. Boyle SC, Liu Z, Kopan R. Notch signaling is required for the formation of mesangial cells from a stromal mesenchyme precursor during kidney development. Development (Cambridge, England). 2014;141(2):346–54.

278. Pepper MS. Transforming growth factor-beta: vasculogenesis, angiogenesis, and vessel wall integrity. Cytokine Growth Factor Rev. 1997;8(1):21–43.

279. Merwin JR, Anderson JM, Kocher O, Van Itallie CM, Madri JA. Transforming growth factor beta 1 modulates extracellular matrix organization and cell-cell junctional complex formation during in vitro angiogenesis. J Cell Physiol. 1990;142(1):117–28.

280. Enenstein J, Waleh NS, Kramer RH. Basic FGF and TGF-beta differentially modulate integrin expression of human microvascular endothelial cells. Exp Cell Res. 1992;203(2):499–503.

281. Takabatake Y, Sugiyama T, Kohara H, Matsusaka T, Kurihara H, Koni PA, et al. The CXCL12 (SDF-1)/CXCR4 axis is essential for the development of renal vasculature. J Am Soc Nephrol (JASN). 2009;20(8):1714–23.

282. Gerety SS, Wang HU, Chen ZF, Anderson DJ. Symmetrical mutant phenotypes of the receptor EphB4 and its specific transmembrane ligand ephrin-B2 in cardiovascular development. Mol Cell. 1999;4(3):403–14.

283. Takahashi T, Takahashi K, Gerety S, Wang H, Anderson DJ, Daniel TO. Temporally compartmentalized expression of ephrin-B2 during renal glomerular development. J Am Soc Nephrol (JASN). 2001;12(12):2673–82.

284. Foo SS, Turner CJ, Adams S, Compagni A, Aubyn D, Kogata N, et al. Ephrin-B2 controls cell motility and adhesion during blood-vessel-wall assembly. Cell. 2006;124(1):161–73.

285. Reidy KJ, Villegas G, Teichman J, Veron D, Shen W, Jimenez J, et al. Semaphorin3a regulates endothelial cell number and podocyte differentiation during glomerular development. Development (Cambridge, England). 2009;136(23):3979–89.

286. Miner JH, Sanes JR. Collagen IV alpha 3, alpha 4, and alpha 5 chains in rodent basal laminae: sequence, distribution, association with laminins, and developmental switches. J Cell Biol. 1994;127(3):879–91.

287. Miner JH, Li C. Defective glomerulogenesis in the absence of laminin alpha5 demonstrates a developmental role for the kidney glomerular basement membrane. Dev Biol. 2000;217(2):278–89.

288. Miner JH, Sanes JR. Molecular and functional defects in kidneys of mice lacking collagen alpha 3(IV): implications for Alport syndrome. J Cell Biol. 1996;135(5):1403–13.

289. Noakes PG, Miner JH, Gautam M, Cunningham JM, Sanes JR, Merlie JP. The renal glomerulus of mice lacking s-laminin/laminin ß2: nephrosis despite molecular compensation by laminin ß1. Nat Genet. 1995;10:400–6.

290. Cebrian C, Borodo K, Charles N, Herzlinger DA. Morphometric index of the developing murine kidney. Dev Dyn. 2004;231(3):601–8.

291. Al-Awqati Q, Goldberg MR. Architectural patterns in branching morphogenesis in the kidney. Kidney Int. 1998;54:1832–42.

292. Bard J. A new role for the stromal cells in kidney development. BioEssays. 1996;18(9):705–7.

293. Loughna S, Landels E, Woolf AS. Growth factor control of developing kidney endothelial cells. Exp Nephrol. 1996;4(2):112–8.

294. Ohuchi H, Hori Y, Yamasaki M, Harada H, Sekine K, Kato S, et al. FGF10 acts as a major ligand for FGF receptor 2 IIIb in mouse multi-organ development. Biochem Biophys Res Commun. 2000;277:643–9.

295. Bonneh-Barkay D, Shlissel M, Berman B, Shaoul E, Admon A, Vlodavsky I, et al. Identification of glypican as a dual modulator of the biological activity of fibroblast growth factors. J Biol Chem. 1997;272:12415–21.

296. Bernfield M, Hinkes MT, Gallo RL. Developmental expression of the syndecans: possible function and regulation. Development (Cambridge, England). 1993;(Suppl):205–12.

297. Davies J, Lyon M, Gallagher J, Garrod D. Sulphated proteoglycan is required for collecting duct growth and branching but not nephron formation during kidney development. Development (Cambridge, England). 1995;121:1507–17.

298. Kispert A, Vainio S, Shen L, Rowitch DH, McMahon AP. Proteoglycans are required for maintenance of Wnt-11 expression in the ureter tips. Development. 1996;122:3627–37.

299. Cano-Gauci DF, Song H, Yang H, McKerlie C, Choo B, Shi W, et al. Glypican-3-deficient mice exhibit developmental overgrowth and some of the renal abnormalities typical of Simpson-Golabi-Behmel syndrome. J Cell Biol. 1999;146:255–64.

300. Jackson SM, Nakato H, Sugiura M, Jannuzi A, Oakes R, Kaluza V, et al. Dally, a drosophila glypican, controls cellular responses to the TGF-ß-related morphogen, Dpp. Development (Cambridge, England). 1997;124:4113–20.

301. Tsuda M, Kamimura K, Nakato H, Archer M, Staatz W, Fox B, et al. The cell-surface proteoglycan *dally* regulates *wingless* signalling in Drosophila. Nature. 1999;400:276–80.

302. Yu J, Carroll TJ, Rajagopal J, Kobayashi A, Ren Q, McMahon AP. A Wnt7b-dependent pathway regulates the orientation of epithelial cell division and establishes the cortico-medullary axis of the mammalian kidney. Development (Cambridge, England). 2009;136(1):161–71.

303. Zhang Z, Pascuet E, Hueber P-A, Chu L, Bichet DG, Lee T-C, et al. Targeted inactivation of EGF receptor inhibits renal collecting duct development and function. J Am Soc Nephrol (JASN). 2010;21(4):573–8.

304. Zhang P, Liégeois NJ, Wong C, Finegold M, Thompson JC, Silverman A, et al. Altered cell differentiation and proliferation in mice lacking p57^{KIP2} indicates a role in Beckwith-Wiedemann syndrome. Nature. 1997;387:151–8.

305. Hatada I, Ohashi H, Fukushima Y, Kaneko Y, Inoue M, Komoto Y, et al. An imprinted gene p57^{KIP2} is

mutated in Beckwith-Wiedemann syndrome. Nat Genet. 1996;14:171–3.

306. Leighton PA, Ingram RS, Eggenschwiler J, Efstratiadis A, Tilghman SM. Disruption of imprinting caused by deletion of the H19 gene region in mice. Nature. 1995;375:34–9.

307. Caspary T, Cleary MA, Perlman EJ, Zhang P, Elledge SJ, Tilghman SM. Oppositely imprinted genes p57(Kip2) and Igf2 interact in a mouse model for Beckwith-Wiedemann syndrome. Genes Dev. 1999;13(23):3115–24.

308. Liu Y, Chattopadhyay N, Qin S, Szekeres C, Vasylyeva T, Mahoney ZX, et al. Coordinate integrin and c-Met signaling regulate Wnt gene expression during epithelial morphogenesis. Development (Cambridge, England). 2009;136(5):843–53.

309. Karner CM, Chirumamilla R, Aoki S, Igarashi P, Wallingford JB, Carroll TJ. Wnt9b signaling regulates planar cell polarity and kidney tubule morphogenesis. Nat Genet. 2009;41(7):793–9.

310. Nagalakshmi VK, Ren Q, Pugh MM, Valerius MT, McMahon AP, Yu J. Dicer regulates the development of nephrogenic and ureteric compartments in the mammalian kidney. Kidney Int. 2011;79(3):317–30.

311. Nagalakshmi VK, Lindner V, Wessels A, Yu J. microRNA-dependent temporal gene expression in the ureteric bud epithelium during mammalian kidney development. Dev Dyn. 2015;244(3):444–56.

312. Raatikainen-Ahokas A, Hytonen M, Tenhunen A, Sainio K, Sariola H. Bmp-4 affects the differentiation of metanephric mesenchyme and reveals an early anterior-posterior axis of the embryonic kidney. Dev Dyn. 2000;217:146–58.

313. Dewulf N, Verschueren K, Lonnoy O, Morén A, Grimsby S, Vande Spiegle K, et al. Distinct spatial and temporal expression patterns of two type 1 receptors for bone morphogenetic proteins during mouse embryogenesis. Endocrinology. 1995;136:2652–63.

314. Mamo TM, Wittern AB, Kleppa MJ, Bohnenpoll T, Weiss AC, Kispert A. BMP4 uses several different effector pathways to regulate proliferation and differentiation in the epithelial and mesenchymal tissue compartments of the developing mouse ureter. Hum Mol Genet. 2017;26(18):3553–63.

315. Tripathi P, Wang Y, Casey AM, Chen F. Absence of canonical Smad signaling in ureteral and bladder mesenchyme causes ureteropelvic junction obstruction. J Am Soc Nephrol (JASN). 2012;23(4):618–28.

316. Yan J, Zhang L, Xu J, Sultana N, Hu J, Cai X, et al. Smad4 regulates ureteral smooth muscle cell differentiation during mouse embryogenesis. PLoS One. 2014;9(8):e104503.

317. Yu J, Carroll TJ, McMahon AP. Sonic hedgehog regulates proliferation and differentiation of mesenchymal cells in the mouse metanephric kidney. Development (Cambridge, England). 2002;129(22):5301–12.

318. Caubit X, Lye CM, Martin E, Core N, Long DA, Vola C, et al. Teashirt 3 is necessary for ureteral

smooth muscle differentiation downstream of SHH and BMP4. Development (Cambridge, England). 2008;135(19):3301–10.

319. Cain JE, Islam E, Haxho F, Blake J, Rosenblum ND. GLI3 repressor controls functional development of the mouse ureter. J Clin Invest. 2011;121(3):1199–206.

320. Bose J, Grotewold L, Ruther U. Pallister-Hall syndrome phenotype in mice mutant for Gli3. Hum Mol Genet. 2002;11(9):1129–35.

321. Weiss AC, Bohnenpoll T, Kurz J, Blank P, Airik R, Lüdtke TH, et al. Delayed onset of smooth muscle cell differentiation leads to hydroureter formation in mice with conditional loss of the zinc finger transcription factor gene Gata2 in the ureteric mesenchyme. J Pathol. 2019;248(4):452–63.

322. Bohnenpoll T, Wittern AB, Mamo TM, Weiss AC, Rudat C, Kleppa MJ, et al. A SHH-FOXF1-BMP4 signaling axis regulating growth and differentiation of epithelial and mesenchymal tissues in ureter development. PLoS Genet. 2017;13(8):e1006951.

323. Niimura F, Labostky PA, Kakuchi J, Okubo S, Yoshida H, Oikawa T, et al. Gene targeting in mice reveals a requirement for angiotensin in the development and maintenance of kidney morphology and growth factor regulation. J Clin Invest. 1995;96:2947–54.

324. Miyazaki Y, Tsuchida S, Nishimura H, Pope JC IV, Harris RC, McKanna JM, et al. Angiotensin induces the urinary peristaltic machinery during the perinatal period. J Clin Invest. 1998;102:1489–97.

325. Vivante A, Kleppa MJ, Schulz J, Kohl S, Sharma A, Chen J, et al. Mutations in TBX18 cause dominant urinary tract malformations via transcriptional dysregulation of ureter development. Am J Hum Genet. 2015;97(2):291–301.

326. Aydoğdu N, Rudat C, Trowe MO, Kaiser M, Lüdtke TH, Taketo MM, et al. TBX2 and TBX3 act downstream of canonical WNT signaling in patterning and differentiation of the mouse ureteric mesenchyme. Development (Cambridge, England). 2018;145(23) https://doi.org/10.1242/dev.171827.

327. Liu J, Sun L, Shen Q, Wu X, Xu H. New congenital anomalies of the kidney and urinary tract and outcomes in Robo2 mutant mice with the inserted piggyBac transposon. BMC Nephrol. 2016;17(1):98.

328. Bohnenpoll T, Weiss AC, Labuhn M, Lüdtke TH, Trowe MO, Kispert A. Retinoic acid signaling maintains epithelial and mesenchymal progenitors in the developing mouse ureter. Sci Rep. 2017;7(1):14803.

329. Bartram MP, Hohne M, Dafinger C, Volker LA, Albersmeyer M, Heiss J, et al. Conditional loss of kidney microRNAs results in congenital anomalies of the kidney and urinary tract (CAKUT). J Mol Med (Berlin, Germany). 2013;91(6):739–48.

330. Humphreys BD, Lin SL, Kobayashi A, Hudson TE, Nowlin BT, Bonventre JV, et al. Fate tracing reveals the pericyte and not epithelial origin

of myofibroblasts in kidney fibrosis. Am J Pathol. 2010;176(1):85–97.

331. Hum S, Rymer C, Schaefer C, Bushnell D, Sims-Lucas S. Ablation of the renal stroma defines its critical role in nephron progenitor and vasculature patterning. PLoS One. 2014;9(2):e88400.

332. Lemley KV, Kriz W. Anatomy of the renal interstitium. Kidney Int. 1991;39(3):370–81.

333. Cullen-McEwen LA, Caruana G, Bertram JF. The where, what and why of the developing renal stroma. Nephron Exp Nephrol. 2005;99(1):e1–8.

334. Quaggin SE, Vanden Heuvel GB, Igarashi P. Pod-1, a mesoderm-specific basic-helix-loop-helix protein expressed in mesenchymal and glomerular epi-thelial cells in the developing kidney. Mech Dev. 1998;71:37–48.

335. Bagherie-Lachidan M, Reginensi A, Pan Q, Zaveri HP, Scott DA, Blencowe BJ, et al. Stromal Fat4 acts non-autonomously with Dchs1/2 to restrict the nephron progenitor pool. Development (Cambridge, England). 2015;142(15):2564–73.

336. Drake KA, Chaney CP, Das A, Roy P, Kwartler CS, Rakheja D, et al. Stromal beta-catenin activation impacts nephron progenitor differentiation in the developing kidney and may contribute to Wilms tumor. Development (Cambridge, England). 2020;147(21) https://doi.org/10.1242/dev.189597.

Disorders of Kidney Formation

8

Norman D. Rosenblum and Indra R. Gupta

Introduction

Congenital anomalies of the kidneys and urinary tract, otherwise known as CAKUT, are classical disorders of development that are the most common cause of renal failure in children [1–3]. These disorders encompass a spectrum of entities including renal agenesis, renal hypodysplasia (RHD), multicystic kidney dysplasia, duplex renal collecting systems, ureteropelvic junction obstruction (UPJO), ureterovesical junction obstruction, megaureter, posterior urethral valves and vesicoureteral reflux (VUR). While congenital disorders like autosomal recessive and autosomal dominant polycystic kidney disease (PKD), nephronophthisis, and heritable nephrotic syndrome could also be considered as disorders of kidney formation, these generally occur later in kidney development as part of terminal cell dif-ferentiation events. However, some of the genes that cause nephronophthisis are also associated with CAKUT. In this chapter, we discuss disorders that arise during the early inductive events that lead to the formation of the kidneys and the urinary tracts. Both tissues arise from a common primordial tissue known as the mesonephric duct and thus, congenital kidney and urinary tract malformations commonly co-occur. In this chapter, we will focus on renal disorders encompassed within CAKUT and discuss their etiology, clinical manifestations and management. Other disorders within CAKUT with significant urinary tract pathology like UPJO, ureterovesical junction obstruction, megaureter, posterior urethral valves and VUR are discussed in other chapters.

Classification and Definition of Renal Malformations

Congenital malformations of the kidney can be defined at the macroscopic level by changes in size, shape, location, or number or microscopically by changes within specific lineages like the ureteric bud, the metanephric mesenchyme, or combinations of both [4]. In clinical practice, most congenital renal malformations are defined grossly using imaging methods like ultrasound and nuclear medicine scans. Sometimes renal tissue is obtained from biopsies or from nephrectomies, and in these cases, histological definitions

N. D. Rosenblum (✉)
Paediatrics, Physiology, and Laboratory Medicine and Pathobiology, Peter Gilgan Centre for Research and Learning, The Hospital for Sick Children, University of Toronto, Toronto, ON, Canada
e-mail: norman.rosenblum@sickkids.ca

I. R. Gupta
Department of Pediatrics, Montreal Children's Hospital, Research Institute of the McGill University Health Centre, McGill University, Montreal, QC, Canada
e-mail: indra.gupta.med@ssss.gouv.qc.ca;
indra.gupta@mcgill.ca

© The Author(s), under exclusive license to Springer Nature Switzerland AG 2023
F. Schaefer, L. A. Greenbaum (eds.), *Pediatric Kidney Disease*,
https://doi.org/10.1007/978-3-031-11665-0_8

of renal hypoplasia, renal dysplasia, and multicystic renal dysplasia can be utilized for classification. One can group congenital malformations of the kidney as follows:

Changes in size
- Renal hypoplasia
- Renal dysplasia

Changes in shape
- Multicystic dysplastic kidney (MCDK)
- Renal fusion

Changes in location
- Renal ectopia
- Renal fusion

Changes in number
- Renal duplication
- Renal agenesis

When induction events do not occur at the right time or location during embryogenesis, the kidneys may fail to form (agenesis, hypoplasia, dysplasia), the kidneys may form, but in the wrong location (ectopia ± hypoplasia/dysplasia), the kidneys may fail to migrate to the correct location (fusion ± hypoplasia/dysplasia) or there may be multiple induction events that arise (duplication). Malformations can be either unilateral or bilateral. Importantly, from animal models and human studies, disorders of renal formation are frequently observed with concurrent lower urinary tract malformations. In these cases, it is not clear if the impairment in induction of the kidney is primary or secondary to urinary tract obstruction. Renal agenesis refers to congenital absence of the kidney and ureter. Typically, renal malformations defined as renal hypoplasia or dysplasia are grossly small in size, defined as less than 2 SD below the mean for kidney length or weight [4–6]. Usually, renal hypoplasia or dysplasia is defined based on the presence of a small hyperechogenic kidney from ultrasound imaging [7]. Simple renal hypoplasia is defined as a small kidney with a reduced number of nephrons and normal architecture. Renal dysplasia is defined by the presence of malformed kidney tissue elements. Characteristic microscopic abnormalities include abnormal differentiation of mesenchymal and epithelial elements, a decreased number of nephrons, loss of corticomedullary differentiation and the presence of dysplastic elements including cartilage and bone (Fig. 8.1). As stated, dysplastic or hypoplastic kidneys are typically small, but can range in size and appear normal or even large due to the presence of multiple cysts or coincident urinary tract obstruction with hydronephrosis. The MCDK is an extreme form of renal dysplasia and is defined grossly as a non-reniform collection of cysts.

In addition to defects in renal formation that affect size, shape, location or number, and tissue patterning, congenital anomalies of the kidneys also encompass defects in the number of nephrons formed. Nephron number in the lower range of that normally observed, but not so low that it would result in renal insufficiency during childhood and/or adolescence, typically manifests in adulthood with hypertension and/or chronic kidney disease (CKD) [8–10].

8 Disorders of Kidney Formation

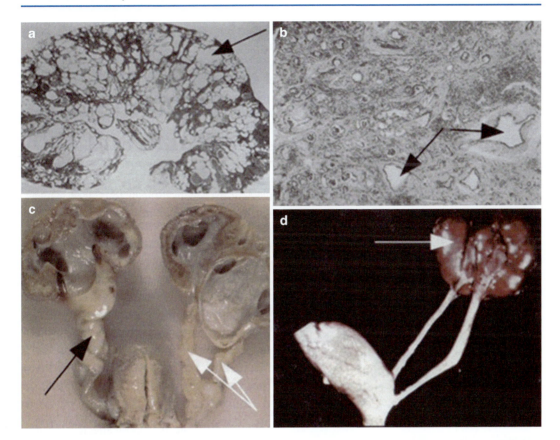

Fig. 8.1 Anatomical features of human renal and lower urinary tract malformations. (**a**) MCDK characterized by numerous cysts (arrow) distorting the renal architecture. (**b**) Dysplastic renal tissue demonstrating lack of recognizable nephron elements, dilated tubules, large amounts of stromal tissue and primitive ducts (arrows) characterized by epithelial tubules with fibromuscular collars. (**c**) Ureteral duplication (right, white arrows) and dilated ureter (left, black arrow) associated with a ureterocele. All ureters are obstructed at the level of the bladder and are associated with hydronephrosis. (**d**) Crossed fused ectopia with fused orthotopic and heterotopic kidneys (arrow)

Epidemiology and Longterm Outcomes of Renal Malformations

The prevalence of renal and urinary tract malformations is 0.3–17 per 1000 liveborn and stillborn infants [11, 12]. Due to their common embryonic origin from the mesonephric duct, lower urinary tract abnormalities are found in about 50% of patients with renal malformations and include VUR (25%), UPJO (11%), and ureterovesical junction obstruction (11%) [13, 14]. Renal malformations are commonly detected in the antenatal period and account for 20–30% of all anomalies detected [15]; upper urinary tract dilatation is the most frequent abnormality that is observed. All major organs are formed between the 4th and 8th week of gestation: the neural tube closes, the aortic arches undergo transformation, the cloacal membrane ruptures, and the kidneys begin to form. Renal malformations are therefore observed in association with non-renal malformations in about 30% of cases [12]. Indeed, there are over 100 multiorgan syndromes associated with renal and urinary tract malformations [16, 17] (Table 8.1).

Bilateral renal agenesis occurs in 1:3000–10,000 births and males are affected more often than females. Unilateral renal agenesis has been reported with a prevalence of 1:1000 autopsies. The incidence of unilateral hypoplasia/dysplasia is 1 in 3000–5000 births (1:3640 for the MCDK) compared to 1 in 10,000 for bilateral dysplasia

Table 8.1 Most frequent syndromes, chromosomal abnormalities and metabolic disorders with renal or urinary tract malformation

Syndromes

Beckwith-Wiedemann

Cerebro-oculo-renal

CHARGE

DiGeorge

Ectrodactyly, ectodermal dysplasia and cleft/lip palates

Ehlers Danlos

Fanconi pancytopenia syndrome

Fraser

Fryns

Meckel

Marfan

MURCS Association

Oculo-auriculo-vertebral (Goldenhar)

Oculo-facial-digital (OFD)

Pallister-Hall

Renal Cyst and Diabetes

Simpson-Golabi-Behmel (SGBS)

Tuberous sclerosis

Townes Brock

VATER

WAGR

Williams Beuren

Zelweger (cerebrohepatorenal)

Chromosomal abnormalities

Trisomy 21

Klinefelter

DiGeorge, 22q11

45, X0 (Turner)

(XXY) Kleinfelter

Tri 9 mosaic, Tri 13, Tri 18, del 4q, del 18q, dup3q, dup 10q

Triploidy

Metabolic disorders

Peroxysomal

Glycosylation defect

Mitochondriopathy

Glutaric aciduria type II

Carnitine palmitoyl transferase II deficiency

[18]. The male to female ratio for bilateral and unilateral renal hypo/dysplasia is 1.32:1 and 1.92:1, respectively [19]. Nine percent of first degree relatives of patients with bilateral renal agenesis or bilateral renal hypoplasia/dysplasia have some type of renal malformation [20]. The incidence of renal ectopia is 1 in 1000 from autopsies, while from clinical studies it is estimated to be less frequent at 1 in 10,000 patients [21]. Males and females are equally affected.

Renal ectopia is bilateral in 10% of cases; when unilateral, there is a slight predilection for the left side. The incidence of fusion anomalies is estimated to be about 1 in 600 infants [22].

While congenital renal malformations are relatively frequent birth defects, they become clinically evident at variable times during life and comprise a wide spectrum of outcomes ranging from no symptoms at all to CKD, which causes early mortality. The range in phenotypic severity makes it extremely difficult to counsel patients with certainty. Melo et al. reported a prevalence of CAKUT of 1.77 per 100 live births (524 cases of CAKUT in 29,653 newborns) in a tertiary care unit and a mortality rate of 24% in those affected (126/524) [11]. Amongst the 524 cases, risk factors for early mortality were the co-existence of non-renal and non-urinary tract organ disease, prematurity, low birth weight, oligohydramnios, and renal involvement (renal agenesis, RHD, multicystic renal dysplasia). Quirino et al. reported on the clinical course of 822 children with prenatally detected CAKUT that were followed for a median time of 43 months [23]. Their results demonstrate that most affected children do well: 29% of the children had urinary tract infection, 2.7% had hypertension, 6% had CKD, and 1.5% died during follow-up. Celedon et al. studied 176 children with chronic renal failure secondary to renal dysplasia, reflux nephropathy or urinary tract obstruction with a minimum of 5 years of follow-up [24]. They noted that patients with a urine albumin to creatinine ratio greater than 200 mg/mmol deteriorated faster compared to those with less than 50 mg/mmol (-6.5 mL/min/1.73 m^2 year vs. -1.5 mL/min/1.73 m^2 year change in estimate glomerular filtration rate [eGFR]). They also observed that those children with more than two febrile urinary tract infections deteriorated faster than those with fewer than two infections (median -3.5 mL/min/1.73 m^2 vs. -2 mL/min/1.73 m^2 year change in eGFR). Similar differences were noted for children with hypertension when compared to those without. Finally, they noted that the rate of decline in eGFR was greater during puberty (-4 mL/min/1.73 m^2/year vs. -1.9 mL/min/1.73 m^2/year change in eGFR). They noted no differences in deterioration of eGFR when comparing children with one or two functioning kidneys. In contrast, Sanna-Cherchi et al. examined the risk of progression to end-stage kidney disease (ESKD) in patients with CAKUT. They found that by 30 years of age, 58 out of 312 patients had initiated dialysis. They also noted that the risk for dialysis was significantly higher for patients with a solitary kidney [25]. The same group reported that patients with bilateral hypo-dysplasia, solitary kidney, or posterior urethral valves with RHD had a higher risk of dialysis requirement at 30 years when compared to patients with unilateral RHD or horseshoe kidney, and the risk was even higher if there was coexistence of VUR. Wuhl et al. compared patients with CAKUT to age-matched patients with other causes of renal failure who were receiving some form of renal replacement therapy (RRT) and registered within the European Dialysis and Transplant Association Registry [26]. Of 212,930 patients ranging in age from 0 to 75 years who commenced RRT, only 2.2% had renal failure secondary to CAKUT. Importantly, the median age for requirement of RRT was 31 years in the CAKUT cohort versus 61 years in the non-CAKUT cohort, suggesting that most children are likely to require dialysis and/or transplantation as adults. CAKUT was the most frequent cause of need for RRT in all pediatric age groups and peaked in incidence in the 15–19-year-old group.

Low birth weight and prematurity are associated with low nephron number and have therefore been studied as surrogate markers of low nephron number. The Helsinki Study followed approximately 20,000 people born between 1924 and 1944 until death or age 86 years and established that low birth weight was a risk factor for CKD in males, whereas prematurity (birth before 34 weeks of gestation) was a risk factor for CKD in females [9]. Similarly, Crump et al. demonstrated that preterm birth, defined as <37 weeks, and extreme preterm birth, defined as <28 weeks, were strongly associated with an increased risk of CKD in childhood and in adulthood [8]. Keller et al. demonstrated that low nephron number is a risk factor for hypertension in middle-aged adults compared with age-, sex-, and race-matched controls without hypertension [10].

Taken together, many questions remain in understanding the long-term outcome of CAKUT, but clearly most children are surviving into adulthood, and thus there is a need for adult nephrologists to understand these disorders.

Abnormal Molecular Signaling in the Malformed Kidney

Human renal development is complete by 34 weeks gestation [4]. Thus, by definition, renal malformation is a problem of disordered renal embryogenesis. The morphologic, cellular, and genetic events that underlie normal renal development are reviewed in Chap. 7. During human kidney development, two primordial tissues, the ureteric bud and the metanephric mesenchyme, undergo epithelial morphogenesis to form the final metanephric kidney [27]. The kidneys and the ureters arise from two epithelial tubes that extend along the length of the embryo, the mesonephric ducts. An epithelial swelling emerges from the mesonephric duct and is known as the ureteric bud. The ureteric bud invades the adjacent undifferentiated mesenchyme and induces the formation of the metanephric mesenchyme. Reciprocal signaling between the ureteric bud and the metanephric mesenchyme induces the ureteric bud to elongate and bifurcate in a process known as branching morphogenesis that ultimately gives rise to the collecting duct system of the adult kidney. The process of ureteric bud branching morphogenesis is critical for kidney development: each ureteric bud tip induces the adjacent ventrally located metanephric mesenchyme to undergo mesenchymal-to-epithelial transition and this determines the final number of nephrons formed *in utero*. Perturbations in ureteric bud outgrowth, branching morphogenesis and mesenchymal-to-epithelial transition are thought to underlie the majority of the malformations described in humans.

Failure of ureteric bud outgrowth and invasion of the metanephric blastema are events antecedent to renal agenesis or severe renal dysplasia.

Studies in the mouse embryo, a model of human renal development, have identified genes that control ureteric bud outgrowth, ureteric bud branching morphogenesis, and mesenchymal-to-epithelial transition. Some of these genes are mutated in human renal malformations also characterized by agenesis or severe dysplasia (reviewed by [28]). If the ureteric bud fails to emerge, the ureter and the kidney do not develop, while if the ureteric bud emerges from an abnormal location, the ureter that forms will not connect to the bladder properly and potentially result in obstruction and/or VUR with a malformed kidney. Indeed, a pathogenic role for abnormal ureteric bud outgrowth from the mesonephric duct was first hypothesized based on the clinical-pathological observation that abnormal insertion of the ureter into the lower urinary tract is frequently associated with a duplex kidney. Moreover, the renal parenchyma associated with the ureter with ectopic insertion into the bladder is frequently dysplastic [29]. The local environment of transcription factors and signalling pathways is therefore critical to the successful formation of an intact kidney and urinary tract. While a large number of transcription factors and ligand-receptor signalling pathways have been identified that regulate kidney development [28, 30], we will focus on the function of a few selected molecules that have been implicated in human congenital renal malformations: *Gdnf-Ret*, *EYA1*, *Six1*, *Sall1*, *Pax2*, *HNF1b*, *Shh*, and components of the renin-angiotensin-system (RAS).

The central ligand-receptor signalling pathway that leads to the outgrowth of the ureteric bud from the mesonephric duct is the GDNF-GFRα1-RET signalling pathway. Glial cell derived neurotrophic factor (GDNF) is a ligand expressed by the metanephric blastema that interacts with the tyrosine kinase receptor, RET, and its co-receptor GFRα1, both expressed on the surface of the mesonephric duct, to initiate outgrowth of the ureteric bud. Mutational inactivation of *Gdnf*, *Gfra1*, or *Ret* in mice causes bilateral renal agenesis due to failure of ureteric bud outgrowth, demonstrating the importance of this pathway [31–34]. Similarly, when GDNF-soaked beads are positioned adjacent to cultured murine mesonephric ducts, multiple ectopic ureteric buds emerge, demonstrating the potency of this signalling pathway [35]. The expression domain of GDNF is therefore tightly regulated in the nephrogenic mesenchyme and the metanephric mesenchyme.

A network of transcription factors promotes *Gdnf* expression: *Eya1*, *Six1*, *Sall1*, and *Pax2*, while *Foxc1* restricts *Gdnf* expression [36]. Another ligand-receptor complex that limits the domain of *Gdnf* expression is the secreted factor SLIT2 and its receptor ROBO2 [37]. *Slit2* is expressed in the mesonephric duct, while *Robo2* is expressed in the nephrogenic mesenchyme Bone morphogenetic protein 4 also negatively regulates the expression domain of *Gdnf* such that the ureteric bud emerges in the correct location [38].

EYA1 is expressed in metanephric mesenchymal cells in the same spatial and temporal pattern as GDNF. Mice with EYA1 deficiency demonstrate renal agenesis and failure of GDNF expression [39]. EYA1 functions in a molecular complex that includes SIX1 and together they translocate to the nucleus to regulate GDNF expression. Therefore, mutational inactivation of *Six1* in mice also results in renal agenesis or severe dysgenesis [40]. Like GDNF, SIX1 and EYA1, SALL1 is expressed in the metanephric mesenchyme prior to and during ureteric bud invasion. Mutational inactivation of *Sall1* in mice causes renal agenesis or severe dysgenesis and a marked decrease in GDNF expression [41]. Thus, EYA1, SIX1 and SALL1 function upstream of GDNF to positively regulate its expression, thereby controlling ureteric bud outgrowth.

PAX2 is another transcription factor that is expressed in the mesonephric duct, the ureteric bud and in metanephric blastema cells induced by ureteric bud branch tips [42]. Mice with a *Pax2* mutation identical in type to that found in humans with renal coloboma syndrome (RCS) exhibit decreased ureteric bud branching and renal hypoplasia. Investigation of the mechanisms controlling abnormal ureteric bud branching in a murine model of RCS (*Pax2^{1Neu}*) revealed that increased ureteric bud cell apoptosis decreases the number of ureteric bud branches and glomeruli formed. Remarkably, rescue of ureteric bud cell apoptosis normalizes the mutant phenotype [43]. *Pax2* appears to function upstream of *Gdnf* since in *Pax2* null mice no *Gdnf* expression is detected and the PAX2 protein can activate the *Gdnf* promoter [44].

PAX2 and HNF1β, another transcription factor, are co-expressed in the mesonephric duct and the ureteric bud lineage. Constitutive inactivation of HNF1β is embryonic-lethal in the mouse at gastrulation prior to the formation of the kidneys, but by using tetraploid and diploid embryo complementation, homozygous mutant embryos were able to proceed past gastrulation. The latter study demonstrated that HNF1β is critical for mesonephric duct integrity, ureteric bud branching morphogenesis, and early nephron formation [45]. Another group conditionally inactivated HNF1β in the proximal tubule, loop of Henle and collecting ducts and noted that null mice had cystic kidneys with cysts arising predominantly from collecting duct and loop of Henle segments [46]. The renal phenotype was severe, leading to death from renal failure in the newborn period. Importantly, cystic kidneys from null animals demonstrated downregulation of uromodulin, *Pkd2*, and *Pkhd1*, suggesting that HNF1β may regulate genes associated with cyst formation [46]. Compound heterozygous mice bearing null alleles for *Pax2* and *Hnf1β* show severe CAKUT phenotypes, including hypoplasia of the kidneys, caudal ectopic aborted ureteric buds, duplex kidneys, megaureters and hydronephrosis [47]. These phenotypes were much more severe than *Pax2* heterozygous null or *Hnf1β* heterozygous null mice, strongly suggesting that *Pax2* and *Hnf1β* genetically interact in a common kidney developmental pathway.

Sonic hedgehog (SHH) is a secreted protein that controls a variety of critical processes during embryogenesis. In mammals, SHH acts to control gene transcription via three members of the GLI family of transcription factors, GLI1, GLI2 and GLI3. A pathogenic role for truncated Gli3 was demonstrated in mice engineered such that the normal *GLI3* allele was replaced with the truncated isoform. These mice are characterized by renal agenesis or dysplasia similar to humans with Pallister Hall Syndrome (PHS) [48]. Subsequent analysis of renal embryogenesis in mice deficient in SHH suggests that the truncated form of GLI3 represses genes like *Pax2* and *Sall1* that are required for the initiation of renal development [49]. Loss of Hedgehog signalling has also been implicated in nonobstructive hydronephrosis and urinary pacemaker dysfunction in mice [50]. *Shh* is expressed in the epithelium of the ureter during embryonic development and signals to the developing ureteric mesenchyme. *Shh* deficiency results in lack of smooth muscle cell differentiation in the ureter and nonobstructive hydronephrosis [51]. Hedgehog signaling is also active in the embryonic metanephric mesenchyme; genetic deficiency of Hedgehog signaling in this spatial domain also results in nonobstructive hydronephrosis but by a different mechanism. In mice so affected, there is loss of pacemaker cell activity in the renal pelvis and ureter [50] The observation that constitutive expression of GLI3 repressor also causes nonobstructive hydronephrosis and that genetic deficiency of *Gli3* in mice with decreased Hedgehog rescues hydronephrosis demonstrates the critical role of GLI3 repressor downstream of Hedgehog signaling. Interestingly, some patients with Pallister Hall Syndrome manifest hydronephrosis, although the underlying mechanisms in these patients are unclear.

Analysis of mice with constitutive activation of Hedgehog signaling and human ureter tissues, implicates Hedgehog signaling in the pathogenesis of UPJO. Mice with deficiency of *Patched1*, a cell surface receptor that inhibits Hedgehog signaling, in renal progenitors that give rise to both nephrogenic and stromal cells are characterized by UPJO due to formation of an ectopic cluster of stromal cells that block the UPJ. Analysis of obstructing ureteric tissue in infants and children with congenital UPJO demonstrated upregulation of hedgehog signaling effectors and stromal genes, suggesting that increased hedgehog signaling may contribute to the pathogenesis of human UPJO, as well [52].

In postnatal renal physiology, the RAS plays a critical role in fluid and electrolyte homeostasis and in the control of blood pressure. Renin cleaves angiotensinogen (AGT) to generate angiotensin (Ang) I which is cleaved by angiotensin-converting enzyme (ACE) to yield Ang II. Ang II is the main effector peptide growth factor of the RAS and acts on two major receptors: AT1R and AT2R. The role of the RAS during kidney development appears to differ somewhat in humans versus rodents, but the metanephric kidney expresses all components of the pathway in both species. Ang is expressed in the ureteric bud lineage and the stromal mesenchyme, while renin is expressed by mesenchymal cells destined to form vascular precursors in the kidney. ACE is expressed slightly later during kidney development in differentiated mesenchymal structures including glomeruli, proximal tubules and collecting ducts. The receptors AT1R and AT2R are expressed in the ureteric bud lineage and in metanephric mesenchymal cells [53]. Mutations of *AGT*, *renin*, *ACE*, or *AT1R* all result in CAKUT phenotypes in the mouse that are characterized by renal malformations with hypoplasia of the medulla and the papillae and hydronephrosis [54]. Mice with mutations in *ATR2* also exhibit CAKUT, but a wider range of phenotypes is observed that includes renal hypo/dysplasia, duplicated collecting systems, VUR, and hydronephrosis [55]. Importantly, genetic inactivation of the RAS pathway in mice does not result in renal tubular dysgenesis (RTD) as observed in humans with similar mutations. It is postulated this may be due to differences between the species: in humans, RAS activity (renin and ANG II levels) peaks during fetal life while nephrogenesis is occurring, while in rodents, RAS activity peaks postnatally from weeks 2–6, when nephrogenesis has ceased. These temporal differences likely explain the lack of concordance between genetic mouse models and affected humans [56].

Ureteric bud branching and modelling of the lower urinary tract with its insertion into the bladder is also controlled by vitamin A and its signaling effectors [57, 58]. Expression of RET, the receptor for GDNF, is controlled by members of the retinoic acid receptor family of transcription factors that function in the vitamin A signaling pathway. These members, including RAR alpha and RAR beta2, are expressed in stromal cells surrounding *Ret*-expressing ureteric bud branch tips [58, 59]. Mice deficient in these receptors exhibit fewer ureteric bud branches and diminished expression of *Ret*. These observations are consistent with the finding that vitamin A deficiency during pregnancy causes renal hypoplasia in the rat fetus [60]. A similar observation has been noted in a human study where maternal vitamin A deficiency was associated with congenital renal malformation [61].

In summary, genetic and nutritional factors like vitamin A and folic acid [61–63] interact to control ureteric bud outgrowth, ureteric bud branching, nephrogenesis, and ureter formation. The number of nephrons is likely determined by a complex combination of factors including genetic variants, environmental events and stochastic factors. This could explain the variable number of nephrons in humans, ranging from approximately 230,000 to 1,800,000 [64]. Loss-of-function mutations in developmental genes can impair nephron formation *in utero* and depending on the magnitude of this effect, renal insufficiency may present at birth, childhood, adolescence or adulthood. Despite evidence in animals that depletion of protein, total calories or micronutrients causes renal hypoplasia, their contribution to human CAKUT remains unclear and an important area of future investigation.

Human Renal Malformations with a Defined Genetic Etiology

In humans, congenital renal malformations are more frequently sporadic than familial in occurrence. This may be due to the fact that infants with severe renal malformations have only recently survived; prior to the late 1970s, chronic dialysis was not offered as a therapy for children, and this continues to be the case in much of the developing world because of a lack of resources. Therefore, it is only in the past 30 years that children with congenital renal malformations have survived and been able to reproduce and potentially transmit deleterious gene mutations.

Therefore, congenital renal malformations appear as sporadic events over time. Genetic haploinsufficiency for many of the aforementioned transcription factors (*EYA1*, *SIX1*, *PAX2*, etc.) can result in a severe renal developmental phenotype, therefore *de novo* heterozygous mutations continue to arise. However, as reported by others, incomplete penetrance with variable expressivity is frequently observed in genetic studies of CAKUT, especially in relation to many of the transcription factors described previously [65]. Congenital renal malformations can occur in isolation, as part of CAKUT, or as part of a syndrome with organ malformations. Importantly, familial cases and extra-renal symptoms are sometimes unrecognized if carefully phenotyping is not performed. A careful evaluation of family history reveals a clustering of isolated or syndromic urinary tract and renal malformations in more than 10% of the cases [66]. Knowledge of the most frequent syndromes, a careful clinical examination and appropriately selected investigations are critical to the clinical approach to these disorders.

Mutations in more than 30 genes have been identified in children with renal development anomalies, generally as part of a multiorgan syndrome (Table 8.2). Some of these syndromes and their associated genes are described here or in some recent reviews [16, 17]. The most frequent syndromes in which renal malformations are encountered are listed in Tables 8.1 and 8.2. For a

Table 8.2 Human gene mutations exhibiting defects in renal morphogenesis

Primary disease	Gene(s)	Kidney phenotype	References
Alagille syndrome	*JAGGED1, NOTCH2*	Cystic dysplasia	[177–179]
Apert syndrome (overlaps with Pfeiffer syndrome and Crouzon syndrome)	*FGFR2, FGFR1*	Hydronephrosis, VUR	[180, 181]
Beckwith-Wiedemann syndrome	*CDKN1C(p57^{KIP2}), H19, LIT1, NSD1*	Medullary dysplasia, nephromegaly, collecting duct abnormalities, cysts, VUR, hydronephrosis, Wilms tumor	[182, 183]
Branchio-Oto-Renal (BOR) syndrome	*EYA1, SIX1, SIX5*	Unilateral or bilateral agenesis/dysplasia, hypoplasia, collecting system anomalies	[79, 80, 184]
Campomelic dysplasia	*SOX9*	Dysplasia, hydronephrosis	[185, 186]
Duane Radial Ray (Okihiro) syndrome	*SALL4*	UNL agenesis, VUR, malrotation, cross-fused ectopia, pelviectasis	[187]
Fraser syndrome	*FRAS1, GRIP1, FREM2, FREM1*	Agenesis, dysplasia, CAKUT	[188, 189–191]
Hypoparathyroidism, sensorineural deafness and renal anomalies (HDR) syndrome	*GATA3*	Dysplasia, VUR, CAKUT, mesangioproliferative glomerulonephritis	[192, 193]
Kallmann syndrome	*KAL1, FGFR1, FGF8, PROK2, PROK2R, CHD7, NELF, HS6ST1*	Agenesis	[133, 194]
Mammary-Ulnar syndrome	*TBX3*	Dysplasia	[195]
Pallister-Hall syndrome	*GLI3*	Dysplasia	[49, 196]
Renal-Coloboma syndrome	*PAX2*	Hypoplasia, vesicoureteral reflux	[109]
Renal tubular dysgenesis	RAS components, *REN, AGT, AGTR1, ACE*	Tubular dysplasia	[139]
Renal cysts and diabetes syndrome	*HNF1β*	Dysplasia, hypoplasia	[197]
Simpson-Golabi Behmel syndrome	*GPC3*	Medullary dysplasia	[198]
Smith Lemli Opitz syndrome	*DHCR7*	Agenesis, dysplasia	[199]
Townes-Brock syndrome	*SALL1*	Hypoplasia, dysplasia, VUR	[91]
Zellweger syndrome	*PEX1*	VUR, cystic dysplasia	[200]

complete list of syndromes featuring renal malformations, the reader is referred to McKusick's Online Mendelian Inheritance in Man.[1]

For most children with renal malformations, neither a syndrome nor a Mendelian pattern of inheritance is obvious. However, genetic studies incorporating chromosomal microarrays, targeted gene panels or whole exome sequencing (WES) have identified a genetic cause for the renal malformation in anywhere from 5% to 30% of cases [16]. One of the first such studies of 100 patients with RHD and renal insufficiency demonstrated that 15% had mutations in two transcription factors [65]: *TCF2* (HNF1β) (especially in the subset with kidney cysts) and *PAX2*. *EYA1* and *SALL1* mutations were found in single cases. Some of the mutations that were identified in these genes were *de novo* mutations explaining the sporadic appearance of RHD. Careful analysis of patients with *TCF2* and *PAX2* mutations revealed the presence of extrarenal symptoms in only half, supporting previous reports that *TCF2* and *PAX2* mutations can be responsible for isolated renal tract anomalies or at least CAKUT malformations with minimal extrarenal features [67, 68]. This study demonstrates that subtle extrarenal symptoms in syndromal RHD can easily be missed. Genetic testing in children with RHD should be preceded by a thorough clinical evaluation for extrarenal symptoms, including eye, ear, and metabolic anomalies. The presence of nonrenal anomalies increases the likelihood of detecting a specific genetic abnormality (Table 8.5). In addition, mutations in genes that are usually associated with syndromes can occur in patients with isolated RHD.

The GDNF/RET Signaling Pathway

The proto-oncogene *RET*, a tyrosine kinase receptor, and its ligand, GDNF, play a pivotal role during early nephrogenesis and enteric nervous system development. Activating *RET* mutations cause multiple endocrine neoplasia, whereas inactivating mutations lead to Hirschsprung disease. A number of human studies have demonstrated that patients with CAKUT have mutations in the RET/GDNF signaling pathway [69–72]. A study of 122 patients with CAKUT identified heterozygous deleterious sequence variants in *GDNF* or *RET* in 6/122 patients, 5%, while another group screened 749 families from all over the world and identified 3 families with heterozygous mutations in RET [69, 73]. Similar findings have been reported in studies of fetuses with bilateral or unilateral renal agenesis [70, 71].

Branchio-Oto-Renal Syndrome

The association of branchial (B), otic (O) and renal (R) anomalies was first described by Fraser and Melnick [74, 75]. Major diagnostic criteria consist of hearing loss (95%), branchial defects (49–69%), ear pits (83%) and renal anomalies (38–67%) [76, 77]. The association of these three major features defines the classical BOR syndrome (OMIM # 113650). Yet, many patients have only one or two of these major features in association with other minor features such as external ear anomalies, preauricular tags or other facial abnormalities (Table 8.3). Hearing loss can be conductive, sensorineural, or mixed.

The frequency of BOR syndrome has been estimated to be 1 in 40,000 births [78]. The transmission is autosomal dominant with incomplete penetrance and variable expressivity. Renal malformations include unilateral or bilateral renal agenesis, hypodysplasia as well as malformation of the lower urinary tract including VUR, pyeloureteral obstruction, and ureteral duplication. Different renal malformations can be observed in

Table 8.3 Major and minor criteria for the diagnosis of BOR syndrome

Major features	Minor features
Deafness	External ear anomalies
Branchial anomalies	Preauricular tags
Preauricular pits	Other facial anomalies
Renal malformations	Cataracts
	Lacrimal duct stenosis

[1] http://www.ncbi.nlm.nih.gov/.

the same family; moreover, some individuals have normal kidneys (BO syndrome, OMIM 120502). Other infrequent abnormalities have been described in patients with the BOR syndrome. These include aplasia of the lacrimal ducts, congenital cataracts and anterior segment anomalies [74, 75]. Characteristic temporal bone findings include cochlear hypoplasia (4/5 of normal size with only 2 turns), dilation of the vestibular aqueduct, bulbous internal auditory canals, deep posterior fossae, and acutely angled promontories [77].

Approximately 40% of patients with BOR syndrome have a mutation in *EYA1* [76]. Mutations in in *SIX1*, *SIX5*, and *SALL1* have also been identified in patients with BOR syndrome, but at lower frequencies [79–81]. Both EYA1 and SIX1 are co-expressed in the developing otic, branchial and renal tissue, where they function in a transcriptional complex that regulates cell proliferation and cell survival [82, 83]. EYA1 and SIX1 control the expression of PAX2 and GDNF in the metanephric mesenchyme [84]. The EYA1 protein contains a highly conserved region called the *eyes absent* homologous region encoded within exons 9–16, which is the site of most mutations identified to date.

A reasonable approach is to perform genetic analysis in families in which at least one member fulfils the criteria for classical BOR syndrome (Table 8.3). Investigations should include a family history, and examination of relatives to look for preauricular pits, lacrimal duct stenosis, and branchial fistulae and/or cysts. Hearing studies and renal ultrasound should be done in all first-degree relatives.

Molecular testing can confirm the diagnosis and provide genetic recurrence risk information to families. However, variability of the phenotype even with the same mutation does not permit accurate prediction of the disease severity. Within the same family, a given mutation may be associated with renal malformation in some individuals, but not in others. This discrepancy might be explained by stochastic factors that impact the formation of the kidneys or by other unlinked genetic events that may act in synergy with the EYA1 protein during nephrogenesis.

Townes-Brocks Syndrome and VATER/VACTERL Associations

Townes-Brocks syndrome (TBS) is an autosomal dominant malformation syndrome usually defined by a triad of anomalies including imperforate anus, dysplastic ears, and thumb malformations [85]. A wide spectrum of additional features includes renal malformations, congenital heart defects, hand and foot malformations, hearing loss, and eye anomalies [86, 87]. Intelligence is usually normal. REAR Syndrome (renal-ear-anal-radial) has also been used to describe this condition [88]. Its incidence is reported to be 1:250,000 live births [89]. The presentation of TBS is highly variable within and between affected families. Importantly, *SALL1*, is the only gene implicated in TBS and it encodes a C_2H_2 zinc finger transcription factor that is required for the normal development of the limbs, nervous system, ears, anus, heart and kidneys [90, 91].

The detection rate of *SALL1* mutations in patients with TBS appears to be higher when malformations of the hands, the ears, and the anus are present [92]. However genetic testing is further complicated by the fact that the phenotypic features of TBS can resemble other disorders like VACTERL association, Goldenhar syndrome, Oculo-Auriculo-Vertebral spectrum, Pallister-Hall syndrome and even BOR syndrome. TBS features overlap those seen in the VACTERL association (anal, radial and renal malformations). In contrast to VACTERL association, TBS is associated with ear anomalies and deafness and it is not characterized by tracheo-oesophageal fistula or vertebral anomalies.

VACTERL association is defined by the presence of at least three of the following congenital malformations: vertebral anomalies, anal atresia, cardiac defects, tracheo-esophageal defects, renal malformations, and limb anomalies [93]. It is reported to occur in 1:10,000–40,000 of all live births. Renal anomalies are reported in 50–80% of patients and include unilateral or bilateral renal agenesis, horseshoe kidney, cystic kidneys, and dysplastic kidneys; they can be accompanied by urinary tract and genital defects [93, 94]. Ninety percent of VACTERL cases appear to be sporadic with little evidence of heritability [93]. In a subset of patients there is evidence of heritability [93, 95, 96], and genes that interact with the Sonic Hedgehog pathway have been implicated [97, 98]. The presence of a single umbilical artery on ultrasound has been associated with a variety of congenital birth defects, including VACTERL syndrome [99]. It has been hypothesized that the single umbilical artery is a risk factor for a placental defect that may affect nutrient supply for multiple organs simultaneously during development [100].

An important diagnosis to consider in patients suspected to have VACTERL syndrome is Fanconi's anemia. Patients with Fanconi's anemia can phenocopy VACTERL syndrome, but also exhibit bone marrow failure manifest as pancytopenia. They can also develop malignancies like acute myelogenous leukemia secondary to their propensity for chromosomal instability manifest as spontaneous cytogenetic aberrations. Patients with Fanconi's anemia also frequently demonstrate skin pigmentation (café au lait spots), microcephaly, growth retardation and microphthalmia. There are at least nine different gene mutations implicated in Fanconi's anemia and they are inherited as X-linked or recessive disorders. It has been reported that approximately 5% of patients with confirmed Fanconi's anemia have features consistent with VACTERL syndrome [101]. Therefore, the diagnosis of Fanconi's anemia needs to be carefully considered in all patients with VACTERL syndrome and confirmed if needed by performing chromosomal breakage studies [101].

Renal-Coloboma Syndrome

Renal Coloboma Syndrome (RCS) (also named papillo-renal syndrome) is an autosomal dominant disorder characterized by the association of renal hypoplasia, VUR and optic nerve coloboma from a mutation in *PAX2* [102]. The prevalence of the syndrome is unknown, but approximately 100 families have been reported [103]. A wide range of renal malformations are observed in RCS. Oligomeganephronic hypoplasia, renal dysplasia and VUR are the most frequent malformations, but multicystic dysplasia [104] and UPJO have also been described [104]. Similarly, the ocular phenotype is extremely variable. The most common finding is an optic disc pit associated with vascular abnormalities and cilio-retinal arteries, with mild visual impairment limited to blind spot enlargement, the "morning glory" anomaly [105]. In other cases, the only ocular anomaly is optic nerve dysplasia with an abnormal vessel pattern and no functional consequence (Fig. 8.2). In contrast, a large coloboma of the

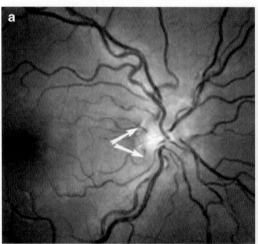
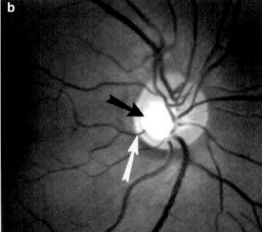

Fig. 8.2 Optic disc appearance in two patients with Renal Coloboma Syndrome and PAX2 mutations: (**a**) Characteristic features of optic disk coloboma with a deep temporal excavation (arrowheads). (**b**) The optic disk is dysplastic with thickening (arrow) and emergence of abnormal vessels ("morning glory anomaly")

optic nerve or of the choroid and retina and the morning glory anomaly can be responsible for a severe visual impairment [106]. Coloboma and the related anomalies are probably the consequence of an incomplete closure of the embryonic fissure of the optic cup. Other extrarenal manifestations can include sensorineural hearing loss, joint laxity, Arnold-Chiari malformation and seizures of unknown cause [107, 108]. In addition to its expression in the developing kidney and in the optic fissure, *PAX2* is also expressed in the hindbrain during its development. However, neurological symptoms are not usually present in RCS.

PAX2 is a transcription factor of the paired-box family of homeotic genes that is expressed in the mesonephros and in the metanephros during renal development. In 1995, Sanyanusin et al reported heterozygous mutations in two RCS families [109]. Since then, more than 30 mutations have been reported, most of them lying in exons 2–4 that encode the paired domain that binds to DNA or in exons 7–9 that encode the transactivation domain [103]. Other gene(s) are probably also responsible for this syndrome since *PAX2* mutations are not found in approximately 50% of RCS patients. Importantly the RCS phenotype is highly variable, even in patients harboring the same *PAX2* mutation, suggesting that modifier genes might be implicated.

Optic nerve coloboma occurs frequently as an isolated anomaly or as a feature of many other multiorgan syndromes such as the CHARGE association, the COACH syndrome and the acro-renal-ocular syndrome. As optic nerve coloboma and the related disorders can be easily misdiagnosed, it is likely that the prevalence of RCS is underestimated. It is wise to examine the fundus in every patient with RHD, and conversely to perform renal ultrasound and serum creatinine in every patient with optic nerve coloboma.

Even in the absence of optic nerve colobomas, mutations in *PAX2* are one of the more common genetic causes of RHD [65] and they also appear to be associated with low nephron number. Barua et al. described families diagnosed with FSGS anywhere from 7 to 68 years of age due to dominantly inherited mutations in *PAX2*. One patient

had a kidney biopsy sample that exhibited glomerulomegaly, which could be secondary to low nephron endowment at birth [110]. Some of the affected individuals had imaging studies that revealed other CAKUT phenotypes including small kidneys and hydronephrosis. Vivante et al. identified heterozygous mutations in *PAX2* in three families and one child with steroid-resistant nephrotic syndrome [111]. The patients developed their steroid-resistant nephrotic syndrome or FSGS either during infancy or in adolescence. Here again, the FSGS lesion could be secondary to low nephron endowment at birth.

Renal Cyst and Diabetes Syndrome

Mutations in the *TCF2* gene encoding the transcription factor HNF1β were initially found in patients with maturity onset diabetes of the young, type 5 (MODY5), an autosomal dominant disorder [112, 113]. Diabetes mellitus is present in approximately 60% of all the cases reported, usually occurs before 25 years of age, and is often associated with pancreatic atrophy [114–116]. In some patients, a subclinical deficiency of pancreatic exocrine functions has been demonstrated. Additional features have been described, including a wide spectrum of renal phenotypes (Table 8.4). The presence of cysts is the most consistent feature of the renal phenotype, leading

Table 8.4 Renal cyst and diabetes syndrome

Main features[a]
Fetal large hyperechoic kidneys
Renal hypodysplasia with cortical microcysts
Diabetes mellitus (MODY type 5)
Occasional features
Genital malformations
Female: vaginal aplasia, rudimentary or bicornuate uterus
Male: epididymal cysts, atresia of the vas deferens, asthenospermia, hypospadias
Hyperuricemia, rarely gout (reduced uric acid fraction excretion)
Hypomagnesemia
Moderate elevation of liver enzymes
Subclinical defect of exocrine pancreatic functions

[a] Age at onset and severity of these symptoms are highly variable

to the name, "Renal Cysts and Diabetes (RCAD) Syndrome". The cysts are usually cortical, bilateral, and small [68]. Mutations in the *TCF2* gene have also been found in association with a variety of isolated renal development disorders such as RHD, MCDKs, renal agenesis, horseshoe kidneys, UPJO as well as clubbing and tiny diverticula of the calyces [117–119]. The most specific finding when histology is available is the presence of cortical glomerular cysts with dilatation of the Bowman spaces (glomerulocystic dysplasia) [120]. Other nonspecific lesions such as cystic renal dysplasia, interstitial fibrosis or oligomeganephronia have also been reported. Antenatal presentations with enlarged hyperechoic kidneys or macroscopic cysts can occur [118, 121].

Various genital tract malformations have been reported mostly in females. These include vaginal aplasia, rudimentary uterus, bicornuate uterus, uterus didelphys and double vagina. In males, hypospadias, epididymal cysts, and agenesis of the vas deferens have been reported [114]. These genital anomalies have been described in approximately 10–15% of patients with *TCF2* mutations, but these malformations might be underestimated especially in paediatric reports. Reduced fractional excretion of uric acid (<15%) and moderate hyperuricemia is observed in some cases and is usually asymptomatic. The hyperuricemia is thought to reflect altered urate transport by the kidney and impaired glomerular filtration [114]. Serum hypomagnesemia has also been reported and this may be due to the fact that HNF1b regulates FXYD2 that is needed for distal tubule reabsorption of magnesium [122]. A similar mechanism may explain the altered urate transport observed in these patients since HNF1b can activate the promoter of URAT1 that regulates urate transport in the proximal tubule [123]. Moderate elevation of liver enzymes is a common finding, but severe hepatopathy has not been reported.

HNF1β is a homeobox-containing basic helix-turn-helix transcription factor, which is involved in the development of the pancreas, the kidneys, the liver and intestine. More than 50 mutations have been reported, most of which are located in the first four exons that encode the DNA-binding domain. In more than one-third of the cases, the gene is entirely deleted [68, 115, 123]. Such alterations are not detected by conventional amplification and screening methods. Importantly, deletions are infrequently transmitted by the parents but appear *de novo* in the proband. Analysis of *TCF2* can thus be recommended not only in patients with a family history of RCAD syndrome but also in cases with renal cysts when polycystic disease or nephronophthisis are unlikely. The presence of cortical bilateral cysts is probably the most typical finding. Reduced uric acid fractional excretion, elevation of liver enzymes, hypomagnesemia, glucose intolerance and abnormalities of the genital tract should be systemically sought and *TCF2* analyzed if one of these symptoms is present. As observed in other syndromes, phenotypic variability can be observed between families and also in family members with the same mutation, suggesting a role for environmental and genetic factors.

Longitudinal follow-up of genetically proven HNF1β nephropathy has been reported in a group of 62 children and adolescents, of whom 87% were diagnosed with bilateral renal dysplasia. Among these patients, 74% and 16% had visible bilateral or unilateral cysts, respectively, at the end of an average of 4 years of follow-up [124]. During this period, 28% of patients had an increase in cyst number, which was associated with a greater decline in GFR compared to patients without an increase in cyst number. Eight percent of patients developed ESKD at a median age of 15 months. Hypomagnesemia was present in 19 of 52 patients evaluated by a median age of 1 year, while recurrent hyperglycemia was observed in 4 of 50 evaluated patients. Increased uric acid was detected in 37% of patients. HNF1β mutations were varied in type, were familial or de novo, and were not correlated with phenotype. The issue of which patients should be screened for a mutation in *HNF1β* has been investigated in a cohort of 433 pediatric patients with known *HNF1β* status and CAKUT using a 17-item weighted score inclusive of abnormalities in renal, pancreatic, genital, electrolyte, and liver function as well as family history. A score of ≥8 was reported to have a sensitivity of 98.2%, specificity of 41.1%, positive predictive value of 19.8% and a negative predictive value 99.4% [125]. The possible utility of this scoring system, particularly in predicting absence of a HNF1β mutation, needs to be validated in other cohorts with HNF1β-associated disease.

Kallmann Syndrome

Kallmann syndrome (KS) is defined by the presence of hypogonadotropic hypogonadism and deficiency of the sense of smell (anosmia or hyposmia) [126]. Some affected individuals exhibit unilateral renal agenesis, cleft lip and/or palate, selective tooth agenesis, bimanual synkinesis and hearing impairment [127]. Other CAKUT phenotypes including duplex systems, hydronephrosis, and VUR have been rarely reported. Anosmia/hyposmia is related to the absence or hypoplasia of the olfactory bulbs and tracts. Hypogonadism is due to a deficiency in gonadotropin-releasing hormone (GnRH). The GnRH-synthesizing neurons migrate during development from the olfactory epithelium to the forebrain along the olfactory nerve pathway [128]. KS is genetically heterogeneous with at least 8 genes reported including *KAL1*, an X-chromosome encoded gene that gives rise to the extracellular matrix protein anosmin-1 [129], *FGF8* (Fibroblast growth factor 8) [130], *FGFR1* (Fibroblast Growth Factor Receptor 1) [131], *PROK2* (prokinectin-2) and *PROKR2* (prokinectin-2 receptor) [132], *CHD7, NELF,* and *HS6ST1* [133]. Chromodomain helicase DNA-binding protein 7 (CHD7) is a transcriptional regulator that binds to enhancer elements in the nucleus. It is implicated in CHARGE syndrome, that is characterized by choanal atresia, malformations of the heart, the inner ear, and the retina, and in Kallmann syndrome. In the largest study to date of 219 patients with Kallmann syndrome, mutations were most commonly observed in the FGF pathway (either FGF8 or FGFR1), in KAL1, in the PROK2/PROKR2 pathway and in CHD7 [133]. Importantly in this study, unilateral renal agenesis was only observed in patients with

KAL1 mutations (reported in 18%, 3/17), or in patients with no mutation in the above-mentioned 8 genes, where the frequency was similar at 17% (4/23). Patients with *KAL1* mutations are typically male since the disorder is X-linked and they demonstrate a much more severe reproductive phenotype compared to patients with other mutations with small testes, absent puberty, and micropenis. Females with KAL1 mutations typically present with partial pubertal development manifesting as spontaneous breast development in the absence of hormonal treatment. KAL1 is expressed in the developing human metanephric kidney at 11 weeks of gestation [134].

Renal Tubular Dysgenesis and Mutations of RAS System Elements

The differential diagnosis of oligohydramnios with neonatal renal failure includes a spectrum of diagnoses including bilateral renal dysplasia, posterior urethral valves, and PKD. All of these diagnoses are detectable and distinguishable on antenatal ultrasound imaging of the kidneys and the urinary tracts. The presence of normal kidneys on antenatal ultrasound in combination with oligo- or anhydramnios should strongly suggest the diagnosis of RTD [135]. RTD is a severe perinatal disorder characterized by absence or paucity of differentiated proximal tubules, early severe oligohydramnios, and perinatal death. The latter is usually due to pulmonary hypoplasia and skull ossification defects [136]. This condition has also been described in clinical conditions associated with renal ischemia, including the twin–twin transfusion syndrome, major cardiac malformations, severe liver diseases, fetal or infantile renal artery stenosis [137] and in fetuses that are exposed *in utero* to ACE inhibitors, Ang II receptor antagonists [138] or non-steroidal anti-inflammatory medications [135]. All of these environmental insults are postulated to lead to chronic hypoperfusion of the fetal kidneys with upregulation of the RAS. The absence or paucity of proximal tubules is believed to be secondary to chronic renal hypoperfusion [56]. Mutations in the genes which encode components of the RAS have been identified in some families [139]. Mutations in the *ACE* gene are seen in 65.5 % of cases, while mutations in the *renin (REN)* are observed in 20 % of cases. Mutations in *AGT* and in the *AGT type I receptor (ATR1)* occur much less frequently [56]. It has been suggested that if there is no expression of the renin protein on immunohistochemistry of the kidneys, then the *renin* gene should first be assessed. Similarly, the plasma renin activity should be measured in the newborn with suspected genetic RTD and if elevated, this should prompt an analysis of genes downstream of the *REN* gene [140].

CHD1L, CHD7 and CHARGE Syndrome

Chromodomain helicase DNA binding protein 1-like protein, CHD1L, belongs to the Snf2 family of helicase-related ATP-hydrolyzing proteins and contains a helicase-like region that is similar to other family members, such as CHD7 which is the major gene that causes CHARGE syndrome. CHARGE syndrome is characterized by Colobomas, Heart defects, choanal Atresia, Retarded growth and development, Genital hypoplasia, and Ear anomalies with deafness. CHARGE syndrome is associated with CAKUT phenotypes including horseshoe kidneys, renal agenesis, VUR and renal cysts [141]. Chromatin-remodelling and -modifying enzymes like CHD1L and CHD7 are predicted to play key roles in differentiation, development and tumour pathogenesis via effects on chromatin structure and accessibility. Brockeschmidt et al. screened 85 patients with CAKUT and identified 3 patients with heterozygous missense variants in CHD1L [142]. The same paper reported that CHD1L was expressed in early ureteric bud and comma- and S-shaped structures during human kidney development. In the postnatal human kidney, CHD1L was expressed in the cytoplasm of tubular cells in all nephron segments. Similarly, Hwang et al. reported that 5 out of 650 families had heterozygous mutations in CHD1L: the affected individuals had a spectrum of CAKUT phenotypes including renal dysplasia, posterior urethral

valves, UVJ obstruction and horseshoe kidneys [73]. It is not yet known if these patients will also be at greater risk for malignancies given that CHD1L is known to be an oncogene in hepatocellular carcinoma [143].

DSTYK and CAKUT

DSTYK is a dual serine-threonine and tyrosine protein kinase that is co-expressed with fibroblast growth factor receptors in the developing mouse and human kidney in both metanephric mesenchyme and ureteric bud cells. Sanna-Cherchi et al. discovered that 7/311 patients with CAKUT had heterozygous mutations in this gene [144]. The CAKUT phenotypes observed in these patients included UPJO, VUR, and RHD.

Copy Number Variants, CAKUT and Neuropsychiatric Disorders

Copy number variants are stretches of DNA that are larger than 1 kb in length with the potential to contribute to functional variation and disease. Rare CNVs have been implicated in neuropsychiatric and craniofacial syndromes, and in syndromes with CAKUT [145, 146]. Sanna-Cherchi et al. examined the burden of rare CNVs in individuals with congenital renal malformations and identified disease-causing CNVs and potentially pathogenic CNVs in 10% and 6%, respectively, of the 522 affected individuals analyzed. This burden of CNVs in CAKUT was compared to 0.2% in population controls [146]. A subsequent analysis of 2824 individuals with CAKUT highlighted an increased prevalence of large, rare, exonic CNVs compared to population-based controls [147]. In this study, genomic abnormalities were identified in 4% of patients with the majority within six pathogenic loci including chromosome 17q12 (RCAD Syndrome), 22q11.2 (DiGeorge Syndrome), 16p11.2, 1q21.1, 4p- (Wolf-Hirschhorn Syndrome), and 16p13.11. In addition, 90% of the CNVs associated with congenital renal malformations were previously reported to predispose to developmental delay or

8 Disorders of Kidney Formation

neuropsychiatric disease, suggesting that there are shared pathways implicated in renal and central nervous system development. Similarly, Handrigan et al. demonstrated that copy number variants at chromosome 16q24.2 are associated with autism spectrum disorder, intellectual disability, and congenital renal malformations [145].

Environmental Factors and Renal Malformations

As mentioned earlier in this chapter, genetic causes of CAKUT can be identified in at most 30% of all cases, which suggests that environmental factors or epigenetic factors explain the remaining cases (Table 8.5). Epigenetics refers to changes in gene expression rather than changes in the gene sequence itself and usually arises from DNA methylation and histone modifications that can silence or enhance gene expression. Maternal obesity and diabetes are major risk factors for CAKUT. From questionnaire data of 562 parents of children with CAKUT, maternal obesity was more highly associated with duplex kidneys and VUR, while maternal diabetes was particularly associated with posterior urethral

Table 8.5 Clinical indications to search for a renal anomaly

Exposure to teratogens
ACE inhibitors and Angiotensin receptor blockers
Alcohol
Alkylating agents
Cocaine
Folic acid antagonists
Vitamin A congeners
Maternal diabetes
Findings on physical examination
High imperforate or anteriorly positioned anus
Abnormal external genitalia
Supernumerary nipples
Preauricular pits and ear tags, cervical cysts or fistula
Hearing loss
Aniridia
Coloboma or optic disc dysplasia
Hemihypertrophy
Single umbilical artery
Other
Hyperglycemia

valves [148]. Dart et al. demonstrated that pregestational diabetes was significantly associated with CAKUT (odds ratio, 1.67; 95% confidence interval, 1.14–2.46), which implies a 67% increased chance of CAKUT in the children of mothers with pregestational diabetes compared to the general population (8.3 vs. 5.0 per 1000 births, respectively) [149]. These findings in humans are strongly supported by animal models in which the pregnant dam has diabetes. Animal models have also shown that maternal undernutrition and uteroplacental insufficiency are risk factors for impaired nephrogenesis and CAKUT. Maternal use of medications, alcohol and illicit drugs like cocaine are also risk factors for impaired nephrogenesis and CAKUT. Maternal use of RAS inhibitors such as ACE inhibitors, Ang II receptor blockers and direct renin inhibitors during pregnancy have been linked to an increased risk of fetopathy in humans. The majority of children manifest hyperechogenic and enlarged kidneys with proximal tubular dysplasia, thickening of arterial walls and multiple small cysts [150, 151]. Maternal supplementation with folate may also decrease the risk of CAKUT. CAKUT phenotypes have been observed in infants exposed to folic acid antagonists *in utero*, such as carbamazepine, phenytoin, primidone, phenobarbital or valproic acid, suggesting that folate is important for kidney and urinary tract development [63, 152]. Fertility treatment with in vitro fertilization or intrauterine semination are also risk factors for CAKUT, possibly through epigenetic effects on the developing zygote. Identifying the environmental risk factors that predispose to CAKUT needs to be addressed in future research.

Clinical Approach to Renal Malformation

The majority of renal malformations are now diagnosed antenatally, largely because of the widespread use and sensitivity of fetal ultrasound. The sensitivity of prenatal ultrasound screening for renal malformations is about 82% and the mean time at which these malformations are detected is 23 weeks gestation [12]. In general, urinary tract malformations detected antenatally are isolated and present as mild hydronephrosis with no therapeutic consequences. Parents should be reassured. In contrast, bilateral forms of renal agenesis, severe dysgenesis, bilateral ureteric obstruction, or obstruction of the bladder outlet or the urethra can cause severe oligohydramnios as early as 18 weeks. Because amniotic fluid is critical to lung development, oligohydramnios as early as the second trimester can result in lung hypoplasia, a potentially fatal disorder. The oligohydramnios sequence, termed Potter's syndrome, in its most severe form consists of a typical facial appearance characterized by epicanthal folds, recessed chin, posteriorly rotated, flattened ears and flattened nose, as well as decreased fetal movement, musculoskeletal features including clubfoot and clubhand, hip dislocation, joint contractures and pulmonary hypoplasia. The renal prognosis can be evaluated antenatally. Poor outcome can be predicted when there is severe oligohydramnios, and small and hyperechogenic kidneys. Normative data on kidney dimensions including kidney length from antenatal ultrasound imaging is available from the 15th week of gestation and can be used to determine if a kidney is small, suggesting some type of renal dysplasia, or increased in size, as observed in autosomal recessive PKD (ARPKD) or autosomal dominant PKD (ADPKD) [153]. Indeed, fetal renal hyperechogenicity with renal cysts suggests the fetus may have ARPKD, ADPKD or a mutation in *HNF1B*. If there is concurrent severe oligohydramnios, then ARPKD is the most likely diagnosis. Amniotic fluid analysis may be of help in some cases if the fetus is suspected to have a trisomy. Trisomy 21, 18, and 13 are all associated with CAKUT [154–156]. Antenatal diagnosis and assessment of the renal prognosis are important for consideration of early termination in cases of fatal (or eventually severe renal disease) and to prepare parents and medical staff for the likelihood of neonatal renal insufficiency. Other organ malformations should be sought carefully and, if detected, a karyotype should be done. Some authors have suggested that fetal urine analysis may be helpful to determine fetal renal prognosis and to decide on *in utero* therapy if congenital lower urinary tract obstruction is noted. Morris et al. performed a systematic review of the literature on fetal urine analysis and concluded that none of the analytes examined had sufficient accuracy to predict poor postnatal renal function [157].

Oligo/anhydramnios from CAKUT is associated with a high incidence of fetal death *in utero*, severe pulmonary hypoplasia, umbilical cord compression and perinatal asphyxia. The earlier that renal oligohydramnios (ROH) is identified in the pregnancy, the more severe the pulmonary hypoplasia [158, 159]. Pulmonary hypoplasia is defined as deficiency in the number of lung cells, airways and alveoli, leading to a reduced surface area for gas exchange. Postnatally, pulmonary hypoplasia is suspected in cases of ROH when there is respiratory failure with the need for high ventilatory support and the chest x-ray reveals a bell-shaped chest, an elevated diaphragm, and/or pneumomediastinum or pneumothorax. Ultrasound and MRI have been used to assess lung volumes antenatally, but there is no consensus on whether they are reliable predictors of pulmonary hypoplasia postnatally. Therefore, it remains difficult to predict pulmonary prognosis postnatally.

When isolated CAKUT or CAKUT with other organ defects is diagnosed in the fetus, genetic counseling and referral to a multidisciplinary team should be offered. An individualized approach that is in accordance with the parental wishes for more information is advised [160]. A screen for gross chromosomal abnormalities can be performed using a chromosomal microarray from the amniotic fluid (if less than 25 weeks) or from fetal blood (greater than 25 weeks or severe oligohydramnios). If the chromosomal microarray is normal, then a targeted gene panel or WES on the parents and the fetus could be considered. Given the incomplete penetrance and variable expressivity of many mutations implicated in CAKUT, it remains to be demonstrated whether targeted gene panels or WES are beneficial for antenatal decision-making.

The clinical presentation of renal malformation in the postnatal period is dependent on the amount of functioning renal mass, the presence of bilateral urinary tract obstruction and the occurrence of urinary tract infection. Bilateral renal agenesis or severe dysplasia is likely to present soon after birth with decreased renal function. This may be accompanied by oliguria. Alternatively, patients may present with a flank mass or an asymptomatic abnormality detected by renal imaging.

A detailed history and careful physical examination should be carried out on all infants with an antenatally detected renal malformation. An early (within 24 h of life) renal ultrasound is recommended for newborns with a history of oligohydramnios, progressive antenatal hydronephrosis, distended bladder on antenatal sonograms, and bilateral severe hydroureteronephrosis. In male infants, a distended bladder and bilateral hydroureteronephrosis may be secondary to posterior urethral valves, a condition which requires immediate renal imaging and clinical intervention. In general, unilateral anomalies do not require urgent investigation after birth. Renal ultrasound for unilateral hydronephrosis is not recommended within the first 72 h of life because urine output gradually increases over the first 24–48 h of life as renal plasma flow and glomerular filtration rate increase [161]. Thus, the degree of urinary tract dilatation can be underestimated during this period of transition.

A careful examination of the genitalia and the position of the anus are part of the initial assessment since CAKUT can occur in the context of cloacal malformations and with genital tract defects in females and males. The mesonephric duct gives rise to the developing kidneys, urinary tracts and the male genital tracts; therefore, a careful examination of the testes, the epididymis, and the ductus deferens is important. Congenital epididymal cysts are the most frequent anomaly noted in association with mesonephric duct anomalies and are usually asymptomatic. Other male genital duct anomalies that may occur in the context of CAKUT include an absent, ectopic or duplicated ductus deferens. Seminal vesicle cysts may also arise and typically present after puberty as pelvic pain or with urinary symptoms like dysuria, polyuria, or urinary retention [162].

Adjacent to the mesonephric ducts are the paired Müllerian or paramesonephric ducts that give rise to the fallopian tubes, the uterus, the cervix, and the upper two thirds of the vagina. Because Müllerian duct development is tightly linked to the growth and elongation of the mesonephric ducts, CAKUT is also observed with concurrent female Müllerian duct anomalies. Indeed, the Mayer-Rokitansky-Kuster-Hauser syndrome describes women with normal female external genitalia, but Müllerian duct anomalies that include aplasia of the uterus, the cervix, and the upper vagina. In a large cohort of 284 women with this syndrome, roughly 30% of them had associated CAKUT anomalies including renal agenesis, horseshoe kidney, ectopic kidney, and urinary tract defects including duplications [163]. Females with Müllerian ducts anomalies are typically discovered because of primary amenorrhea, dyspareunia, infertility, and/or obstetric complications [164]. In females with CAKUT and a suspected Müllerian duct anomaly, MRI imaging may be indicated to define the anatomical defect with better precision.

Clinical Approach to Specific Malformations

Unilateral Renal Agenesis

A diagnosis of unilateral renal agenesis depends on the certainty that a second kidney does not exist in the pelvis or some other ectopic location. Since absence of one kidney induces compensatory hypertrophy in the existing kidney, the presence of a large kidney on one side suggests the possibility of unilateral renal agenesis. Interestingly, compensatory hypertrophy has been observed to begin as early as 20 weeks of gestation: van Vuuren et al. examined 67 fetuses with a diagnosis of MCDK or unilateral renal agenesis and noted that 87% of the cases of MCDK and 100% of the cases of unilateral renal agenesis exhibited compensatory hypertrophy of the contralateral kidney with kidney length greater than the 95th percentile for gestational age [165]. Since unilateral agenesis is associated with contralateral urinary tract abnormalities including UPJO and VUR in 20–40% of the cases [166, 167], imaging of the contralateral side is suggested. Management of affected patients involves determining the functional status of the contralateral kidney. If the contralateral kidney is normal, the long-term renal functional outcome is usually excellent, although a recent study suggests that some patients may in fact have a poor long-term outcome and require dialysis [25]. It is therefore reasonable to propose that individuals with a single functioning kidney should have their blood pressure measured, urine tested for protein, and renal function measured periodically throughout life. While some have suggested that children with single kidneys should avoid contact/collision sports, at least one study suggests that kidney injuries occur much less frequently than other organ injuries, and thus sports restriction may not be indicated solely on the basis of having a single kidney [168].

Renal Hypoplasia

Unless associated with other malformations, renal hypoplasia can be asymptomatic. Unilateral hypoplasia is often discovered as an incidental finding during an abdominal sonogram or other imaging study. In contrast, patients with bilateral renal hypoplasia are at risk for decreased renal function and CKD.

Renal Dysplasia

The dysplastic kidney is generally smaller than normal. However, cystic elements can contribute to large kidney size, the most extreme example being the MCDK (see below). During the antenatal period, unilateral disease is likely to be discovered as an incidental finding. This may also be the case for bilateral renal dysplasia unless it is associated with oligohydramnios. After birth, bilateral renal dysplasia may limit GFR, causing renal failure that is usually progressive. Postnatal ultrasonography of the dysplastic kidney is characterized by small size, increased echogenicity, loss of corticomedullary differentiation and cortical cysts. Renal dysplasia is strongly associated with dilatation of the upper and lower urinary tract from VUR, posterior urethral valves, and/or other urinary tract obstruction [169]. Accordingly,

imaging of the lower urinary tract should be performed to determine whether these abnormalities are present.

Multicystic Dysplastic Kidney

The MCDK presents by ultrasonography as a large cystic non-reniform mass in the renal fossa and by palpation as a flank mass. The MCDK is nonfunctional, a condition that can be demonstrated by imaging with MAG3 or DTPA radionuclide scanning. The MCDK is usually unilateral. If bilateral, it is fatal. Complications of MCDK include hypertension (0.01–0.1%). Wilms tumour and renal cell carcinoma have also been described in MCDK, but the incidence of malignant complications is not significantly different from the general population [170]. In 25% of cases, the contralateral urinary tract is abnormal. Contralateral abnormalities can include rotational or positional anomalies, renal hypoplasia, VUR and UPJO [18]. Contralateral UPJO occurs in 5–10% of cases.

Gradual reduction in renal size and eventual resolution of the mass of the MCDK is common. At two years, an involution in size by ultrasound has been noted in up to 60% of the affected kidneys. Complete disappearance of the MCDK can occur in a minority of patients (3–4%) by the time of birth, and in 20–25% by two years. Increase in the size of MCDK can be seen in some cases. Several reports suggest that if the kidney length of the MCDK is less than 6.2 cm on the initial postnatal US, then complete resolution is likely to occur [171, 172]. The contralateral kidney usually shows compensatory hypertrophy by ultrasound evaluation. If the contralateral kidney does not show hypertrophy, it could be hypoplastic.

Management of patients with MCDK has shifted from routine nephrectomy in the past, to observation and medical therapy. Because of the risk of associated anomalies in the contralateral kidney, the possibility of VUR should be evaluated and blood pressure should be measured. For children with isolated MCDK and a contralateral kidney that is structurally normal with compensatory hypertrophy, the prognosis is excellent. While there exist no evidence-based guidelines for long-term follow-up of these children, a review of published evidence and expert opinion supports serial investigation by ultrasound and urinalysis within the first two years of life to monitor MCDK involution and contralateral renal growth, and then very intermittent examination of renal growth, blood pressure and urine protein excretion through the end of puberty [173]. For the small number of patients with unilateral MCDK who develop hypertension, estimated to be 5.4 out of 1000 children [170], medical therapy is usually effective. Nephrectomy may be curative in resistant cases.

Renal Ectopia

Normally, the kidneys lie on either side of the spine in the lumbar region and are located in the retroperitoneal renal fossae. Rapid caudal growth during embryogenesis results in migration of the developing kidney from the pelvis to the retroperitoneal renal fossa. With ascension, comes a 90° rotation from a horizontal to a vertical position with the renal hilum finally directed medially. Migration and rotation are complete by 8 weeks of gestation.

Simple congenital ectopy refers to a low-lying kidney that failed to ascend normally. It most commonly lies over the pelvic brim or in the pelvis and is termed a pelvic kidney. Less commonly, the kidney may lie on the contralateral side of the body, a state that is termed crossed ectopy without fusion. Clinical presentation can be asymptomatic or symptomatic. Asymptomatic presentation is when the ectopic kidney has been diagnosed coincidentally such as might occur during routine antenatal sonography. Symptomatic presentation occurs with urinary tract infections. Symptoms such as abdominal pain or fever may occur. On examination, an abdominal mass may be palpable. Other presenting features include hematuria, incontinence, renal insufficiency and hypertension [21]. A high incidence of urological abnormalities has been associated with renal ectopia. VUR is the most common, occurring in 20% of crossed renal ectopia and 30% of simple renal ectopia. In bilateral simple renal ectopia, there is a higher incidence of VUR, occurring in 70% of cases. Other associated urological abnormalities include contralateral renal dysplasia (4%), cryptorchidism (5%) and hypospadias (5%) [21]. Reduced renal function is commonly observed by radionuclide scan in the ectopic kidney. Female genital anomalies such as agenesis of the uterus and vagina [174] or unicornuate uterus [175] have also been associated with ectopic kidneys. Other anomalies described include adrenal, cardiac and skeletal anomalies. Clinical assessment should therefore include a careful physical examination for other anomalies. Renal ultrasonography will help with diagnosis and defining the underlying anatomy. A VCUG should be undertaken, particularly if there is hydronephrosis, given the risk of VUR and obstruction. A DMSA scan is also recommended to assess for differential renal function.

Renal Fusion

Renal fusion is defined as the fusion of two kidneys. The most common fusion anomaly is the horseshoe kidney, in which fusion occurs at one pole of each kidney, usually the lower pole. The fused kidney may lie in the midline (symmetric horseshoe kidney) or the fused part may lie lateral to the midline (asymmetric horseshoe kidney). In a crossed fused ectopic kidney, the kidney from one side has crossed the midline to fuse with the kidney on the other side. Fusion is thought to occur before the kidneys ascend from the pelvis to their normal dorsolumbar position. This is usually between the fourth to ninth week of gestation. As a result, fusion anomalies seldom assume the high position of normal kidneys. The blood supply may therefore come from vessels such as the iliac arteries. Abnormal rotation is also associated with early fusion of the developing kidneys. The pelvis of each kidney lies anteriorly and the ureter, therefore, traverses over the isthmus of a horseshoe kidney or the anterior surface of the fused kidney. Ureteric compression may occur due to external compression by a traversing aberrant artery. The majority of patients are asymptomatic. Some, however, develop obstruction which presents with loin pain, hematuria and may be associated with urinary tract infections due to urinary stasis or VUR. Renal calculi may occur in up to 20% of cases [176].

Other associated urological anomalies include ureteral duplication, ectopic ureter and retrocaval ureter. Genital anomalies such as bicornuate and/or septate uterus, hypospadias, and undescended testis have also been described. Associated non-renal anomalies involve the gastrointestinal tract (anorectal malformations such as imperforate anus, malrotation, and Meckel diverticulum) the central nervous system (neural tube defects), and the skeleton (rib defects, clubfoot, or congenital hip dislocation). Investigations should include static imaging (renal ultrasound) and functional imaging (DMSA scan) and a VCUG.

References

1. Annual report 2011. Available from: https://naprtcs.org/registries/annual-report.
2. Ardissino G, Dacco V, Testa S, Bonaudo R, Claris-Appiani A, Taioli E, et al. Epidemiology of chronic renal failure in children: data from the ItalKid project. Pediatrics. 2003;111(4 Pt 1):e382–7.
3. Harambat J, van Stralen KJ, Kim JJ, Tizard EJ. Epidemiology of chronic kidney disease in children. Pediatr Nephrol. 2012;27(3):363–73.
4. Potter EL. Normal and abnormal development of the kidney. Chicago: Year Book Medical Publishers; 1972.
5. Dinkel E, Ertel M, Dittrich M, Peters H, Berres M, Schulte-Wissermann H. Kidney size in childhood. Sonographical growth charts for kidney length and volume. Pediatr Radiol. 1985;15(1):38–43.
6. Han BK, Babcock DS. Sonographic measurements and appearance of normal kidneys in children. AJR Am J Roentgenol. 1985;145(3):611–6.
7. Montini G, Busutti M, Yalcinkaya F, Woolf AS, Weber S, European Society for Paediatric Nephrology Working Group on Congenital Anomalies of the Kidney, et al. A questionnaire survey of radiological diagnosis and management of renal dysplasia in children. J Nephrol. 2018;31(1):95–102.
8. Crump C, Sundquist J, Winkleby MA, Sundquist K. Preterm birth and risk of chronic kidney disease from childhood into mid-adulthood: national cohort study. BMJ. 2019;365:l1346.
9. Eriksson JG, Salonen MK, Kajantie E, Osmond C. Prenatal growth and CKD in older adults: longitudinal findings from the Helsinki Birth Cohort Study, 1924-1944. Am J Kidney Dis. 2018;71(1):20–6.
10. Keller G, Zimmer G, Mall G, Ritz E, Amann K. Nephron number in patients with primary hypertension. N Engl J Med. 2003;348(2):101–8.
11. Melo BF, Aguiar MB, Bouzada MC, Aguiar RL, Pereira AK, Paixao GM, et al. Early risk fac-

tors for neonatal mortality in CAKUT: analysis of 524 affected newborns. Pediatr Nephrol. 2012;27(6):965–72.
12. Wiesel A, Queisser-Luft A, Clementi M, Bianca S, Stoll C, Group ES. Prenatal detection of congenital renal malformations by fetal ultrasonographic examination: an analysis of 709,030 births in 12 European countries. Eur J Med Genet. 2005;48(2):131–44.
13. Jain S, Chen F. Developmental pathology of congenital kidney and urinary tract anomalies. Clin Kidney J. 2019;12(3):382–99.
14. Piscione TD, Rosenblum ND. The malformed kidney: disruption of glomerular and tubular development. Clin Genet. 1999;56(5):341–56.
15. Queisser-Luft A, Stolz G, Wiesel A, Schlaefer K, Spranger J. Malformations in newborn: results based on 30,940 infants and fetuses from the Mainz congenital birth defect monitoring system (1990-1998). Arch Gynecol Obstet. 2002;266(3):163–7.
16. Sanna-Cherchi S, Westland R, Ghiggeri GM, Gharavi AG. Genetic basis of human congenital anomalies of the kidney and urinary tract. J Clin Invest. 2018;128(1):4–15.
17. van der Ven AT, Vivante A, Hildebrandt F. Novel insights into the pathogenesis of monogenic congenital anomalies of the kidney and urinary tract. J Am Soc Nephrol. 2018;29(1):36–50.
18. Winyard P, Chitty L. Dysplastic and polycystic kidneys: diagnosis, associations and management. Prenat Diagn. 2001;21(11):924–35.
19. Harris J, Robert E, Kallen B. Epidemiologic characteristics of kidney malformations. Eur J Epidemiol. 2000;16(11):985–92.
20. Roodhooft AM, Birnholz JC, Holmes LB. Familial nature of congenital absence and severe dysgenesis of both kidneys. N Engl J Med. 1984;310(21):1341–5.
21. Guarino N, Tadini B, Camardi P, Silvestro L, Lace R, Bianchi M. The incidence of associated urological abnormalities in children with renal ectopia. J Urol. 2004;172(4 Pt 2):1757–9; discussion 9.
22. Weizer AZ, Silverstein AD, Auge BK, Delvecchio FC, Raj G, Albala DM, et al. Determining the incidence of horseshoe kidney from radiographic data at a single institution. J Urol. 2003;170(5):1722–6.
23. Quirino IG, Diniz JS, Bouzada MC, Pereira AK, Lopes TJ, Paixao GM, et al. Clinical course of 822 children with prenatally detected nephrouropathies. Clin J Am Soc Nephrol. 2012;7(3):444–51.
24. Gonzalez Celedon C, Bitsori M, Tullus K. Progression of chronic renal failure in children with dysplastic kidneys. Pediatr Nephrol. 2007;22(7):1014–20.
25. Sanna-Cherchi S, Ravani P, Corbani V, Parodi S, Haupt R, Piaggio G, et al. Renal outcome in patients with congenital anomalies of the kidney and urinary tract. Kidney Int. 2009;76(5):528–33.
26. Wuhl E, van Stralen KJ, Verrina E, Bjerre A, Wanner C, Heaf JG, et al. Timing and outcome of renal replacement therapy in patients with congenital mal-

formations of the kidney and urinary tract. Clin J Am Soc Nephrol. 2013;8(1):67–74.

27. Costantini F. Genetic controls and cellular behaviors in branching morphogenesis of the renal collecting system. Wiley Interdiscip Rev Dev Biol. 2012;1(5):693–713.

28. Chai OH, Song CH, Park SK, Kim W, Cho ES. Molecular regulation of kidney development. Anat Cell Biol. 2013;46(1):19–31.

29. Schwarz RD, Stephens FD, Cussen LJ. The pathogenesis of renal dysplasia. II. The significance of lateral and medial ectopy of the ureteric orifice. Invest Urol. 1981;19(2):97–100.

30. Hu MC, Rosenblum ND. Genetic regulation of branching morphogenesis: lessons learned from loss-of-function phenotypes. Pediatr Res. 2003;54(4):433–8.

31. Enomoto H, Araki T, Jackman A, Heuckeroth RO, Snider WD, Johnson EM Jr, et al. GFR alpha1-deficient mice have deficits in the enteric nervous system and kidneys. Neuron. 1998;21(2):317–24.

32. Pichel JG, Shen L, Sheng HZ, Granholm AC, Drago J, Grinberg A, et al. Defects in enteric innervation and kidney development in mice lacking GDNF. Nature. 1996;382(6586):73–6.

33. Schuchardt A, D'Agati V, Larsson-Blomberg L, Costantini F, Pachnis V. Defects in the kidney and enteric nervous system of mice lacking the tyrosine kinase receptor Ret. Nature. 1994;367(6461):380–3.

34. Schuchardt A, D'Agati V, Pachnis V, Costantini F. Renal agenesis and hypodysplasia in ret-k-mutant mice result from defects in ureteric bud development. Development. 1996;122(6):1919–29.

35. Maeshima A, Sakurai H, Choi Y, Kitamura S, Vaughn DA, Tee JB, et al. Glial cell-derived neurotrophic factor independent ureteric bud outgrowth from the Wolffian duct. J Am Soc Nephrol. 2007;18(12):3147–55.

36. Kume T, Deng K, Hogan BL. Murine forkhead/winged helix genes Foxc1 (Mf1) and Foxc2 (Mfh1) are required for the early organogenesis of the kidney and urinary tract. Development. 2000;127(7):1387–95.

37. Grieshammer U, Le M, Plump AS, Wang F, Tessier-Lavigne M, Martin GR. SLIT2-mediated ROBO2 signaling restricts kidney induction to a single site. Dev Cell. 2004;6(5):709–17.

38. Miyazaki Y, Oshima K, Fogo A, Hogan BL, Ichikawa I. Bone morphogenetic protein 4 regulates the budding site and elongation of the mouse ureter. J Clin Invest. 2000;105(7):863–73.

39. Xu PX, Adams J, Peters H, Brown MC, Heaney S, Maas R. Eya1-deficient mice lack ears and kidneys and show abnormal apoptosis of organ primordia. Nat Genet. 1999;23(1):113–7.

40. Xu PX, Zheng W, Huang L, Maire P, Laclef C, Silvius D. Six1 is required for the early organogenesis of mammalian kidney. Development. 2003;130(14):3085–94.

41. Nishinakamura R, Matsumoto Y, Nakao K, Nakamura K, Sato A, Copeland NG, et al. Murine homolog of SALL1 is essential for ureteric bud invasion in kidney development. Development. 2001;128(16):3105–15.

42. Dressler GR, Deutsch U, Chowdhury K, Nornes HO, Gruss P. Pax2, a new murine paired-box-containing gene and its expression in the developing excretory system. Development. 1990;109(4):787–95.

43. Dziarmaga A, Eccles M, Goodyer P. Suppression of ureteric bud apoptosis rescues nephron endowment and adult renal function in Pax2 mutant mice. J Am Soc Nephrol. 2006;17(6):1568–75.

44. Brophy PD, Ostrom L, Lang KM, Dressler GR. Regulation of ureteric bud outgrowth by Pax2-dependent activation of the glial derived neurotrophic factor gene. Development. 2001;128(23):4747–56.

45. Lokmane L, Heliot C, Garcia-Villalba P, Fabre M, Cereghini S. vHNF1 functions in distinct regulatory circuits to control ureteric bud branching and early nephrogenesis. Development. 2010;137(2):347–57.

46. Gresh L, Fischer E, Reimann A, Tanguy M, Garbay S, Shao X, et al. A transcriptional network in polycystic kidney disease. EMBO J. 2004;23(7):1657–68.

47. Paces-Fessy M, Fabre M, Lesaulnier C, Cereghini S. Hnf1b and Pax2 cooperate to control different pathways in kidney and ureter morphogenesis. Hum Mol Genet. 2012;21(14):3143–55.

48. Bose J, Grotewold L, Ruther U. Pallister-Hall syndrome phenotype in mice mutant for Gli3. Hum Mol Genet. 2002;11(9):1129–35.

49. Hu MC, Mo R, Bhella S, Wilson CW, Chuang PT, Hui CC, et al. GLI3-dependent transcriptional repression of Gli1, Gli2 and kidney patterning genes disrupts renal morphogenesis. Development. 2006;133(3):569–78.

50. Cain JE, Islam E, Haxho F, Blake J, Rosenblum ND. GLI3 repressor controls functional development of the mouse ureter. J Clin Invest. 2011;121(3):1199–206.

51. Yu J, Carroll TJ, McMahon AP. Sonic hedgehog regulates proliferation and differentiation of mesenchymal cells in the mouse metanephric kidney. Development. 2002;129(22):5301–12.

52. Sheybani-Deloui S, Chi L, Staite MV, Cain JE, Nieman BJ, Henkelman RM, et al. Activated hedgehog-GLI signaling causes congenital ureteropelvic junction obstruction. J Am Soc Nephrol. 2018;29(2):532–44.

53. Yosypiv IV. Renin-angiotensin system in ureteric bud branching morphogenesis: implications for kidney disease. Pediatr Nephrol. 2014;29(4):609–20.

54. Yosypiv IV. Renin-angiotensin system in ureteric bud branching morphogenesis: insights into the mechanisms. Pediatr Nephrol. 2011;26(9):1499–512.

55. Nishimura H, Yerkes E, Hohenfellner K, Miyazaki Y, Ma J, Hunley TE, et al. Role of the angiotensin type 2 receptor gene in congenital anomalies of the kidney and urinary tract, CAKUT, of mice and men. Mol Cell. 1999;3(1):1–10.

56. Gubler MC, Antignac C. Renin-angiotensin system in kidney development: renal tubular dysgenesis. Kidney Int. 2010;77(5):400–6.

57. Batourina E, Choi C, Paragas N, Bello N, Hensle T, Costantini FD, et al. Distal ureter morphogenesis depends on epithelial cell remodeling mediated by vitamin A and Ret. Nat Genet. 2002;32(1):109–15.

58. Batourina E, Gim S, Bello N, Shy M, Clagett-Dame M, Srinivas S, et al. Vitamin A controls epithelial/mesenchymal interactions through Ret expression. Nat Genet. 2001;27(1):74–8.

59. Mendelsohn C, Batourina E, Fung S, Gilbert T, Dodd J. Stromal cells mediate retinoid-dependent functions essential for renal development. Development. 1999;126(6):1139–48.

60. Lelievre-Pegorier M, Vilar J, Ferrier ML, Moreau E, Freund N, Gilbert T, et al. Mild vitamin A deficiency leads to inborn nephron deficit in the rat. Kidney Int. 1998;54(5):1455–62.

61. Goodyer P, Kurpad A, Rekha S, Muthayya S, Dwarkanath P, Iyengar A, et al. Effects of maternal vitamin A status on kidney development: a pilot study. Pediatr Nephrol. 2007;22(2):209–14.

62. Czeizel AE, Dobo M, Vargha P. Hungarian cohort-controlled trial of periconceptional multivitamin supplementation shows a reduction in certain congenital abnormalities. Birth Defects Res A Clin Mol Teratol. 2004;70(11):853–61.

63. Hernandez-Diaz S, Werler MM, Walker AM, Mitchell AA. Folic acid antagonists during pregnancy and the risk of birth defects. N Engl J Med. 2000;343(22):1608–14.

64. Nyengaard JR, Bendtsen TF. Glomerular number and size in relation to age, kidney weight, and body surface in normal man. Anat Rec. 1992;232(2):194–201.

65. Weber S, Moriniere V, Knuppel T, Charbit M, Dusek J, Ghiggeri GM, et al. Prevalence of mutations in renal developmental genes in children with renal hypodysplasia: results of the ESCAPE study. J Am Soc Nephrol. 2006;17(10):2864–70.

66. Schwaderer AL, Bates CM, McHugh KM, McBride KL. Renal anomalies in family members of infants with bilateral renal agenesis/adysplasia. Pediatr Nephrol. 2007;22(1):52–6.

67. Salomon R, Tellier AL, Attie-Bitach T, Amiel J, Vekemans M, Lyonnet S, et al. PAX2 mutations in oligomeganephronia. Kidney Int. 2001;59(2):457–62.

68. Ulinski T, Lescure S, Beaufils S, Guigonis V, Decramer S, Morin D, et al. Renal phenotypes related to hepatocyte nuclear factor-1beta (TCF2) mutations in a pediatric cohort. J Am Soc Nephrol. 2006;17(2):497–503.

69. Chatterjee R, Ramos E, Hoffman M, VanWinkle J, Martin DR, Davis TK, et al. Traditional and targeted exome sequencing reveals common, rare and novel functional deleterious variants in RET-signaling complex in a cohort of living US patients with urinary tract malformations. Hum Genet. 2012;131(11):1725–38.

70. Jeanpierre C, Mace G, Parisot M, Moriniere V, Pawtowsky A, Benabou M, et al. RET and GDNF mutations are rare in fetuses with renal agenesis or other severe kidney development defects. J Med Genet. 2011;48(7):497–504.

71. Skinner MA, Safford SD, Reeves JG, Jackson ME, Freemerman AJ. Renal aplasia in humans is associated with RET mutations. Am J Hum Genet. 2008;82(2):344–51.

72. Yang Y, Houle AM, Letendre J, Richter A. RET Gly691Ser mutation is associated with primary vesicoureteral reflux in the French-Canadian population from Quebec. Hum Mutat. 2008;29(5):695–702.

73. Hwang DY, Dworschak GC, Kohl S, Saisawat P, Vivante A, Hilger AC, et al. Mutations in 12 known dominant disease-causing genes clarify many congenital anomalies of the kidney and urinary tract. Kidney Int. 2014;85(6):1429–33.

74. Fraser FC, Ling D, Clogg D, Nogrady B. Genetic aspects of the BOR syndrome—branchial fistulas, ear pits, hearing loss, and renal anomalies. Am J Med Genet. 1978;2(3):241–52.

75. Melnick M, Bixler D, Silk K, Yune H, Nance WE. Autosomal dominant branchiootorenal dysplasia. Birth Defects Orig Artic Ser. 1975;11(5):121–8.

76. Chang EH, Menezes M, Meyer NC, Cucci RA, Vervoort VS, Schwartz CE, et al. Branchio-oto-renal syndrome: the mutation spectrum in EYA1 and its phenotypic consequences. Hum Mutat. 2004;23(6):582–9.

77. Chen A, Francis M, Ni L, Cremers CW, Kimberling WJ, Sato Y, et al. Phenotypic manifestations of branchio-oto-renal syndrome. Am J Med Genet. 1995;58(4):365–70.

78. Fraser FC, Sproule JR, Halal F. Frequency of the branchio-oto-renal (BOR) syndrome in children with profound hearing loss. Am J Med Genet. 1980;7(3):341–9.

79. Hoskins BE, Cramer CH, Silvius D, Zou D, Raymond RM, Orten DJ, et al. Transcription factor SIX5 is mutated in patients with branchio-oto-renal syndrome. Am J Hum Genet. 2007;80(4):800–4.

80. Kochhar A, Orten DJ, Sorensen JL, Fischer SM, Cremers CW, Kimberling WJ, et al. SIX1 mutation screening in 247 branchio-oto-renal syndrome families: a recurrent missense mutation associated with BOR. Hum Mutat. 2008;29(4):565.

81. Krug P, Moriniere V, Marlin S, Koubi V, Gabriel HD, Colin E, et al. Mutation screening of the EYA1, SIX1, and SIX5 genes in a large cohort of patients harboring branchio-oto-renal syndrome calls into question the pathogenic role of SIX5 mutations. Hum Mutat. 2011;32(2):183–90.

82. Li X, Oghi KA, Zhang J, Krones A, Bush KT, Glass CK, et al. Eya protein phosphatase activity regulates Six1-Dach-Eya transcriptional effects in mammalian organogenesis. Nature. 2003;426(6964):247–54.

83. Ruf RG, Xu PX, Silvius D, Otto EA, Beekmann F, Muerb UT, et al. SIX1 mutations cause branchio-oto-renal syndrome by disruption of EYA1-SIX1-

DNA complexes. Proc Natl Acad Sci U S A. 2004;101(21):8090–5.

84. Sajithlal G, Zou D, Silvius D, Xu PX. Eya 1 acts as a critical regulator for specifying the metanephric mesenchyme. Dev Biol. 2005;284(2):323–36.

85. Miller EM, Hopkin R, Bao L, Ware SM. Implications for genotype-phenotype predictions in Townes-Brocks syndrome: case report of a novel SALL1 deletion and review of the literature. Am J Med Genet A. 2012;158A(3):533–40.

86. O'Callaghan M, Young ID. The Townes-Brocks syndrome. J Med Genet. 1990;27(7):457–61.

87. Townes PL, Brocks ER. Hereditary syndrome of imperforate anus with hand, foot, and ear anomalies. J Pediatr. 1972;81(2):321–6.

88. Kurnit DM, Steele MW, Pinsky L, Dibbins A. Autosomal dominant transmission of a syndrome of anal, ear, renal, and radial congenital malformations. J Pediatr. 1978;93(2):270–3.

89. Martinez-Frias ML, Bermejo Sanchez E, Arroyo Carrera I, Perez Fernandez JL, Pardo Romero M, Buron Martinez E, et al. [The Townes-Brocks syndrome in Spain: the epidemiological aspects in a consecutive series of cases]. An Esp Pediatr. 1999;50(1):57–60.

90. Kohlhase J. SALL1 mutations in Townes-Brocks syndrome and related disorders. Hum Mutat. 2000;16(6):460–6.

91. Kohlhase J, Wischermann A, Reichenbach H, Froster U, Engel W. Mutations in the SALL1 putative transcription factor gene cause Townes-Brocks syndrome. Nat Genet. 1998;18(1):81–3.

92. Marlin S, Blanchard S, Slim R, Lacombe D, Denoyelle F, Alessandri JL, et al. Townes-Brocks syndrome: detection of a SALL1 mutation hot spot and evidence for a position effect in one patient. Hum Mutat. 1999;14(5):377–86.

93. Solomon BD, Pineda-Alvarez DE, Raam MS, Bous SM, Keaton AA, Velez JI, et al. Analysis of component findings in 79 patients diagnosed with VACTERL association. Am J Med Genet A. 2010;152A(9):2236–44.

94. Rittler M, Paz JE, Castilla EE. VACTERL association, epidemiologic definition and delineation. Am J Med Genet. 1996;63(4):529–36.

95. Brown AK, Roddam AW, Spitz L, Ward SJ. Oesophageal atresia, related malformations, and medical problems: a family study. Am J Med Genet. 1999;85(1):31–7.

96. van Rooij IA, Wijers CH, Rieu PN, Hendriks HS, Brouwers MM, Knoers NV, et al. Maternal and paternal risk factors for anorectal malformations: a Dutch case-control study. Birth Defects Res A Clin Mol Teratol. 2010;88(3):152–8.

97. Garcia-Barcelo MM, Wong KK, Lui VC, Yuan ZW, So MT, Ngan ES, et al. Identification of a HOXD13 mutation in a VACTERL patient. Am J Med Genet A. 2008;146A(24):3181–5.

98. Stankiewicz P, Sen P, Bhatt SS, Storer M, Xia Z, Bejjani BA, et al. Genomic and genic deletions of the FOX gene cluster on 16q24.1 and inactivating mutations of FOXF1 cause alveolar capillary dysplasia and other malformations. Am J Hum Genet. 2009;84(6):780–91.

99. Tongsong T, Wanapirak C, Piyamongkol W, Sudasana J. Prenatal sonographic diagnosis of VATER association. J Clin Ultrasound. 1999;27(7):378–84.

100. Murphy-Kaulbeck L, Dodds L, Joseph KS, Van den Hof M. Single umbilical artery risk factors and pregnancy outcomes. Obstet Gynecol. 2010;116(4):843–50.

101. Faivre L, Portnoi MF, Pals G, Stoppa-Lyonnet D, Le Merrer M, Thauvin-Robinet C, et al. Should chromosome breakage studies be performed in patients with VACTERL association? Am J Med Genet A. 2005;137(1):55–8.

102. Weaver RG, Cashwell LF, Lorentz W, Whiteman D, Geisinger KR, Ball M. Optic nerve coloboma associated with renal disease. Am J Med Genet. 1988;29(3):597–605.

103. Bower M, Salomon R, Allanson J, Antignac C, Benedicenti F, Benetti E, et al. Update of PAX2 mutations in renal coloboma syndrome and establishment of a locus-specific database. Hum Mutat. 2012;33(3):457–66.

104. Fletcher J, Hu M, Berman Y, Collins F, Grigg J, McIver M, et al. Multicystic dysplastic kidney and variable phenotype in a family with a novel deletion mutation of PAX2. J Am Soc Nephrol. 2005;16(9):2754–61.

105. Dureau P, Attie-Bitach T, Salomon R, Bettembourg O, Amiel J, Uteza Y, et al. Renal coloboma syndrome. Ophthalmology. 2001;108(10):1912–6.

106. Parsa CF, Silva ED, Sundin OH, Goldberg MF, De Jong MR, Sunness JS, et al. Redefining papillorenal syndrome: an underdiagnosed cause of ocular and renal morbidity. Ophthalmology. 2001;108(4):738–49.

107. Eccles MR, Schimmenti LA. Renal-coloboma syndrome: a multi-system developmental disorder caused by PAX2 mutations. Clin Genet. 1999;56(1):1–9.

108. Schimmenti LA, Cunliffe HE, McNoe LA, Ward TA, French MC, Shim HH, et al. Further delineation of renal-coloboma syndrome in patients with extreme variability of phenotype and identical PAX2 mutations. Am J Hum Genet. 1997;60(4):869–78.

109. Sanyanusin P, Schimmenti LA, McNoe LA, Ward TA, Pierpont ME, Sullivan MJ, et al. Mutation of the PAX2 gene in a family with optic nerve colobomas, renal anomalies and vesicoureteral reflux. Nat Genet. 1995;9(4):358–64.

110. Barua M, Stellacci E, Stella L, Weins A, Genovese G, Muto V, et al. Mutations in PAX2 associate with adult-onset FSGS. J Am Soc Nephrol. 2014;25(9):1942–53.

111. Vivante A, Chacham OS, Shril S, Schreiber R, Mane SM, Pode-Shakked B, et al. Dominant PAX2 mutations may cause steroid-resistant nephrotic

165. van Vuuren SH, van der Doef R, Cohen-Overbeek TE, Goldschmeding R, Pistorius LR, de Jong TP. Compensatory enlargement of a solitary functioning kidney during fetal development. Ultrasound Obstet Gynecol. 2012;40(6):665–8.

166. Cascio S, Paran S, Puri P. Associated urological anomalies in children with unilateral renal agenesis. J Urol. 1999;162(3 Pt 2):1081–3.

167. Kaneyama K, Yamataka A, Satake S, Yanai T, Lane GJ, Kaneko K, et al. Associated urologic anomalies in children with solitary kidney. J Pediatr Surg. 2004;39(1):85–7.

168. Grinsell MM, Butz K, Gurka MJ, Gurka KK, Norwood V. Sport-related kidney injury among high school athletes. Pediatrics. 2012;130(1):e40–5.

169. Shibata S, Nagata M. Pathogenesis of human renal dysplasia: an alternative scenario to the major theories. Pediatr Int. 2003;45(5):605–9.

170. Narchi H. Risk of hypertension with multicystic kidney disease: a systematic review. Arch Dis Child. 2005;90(9):921–4.

171. Hains DS, Bates CM, Ingraham S, Schwaderer AL. Management and etiology of the unilateral multicystic dysplastic kidney: a review. Pediatr Nephrol. 2009;24(2):233–41.

172. Rabelo EA, Oliveira EA, Silva GS, Pezzuti IL, Tatsuo ES. Predictive factors of ultrasonographic involution of prenatally detected multicystic dysplastic kidney. BJU Int. 2005;95(6):868–71.

173. Jawa NA, Rosenblum ND, Radhakrishnan S, Pearl RJ, Levin L, Matsuda-Abedini M. Choosing wisely: improving the quality of care by reducing unnecessary testing in children with isolated unilateral multicystic dysplastic kidney or solitary kidney. Pediatrics. 2021;148(2):e2020035550.

174. D'Alberton A, Reschini E, Ferrari N, Candiani P. Prevalence of urinary tract abnormalities in a large series of patients with uterovaginal atresia. J Urol. 1981;126(5):623–4.

175. Fedele L, Bianchi S, Agnoli B, Tozzi L, Vignali M. Urinary tract anomalies associated with unicornuate uterus. J Urol. 1996;155(3):847–8.

176. Raj GV, Auge BK, Assimos D, Preminger GM. Metabolic abnormalities associated with renal calculi in patients with horseshoe kidneys. J Endourol. 2004;18(2):157–61.

177. Oda T, Elkahloun AG, Pike BL, Okajima K, Krantz ID, Genin A, et al. Mutations in the human Jagged1 gene are responsible for Alagille syndrome. Nat Genet. 1997;16(3):235–42.

178. Kamath BM, Podkameni G, Hutchinson AL, Leonard LD, Gerfen J, Krantz ID, et al. Renal anomalies in Alagille syndrome: a disease-defining feature. Am J Med Genet A. 2012;158A(1):85–9.

179. McDaniell R, Warthen DM, Sanchez-Lara PA, Pai A, Krantz ID, Piccoli DA, et al. NOTCH2 mutations cause Alagille syndrome, a heterogeneous disorder of the notch signaling pathway. Am J Hum Genet. 2006;79(1):169–73.

180. Wilkie AO, Slaney SF, Oldridge M, Poole MD, Ashworth GJ, Hockley AD, et al. Apert syndrome results from localized mutations of FGFR2 and is allelic with Crouzon syndrome. Nat Genet. 1995;9(2):165–72.

181. Seyedzadeh A, Kompani F, Esmailie E, Samadzadeh S, Farshchi B. High-grade vesicoureteral reflux in Pfeiffer syndrome. Urol J. 2008;5(3):200–2.

182. Hatada I, Ohashi H, Fukushima Y, Kaneko Y, Inoue M, Komoto Y, et al. An imprinted gene p57KIP2 is mutated in Beckwith-Wiedemann syndrome. Nat Genet. 1996;14(2):171–3.

183. Goldman M, Smith A, Shuman C, Caluseriu O, Wei C, Steele L, et al. Renal abnormalities in beckwith-wiedemann syndrome are associated with 11p15.5 uniparental disomy. J Am Soc Nephrol. 2002;13(8):2077–84.

184. Abdelhak S, Kalatzis V, Heilig R, Compain S, Samson D, Vincent C, et al. Clustering of mutations responsible for branchio-oto-renal (BOR) syndrome in the eyes absent homologous region (eyaHR) of EYA1. Hum Mol Genet. 1997;6(13):2247–55.

185. Houston CS, Opitz JM, Spranger JW, Macpherson RI, Reed MH, Gilbert EF, et al. The campomelic syndrome: review, report of 17 cases, and follow-up on the currently 17-year-old boy first reported by Maroteaux et al in 1971. Am J Med Genet. 1983;15(1):3–28.

186. Wagner T, Wirth J, Meyer J, Zabel B, Held M, Zimmer J, et al. Autosomal sex reversal and campomelic dysplasia are caused by mutations in and around the SRY-related gene SOX9. Cell. 1994;79(6):1111–20.

187. Sakaki-Yumoto M, Kobayashi C, Sato A, Fujimura S, Matsumoto Y, Takasato M, et al. The murine homolog of SALL4, a causative gene in Okihiro syndrome, is essential for embryonic stem cell proliferation, and cooperates with Sall1 in anorectal, heart, brain and kidney development. Development. 2006;133(15):3005–13.

188. McGregor L, Makela V, Darling SM, Vrontou S, Chalepakis G, Roberts C, et al. Fraser syndrome and mouse blebbed phenotype caused by mutations in FRAS1/Fras1 encoding a putative extracellular matrix protein. Nat Genet. 2003;34(2):203–8.

189. Alazami AM, Shaheen R, Alzahrani F, Snape K, Saggar A, Brinkmann B, et al. FREM1 mutations cause bifid nose, renal agenesis, and anorectal malformations syndrome. Am J Hum Genet. 2009;85(3):414–8.

190. Jadeja S, Smyth I, Pitera JE, Taylor MS, van Haelst M, Bentley E, et al. Identification of a new gene mutated in Fraser syndrome and mouse myelencephalic blebs. Nat Genet. 2005;37(5):520–5.

191. Vogel MJ, van Zon P, Brueton L, Gijzen M, van Tuil MC, Cox P, et al. Mutations in GRIP1 cause Fraser syndrome. J Med Genet. 2012;49(5):303–6.

192. Peco-Antic A, Bogdanovic R, Paripovic D, Paripovic A, Kocev N, Golubovic E, et al. Epidemiology of

chronic kidney disease in children in Serbia. Nephrol Dial Transplant. 2012;27(5):1978–84.

193. Chenouard A, Isidor B, Allain-Launay E, Moreau A, Le Bideau M, Roussey G. Renal phenotypic variability in HDR syndrome: glomerular nephropathy as a novel finding. Eur J Pediatr. 2013;172(1):107–10.

194. Franco B, Guioli S, Pragliola A, Incerti B, Bardoni B, Tonlorenzi R, et al. A gene deleted in Kallmann's syndrome shares homology with neural cell adhesion and axonal path-finding molecules. Nature. 1991;353(6344):529–36.

195. Bamshad M, Lin RC, Law DJ, Watkins WC, Krakowiak PA, Moore ME, et al. Mutations in human TBX3 alter limb, apocrine and genital development in ulnar-mammary syndrome. Nat Genet. 1997;16(3):311–5.

196. Kang S, Graham JM Jr, Olney AH, Biesecker LG. GLI3 frameshift mutations cause autosomal dominant Pallister-Hall syndrome. Nat Genet. 1997;15(3):266–8.

197. Bohn S, Thomas H, Turan G, Ellard S, Bingham C, Hattersley AT, et al. Distinct molecular and morphogenetic properties of mutations in the human HNF1beta gene that lead to defective kidney development. J Am Soc Nephrol. 2003;14(8):2033–41.

198. Pilia G, Hughes-Benzie RM, MacKenzie A, Baybayan P, Chen EY, Huber R, et al. Mutations in GPC3, a glypican gene, cause the Simpson-Golabi-Behmel overgrowth syndrome. Nat Genet. 1996;12(3):241–7.

199. Tint GS, Irons M, Elias ER, Batta AK, Frieden R, Chen TS, et al. Defective cholesterol biosynthesis associated with the Smith-Lemli-Opitz syndrome. N Engl J Med. 1994;330(2):107–13.

200. Preuss N, Brosius U, Biermanns M, Muntau AC, Conzelmann E, Gartner J. PEX1 mutations in complementation group 1 of Zellweger spectrum patients correlate with severity of disease. Pediatr Res. 2002;51(6):706–14.

Part III

Ciliopathies

Ciliopathies: Their Role in Pediatric Kidney Disease

9

Miriam Schmidts and Philip L. Beales

Cilia in the Historic Context

Cilia are evolutionarily well conserved, hair-like structures projecting from the surface of most cells in vertebrates and are broadly divided into motile and non-motile cilia. While non-motile cilia can be found as single organelles on most cells in mammals, the occurrence of motile cilia in bundles of multiple (hundreds) is restricted to certain tissues in vertebrates such as the respiratory tract, the reproductive system (epididymidis and oviduct), the ependyma lining the brain ventricles and the embryonic node where they are involved in fluid movement and mucociliary clearance. Also, the flagellum of mammalian sperm has a very similar structure to motile cilia. In vertebrate photoreceptor cells within the ret-ina, a modified ciliary structure called "connecting cilium" links inner and outer segment of those cells. See Figs. 9.1a–c and 9.2a–k for examples of cilia visualisation.

Although the existence of cilia has been described as early as the 1800s by Purkinje and Valentin [3, 4], their significance for mammalian development, organ maintenance and clinical disease has only been fully appreciated in the last two decades. Cilia were regarded as functionless cellular extensions for many years as no link between this organelle and human disease was made despite the fact that dextrocardia had already been visualised by Leonardo da Vinci in the fifteenth century and in 1793, the Scottish pathologist Matthew Baillie mentioned situs inversus in his book *The Morbid Anatomy of Some of the Most Important Parts of the Human Body*. As published by Afzelius in 1979 [5], we realise today that situs abnormalities result from (mainly motile) ciliary dysfunction in the embryonic node. The function of non-motile, so called primary cilia remained elusive for even longer; however, when "rediscovered," their role in (cystic) kidney disease was one of the initial ciliary functions acknowledged [6, 7], Since then, a large number of (inherited) human diseases have been identified to result from ciliary malfunction [8–10]. See Table 9.1 for a summary of ciliary diseases with renal involvement and their underlying genetic cause.

M. Schmidts (✉)
Department of Pediatrics, Genetics Division, Center for Pediatrics and Adolescent Medicine, University Hospital Freiburg, Freiburg, Germany

Department of Human Genetics, Genome Research, Radboud University Hospital Nijmegen, Nijmegen, The Netherlands
e-mail: miriam.schmidts@radboudumc.nl

P. L. Beales
Department of Genetics and Genomics Medicine, Institute of Child Health, University College London, London, UK
e-mail: p.beales@ucl.ac.uk

© The Author(s), under exclusive license to Springer Nature Switzerland AG 2023
F. Schaefer, L. A. Greenbaum (eds.), *Pediatric Kidney Disease*,
https://doi.org/10.1007/978-3-031-11665-0_9

Table 9.1 (continued)

Disease	Renal phenotype	Retinopathy	Skeletal phenotype	Obesity	Developmental delay	Situs inversus	Other	Gene
BBS	~30%, mainly NPHP-like, rarely cystic	+	Often polydactyly	Always	Very often	Rarely	Hypogonoadism	BBS1, BBS2, BBS3 (ARL6), BBS4, BBS5, BBS6 (MKKS), BBS7, BBS8 (TTC8), BBS9, BBS10, BBS11 (TRIM32), BBS13 (MKS1), BBS14 (CEP290), BBS15 (C2ORF86), BBS17 (LZTFL1), BBS18 (BBIP1), BBS19 (IFT27)
Alstrom syndrome	Often	+	–	Always	–	–	Frequent cardiomyopathy, sensorineural hearing loss, hepatic disease	Alms1
Meckel-Gruber syndrome	Often; NPHP like or cystic	na	Often orofacial clefting		na (early lethality)	Sometimes	Occipital encephalocele	MKS1, MKS2 (TMEM216), MKS3 (TMEM67), MKS4 (CEP290), MKS5 (RPGRIP1L), MKS6 (CC2D2A), MKS7 (NPHP3), MKS8 (TCTN2), MKS9 (B9D1), MKS10 (B9D2), MKS11 (TMEM231)
Orofacial digital syndrome (OFD)	Renal malformations	Usually not	Often polysyndactyly, orofacial clefting	–		Rarely	Lobulated tongue, heart defects, agenesis of the corpus callosum, conductive hearing loss, cerebellar atrophy described	OFD1 (CXORF5), TCTN3, C5orf42, DDX59

9 Ciliopathies: Their Role in Pediatric Kidney Disease

Short rib-polydactyly syndrome (SRPS)	Often; NPHP-like or cystic	Usually not evident	Often polydactyly, short ribs, shortened long bones, brachydactyly, abnormal pelvis configuration, sometimes orofacial clefting	–	na (early lethality)	Rarely	Always lethal perinatally due to cardiorespiratory insufficiency	DYNC2H1, NEK1, WDR60, WDR34, WDR35
Jeune asphyxiating thoracic dystrophy (JATD)	<30%, mainly NPHP-like, rarely cystic	Rarely	Short ribs, short long bones, rarely polydactyly, abnormal pelvis configuration, scoliosis, cone shaped epiphyses	Single cases	–	–	Sometimes retinal degeneration, mainly in cases with renal disease;	DYNC2H1, WDR34, WDR60, IFT80, IFT172, IFT140, WDR19 (IFT144), TTC21B (IFT139), CSPP1
Mainzer-Saldino-syndrome (MSS)	Always; mainly NPHP-like, rarely cystic	Always	(Mildly) shortened ribs, cone shaped epiphyses	–	Single cases	Not described	Always retinal degeneration	IFT140, IFT172
Sensenbrenner syndrome (CED)	Very often; mainly NPHP-like	Often	(Mildly) shortened ribs, brachydactyly, craniosynostosis	–	Sometimes	Usually not	Thin and sparse growing hair, nail dysplasia (ectodermal defects), heart defects	IFT122, WDR19 (IFT144), IFT43, WDR35

Ciliary Ultrastructure

The ciliary research field originates from the protozoan flagellar research undertaken since the 1950s and was therefore initially more focussed on motile cilia, possibly also because those were easier to detect due to their moving features. Electron microscopy is an essential imaging technique for visualisation these cilia also lack the central pair (9 + 0 structure). In motile cilia, so-called inner and outer dynein arms extend from the outer microtubule pairs and those outer pairs are connected to the central pair via radial spokes. This complex construction enables sliding of the microtubules generating ciliary movement. Dynein arms and radial spokes are absent from non-motile primary ciliary.

This ciliary *axoneme* is anchored to and extends from the *basal body* which itself lies within the cytosol and is derived from the mother centriole after cell division. Along its vertical axis, the primary cilium can be structurally divided into different sub-compartments: *the ciliary tip, the ciliary body, the ciliary necklace* [11], *the transition zone* [12], *the so-called inversin compartment* [13] *and the basal body* [14, 15]. The specialise cellular plasma membrane at the ciliary insertion site is referred to as the *ciliary pocket* (Fig. 9.3 for a schematic of ciliary structures). As cilia lack organelles such as endoplasmatic reticulum and Golgi and therefore no protein synthesis occurs within the cilium, all ciliary proteins are produced within the cellular cytosol, and transported to the cilium. Within the

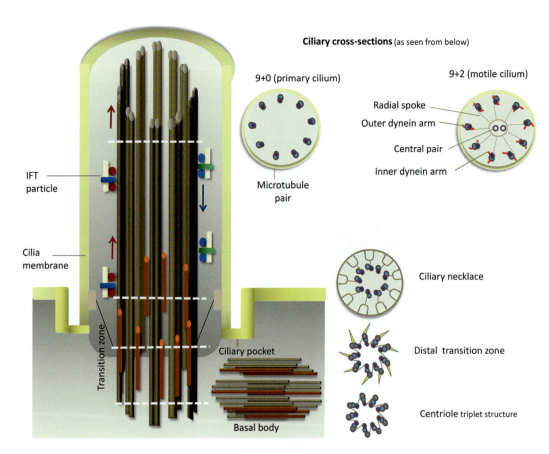

Fig. 9.3 Simplified schematic of the ciliary ultrastructure

cilium, so called **Intra flagellar Transport** (**IFT**) enables protein trafficking from the ciliary base to the tip and vice versa (Fig. 9.3 for a schematic of ciliary ultrastructure and Fig. 9.4 for a schematic of IFT). Figure 9.5a–c shows a schematic of ciliary protein complex localisation and IFT defects are visualised in Fig. 9.6a, b.

Although cilia extend from the cell body and are surrounded by specialised plasma membrane forming the " *ciliary membrane*," cilia represent a distinct cellular compartment with the so called " *transition zone*" which acting as a barrier between the cilium and the rest of the cell [22, 23]. At the transition zone, the microtubule trip-

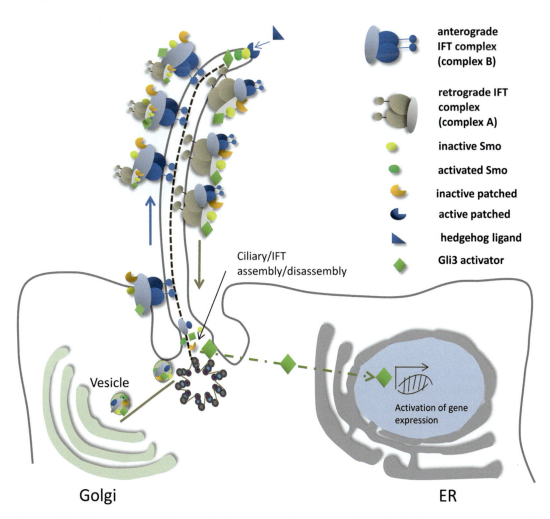

Fig. 9.4 Simplified schematic of Intraflagellar Transport (IFT) and it's relation to hedgehog signalling. Hedgehog signalling pathway components such as smoothened (smo) and patched localise to the cilium and require anterograde IFT to localise to the ciliary tip where binding of the hedgehog ligand (*blue triangle*) activates the smoothened inhibitor patched (*orange*) which in turn releases smoothened (*yellow*). Activated smoothened (*green ball*) releases GLI3 activator from its inhibitor SUFU (not shown). Gli3 activator (*green rectangle*) requires retrograde IFT to translocate to the nucleus where it activates genes involved in chondrogenic and osteogenic differentiation [16–19]

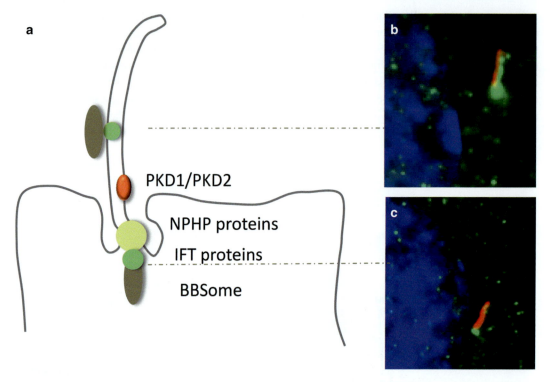

Fig. 9.5 (a–c) Localisation of major ciliary protein complexes. (**a**) Schematic of protein-complex localisation: While Bardet-Biedl-Syndrome (BBS) proteins and intraflagellar transport (IFT) proteins are detected both at the ciliary base and along the ciliary axoneme, many proteins encoded by genes mutated in nephronophthisis localise to the ciliary transition zone. (**b**) Immunofluorescence image of axonemal IFT140 localisation (*green*). (**c**) Immunofluorescence image of IFT140 localisation at the base of the cilium (*green*). The ciliary axoneme is marked in *red* using anti-acetylated tubulin antibody. ((**b**, **c**) Used with permission of John Wiley and Sons from Schmidts et al. [20])

lets of the basal body transform into the axonemal microtubule doublets. As the protein and lipid composition of the ciliary axoneme and ciliary membrane is distinct from the cell body, selective recruitment of components and transport of those components into the cilium is required. How this is precisely undertaken is still unclear, but some progress in understanding has been made in recent years. Interestingly, the connecting cilium of retinal photoreceptors is very similar in its structure to the ciliary transition zone and many proteins encoded by genes found to carry mutations leading to nephronophthisis (often with retinal degeneration) localise to the ciliary transition zone as well as the photoreceptor connecting cilium. This implicates a function of these proteins in "gate keeping" (between cytosol and ciliary axoneme as well as between inner and outer photoreceptor segment) [12, 23]. Two highly specialised areas occur within the ciliary membrane: the *ciliary necklace*, initially described by Gilula and Satir [11] where the microtubules of the basal body are connected to the plasma membrane and the base of a plasma membrane invagination around the proximal ciliary axoneme, the ciliary pocket [24]. The "*inversin compartment*" is found in the proximal ciliary region the ciliary necklace, the transitional zone and the basal body [13]. Mutations in *INVS* encoding Inversin cause nephronophthisis type 2. Please also refer to the nephronophthisis chapter of this book (Chap. 13) for details.

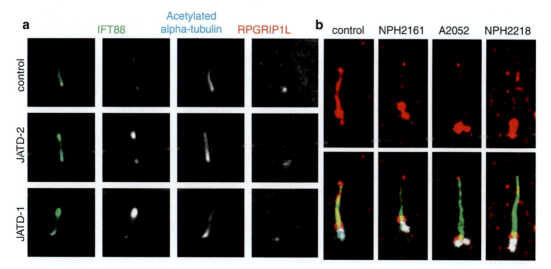

Fig. 9.6 (**a**, **b**) Visualisation of disturbed intraflagellar transport by immunofluorescence. (**a**) Compared with controls, IFT88 accumulates in distal ends of cilia in fibroblasts from Jeune Syndrome patients (JATD-1 and -2) carrying mutations in the dynein-2 complex protein dync2h1 leading to impaired retrograde intraflagellar transport (IFT). Cells were stained with anti-IFT88 (*green*); anti-acetylated α tubulin (marker for the ciliary axoneme, *cyan*); and anti-RPGRIP1L (marker for the ciliary base, *red*) (reprinted with permission from [21]). (**b**) Fibroblasts of patients with biallelic mutations in the anterograde IFT component IFT172 show decreased axonemal and increased basal body staining of IFT140 (*red*) compared to controls. The ciliary axoneme is marked with anti-acetylated-tubulin antibody (*green*), basal bodies are marked in *blue* using anti-g-tubulin antibody. (Reprinted with permission from Exome sequencing identifies DYNC2H1 mutations as a common cause of asphyxiating thoracic dystrophy (Jeune syndrome) without major polydactyly, renal or retinal involvement. (**a**) Used with permission of BMJ Publishing Group from Schmidts et al. [21]; (**b**) Halbritter et al. [1])

Ciliary Assembly

As described above, proteins necessary to build a cilium cannot be synthesized within the cilium but have to be transported to the building site. How exactly ciliary components get to the cilium and the precise process of the transformation of the mother centriole (the older of the two centrioles) into a basal body from where the cilium is assembled has not been understood in all its depth to date. Ciliogenesis is tightly linked to the cell cycle: dividing cells do not exhibit a cilium, cilia are only observed during the G1 cell cycle phase or when cells are quiescent. At least some ciliary proteins seem to reach the ciliary building site by vesicular transport: ciliary vesicles (post-Golgi vesicles) traffic close to the ciliary building site and merge there with the plasma membrane [25]. In this process of sorting membrane proteins to cilia, Bardet-Biedl syndrome proteins have been shown to be essential in assembling a coat that traffics membrane proteins to the cilium [26, 27]. Ciliogenesis is thought to start with the basal body docking to ciliary vesicles which then fuse with the plasma membrane, probably at the site of the ciliary pocket [28–32]. One of the proteins promoting this process has been identified as CEP164 and mutations in the *CEP164* gene cause nephronophthisis in humans [33, 34]. The fact that primary cilia and flagella only ever extend from the mother centriole could be due to the lack of subdistal appendages at the daughter centriole which seem to play a crucial role in anchoring the basal body to the plasma membrane [35]. Cilia stability seems to also depend on posttranslational modification of tubulin, including acetylation [36, 37], glutamylation [38, 39] and farnesylation. The latter seems of particular importance as Thomas et al. identified a homozygous *PDE6D* mutation Joubert syndrome which impaired the targeting of another known joubert protein, INPP5E to the cilium [40].

Cilia and Cell Cycle

As indicated above, ciliogenesis is interlinked with the cell cycle: dividing cells do not normally exhibit cilia, those only become visible after the cell's exit from cell cycle. When cells divide, one centrosome stays within the mother cell while the other can be found in the daughter cell. After cell division, the centrioles duplicate and the original centrioles from which duplication occurs are referred to as "mother centrioles." Once a cell has left cell cycle again, the cilium is built from this mother centriole [41]. When cells re-enter the cell cycle, cilia need to be disassembled which seems to be initiated by Percentrin-1 (PCM1) mediated recruitment of Polo-like kinase 1 (Plk1) to the pericentriolar material [42, 43]. While it has been accepted for many decades that ciliogenesis is linked to mitotic exit of the cell, the possibility that cilia themselves might influence cell cycle progression has only been recently taken into account. For example, the IFT protein Ift88 seems required for spindle orientation during mitosis [44]. Lack of Ift88 in mice leads to a polycystic kidney phenotype [7] and as for cystic renal phenotypes in humans, it remains controversial to which extent and at what time point cellular hyperproliferation contributes to the initiation and/or progression of disease [45]. The INPP5E protein (genetic mutations can cause a Joubert phenotype with renal disease) and the tumor suppressor protein VHL (mutations in the VHL gene cause Von-Hippel-Lindau syndrome which is associated with cystic renal disease) are both involved in stabilising cilia by inhibiting AURKA triggered ciliary disassembly for cell-cycle re-entry [46–48]. The question how cilia influence cell cycle, how they are influenced by cell cycle and how this contributes to ciliopathy, especially polycystic phenotypes, is difficult to resolve as proteins encoded by genes mutated in ciliopathy subjects often have multiple extra-ciliary functions which might influence cell-cycle progression independently of the cilium. For example, several genes mutated in subjects with nephronophthisis such as *ZNF423*, *CEP164* and *NEK8* have been linked to DNA damage repair and therefore directly to cell cycle progression [34, 49]. It is, however, of note that, except for VHL, no increased rate of malignancies has been demonstrated for humans affected by ciliopathies to date.

Intraflagellar Transport (IFT)

Transport of ciliary proteins along the axoneme is undertaken via IFT, an energy dependent process. Kosminski et al. were the first to notice this process in 1993 [50]. IFT is a highly conserved transport mechanism along cilia and flagellae from the green algae *Chlamydomonas* to vertebrates and mammals including humans. Building a cilium from the base to the tip is largely dependent on anterograde IFT [51]. Counter-intuitively, the anterograde IFT complex transporting proteins from the ciliary base to the tip is named "complex B" while the complex enabling retrograde transport from the ciliary tip back to the base is called "complex A." Motor for the anterograde complex is kinesin-2 while the cytoplasmic dynein-2 complex enables transport from the ciliary tip back to the base. Although named "cytoplasmic dynein," the latter complex localises to the ciliary axoneme and should not be confused with the cytoplasmic dynein-1 complex which enables transport along microtubules within the cell body and along neuronal axons. The precise composition of the dynein-2 complex has still not been completely elucidated; however, it is assumed that it resembles dynein-1 complex, a homodimer consisting of two heavy chains, two light-intermediate chains, two intermediate chains and two light chains. IFT-complex A and B are multiprotein assemblies functioning as an adaptor system between the motor complexes and cargo. As IFT-A complex proteins and the dynein-2 complex have to be brought up to the ciliary tip before they can fulfill their function in retrograde transport back from the tip to the base and vice versa, kinesin-2 and IFT complex B must be transported back to the base after they have reached the ciliary tip, it is evident that both complexes must be transported as cargo by each other [25, 52, 53]. Knockout mice for the kinesin-2 component *Kif3a*, the dynein-2 motor heavy chain *Dync2h1* or IFT components often exhibit fewer or shorter cilia and are lethal around midgestation, indicating the fundamental role of these highly conserved proteins during development [43]. Kidney specific gene disruption or hypomorphic mutations often cause renal cysts in mice [7, 54, 55]. Human mutations in genes encoding dynein-2 complex components and IFT particles mainly cause ciliary chondrodysplasias with variable extraskeletal involvement [1, 20, 21, 56–69] and mutations in the IFT-A component *TTC21B/IFT139* and in the IFT-B component *IFT27* were recently identified in Bardet-Biedl-Syndrome [68, 70]. For more details also see the human disease section below and Fig. 9.4 for a schematic of IFT and its relation to hedgehog signalling.

Ciliary Signalling Pathways

Single non-motile (primary) cilia are considered sensory organelles involved in multiple signalling pathways transducing both signals from the cellular surroundings to the cells as well as modifying cell signalling pathways within the cell [71, 72]. As mentioned above, cilia and ciliary proteins have been highly conserved throughout evolution and mutations in genes encoding ciliary components often result in complex developmental defects in vertebrates. This can be attributed to disturbances of fundamental signalling pathways essential for embryogenesis, organogenesis and proper tissue maintenance.

Hedgehog Signalling

The best explored cilia-regulated cellular pathway is hedgehog signalling [16, 17, 73]. Hedgehog signalling crucially influences chondrogenic (and subsequently osteogenic) proliferation and differentiation [74]. Mouse models of ciliary chondrodysplasias, e.g., knockout mice for *Evc* (mutations in the EVC1 and EVC2 gene cause Ellis-van Creveld-Syndrome in humans), *Dync2h1* and *Ift80* (associated with Jeune Syndrome and Short-Rib-Polydactyly Syndrome

type III in humans) indicate that IFT defects lead to imbalances in the hedgehog signalling pathway [18, 75, 76]. Lack of hedgehog signal transduction leads to decreased chondrogenic proliferation and imbalanced chondrogenic differentiation at the growth plates which impairs bone growth. As a result' mice, as well as human subjects with mutations in these genes as well as in *IFT144/WDR19*, exhibit shortened ribs and long bones. Lack of Ift80 or Ift144 also induces polydactyly in mice, a hallmark of dysregulated hedgehog signalling [18, 75–77].

The hedgehog signaling pathway operates via ciliary trafficking: the pathway components smoothened (smo) and patched move via anterograde IFT to the ciliary tip, where smo becomes activated and releases GLI3 activator. The latter is subsequently transported back to the base of the cilium via retrograde IFT and enters the cell body and nucleus where it activates genes regulating chondrogenic and osteogenic differentiation and proliferation (simplified schematic in Fig. 9.4).

Apart from altered bone growth, impaired hedgehog signalling leads to complex developmental defects in mammals including polydactyly, heart defects, midline defects such as clefting and holoprosencephaly. Renal abnormalities, especially ectopic kidneys but also cystic-dysplastic changes, can also be observed in mice [78] and human subjects affected by Smith-Lemli-Opitz syndrome, a condition thought to result from altered hedgehog signalling due to a cholesterol biosynthesis defect [79]. However, neither human subjects with *IFT80*- nor *EVC1/EVC2* mutation nor the corresponding mouse models exhibit a renal phenotype. On the other hand, human subjects with mutations in other IFT genes such as *WDR19/IFT144*, *TTC21B/IFT139*, *IFT140*, *IFT43*, *WDR35* or *IFT172* genes are affected by childhood-onset cystic or nehronopthisis-like renal disease [1, 20, 64, 65, 67–69], and in knockout mouse models for *IFT140* or *IFT172*, early onset cystic (dysplastic) kidney disease is observed [55, 80]. While it seems likely that the skeletal phenotype observed in those subjects is due to imbalances in the hedgehog pathway secondary to IFT defects, this does not necessarily apply to the renal phenotype as no changes in the hedgehog pathway were noted in kidneys from *Ift140* knockout mice prior to the onset of cystogenesis [55].

Wnt Signalling and Planar Cell Polarity (PCP)

The role of cilia and ciliary proteins in regulating wnt signalling is subject of an ongoing discussion recently reviewed by Wallingford and Mitchell [81]. Wnt signalling can be roughly divided into a so-called "canonical" pathway branch involving wnt/beta-catenin and a so called "non-canonical" or planar cell polarity (PCP) branch. Canonical Wnt/beta-catenin dependent signalling occurs after extracellular wnt ligand binds to transmembrane Frizzled receptors which stabilize beta-catenin. Beta-catenin subsequently localises to the nucleus to activate further target genes [82]. The non-canonical or PCP pathway is mediated via Frizzled and the large transmembrane proteins Vangl2 and Celsr and involves cytoplasmic regulatory proteins such as Dishevelled (Dvl). PCP describes the process of orientation of cells and their structures along an axis in an epithelial plane in a coordinated manner [83]. Classical PCP readouts exist for all species from *drosophila* flies over *xenopus* frogs to mammals, including orientation of hair on the fly wing, convergent extension (axis elongation by cell intercalation) of the anterior-posterior body axis of frog embryos and orientation of hair cells in the inner ear of mice.

The first indication that proteins encoded by genes defective in human ciliopathies play a role in PCP came from Bardet-Biedl-Syndrome mouse models displaying typical PCP-related defects in the cochlea [84]. Further initial experiments suggested that the ciliary protein encoded by *NPHP2, Inversin (Invs)*, inhibits Dvl-mediated transduction of the canonical wnt pathway while promoting a shift towards PCP signalling [85], proposing that Inversin might act as a switch between canonical and non-canonical/PCP Wnt signalling [85]. This would imply that in an inversin-deficient state such as in nephronophthi-

sis patients with Inversin mutations, non-canonical wnt signalling might be expanded and PCP signalling reduced. In line with the assumption that cilia might act as a negative regulator of canonical wnt signalling, increased canonical wnt signalling was found in cells deficient for Bardet-Biedl-Syndrome proteins BBS1, BBS4 and MKKS and the anterograde IFT motor protein KIF3A [86], in mice mutant for *Kif3a, Ift88* and *Ofd1* [87] as well as in kidney-specific *Ift20* knockout mice exhibiting a cystic renal phenotype [88]. However, no abnormalities in wnt signalling were found by Ocbina et al. in the absence of cilia in mice mutant for *Kif3a, Ift88, Ift72* [89] and in *ift88* zebrafish mutants [90]. The relationship between cilia and wnt signalling therefore remains unclear.

Loss of ciliary proteins such as Ift88 and *Kif3a* in mice results in developmental defects resembling those expected for loss of PCP including mis-orientated inner ear kinocilia [91]. Also, renal tubules elongate during development using a process strongly resembling convergent extension, depending on the non-canonical wnt ligand *Wnt9b*, where loss of Wnt9b leads to renal cyst formation [92]. Furthermore, *Ift20* disruption in mice causes cystic renal disease and in those kidneys, mitotic spindle mis-orientation has been described [88]. As mis-orientated mitotic spindles could affect orientated cell division (OCD), and OCD is the basis for planar cell polarity and necessary for postnatal tubule elongation, loss of OCD might contribute to cystic phenotypes [93]. This is supported by observations in Kif3a, Pkd1, Tsc1/2 and Hnf1b-deficient mice [94–96]. Last, the wnt-regulator Dvl might also control apical docking and planar polarisation of basal bodies from which cilia extend in epithelial cells [97]. Ciliary polarity, which in turn could potentially define cellular polarity, is influenced by the anaphase promoting complex APC/C [98]. These findings, together with the suggestion that the nephronophthisis protein Inversin might act as a switch from canonical wnt towards PCP signalling [85], has led to the hypothesis that cystic and NPHP-phenotypes observed in ciliopathies might result from disturbed PCP. However, loss of OCD and/or PCP might not be the cyst-initiating event as mice mutant for the murine homologue of PKHD1, the Fibrocystin gene causing ARPKD in humans, do not develop cysts despite disrupted OCD [99]. Moreover, cysts can be present despite normal OCD as shown in mice lacking IFT140 in the kidneys [55]. Recent work in the Xenopus model suggests nevertheless that tubular morphogenesis requires planar cell polarity (PCP) and non-canonical Wnt signalling [100].

Flow Hypothesis, Ca-Signalling/Mechanosensation and mTOR

In 2001, Praetorius and Spring observed increased intracellular calcium levels after flow induced bending of primary cilia on canine kidney cells [101] and subsequently demonstrated that loss of cilia abolishes the flow-induced calcium influx [102]. This was subsequently confirmed in mice with ciliary defects due to *Ift88* deficiency [103]. The *Polycystin-1* and *Polycystin-2* (*PKD1* and *PKD2*) genes, mutated in subjects with ADPKD, are thought to play a role in this mechanosensation and calcium influx process [104, 105]. However, loss of mechanosensation and/or flow induced calcium influx alone is probably not sufficient to cause cystic kidney disease and Polycystin-1, although required for maintenance of tubular morphology in the long run, does not appear essential in the short or intermediate term. Possibly a second exogenous harmful event such as kidney injury is required for cyst formation in the long term [93]. How lack of flow and subsequently reduced calcium influx might lead to cystogenesis has not been clearly established. Delayed or reduced clearance of intracellular cAMP may be involved as accumulation of cAMP was noticed in cystic renal tissue [106]. This in turn might lead to increased MAP kinase signalling stimulating both cell proliferation and fluid secretion into the cyst lumen. Interestingly, fluid flow also induces phosphorylation of a key regulator of cardiac hypertrophy, histone deacetylase 5 (HDAC5) via polycystin-mediated mechanosensation. This leads to myocyte enhancer factor 2C (MEF2C)-dependent transcriptional events in the nucleus and kidney-specific knockout of *Mef2c* results in extensive renal tubule dilatation and cysts whereas *Hdac5* heterozygosity or treatment with an HDAC inhibitor reduces cyst formation in *Pkd2−/−* mouse embryos, indicating a potential treatment target [107].

Based on the observations that human subjects with tuberous sclerosis due to *TSC2* mutations develop cystic renal disease, TSC2 (Tuberin) is considered a negative regulator of mTor signalling [108], Polycystin-1 interacts with Tuberin and mTor activity is elevated in cystic tissues [109, 110], a hypothesis evolved that mTor signalling might be involved in the initiation and/or progression of cystic renal disease and that inhibition of such signalling could delay disease progression. However, while in a rodent model the mTORC1 inhibitor Rapamycin significantly delayed cyst progression [111], a clinical trial using everolimus in human PKD subjects ended with disappointing results: despite slowing down cyst expansion, renal function was not better preserved in everolimus treated subjects compared to controls. Possibly the administered dose was insufficient or more likely, the timepoint of treatment initiation was chosen too late with regards to the disease course to achieve stabilisation of renal function [112]. Nevertheless, mTor signalling seems to play a role in progression of cystic kidney disease and is potentially connected to flow-induced cilia bending: when cells are grown in a flow chamber, flow leads to Lkb1 induced mTor inhibition resulting in smaller cell size [113]. Flow might further regulate cilia length, potentially also through mTor signalling as cilia length is reduced under flow and increased within cysts where flow is absent [95]. Likewise, mTor inhibitors seem to decrease cilia length reflecting the effects of flow [93, 114].

Yap-Hippo Signalling

The hippo-signalling pathway has emerged in recent years as an important pathway controlling cell and organ growth, stem cell function, regeneration functions and tumor suppression. Dysregulation of hippo signalling was initially noticed to lead to initiation and maintenance of cancerous growth [115]. More recently evidence for this pathway has emerged indicating its fundamental role for developmental processes, including kidney and eye development in mammals. Knockout mice for one of the main pathway components, *Yes-associated protein-1* (*Yap1*), die during early gestation with major developmental defects including yolk sack and axis elongation defects [116] while heterozygous *YAP1* loss of function mutations lead to optic fissure closure defects and possibly also cleft-lip palate, hearing loss, learning difficulties and hematuria with incomplete penetrance in humans [117]. More importantly, inactivation of another major pathway molecule, TAZ, in mice leads to polycystic kidneys (glomerulocystic disease), severe urinary concentrating defects and pulmonary emphysema [118, 119]. The renal phenotype partially resembles that of nephronophthisis patients. Further, NPHP3, NPHP4 and NPHP9/NEK8, products of genes mutated in subjects with nephronophthisis and Meckel-Gruber Syndrome, seem to be involved in Hippo-pathway regulation [120–122]. It is of note, however, that YAP1 is not only directly implicated in the hippo signalling pathway but also modulates WNT signalling via β-catenin-interaction [123], BMP signalling via interaction with Smad7 [124] as well as NOTCH signalling through up-regulation of *JAG1* [125] so that the observed developmental defects in patients with *YAP1* mutations are probably not solely effects of impaired hippo signalling. Moreover, *YAP1* itself is up-regulated by hedgehog signalling [126] raising the possibility that disturbed hedgehog signalling in ciliopathy/nephronophthisis subjects might contribute to the observed abnormalities in hippo signalling.

The substantial cross-talk between major developmental signalling pathways including wnt, hedgehog, hippo, notch and mTor [127] leaves the actual molecular basis of a developmental defect such as nephronophthisis uncertain. Nonetheless, in view of the clear renal phenotype observed in TAZ-deficient mice and well established protein-protein interactions between NPHP proteins and TAZ, dysregulated hippo signalling is one of the best candidates so far regarding the primary molecular pathomechanism leading to nephronophthisis like disorders.

Other Cilia Associated Cell Signalling Pathways

Excellent overviews of how the cilium orchestrates cellular signalling pathways during development and tissue repair have been provided by Christensen et al. [128] and Satir et al. [129]. Due to space constraints, not all pathways can be discussed here in detail so we will only scratch the surface of the relationship between cilia and TGF-beta signalling. Clathrin-dependent endocytosis governs TGF-beta signalling and interestingly, TGF-β receptors localise to endocytotic vesicles at the ciliary base and to the ciliary tip in vitro. Activation of SMAD2/3 at the ciliary base has been observed. TGF-β signalling seems to be reduced in the absence of cilia in fibroblasts lacking Ift88 suggesting that cilia might regulate TGF-β signalling and that the cilium could represent a compartment for clathrin-dependent endocytotic regulation of signal transduction [130]. Increased TGF-beta signalling has been associated with increased interstitial fibrosis in progressive renal dysfunction in ADPKD and other renal conditions. Most interestingly, the PPAR-γ agonist rosiglitazone, reversing a downstream effect of TGFß, was nephro-protective and prolonged survival in an ADPKD rodent model via inhibition of TGF-ß induced renal fibrosis [131]. If this effect is also applicable to humans remains to be established.

Cilia in Renal Disease

The clinical aspects of human ciliopathies with renal involvement are discussed in more detail in the polycystic kidney disease and nephronophthisis chapters of this book (Chaps. 12 and 13, respectively). We will here give a short introduction and overview, mainly focusing on conditions resulting from mutations in IFT and BBS genes. Please also see Table 9.1 for a summary of ciliopathies with renal involvement.

Polycystic Kidney Disease (ADPKD and ARPKD)

The classic ciliary polycystic renal diseases are represented by autosomal dominant polycystic kidney disease (ADPKD) and autosomal recessive polycystic kidney disease (ARPKD). The hallmark of both diseases is extensive cystic enlargement of both kidneys. ADPKD is one of the most common monogenetic disorders with an incidence of 1 in 600–800 live births in the western world and clinical signs of ADPKD usually become manifest in adulthood [132]. In affected subjects, heterozygous mutations in either PKD1 or PKD2, encoding for Polycystin 1 and Polycystin 2, have been identified and it is common belief that a second acquired somatic mutation is necessary for the initiation of cystogenesis ("second hit hypothesis"). Gene dosage at least of PKD1 probably plays a role for the severity of the phenotype, which rarely can mimic ARPKD [133].

With a frequency of 1:20,000 live births, ARPKD is a lot less common than ADPKD and is inherited in an autosomal-recessive manner. Two mutated germline alleles are present from the very beginning causing a very early disease onset due to loss of Fibrocystin function, the protein encoded by the *PKHD1* gene. Increased renal echogeneity and cysts are usually present prenatally and biliary dysgenesis resulting in intrahepatic bile duct dilatation and congenital hepatic fibrosis (Caroli disease) occurs frequently. Fibrocystin co-localises with PKD2 at the ciliary axoneme and the ciliary base; however, its exact function has remained elusive [134].

As outlined above, flow mediated ciliary bending might activate calcium influx and it has been suggested that PKD1 and PKD2 proteins together function as a Ca^{2+}-permeable receptor channel complex [104, 135, 136]. Further, Polycystins interact with the tuberous sclerosis protein Tuberin which is known to influence mTor signalling and the mTor pathway was found to be overactivated in cystic epithelia from Polycystin-deficient kidneys. However, despite major efforts over the past two decades, the exact pathomechanism for cystogenesis in ADPKD and ARPKD remains to be defined and to date, efficient pharmacological treatment remains to be developed. For more details on ciliary signalling pathways please refer to the above sections and the polycystic kidney disease chapter of this book, Chap. 12.

Syndromal Nephronophthisis (NPHP)

For a detailed description of Nephronophthisis, including isolated Nephronophthisis, Joubert Syndrome, Senior-Loken Syndrome and Cogan Syndrome, please refer Chap. 13. Nephronophthisis can be translated as "vanishing nephrons" or "vanishing kidney" and in contrast to ADPKD and ARPKD, where increasing numbers of cysts and increasing cyst volumes lead to larger kidneys, in subjects affected by NPHP or NPHP-like renal disease kidneys appear normal or small in size, often with increased echogenicity in ultrasound images. Many genes have been identified to date causing either isolated NPHP or NPHP combined with extrarenal symptoms which could be described as "syndromal" NPHP. These extrarenal symptoms include retinal degeneration, cerebellar malformations, skeletal dysplasia including polydactyly, situs inversus, obesity and learning difficulties. There is excessive genetic and phenotypic heterogeneity, meaning that not only the clinical symptoms overlap between different syndromes with NPHP- or NPHP-like renal phenotypes but also mutations in one and the same gene can cause different phenotypes. We will focus in this chapter on selected phenotypes of "syndromal NPHP" including Bardet-Biedl-Syndrome resulting from mutations in BBS genes and ciliary skeletal dysplasias such as Short-rib polydactyly syndrome (SRPS), Jeune Syndrome (JATD), Mainzer-Saldino Syndrome and Sensenbrenner Syndrome (CED), consequences of impaired intraflagellar transport (IFT).

Bardet-Biedl-Syndrome (LMBBS, BBS)

Among the first human ciliopathy diseases recognised as such was Bardet-Biedl-Syndrome (BBS,

Laurence-Moon-Bardet-Biedl-Syndrome, LMBBS) and therefore this condition is often referred as an example of a classical complex developmental phenotype resulting from hereditary cilia malfunction. The main features of BBS are polydactyly, developmental delay, obesity, retinal degeneration, cystic or, more commonly, NPHP-like renal disease and hypogenitalism [137]. BBS is very rare with an estimated frequency varying between 1:160,000 in northern European populations to 1:13,500 and 1:17,500 in isolated consanguineous communities such as in Kuwait and Newfoundland. Like other ciliopathies, BBS is a genetically very heterogeneous disease with mutations in 19 genes identified to date and there is considerable genetic and phenotypic overlap (especially regarding eyes and kidneys) with other ciliopathies such as Meckel-Gruber-Syndrome and Senior-Loken-syndrome. Perinatally, BBS can be difficult to distinguish from McKusick-Kaufman syndrome if polydactyly and hydrometrocolpos are present [138]. Although BBS represents an autosomal-recessive condition, in individual cases more than two mutated alleles at two different loci have been found to be necessary to cause the phenotype ("triallelic inheritance") [139, 140]. However, the vast majority of cases are inherited in the classical recessive manner [141]. Nevertheless, several "modifier" genes have been described which may influence the phenotype. While genotype-phenotype correlations have proven difficult to establish, mutations in certain genes seem to predispose for more severe kidney involvement. Mutations in *BBS6*, *BBS10* and *BBS12* are associated with renal disease at an overall frequency of 30–86%; however, this includes minor anomalies and the majority of patients do not progress to renal failure [142].

While some of the proteins encoded by genes mutated in BBS localise to the ciliary transition zone (e.g., CEP290), others localise further proximal to the basal body area and axonemal localisation has been observed as well. BBS proteins seem to form two different major protein complexes: the so-called BBSome and the BBS chaperone complex where the formation of the BBSome requires the function of the BBS chaperone complex. Data from mouse and zebrafish models indicate a role for BBS genes in intracellular and intraflagellar trafficking of ciliary components. Therefore, although the BBSome does not seem to be required for ciliary assembly itself, due to its trafficking function specific signalling receptors and transmembrane proteins no longer reach the cilium in subjects affected by BBS, leading to organ-specific signalling abnormalities and subsequently the characteristic developmental defects [26, 143, 144]. While the loss of function of BBS and IFT proteins conceivably leads to retinal degeneration due to impaired transport of molecules such as rhodopsin along the connecting cilium between the inner and outer segments of photoreceptor cells, the mechanism for (NPHP-like) renal disease in BBS and IFT-related diseases as largely remains elusive. As discussed above, imbalances in the hippo signalling pathway seem to play a role in classical nephronophthisis. To which extent this applies to BBS has not yet been investigated. While polydactyly in BBS as well as indirectly IFT-dependent disorders point towards a hedgehog-based mechanism at least for the skeletal phenotype, a contribution of misregulated hedgehog signalling to the renal phenotype has yet to be proven. Clinical hallmarks of BBS are shown in Fig. 9.7a–h.

Alström Syndrome

Alström syndrome is a very rare autosomal-recessive ciliopathy occurring with a frequency of 1:500,000–1:1,000,000 but can be more common amongst consanguineous populations. Over 100 mutations in a single large gene, *Alms1*, have been published to date. Clinical characteristics include obesity, retinal dysfunction, cardiomyopathy, hearing loss, hepatic involvement, renal disease and hypogonadism, resembling the BBS phenotype; however, with higher lethality due to cardiac complications [146]. In contrast to BBS, polydactyly and developmental delay are not common features. The Alms1 protein localises to the base of the cilium [147] and knockdown of *Alms1* in kidney epithelial cells in vitro causes

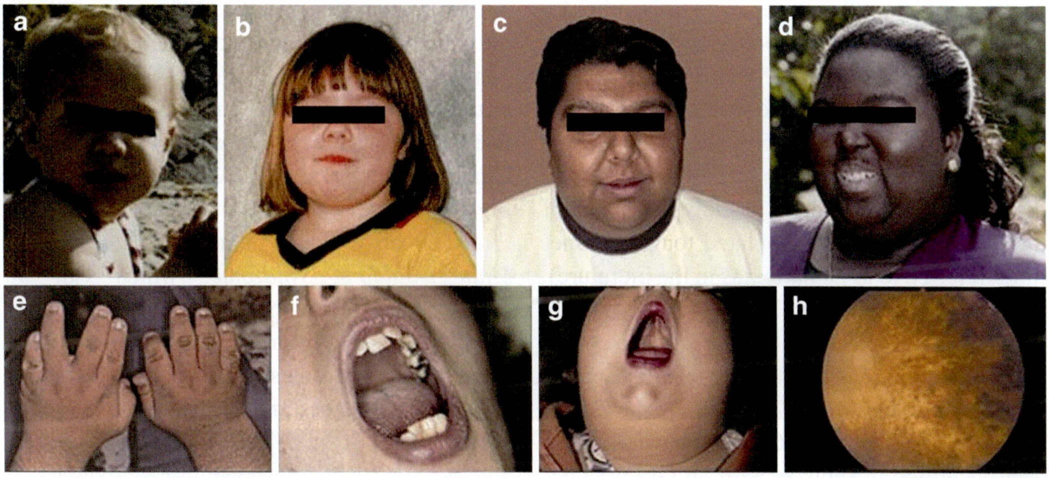

Fig. 9.7 (**a–h**) Clinical hallmarks of Bardet-Biedl-Syndrome (BBS). (**a–d**) Dysmorphic facial features including a flat nasal bridge, retrognathia, small mouth, malar hypoplasia, deep-set eyes, downward slanting palpebral fissures, hypertelorism (**e**) Brachydactyly and scars from removal of accessory digits. (**f, g**) High arched palate and dental crowding. (**h**) Rod-cone dystrophy in fundoscopy. (Used with permission of Nature Publishing Group from Forsythe and Beales [145])

shortened cilia and seems to abrogate calcium influx in response to mechanical stimuli. In a mouse model of Alström syndrome, loss of cilia from the kidney proximal tubules was observed [148]. *Alms1*-disrupted mice also recapitulate the neurosensory deficits observed in humans with Alström Syndrome and their cochleae display signs of disturbed planar cell polarity abnormal orientation of hair cell stereociliary bundles which seemed to be prematurely lost when the mice grow older [149]. Alms1 has further been implicated in cell cycle control, and intracellular transport as well as the recycling endosome pathway [150]. To which extent disturbance any of these processes contributes to the renal phenotype still requires further investigation.

Joubert-Syndrome Related Disorders (JSRD)

Joubert syndrome (JS) is a very rare neurodevelopmental, mostly autosomal recessive but rarely X-linked disorder characterised by the so-called molar tooth sign (MTS). MTS represents a complex midbrain-hindbrain malformation visible on brain imaging. Anatomical correlate is hypodysplasia of the cerebellar vermis, abnormally deep interpeduncular fossa at the level of the isthmus and upper pons, and horizontalized, thickened and elongated superior cerebellar peduncles [151]. The estimated incidence is 1/80,000–1/100,000 live births. Clinically, neurological features such hypotonia at birth, ataxia, developmental delay, abnormal eye movements and neonatal breathing dysregulation are predominant but multiple extra-neurological symptoms occur. JS and Joubert Syndrome related disorders (JSRD) can be classified in six phenotypic subgroups: isolated JS; JS with ocular defect; JS with renal defect; JS with oculo-renal defects; JS with hepatic defect and JS with orofaciodigital defects.

JS/JSRD are genetically heterogeneous and there is marked phenotypical variability even within families. JS with renal defect (JS-R) is characterized by additional juvenile nephronophthisis but no retinal disease and mainly caused by mutations in *NPHP* and *RPGRIP1L*. JS with oculo-renal defects (JS-OR) occurs mainly due to mutations in *CEP290*, a transition zone protein encoding gene also found defective in BBS. Mutations in *TMEM67*, a gene also found to cause Meckel-Gruber Syndrome, have

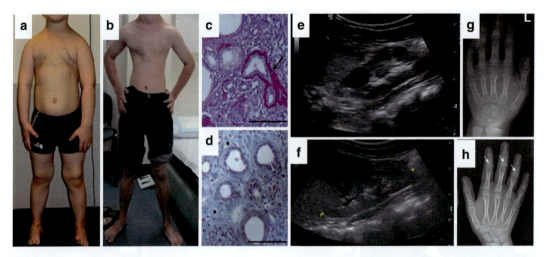

Fig. 9.9 (**a–h**) Clinical hallmarks of Mainzer-Saldino-Syndrome. (**a**, **b**) Mildly narrowed thorax. (**c**, **d**) Histological pictures of a renal biopsy. (**e**, **f**) Ultrasound images showing increased echogeneity and small renal cysts. (**g**, **h**) Cone shaped epiphyses. ((**b–h**) Used with permission of Elsevier from Perrault et al. [69]; (**a**, **e–g**) Used with permission of John Wiley and Sons from Schmidts et al. [20])

In humans affected by SRPS, kidney function cannot be followed due to neonatal death from respiratory failure, but mice carrying mutations in *Nek1* exhibit cystic renal disease [162]. Nek1 binds to the kinesin-2 component Kif3a [163], and kidney specific loss of Kif3a causes cystic disease [54]. Moreover, NEK1 and TAZ proteins interact physically to maintain normal levels of Polycystin 2 [164], so it seems possible that surviving patients would present with cystic or nephronophthisis-like renal involvement. Surprisingly, while impaired function of IFT proteins and Kif3a results in cystic kidney disease in mice, the combined knockout of *Kif3a* and *Pkd1* resulted in a milder rather than more severe phenotype, suggesting the existence of a cilia-dependent, as yet unidentified cyst growth promoting pathway [165]. No human mutations have been identified in *KIF3A* or other components of the kinesin-2 complex to date; presumably such mutations would lead to an early embryonic lethal phenotype.

Although mutations in some genes seem to be able to cause both JATD and *Sensenbrenner-Syndrome/CED* as mentioned above, the clinical phenotype is slightly different in CED where additional ectodermal defects such as dysplastic finger- and toe-nail, sparse and slow growing hair and teeth abnormalities are frequently observed. The thoracic phenotype is usually milder than in JATD and polydactyly not usually observed; however, craniosynostosis has been described and human subjects frequently present with renal involvement [166]. Clinical hallmarks of Sensenbrenner syndrome are shown in Fig. 9.10a–c.

While the skeletal features observed in skeletal chondrodysplasias, especially polydactyly, point towards imbalances in the hedgehog pathway as a molecular origin of disease, the molecular pathogenesis of renal disease in subjects with IFT and dynein-2 mutations has remained elusive as neither hedgehog- nor wnt signalling defects could be established as causative for the kidney phenotype in mouse models (see the IFT and Hedgehog Signalling sections of this chapter for more details). However, given the NPHP-like phenotype observed, hippo signalling might be a good candidate pathway leading to the renal phenotype in this group of ciliopathies.

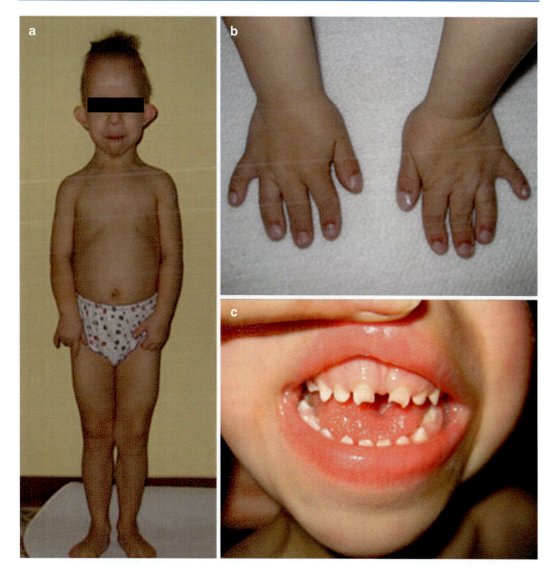

Fig. 9.10 (a–c) Clinical hallmarks of Sensenbrenner Syndrome (CED). Four-year-old girl displaying short extremities, mildly shortened and narrowed thorax, thin sparse hair, dolichocephaly, prominent forehead, full, hypertelorism, small flat nose, prominent auricles (**a**). (**b**) Brachydactyly. (**c**) Small abnormally shaped teeth. (Used with permission of Elsevier from Walczak-Sztulpa et al. [63])

Summary and Conclusion

Cilia are antenna-like structures projecting from most cells and hundreds of years after their first notion, we begin to acknowledge some of their essential function in human development, including the kidney. Extensive phenotypic and genetic heterogeneity has created a slightly chaotic picture of ciliopathies in the past and many aspects of these complex inherited conditions have remained unclear. Despite linking ciliopathies to imbalances in multiple fundamental cell signalling pathways, the molecular basis of disease, especially kidney mal-development, is still largely elusive to date.

Acknowledgments We apologize to all colleagues whose findings could not be cited due to space constraints. Miriam Schmidts and Philip L. Beales acknowledge funding from the Dutch Kidney Foundation, DKF (KOUNCII, CP11.18). Miriam Schmidts is funded by an Action Medical Research UK Clinical Training Fellowship (RTF-1411) and Philip L. Beales receives funding from the European Community's Seventh Framework Programme FP7/2009; 241955, SYSCILIA, the Wellcome Trust and is an NIHR Senior Investigator.

References

1. Halbritter J, Bizet AA, Schmidts M, Porath JD, Braun DA, Gee HY, et al. Defects in the IFT-B component IFT172 cause Jeune and Mainzer-Saldino syndromes in humans. Am J Hum Genet. 2013;93(5):915–25.
2. Westhoff JH, Giselbrecht S, Schmidts M, Schindler S, Beales PL, Tonshoff B, et al. Development of an automated imaging pipeline for the analysis of the zebrafish larval kidney. PLoS One. 2013;8(12):e82137.
3. Wheatley DN. Landmarks in the first hundred years of primary (9 + 0) cilium research. Cell Biol Int. 2005;29(5):333–9.
4. Purkyně JE, Valentin GG. De phaenomeno generali et fundamentali motus vibratorii continui in membranis cum externis tum internis animalium plurimorum et superiorum et inferiorum ordinum obvii: commentatio physiologica. Wratislaviae: Sumptibus A. Schulz; 1835.
5. Afzelius BA. The immotile-cilia syndrome and other ciliary diseases. Int Rev Exp Pathol. 1979;19:1–43.
6. Murcia NS, Richards WG, Yoder BK, Mucenski ML, Dunlap JR, Woychik RP. The oak ridge polycystic kidney (orpk) disease gene is required for left-right axis determination. Development. 2000;127(11):2347–55.
7. Pazour GJ, Dickert BL, Vucica Y, Seeley ES, Rosenbaum JL, Witman GB, et al. Chlamydomonas IFT88 and its mouse homologue, polycystic kidney disease gene tg737, are required for assembly of cilia and flagella. J Cell Biol. 2000;151(3):709–18.
8. Fliegauf M, Benzing T, Omran H. When cilia go bad: cilia defects and ciliopathies. Nat Rev Mol Cell Biol. 2007;8(11):880–93.
9. Baker K, Beales PL. Making sense of cilia in disease: the human ciliopathies. Am J Med Genet C: Semin Med Genet. 2009;151C(4):281–95.
10. Hildebrandt F, Benzing T, Katsanis N. Ciliopathies. N Engl J Med. 2011;364(16):1533–43.
11. Gilula NB, Satir P. The ciliary necklace. A ciliary membrane specialization. J Cell Biol. 1972;53(2):494–509.
12. Fliegauf M, Horvath J, von Schnakenburg C, Olbrich H, Muller D, Thumfart J, et al. Nephrocystin specifically localizes to the transition zone of renal and respiratory cilia and photoreceptor connecting cilia. J Am Soc Nephrol. 2006;17(9):2424–33.
13. Shiba D, Yamaoka Y, Hagiwara H, Takamatsu T, Hamada H, Yokoyama T. Localization of Inv in a distinctive intraciliary compartment requires the C-terminal ninein-homolog-containing region. J Cell Sci. 2009;122(Pt 1):44–54.
14. Wheatley DN. Cilia and centrioles of the rat adrenal cortex. J Anat. 1967;101(Pt 2):223–37.
15. Wheatley DN. Primary cilia in normal and pathological tissues. Pathobiology. 1995;63(4):222–38.
16. Goetz SC, Ocbina PJ, Anderson KV. The primary cilium as a hedgehog signal transduction machine. Methods Cell Biol. 2009;94:199–222.
17. Huangfu D, Liu A, Rakeman AS, Murcia NS, Niswander L, Anderson KV. Hedgehog signalling in the mouse requires intraflagellar transport proteins. Nature. 2003;426(6962):83–7.
18. Ruiz-Perez VL, Blair HJ, Rodriguez-Andres ME, Blanco MJ, Wilson A, Liu YN, et al. Evc is a positive mediator of Ihh-regulated bone growth that localises at the base of chondrocyte cilia. Development. 2007;134(16):2903–12.
19. Quinlan RJ, Tobin JL, Beales PL. Modeling ciliopathies: primary cilia in development and disease. Curr Top Dev Biol. 2008;84:249–310.
20. Schmidts M, Frank V, Eisenberger T, Al Turki S, Bizet AA, Antony D, et al. Combined NGS approaches identify mutations in the intraflagellar transport gene IFT140 in skeletal ciliopathies with early progressive kidney disease. Hum Mutat. 2013;34(5):714–24.
21. Schmidts M, Arts HH, Bongers EM, Yap Z, Oud MM, Antony D, et al. Exome sequencing identifies DYNC2H1 mutations as a common cause of asphyxiating thoracic dystrophy (Jeune syndrome) without major polydactyly, renal or retinal involvement. J Med Genet. 2013;50(5):309–23.
22. Williams CL, Li C, Kida K, Inglis PN, Mohan S, Semenec L, et al. MKS and NPHP modules cooperate to establish basal body/transition zone membrane associations and ciliary gate function during ciliogenesis. J Cell Biol. 2011;192(6):1023–41.
23. Reiter JF, Blacque OE, Leroux MR. The base of the cilium: roles for transition fibres and the transition zone in ciliary formation, maintenance and compartmentalization. EMBO Rep. 2012;13(7):608–18.
24. Rohatgi R, Snell WJ. The ciliary membrane. Curr Opin Cell Biol. 2010;22(4):541–6.
25. Rosenbaum J. Intraflagellar transport. Curr Biol. 2002;12(4):R125.
26. Nachury MV, Loktev AV, Zhang Q, Westlake CJ, Peranen J, Merdes A, et al. A core complex of BBS proteins cooperates with the GTPase Rab8 to promote ciliary membrane biogenesis. Cell. 2007;129(6):1201–13.
27. Jin H, White SR, Shida T, Schulz S, Aguiar M, Gygi SP, et al. The conserved Bardet-Biedl syndrome proteins assemble a coat that traffics membrane proteins to cilia. Cell. 2010;141(7):1208–19.

28. Poole CA, Flint MH, Beaumont BW. Analysis of the morphology and function of primary cilia in connective tissues: a cellular cybernetic probe? Cell Motil. 1985;5(3):175–93.

29. Sorokin S. Centrioles and the formation of rudimentary cilia by fibroblasts and smooth muscle cells. J Cell Biol. 1962;15:363–77.

30. Rattner JB, Sciore P, Ou Y, van der Hoorn FA, Lo IK. Primary cilia in fibroblast-like type B synoviocytes lie within a cilium pit: a site of endocytosis. Histol Histopathol. 2010;25(7):865–75.

31. Ghossoub R, Molla-Herman A, Bastin P, Benmerah A. The ciliary pocket: a once-forgotten membrane domain at the base of cilia. Biol Cell. 2011;103(3):131–44.

32. Avasthi P, Marshall WF. Stages of ciliogenesis and regulation of ciliary length. Differentiation. 2012;83(2):S30–42.

33. Schmidt KN, Kuhns S, Neuner A, Hub B, Zentgraf H, Pereira G. Cep164 mediates vesicular docking to the mother centriole during early steps of ciliogenesis. J Cell Biol. 2012;199(7):1083–101.

34. Chaki M, Airik R, Ghosh AK, Giles RH, Chen R, Slaats GG, et al. Exome capture reveals ZNF423 and CEP164 mutations, linking renal ciliopathies to DNA damage response signaling. Cell. 2012;150(3):533–48.

35. Kim S, Dynlacht BD. Assembling a primary cilium. Curr Opin Cell Biol. 2013;25(4):506–11.

36. Shida T, Cueva JG, Xu Z, Goodman MB, Nachury MV. The major alpha-tubulin K40 acetyltransferase alphaTAT1 promotes rapid ciliogenesis and efficient mechanosensation. Proc Natl Acad Sci U S A. 2010;107(50):21517–22.

37. Kalebic N, Sorrentino S, Perlas E, Bolasco G, Martinez C, Heppenstall PA. alphaTAT1 is the major alpha-tubulin acetyltransferase in mice. Nat Commun. 2013;4:1962.

38. O'Hagan R, Barr MM. Regulation of tubulin glutamylation plays cell-specific roles in the function and stability of sensory cilia. Worm. 2012;1(3):155–9.

39. Pathak N, Obara T, Mangos S, Liu Y, Drummond IA. The zebrafish fleer gene encodes an essential regulator of cilia tubulin polyglutamylation. Mol Biol Cell. 2007;18(11):4353–64.

40. Thomas S, Wright KJ, Le Corre S, Micalizzi A, Romani M, Abhyankar A, et al. A homozygous PDE6D mutation in Joubert syndrome impairs targeting of farnesylated INPP5E protein to the primary cilium. Hum Mutat. 2014;35(1):137–46.

41. Paridaen JT, Wilsch-Brauninger M, Huttner WB. Asymmetric inheritance of centrosome-associated primary cilium membrane directs ciliogenesis after cell division. Cell. 2013;155(2):333–44.

42. Wang G, Chen Q, Zhang X, Zhang B, Zhuo X, Liu J, et al. PCM1 recruits Plk1 to the pericentriolar matrix to promote primary cilia disassembly before mitotic entry. J Cell Sci. 2013;126(Pt 6):1355–65.

43. Norris DP, Grimes DT. Mouse models of ciliopathies: the state of the art. Dis Model Mech. 2012;5(3):299–312.

44. Delaval B, Bright A, Lawson ND, Doxsey S. The cilia protein IFT88 is required for spindle orientation in mitosis. Nat Cell Biol. 2011;13(4):461–8.

45. Pan J, Seeger-Nukpezah T, Golemis EA. The role of the cilium in normal and abnormal cell cycles: emphasis on renal cystic pathologies. Cell Mol Life Sci. 2013;70(11):1849–74.

46. Bielas SL, Silhavy JL, Brancati F, Kisseleva MV, Al-Gazali L, Sztriha L, et al. Mutations in INPP5E, encoding inositol polyphosphate-5-phosphatase E, link phosphatidyl inositol signaling to the ciliopathies. Nat Genet. 2009;41(9):1032–6.

47. Jacoby M, Cox JJ, Gayral S, Hampshire DJ, Ayub M, Blockmans M, et al. INPP5E mutations cause primary cilium signaling defects, ciliary instability and ciliopathies in human and mouse. Nat Genet. 2009;41(9):1027–31.

48. Xu J, Li H, Wang B, Xu Y, Yang J, Zhang X, et al. VHL inactivation induces HEF1 and Aurora kinase A. J Am Soc Nephrol. 2010;21(12):2041–6.

49. Choi HJ, Lin JR, Vannier JB, Slaats GG, Kile AC, Paulsen RD, et al. NEK8 links the ATR-regulated replication stress response and S phase CDK activity to renal ciliopathies. Mol Cell. 2013;51(4):423–39.

50. Kozminski KG, Johnson KA, Forscher P, Rosenbaum JL. A motility in the eukaryotic flagellum unrelated to flagellar beating. Proc Natl Acad Sci U S A. 1993;90(12):5519–23.

51. Cole DG, Diener DR, Himelblau AL, Beech PL, Fuster JC, Rosenbaum JL. Chlamydomonas kinesin-II-dependent intraflagellar transport (IFT): IFT particles contain proteins required for ciliary assembly in Caenorhabditis elegans sensory neurons. J Cell Biol. 1998;141(4):993–1008.

52. Pazour GJ, Rosenbaum JL. Intraflagellar transport and cilia-dependent diseases. Trends Cell Biol. 2002;12(12):551–5.

53. Cole DG, Snell WJ. SnapShot: intraflagellar transport. Cell. 2009;137(4):784–e1.

54. Lin F, Hiesberger T, Cordes K, Sinclair AM, Goldstein LS, Somlo S, et al. Kidney-specific inactivation of the KIF3A subunit of kinesin-II inhibits renal ciliogenesis and produces polycystic kidney disease. Proc Natl Acad Sci U S A. 2003;100(9):5286–91.

55. Jonassen JA, SanAgustin J, Baker SP, Pazour GJ. Disruption of IFT complex A causes cystic kidneys without mitotic spindle misorientation. J Am Soc Nephrol. 2012;23(4):641–51.

56. Dagoneau N, Goulet M, Genevieve D, Sznajer Y, Martinovic J, Smithson S, et al. DYNC2H1 mutations cause asphyxiating thoracic dystrophy and short rib-polydactyly syndrome, type III. Am J Hum Genet. 2009;84(5):706–11.

57. Beales PL, Bland E, Tobin JL, Bacchelli C, Tuysuz B, Hill J, et al. IFT80, which encodes a conserved intraflagellar transport protein, is mutated in

58. Merrill AE, Merriman B, Farrington-Rock C, Camacho N, Sebald ET, Funari VA, et al. Ciliary abnormalities due to defects in the retrograde transport protein DYNC2H1 in short-rib polydactyly syndrome. Am J Hum Genet. 2009;84(4):542–9.

59. Baujat G, Huber C, El Hokayem J, Caumes R, Do Ngoc Thanh C, David A, et al. Asphyxiating thoracic dysplasia: clinical and molecular review of 39 families. J Med Genet. 2013;50(2):91–8.

60. McInerney-Leo AM, Schmidts M, Cortes CR, Leo PJ, Gener B, Courtney AD, et al. Short-rib polydactyly and Jeune syndromes are caused by mutations in WDR60. Am J Hum Genet. 2013;93(3):515–23.

61. Schmidts M, Vodopiutz J, Christou-Savina S, Cortes CR, McInerney-Leo AM, Emes RD, et al. Mutations in the gene encoding IFT dynein complex component WDR34 cause Jeune asphyxiating thoracic dystrophy. Am J Hum Genet. 2013;93(5):932–44.

62. Huber C, Wu S, Kim AS, Sigaudy S, Sarukhanov A, Serre V, et al. WDR34 mutations that cause short-rib polydactyly syndrome type III/severe asphyxiating thoracic dysplasia reveal a role for the NF-kappaB pathway in cilia. Am J Hum Genet. 2013;93(5):926–31.

63. Walczak-Sztulpa J, Eggenschwiler J, Osborn D, Brown DA, Emma F, Klingenberg C, et al. Cranioectodermal dysplasia, Sensenbrenner syndrome, is a ciliopathy caused by mutations in the IFT122 gene. Am J Hum Genet. 2010;86(6):949–56.

64. Bredrup C, Saunier S, Oud MM, Fiskerstrand T, Hoischen A, Brackman D, et al. Ciliopathies with skeletal anomalies and renal insufficiency due to mutations in the IFT-A gene WDR19. Am J Hum Genet. 2011;89(5):634–43.

65. Gilissen C, Arts HH, Hoischen A, Spruijt L, Mans DA, Arts P, et al. Exome sequencing identifies WDR35 variants involved in Sensenbrenner syndrome. Am J Hum Genet. 2010;87(3):418–23.

66. Mill P, Lockhart PJ, Fitzpatrick E, Mountford HS, Hall EA, Reijns MA, et al. Human and mouse mutations in WDR35 cause short-rib polydactyly syndromes due to abnormal ciliogenesis. Am J Hum Genet. 2011;88(4):508–15.

67. Arts HH, Bongers EM, Mans DA, van Beersum SE, Oud MM, Bolat E, et al. C14ORF179 encoding IFT43 is mutated in Sensenbrenner syndrome. J Med Genet. 2011;48(6):390–5.

68. Davis EE, Zhang Q, Liu Q, Diplas BH, Davey LM, Hartley J, et al. TTC21B contributes both causal and modifying alleles across the ciliopathy spectrum. Nat Genet. 2011;43(3):189–96.

69. Perrault I, Saunier S, Hanein S, Filhol E, Bizet AA, Collins F, et al. Mainzer-Saldino syndrome is a ciliopathy caused by IFT140 mutations. Am J Hum Genet. 2012;90(5):864–70.

70. Aldahmesh MA, Li Y, Alhashem A, Anazi S, Alkuraya H, Hashem M, et al. IFT27, encoding a small GTPase component of IFT particles, is mutated in a consanguineous family with Bardet-Biedl syndrome. Hum Mol Genet. 2014;23(12):3307–15.

71. Eggenschwiler JT, Anderson KV. Cilia and developmental signaling. Annu Rev Cell Dev Biol. 2007;23:345–73.

72. Goetz SC, Anderson KV. The primary cilium: a signalling centre during vertebrate development. Nat Rev Genet. 2010;11(5):331–44.

73. Huangfu D, Anderson KV. Cilia and hedgehog responsiveness in the mouse. Proc Natl Acad Sci U S A. 2005;102(32):11325–30.

74. Kronenberg HM. Developmental regulation of the growth plate. Nature. 2003;423(6937):332–6.

75. Ocbina PJ, Eggenschwiler JT, Moskowitz I, Anderson KV. Complex interactions between genes controlling trafficking in primary cilia. Nat Genet. 2011;43(6):547–53.

76. Rix S, Calmont A, Scambler PJ, Beales PL. An Ift80 mouse model of short rib polydactyly syndromes shows defects in hedgehog signalling without loss or malformation of cilia. Hum Mol Genet. 2011;20(7):1306–14.

77. Ashe A, Butterfield NC, Town L, Courtney AD, Cooper AN, Ferguson C, et al. Mutations in mouse Ift144 model the craniofacial, limb and rib defects in skeletal ciliopathies. Hum Mol Genet. 2012;21(8):1808–23.

78. Hu MC, Mo R, Bhella S, Wilson CW, Chuang PT, Hui CC, et al. GLI3-dependent transcriptional repression of Gli1, Gli2 and kidney patterning genes disrupts renal morphogenesis. Development. 2006;133(3):569–78.

79. Kelley RI, Hennekam RC. The Smith-Lemli-Opitz syndrome. J Med Genet. 2000;37(5):321–35. [Review].

80. Friedland-Little JM, Hoffmann AD, Ocbina PJ, Peterson MA, Bosman JD, Chen Y, et al. A novel murine allele of intraflagellar transport protein 172 causes a syndrome including VACTERL-like features with hydrocephalus. Hum Mol Genet. 2011;20(19):3725–37.

81. Wallingford JB, Mitchell B. Strange as it may seem: the many links between Wnt signaling, planar cell polarity, and cilia. Genes Dev. 2011;25(3):201–13.

82. van Amerongen R, Nusse R. Towards an integrated view of Wnt signaling in development. Development. 2009;136(19):3205–14.

83. Vladar EK, Antic D, Axelrod JD. Planar cell polarity signaling: the developing cell's compass. Cold Spring Harb Perspect Biol. 2009;1(3):a002964.

84. Ross AJ, May-Simera H, Eichers ER, Kai M, Hill J, Jagger DJ, et al. Disruption of Bardet-Biedl syndrome ciliary proteins perturbs planar cell polarity in vertebrates. Nat Genet. 2005;37(10):1135–40.

85. Simons M, Gloy J, Ganner A, Bullerkotte A, Bashkurov M, Kronig C, et al. Inversin, the gene product mutated in nephronophthisis type II, functions as a molecular switch between Wnt signaling pathways. Nat Genet. 2005;37(5):537–43.

86. Gerdes JM, Liu Y, Zaghloul NA, Leitch CC, Lawson SS, Kato M, et al. Disruption of the basal body compromises proteasomal function and perturbs intracellular Wnt response. Nat Genet. 2007;39(11):1350–60.
87. Corbit KC, Shyer AE, Dowdle WE, Gaulden J, Singla V, Chen MH, et al. Kif3a constrains beta-catenin-dependent Wnt signalling through dual ciliary and non-ciliary mechanisms. Nat Cell Biol. 2008;10(1):70–6.
88. Jonassen JA, San Agustin J, Follit JA, Pazour GJ. Deletion of IFT20 in the mouse kidney causes misorientation of the mitotic spindle and cystic kidney disease. J Cell Biol. 2008;183(3):377–84.
89. Ocbina PJ, Tuson M, Anderson KV. Primary cilia are not required for normal canonical Wnt signaling in the mouse embryo. PLoS One. 2009;4(8):e6839.
90. Huang P, Schier AF. Dampened hedgehog signaling but normal Wnt signaling in zebrafish without cilia. Development. 2009;136(18):3089–98.
91. Jones C, Roper VC, Foucher I, Qian D, Banizs B, Petit C, et al. Ciliary proteins link basal body polarization to planar cell polarity regulation. Nat Genet. 2008;40(1):69–77.
92. Karner CM, Chirumamilla R, Aoki S, Igarashi P, Wallingford JB, Carroll TJ. Wnt9b signaling regulates planar cell polarity and kidney tubule morphogenesis. Nat Genet. 2009;41(7):793–9.
93. Kotsis F, Boehlke C, Kuehn EW. The ciliary flow sensor and polycystic kidney disease. Nephrol Dial Transplant. 2013;28(3):518–26.
94. Patel V, Li L, Cobo-Stark P, Shao X, Somlo S, Lin F, et al. Acute kidney injury and aberrant planar cell polarity induce cyst formation in mice lacking renal cilia. Hum Mol Genet. 2008;17(11):1578–90.
95. Bonnet CS, Aldred M, von Ruhland C, Harris R, Sandford R, Cheadle JP. Defects in cell polarity underlie TSC and ADPKD-associated cystogenesis. Hum Mol Genet. 2009;18(12):2166–76.
96. Verdeguer F, Le Corre S, Fischer E, Callens C, Garbay S, Doyen A, et al. A mitotic transcriptional switch in polycystic kidney disease. Nat Med. 2010;16(1):106–10.
97. Park TJ, Mitchell BJ, Abitua PB, Kintner C, Wallingford JB. Dishevelled controls apical docking and planar polarization of basal bodies in ciliated epithelial cells. Nat Genet. 2008;40(7):871–9.
98. Ganner A, Lienkamp S, Schafer T, Romaker D, Wegierski T, Park TJ, et al. Regulation of ciliary polarity by the APC/C. Proc Natl Acad Sci U S A. 2009;106(42):17799–804.
99. Nishio S, Tian X, Gallagher AR, Yu Z, Patel V, Igarashi P, et al. Loss of oriented cell division does not initiate cyst formation. J Am Soc Nephrol. 2010;21(2):295–302.
100. Lienkamp SS, Liu K, Karner CM, Carroll TJ, Ronneberger O, Wallingford JB, Walz G. Vertebrate kidney tubules elongate using a planar cell polarity-dependent, rosette-based mechanism of convergent

extension. Nat Genet. 2012;44(12):1382–7. https://doi.org/10.1038/ng.2452.
101. Praetorius HA, Spring KR. Bending the MDCK cell primary cilium increases intracellular calcium. J Membr Biol. 2001;184(1):71–9.
102. Praetorius HA, Spring KR. Removal of the MDCK cell primary cilium abolishes flow sensing. J Membr Biol. 2003;191(1):69–76.
103. Liu W, Murcia NS, Duan Y, Weinbaum S, Yoder BK, Schwiebert E, et al. Mechanoregulation of intracellular Ca2+ concentration is attenuated in collecting duct of monocilium-impaired orpk mice. Am J Physiol Renal Physiol. 2005;289(5):F978–88.
104. Nauli SM, Alenghat FJ, Luo Y, Williams E, Vassilev P, Li X, et al. Polycystins 1 and 2 mediate mechanosensation in the primary cilium of kidney cells. Nat Genet. 2003;33(2):129–37.
105. Xu C, Rossetti S, Jiang L, Harris PC, Brown-Glaberman U, Wandinger-Ness A, et al. Human ADPKD primary cyst epithelial cells with a novel, single codon deletion in the PKD1 gene exhibit defective ciliary polycystin localization and loss of flow-induced Ca2+ signaling. Am J Physiol Renal Physiol. 2007;292(3):F930–45.
106. Cowley BD Jr. Calcium, cyclic AMP, and MAP kinases: dysregulation in polycystic kidney disease. Kidney Int. 2008;73(3):251–3.
107. Xia S, Li X, Johnson T, Seidel C, Wallace DP, Li R. Polycystin-dependent fluid flow sensing targets histone deacetylase 5 to prevent the development of renal cysts. Development. 2010;137(7):1075–84.
108. Inoki K, Li Y, Zhu T, Wu J, Guan KL. TSC2 is phosphorylated and inhibited by Akt and suppresses mTOR signalling. Nat Cell Biol. 2002;4(9):648–57.
109. Shillingford JM, Murcia NS, Larson CH, Low SH, Hedgepeth R, Brown N, et al. The mTOR pathway is regulated by polycystin-1, and its inhibition reverses renal cystogenesis in polycystic kidney disease. Proc Natl Acad Sci U S A. 2006;103(14):5466–71.
110. Distefano G, Boca M, Rowe I, Wodarczyk C, Ma L, Piontek KB, et al. Polycystin-1 regulates extracellular signal-regulated kinase-dependent phosphorylation of tuberin to control cell size through mTOR and its downstream effectors S6K and 4EBP1. Mol Cell Biol. 2009;29(9):2359–71.
111. Tao Y, Kim J, Schrier RW, Edelstein CL. Rapamycin markedly slows disease progression in a rat model of polycystic kidney disease. J Am Soc Nephrol. 2005;16(1):46–51.
112. Walz G, Budde K, Mannaa M, Nurnberger J, Wanner C, Sommerer C, et al. Everolimus in patients with autosomal dominant polycystic kidney disease. N Engl J Med. 2010;363(9):830–40.
113. Boehlke C, Kotsis F, Patel V, Braeg S, Voelker H, Bredt S, et al. Primary cilia regulate mTORC1 activity and cell size through Lkb1. Nat Cell Biol. 2010;12(11):1115–22.
114. Yuan S, Li J, Diener DR, Choma MA, Rosenbaum JL, Sun Z. Target-of-rapamycin complex 1 (Torc1) signaling modulates cilia size and function through

114. protein synthesis regulation. Proc Natl Acad Sci U S A. 2012;109(6):2021–6.

115. Johnson R, Halder G. The two faces of Hippo: targeting the Hippo pathway for regenerative medicine and cancer treatment. Nat Rev Drug Discov. 2014;13(1):63–79.

116. Morin-Kensicki EM, Boone BN, Howell M, Stonebraker JR, Teed J, Alb JG, et al. Defects in yolk sac vasculogenesis, chorioallantoic fusion, and embryonic axis elongation in mice with targeted disruption of Yap65. Mol Cell Biol. 2006;26(1):77–87.

117. Williamson KA, Rainger J, Floyd JA, Ansari M, Meynert A, Aldridge KV, et al. Heterozygous loss-of-function mutations in YAP1 cause both isolated and syndromic optic fissure closure defects. Am J Hum Genet. 2014;94(2):295–302.

118. Hossain Z, Ali SM, Ko HL, Xu J, Ng CP, Guo K, et al. Glomerulocystic kidney disease in mice with a targeted inactivation of Wwtr1. Proc Natl Acad Sci U S A. 2007;104(5):1631–6.

119. Makita R, Uchijima Y, Nishiyama K, Amano T, Chen Q, Takeuchi T, et al. Multiple renal cysts, urinary concentration defects, and pulmonary emphysematous changes in mice lacking TAZ. Am J Physiol Renal Physiol. 2008;294(3):F542–53.

120. Habbig S, Bartram MP, Muller RU, Schwarz R, Andriopoulos N, Chen S, et al. NPHP4, a cilia-associated protein, negatively regulates the Hippo pathway. J Cell Biol. 2011;193(4):633–42.

121. Frank V, Habbig S, Bartram MP, Eisenberger T, Veenstra-Knol HE, Decker C, et al. Mutations in NEK8 link multiple organ dysplasia with altered Hippo signalling and increased c-MYC expression. Hum Mol Genet. 2013;22(11):2177–85.

122. Habbig S, Bartram MP, Sagmuller JG, Griessmann A, Franke M, Muller RU, et al. The ciliopathy disease protein NPHP9 promotes nuclear delivery and activation of the oncogenic transcriptional regulator TAZ. Hum Mol Genet. 2012;21(26):5528–38.

123. Rosenbluh J, Nijhawan D, Cox AG, Li X, Neal JT, Schafer EJ, et al. Beta-catenin-driven cancers require a YAP1 transcriptional complex for survival and tumorigenesis. Cell. 2012;151(7):1457–73.

124. Aragon E, Goerner N, Xi Q, Gomes T, Gao S, Massague J, et al. Structural basis for the versatile interactions of Smad7 with regulator WW domains in TGF-beta pathways. Structure. 2012;20(10):1726–36.

125. Tschaharganeh DF, Chen X, Latzko P, Malz M, Gaida MM, Felix K, et al. Yes-associated protein up-regulates jagged-1 and activates the notch pathway in human hepatocellular carcinoma. Gastroenterology. 2013;144(7):1530–42.e12.

126. Fernandez LA, Northcott PA, Dalton J, Fraga C, Ellison D, Angers S, et al. YAP1 is amplified and up-regulated in hedgehog-associated medulloblastomas and mediates sonic hedgehog-driven neural precursor proliferation. Genes Dev. 2009;23(23):2729–41.

127. Shimobayashi M, Hall MN. Making new contacts: the mTOR network in metabolism and signalling crosstalk. Nat Rev Mol Cell Biol. 2014;15(3):155–62.

128. Christensen ST, Pedersen SF, Satir P, Veland IR, Schneider L. The primary cilium coordinates signaling pathways in cell cycle control and migration during development and tissue repair. Curr Top Dev Biol. 2008;85:261–301.

129. Satir P, Pedersen LB, Christensen ST. The primary cilium at a glance. J Cell Sci. 2010;123(Pt 4):499–503.

130. Clement CA, Ajbro KD, Koefoed K, Vestergaard ML, Veland IR, Henriques de Jesus MP, et al. TGF-beta signaling is associated with endocytosis at the pocket region of the primary cilium. Cell Rep. 2013;3(6):1806–14.

131. Liu Y, Dai B, Xu C, Fu L, Hua Z, Mei C. Rosiglitazone inhibits transforming growth factor-beta1 mediated fibrogenesis in ADPKD cyst-lining epithelial cells. PLoS One. 2011;6(12):e28915.

132. Guay-Woodford LM. Renal cystic diseases: diverse phenotypes converge on the cilium/centrosome complex. Pediatr Nephrol. 2006;21(10):1369–76.

133. Kleffmann J, Frank V, Ferbert A, Bergmann C. Dosage-sensitive network in polycystic kidney and liver disease: multiple mutations cause severe hepatic and neurological complications. J Hepatol. 2012;57(2):476–7.

134. Harris PC, Torres VE. Polycystic kidney disease. Annu Rev Med. 2009;60:321–37.

135. Mochizuki T, Wu G, Hayashi T, Xenophontos SL, Veldhuisen B, Saris JJ, et al. PKD2, a gene for polycystic kidney disease that encodes an integral membrane protein. Science. 1996;272(5266):1339–42.

136. Hughes J, Ward CJ, Peral B, Aspinwall R, Clark K, San Millan JL, et al. The polycystic kidney disease 1 (PKD1) gene encodes a novel protein with multiple cell recognition domains. Nat Genet. 1995;10(2):151–60.

137. Beales PL, Elcioglu N, Woolf AS, Parker D, Flinter FA. New criteria for improved diagnosis of Bardet-Biedl syndrome: results of a population survey. J Med Genet. 1999;36(6):437–46.

138. Forsythe E, Beales PL. Bardet-Biedl syndrome. Eur J Hum Genet. 2013;21(1):8–13.

139. Katsanis N, Ansley SJ, Badano JL, Eichers ER, Lewis RA, Hoskins BE, et al. Triallelic inheritance in Bardet-Biedl syndrome, a Mendelian recessive disorder. Science. 2001;293(5538):2256–9.

140. Eichers ER, Lewis RA, Katsanis N, Lupski JR. Triallelic inheritance: a bridge between Mendelian and multifactorial traits. Ann Med. 2004;36(4):262–72.

141. Redin C, Le Gras S, Mhamdi O, Geoffroy V, Stoetzel C, Vincent MC, et al. Targeted high-throughput sequencing for diagnosis of genetically heterogeneous diseases: efficient mutation detection in Bardet-Biedl and Alstrom syndromes. J Med Genet. 2012;49(8):502–12.

142. Imhoff O, Marion V, Stoetzel C, Durand M, Holder M, Sigaudy S, et al. Bardet-Biedl syndrome: a study of the renal and cardiovascular phenotypes in a French cohort. Clin J Am Soc Nephrol. 2011;6(1):22–9.

143. Sheffield VC. The blind leading the obese: the molecular pathophysiology of a human obesity syndrome. Trans Am Clin Climatol Assoc. 2010;121:172–81; discussion 81–2.

144. Nachury MV, Seeley ES, Jin H. Trafficking to the ciliary membrane: how to get across the periciliary diffusion barrier? Annu Rev Cell Dev Biol. 2010;26:59–87.

145. Forsythe E, Beales PL. Bardet Biedl syndrome. Eur J Hum Genet. 2012;21:8–13.

146. Marshall JD, Maffei P, Beck S, Barrett TG, Paisey R, Naggert JK. Clinical utility gene card for: Alstrom syndrome—update 2013. Eur J Hum Genet. 2013;21(11) https://doi.org/10.1038/ejhg.2013.61.

147. Hearn T, Spalluto C, Phillips VJ, Renforth GL, Copin N, Hanley NA, et al. Subcellular localization of ALMS1 supports involvement of centrosome and basal body dysfunction in the pathogenesis of obesity, insulin resistance, and type 2 diabetes. Diabetes. 2005;54(5):1581–7.

148. Li G, Vega R, Nelms K, Gekakis N, Goodnow C, McNamara P, et al. A role for Alstrom syndrome protein, alms1, in kidney ciliogenesis and cellular quiescence. PLoS Genet. 2007;3(1):e8.

149. Jagger D, Collin G, Kelly J, Towers E, Nevill G, Longo-Guess C, et al. Alstrom syndrome protein ALMS1 localizes to basal bodies of cochlear hair cells and regulates cilium-dependent planar cell polarity. Hum Mol Genet. 2011;20(3):466–81.

150. Collin GB, Marshall JD, King BL, Milan G, Maffei P, Jagger DJ, et al. The Alstrom syndrome protein, ALMS1, interacts with alpha-actinin and components of the endosome recycling pathway. PLoS One. 2012;7(5):e37925.

151. Maria BL, Quisling RG, Rosainz LC, Yachnis AT, Gitten J, Dede D, et al. Molar tooth sign in Joubert syndrome: clinical, radiologic, and pathologic significance. J Child Neurol. 1999;14(6):368–76.

152. Brancati F, Dallapiccola B, Valente EM. Joubert syndrome and related disorders. Orphanet J Rare Dis. 2010;5:20.

153. Iannicelli M, Brancati F, Mougou-Zerelli S, Mazzotta A, Thomas S, Elkhartoufi N, et al. Novel TMEM67 mutations and genotype-phenotype correlates in meckelin-related ciliopathies. Hum Mutat. 2010;31(5):E1319–31.

154. Valente EM, Dallapiccola B, Bertini E. Joubert syndrome and related disorders. Handb Clin Neurol. 2013;113:1879–88.

155. Lopez E, Thauvin-Robinet C, Reversade B, Khartoufi NE, Devisme L, Holder M, et al. C5orf42 is the major gene responsible for OFD syndrome type VI. Hum Genet. 2014;133(3):367–77.

156. Betleja E, Cole DG. Ciliary trafficking: CEP290 guards a gated community. Curr Biol. 2010;20(21):R928–31.

157. Huber C, Cormier-Daire V. Ciliary disorder of the skeleton. Am J Med Genet C: Semin Med Genet. 2012;160C(3):165–74.

158. El Hokayem J, Huber C, Couve A, Aziza J, Baujat G, Bouvier R, et al. NEK1 and DYNC2H1 are both involved in short rib polydactyly Majewski type but not in Beemer Langer cases. J Med Genet. 2012;49(4):227–33.

159. Cavalcanti DP, Huber C, Sang KH, Baujat G, Collins F, Delezoide AL, et al. Mutation in IFT80 in a fetus with the phenotype of Verma-Naumoff provides molecular evidence for Jeune-Verma-Naumoff dysplasia spectrum. J Med Genet. 2011;48(2):88–92.

160. Thiel C, Kessler K, Giessl A, Dimmler A, Shalev SA, von der Haar S, et al. NEK1 mutations cause short-rib polydactyly syndrome type majewski. Am J Hum Genet. 2011;88(1):106–14.

161. Chen Y, Chen CF, Riley DJ, Chen PL. Nek1 kinase functions in DNA damage response and checkpoint control through a pathway independent of ATM and ATR. Cell Cycle. 2011;10(4):655–63.

162. Upadhya P, Birkenmeier EH, Birkenmeier CS, Barker JE. Mutations in a NIMA-related kinase gene, Nek1, cause pleiotropic effects including a progressive polycystic kidney disease in mice. Proc Natl Acad Sci U S A. 2000;97(1):217–21.

163. Surpili MJ, Delben TM, Kobarg J. Identification of proteins that interact with the central coiled-coil region of the human protein kinase NEK1. Biochemistry. 2003;42(51):15369–76.

164. Yim H, Sung CK, You J, Tian Y, Benjamin T. Nek1 and TAZ interact to maintain normal levels of polycystin 2. J Am Soc Nephrol. 2011;22(5):832–7.

165. Ma M, Tian X, Igarashi P, Pazour GJ, Somlo S. Loss of cilia suppresses cyst growth in genetic models of autosomal dominant polycystic kidney disease. Nat Genet. 2013;45(9):1004–12.

166. Arts HH, Knoers NV. Current insights into renal ciliopathies: what can genetics teach us? Pediatr Nephrol. 2013;28(6):863–74.

Polycystic Kidney Disease: ADPKD and ARPKD

10

Max Christoph Liebau, Djalila Mekahli, and Carsten Bergmann

Introduction

Polycystic kidney diseases (PKD) are among the most common causes of chronic kidney disease (CKD) and end stage kidney disease (ESKD) both in children and adults [1]. The two main forms of genetic cystic kidney disorders are Autosomal Dominant and Autosomal Recessive Polycystic Kidney Disease (ADPKD and ARPKD). ADPKD is a disorder mainly manifesting at adult ages and is oligosymptomatic in childhood, although it is nowadays accepted that cysts may be present even prenatally and early pediatric involvement raises increased attention [1, 2]. In contrast, ARPKD is usually presenting in early childhood. However, mild phenotypes with disease onset at adult age have been reported anecdotally [1, 3, 4]. Recent cell biological and clinical research approaches have considerably expanded our knowledge on both PKDs. Still, many important questions remain to be solved. This chapter aims to give an overview of the current knowledge of ADPKD and ARPKD with a special focus on pediatric clinical aspects. For genetics we focus on the main genes, but would like to emphasize that there is a growing list of genes that when mutated may mimic ADPKD or ARPKD.

M. C. Liebau (✉)
Department of Pediatrics, University Hospital Cologne, University of Cologne, Cologne, Germany

Center for Family Health, Cologne, Germany

Center for Rare Diseases, Cologne, Germany

Center for Molecular Medicine, Cologne, Germany
e-mail: max.liebau@uk-koeln.de

D. Mekahli
Department of Pediatric Nephrology and Organ Transplantation, University Hospitals Leuven, Leuven, Belgium

PKD Research Group, Laboratory of Pediatrics, Department of Development and Regeneration, KU Leuven, Leuven, Belgium
e-mail: Djalila.mekahli@uzleuven.be

C. Bergmann
Medizinische Genetik Mainz, Limbach Genetics, Mainz, Germany

Department of Medicine IV (Nephrology), Faculty of Medicine, Medical Center-University of Freiburg, Freiburg, Germany
e-mail: carsten.bergmann@medgen-mainz.de;
carsten.bergmann@uniklinik-freiburg.de

Classification and Differential Diagnosis of Cystic Kidney Diseases

In their seminal studies, Osathanondh and Potter systematically classified cystic kidney diseases into four distinct types [5]. While this historical classification has had a great impact for concise pathoanatomical description, it is hard to reconcile with our current understanding of clinical and genetic entities. Accurate diagnosis is essen-

© The Author(s), under exclusive license to Springer Nature Switzerland AG 2023
F. Schaefer, L. A. Greenbaum (eds.), *Pediatric Kidney Disease*,
https://doi.org/10.1007/978-3-031-11665-0_10

tial both in the management of patients with PKD and in counselling their families. Notably, cystic kidneys are an important feature of numerous genetic syndromes, including both dominant disorders like tuberous sclerosis complex (TSC) and recessively inherited diseases such as Joubert syndrome.

Clinical Aspects Guiding Diagnosis in Patients with Kidney Cysts

The differential diagnosis of cysts in the kidney is broad and in addition to ARPKD and ADPKD includes, e.g. single simple cysts, multicystic dysplastic kidneys and cystic dysplasia, nephronophthisis and other ciliopathies, as well as *HNF1B*-nephropathy or TSC. Six straightforward questions that can be answered by the patient and sonographic examination may be helpful to narrow down a potential clinical diagnosis [6].

In a first general consideration, it is important to differentiate a **kidney with a single or a few cysts from a cystic kidney**. Simple kidney cysts are fairly common in elderly persons [7] and usually do not impose problems or require treatment. However, simple cysts are not common in young children and even a single cyst should raise suspicion in pediatric patients. **Family history** is important. Whereas only 10–20% of ADPKD patients lack a family history [8], ARPKD and nephronophthisis (NPH) are usually inherited recessively with healthy parents and are found more frequently in offspring of consanguineous couples. Kidney ultrasound in the parents or grandparents is a useful investigation in the evaluation of a child with early-onset cystic kidney disease of unknown origin. A third important question addresses the **age of the patient** at the time of clinical presentation. ARPKD fetuses and a minor subset of ADPKD patients may be identified with oligo- or anhydramnios already during pregnancy. Juvenile nephronophthisis (NPH) classically presents with polyuria and polydipsia in school children. Most ADPKD patients are adults. While cysts in the kidney may appear during childhood or even prenatally in ADPKD and

can be found by ultrasound, most children do not yet show clinical symptoms. Fourthly, the **localization of cysts** may give a hint. Cysts in NPH are found at the cortico-medullary border, whereas in ADPKD cysts localize to all parts of the kidney. **Kidney and cyst size** can also point to the correct diagnosis. Kidneys in NPH tend to be normal-sized or small, whereas ARPKD and ADPKD kidneys are large. Cysts are typically tiny in early stages of ARPKD, but may resemble large ADPKD macrocysts during the course of the disease. Finally, cystic kidney disorders may be accompanied by **extra-renal symptoms**, such as retinitis pigmentosa presenting with initial night blindness later progressing to almost complete loss of vision in case of syndromes accompanied by NPH, liver cysts in ADPKD and congenital hepatic fibrosis in ARPKD.

With these six pieces of information at hand, a potential diagnosis can be made clinically in many cases. Nonetheless, clinical diagnosis can be challenging due to overlapping syndromes and symptoms, and establishing a confirmatory genetic diagnosis can be helpful.

General Considerations on Genetic Diagnostics for Polycystic Kidney Disease

Marquardt first postulated genetic heterogeneity of polycystic kidney diseases when stating in 1935: "In surviving individuals, cystic kidneys are inherited dominantly. In non-viable individuals, cystic kidneys are recessive." [9]. It took more than 35 years from that point of view before Blyth and Ockenden demonstrated in a systematic analysis that age at presentation alone is not a reliable criterion for defining genetic heterogeneity [10].

Indications for genetic testing and recommendations for preferred testing strategies have changed significantly over recent years. In all patients with PKD manifesting prenatally or in early childhood, genetic testing is highly recommended as a first-line diagnostic procedure as part of the initial patient evaluation [11]. Testing is not required in children with a single cyst, absent extra-renal anomalies and a negative family history of ADPKD, but may be indicated in children with progressive disease indicated by kidney cysts increasing in size or number.

Genetic testing may be recommended due to the following aspects: The high gene detection rate in cystic kidney diseases allows to rapidly establish a definite diagnosis and avoid a "diagnostic odyssey" with unnecessary diagnostic measures for the majority of patients. To establish a definite diagnosis often is of **psychological benefit** for patients and families. Knowledge of the genotype may point to renal and **extra-renal comorbidities**, which would otherwise have taken considerably longer to diagnose and may benefit from early detection and disease monitoring (e.g. diabetes mellitus in *HNF1B* disease). Valid information on the recurrence **risk for future children** or other family members is only possible with knowledge of the genotype. The genotype can also be relevant for the inclusion of patients in clinical trials and the future choice of treatment options (see below).

Professional genetic counseling is highly recommended due to variable expressivity and the variety of extra-renal features seen in patients with cystic kidneys. It can also address the complex aspects of prenatal testing and pre-implantation diagnostics in line with regional practices and regulations. Given the large clinical and genetic heterogeneity and vast pleiotropy, a **comprehensive gene testing** approach is recommended for cystic kidney diseases. A stepwise approach might only be indicated in a minority of patients in which there is clear phenotypic evidence for a specific disease, such as von Hippel-Lindau syndrome for which only one single (small) gene is known and variant detection rate is high.

Whatever primary strategy is chosen, an expanded gene panel or exome sequencing, the testing approach should be able to detect copy-number variations (CNVs) (e.g., deletions account for 50% of anomalies in *HNF1B*) and to cover complex genomic regions such as in *PKD1* [12]. Analysis of the *PKD1* gene is most complicated and needs expert knowledge due to genomic duplication of the first 33 exons at six other sites

on chromosome 16p. Many of these pseudogenes are expressed as mRNA transcripts, but probably do not encode proteins. Both *PKD1* and *PKD2* variants are scattered throughout the genes' coding regions exhibiting marked allelic heterogeneity, with most variants being unique to single families ('private' variants) [1, 8, 13].

Ethical concerns exist on the question whether or not an ADPKD diagnosis should be actively sought in asymptomatic children. This includes genetic screening in addition to ultrasound examination. There is consensus on the need for early monitoring of modifiable risk factors (hypertension, proteinuria) and of early treatment of potential complications in children at risk for ADPKD [14]. As there is currently no established disease-controlling targeted treatment that would need to be started during childhood, it has, however, been argued that one should not take the right of self-determination from these children before these individuals are old enough to decide on their own what they consider best for them. Next to the last KDIGO recommendations, a recent consensus has highlighted the need of counselling these families and involving them in a process of shared decision-making between the child, parents and physicians [14, 15]. An algorithm has been proposed to facilitate the counseling of these ADPKD families in accordance to their own decision [16].

Autosomal Dominant Polycystic Kidney Disease (ADPKD)

Epidemiology and Morphology

ADPKD is the most common inherited kidney disease and one of the commonest Mendelian human disorders overall with a frequency of 1/500–1000 [1, 15, 17]. This approximates to about 12.5 million affected individuals worldwide. ADPKD is among the most common causes of ESKD; about 5–10% of all patients requiring kidney replacement therapy (KRT) as kidney transplant or dialysis are affected by ADPKD. Overall, the disease is a major health care issue of socio-economic interest.

Histopathologically, kidney cysts are fluid-filled epithelia-lined cavities. ADPKD is characterized by the formation and progressive enlargement of kidney cysts from all segments of the nephron and additional kidney fibrosis. In contrast to ARPKD in which the cysts usually remain connected with the tubular lumen, cysts in ADPKD become disconnected from the tubular space. Kidney cysts in ADPKD vary considerably in size and appearance, from a few millimeters to many centimeters (Fig. 10.1).

ADPKD is a systemic disorder with profound extra-renal cystic and non-cystic complications. Their prevalences in adults compared to children are summarized in Table 10.1.

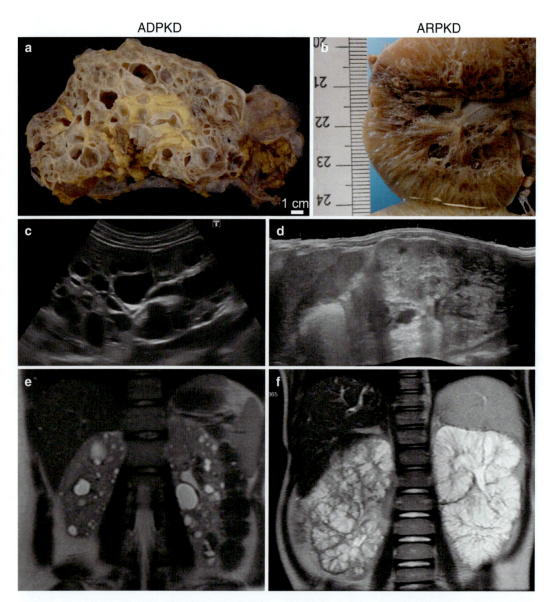

Fig. 10.1 (a) Macroscopic appearance of advanced-stage ADPKD (a) and ARPKD kidneys (b). On cut section, multiple cysts in the cortex and medulla can be seen that vary considerably in size and appearance, from a few millimetres to diameters of many centimeters in the ADPKD kidney, while ubiquitous small dilatations can be seen in the ARPKD kidney. These findings can also be recapitulated by ultrasound (c, d) and T2-weighted magnetic resonance imaging (MRI; e, f). (From Liebau and Serra [6] with permission)

Table 10.1 Extra-renal manifestations of ADPKD (according to [2, 198])

Manifestation	Prevalence in adults	Prevalence in children
Hepatic cysts	>90%	<5%
Arterial hypertension	Up to 70%	20–35%
Left ventricular hypertrophy	Up to 70%	
Valvular abnormalities	Up to 20%	12%
Intracranial aneurysm	6–16%	Rare
Abdominal aorta aneurysm	5–10%	
Diverticula	Up to 40%	
Hernias	Up to 45%	16%
Bronchiectasis	Up to 37%	
Genitourinary cysts	39–60%	
Depression	Up to 60%	
Pain	Up to 60%	10–20%

Clinical Course

Kidney Function

The kidneys are usually in the center of disease burden in ADPKD. A common classification differentiates a PKD1 subtype of patients with variants in the *PKD1* gene from a PKD2 subtype of patients with variants in *PKD2* [1]. ESKD presents in about 50% of ADPKD patients by the age of 60 years. On average, PKD2 is regarded to be significantly milder than PKD1 with a 20 years later median age of onset of ESKD (58.1 vs. 79.9 years) and a lower prevalence of arterial hypertension and urinary tract infections [1, 18].

Diagnosis by Imaging and Emerging Imaging Markers Predicting Clinical Courses

ADPKD diagnosis is usually established by ultrasound. Whereas 95% of patients exhibit characteristic ultrasonographic features at 20 years and almost all patients at 30 years of age, the proportion of affected children that can be identified by ultrasound is less clear. Even a single kidney cyst in a pediatric patient should raise suspicion and result in a diagnostic work-up encompassing a careful record of family and medical history, physical examination and, where required, further abdominal imaging [7, 14]. As novel treatment approaches are emerging it may become more important to identify ADPKD patients at an early stage of disease [16]. Various early markers of kidney disease are under investigation [19]. Approximately 60% of children younger than 5 years with a *PKD1* variant and 75–80% of those aged 5–18 years have kidney cysts detectable by ultrasound [20]. In the early 1990s, Bear et al. proposed a false negative diagnosis rate by ultrasound of about 35% below the age of 10 years [21]. The false positive yield of ultrasound is considered extremely low since simple cysts are extremely rare in childhood [22]. Ravine et al. found nil prevalence of cysts in healthy individuals aged 15–29 years [23].

Especially in children with a family history, ADPKD will be the most likely underlying condition for a child with kidney cysts. In adults aged ≤39 years with a family history of ADPKD, the diagnosis of ADPKD can be established by the presence of three uni- or bilateral kidney cysts [24]. Two cysts on each side for patients aged 40–59 years and four cysts on each side for patients aged >60 years make ADPKD the very likely diagnosis according to the modified Ravine criteria. The presence of less than two cysts in persons at risk aged >40 years practically excludes ADPKD. In 420 children with a family history of ADPKD, ultrasound screening detected kidney cysts in 46% of individuals at the age of 15 years [25].

Children affected by ADPKD also exhibit enlarged kidneys with an increased rate of kidney growth. ADPKD children who are hypertensive have larger kidneys than normotensive patients [26–28].

Magnetic resonance imaging (MRI) and computed tomography (CT) have higher detection rates, especially of small cysts. Given this, MRI may be a helpful tool to discover small cysts, e.g. to detect affected persons prior to living kidney donation, but unmodified application of the Ravine criteria to MRI and CT data would frequently yield false-positive results [29, 30]. Novel high-resolution ultrasound equipment may also be more sensitive in detecting small cysts. New reference datasets have therefore been established for MRI-based cyst detection, revealing at least one cyst in about 60% of healthy adults [30]. Men appear to have more cysts than women and cysts grow with age by size and number.

A study by the CRISP (Consortium for Radiologic Imaging Studies of Polycystic Kidney Disease) consortium on ADPKD patients suggested that total kidney volume (TKV) as measured by MRI predicts kidney function decline in ADPKD. Total TKV values should be standardized to body height, especially in children. Height-adjusted TKV is considered to be a reasonably likely surrogate parameter for disease severity in ADPKD, even before kidney function declines [6].

The CRISP consortium used annual MRI as well as GFR measurements to monitor kidney and cyst volume in 232 young ADPKD patients with a GFR of >60 mL/min/1.73 m^2 over a period of 3 and 8 years [31]. The progression of cyst growth and kidney volume occurred prior to functional impairment. Rapid kidney growth was associated with faster decline in kidney function and lower kidney blood flow [31, 32]. Kidney blood flow and age as well as gender, hypertension, and kidney volume predicted the loss of kidney function [33]. In addition to height-adjusted TKV, novel radiomics approaches like image texture analysis may become an important tools to monitor the disease course and the response to interventions and to predict kidney function decline in ADPKD [34].

The applicability of MRI and CT for disease monitoring in children is limited. MRI requires sedation, and CT is associated with high radiation exposure. For daily clinical work, ultrasound remains the method of choice [6, 7], even more so as the resolution of modern ultrasound equipment is excellent. Recently, Breysem et al. validated 3D ultrasound for measuring TKV in children compared to the 2D ultrasound ellipsoid method and MRI-based volumetry in a pediatric ADPKD cohort [35]. 3D ultrasound manual contouring volumetry outperformed the 2D ellipsoid method and was comparable with MRI volumetry in children, especially for smaller kidneys. While these findings require further validation, 3D-ultrasound holds promise as a potential alternative to MRI in pediatric imaging assessment.

Early-Onset ADPKD and Clinical Spectrum of Kidney Disease in Pediatric ADPKD

Clinical symptoms of ADPKD usually do not arise before the fourth to fifth decade of life. However, there is striking phenotypic variability not only between but even within families, indicating that modifying genes, environmental factors and/or other mechanisms considerably influence the clinical course in ADPKD [36, 37]. In line with this, a small proportion of ADPKD patients presents with an early-manifesting clinical course [1]. Early manifestation in ADPKD is usually defined as clinical symptoms (e.g., arterial hypertension, proteinuria, impaired urinary concentration, impaired kidney function) occurring before the age of 15 years. Among these are cases with significant peri-/neonatal morbidity and mortality, sometimes indistinguishable from those with severe ARPKD [2]. Conflicting data exist on the precise incidence of early-manifesting ADPKD cases. While most authors propose a figure of about 2%, Sweeney and Avner suggested a prevalence of up to 5% [38, 39]. Given the prevalence rates for ADPKD (1/400–1000) and ARPKD (1/20,000), it is plausible that the total number of patients with early-onset ADPKD seen in pediatric nephrology clinics may be comparable to those of the children with ARPKD. A subset of these ADPKD patients may resemble ARPKD. Importantly, variants in *TCF2/HNF1B*, which initially were mainly found in children with bilateral cystic dysplasia [40], can also result in PKD-mimicking phenotypes [11, 41].

Longitudinal studies in children with ADPKD demonstrated that severe kidney enlargement at young age and hypertension are risk factors for accelerated kidney growth [14, 26, 27, 42]. Many clinical symptoms such as pain, hematuria, proteinuria, stones and hypertension are associated with large kidney size. Furthermore, a large cyst number in early childhood is a predictor for faster progression of structural anomalies.

Intriguingly, in children with ADPKD, kidney involvement is commonly asymmetric (including asymmetric kidney enlargement) and even limited to one kidney in a small minority of cases at early stages of the disease [43]. As in ARPKD, the kidneys can present as large and hyperechoic bilateral masses with decreased corticomedullary differentiation [44, 45]. Unlike ARPKD, ADPKD kidneys are frequently characterized by greatly variable macrocysts (up to several centimeters in diameter) even in small children [6, 7].

Gross hematuria is a risk factor for the progression of kidney disease [46, 47]. Hematuria is not common in children and occurs in only about 10% of ADPKD children at a mean age of 9 years [26].

Arterial Hypertension

Arterial hypertension is common in pediatric ADPKD patients even in the presence of normal kidney function and particularly in children with very early onset ADPKD [47]. Hypertension should be diagnosed as early as possible and be treated aggressively [14, 15].

Cardiovascular disease represents the main cause of mortality in ADPKD. The onset of hypertension before age 35 years constitutes an important prognostic factor of rapid disease progression [46]. In children with ADPKD the prevalence of hypertension is between 20% and 40% [14, 48, 49]. 24-Hour ambulatory blood pressure monitoring (ABPM) represents the gold standard in evaluating hypertension in pediatric populations. ABPM in children with ADPKD revealed isolated nocturnal hypertension with normal daytime blood pressure in 16–18% of patients [11, 48].

The precise pathogenesis of hypertension in PKD still remains to be elucidated. It has been hypothesized that cyst expansion results in intrarenal activation of the renin-angiotensin-aldosterone system (RAAS) with stimulation of cyst growth, fibrosis, and hypertension [50].

Extra-Renal Manifestations

Intracerebral aneurysms (ICAs) are an important, specific cardiovascular comorbidity in ADPKD and are associated with a five-fold higher prevalence than in the general population. The risk to develop ICAs is higher in patients with a family history of ADPKD–associated ICA or subarachnoid hemorrhage (22% versus 6%) [51].

However, PKD associated intracranial aneurysms are extremely unusual in childhood and routine screening is not recommended [52].

Simple, mostly solitary hepatic cysts are common with a prevalence of 2.5–10% in the general population [53]. Women may be more often and more severely affected, especially those who used estrogens, had multiple pregnancies or both [54, 55]. Hepatic cysts can be predominant with multiple cysts throughout the liver in the presence of very few kidney cysts. Atypical or alternate disease including *GANAB*, *ALG9* variants in the case of liver cysts or *HNF1B* with significant pancreatic involvement are also to be considered [56].

Other anomalies may occur including mitral valve prolapse (usually without clinical significance), left ventricular hypertrophy, aneurysms of the abdominal aorta, diverticular disease, hernia, chronic back pain, cystic lesions in the genitourinary tract, the pancreas and the lung, hematuria, urinary tract infection, kidney stones, deregulated phosphate homeostasis, and arachnoidal cysts as well as pain and depression [18, 54] (Table 10.1). Extra-renal manifestations overall are rare in children with ADPKD.

ADPKD Genetics

As the name implies, ADPKD is transmitted in an autosomal dominant fashion, i.e., virtually all individuals who inherit a mutated *PKD1* or *PKD2* germline allele will develop kidney cysts by age 30–40. The majority of ADPKD patients are adults who carry a germline variant in the *PKD1* gene on chromosome 16p13.3 (~80%). About 10–15% harbor a variant in the *PKD2* gene on chromosome 4q21 [1, 18]. The majority of patients with ADPKD are explained by heterozygous variants in either *PKD1* or *PKD2*. However, there is a growing list of genes that when mutated either mimic ADPKD or give rise to more atypical ADPKD phenotypes (*GANAB*, *DNAJB11*, *HNF1β*, *PKHD1*, *DZIP1L*, *TSC1/2*, *VHL*, *ALG9*, *IFT140*, *OFD1* in women, etc.).

Remarkably, ADPKD variants can occur *de novo* without a family history. This frequently results in some kind of mosaicism and the clinical course may be atypical. In patients with early and severe disease manifestations (discussed in greater detail above), pathogenic *PKD1* variants can affect both disease alleles in a recessive mode of inheritance.

PKD1 and *PKD2* Genes and Their Encoded Polycystin-1 and -2 Proteins

PKD1 is a large gene with a longest open reading frame transcript of 46 exons predicted to encode a 4302 aa multidomain integral membrane glycoprotein (polycystin-1). *PKD2* has 15 exons encoding a 5.3 kb transcript that is translated into a 968 aa protein (polycystin-2). In keeping with the systemic nature of ADPKD, the two polycystins are widely expressed in tissues. The expression of polycystin-1 and -2 is developmentally regulated with highest levels during late fetal and early neonatal life. Intra-renal expression is highest in distal tubule and collecting duct epithelial cells. Notably, the majority of cysts in ADPKD originate from collecting ducts.

Although the two-hit model of tumorigenesis is too simplistic, it may still provide a reasonable basis of our understanding of ADPKD. According to this data, second-hit variant and resulting loss of heterozygosity has been proposed as the mechanism underlying cyst formation in ADPKD. The considerable intrafamilial phenotypic variation, focal cyst formation with evidence of epithelial cell clonality within individual cysts, as well as the detection of somatic variants in cells lining kidney and liver cysts are all in keeping with this theory [57–61]. However, numerous findings rule out the two-hit model of a germline variant on one allele and a somatic variant on the other as the sole cause of cystogenesis. Patients and mice have been described that carry germline variants in both *PKD1* and *PKD2* (double-heterozygotes) and, thus, are to be regarded as "homozygously" affected in every cell of the organism [62, 63]. In contradiction to a simple two-hit theory, not every renal tubular cell or nephron in these individuals may give rise to a cyst. Therefore, the second-hit variant to the other *PKD* gene may act as a modifying factor that boosts the risk of cyst development and/or drives cyst progression, rather than initiating cyst

events [64]. As regards mechanisms underlying cystogenesis, it is worth noting that increased as well as decreased polycystin-1 expression may result in cyst formation [1, 65, 66]. Haploinsufficiency of *Pkd1* itself has been demonstrated to suffice to elicit a cystic phenotype [67]. Finally, the timepoint of *Pkd1* inactivation crucially determines the severity of the cystic phenotype in mice [68]. Ischemia [69–71], nephrotoxic injury [72] and immunological events involving, e.g. macrophages [73, 74] may affect cystogenesis and it has been suggested that these events might represent a required third or even further additional hit [75].

Polycystin-1 and polycystin-2 are glycosylated integral membrane proteins (Fig. 10.2). Polycystin-2 has six transmembrane passes with cytoplasmic N- and C-termini. It is believed to function as a divalent cation channel, particularly involved in cellular Ca^{2+} signalling, belonging to the transient receptor potential (TRP) protein superfamily [76].

Polycystin-1 is a huge integral membrane glycoprotein with an extensive amino-terminal extracellular region, 11 transmembrane passes, and a short 200-amino acid cytoplasmic carboxy-terminus. The intracellular C-terminus is supposed to mediate protein interactions, by, e.g., a heterotrimeric G-protein activation site and a coiled-coil domain that interacts with the C-terminus of polycystin-2. The large extracellular portion of polycystin-1 contains numerous structural motifs, which are putatively involved in protein-protein or protein-carbohydrate interactions. It has been proposed that polycystin-1 and polycystin-2 form a chemo- and mechano-sensing protein complex which senses fluid flow in the renal tubule and controls cell growth and differentiation [1]. Bending of the primary cilia leads to an increase in intracellular calcium potentially via a polycystin-1-dependent mechanism [77, 78] and the ratio of polycystin-1 to polycystin-2 regulates pressure sensing [79]. However, the exact mechanisms remain unknown [80, 81]. Polycystin-1 is involved in the regulation of multiple intracellular signalling pathways [1, 82–85]. Hogan et al. found urinary exosomes with abundant expression of polycystin-1, poly-

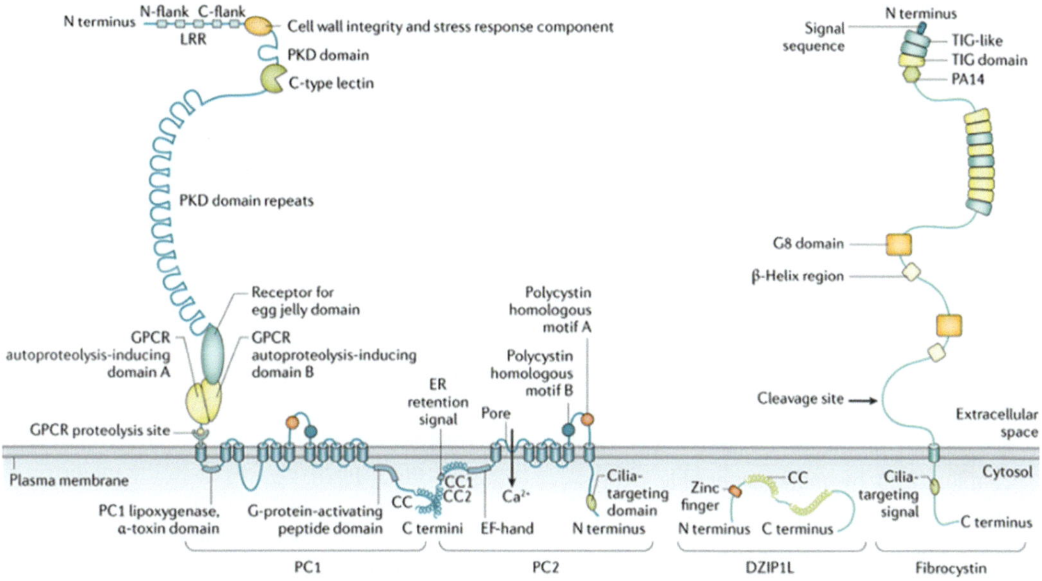

10 Polycystic Kidney Disease: ADPKD and ARPKD

Fig. 10.2 Structures of polycystin-1, polycystin-2, polyductin/fibrocystin and DZIP1L. (From Bergmann et al. [1] with permission)

cystin-2 and the ARPKD protein fibrocystin among others, which may point to a role in paracrine signalling [86].

PKD1/PKD2 Variant Spectrum and Routine Diagnostic Testing

Genotype-Phenotype Correlations

The wide range of age at attainment of ESKD observed within families illustrates the limitations of simple genotype-phenotype correlation analysis. There is no evidence for any sex influence in *PKD1*, however, females affected by *PKD2* were found to have a significantly longer median survival (71.0 vs. 67.3 years) than males. Another study corroborated these findings by a later mean age of onset of ESKD (76.0 vs. 68.1 years) in *PKD2* females [87, 88].

While no genotype-phenotype correlations have been identified for *PKD2* [8, 89], certain associations have been established in *PKD1*. Patients with a truncating variant have a more severe course than patients carrying a missense variant [90, 91]. *PKD1* missense variants however still go along with a more severe phenotype than *PKD2* variants. In addition, the presence of variants in multiple PKD genes can result in a

more severe phenotype [92]. These patients were found to carry variants in PKD genes including *HNF1B* or a variant *in trans* affecting the other *PKD1* allele in addition to the expected germline variant [92]. However, this mechanism is unlikely to explain all cases with early-onset ADPKD. Variants 5′ to the median are associated with a slightly earlier age at onset of ESKD (53 vs. 56 years) [93]. Moreover, the median position of the *PKD1* variant was found to be located further 5′ in families with a vascular phenotype of intracranial aneurysms and subarachnoid haemorrhage [94]. At the population level phenotype findings do predict eGFR endpoints and ESKD, with genotype improving the predictive value of imaging findings and vice versa [95]. However, for genetic counselling and the prediction of the outcome of an individual patient, these genotype-phenotype correlations are only of limited value [96].

Data on families with early-manifesting offspring support a common familial modifying background for early and severe disease expression, but the underlying mechanisms are still controversial and may include anticipation, imprinting, and the segregation of modifying genes. Segregation of modifying alleles inherited from the unaffected parent is an intriguing possibility [97] further supported by the low incidence of *in utero* presentation of ADPKD in second degree relatives. The mechanisms underlying early-onset ADPKD still require further examination [98].

Tuberous Sclerosis Complex and Contiguous TSC2–PKD1 Gene Deletion Syndrome: Important Differential Diagnoses of Cystic Kidney Disease

Tuberous sclerosis complex (TSC) is an autosomal dominant genetic syndrome characterized by marked variable expressivity and hamartomatous lesions in the brain, heart, lung, skin and kidney. Around 90% of patients suffer from epilepsy, and half exhibit cognitive impairment, autism or other behavioural disorders. Additional clinical manifestations of TSC may include sclerotic bone lesions, renal cell carcinoma (RCC) and neuroendocrine tumours [99]. Cutaneous manifestations also frequently occur with TSC and include, for example, "white spots", facial angiofibromas and peri-/subungual fibromas. About 80–90% of TSC patients have renal manifestations by adulthood, representing the second most significant cause of morbidity and mortality in all ages combined, and the most common cause of mortality after the age of 30 years. Renal lesions in TSC consist of renal cysts, angiomyolipomas (AML), fat-poor lesions, and RCC, causing CKD. There is a clear correlation between the presence of renal abnormalities (AML and renal cysts) and age. Renal lesions are observed in 38–55% of affected children at preschool age, increasing to 75–80% at school age and reaching 86–100% in adults [100]. Renal AML develop in up to 80% of individuals with TSC and appear typically first in childhood and then tend to grow during adolescence and into adulthood. The main complication of AML is retroperitoneal hemorrhage, which can be fatal due to the associated blood loss, pain, renal insufficiency, and arterial hypertension. Approximately 35–50% of patients with TSC develop multiple renal cysts [100, 101].

The incidence of TSC is 1 in 6000–10,000 live births, and its prevalence is independent of population, ethnicity and sex. TSC is caused by germline loss-of-function variants in *TSC1* (OMIM 605284; located on chromosome 9q34) or *TSC2* (OMIM 191092; located on chromosome 16p13.3), genes that encode hamartin and tuberin, respectively [101]. In the majority of patients, variants in these two genes arise *de novo*, however, the patients themselves who carry a pathogenic *de novo* variant in *TSC1* or *TSC2* bear a 50% risk to transmit the variant to their offspring. The two proteins hamartin and tuberin form a complex that negatively regulates mechanistic target of rapamycin (mTOR) complex 1 (mTORC1), a master regulator of cellular biosynthesis. Loss of the hamartin–tuberin complex results in aberrant activation of mTORC1, which promotes cell proliferation and differentiation. TSC-related cysts are thought to arise as a result of a second-hit variant in *TSC1* or *TSC2* in the renal epithelium, although genetic studies have yet to confirm this hypothesis [102].

A subset of patients carries a deletion encompassing the adjacent *TSC2* and *PKD1* genes (OMIM 600273, on chromosome 16p13) ("contiguous *TSC2–PKD1* gene deletion syndrome"). This disease was first reported by Brook–Carter et al. in 1994 with a variety of phenotypes dominated by severe, very early-onset of ADPKD and occurs in ~2–5% of TSC patients, resulting in significant kidney insufficiency already from childhood [102, 103]. Data on children diagnosed with the contiguous gene syndrome (*TSC2-PKD1*) and their long-term outcome are scarce and currently no data on the epidemiology nor recommendations for the diagnostics, follow-up and treatment of *TSC2-PKD1* are available. The global ADPedKD initiative (www.ADPedKD.org) aims to remedy this paucity of information by collecting information on this subgroup [104].

The expansion of knowledge of the pathogenesis of TSC and the identification of the *TSC1* and *TSC2* genes and their proteins, the hamartin–tuberin complex led to the approval of mTORC1 inhibitors (also termed rapalogues), such as sirolimus and everolimus, for the treatment of the progression of subependymal giant cell astrocytomas, angiomyolipomas, skin lesions, epilepsy and lymphangioleiomyomatosis. In contrast, the efficacy of these agents in the treatment of TSC-associated renal cystic disease has not yet been fully evaluated [102].

Autosomal Recessive Polycystic Kidney Disease (ARPKD)

Epidemiology and Morphology

ARPKD is much rarer than its dominant counterpart with a proposed incidence among Caucasians of about 1 in 20,000 live births corresponding to a carrier frequency of approximately 1:70 in non-isolated populations [1, 105]. The exact incidence is unknown since published studies vary in the cohorts of patients examined (e.g., autopsied patients vs. moderately affected patients followed by pediatricians), and some severely affected babies may die perinatally without a definitive diagnosis. Isolated populations may have a higher prevalence. A recent study calculated an estimated annualized incidence of ARPKD in the USA to be 1:26,485 live births [106].

Macroscopically, the cut surface of ARPKD kidneys demonstrates the cortical extension of fusiform or cylindrical spaces arranged radially throughout the kidney parenchyma from medulla to cortex (Fig. 10.1). Histologic changes in ARPKD can vary depending on the age of presentation and the extent of cystic involvement. Invariable histological manifestations are fusiform dilations of renal collecting ducts and distal tubuli lined by columnar or cuboidal epithelium that usually remain in contact with the urinary system (unlike ADPKD), whereas glomerular cysts or dysplastic elements (e.g., cartilage, etc.) are usually not evident in ARPKD kidneys (Fig. 10.3). During early fetal development, a transient phase of proximal tubular cyst formation has been identified that can also be observed in various mouse models but is largely absent by birth [1, 107, 108]. With advancing clinical course and development of larger kidney cysts accompanied by interstitial fibrosis, ARPKD kidney structure may increasingly resemble the pattern observed in ADPKD.

Liver changes are obligatory for ARPKD and characterized by dysgenesis of the hepatic portal triad attributable to defective remodelling of the ductal plate with hyperplastic biliary ducts and congenital hepatic fibrosis (CHF) (Fig. 10.4). These hepatobiliary changes, subsumed as ductal plate malformation (DPM), are present from early embryonic development (first trimester) on and lead to progressive portal fibrosis [109]. At later stages, fibrous septa may link different portal tracts by intersecting the hepatic parenchyma often leading to portal hypertension. However, the remaining liver parenchyma usually develops normally and hepatocellular function initially often remains stable [110, 111]. As discussed for ADPKD, liver cysts usually arise from DPM and biliary ectasia, with transitions to extensive dilations of both intra- and extrahepatic bile ducts resembling Caroli's disease/syndrome.

Although ARPKD can be reliably diagnosed pathoanatomically, histology has lost relevance for daily clinical work with the increasing availability of genetic workup [11, 112, 113].

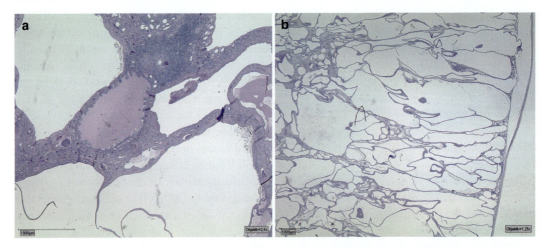

Fig. 10.3 Histological findings in ADPKD (**a**) and ARPKD (**b**) kidneys. ADPKD kidneys show a higher degree of tubuolinterstitial fibrosis. Fusiform dilations of renal collecting ducts and distal tubuli lined by columnar or cuboidal epithelium can be observed in ARPKD. These dilated collecting ducts run perpendicular to the renal capsule

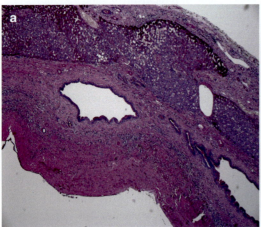
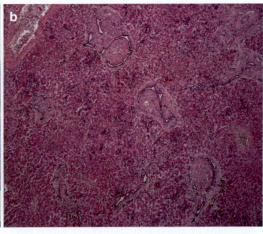

Fig. 10.4 Histological liver findings. Hepatic cysts (**a**) and the obligatory hepatobiliary changes in ARPKD subsumed as ductal plate malformation (DPM, **b**) characterized by dysgenesis of the hepatic portal triad with hyperplastic biliary ducts and congenital hepatic fibrosis (CHF)

Clinical Course and Prenatal Diagnosis

ARPKD is typically an infantile disease characterized by hepatorenal fibrocystic changes. Patients frequently present with pre- or perinatal detection of massively enlarged kidneys (Fig. 10.1, Table 10.2). Parents are typically not affected. In severely affected fetuses, oligo- or anhydramnios may develop that can result in pulmonary hypoplasia with severe perinatal respiratory disease. Despite dramatic advances in neonatal and intensive care over the past decades, the short-term mortality of ARPKD remains substantial. In less-severely affected children, progression of CKD is slow, resulting in an overall need for KRT in about 40–50% of patients in young adulthood [3, 114]. There is obligatory hepatic involvement in ARPKD resulting in portal hypertension and a risk of cholangitis.

10 Polycystic Kidney Disease: ADPKD and ARPKD

Table 10.2 Clinical manifestations of ARPKD and ADPKD

	ARPKD	ADPKD
Incidence	1:20,000	1:500–1:1000
Macroscopic renal findings	Symmetrical, massively enlarged, reniform kidneys	Symmetrical, enlarged, reniform kidneys
Localization of renal cysts	Mainly dilated collecting ducts and distal tubuli	Cysts derived from all parts of nephron
Ultrasound and diameter of renal cysts	Increased echogenicity of renal parenchyma. "Salt-and-pepper"-pattern. Small, sometimes invisible cysts (<2 mm). More ADPKD-like pattern with avancing age	Cysts of different sizes in cortex and medulla. Usually several large cysts
Hepatic pathology	Mandatory: Ductal plate malformation/congenital hepatic fibrosis with hyperplastic biliary ducts and portal fibrosis (may impress as Caroli syndrome)	"Liver cysts". Common in adults, rare in children. Occasionally ductal plate malformation/congenital hepatic fibrosis
Associated anomalies	Lung hypoplasia. Rarely pancreatic cysts. Single case reports of intracranial aneurysms	Pancreatic cysts and/or cysts in other epithelial organs. Familiarly clustered intracranial aneurysms, abdominal aorta aneurysms. Diverticula. Hernia. Bronchiectasis
Main clinical manifestations	Neonatal respiratory distress/failure due to pulmonary hypoplasia. Renal insufficiency. Portal hypertension. Hyponatremia. Hypertension	Arterial hypertension. Proteinuria. Hematuria. Arterial hypertension. Renal insufficiency. Pain
Risk for siblings	25%	50% (except in rare cases of spontaneous mutation with virtually no risk)
Risk for own children	<1% (unless unaffected parent is related to affected partner, or ARPKD is known in the unaffected partner's family)	50% (also for patients with spontaneous mutations)
Manifestation in affected family members	About 20% gross intrafamilial variability	Often similar within the same family
Parental kidneys	No alterations	Usually one affected parent (unless parents are <30 years or in case of spontaneous mutation)
Prognosis	Substantial mortality in patients with neonatal respiratory distress. Severe complications due to portal hypertension	Median age of end stage renal disease: 58.1 years (PKD1) vs. 79.9 years (PKD2)

Overall, the clinical spectrum is variable [115]. Notably, early studies differed widely by their selection criteria and their mode of data analysis, thus hampering direct comparison. Longitudinal registry studies with detailed characterization of patient courses have recently been established and provided important insights [106, 116]. Treatment in ARPKD remains largely symptomatic and opinion-based, although first consensus expert recommendations have been established [112].

Diagnosis by Imaging

Ultrasound remains the method of choice to diagnose children with ARPKD. Bilateral large and hyperechogenic kidneys with poor corticomedullary differentiation are the typical finding. Cysts are usually fusiform and tiny (<2 mm in diameter) and may impose as a 'pepper-salt' pattern on ultrasound. Macrocysts are uncommon in small infants, although they may be observed in advanced disease stages when ARPKD and ADPKD may become hard to differentiate by their sonographic appearance [7, 117–119]. In a large collection of ARPKD patients, 92% of ARPKD patients had a kidney length at or above the 97th centile for age [120]. In no case the kidney size was decreased and SD scores ranged from 0 to 17. In contrast to ADPKD, clear correlations were neither observed between kidney length and kidney function nor between kidney length and duration of the disease. Various studies have found a relative decrease of kidney length during the course of the disease but numbers overall remain small and methods to quantify and standardize kidney size differed [121–124]. A recent study on 456 ARPKD patients from the international ARPKD registry study ARegPKD (www.ARegPKD.org) confirmed this finding but also revealed that height-adjusted estimated TKV remained rather stable over time [125]. Overall, there was an inverse relationship of height-adjusted estimated TKV with kidney function but with substantial variability. However, there was a clear correlation of early height-adjusted TKV (in the first 18 months) with poor kidney prognosis in childhood and adolescence (94% 10-year kidney survival for lowest quartile vs. 20% for highest quartile; Fig. 10.5) [125].

Typical ultrasound findings of the liver and portal hypertension in ARPKD include hepatomegaly, increased liver echogenicity, inhomogeneous liver parenchyma, liver cysts and dilated bile ducts, enlarged left liver lobes and splenomegaly [3, 111]. Some studies suggest that liver elastography, either by, e.g. magnet resonance techniques or by ultrasound Acoustic Radiation Force Impulse especially of the left liver lobe may be helpful in identifying liver fibrosis in patients with ARPKD [126–129]. In one cross-sectional study liver magnetic resonance elastography and ultrasound elastography measurement were strongly correlated and magnetic resonance elastography showed 78% sensitivity and 93% specificity to distinguish ARPKD and control groups at a proposed cut-off of 2.48 kPa [128]. Longitudinal data will be required to evaluate the prognostic value of these measurements for liver outcome.

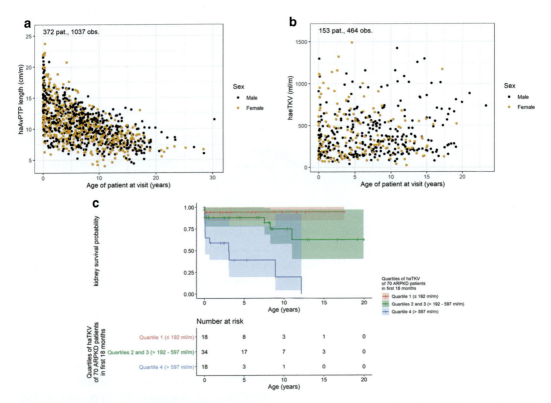

Fig. 10.5 Development of height-adjusted pole-to-pole length (**a**) and height-adjusted total kidney volume (**b**) in relation to age and kidney survival in patients in the different quartiles of height-adjusted total kidney volume (**c**). (Modified from [125])

Perinatal Disease and Mortality

Overall, the majority of cases are identified late in pregnancy or at birth. As many as 30% of affected neonates have been reported to die shortly after birth from respiratory insufficiency. Early detection of oligohydramnios seems to be associated with worse outcome [130]. In severe cases fetuses may display a "Potter" oligohydramnios phenotype with pulmonary hypoplasia (Fig. 10.6), a characteristic facies, and contracted limbs with club feet. A study performed from 2010 to 2014 in the ultrasound estimated neonatal survival to be almost 80% [106]. Advances in neonatal intensive care and improvements in kidney replacement therapies have increased the survival rates of ARPKD patients, with most of them reaching adult age. In a large study of almost 200 ARPKD patients with known *PKHD1* variant status, survival rates among those patients who survived the first month of life were 94% at 5 years and 92% at 10 years of age [120]. Kidney failure is rarely a cause of neonatal demise. In non-oliguric ARPKD neonates hyponatremia, considered to be related to defective urine concentration, is often present in the newborn period, but this complication usually resolves over time [4, 120, 131].

Kidney Disease

In a recent European study on 304 patients with ARPKD KRT was required in 25–30% of patients by the age of 15 years [114]. In another analysis 40% of young adult patients with ARPKD were on KRT [3].

Several antenatal and perinatal risk factors for dialysis dependency in early life have been identified. The presence of oligohydramnios or anhydramnios, prenatal kidney enlargement, a low Apgar score, and the need for postnatal breathing support were independently associated with an increased risk of requiring chronic dialysis [132]. The likelihood of early dialysis varied from 1.5% for patients without prenatal sonographic anomalies to 32% in patients with documented oligohydramnios or anhydramnios, kidney cysts, and enlarged kidneys (Table 10.3).

CKD with an eGFR <75% of age-adjusted normal ranges was first detected at a mean age of 4 years in a previous survey among pediatric nephrology units [120]. Infants with ARPKD may have a transient improvement in their glomerular filtration rate (GFR) due to kidney maturation in the first months of life. Subsequently, a progressive but highly variable decrease in kidney function occurs. In a small cohort of children with

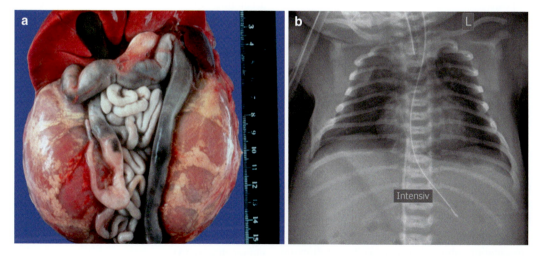

Fig. 10.6 Abdominal situs of an ARPKD patient with symmetrically enlarged kidneys that maintain their reniform configuration (**a**) and chest X-ray of a patient with pulmonary hypoplasia due to ARPKD (**b**)

Table 10.3 Multivariate cox model of pre-, peri- and postnatal predictors of necessity of kidney replacement therapy within the first year of life. Model based predicted probabilities for kidney replacement therapy within 12 and months after birth (modified from [132])

Parameter	Hazard ratio	95% CI Lower	Upper	p
Sex	0.925	0.462	1.850	0.825
Oligo/anhydramnios	4.473	1.295	15.449	0.018
Prenatal enlarged kidneys	3.177	1.087	9.282	0.035
Vaginal delivery	1.271	0.584	2.765	0.545
Gestational age at birth (weeks)	1.121	0.917	1.371	0.265
Birth weight SDS	1.291	1.031	1.618	0.026
Apgar 10′	0.748	0.564	0.991	0.043
Assisted breathing and/or ventilation	6.994	1.536	31.845	0.012

Prenatal symptom combination	Probability of dialysis within 12 months after birth (95% confidence interval)
No prenatal abnormalities	0.015 (0.005–0.041)
Enlarged kidneys	0.033 (0.006–0.155)
Renal cysts	0.034 (0.008–0.135)
Enlarged kidneys and renal cysts	0.071 (0.021–0.215)
Oligo/anhydramnios	0.087 (0.032–0.214)
Oligo/anhydramnios and enlarged kidneys	0.174 (0.055–0.431)
Oligo/anhydramnios and renal cysts	0.178 (0.047–0.486)
Oligo/anhydramnios and enlarged kidneys and renal cysts	0.323 (0.222–0.445)

ARPKD the annual GFR decline was 1.4 mL/min/1.73 m^2 (−6%) and rates of GFR decline in ARPKD patients were not significantly different from children with other causes of CKD [133].

In a cohort in the US, patients with perinatal presentation showed worse kidney follow-up than those with non-perinatal presentation [121]. While 25% of the perinatally symptomatic patients required kidney replacement therapy by the age of 11 years, 25% of the non-perinatal patients required kidney transplantation by age 32 years. Also, corticomedullary involvement on high resolution ultrasound was associated with worse kidney function in comparison with medullary involvement only in this specific cohort. Kidney volume correlated inversely with function, although with wide variability [121].

Liver Disease

In keeping with the generally prolonged survival in ARPKD, for many patients the hepatobiliary complications come to dominate the clinical picture [3, 124]. Interdisciplinary management by pediatric nephrologists and hepatologists is essential for optimal management of ARPKD from early life onward [4].

While hepatocellular function is usually preserved, these individuals develop sequelae of portal hypertension and may present with hematemesis or melena due to bleeding oesophageal varices and/or hypersplenism with consequent pancytopenia. Typical hepatic manifestations usually present later than classic kidney involvement [3, 110, 131], although complications of portal hypertension may occur early in life [134].

A serious, potentially lethal complication in ARPKD especially after kidney transplantation is ascending suppurative cholangitis that may cause fulminant hepatic failure [135–137]. Cholangitis always requires diligent evaluation with aggressive antimicrobial treatment. Noteworthy, ARPKD patients may not display the full picture of clinical and laboratory findings of cholangitis; thus, every patient with unexplained recurrent sepsis, particularly with gram-negative organisms, should be critically evaluated for this diagnosis [110, 138, 139].

A recent study on 49 young adults with ARPKD characterized the clinical phenotype in this age group and identified prominent liver involvement. ARPKD should also be considered as a differential diagnosis in adults with cystic kidney disease [3].

Adult ARPKD patients beyond the age of 40 years may have a slightly increased risk to develop hepatic tumors, especially cholangiocarcinoma [140, 141].

Additional Extra-Renal Manifestations

Studies have also described additional extra-renal clinical aspects. Arterial hypertension is a very common finding, affects up to 80% of children with ARPKD and usually develops in the first few months of life (Table 10.2). Arterial hypertension may be very pronounced in ARPKD. It was recently shown that children with ARPKD show high rates of abnormal left ventricular geometry with systolic mechanical dysfunction [142].

There have been various reports of patients with both intracranial and extracranial aneurysms [143].

Neurocognitive function and growth in ARPKD children appear to be comparable to children with other causes of CKD [144, 145].

Pulmonary tests in the follow-up of a subgroup were within normal references suggesting good long-term pulmonary outcome [146].

Genetics

PKHD1 is the major, but not the only gene for ARPKD. Variants in an increasing number of other genes such as *PKD1, PKD2, HNF1B, DZIP1L, CYS1* can mimic the disease and lead to an ARPKD-like phenotype [64]. *PKHD1* variant analysis is characterized by vast allelic heterogeneity and a huge number of private variants and missense changes.

PKHD1 Gene and Polyductin/ Fibrocystin Protein

The *PKHD1* gene is highly expressed in fetal and adult kidney, at lower levels in liver, and weakly in other tissues including pancreas, arterial walls and the lung [147]. *PKHD1* is amongst the largest disease genes in the human genome, extending over a genomic segment of at least 470 kb and including a minimum of 86 exons. *PKHD1* undergoes a complex and extensive pattern of alternative splicing, generating transcripts of highly variable size. The longest *PKHD1* transcript contains 67 exons encoding a protein of 4074 amino acids.

The predicted full-length protein (termed fibrocystin or polyductin) represents an integral membrane protein with a single transmembrane (TM)-spanning segment, and a short cytoplasmic C-terminal tail (Fig. 10.7). Based on the structural features of the deduced protein and on the human ARPKD phenotype, fibrocystin might be involved in cellular adhesion, repulsion and proliferation. In addition, the domain and structural analyses suggest that the potential *PKHD1* gene products may be involved in intercellular signalling and function as receptor, ligand and/or membrane-associated enzyme [1].

In common with most other cystoproteins, fibrocystin has been identified at primary cilia with concentration in the basal body area [148–151]. As part of acquisition of epithelial polarity during kidney development, fibrocystin becomes localized to the apical zone of nephron precursor cells and subsequently to the basal bodies at the origin of primary cilia in fully differentiated epithelial cells. Its peculiar subcellular localization and suggested proteins interactions point to a role of fibrocystin in centrosomal, mitochondrial or cilia-associated function. There is evidence for overlapping functions with, e.g. polycystin-1 [1, 152–154]. In addition, there is preliminary evidence of fibrocystin isoproteins which may be secreted in exosomes and undergo posttranslational processing [86, 152, 155, 156].

The number of alternative *PKHD1* transcripts that are actually translated into protein is as yet unknown. The distribution of variants over the entire *PKHD1* gene suggests that the longest transcript is necessary for proper fibrocystin function in kidney and liver. Thus, it might be proposed that a critical amount of the full-length protein is required for normal function.

Genotype-Phenotype Correlations

The analysis of genotype-phenotype correlations for *PKHD1* is hampered by multiple allelism and the high rate of different compound heterozygotes. Until recently, genotype-phenotype correlations were largely limited to the type (truncating/non-truncating) and allelic distribution (homozygous/compound heterozygous) of the variants.

Almost all patients carrying two truncating variants display a very severe phenotype although more recently it was shown that some patients may survive [114, 132, 157, 158]. Patients with at least one missense variant tend to be less severely affected and are more likely to survive the neonatal period. However, missense changes can clinically impress as severe as truncating variants. No significant clinical differences could be observed between patients with two missense variants and those patients harboring a truncating variant *in trans*; thus, the milder variant obviously defines the phenotype. Loss of function probably explains the rather uniform phenotype and early demise of many patients with two null alleles. Phenotypic diversity also reflects the variable extent to which different *PKHD1* missense variants might compromise the function and/or abundance of the mutant protein. Complex transcriptional profiles may play a further role in defining the patient's phenotype [158, 159].

Recently, the localization of a specific missense variant was shown to be of additional relevance for the phenotype. In a cohort of 304 patients, patients with two missense variants affecting amino acids 709-1837 of fibrocystin or a missense variant in this region and a null variant less frequently developed chronic kidney failure than other subgroups. Missense variants affecting amino acids 1838-2624 showed better hepatic outcome. Variants affecting amino acids 2625-4074 of fibrocystin were associated with a more severe hepatic phenotype [114].

The aspect of renal-hepatobiliary morbidity patterns in ARPKD has repetitively been discussed [111, 120, 131]. Many patients show uniform disease progression, but individual ARPKD patients present with an organ-specific phenotype. The observations that different variant localizations are associated with specific kidney and liver disease courses opens novel paths to understand the underlying pathophysiology [114].

Phenotypes cannot yet be fully explained on the basis of the *PKHD1* genotype but likely depend on mutational load for an individual patient, epigenetic factors (e.g., alternative splic-

ing), and environmental influences [1]. Such modifiers will probably have their greatest impact on the phenotype in the setting of hypomorphic missense changes and may explain some of the clinical variability.

Phenotypic Variability Among Affected Siblings

For about 20% of pedigrees gross intrafamilial phenotypic variability with peri-/neonatal demise in one and survival into childhood or even adulthood in another affected sibling have been described [160]. An even higher proportion of 20 out of 48 sibships (42%) was observed among families with at least one neonatal survivor per family [120]. Likewise, data from the ARegPKD dataset suggest a rather limited variability of kidney function decline and hepatic symptoms in the clinical courses of patients surviving the neonatal period. With regards to genetic counselling this rate is alarming [161]. Of course, phenotype categorization into 'severe' and 'moderate' is a simplified and artificial view given the considerably better prognosis for patients surviving the most critical neonatal period. Also, the survival chance of an affected neonate might depend on available intensive care facilities and parental awareness of ARPKD risk. Hence, caution should be warranted in predicting the clinical outcome of a further affected child.

Prenatal Diagnosis

As previously pointed out the diagnosis is frequently identified antenatally. In view of the recurrence risk of 25%, the oftentimes devastating course of early manifestations of ARPKD and a usually similar clinical course among affected siblings, many parents of ARPKD children seek early and reliable prenatal diagnosis (PND) to guide future family planning. Frequently, ARPKD patients are identified by ultrasound only late in pregnancy or at birth. Therefore, an early and reliable PND for ARPKD in "at risk" families is feasible by molecular genetic analysis [147, 162, 163] as the basis for PND and genetic counselling according to local regulations.

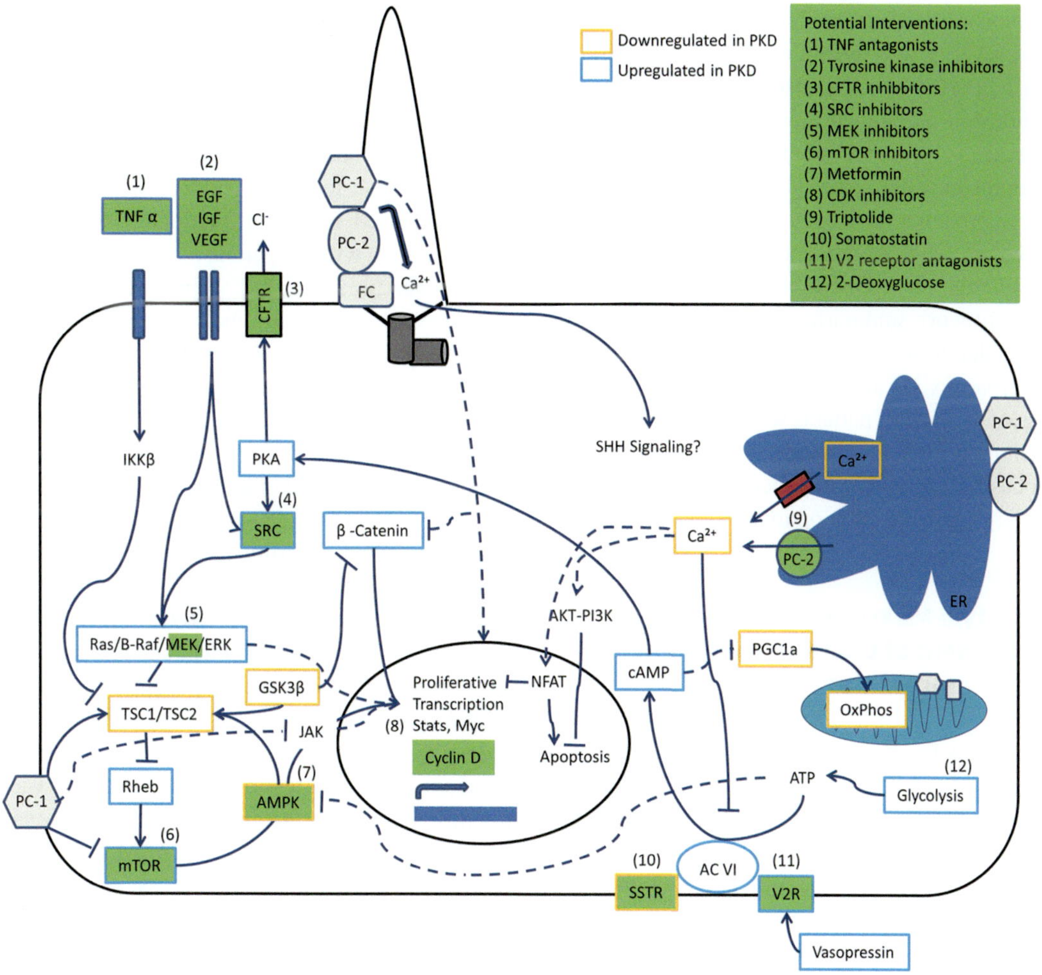

Fig. 10.7 Schematic presentation of polycystin-associated signalling pathways and potential pharmacological targets. Polycystin-1 (PC-1), polycystin-2 (PC-2), and fibrocystin/polyductin (FC) are located in primary cilia. PC2 is also located in the endoplasmic reticulum. The ciliary polycystin complex regulates ciliary calcium signals that may lead to calcium-induced calcium release from the endoplasmic reticulum. Reduction of calcium enhances cAMP accumulation, that is furthermore supported by activation of V2-receptors (V2R) but may be inhibited by activation of the somatostatin receptor (SSTR). cAMP stimulates chloride-driven fluid secretion. In PKD cAMP also stimulates cell proliferation in an src-, Ras-, and B-raf–dependent manner. Finally, Mammalian target of rapamycin (mTOR) is activated in cyst-lining PKD epithelia. *AC-VI* adenylyl cyclase type VI, *ATP* adenosine triphosphate, *CFTR* cystic fibrosis transmembrane conductance regulator, *ER* endoplasmic reticulum, *ERK* extracellular signal–regulated kinase, *MEK* mitogen-activated protein kinase kinase, *PKA* protein kinase A, *EGF* epidermal growth factor, *IGF* insulin-like growth factors, *VEGF* vascular endothelial growth factor, *CFTR* cystic fibrosis transmembrane conductance regulator, *AMPK* AMP-activated protein kinase, *SHH* sonic hedgehog signaling

Therapeutic Management

Currently, there is no curative treatment option for patients affected by PKDs to ameliorate or even regress the clinical course. However, given the insights into cell biology and dysregulated intracellular signaling pathways in different PKDs, novel treatment approaches in ADPKD have been suggested [164]. Using different rodent models, various research groups have published promising data on treatment of PKD. Interestingly, the severity and dynamics of cystic kidney disease in orthologous mouse models varies widely. Choosing preclinical models that mimic human disease is utmost relevant when testing potential therapeutic approaches [165]. Multiple therapeutic approaches have been identified in preclinical models. As a consequence, several clinical trial programs for ADPKD have been established. Recent work summarizes the pathophysiological considerations underlying those novel treatment approaches [1] and current state-of-the-art management in adult patients with ADPKD [164]. We will therefore only provide a brief overview here, focusing on pediatric aspects of available and emerging therapeutic options.

Lifestyle Measures, Pediatric Treatment of CKD and Treatment of Co-morbidities

The basis for treatment of PKD and CKD lies in the strict application of symptomatic measures [164]. **Dietary sodium restriction, sufficient physical activity and normalization of the body mass index** should be implemented as initial approach for patients diagnosed or at-risk for ADPKD. Based on the role of vasopressin in ADPKD, **increased water intake** has been suggested in order to suppress endogenous vasopressin concentration and thereby reduce kidney cyst growth targeting a goal urine osmolality below 280 mOsm/kg H_2O [166]. Ongoing controlled trials to evaluate the impact of high water intake on TKV are in progress [167]. In addition, high fluid intake might also be generally beneficial to reduce the risk of nephrolithiasis and UTI in ADPKD. Low salt intake and maintenance of a normal body mass index would be also recommended in view of the increased risk of hypertension and cardiovascular comorbidities in children with ADPKD [14, 164]. Last but not least, **avoidance of smoking and potentially nephrotoxic drugs** including nonsteroidal anti-inflammatory drugs is also appropriate. Extra-renal co-morbidities require adequate treatment. For this chapter we will focus on aspects concerning liver disease.

Blood Pressure Control

Blood pressure control is essential in PKD patients. While blood pressure control is a critical aspect of CKD management in general in both children and adults, hypertension is a key modifiable risk factor in children with ADPKD [14]. Increased TKV and fractional cyst volume is associated with hypertension and decreased eGFR over time [27, 28]. When lifestyle measures remain insufficient, the first line pharmacologic treatment will be the inhibition of RAAS.

The HALT-PKD trials compared the combination of ACE inhibition (ACEI) with an angiotensin receptor blocker to ACEI alone in adult patients with an eGFR of either >60 or 25–60 mL/min/1.73 m^2 as well as standard blood pressure with low blood pressure targets in early-stage patients. Altogether more than 1000 ADPKD patients were enrolled [168, 169]. In these trials rigorous blood pressure control showed benefits over standard blood pressure control in early ADPKD in terms of a reduced increase in total kidney volume, a greater decline in left ventricular mass index and less albuminuria. eGFR was not different among the groups. The international consensus guidelines for pediatric ADPKD recommend at least annual blood pressure measurements for children at-risk of or diagnosed with ADPKD, with a preference for periodic 24-h ambulatory blood pressure monitoring due to the increased risk of masked hypertension. Blood pressure should be maintained below the 75th percentile (or <125/72 mmHg from age 16 years) [14]. It was suggested that lowering blood pressure even below the 50th percentile (or <120/70 mmHg from age 16 years) might provide additional long-term benefit in hypertensive children with ADPKD. Targeting the 50th–75th percentile blood pressure would be the ideal goals for hypertensive children with ADPKD [14, 16].

While formal recommendations for children with ARPKD are lacking, it is reasonable to apply the same treatment targets in the ARPKD population. Hypertension can be difficult to control in ARPKD children and may require multi-drug treatment. Hypertension needs early and aggressive treatment with careful blood pressure monitoring to prevent sequelae of hypertension (e.g., cardiac hypertrophy, congestive heart failure) and deterioration of kidney function [110]. The pathophysiology of hypertension in ARPKD is not clearly understood but may involve dysregulation of renal sodium transport and activation of the RAS [170, 171] leading to increased intravascular volume [172]. It is therefore important to point out that hyponatremia in ARPKD can be considered to be an effect of excess water retention rather than sodium loss. Thus, general principles of handling hyponatremia apply. Feeding may need to be concentrated to minimize fluid intake [11, 112]. Sodium supplementation may increase hypertension. RAS antagonists (ACE inhibitors or AT1 receptor blockers) are regarded the treatment of choice [112]. Moreover, it has been proposed that the epithelial sodium channel blocker amiloride can be used to decrease intracellular cAMP concentrations that may result in Pseudo-Liddle syndrome [173].

Management of CKD and ESKD in Pediatric PKD Patients

The management of children with PKD with declining kidney function should follow the standard guidelines established for chronic kidney failure in other pediatric patients. Both peritoneal dialysis (PD) and hemodialysis are successfully used in ARPKD neonates and infants. PD has been recommended as the chronic modality of choice for infants with ESKD as nutrition can be optimized and vascular access can be preserved for later use [174]. Maintenance PD can be used in young ARPKD children with only minor modifications compared to other inborn kidney diseases [175]. Kidney transplantation is the treatment of choice for individuals with ESKD. In case of massively enlarged kidneys, native nephrectomies may be warranted to allow allograft placement.

ARPKD is one of the two major indications for combined liver and kidney transplantation (CLKTx) during childhood, next to primary hyperoxaluria that is discussed in detail elsewhere in this book [176, 177]. The best timing and strategy for combined transplantation is still a matter of debate and usually requires individualized

decision-making. Recurrent cholangitis and evidence of severe portal hypertension may be indications for combined liver and kidney transplantation in ARPKD [137, 140, 176, 178]. Organ survival after CLKTx in ARPKD is good, but data from the ESPN-ERA/EDTA registry suggested higher mortality in ARPKD patients undergoing CLKTx in comparison to patients undergoing isolated kidney transplantation [137].

Functional consequences of CKD are rarely a clinical problem in children with ADPKD. In cases with VEO-ADPKD the same general principles apply as in ARPKD and other causes of pediatric CKD.

Management of Liver Disease

Liver cysts in ADPKD only rarely result in clinical problems and complications appear much less common than complications of kidney cysts. Usually, hepatic, pancreatic, or ovarian cysts are not observed before puberty [47]. Massive liver enlargement secondary to hepatic cysts may result in disabling discomfort. These individuals may benefit from percutaneous sclerotherapy when one or a few large cysts are present. Occasionally, more aggressive surgical intervention with fenestration, partial hepatectomy or even liver transplantation may be required [179]. Furthermore, as discussed below somatostatin analogues are under investigation for hepatic cysts.

Cholangitis is a prominent co-morbidity in ARPKD and always requires diligent evaluation with aggressive antimicrobial treatment.

Primary management of variceal bleeding in ARPKD may include endoscopic approaches, such as sclerotherapy or variceal banding. In some patients, portosystemic shunting or liver-kidney transplantation (sequential or combined) can be considered as a viable therapeutic option; however, since ammonia is cleared by the kidneys, impaired kidney function in ARPKD patients makes portosystemic shunting less attractive. Transjugular intrahepatic portosystemic shunt (TIPS) has been used in pediatric patients as a feasible and effective treatment alternative for surgical shunting but hepatic encephalopathy may be a problem [180, 181].

focus on a potential role of somatostatin analogues for the treatment of polycystic liver disease.

mTOR Inhibition and Other Targeted Therapy of Cellular Metabolism

mTOR activation has been observed in the cyst epithelium of ADPKD kidneys. After promising results in animal models [1], different trials studied mTOR inhibition in ADPKD. The two large trials on mTOR inhibition in ADPKD did not deliver a therapeutic breakthrough [195, 196]. mTOR inhibitors might still be an option in selected patients with ADPKD or if administered in combination with other agents or in a tubule-specific way.

In addition to mTOR inhibitors, inhibition of glycolysis, activation of AMPK through Metformin, PPAR-α activation or Sirtuin inhibition are additional pharmacological strategies that are currently under investigation [85].

Dietary Intervention

Dietary interventions are an interesting emerging therapeutic strategy in addition to pharmacological approaches based on observations that PKD proteins may be involved in the regulation of cellular metabolism [85]. Moderate food or caloric restriction has shown positive effects on kidney volume in preclinical models. Importantly, obesity is a known risk factor for rapid disease progression in ADPKD. In addition to caloric restriction, time restricted feeding and ketogenic diet as well as the addition of β-hydroxybutyrate to normal chow have shown promising effects in preclinical mouse, rat and cat models of PKD [197]. Pilot clinical trials have recently been initiated.

Acknowledgments CB holds a part-time faculty appointment at the University of Freiburg in addition to his employment with the Limbach Group for which he heads and manages Limbach Genetics. His research lab receives support from the Deutsche Forschungsgemeinschaft (DFG) (BE 3910/8-1, BE 3910/9-1, and Collaborative Research Center SFB 1453—Project-ID 431984000) and the Federal Ministry of Education and Research (BMBF, 01GM1903I and 01GM1903G). MCL was supported the Deutsche Forschungsgemeinschaft (DFG) (Li 2397/5-1) and the

Federal Ministry of Education and Research (BMBF, 01GM1515E and 01GM1903B). MCL was also supported by the Köln Fortune and the GEROK program of the medical faculty of the University of Cologne), the Marga and Walter Boll-Stiftung, the European Society for Paediatric Nephrology (ESPN 2014.2; ESPN 2016.3) and the PKD Familiäre Zystennieren e.V. (PKD Foundation).

We thank Heike Göbel and Uta Drebber (both Institute for Pathology, University Hospital of Cologne), Andreas Serra (Zürich, Switzerland), Bernd Hoppe (Bonn, Germany), and Lisa Guay-Woodford (Washington, USA) for providing picture material.

References

1. Bergmann C, Guay-Woodford LM, Harris PC, et al. Polycystic kidney disease. Nat Rev Dis Primer. 2018;4:50. https://doi.org/10.1038/s41572-018-0047-y.
2. De Rechter S, Bammens B, Schaefer F, et al. Unmet needs and challenges for follow-up and treatment of autosomal dominant polycystic kidney disease: the paediatric perspective. Clin Kidney J. 2018;11:i14–26. https://doi.org/10.1093/ckj/sfy088.
3. Burgmaier K, Kilian S, Bammens B, et al. Clinical courses and complications of young adults with autosomal recessive polycystic kidney disease (ARPKD). Sci Rep. 2019;9:7919. https://doi.org/10.1038/s41598-019-43488-w.
4. Liebau MC. Early clinical management of autosomal recessive polycystic kidney disease. Pediatr Nephrol Berl Ger. 2021;36:3561–70. https://doi.org/10.1007/s00467-021-04970-8.
5. Osathanondh V, Potter EL. Pathogenesis of polycystic kidneys. Type 4 due to urethral obstruction. Arch Pathol. 1964;77:502–9.
6. Liebau MC, Serra AL. Looking at the (w)hole: magnet resonance imaging in polycystic kidney disease. Pediatr Nephrol Berl Ger. 2013;28:1771–83. https://doi.org/10.1007/s00467-012-2370-y.
7. Gimpel C, Avni EF, Breysem L, et al. Imaging of kidney cysts and cystic kidney diseases in children: an International Working Group Consensus Statement. Radiology. 2019;290:769–82. https://doi.org/10.1148/radiol.2018181243.
8. Harris PC, Rossetti S. Determinants of renal disease variability in ADPKD. Adv Chronic Kidney Dis. 2010;17:131–9. https://doi.org/10.1053/j.ackd.2009.12.004.
9. Marquardt W. Cystennieren, Cystenleber, und Cystenpancreas bei zwei Geschwistern. 1935.
10. Blyth H, Ockenden BG. Polycystic disease of kidney and liver presenting in childhood. J Med Genet. 1971;8:257–84.
11. Gimpel C, Avni FE, Bergmann C, et al. Perinatal diagnosis, management, and follow-up of cystic renal diseases: a clinical practice recommendation with systematic literature reviews. JAMA

Pediatr. 2018;172:74–86. https://doi.org/10.1001/jamapediatrics.2017.3938.

12. Ali H, Al-Mulla F, Hussain N, et al. PKD1 duplicated regions limit clinical utility of whole exome sequencing for genetic diagnosis of autosomal dominant polycystic kidney disease. Sci Rep. 2019;9:4141. https://doi.org/10.1038/s41598-019-40761-w.

13. Rossetti S, Consugar MB, Chapman AB, et al. Comprehensive molecular diagnostics in autosomal dominant polycystic kidney disease. J Am Soc Nephrol (JASN). 2007;18:2143–60. https://doi.org/10.1681/ASN.2006121387.

14. Gimpel C, Bergmann C, Bockenhauer D, et al. International consensus statement on the diagnosis and management of autosomal dominant polycystic kidney disease in children and young people. Nat Rev Nephrol. 2019;15:713–26. https://doi.org/10.1038/s41581-019-0155-2.

15. Chapman AB, Devuyst O, Eckardt K-U, et al. Autosomal-dominant polycystic kidney disease (ADPKD): executive summary from a kidney disease: improving global outcomes (KDIGO) controversies conference. Kidney Int. 2015;88:17–27. https://doi.org/10.1038/ki.2015.59.

16. Gimpel C, Bergmann C, Mekahli D. The wind of change in the management of autosomal dominant polycystic kidney disease in childhood. Pediatr Nephrol Berl Ger. 2021; https://doi.org/10.1007/s00467-021-04974-4.

17. Wilson PD. Polycystic kidney disease. N Engl J Med. 2004;350:151–64. https://doi.org/10.1056/NEJMra022161.

18. Cornec-Le Gall E, Alam A, Perrone RD. Autosomal dominant polycystic kidney disease. Lancet Lond Engl. 2019;393:919–35. https://doi.org/10.1016/S0140-6736(18)32782-X.

19. Benz EG, Hartung EA. Predictors of progression in autosomal dominant and autosomal recessive polycystic kidney disease. Pediatr Nephrol Berl Ger. 2021;36:2639–58. https://doi.org/10.1007/s00467-020-04869-w.

20. Gabow PA, Kimberling WJ, Strain JD, et al. Utility of ultrasonography in the diagnosis of autosomal dominant polycystic kidney disease in children. J Am Soc Nephrol (JASN). 1997;8:105–10.

21. Bear JC, Parfrey PS, Morgan JM, et al. Autosomal dominant polycystic kidney disease: new information for genetic counselling. Am J Med Genet. 1992;43:548–53. https://doi.org/10.1002/ajmg.1320430309.

22. McHugh K, Stringer DA, Hebert D, Babiak CA. Simple renal cysts in children: diagnosis and follow-up with US. Radiology. 1991;178:383–5. https://doi.org/10.1148/radiology.178.2.1987597.

23. Ravine D, Gibson RN, Donlan J, Sheffield LJ. An ultrasound renal cyst prevalence survey: specificity data for inherited renal cystic diseases. Am J Kidney Dis. 1993;22:803–7.

24. Pei Y, Obaji J, Dupuis A, et al. Unified criteria for ultrasonographic diagnosis of ADPKD. J Am Soc

25. Reed B, Nobakht E, Dadgar S, et al. Renal ultrasonographic evaluation in children at risk of autosomal dominant polycystic kidney disease. Am J Kidney Dis. 2010;56:50–6. https://doi.org/10.1053/j.ajkd.2010.02.349.

26. Fick-Brosnahan GM, Tran ZV, Johnson AM, et al. Progression of autosomal-dominant polycystic kidney disease in children. Kidney Int. 2001;59:1654–62. https://doi.org/10.1046/j.1523-1755.2001.0590051654.x.

27. Cadnapaphornchai MA, McFann K, Strain JD, et al. Prospective change in renal volume and function in children with ADPKD. Clin J Am Soc Nephrol (CJASN). 2009;4:820–9. https://doi.org/10.2215/CJN.02810608.

28. Cadnapaphornchai MA, Masoumi A, Strain JD, et al. Magnetic resonance imaging of kidney and cyst volume in children with ADPKD. Clin J Am Soc Nephrol (CJASN). 2011;6:369–76. https://doi.org/10.2215/CJN.03780410.

29. Chapman AB, Wei W. Imaging approaches to patients with polycystic kidney disease. Semin Nephrol. 2011;31:237–44. https://doi.org/10.1016/j.semnephrol.2011.05.003.

30. Nascimento AB, Mitchell DG, Zhang XM, et al. Rapid MR imaging detection of renal cysts: age-based standards. Radiology. 2001;221:628–32. https://doi.org/10.1148/radiol.2213010178.

31. Grantham JJ, Torres VE, Chapman AB, et al. Volume progression in polycystic kidney disease. N Engl J Med. 2006;354:2122–30. https://doi.org/10.1056/NEJMoa054341.

32. Torres VE, King BF, Chapman AB, et al. Magnetic resonance measurements of renal blood flow and disease progression in autosomal dominant polycystic kidney disease. Clin J Am Soc Nephrol (CJASN). 2007;2:112–20. https://doi.org/10.2215/CJN.00910306.

33. Chapman AB. Approaches to testing new treatments in autosomal dominant polycystic kidney disease: insights from the CRISP and HALT-PKD studies. Clin J Am Soc Nephrol (CJASN). 2008;3:1197–204. https://doi.org/10.2215/CJN.00060108.

34. Kline TL, Korfiatis P, Edwards ME, et al. Image texture features predict renal function decline in patients with autosomal dominant polycystic kidney disease. Kidney Int. 2017;92:1206–16. https://doi.org/10.1016/j.kint.2017.03.026.

35. Breysem L, De Rechter S, De Keyzer F, et al. 3DUS as an alternative to MRI for measuring renal volume in children with autosomal dominant polycystic kidney disease. Pediatr Nephrol Berl Ger. 2018;33:827–35. https://doi.org/10.1007/s00467-017-3862-6.

36. Paterson AD, Magistroni R, He N, et al. Progressive loss of renal function is an age-dependent heritable trait in type 1 autosomal dominant polycystic kidney disease. J Am Soc Nephrol (JASN). 2005;16:755–62. https://doi.org/10.1681/ASN.2004090758.

37. Persu A, Duyme M, Pirson Y, et al. Comparison between siblings and twins supports a role for modifier genes in ADPKD. Kidney Int. 2004;66:2132–6. https://doi.org/10.1111/j.1523-1755.2004.66003.x.

38. Sweeney WE Jr, Avner ED. Diagnosis and management of childhood polycystic kidney disease. Pediatr Nephrol Berl Ger. 2011;26:675–92. https://doi.org/10.1007/s00467-010-1656-1.

39. Sweeney WE Jr, Avner ED. Molecular and cellular pathophysiology of autosomal recessive polycystic kidney disease (ARPKD). Cell Tissue Res. 2006;326:671–85. https://doi.org/10.1007/s00441-006-0226-0.

40. Ulinski T, Lescure S, Beaufils S, et al. Renal phenotypes related to hepatocyte nuclear factor-1beta (TCF2) mutations in a pediatric cohort. J Am Soc Nephrol (JASN). 2006;17:497–503. https://doi.org/10.1681/ASN.2005101040.

41. Faguer S, Bouissou F, Dumazer P, et al. Massively enlarged polycystic kidneys in monozygotic twins with TCF2/HNF-1beta (hepatocyte nuclear factor-1beta) heterozygous whole-gene deletion. Am J Kidney Dis. 2007;50:1023–7. https://doi.org/10.1053/j.ajkd.2007.06.016.

42. Shamshirsaz AA, Shamshirsaz A, Reza Bekheirnia M, et al. Autosomal-dominant polycystic kidney disease in infancy and childhood: progression and outcome. Kidney Int. 2005;68:2218–24. https://doi.org/10.1111/j.1523-1755.2005.00678.x.

43. Fick-Brosnahan G, Johnson AM, Strain JD, Gabow PA. Renal asymmetry in children with autosomal dominant polycystic kidney disease. Am J Kidney Dis. 1999;34:639–45. https://doi.org/10.1016/S0272-6386(99)70387-2.

44. Digby EL, Liauw J, Dionne J, et al. Etiologies and outcomes of prenatally diagnosed hyperechogenic kidneys. Prenat Diagn. 2021;41:465–77. https://doi.org/10.1002/pd.5883.

45. Yulia A, Napolitano R, Aiman A, et al. Perinatal and infant outcome of fetuses with prenatally diagnosed hyperechogenic kidneys. Ultrasound Obstet Gynecol. 2021;57:953–8. https://doi.org/10.1002/uog.22121.

46. Chebib FT, Torres VE. Assessing risk of rapid progression in autosomal dominant polycystic kidney disease and special considerations for disease-modifying therapy. Am J Kidney Dis. 2021;78:282–92. https://doi.org/10.1053/j.ajkd.2020.12.020.

47. Cadnapaphornchai MA. Autosomal dominant polycystic kidney disease in children. Curr Opin Pediatr. 2015;27:193–200. https://doi.org/10.1097/MOP.0000000000000195.

48. Massella L, Mekahli D, Paripović D, et al. Prevalence of hypertension in children with early-stage ADPKD. Clin J Am Soc Nephrol (CJASN). 2018;13:874–83. https://doi.org/10.2215/CJN.11401017.

49. Marlais M, Cuthell O, Langan D, et al. Hypertension in autosomal dominant polycystic kidney disease: a meta-analysis. Arch Dis Child. 2016;101:1142–7. https://doi.org/10.1136/archdischild-2015-310221.

50. Cadnapaphornchai MA. Hypertension in children with autosomal dominant polycystic kidney disease (ADPKD). Curr Hypertens Rev. 2013;9:21–6. https://doi.org/10.2174/1573402111309010004.

51. Pirson Y, Chauveau D, Torres V. Management of cerebral aneurysms in autosomal dominant polycystic kidney disease. J Am Soc Nephrol (JASN). 2002;13:269–76.

52. Walker EYX, Marlais M. Should we screen for intracranial aneurysms in children with autosomal dominant polycystic kidney disease? Pediatr Nephrol Berl Ger. 2022; https://doi.org/10.1007/s00467-022-05432-5.

53. Cheung J, Scudamore CH, Yoshida EM. Management of polycystic liver disease. Can J Gastroenterol. 2004;18:666–70.

54. Pirson Y. Extrarenal manifestations of autosomal dominant polycystic kidney disease. Adv Chronic Kidney Dis. 2010;17:173–80. https://doi.org/10.1053/j.ackd.2010.01.003.

55. Gevers TJG, Drenth JPH. Diagnosis and management of polycystic liver disease. Nat Rev Gastroenterol Hepatol. 2013;10:101–8. https://doi.org/10.1038/nrgastro.2012.254.

56. Cornec-Le Gall E, Torres VE, Harris PC. Genetic complexity of autosomal dominant polycystic kidney and liver diseases. J Am Soc Nephrol (JASN). 2018;29:13–23. https://doi.org/10.1681/ASN.2017050483.

57. Koptides M, Mean R, Demetriou K, et al. Genetic evidence for a trans-heterozygous model for cystogenesis in autosomal dominant polycystic kidney disease. Hum Mol Genet. 2000;9:447–52.

58. Qian F, Watnick TJ, Onuchic LF, Germino GG. The molecular basis of focal cyst formation in human autosomal dominant polycystic kidney disease type I. Cell. 1996;87:979–87.

59. Watnick T, He N, Wang K, et al. Mutations of PKD1 in ADPKD2 cysts suggest a pathogenic effect of trans-heterozygous mutations. Nat Genet. 2000;25:143–4. https://doi.org/10.1038/75981.

60. Zhang Z, Bai H, Blumenfeld J, et al. Detection of PKD1 and PKD2 somatic variants in autosomal dominant polycystic kidney cyst epithelial cells by whole-genome sequencing. J Am Soc Nephrol (JASN). 2021; https://doi.org/10.1681/ASN.2021050690.

61. Wills ES, Cnossen WR, Veltman JA, et al. Chromosomal abnormalities in hepatic cysts point to novel polycystic liver disease genes. Eur J Hum Genet (EJHG). 2016;24:1707–14. https://doi.org/10.1038/ejhg.2016.97.

62. Pei Y, Paterson AD, Wang KR, et al. Bilineal disease and trans-heterozygotes in autosomal dominant polycystic kidney disease. Am J Hum Genet. 2001;68:355–63.

63. Wu G, Tian X, Nishimura S, et al. Trans-heterozygous Pkd1 and Pkd2 mutations modify

expression of polycystic kidney disease. Hum Mol Genet. 2002;11:1845–54.

64. Bergmann C. ARPKD and early manifestations of ADPKD: the original polycystic kidney disease and phenocopies. Pediatr Nephrol Berl Ger. 2015;30:15–30. https://doi.org/10.1007/s00467-013-2706-2.

65. Thivierge C, Kurbegovic A, Couillard M, et al. Overexpression of PKD1 causes polycystic kidney disease. Mol Cell Biol. 2006;26:1538–48. https://doi.org/10.1128/MCB.26.4.1538-1548.2006.

66. Happé H, Peters DJM. Translational research in ADPKD: lessons from animal models. Nat Rev Nephrol. 2014;10:587–601. https://doi.org/10.1038/nrneph.2014.137.

67. Lantinga-van Leeuwen IS, Dauwerse JG, Baelde HJ, et al. Lowering of Pkd1 expression is sufficient to cause polycystic kidney disease. Hum Mol Genet. 2004;13:3069–77. https://doi.org/10.1093/hmg/ddh336.

68. Piontek K, Menezes LF, Garcia-Gonzalez MA, et al. A critical developmental switch defines the kinetics of kidney cyst formation after loss of Pkd1. Nat Med. 2007;13:1490–5. https://doi.org/10.1038/nm1675.

69. Bastos AP, Piontek K, Silva AM, et al. Pkd1 haploinsufficiency increases renal damage and induces microcyst formation following ischemia/reperfusion. J Am Soc Nephrol (JASN). 2009;20:2389–402. https://doi.org/10.1681/ASN.2008040435.

70. Patel V, Li L, Cobo-Stark P, et al. Acute kidney injury and aberrant planar cell polarity induce cyst formation in mice lacking renal cilia. Hum Mol Genet. 2008;17:1578–90. https://doi.org/10.1093/hmg/ddn045.

71. Takakura A, Contrino L, Zhou X, et al. Renal injury is a third hit promoting rapid development of adult polycystic kidney disease. Hum Mol Genet. 2009;18:2523–31. https://doi.org/10.1093/hmg/ddp147.

72. Happé H, Leonhard WN, van der Wal A, et al. Toxic tubular injury in kidneys from Pkd1-deletion mice accelerates cystogenesis accompanied by dysregulated planar cell polarity and canonical Wnt signaling pathways. Hum Mol Genet. 2009;18:2532–42. https://doi.org/10.1093/hmg/ddp190.

73. Karihaloo A, Koraishy F, Huen SC, et al. Macrophages promote cyst growth in polycystic kidney disease. J Am Soc Nephrol (JASN). 2011;22:1809–14. https://doi.org/10.1681/ASN.2011010084.

74. Swenson-Fields KI, Vivian CJ, Salah SM, et al. Macrophages promote polycystic kidney disease progression. Kidney Int. 2013;83:855–64. https://doi.org/10.1038/ki.2012.446.

75. Weimbs T. Third-hit signaling in renal cyst formation. J Am Soc Nephrol (JASN). 2011;22:793–5. https://doi.org/10.1681/ASN.2011030284.

76. Hofherr A, Köttgen M. TRPP channels and polycystins. Adv Exp Med Biol. 2011;704:287–313. https://doi.org/10.1007/978-94-007-0265-3_16.

77. Nauli SM, Alenghat FJ, Luo Y, et al. Polycystins 1 and 2 mediate mechanosensation in the primary cilium of kidney cells. Nat Genet. 2003;33:129–37. https://doi.org/10.1038/ng1076.

78. Praetorius HA, Spring KR. Bending the MDCK cell primary cilium increases intracellular calcium. J Membr Biol. 2001;184:71–9.

79. Sharif-Naeini R, Folgering JHA, Bichet D, et al. Polycystin-1 and -2 dosage regulates pressure sensing. Cell. 2009;139:587–96. https://doi.org/10.1016/j.cell.2009.08.045.

80. Ta CM, Vien TN, Ng LCT, DeCaen PG. Structure and function of polycystin channels in primary cilia. Cell Signal. 2020;72:109626. https://doi.org/10.1016/j.cellsig.2020.109626.

81. Delling M, DeCaen PG, Doerner JF, et al. Primary cilia are specialized calcium signalling organelles. Nature. 2013;504:311–4. https://doi.org/10.1038/nature12833.

82. Douguet D, Patel A, Honoré E. Structure and function of polycystins: insights into polycystic kidney disease. Nat Rev Nephrol. 2019;15:412–22. https://doi.org/10.1038/s41581-019-0143-6.

83. Hardy E, Tsiokas L. Polycystins as components of large multiprotein complexes of polycystin interactors. Cell Signal. 2020;72:109640. https://doi.org/10.1016/j.cellsig.2020.109640.

84. Strubl S, Torres JA, Spindt AK, et al. STAT signaling in polycystic kidney disease. Cell Signal. 2020;72:109639. https://doi.org/10.1016/j.cellsig.2020.109639.

85. Haumann S, Müller R-U, Liebau MC. Metabolic changes in polycystic kidney disease as a potential target for systemic treatment. Int J Mol Sci. 2020;21 https://doi.org/10.3390/ijms21176093.

86. Hogan MC, Manganelli L, Woollard JR, et al. Characterization of PKD protein-positive exosome-like vesicles. J Am Soc Nephrol (JASN). 2009;20:278–88. https://doi.org/10.1681/ASN.2008060564.

87. Magistroni R, He N, Wang K, et al. Genotype-renal function correlation in type 2 autosomal dominant polycystic kidney disease. J Am Soc Nephrol (JASN). 2003;14:1164–74.

88. Cho Y, Tong A, Craig JC, et al. Establishing a Core outcome set for autosomal dominant polycystic kidney disease: report of the standardized outcomes in nephrology-polycystic kidney disease (SONG-PKD) consensus workshop. Am J Kidney Dis. 2021;77:255–63. https://doi.org/10.1053/j.ajkd.2020.05.024.

89. Hateboer N, Veldhuisen B, Peters D, et al. Location of mutations within the PKD2 gene influences clinical outcome. Kidney Int. 2000;57:1444–51. https://doi.org/10.1046/j.1523-1755.2000.00989.x.

90. Cornec-Le Gall E, Audrézet M-P, Chen J-M, et al. Type of PKD1 mutation influences renal outcome in ADPKD. J Am Soc Nephrol (JASN). 2013;24:1006–13. https://doi.org/10.1681/ASN.2012070650.

91. Cornec-Le Gall E, Audrézet M-P, Rousseau A, et al. The PROPKD score: a new algorithm to predict renal survival in autosomal dominant polycystic kidney

disease. J Am Soc Nephrol (JASN). 2016;27:942–51. https://doi.org/10.1681/ASN.2015010016.

92. Bergmann C, von Bothmer J, Ortiz Brüchle N, et al. Mutations in multiple PKD genes may explain early and severe polycystic kidney disease. J Am Soc Nephrol (JASN). 2011;22:2047–56. https://doi.org/10.1681/ASN.2010101080.

93. Rossetti S, Burton S, Strmecki L, et al. The position of the polycystic kidney disease 1 (PKD1) gene mutation correlates with the severity of renal disease. J Am Soc Nephrol (JASN). 2002;13:1230–7.

94. Rossetti S, Chauveau D, Kubly V, et al. Association of mutation position in polycystic kidney disease 1 (PKD1) gene and development of a vascular phenotype. Lancet. 2003;361:2196–201. https://doi.org/10.1016/S0140-6736(03)13773-7.

95. Lavu S, Vaughan LE, Senum SR, et al. The value of genotypic and imaging information to predict functional and structural outcomes in ADPKD. JCI Insight. 2020;5 https://doi.org/10.1172/jci.insight.138724.

96. Durkie M, Chong J, Valluru MK, et al. Biallelic inheritance of hypomorphic PKD1 variants is highly prevalent in very early onset polycystic kidney disease. Genet Med. 2021;23:689–97. https://doi.org/10.1038/s41436-020-01026-4.

97. Fain PR, McFann KK, Taylor MRG, et al. Modifier genes play a significant role in the phenotypic expression of PKD1. Kidney Int. 2005;67:1256–67. https://doi.org/10.1111/j.1523-1755.2005.00203.x.

98. Snoek R, Stokman MF, Lichtenbelt KD, et al. Preimplantation genetic testing for monogenic kidney disease. Clin J Am Soc Nephrol (CJASN). 2020;15:1279–86. https://doi.org/10.2215/CJN.03550320.

99. De Waele L, Lagae L, Mekahli D. Tuberous sclerosis complex: the past and the future. Pediatr Nephrol Berl Ger. 2015;30:1771–80. https://doi.org/10.1007/s00467-014-3027-9.

100. Janssens P, Van Hoeve K, De Waele L, et al. Renal progression factors in young patients with tuberous sclerosis complex: a retrospective cohort study. Pediatr Nephrol Berl Ger. 2018;33:2085–93. https://doi.org/10.1007/s00467-018-4003-6.

101. Northrup H, Aronow ME, Bebin EM, et al. Updated international tuberous sclerosis complex diagnostic criteria and surveillance and management recommendations. Pediatr Neurol. 2021;123:50–66. https://doi.org/10.1016/j.pediatrneurol.2021.07.011.

102. Lam HC, Siroky BJ, Henske EP. Renal disease in tuberous sclerosis complex: pathogenesis and therapy. Nat Rev Nephrol. 2018;14:704–16. https://doi.org/10.1038/s41581-018-0059-6.

103. Shang S, Mei Y, Wang T, et al. Diagnosis and genotype-phenotype correlation in patients with PKD1/TSC2 contiguous gene deletion syndrome. Clin Nephrol. 2022; https://doi.org/10.5414/CN110476.

104. De Rechter S, Bockenhauer D, Guay-Woodford LM, et al. ADPedKD: a global online platform on the management of children with ADPKD. Kidney Int Rep. 2019;4:1271–84. https://doi.org/10.1016/j.ekir.2019.05.015.

105. Guay-Woodford LM. Autosomal recessive polycystic kidney disease: the prototype of the hepato-renal fibrocystic diseases. J Pediatr Genet. 2014;3:89–101. https://doi.org/10.3233/PGE-14092.

106. Alzarka B, Morizono H, Bollman JW, et al. Design and implementation of the hepatorenal fibrocystic disease core center clinical database: a centralized resource for characterizing autosomal recessive polycystic kidney disease and other hepatorenal fibrocystic diseases. Front Pediatr. 2017;5:80. https://doi.org/10.3389/fped.2017.00080.

107. Nakanishi K, Sweeney WE Jr, Zerres K, et al. Proximal tubular cysts in fetal human autosomal recessive polycystic kidney disease. J Am Soc Nephrol (JASN). 2000;11:760–3.

108. Denamur E, Delezoide A-L, Alberti C, et al. Genotype-phenotype correlations in fetuses and neonates with autosomal recessive polycystic kidney disease. Kidney Int. 2010;77:350–8. https://doi.org/10.1038/ki.2009.440.

109. Wehrman A, Kriegermeier A, Wen J. Diagnosis and management of hepatobiliary complications in autosomal recessive polycystic kidney disease. Front Pediatr. 2017;5:124. https://doi.org/10.3389/fped.2017.00124.

110. Büscher R, Büscher AK, Weber S, et al. Clinical manifestations of autosomal recessive polycystic kidney disease (ARPKD): kidney-related and non-kidney-related phenotypes. Pediatr Nephrol Berl Ger. 2014;29:1915–25. https://doi.org/10.1007/s00467-013-2634-1.

111. Gunay-Aygun M, Font-Montgomery E, Lukose L, et al. Characteristics of congenital hepatic fibrosis in a large cohort of patients with autosomal recessive polycystic kidney disease. Gastroenterology. 2013;144:112–121.e2. https://doi.org/10.1053/j.gastro.2012.09.056.

112. Guay-Woodford LM, Bissler JJ, Braun MC, et al. Consensus expert recommendations for the diagnosis and management of autosomal recessive polycystic kidney disease: report of an international conference. J Pediatr. 2014;165:611–7. https://doi.org/10.1016/j.jpeds.2014.06.015.

113. Bergmann C. Genetics of autosomal recessive polycystic kidney disease and its differential diagnoses. Front Pediatr. 2017;5:221. https://doi.org/10.3389/fped.2017.00221.

114. Burgmaier K, Brinker L, Erger F, et al. Refining genotype-phenotype correlations in 304 patients with autosomal recessive polycystic kidney disease and PKHD1 gene variants. Kidney Int. 2021;100:650–9. https://doi.org/10.1016/j.kint.2021.04.019.

115. Adeva M, El-Youssef M, Rossetti S, et al. Clinical and molecular characterization defines a broadened spectrum of autosomal recessive polycystic kidney disease (ARPKD). Medicine (Baltimore).

2006;85:1–21. https://doi.org/10.1097/01.md.0000200165.90373.9a.

116. Ebner K, Feldkoetter M, Ariceta G, et al. Rationale, design and objectives of ARegPKD, a European ARPKD registry study. BMC Nephrol. 2015;16:22. https://doi.org/10.1186/s12882-015-0002-z.

117. Nahm A-M, Henriquez DE, Ritz E. Renal cystic disease (ADPKD and ARPKD). Nephrol Dial Transplant. 2002;17:311–4.

118. Nicolau C, Torra R, Badenas C, et al. Sonographic pattern of recessive polycystic kidney disease in young adults. Differences from the dominant form. Nephrol Dial Transplant. 2000;15:1373–8.

119. Vester U, Kranz B, Hoyer PF. The diagnostic value of ultrasound in cystic kidney diseases. Pediatr Nephrol Berl Ger. 2010;25:231–40. https://doi.org/10.1007/s00467-008-0981-0.

120. Bergmann C, Senderek J, Windelen E, et al. Clinical consequences of PKHD1 mutations in 164 patients with autosomal-recessive polycystic kidney disease (ARPKD). Kidney Int. 2005;67:829–48. https://doi.org/10.1111/j.1523-1755.2005.00148.x.

121. Gunay-Aygun M, Font-Montgomery E, Lukose L, et al. Correlation of kidney function, volume and imaging findings, and PKHD1 mutations in 73 patients with autosomal recessive polycystic kidney disease. Clin J Am Soc Nephrol (CJASN). 2010;5:972–84. https://doi.org/10.2215/CJN.07141009.

122. Avni FE, Guissard G, Hall M, et al. Hereditary polycystic kidney diseases in children: changing sonographic patterns through childhood. Pediatr Radiol. 2002;32:169–74.

123. Blickman JG, Bramson RT, Herrin JT. Autosomal recessive polycystic kidney disease: long-term sonographic findings in patients surviving the neonatal period. AJR Am J Roentgenol. 1995;164:1247–50. https://doi.org/10.2214/ajr.164.5.7717240.

124. Abdul Majeed N, Font-Montgomery E, Lukose L, et al. Prospective evaluation of kidney and liver disease in autosomal recessive polycystic kidney disease-congenital hepatic fibrosis. Mol Genet Metab. 2020;131:267–76. https://doi.org/10.1016/j.ymgme.2020.08.006.

125. Burgmaier K, Kilian S, Arbeiter K, et al. Early childhood height-adjusted total kidney volume as a risk marker of kidney survival in ARPKD. Sci Rep. 2021;11:21677. https://doi.org/10.1038/s41598-021-00523-z.

126. Hartung EA, Wen J, Poznick L, et al. Ultrasound elastography to quantify liver disease severity in autosomal recessive polycystic kidney disease. J Pediatr. 2019;209:107–115.e5. https://doi.org/10.1016/j.jpeds.2019.01.055.

127. Luoto TT, Koivusalo AI, Pakarinen MP. Long-term outcomes and health perceptions in pediatric-onset portal hypertension complicated by varices. J Pediatr Gastroenterol Nutr. 2020;70:628–34. https://doi.org/10.1097/MPG.0000000000002643.

128. Hartung EA, Calle-Toro JS, Lopera CM, et al. Magnetic resonance elastography to quantify liver disease severity in autosomal recessive polycystic kidney disease. Abdom Radiol N Y. 2021;46:570–80. https://doi.org/10.1007/s00261-020-02694-1.

129. Wicher D, Jankowska I, Lipiński P, et al. Transient elastography for detection of liver fibrosis in children with autosomal recessive polycystic kidney disease. Front Pediatr. 2018;6:422. https://doi.org/10.3389/fped.2018.00422.

130. Mehler K, Beck BB, Kaul I, et al. Respiratory and general outcome in neonates with renal oligohydramnios—a single-centre experience. Nephrol Dial Transplant. 2011;26:3514–22. https://doi.org/10.1093/ndt/gfr046.

131. Guay-Woodford LM, Desmond RA. Autosomal recessive polycystic kidney disease: the clinical experience in North America. Pediatrics. 2003;111:1072–80.

132. Burgmaier K, Kunzmann K, Ariceta G, et al. Risk factors for early dialysis dependency in autosomal recessive polycystic kidney disease. J Pediatr. 2018;199:22–28.e6. https://doi.org/10.1016/j.jpeds.2018.03.052.

133. Dell KM, Matheson M, Hartung EA, et al. Kidney disease progression in autosomal recessive polycystic kidney disease. J Pediatr. 2016;171:196–201.e1. https://doi.org/10.1016/j.jpeds.2015.12.079.

134. Wicher D, Grenda R, Teisseyre M, et al. Occurrence of portal hypertension and its clinical course in patients with molecularly confirmed autosomal recessive polycystic kidney disease (ARPKD). Front Pediatr. 2020;8:591379. https://doi.org/10.3389/fped.2020.591379.

135. Davis ID, Ho M, Hupertz V, Avner ED. Survival of childhood polycystic kidney disease following renal transplantation: the impact of advanced hepatobiliary disease. Pediatr Transplant. 2003;7:364–9. https://doi.org/10.1034/j.1399-3046.2003.00094.x.

136. Khan K, Schwarzenberg SJ, Sharp HL, et al. Morbidity from congenital hepatic fibrosis after renal transplantation for autosomal recessive polycystic kidney disease. Am J Transplant. 2002;2:360–5. https://doi.org/10.1034/j.1600-6143.2002.20412.x.

137. Mekahli D, van Stralen KJ, Bonthuis M, et al. Kidney versus combined kidney and liver transplantation in young people with autosomal recessive polycystic kidney disease: data from the European Society for Pediatric Nephrology/European Renal Association-European Dialysis and Transplant (ESPN/ERA-EDTA) Registry. Am J Kidney Dis. 2016;68:782–8. https://doi.org/10.1053/j.ajkd.2016.06.019.

138. Gunay-Aygun M, Avner ED, Bacallao RL, et al. Autosomal recessive polycystic kidney disease and congenital hepatic fibrosis: summary statement of a first National Institutes of Health/Office of Rare Diseases conference. J Pediatr. 2006;149:159–64. https://doi.org/10.1016/j.jpeds.2006.03.014.

139. Kashtan CE, Primack WA, Kainer G, et al. Recurrent bacteremia with enteric pathogens in recessive poly-

140. Telega G, Cronin D, Avner ED. New approaches to the autosomal recessive polycystic kidney disease patient with dual kidney-liver complications. Pediatr Transplant. 2013;17:328–35. https://doi.org/10.1111/petr.12076.

141. Turkbey B, Ocak I, Daryanani K, et al. Autosomal recessive polycystic kidney disease and congenital hepatic fibrosis (ARPKD/CHF). Pediatr Radiol. 2009;39:100–11. https://doi.org/10.1007/s00247-008-1064-x.

142. Chinali M, Lucchetti L, Ricotta A, et al. Cardiac abnormalities in children with autosomal recessive polycystic kidney disease. Cardiorenal Med. 2019;9:180–9. https://doi.org/10.1159/000496473.

143. Gately R, Lock G, Patel C, et al. Multiple cerebral aneurysms in an adult with autosomal recessive polycystic kidney disease. Kidney Int Rep. 2021;6:219–23. https://doi.org/10.1016/j.ekir.2020.10.001.

144. Hartung EA, Matheson M, Lande MB, et al. Neurocognition in children with autosomal recessive polycystic kidney disease in the CKiD cohort study. Pediatr Nephrol Berl Ger. 2014;29:1957–65. https://doi.org/10.1007/s00467-014-2816-5.

145. Hartung EA, Dell KM, Matheson M, et al. Growth in children with autosomal recessive polycystic kidney disease in the CKiD cohort study. Front Pediatr. 2016;4:82. https://doi.org/10.3389/fped.2016.00082.

146. Jahnukainen T, Kirjavainen T, Luoto T, et al. Long-term pulmonary function in children with recessive polycystic kidney disease. Arch Dis Child. 2015;100:944–7. https://doi.org/10.1136/archdischild-2015-308451.

147. Ward CJ, Hogan MC, Rossetti S, et al. The gene mutated in autosomal recessive polycystic kidney disease encodes a large, receptor-like protein. Nat Genet. 2002;30:259–69. https://doi.org/10.1038/ng833.

148. Menezes LFC, Cai Y, Nagasawa Y, et al. Polyductin, the PKHD1 gene product, comprises isoforms expressed in plasma membrane, primary cilium, and cytoplasm. Kidney Int. 2004;66:1345–55. https://doi.org/10.1111/j.1523-1755.2004.00844.x.

149. Wang S, Luo Y, Wilson PD, et al. The autosomal recessive polycystic kidney disease protein is localized to primary cilia, with concentration in the basal body area. J Am Soc Nephrol (JASN). 2004;15:592–602.

150. Ward CJ, Yuan D, Masyuk TV, et al. Cellular and subcellular localization of the ARPKD protein; fibrocystin is expressed on primary cilia. Hum Mol Genet. 2003;12:2703–10. https://doi.org/10.1093/hmg/ddg274.

151. Zhang M-Z, Mai W, Li C, et al. PKHD1 protein encoded by the gene for autosomal recessive polycystic kidney disease associates with basal bodies and primary cilia in renal epithelial cells. Proc Natl Acad Sci U S A. 2004;101:2311–6.

152. Garcia-Gonzalez MA, Menezes LF, Piontek KB, et al. Genetic interaction studies link autosomal dominant and recessive polycystic kidney disease in a common pathway. Hum Mol Genet. 2007;16:1940–50. https://doi.org/10.1093/hmg/ddm141.

153. Olson RJ, Hopp K, Wells H, et al. Synergistic genetic interactions between Pkhd1 and Pkd1 result in an ARPKD-like phenotype in murine models. J Am Soc Nephrol. 2019;30:2113–27. https://doi.org/10.1681/ASN.2019020150.

154. Dafinger C, Mandel AM, Braun A, et al. The carboxy-terminus of the human ARPKD protein fibrocystin can control STAT3 signalling by regulating SRC-activation. J Cell Mol Med. 2020;24:14633–8. https://doi.org/10.1111/jcmm.16014.

155. Hiesberger T, Gourley E, Erickson A, et al. Proteolytic cleavage and nuclear translocation of fibrocystin is regulated by intracellular Ca2+ and activation of protein kinase C. J Biol Chem. 2006;281:34357–64. https://doi.org/10.1074/jbc.M606740200.

156. Bakeberg JL, Tammachote R, Woollard JR, et al. Epitope-tagged Pkhd1 tracks the processing, secretion, and localization of fibrocystin. J Am Soc Nephrol (JASN). 2011;22:2266–77. https://doi.org/10.1681/ASN.2010111173.

157. Ebner K, Dafinger C, Ortiz-Bruechle N, et al. Challenges in establishing genotype-phenotype correlations in ARPKD: case report on a toddler with two severe PKHD1 mutations. Pediatr Nephrol Berl Ger. 2017;32:1269–73. https://doi.org/10.1007/s00467-017-3648-x.

158. Frank V, Zerres K, Bergmann C. Transcriptional complexity in autosomal recessive polycystic kidney disease. Clin J Am Soc Nephrol (CJASN). 2014;9:1729–36. https://doi.org/10.2215/CJN.00920114.

159. Boddu R, Yang C, O'Connor AK, et al. Intragenic motifs regulate the transcriptional complexity of Pkhd1/PKHD1. J Mol Med Berl Ger. 2014;92:1045–56. https://doi.org/10.1007/s00109-014-1185-7.

160. Deget F, Rudnik-Schöneborn S, Zerres K. Course of autosomal recessive polycystic kidney disease (ARPKD) in siblings: a clinical comparison of 20 sibships. Clin Genet. 1995;47:248–53.

161. Ajiri et al. Phenotypic variability in siblings with autosomal recessive polycystic kidney disease. Kidney Int Rep. 2022;7(7):1643–52. https://doi.org/10.1016/j.ekir.2022.04.095. eCollection. PMID: 35812281.

162. Onuchic LF, Furu L, Nagasawa Y, et al. PKHD1, the polycystic kidney and hepatic disease 1 gene, encodes a novel large protein containing multiple immunoglobulin-like plexin-transcription-factor domains and parallel beta-helix 1 repeats. Am J Hum Genet. 2002;70:1305–17. https://doi.org/10.1086/340448.

163. Zerres K, Senderek J, Rudnik-Schöneborn S, et al. New options for prenatal diagnosis in autosomal recessive polycystic kidney disease by mutation anal-

164. Chebib FT, Torres VE. Recent advances in the management of autosomal dominant polycystic kidney disease. Clin J Am Soc Nephrol (CJASN). 2018;13:1765–76. https://doi.org/10.2215/CJN.03960318.

165. Watnick T, Germino GG. mTOR inhibitors in polycystic kidney disease. N Engl J Med. 2010;363:879–81. https://doi.org/10.1056/NEJMe1006925.

166. Wang CJ, Creed C, Winklhofer FT, Grantham JJ. Water prescription in autosomal dominant polycystic kidney disease: a pilot study. Clin J Am Soc Nephrol (CJASN). 2011;6:192–7. https://doi.org/10.2215/CJN.03950510.

167. Wong ATY, Mannix C, Grantham JJ, et al. Randomised controlled trial to determine the efficacy and safety of prescribed water intake to prevent kidney failure due to autosomal dominant polycystic kidney disease (PREVENT-ADPKD). BMJ Open. 2018;8:e018794. https://doi.org/10.1136/bmjopen-2017-018794.

168. Schrier RW, Abebe KZ, Perrone RD, et al. Blood pressure in early autosomal dominant polycystic kidney disease. N Engl J Med. 2014; https://doi.org/10.1056/NEJMoa1402685.

169. Torres VE, Abebe KZ, Chapman AB, et al. Angiotensin blockade in late autosomal dominant polycystic kidney disease. N Engl J Med. 2014; https://doi.org/10.1056/NEJMoa1402686.

170. Goto M, Hoxha N, Osman R, Dell KM. The renin-angiotensin system and hypertension in autosomal recessive polycystic kidney disease. Pediatr Nephrol Berl Ger. 2010;25:2449–57. https://doi.org/10.1007/s00467-010-1621-z.

171. Goto M, Hoxha N, Osman R, et al. Renin-angiotensin system activation in congenital hepatic fibrosis in the PCK rat model of autosomal recessive polycystic kidney disease. J Pediatr Gastroenterol Nutr. 2010;50:639–44. https://doi.org/10.1097/MPG.0b013e3181cc80e4.

172. Kaplan BS, Fay J, Shah V, et al. Autosomal recessive polycystic kidney disease. Pediatr Nephrol Berl Ger. 1989;3:43–9.

173. Veizis EI, Carlin CR, Cotton CU. Decreased amiloride-sensitive Na+ absorption in collecting duct principal cells isolated from BPK ARPKD mice. Am J Physiol Renal Physiol. 2004;286:F244–54. https://doi.org/10.1152/ajprenal.00169.2003.

174. Zurowska AM, Fischbach M, Watson AR, et al. Clinical practice recommendations for the care of infants with stage 5 chronic kidney disease (CKD5). Pediatr Nephrol Berl Ger. 2013;28:1739–48. https://doi.org/10.1007/s00467-012-2300-z.

175. Akarkach A, Burgmaier K, Sander A, et al. Maintenance peritoneal dialysis in children with autosomal recessive polycystic kidney disease: a comparative cohort study of the International Pediatric Peritoneal Dialysis Network Registry. Am J Kidney Dis. 2020;75:460–4. https://doi.org/10.1053/j.ajkd.2019.10.009.

176. Brinkert F, Lehnhardt A, Montoya C, et al. Combined liver-kidney transplantation for children with autosomal recessive polycystic kidney disease (ARPKD): indication and outcome. Transpl Int. 2013;26:640–50. https://doi.org/10.1111/tri.12098.

177. Jalanko H, Pakarinen M. Combined liver and kidney transplantation in children. Pediatr Nephrol Berl Ger. 2013; https://doi.org/10.1007/s00467-013-2487-7.

178. Büscher R, Büscher AK, Cetiner M, et al. Combined liver and kidney transplantation and kidney after liver transplantation in children: indication, postoperative outcome, and long-term results. Pediatr Transplant. 2015;19:858–65. https://doi.org/10.1111/petr.12595.

179. Abu-Wasel B, Walsh C, Keough V, Molinari M. Pathophysiology, epidemiology, classification and treatment options for polycystic liver diseases. World J Gastroenterol (WJG). 2013;19:5775–86. https://doi.org/10.3748/wjg.v19.i35.5775.

180. Ghannam JS, Cline MR, Hage AN, et al. Technical success and outcomes in pediatric patients undergoing transjugular intrahepatic portosystemic shunt placement: a 20-year experience. Pediatr Radiol. 2019;49:128–35. https://doi.org/10.1007/s00247-018-4267-9.

181. Verbeeck S, Mekhali D, Cassiman D, et al. Long-term outcome of transjugular intrahepatic portosystemic shunt for portal hypertension in autosomal recessive polycystic kidney disease. Dig Liver Dis. 2018;50:707–12. https://doi.org/10.1016/j.dld.2018.03.009.

182. Burgmaier K, Brandt J, Shroff R, et al. Gastrostomy tube insertion in pediatric patients with autosomal recessive polycystic kidney disease (ARPKD): current practice. Front Pediatr. 2018;6:164. https://doi.org/10.3389/fped.2018.00164.

183. Arbeiter A, Büscher R, Bonzel K-E, et al. Nephrectomy in an autosomal recessive polycystic kidney disease (ARPKD) patient with rapid kidney enlargement and increased expression of EGFR. Nephrol Dial Transplant. 2008;23:3026–9. https://doi.org/10.1093/ndt/gfn288.

184. Bean SA, Bednarek FJ, Primack WA. Aggressive respiratory support and unilateral nephrectomy for infants with severe perinatal autosomal recessive polycystic kidney disease. J Pediatr. 1995;127:311–3. https://doi.org/10.1016/S0022-3476(95)70318-7.

185. Beaunoyer M, Snehal M, Li L, et al. Optimizing outcomes for neonatal ARPKD. Pediatr Transplant. 2007;11:267–71. https://doi.org/10.1111/j.1399-3046.2006.00644.x.

186. Shukla AR, Kiddoo DA, Canning DA. Unilateral nephrectomy as palliative therapy in an infant with autosomal recessive polycystic kidney disease. J Urol. 2004;172:2000–1.

187. Spechtenhauser B, Hochleitner BW, Ellemunter H, et al. Bilateral nephrectomy, peritoneal dialysis and subsequent cadaveric renal transplantation for treatment of renal failure due to

polycystic kidney disease requiring continuous ventilation. Pediatr Transplant. 1999;3:246–8. https://doi.org/10.1034/j.1399-3046.1999.00030.x.

188. Burgmaier K, Ariceta G, Bald M, et al. Severe neurological outcomes after very early bilateral nephrectomies in patients with autosomal recessive polycystic kidney disease (ARPKD). Sci Rep. 2020;10:16025. https://doi.org/10.1038/s41598-020-71956-1.

189. Torres VE, Chapman AB, Devuyst O, et al. Tolvaptan in patients with autosomal dominant polycystic kidney disease. N Engl J Med. 2012;367:2407–18. https://doi.org/10.1056/NEJMoa1205511.

190. Torres VE, Chapman AB, Devuyst O, et al. Multicenter, open-label, extension trial to evaluate the long-term efficacy and safety of early versus delayed treatment with tolvaptan in autosomal dominant polycystic kidney disease: the TEMPO 4:4 trial. Nephrol Dial Transplant. 2018;33:477–89. https://doi.org/10.1093/ndt/gfx043.

191. Torres VE, Chapman AB, Devuyst O, et al. Tolvaptan in later-stage autosomal dominant polycystic kidney disease. N Engl J Med. 2017;377:1930–42. https://doi.org/10.1056/NEJMoa1710030.

192. Schaefer F, Mekahli D, Emma F, et al. Tolvaptan use in children and adolescents with autosomal dominant polycystic kidney disease: rationale and design of a two-part, randomized, double-blind, placebo-controlled trial. Eur J Pediatr. 2019;178:1013–21. https://doi.org/10.1007/s00431-019-03384-x.

193. Mekahli D, Guay-Woodford LM, Cadnapaphornchai M, et al. Randomized, placebo-controlled, phase 3b trial of tolvaptan in the treatment of children and adolescents with autosomal dominant polycystic kidney disease (ADPKD): 1-year data. https://espn2021.org/abstracts/abstract.php?bid=79. Accessed 29 Jan 2022.

194. Griffiths J, Mills MT, Ong AC. Long-acting somatostatin analogue treatments in autosomal dominant polycystic kidney disease and polycystic liver disease: a systematic review and meta-analysis. BMJ Open. 2020;10:e032620. https://doi.org/10.1136/bmjopen-2019-032620.

195. Serra AL, Poster D, Kistler AD, et al. Sirolimus and kidney growth in autosomal dominant polycystic kidney disease. N Engl J Med. 2010;363:820–9. https://doi.org/10.1056/NEJMoa0907419.

196. Walz G, Budde K, Mannaa M, et al. Everolimus in patients with autosomal dominant polycystic kidney disease. N Engl J Med. 2010;363:830–40. https://doi.org/10.1056/NEJMoa1003491.

197. Torres JA, Kruger SL, Broderick C, et al. Ketosis ameliorates renal cyst growth in polycystic kidney disease. Cell Metab. 2019;30:1007–1023.e5. https://doi.org/10.1016/j.cmet.2019.09.012.

198. Luciano RL, Dahl NK. Extra-renal manifestations of autosomal dominant polycystic kidney disease (ADPKD): considerations for routine screening and management. Nephrol Dial Transplant. 2014;29:247–54. https://doi.org/10.1093/ndt/gft437.

Nephronophthisis and Autosomal Dominant Tubulointerstitial Kidney Disease (ADTKD)

11

Jens König and Heymut Omran

The Nephronophthisis complex

The nephronophthisis complex comprises a clinically and genetically heterogeneous group of tubulointerstitial cystic disorders with an autosomal recessive inheritance pattern. It represents the most frequent genetic cause of end-stage kidney disease (ESKD) in children and young adults. Nephronophthisis can be accompanied by anomalies in other organs, e.g. liver, pancreas, central nervous system, eyes and bones. There are several well described complex clinical syndromes that can feature the renal picture of nephronophthisis, including Senior-Løken-syndrome, Joubert syndrome, COACH syndrome, Jeune syndrome, Sensenbrenner syndrome, Meckel-Gruber syndrome and others. Because of the extended clinical as well as genetic overlap, the term *nephronophthisis complex* has been introduced. However, phenotypic variability as well as the polygenic background complicate the timely establishment of the correct diagnosis.

Nephronophthisis

Nephronophthisis literally means "damage of the nephrons". 1951 Fanconi et al. introduced the term *familial juvenile nephronophthisis* to describe a disease characterized by autosomal recessive inheritance, a defect in urinary concentrating capacity, severe anaemia and progressive renal failure that leads to death before puberty [1, 2]. The incidence ranges from 1:1,000,000 in the US to 1:50,000 in Europe. To date, variants have been identified in 25 genes (Fig. 11.1) encoding nephrocystin proteins that localize to primary cilia, basal bodies and centrosomes. Thus, nephronophthisis (NPH) belongs to a group of rare hereditary disorders referred to as ciliopathies. Mutations in these genes lead to renal as well as extrarenal disease manifestations [3].

The clinical hallmarks of NPH are a reduced urinary concentrating capacity presenting as polyuria and polydipsia with regular fluid intake at night and slowly progressive chronic kidney failure. Other clinical manifestations comprise growth retardation, anaemia and persisting primary or secondary enuresis. However, these features are only facultative findings. Urine analyses usually do not show any characteristic abnormalities. Proteinuria and arterial hypertension are no typical findings before the onset of end-stage kidney failure. On ultrasound, patients generally show normal or small-sized kidneys with increased echogenicity and a loss of cortico-

J. König (✉) · H. Omran
Department of General Pediatrics, University Children's Hospital Muenster, Münster, Germany
e-mail: Jens.koenig@ukmuenster.de;
Heymut.Omran@ukmuenster.de

© The Author(s), under exclusive license to Springer Nature Switzerland AG 2023
F. Schaefer, L. A. Greenbaum (eds.), *Pediatric Kidney Disease*,
https://doi.org/10.1007/978-3-031-11665-0_11

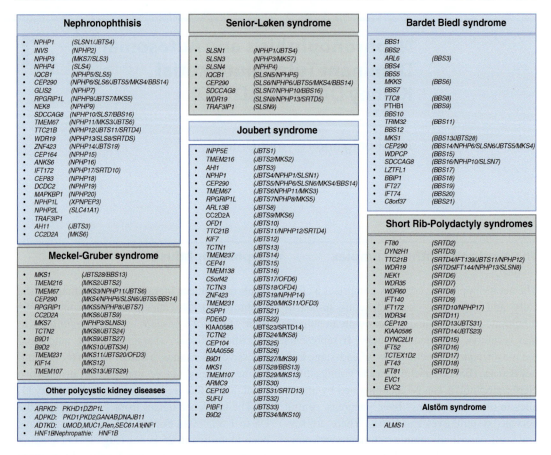

Fig. 11.1 Genetic overview on hereditary cystic kidney diseases

medullary differentiation. Cysts, which are typically located at the cortico-medullary junction, often only occur late in the disease process [4] and are not an obligatory finding (Fig. 11.2). In contrast to other hereditary cystic kidney diseases such as polycystic kidney diseases (ADPKD and ARPKD), HNF1B nephropathy or Bardet-Biedl syndrome, prenatal cystic presentation is untypical and limited to infantile NPH [5]. Because of the lack of disease-specific clinical features and the slow progress, still about 15% of patients are only diagnosed when ESKD has already been reached.

In the past, kidney biopsy has been used for the diagnosis of NPH. Histology is characterized by disintegrated tubular basement membranes, tubular atrophy and cyst formation, as well as a sclerosing tubulointerstitial nephropathy accompanied by lymphocyte infiltrates [6, 7]. Since cortico-medullary cysts only occur late in the disease process [8], they are no obligatory finding and thus no hallmark of the disease. Nowadays, against the backdrop of the availability of rapid and targeted molecular genetic analysis, kidney biopsy for the diagnosis of NPH is largely obsolete and should be limited to cases in which his-

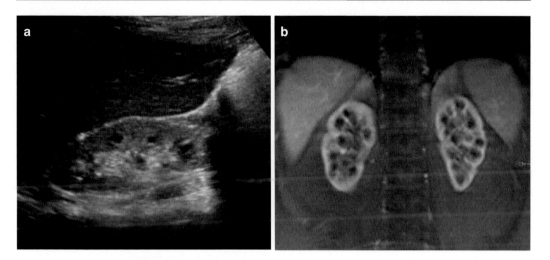

Fig. 11.2 Ultrasound (**a**) and MRI (**b**) presentation of the kidneys in a patient with classical juvenile nephronophthisis. Please note that despite the prominent cysts at the cortico-medullary junction, these are no obligatory finding

tology is needed to rule out other differential diagnoses (e.g. tubulointerstitial nephritis).

Genetics

To date, 25 genes have been identified to be associated with NPH (Fig. 11.1). Yet, about 40% of all cases still remain genetically unsolved. While *NPHP1* defects account for 20–60% of NPH cases, each of the remaining genes makes up for 1% or less of all cases [9].

Most gene products (so called nephrocystins) affected by *NPHP* gene mutations are located at the ciliary base and transition zone of primary cilia excerpting a kind of gate keeper function controlling transport processes from the cytoplasm into the cilium and vice versa [10]. Primary cilia are evolutionarily conserved, membrane-bound, microtubular projections protruding from the cell surface. They are found on virtually all cell types in the human body and play an essential role in transducing signaling information from the extracellular milieu into the cell. Only recently mutations in *NPHP1L* und *NPHP2L* have been identified, genes that encode mitochondrial rather than ciliary proteins [11].

Based on functional interaction studies, currently four distinct nephrocystin modules have been described: the NPHP 1-4-8 module, the NPHP 2-3-9-ANKS6 module, the NPHP5-6 module and the MKS module. These nephrocystin modules are related to different signaling pathways including the Wnt pathway, Hedgehog pathway, Hippo pathway, DNA damage response (DDR) pathway, mTOR pathway, the intracellular calcium and the cAMP signaling pathway [9].

Genotype-Phenotype Correlation

Depending on the onset of ESKD, three clinical subtypes of NPH have been defined: Infantile, juvenile, and adolescent NPH. The so called "classical juvenile NPH" is by far the most common entity, leading to ESKD at a median age of 13 years [4, 12]. In infantile NPH ESKD is reached very early in life (median age 8 months) whereas in adolescent forms kidney function is usually preserved until adulthood (median age 19 years).

Large homozygous deletions of approximately 290 kb involving the *NPHP1* locus on chromosome 2q12-q13 are the main genetic cause of the classical juvenile NPH accounting for up to 60% of patients. Only some patients carry point mutations or compound heterozygous variants [13, 14]. Homozygous *NPHP1* deletions have also been reported in adults who developed ESKD between 27 and 60 years of age [15].

Other genetic defects primarily associated with adolescent NPH comprise *NPHP3, NPHP4* and *NPHP9/NEK8*. While the kidney phenotype and clinical course described above is very similar for most NPH variants, this does not apply to infantile NPH, which typically already presents in utero or early infancy with enlarged cystic kidneys, arterial hypertension and ESKD before the age of 4 years. Histologically, infantile NPH differs from juvenile NPH by a cortical rather than medullary cyst location and the absence of typical tubular basement membrane changes [16]. Mutations in *NPHP2/INV* (9q22-q31) were the first molecular defects identified in infantile NPH, often associated with laterality defects like *situs inversus* and congenital heart defects [17]. Subsequently, mutations in various other genes were identified to cause infantile NPH, i.e. *NPHP3, NPHP12/TTC21B, NPHP14/ZNF423* and *NPHP18/CEP83* [9].

Detailed information about all NPH-related genes identified so far and their clinical implications is given in Table 11.1.

Life table analyses demonstrate the impact of the underlying genetic defect on renal survival. While loss-of-function mutations in *NPHP3* go along with a >50% chance of ESKD before the age of 4 years, so called hypomorphic mutations in the same gene were found to be responsible for an adolescent type of NPH. Kidney failure in the vast majority of *NPHP1* deletion carriers occurs in a narrow time slot between 7 to 16 years of age. Renal survival curves of individuals suffering from *NPHP4* variants resemble those of *NPHP1* carriers, yet with a slower progression and a fraction of 25% patients with preserved renal function at 30 years of age [4].

Extra-renal Disease Manifestations

Owing to the ubiquitous presence of primary cilia and depending on the underlying molecular defect, the clinical presentation of NPH is not necessarily limited to the kidneys but can be associated with extra-renal disease manifestations. Standardized phenotypic surveys revealed extrarenal manifestations in approx. 20–40% of affected individuals, exceeding previous incidence estimates [4]. The clinical spectrum encompasses ophthalmological abnormalities (oculomotor apraxia, retinitis pigmentosa, Leber amaurosis), hepatic fibrosis, neurologic disorders, chronic lung and upper airway infections as well as skeletal defects (Fig. 11.3). Less frequently, laterality defects, genital anomalies, congenital heart defects and endocrine dysfunctions (e.g. hypogonadism, short stature, obesity) are observed. In addition, NPH resembles the kidney phenotype of various mulivisceral ciliopathies described in detail below:

Senior-Løken Syndrome

The term Senior-Løken syndrome denotes the association of NPH and retinal degeneration [18, 19]. Two variants of retinal disorders have been described:

Leber congenital amaurosis (LCA), the most severe variant, is a clinically and genetically heterogeneous retinal disorder that occurs in infancy and is accompanied by profound visual loss, nystagmus, poor pupillary reflexes, and either a normal retina or varying degrees of atrophy and pigmentary changes [19–21]. Affected children exhibit the so-called oculodigital sign characterized by poking, rubbing and pressing of the eyes in order to mechanically stimulate the retina. The electroretinogram is extinguished or severely reduced [22]. All but one form of Leber congenital amaurosis is inherited as an autosomal recessive trait. LCA is a disorder of photoreceptors, caused by failed transport of rhodopsin and a loss of outer segments of the photoreceptor resulting in its ultimate cell death.

Although LCA is a clinical diagnosis, molecular testing is currently available for many different genes, including several genes that can be associated with NPH such as *IQCB1/NPHP5* and *CEP290/NPHP6* [23] (Fig. 11.1). So far, all reported Senior-Løken patients with underlying *IQCB1/NPHP5* mutations presented with early severe retinal degeneration (Leber congenital amaurosis) [23]. Conversely, genetic testing for *IQCB1/NPHP5* variations in patients with a late or mild ocular manifestation does not appear to be very promising. The onset of ESKD in this

Table 11.1 Clinical presentation of genetic defects associated with NPH and NPH-related ciliopathies

Gene	OMIM entry	Age at ESRD	Isolated NPH	Joubert syndrome	Severe retinal degeneration/LCA	Tapeto-retinal degeneration	OMA type Cogan II	Liver fibrosis	Situs inversus	Meckel-Gruber syndrome	Skeletal anomalies	Other symptoms
					NPH associated with extrarenal manifestations							
NPHP1/JBTS4/SLSN1	256100	Juvenile	+	+ (2%)	-	+	+ (2%)	-	-	-	-	-
NPHP2/INVS	602088	Infantile	+	-	+ (10%)	-	-	+	+	-	-	VSD, HT, OH
NPHP3/SLNS3	604387	Infantile/adolescent	+	+	+ (10%)	+	-	+	+	+	-	congenital heart defects
NPHP4	606966	Adolescent	+	-	-	+	+	+	-	-	-	-
NPHP5/IQCB1	609254	Adolescent	-	-	+ (100%)	-	-	-	-	-	-	-
NPHP6/CEP290	610188	Juvenile	-	+	+ (100%)	+	+	+	-	+	-	congenital heart defects, COACH syndrome
NPHP7/Glis2	611498	Juvenile	+	-	-	-	-	-	-	-	-	-
NPHP8/RPGRIP1L/MKS5	611560	Juvenile	+	+	+ (10%)	+	+	+	-	+	-	COACH syndrome, RHYNS-syndrome
NPHP9/NEK8	613824	Infantile	+	-	+ (30%)	-	-	-	-	+	-	-
NPHP10/SDCC8GA	613615	Juvenile	+	-	+	+	-	-	-	-	-	BBS-like
NPHP11/TMEM67/MKS3	613550	Infantile	+	+	-	-	+	+	-	+	-	COACH syndrome; RHYNS-syndrome
NPHP13/WDR19	614377	Juvenile	+	+	+	+	-	+	-	-	+	-
NPHP14/ZNF423	614844	Infantile	-	+	+	-	-	-	+	-	-	-

(continued)

Table 11.1 (continued)

Gene	OMIM entry	Age at ESRD	Isolated NPH	NPH associated with extrarenal manifestations								
				Joubert syndrome	Severe retinal degeneration/ LCA	Tapeto-retinal degeneration	OMA type Cogan II	Liver fibrosis	Situs inversus	Meckel-Gruber syndrome	Skeletal anomalies	Other symptoms
NPHP15/ CEP164	614845	Juvenile	–	+	+	–	–	+	–	–	+	bronchiectasis
NPHP16/ ANKS6	615382	Infantile, juvenile	+	–	–	–	–	+	+	–	–	congenital heart defects
NPHP17/ IFT172	615630	Juvenile	–	+	+	+	–	+	–	–	+	Pituitary hypoplasia
NPHP18/ CEP83	615862	Infantile	+	–	–	+	–	+	–	+	–	Mental retardation, hydrocephalus
NPHP19/ DCDC2	616217	Juvenile	+	–	–	–	–	+	–	–	–	
NPHP20/ MAPKBP1	617271	Juvenile	+	–	–	–	–	–	–	–	–	
NPHP1L/ XPNPEP3	613159	Adult	+	–	–	–	–	–	–	–	–	Myocardiosis, epilepsy
NPHP2L/ SLC41A1	610801	Juvenile	+	–	–	–	–	–	–	–	–	bronchiectasis
TRAF3IP1	616629	Infantil/ juvenile	+	+	+	+	–	+	–	–	+	1 patient BBS-like
AHI1/JBTS3	608629	Juvenile, adult	(+)	+	(+)	(+)	+	–	–	–	+	
CC2D2A/ MKS6	612284	? (no)	no	+	–	–	(+)		–	+	+	COACH syndrome

BBS Bardet Biedl syndrome; *COACH* (cerebellar vermis hypoplasia, oligophrenia [kognitive dysfunction], ataxia, coloboma, hypotonia) syndrome; *OMA* oculomotor apraxia; *LCA* Leber congenital amaurosis; *OH* oligohydramnious; *OMA* okulomotor apraxia type Cogan II

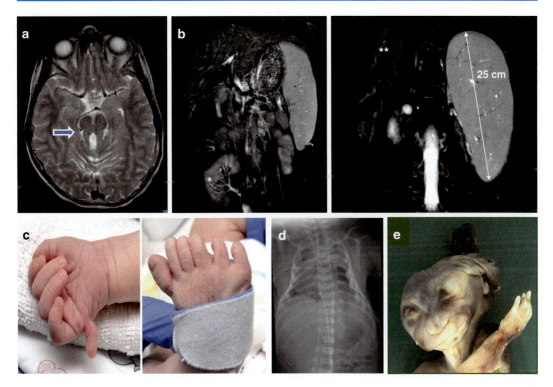

Fig. 11.3 Examples for extra-renal disease manifestations: (**a**) Molar tooth sign in a patient with Joubert syndrome (arrow). (**b**) MRI image showing massive hepatosplenomagly based on congenital hepatic fibrosis in a patient with COACH syndrome; *: transplant kidney; **: transjugular intrahepatic portosystemic shunt (TIPS). (**c**) Postaxial hexadactyly (both feet and hands) in a patient with short-rib polydactyly syndrome. (**d**) Thoracic Hypoplasia in a patient with Jeune syndrome/Jeune Thoracic hypoplasia (JTA). (**e**) Occipital meningoencephalocele and a massively malformed brain resembling anencephaly. (Used with permission of Springer Science + Business Media from Bergmann [33])

cohort however ranges from 6 to 32 years with a median age of 15 years.

A milder retinopathy variant that can also be associated with NPH is referred to as **tapeto-retinal degeneration**. Usually patients suffer from slowly progressive severe tube-like restriction of the visual fields and night blindness. Fundoscopy reveals various degrees of atrophic and pigmentary retinal alterations.

Mutations associated with this milder form of Senior-Løken syndrome have been identified in the following genes: *NPHP1, NPHP4, SDCC8G8, WDR19/IFT144* and *TRAF3IP1*. While *SDCC8G8* localizes to centrosomes and cell-cell-junctions in mammalian renal epithelial cell lines and shows interactions with *NPHP5* and *OFD1, WDR19/IFT144* and *TRAF3IP1* are closely linked to intraflagellar transport processes in cilia. Mutations of all three genes cause kidney cysts in zebrafish models [24].

Joubert Syndrome

Joubert syndrome (JS) is an autosomal recessive multisystem ciliopathy with a predicted incidence of 1:55,000–200,000. Clinically JS is characterized by muscular hypotonia, cerebellar ataxia, unusual eye movements, hyperpnea/apnea in infancy, variable degrees of cognitive impairment, speech ataxia and kidney cyst formation. Additionally, certain dysmorphic features have been described such as hypertelorism, broad forehead and unilateral or bilateral ptosis [25]. There is high phenotypic variability even among family members. Neuroimaging (MRI) plays an essential role in the diagnosis of JS since the "molar tooth sign" is pathognomonic and by definition an essential feature for the diagnosis of JS. It reflects a complex malformation of the midhin brain encompassing cerebellar vermis hypoplasia, increased interpeduncular distance at the pontomesencephalic junction and elongated superior cerebellar peduncles (Fig. 11.3a) [26].

Neurocognitive functioning may range from extremely impaired to almost normal with relative strengths in verbal comprehension and reasoning abilities. Diffuse background slowing in EEG can be found in about one third of patients and is associated with a poorer neurological outcome; however clinical seizures occur in less than 10% of JS patients [27]. A systemic evaluation of the MRI presentation of 110 JS patients revealed the severity of the cerebellar vermis hypoplasia to be associated with the neurodevelopmental outcome [28].

Only about 25% of the patients present an isolated neurological phenotype; the majority of cases is characterized by various phenotypic combinations of additional ocular, kidney and hepatic disease manifestations.

The **ophthalmologic** involvement comprises oculomotor apraxia (78%) with jerking head thrusting and a rotating nystagmus (67%) [29], strabismus (72%) and ptosis (31%). Retinopathy may be present in a subset of patients depending on the underlying genetic defect, with severe forms been associated with *CEP290/NPHP6* and *AHI1* mutations, while in patients with *TMEM67*, *C5orf52* and *KIAA0586* defects no retinal degeneration has been observed so far [25].

Liver disease is observed in 15–45% of JS patients, usually characterized by elevated liver enzymes, increased liver echogenicity and parenchymal stiffness on ultrasound/elastography or splenomegaly). Histopathology resembles the findings seen in ARPKD with ductal plate malformation and portal fibrosis. 15% of patients develop portal hypertension with a need for transjugular intrahepatic portosystemic shunting (TIPS; Fig. 11.3) or liver transplantation. Most patients with severe liver disease carry mutations in the *TMEM67* gene [30].

Kidney involvement is found in 25–30% of JS patients, particularly in those carrying *CEP290/NPHP6*, *TMEM67* and *AHI1* mutations. Most patients display an NPH phenotype with reduced urinary concentrating capacity and slowly progressing GFR decline. Prenatal ultrasound is usually normal and a poor predictor for kidney disease in JS. However, in some patients an ARPKD-like phenotype with enlarged cystic kidneys and early onset hypertension can be observed) [31]. The onset of ESKD ranges from 6–24 years (mean 11.3 ± 4.8 years) and is not necessarily associated with the genotype [32].

So far mutations in 35 different genes are implicated to be causative for JS, which altogether explain 62–94% of the clinical cases [31]. Almost all of these genes show a genetic overlap with other ciliopathy disorders, particularly with Senior-Løken syndrome, COACH syndrome and Meckel-Gruber syndrome. To simplify terminology, the term Joubert syndrome is now used to refer to all patients displaying a molar tooth sign including SLS and COACH syndrome.

For most genes it has proven difficult to identify clear-cut genotype-phenotype correlations. However, for individual genes, such as *CEP290/NPHP6*, the severity of the genetic defect does predict clinical disease severity, with two truncating mutations causing a severe early-onset disorder mimicking a Meckel-Gruber phenotype whereas the presence of at least one missense mutation leads to a milder, late-onset phenotype with limited organ involvement as in NPH [33]. Since *NPHP1* mutations) have also been reported to be a rare cause of JS, the *NPHP1* gene has been referred to as *JBTS4* [29]. However, screening of 117 Joubert syndrome patients revealed *NPHP1* abnormalities only in 2% of cases indicating that this gene is only a minor contributor in the pathogenesis of this disorder [34].

COACH Syndrome

The acronym COACH stands for the clinical key features **c**erebellar vermis hypoplasia, **o**ligophrenia [neurocognitive impairment], **a**taxia, **c**oloboma and congenital **h**epatic fibrosis. COACH syndrome is a rare autosomal recessive disorder that shows substantial overlap with Joubert syndrome and is almost exclusively caused by mutations in the *TMEM67* gene [35]. In contrast to Joubert syndrome, the pathognomonic feature of this syndrome is an obligatory liver involvement caused by the malformation of the embryonic ductal plate resulting in fibrosis of the liver. Elevated liver enzymes, reduced blood flow in the portal vein and splenomegaly secondary to portal hypertension regularly develop during progression of the disease. Liver transplantation is necessary in most cases in the long run.

Chorioretinal colobomas found in the majority of *TMEM67* patients are typically located inferior to the optic nerve and do not impair vision in most patients. Retinal degeneration seems to be no problem in this particular cohort. Kidney involvement however is observed in 50% of the patients presenting with an NPH phenotype. Just recently, an impaired sense of smell (hyposmia) has been described as a so far underdiagnosed clinical feature associated with *TMEM67* mutations that can further compromise the quality of life of affected patients [36].

Meckel Gruber Syndrome

Meckel Gruber syndrome (MKS) is a neonatally lethal dysmorphic disorder affecting multiple organ systems. It follows an autosomal recessive inheritance with a global incidence of approximately 1:135.000 births. Typical clinical features comprise occipital encephalocele (Fig. 11.3e), bilateral cystic kidney dysplasia, hepatobiliary ductal plate malformation and postaxial polydactyly. Associated features might include severe cardiac anomalies, lung hypoplasia, situs inversus, severe malformations of the central nervous system, hydrocephalus, cleft palate, microphthalmia, retinal colobomas, genital disorders and skeletal deformities [37–39]. Survival beyond the neonatal period is unusual, most affected individuals die *in utero* [40]. However, owing to its allelic overlap with Joubert syndrome, rare cases have survived the first few years of life [25]. Prenatal ultrasound documenting the combination of occipital encephalocele, grossly enlarged hyperechogenic kidneys and polydactyly as well as elevated levels of alpha-fetoprotein in amniotic fluid may lead to early diagnosis. Oligohydramnios is common and often results in Potter's sequence featuring typical facial deformities and joint contractures. Prenatal MRI may be helpful to confirm typical additional malformations. Prenatal genetic testing is only useful when positive because the associated genes identified so far only account for 50–60% of cases [25].

Mutations in 13 genes responsible for MKS-like phenotypes have been reported to date: *MKS1, MKS2/TMEM216, MKS3/TMEM67, MKS4/CEP290, MKS5/RPGRIP1L, MKS6/CC2D2A, MKS7/NPHP3, MKS8/TCTN2, MKS9/B9D1, MKS10/B9D2, MKS11/TMEM231, MKS12/KIF14, MKS13/TMEM107.* Besides genetic heterogeneity, there is significant clinical overlap with NPH and Joubert syndrome (Fig. 11.4). Current data suggest that severe truncating mutations cause MKS whereas milder, non-truncating mutations cause Joubert or isolated NPH syndromes [33]. In fact, there are even some families in which one child is diagnosed with Joubert syndrome and another with MKS, indicating that genetic modifiers also influence the clinical phenotype [41].

Congenital Oculomotor Apraxia Type Cogan II

Congenital oculomotor apraxia (COMA) type Cogan II is characterized by the impairment of horizontal voluntary eye movements, ocular attraction movements, and optokinetic nystagmus [42]. Compensation for the defective horizontal eye movements is accomplished by jerky movements of the head. The disease is not progressive, and most older patients compensate the impaired eye movements by an over-shooting thrust of the eyeballs rather than by head jerks. The condition can improve with age. Some individuals with COMA type Cogan II have an increased risk to develop chronic kidney failure due to NPH. Hence, kidney function should be analysed at regular intervals in this condition.

Recently, genetic variants in the *SUFU* gene have been reported as the first disease-specific genetic cause of COMA without associated kidney disease [43]. In addition, genetic variants in different NPHP genes have been reported in association with COMA type Cogan II including *NPHP1, NPHP4, NPHP6/CEP290* and *NPHP8* [44]. Particularly, deletions in *NPHP1* have been

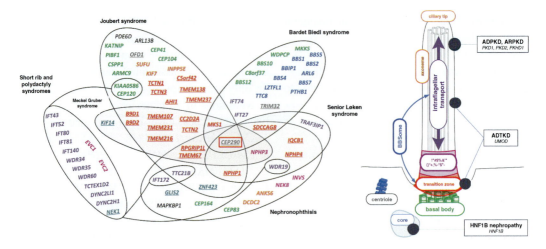

Fig. 11.4 Venn diagram illustrating the genetic and clinical overlap in hereditary renal ciliopathies. Colours indicate the ciliary location of corresponding gene products

described in quite a few affected individuals [4]. However, the vast majority of clinical cases remain genetically unsolved.

Since usually oculomotor apraxia precedes the kidney phenotype by many years but all *NPHP1* deletion carriers developed ESRD in the long run, genetic testing appears to be justified in all patients presenting COMA in early infancy, even though it will only be positive in a minority of patients.

RHYNS Syndrome

RHYNS syndrome was defined in 1997 as the combination of Retinitis pigmentosa, Hypopituitarism, Nephronophthisis and mild Skeletal dysplasia in a 17-year-old man [45]. Four years later, two brothers with a similar clinical picture were reported [46]. Just recently a whole exome sequencing approach revealed biallelic *TMEM67* variants in the index patient reported 20 years before [47].

Previously, growth hormone deficiency associated with an absent, small or ectopic pituitary gland was observed in individual JS patients and associated with variants in the ciliary genes *KIAA0753* and *CELSR2* [48, 49].

Skeletal Ciliopathies

Skeletal ciliopathies represent a distinct group of hereditary disorders clinically characterized by abnormal bone growth resulting in a long narrow chest with short ribs, short stature associated with disproportionately short limbs and polydactyly. Specific disorders in this group include the asphyxiating thoracic dystrophy (Jeune's syndrome), cranioectodermal dysplasia (Sensenbrenner syndrome), Ellis-van Creveld syndrome (EVC) and various types of short rib-polydactyly syndromes (e.g. Mainzer-Saldino syndrome) [50]. Molecular defects in 26 genes have been identified so far mostly encoding components of the ciliary transport machinery [51, 52].

Bone disorders can be accompanied by non-skeletal features including NPH leading to ESKD, cystic kidney disease, congenital hepatic fibrosis, retinal degeneration, neurological abnormalities, cardiac anomalies, cleft lip/palate and other oral defects. Other rare features include fibrocystic changes in the pancreas, ambiguous genitalia, anal atresia, polyhydramnios, malrotation, and hydrops fetalis [25]. Owing to the severity of pulmonary insufficiency associated with asphyxiating thoracic dystrophy, high levels of perinatal lethality are observed. In cranioectodermal dysplasia (Sensenbrenner syndrome) most affected children develop early-onset NPH leading to ESKD in infancy or early childhood [51].

Respiratory Phenotype

Typically, defects of motile cilia are responsible for chronic respiratory problems subsumed under the term primary ciliary dyskinesia (PCD), a clinical entity characterized by impaired mucociliary clearance, chronic respiratory infections and distinctive low nasal nitric oxide (nNO) levels [53]. However, functional assessment of patients with renal ciliopathies revealed that molecular defects classically associated with non-motile ciliopathies can also have an impact on motile ciliary function.

Future Challenges: Genetic and Phenotypic Heterogeneity

Although the clinical characteristics of the different hereditary disease entities appear quite discriminative, there is significant genetic as well as phenotypic overlap that hampers an early diagnosis and individual management [50] (Fig. 11.4). No doubt, the tremendous progress of genetics in the last two decades had major impact on the molecular understanding of NPH-related ciliopathies. However, the new insights also further complicated the clinical situation for physicians dealing with affected individuals: It has become increasingly evident that so far well-defined clinical entities can be caused by mutations in multiple genes. Vice versa, mutations in the same gene can cause very different phenotypes that range from lethal early embryonic multivisceral manifestations to single organ involvement starting in adolescence [33] (Fig. 11.4). This complexity has been attributed to allelic heterogeneity, locus heterogeneity, reduced penetrance, variable expressivity, modifier genes, and/or environmental factors [54]. In clinical terms, this implies that the traditional approach using textbook signs and symptoms to guide diagnosis and management is no longer sufficient [56]. From the patient's perspective, the "diagnostic odyssey" does not necessarily end with the identification of a disease-causing gene defect [55]. Novel approaches are needed that should combine a deep and comprehensive clinical characterization with careful genotyping in order to discover non-obvious phenotypes and to determine precise diagnoses.

Large-scale collaborative efforts linking comprehensive clinical data collection with translational research will be fundamental to identify novel therapeutic targets and develop disease specific treatment approaches. Several national initiatives have started to address these questions, including the German NEOCYST consortium and the Dutch KOUNCIL initiative [57].

Therapy

So far, there is no specific therapy correcting the genetic or functional defects in NPH or NPH-related ciliopathies. Thus, in the early disease stage without kidney impairment, the main goal is the correction of water and electrolyte imbalances by replacing ongoing losses of water and salt due to the reduced urinary concentrating capacity.

The recent molecular insights into the pathogenesis of NPH have lead to potential novel therapeutic strategies addressing various intracellular signalling pathways. Yet, despite promising preclinical results, no clinical trials including NPH patients have been initiated to date.

Once the disease has progressed to ESKD, renal replacement therapy is required and early, if possible pre-emptive transplantation is the therapy of choice. NPH patients are not at risk of recurrence of the primary disease and the outcome of transplantation is excellent.

Autosomal Dominant Tubulointerstitial Kidney Disease (ADTKD)

Autosomal dominant tubulointerstitial kidney diseases (ADTKD) encompass a group of rare disease entities characterized by autosomal dominant inheritance, tubular damage, interstitial fibrosis, the absence of glomerular lesions and a slow progression towards ESKD in late adulthood [58]. Although the clinical and histological presentation may show significant overlap with NPH [59, 60], there are two major differences: NPH refers to autosomal recessive conditions that typically present in childhood and in most cases lead to ESKD before adulthood whereas ADTKD is inherited in an autosomal dominant fashion and typically presents later in life. However, as an exception to this rule even children younger than 10 years can occasionally present clinical symptoms from ADTKD.

Recent data suggest that ADTKD qualifies to be one of the most common genetic disorders in adulthood, accounting for about 5% of genetically caused ESKD cases. So far five genes have been identified in which variants lead to ADTKD: *UMOD*; *REN*; *MUC*; *HNF1B* and *SEC61A1* [61].

disease (MCKD)" was commonly used but fell out of fashion because the occurrence of medullary cysts is not an obligatory feature—in fact most patients with ADTKD show no cysts at all. Another term usually used by paediatric nephrologists was "familial juvenile hyperuricaemic nephropathy (FJHN)", describing a condition that is synonymous to what adult nephrologists called MCKD.

Only recently, the introduction of a gene-based, unifying terminology simplified the communication between disciplines and resulted in an increasing number of reported cases. Of note, following the KDIGO terminology, when an affected gene is identified it should be added as a suffix to the term ADTKD for further subclassification [58, 61]. To date, at least five subtypes can be distinguished (Table 11.2). Yet, about 50–60% of clinical ADTKD cases remain genetically unsolved, pointing to more causative genes to be identified in the future.

Terminology and Classification

In the past, the terminology for this heterogeneous disease complex has been inconsistent and confusing. The term "medullary cystic kidney

Pathophysiology

UMOD encodes uromodulin (previously known as Tamm-Horsfall protein), which is expressed

Table 11.2 Classification of ADTKD

Gene (OMIM-ID; chromosome)	KDIGO terminology	Former terminology	Protein	Protein function
UMOD (*191845; 16q12)	ADTKD-*UMOD*	MCKD2 FJHN	Uromodulin	• Regulates transport and blood pressure • Protection against urinary tract infections • Protection against kidney stones • Regulation of innate immunity
MUC1 (*158340; 1q22)	ADTKD-*MUC1*	MCKD1	Mucin 1	• Protection of epithelial mucus barrier • Immunomodulatory propertiesSignal transduction
HNF1B (*189907; 17q12)	ADTKD-*HNF1B*	–	Hepatocyte nuclear factor 1β	• Transcription factor involved in the development of neural tube, pancreas, gut, liver, lung, kidney and genital tract
REN (*179820; 1q32)	ADTKD-*REN*	–	Preprorenin	• Protease, cleavage of angiotensinogen (renin–angiotensin–aldosterone axis) • Role in nephrogenesis
SEC61A1 (*609213; 3q21.3)	ADTKD-*SEC61A1*	–	Alpha1 subunit of *SEC61*	• Alpha1 subunit of SEC61channel forming translocon complex that mediates transport of signal peptide-containing precursor polypeptides across the ER

Modified from Devuyst O, Olinger E, Weber S, Eckardt KU, Kmoch S, Rampoldi L, Bleyer AJ. Autosomal dominant tubulointerstitial kidney disease Nat Rev. Dis Primers. 2019 Sep 5;5(1):60

exclusively at the luminal side of renal epithelial cells of the thick ascending limb of the loop of Henle. Uromodulin is the most abundant protein in the urine of humans [62]. Studies in *UMOD*-knockout mice suggest that uromodulin has multiple physiological roles, including protection against urinary tract infections and kidney stones by direct binding of either fimbria from Escherichia coli bacteria and preventing the adhesion of these bacteria to urothelial cells or direct binding of calcium oxalate crystals [63, 64]. Furthermore, uromodulin plays an important role in maintaining the water-tight integrity of the thick ascending limb. At the same time, it appears to facilitate the transport of the NaK2Cl-Cotransporter [65] and the ROMK potassium channel to the surface of epithelial cells in the thick ascending limb [66]. Subsequently, in the scenario of defective uromodulin, restricted urinary concentration and mild volume depletion evoke an increased reabsorption of uric acid in the proximal tubule potentially explaining hyperuricemia and gout observed in 25–75% of affected patients [67]. Mutated uromodulin proteins are unable to leave the endoplasmic reticulum, resulting in accumulation of abnormal uromodulin within the epithelial cells, followed by cellular atrophy and death. This might explain the progressive chronic kidney failure of *UMOD* patients.

Mutations in the ***MUC1*** gene on chromosome 1q21 have been identified as causative of what in the past was referred to as medullary cystic kidney disease 1 (MCKD1). The majority of affected individuals show a single cytosine insertion into one variable-number tandem repeat sequence within the *MUC1* coding region. Mucin 1 is expressed intracellularly in the secretory epithelia of multiple organs, e.g. the lungs, the stomach, the intestine and the distal tubule and collecting duct of the kidneys. For so far unexplained reasons, clinical sequelae are limited to the kidneys [61]. Mutations in the *MUC1* gene result in an abnormal mucin 1 protein. The mucin 1 protein seems to play an essential role for the protection of the epithelial mucus barrier but also in signal transduction and immunomodulation. Since knockout studies in mice indicated that mucin 1

is not an essential protein, a dominant negative or gain-of function effect of *MUC1* mutations is discussed [68].

The **hepatocyte nuclear factor 1B** (HNF1B) is a ubiquitous transcription factor mainly involved in the early development of multiple organs, primarily of the neural tube, the pancreas, the gut, the liver, the lungs, the kidneys and the genital tract. Variants in the *HNF1B* gene represent the most important genetic cause of congenital anomalies of the kidney and urinary tract (CAKUT) in children. Its precise prevalence as a cause of ADTKD is hard to determine owing to a high rate of assumed undetected cases and numbers range from 5 to 31% depending on the study cohort [69].

Mutations in the ***REN*** gene leading to ADTKD are extremely rare and have been identified only in about 20 families worldwide. It appears that these mutations result in a disrupted translocation of preprorenin into the endoplasmic reticulum of renin expressing cells. Subsequently, the cleavage of pre-prorenin into prorenin and further into renin is blocked. Renin as part of the renin-angiotensin-aldosterone system (RAAS) has a high impact on nephrogenesis, blood pressure control, thirst regulation and erythropoiesis. As a consequence, ADTKD-*REN* is characterized by early onset low-erythropoietin anaemia and slowly progressive CKD accompanied by arterial hypotension and hyperkalaemia. Anaemia in ADTKD-*REN* resembles that observed in haemodialysis and patients receiving long-term angiotensin converting enzyme (ACE) inhibition, since the RAAS contributes to erythropoietin production [70]. At the same time the accumulation of preprorenin in renal tubular cells leads to apoptosis of these cells [71]. Because renin is essential for nephrogenesis, homozygous mutations of renin cause recessive renal tubular dysgenesis and are almost always incompatible with life [72]. In ADTKD-*REN* however, production of wildtype renin occurs via one allele allowing kidney development [61].

Mutations in the ***SEC61A1*** gene are even rarer and have so far only been reported in two families characterized by congenital anaemia, neutropenia and tubulointerstitial kidney disease as well as another two families with a defect in plasma cell development, recurrent infections and an unknown kidney phenotype [73, 74]. *SEC61A* encodes the alpha 1 subunit of the heterotrimer SEC61, that is part of the ER translocon responsible for the transport of newly synthesized secretory proteins into the endoplasmatic reticulum. Mutations of *SEC61A* lead to aggregation of the altered protein in the ER and by affecting the translocon pore it appears to have a functional impact on post-translational modifications, folding and sorting of various proteins, including renin, uromodulin and mucin1. In addition, alterations in the Ca^{2+} homeostasis and energy metabolism have also been reported [75].

Clinical Presentation

Clinical symptoms are similar in all disease variants and may resemble the phenotype of NPH. Usual findings include slowly progressing chronic kidney disease, bland urine sediment, polyuria due to reduced urinary concentrating capacity and a family history compatible with an autosomal dominant inheritance pattern. If significant proteinuria or hematuria is observed, alternative causes should be ruled out. On ultrasound small cortico-medullary cysts might develop during the course of the disease but these are not a prerequisite for the diagnosis. Kidney size is normal or slightly reduced. Histological findings comprise tubular basement membrane disintegration, tubular atrophy with cyst development, and interstitial round cell infiltration associated with fibrosis resembling the findings observed in "classical" NPH. Thus, imaging and histological findings cannot confirm the diagnosis, and analysis of the clinical and pedigree data is mandatory. A definite diagnosis can be achieved by genetic testing (Table 11.3). However, for economic reasons as well as in view of the methodological difficulties associated with the genetic evaluation of *MUC1* in particular, genetic confirmation is still heavily restricted in adults.

Clinical Presentation of ADTKD-*UMOD*

Patients affected by *UMOD* mutations are typically characterized by juvenile onset of hyperuricemia, gout, and progressive kidney failure. Clinical features of both conditions vary in presence and severity. As mentioned above, the demonstration of kidney cysts is not obligatory and may differ within the same pedigree [76].

In 2004, Scolari et al. reported 205 patients from 31 families with *UMOD* mutations of whom 75% showed hyperuricemia and 65% gout, although in a subset of families neither symptom was observed. Chronic kidney disease was present in 70% of patients, leading to ESKD in 80% of these between 20 and 70 years of age [77]. Comparable findings were reported in a series of 109 patients from 45 families and in an Italian kindred with ten affected individuals, with median ages at ESKD of 54 (range 25–70) [78] and 31 (16–54) years [79], respectively. The clinical course appeared more severe in homozygotes from consanguineous families. In a large Spanish kindred with *UMOD* mutations one individual with recessive (bi-allelic) *UMOD* mutations was identified. The homozygous individual survived to adulthood and presented with an earlier onset of hyperuricemia and faster progression to ESKD than heterozygous individuals [80].

Mild urinary concentrating defects are common and may manifest by persisting enuresis [77]. MRI and ultrasound-based imaging studies on 12 individuals with *UMOD* mutations revealed small kidneys, decreased parenchyma, or cysts in all families. Kidney histology showed microcysts in 4 out of 12 cases and in the others dilated or atrophic tubules, global sclerosis, extensive tubulo-interstitial atrophy with fibrosis, and signs of chronic diffuse inflammation [62].

Clinical Presentation of ADTKD-*MUC1*

In contrast to patients with *UMOD* or *REN* gene mutations, slowly progressive chronic kidney disease is the first and main symptom in patients with *MUC1* mutations. Hyperuricemia and gout, if present at all, develop later in the course of the

11 Nephronophthisis and Autosomal Dominant Tubulointerstitial Kidney Disease (ADTKD)

Table 11.3 Clinical and laboratory findings in autosomal dominant tubulointerstitial kidney disease (ADTKD)

ADTKD type	OMIM entry	Clinical features	Age at ESRD	Laboratory findings	Renal Imaging	Other findings
ADTKD-*UMOD*	603860	• Teenage onset gout • Polyuria/polydipsia • Enuresis	16–70 years. (median 42)	• Hyperuricemia • Low urinary levels of uromodelin	Normal (50%) or small kidneys, corticomedullary cysts (40%), echogenicity ↑ (10%)	Intracellular deposits of uromodelin in thick ascending limb (TAL) of Henle
ADTKD-*MUC1*	174000	• Gout	50–76 years (median 62)	• Hyperuricemia	Normal (50%) or small kidneys, corticomedullary cysts (40%)	Intracellular deposits of MUC1fs in TAL and extra-renal tissue
ADTKD-*REN*	613092	• Childhood anaemia • Mild hypotension • Gout in adolescence	43–68 years (median 57)	• Anaemia • Mild hyperkalaemia • Hyperuricemia • Low to low-normal plasma renin levels	Normal or small echogenic kidneys, no cysts	Reduced renin-staining in juxtraglomerular apparatus
ADTKD-*HNF1B*		• CAKUT • Childhood CKD • Genital abnor-malities in girls • Syndromic features in those with 17q12 deletion	0–?	• Hypomagnesemia • Hyperuricemia • Hypokalaemia • Elevated liver enzymes • MODY	Small to normal echogenic kidneys with cortical and medullary cysts	—
ADTKD-*SEC61A1*		• Intrauterine and postnatal growth retardation • Recurrent abcess formation • Polydactyly	NA	• Congenital anaemia • Leuco-/neutropenia	Normal or small echogenic kidneys, with cortical and medullary cysts	• Cleft palate • Bifid uvula • Mild cognitive impairment

Modified from Devuyst O, Olinger E, Weber S, Eckardt KU, Kmoch S, Rampoldi L, Bleyer AJ. Autosomal dominant tubulointerstitial kidney disease Nat Rev. Dis Primers. 2019 Sep 5;5(1):60

CAKUT Congintal Anomalies of the Kidney and Urinary Tract; *MODY* Maturity Onset Diabetes of the Young

disease. Other clinical manifestations are uncommon. This was illustrated by the examination of six large Cypriot families including 72 affected individuals, in whom *MUC1* was first localized as the causative gene [81]. The disease led to ESKD at a mean age of 54 years, ranging from 36 to 80 years. The annual loss of estimated GFR is comparable in ADTKD-*UMOD* and ADTKD-*MUC1*, amounting to 3–4 mL/min/1.73 m² on average [67]. Arterial hypertension was found in 51% of affected individuals, and strictly related to renal function. Hyperuricemia and gout were no early findings, although the prevalence of hyperuricemia increased at approximately the same rate as in other causes of chronic kidney disease. Cysts were detected sonographically in 40% of tested gene defect carriers. Mainly corticomedullary or medullary, but also cortical cysts were reported. Approximately half of the affected individuals had normal sized kidneys with no cysts, while 11% had small echogenic kidneys without cysts.

In another 23 kindreds with 128 affected individuals, ESKD was reached at a median age of 32 years [82], ranging from 5 to 76 years. Kidney biopsy revealed histological findings identical to those found in "classical" NPH. Hyperuricemia was not a consistent finding and only reported in eight families. Hypertension was present in affected individuals from 13 families.

Clinical Presentation of ADTKD-*Ren*
Patients with *REN* gene variants present a very similar phenotype as *UMOD* patients with early onset gout and development of chronic kidney disease. However, *REN* patients are somewhat older when presenting with gout for the first time (20–30 years) and kidney failure progression is slower. ESKD usually occurs after the age of 40 years. Unlike *UMOD* patients, *REN* mutations lead to additional clinical symptoms caused by the low serum levels of renin and angiotensin. A nearly universal manifestation is the presence of hypoproliferative anaemia (haemoglobin range 7–11 g/dL) in early childhood that often resolves in adolescents, likely due to the increased sex steroid and subsequent erythropoietin production [71]. Additionally, some patients present with

low blood pressure, mild hyperkalemia responsive to fludrocortisone and an increased risk of acute kidney injury in a setting of volume depletion or application of non-steroidal inflammatory drugs.

Clinical Presentation of ADTKD-*HNF1B*
Variants in the *HNF1B* gene represent the most prevalent genetic cause of congenital anomalies of the kidney and urinary tract (CAKUT). Inheritance follows an autosomal dominant trait, but about 50% of patients carry *de novo* mutations with no positive family history. The clinical spectrum is highly heterogeneous and can vary significantly even between family members [83–86].

Initially, *HNF1B* variants have been described in the context of familial forms of maturity onset diabetes mellitus (MODY diabetes). Since many of the affected patients also presented malformations of the kidneys and the urinary tract, the term Renal Cyst and Diabetes Syndrome (RCDS) was introduced to refer to this clinical association [83]. The spectrum of kidney malformations observed in this context is highly variable: The majority of patients present bilateral kidney dysplasia in association with cortically located cysts. However, isolated kidney dysplasia, unilateral multicystic dysplastic kidneys, glomerulocystic changes, various urinary tract malformations and unilateral agenesis of the kidney have also been described. Prenatal ultrasound often reveals hyperechogenic kidneys with or without the evidence of cysts [84–86]. In contrast to ARPKD, kidneys usually are not enlarged, and amniotic fluid is preserved in most cases. Noteworthy, in many girls there is an association with malformations of the female genital tract [89, 90]. Thus, abdominal ultrasound should include a statement on potential genital abnormalities. Vice versa, the additional detection of such malformations increases the probability of an underlying *HNF1B* gene defect significantly.

The term HNF1B nephropathy can be misleading since many patients present a systemic disease rather than an isolated kidney phenotype [87, 88]. In addition to MODY-type diabetes and genital malformations, this primarily concerns hypomagnesemia caused by tubular magnesium loss, hyperuricemia, pancreatic changes and concomitant hepatopathy with elevated liver enzymes. Furthermore, autism spectrum disorders have been observed in some patients [91, 92]. However, extra-renal manifestations are not obligatory findings and might only develop late in the disease process, if at all. Nevertheless, regular screening is recommended. Additionally, owing to its dominant inheritance, genetic counseling and the clinical examination of other family members might be indicated [93].

Regarding kidney function, only a minority of patients experience severe forms with the need of renal replacement therapy in infancy or early childhood. In most children a stable or only slowly declining GFR is observed for many years with preserved kidney function until adolescence at least [94]. However, HNF1B gene defects may be a relevant contributor to chronic kidney disease in adulthood, as has only recently been elucidated [94].

Clinical Presentation of ADTKD-*SEC61A1*

So far only two families with ADTKD-*SEC61A1* have been reported. The phenotype of the first family was characterized by congenital anaemia in conjunction with intrauterine and postnatal growth retardation, cleft palate, bifid uvula, preaxial polydactyly and mild cognitive impairment [73]. In the second family, congenital anaemia was accompanied by neutropenia and recurrent cutaneous abscess formation during childhood. Gout was also a common feature in affected family members; however, growth and cognitive development were normal in this family [74].

Diagnostic Work-Up and Genetic Testing

In the presence of a tubulointerstitial disease with slowly progressive CKD, the first diagnostic step is to rule out disease entities with a higher prevalence by simple measures like urinalysis and ultrasound: While the detection of haematuria and proteinuria indicate glomerular rather than

tubular disease, enlarged kidney volume in combination with cystic lesions should guide the diagnosis to ADPKD in place of ADTKD. Next, family history—if positive at all—should be consistent with dominant inheritance to rule out NPH. Finally, while teenage-onset hyperuricemia and a medical history for gout hint towards underlying *UMOD* mutations, childhood anaemia and arterial hypotension may be clinical indicators for ADTKD-*REN* [61].

Yet, clinical phenotyping will only be able to provide diagnostic clues and neither extensive imaging nor a comprehensive histological work-up are sufficient to pin down a final diagnosis. Interestingly, measurement of reduced urinary uromodulin concentrations as well as negative MUC1 staining in uroepithelial bladder cells have been used to facilitate diagnosis in ADTKD-*UMOD* and ADTKD-*MUC1* individuals, respectively [95, 96]. However, both methods are not routinely accessible.

Thus, for the confirmation of the diagnosis ADTKD, the identification of the underlying genetic defect is mandatory. Although expensive, methodically difficult and so far without clear-cut therapeutic consequences, the confirmation of a molecular diagnosis helps to avoid unnecessary invasive procedures, to guide further extra-renal diagnostics, to provide personal counselling and to evaluate family members as potential kidney donors [61]. However, it should be pointed out that genetic testing of asymptomatic children for conditions in which there is no specific treatment is generally discouraged [97].

Therapy

As in NPH, there is no specific therapy correcting the genetic or functional defects in ADTKD so far. Symptomatic treatment strategies include the management of hyperuricemia, gout and progressive kidney failure. Hyperuricemia should be treated with allopurinol or other urate-lowering medication to avoid tophus development. However, whether this treatment also slows down the decline of kidney function is still under debate [98].

CKD management should include blood pressure control, correction of electrolyte abnormalities, free water supply to compensate for urinary concentration defects, cautious use of diuretics due to the associated risk of salt loss and hyperuricemia as well as a general avoidance of NSAIDs. Whether or not angiotensin receptor inhibition can be nephroprotective in this particular non-proteinuric cohort still needs to be elucidated. However, if angiotensin receptor blockers are used, losartan is the drug of choice in patients with hyperuricaemia since this compound increases urinary urate excretion [99].

Children with ADTKD-*HNF1B* and ADTKD-*REN* disease are likely to benefit from early management by neonatologists and paediatric nephrologists, including postnatal ventilation and circulation management as well as neonatal dialysis when required [58].

In ESKD, kidney transplantation is the method of choice for ADTKD patients since the disease does not recur in transplanted kidneys. Genetic testing for family members of patients with ADTKD is mandatory before a living donation.

Acknowledgements We would like to graciously acknowledge Andrea Titieni, Joachim Gerß and Carsten Bergmann for their contribution of figures and clinical pictures.

References

1. Fanconi G, Hanhart E, von Albertini A, Uhlinger E, Dolivo G, Prader A. Die familiäre juvenile Nephronophthise. Helv Paediatr Acta. 1951;6:1–49.
2. Smith C, Graham J. Congenital medullary cysts of kidneys with severe refractory anemia. Am J Dis Child. 1945;69:369–77.
3. Titieni A, König J. Nephronophthise und assoziierte Ziliopathien. Medgen. 2018;30:461–8.
4. König J, Kranz B, König S, Schlingmann KP, Titieni A, Tönshoff B, Habbig S, Pape L, Häffner K, Hansen M, Büscher A, Bald M, Billing H, Schild R, Walden U, Hampel T, Staude H, Riedl M, Gretz N, Lablans M, Bergmann C, Hildebrandt F, Omran H, Konrad M. Phenotypic spectrum of children with nephronophthisis and related ciliopathies. Clin J Am Soc Nephrol. 2017;12(12):1974–83.
5. Srivastava S, Molinari E, Raman S, Sayer JA. Many genes-one disease? Genetics of nephronophthisis (NPHP) and NPHP-associated disorders. Front Pediatr. 2017;5:287.
6. Waldherr R, Lennert T, Weber HP, Fodisch HJ, Scharer K. The nephronophthisis complex. A clinicopathologic study in children. Virchows Arch [Pathol Anat]. 1982;394:235–54.
7. Zollinger HU, Mihatsch MJ, Edefonti A, Gaboardi F, Imbasciati E, Lennert T. Nephronophthisis (medullary cystic disease of the kidney). A study using electron microscopy, immunofluorescence, and a review of the morphological findings. Helv Paediatr Acta. 1980;35:509–30.
8. Blowey DL, Querfeld U, Geary D, Warady BA, Alon U. Ultrasound findings in juvenile nephronophthisis. Pediatr Nephrol. 1996;10:22–4.
9. Luo F, Tao YH. Nephronophthisis: a review of genotype-phenotype correlation. Nephrology (Carlton). 2018;23(10):904–11.
10. Omran H. NPHP proteins: gatekeepers of the ciliary compartment. J Cell Biol. 2010;190(5):715–7.
11. Simms RJ, Eley L, Sayer JA. Nephronophthisis. Eur J Hum Genet. 2009;17(4):406–16.
12. Hildebrandt F, Strahm B, Nothwang HG, Gretz N, Schnieders B, Singh-Sawhney I, Kutt R, Vollmer M, Brandis M. Molecular genetic identification of families with juvenile nephronophthisis type 1: rate of progression to renal failure. APN Study Group. Arbeitsgemeinschaft fuer Paediatrische Nephrologie. Kidney Int. 1997b;51:261–9.
13. Konrad M, Saunier S, Heidet L, Silbermann F, Benessy F, Calado J, Le Paslier D, Broyer M, Gubler MC, Antignac C. Large homozygous deletions of the 2q13 region are a major cause of juvenile nephronophthisis. Hum Mol Genet. 1996;5:367–71.
14. Hildebrandt F, Rensing C, Betz R, Sommer U, Birnbaum S, Imm A, Omran H, Leipoldt M, Otto E. Arbeitsgemeinschaft fuer Paediatrische Nephrologie (APN) Study Group: establishing an algorithm for molecular genetic diagnostics in 127 families with juvenile nephronophthisis. Kidney Int. 2001;59(2):434–45.
15. Snoek R, van Setten J, Keating BJ, et al. NPHP1 (Nephrocystin-1) gene deletions cause adult-onset ESRD. J Am Soc Nephrol. 2018;29:1772–9.
16. Gagnadoux MF, Bacri JL, Broyer M, Habib R. Infantile chronic tubulo-interstitial nephritis with cortical microcysts: variant of nephronophthisis or new disease entity? Pediatr Nephrol. 1989;3:50–5.
17. Otto EA, Schermer B, Obara T, O'Toole JF, Hiller KS, Mueller AM, Ruf RG, Hoefele J, Beekmann F, Landau D, Foreman JW, Goodship JA, Strachan T, Kispert A, Wolf MT, Gagnadoux MF, Nivet H, Antignac C, Walz G, Drummond IA, Benzing T, Hildebrandt F. Mutations in INVS encoding inversin cause nephronophthisis type 2, linking renal cystic disease to the function of primary cilia and left-right axis determination. Nat Genet. 2003;34:413–20.
18. Senior B, Friedmann AI, Braudo JL. Juvenile familial nephropathy with tapetoretinal degeneration:

18. a new oculo-renal dystrophy. Am J Opthalmol. 1961;52:625–33.

19. Leber T. Über Retinitis pigmentosa und angeborene Amaurose. Arch Ophthalmol. 1869;15:1–25.

20. Leber T. Über anormale Formen der Retinitis pigmentosa. Arch Ophthalmol. 1871;17:314–41.

21. François J. Leber's congenital tapeto-retinal degeneration. Int Ophthalmol Clin. 1968;8:929–47.

22. Franceschetti A, Dieterle P. L'importance diagnostique de l'éléctro-rétinogramme dans le dégénérescences tapéto-rétinennes avec rétrécissement du champ visuel et héméralopie. Conf Neurol. 1954;14:184–6.

23. Otto EA, Loeys B, Khanna H, Hellemans J, Sudbrak R, Fan SL, Muerb U, O'Toole JF, Helou J, Attanasio M, et al. Nephrocystin-5, a ciliary IQ domain protein, is mutated in Senior-Loken syndrome and interacts with RPGR and calmodulin. Nat Genet. 2005;37:282–8.

24. Adamiok-Ostrowska A, Piekiełko-Witkowska A. Ciliary genes on renal cystic diseases. Cells. 2020;9(4):907.

25. Grochowsky A, Gunay-Aygun M. Clinical characteristics of individual organ system disease in non-motile ciliopathies. Transl Sci Rare Dis. 2019;4(1–2):1–23.

26. Maria BL, Quisling RG, Rosainz LC, Yachnis AT, Gitten JC, Dede DE, Fennell E. Molar tooth sign in Joubert syndrome: clinical, radiologic, and pathologic significance. J Child Neurol. 1999;14:368–76.

27. Summers AC, Snow J, Wiggs E, Liu AG, Toro C, Poretti A, et al. Neuropsychological phenotypes of 76 individuals with Joubert syndrome evaluated at a single center. Am J Med Genet A. 2017;173(7):1796–812.

28. Poretti A, Snow J, Summers AC, Tekes A, Huisman T, Aygun N, et al. Joubert syndrome: neuroimaging findings in 110 patients in correlation with cognitive function and genetic cause. J Med Genet. 2017;54(8):521–9.

29. Parisi MA, Bennett CL, Eckert ML, Dobyns WB, Gleeson JG, Shaw DWW, McDonald R, Eddy A, Chance PF, Glass IA. The NPHP1 gene deletion associated with juvenile nephronophthisis is present in a subset of individuals with Joubert syndrome. Am J Hum Genet. 2004;75:82–91.

30. Strongin A, Heller T, Doherty D, Glass IA, Parisi MA, Bryant J, et al. Characteristics of liver disease in 100 individuals with joubert syndrome prospectively evaluated at a single center. J Pediatr Gastroenterol Nutr. 2018;66(3):428–35.

31. Parisi MA. The molecular genetics of Joubert syndrome and related ciliopathies: the challenges of genetic and phenotypic heterogeneity. Transl Sci Rare Dis. 2019;4(1–2):25–49.

32. Fleming LR, Doherty DA, Parisi MA, Glass IA, Bryant J, Fischer R, et al. Prospective evaluation of kidney disease in joubert syndrome. Clin J Am Soc Nephrol. 2017;12(12):1962–73.

33. Bergmann C. Educational paper: ciliopathies. Eur J Pediatr. 2012;171(9):1285–300.

34. Parisi MA, Doherty D, Eckert ML, Shaw DW, Ozyurek H, Aysun S, Giray O, Al Swaid A, Al Shahwan S, Dohayan N, Bakhsh E, Indridason OS, Dobyns WB, Bennett CL, Chance PF, Glass IA. AHI1 mutations cause both retinal dystrophy and renal cystic disease in Joubert syndrome. J Med Genet. 2006;43:334–9.

35. Doherty D, Parisi MA, Finn LS, Gunay-Aygun M, Al-Mateen M, Bates D, Clericuzio C, Demir H, Dorschner M, van Essen AJ, Gahl WA, Gentile M, Gorden NT, Hikida A, Knutzen D, Ozyurek H, Phelps I, Rosenthal P, Verloes A, Weigand H, Chance PF, Dobyns WB, Glass IA. Mutations in 3 genes (MKS3, CC2D2A and RPGRIP1L) cause COACH syndrome (Joubert syndrome with congenital hepatic fibrosis). J Med Genet. 2010;47(1):8–21.

36. Dahmer-Heath M, Schriever V, Kollmann S, Schleithoff C, Titieni A, Cetiner M, Patzer L, Tönshoff B, Hansen M, Pennekamp P, Gerß J, Konrad M, König J. Systematic evaluation of olfaction in patients with hereditary cystic kidney diseases/renal ciliopathies. J Med Genet. 2020.

37. Hartill V, Szymanska K, Sharif SM, Wheway G, Johnson CA. Meckel-gruber syndrome: an update on diagnosis, clinical management, and research advances. Front Pediatr. 2017;5:244.

38. Salonen R. The meckel syndrome: clinicopathological findings in 67 patients. Am J Med Genet. 1984;18(4):671–89.

39. Sergi C, Adam S, Kahl P, Otto HF. Study of the malformation of ductal plate of the liver in Meckel syndrome and review of other syndromes presenting with this anomaly. Pediatr Dev Pathol. 2000;3(6):568–83.

40. Alexiev BA, Lin X, Sun CC, Brenner DS. Meckel-Gruber syndrome: pathologic manifestations, minimal diagnostic criteria, and differential diagnosis. Arch Pathol Lab Med. 2006;130(8):1236–8.

41. Sattar S, Gleeson JG. The ciliopathies in neuronal development: a clinical approach to investigation of Joubert syndrome and Joubert syndrome-related disorders. Dev Med Child Neurol. 2011;53(9):793–8.

42. Cogan DG. Heredity of congenital ocular motor apraxia. Trans Am Acad Ophthal Otolaryng. 1972;76:60–3.

43. Schröder S, Li Y, Yigit G, Altmüller J, Bader I, Bevot A, Biskup S, Dreha-Kulaczewski S, Christoph Korenke G, Kottke R, Mayr JA, Preisel M, Toelle SP, Wente-Schulz S, Wortmann SB, Hahn H, Boltshauser E, Uhmann A, Wollnik B, Brockmann K. Heterozygous truncating variants in SUFU cause congenital ocular motor apraxia. Genet Med. 2020;23(2):341–51.

44. Betz R, Rensing C, Otto E, Mincheva A, Zehnder D, Lichter P, Hildebrandt F. Children with ocular motor apraxia type Cogan carry deletions in the gene (NPHP1) for juvenile nephronophthisis. J Pediatr. 2000;136(6):828–31.

45. Di Rocco M, Picco P, Arslanian A, et al. Retinitis pigmentosa, hypopituitarism, nephronophthisis, and mild skeletal dysplasia (RHYNS): a new syndrome? Am J Med Genet. 1997;73:1–4.

46. Hedera P, Gorski JL. Retinitis pigmentosa, growth hormone deficiency, and acromelic skeletal dysplasia in two brothers: possible familial RHYNS syndrome. Am J Med Genet. 2001;101:142–5.

47. Brancati F, Camerota L, Colao E, Vega-Warner V, Zhao X, Zhang R, Bottillo I, Castori M, Caglioti A, Sangiuolo F, Novelli G, Perrotti N, Otto EA, Undiagnosed Disease Network Italy. Biallelic variants in the ciliary gene TMEM67 cause RHYNS syndrome. Eur J Hum Genet. 2018;26(9):1266–71.

48. Stephen J, Vilboux T, Mian L, et al. Mutations in KIAA0753 cause Joubert syndrome associated with growth hormone deficiency. Hum Genet. 2017;136:399–08.

49. Vilboux T, Malicdan MC, Roney JC, et al. CELSR2, encoding a planar cell polarity protein, is a putative gene in Joubert syndrome with cortical heterotopia, microophthalmia, and growth hormone deficiency. Am J Med Genet A. 2017;173:661–6.

50. Braun DA, Hildebrandt F. Ciliopathies Cold Spring Harb Perspect Biol. 2017;9(3):a028191.

51. Zhang W, Taylor SP, Ennis HA, Forlenza KN, Duran I, Li B, Sanchez JAO, Nevarez L, Nickerson DA, Bamshad M, University of Washington Center for Mendelian Genomics, Lachman RS, Krakow D, Cohn DH. Expanding the genetic architecture and phenotypic spectrum in skeletal ciliopathies. Hum Mutat. 2018;39(1):152–66.

52. Arts H, Knoers N. Cranioectodermal dysplasia. In: Adam MP, Ardinger HH, Pagon RA, Wallace SE, LJH B, Stephens K, Amemiya A, editors. GeneReviews®. Seattle, WA, University of Washington, Seattle; 2013. p. 1993–2020.

53. Wallmeier J, Nielsen KG, Kuehni CE, Lucas JS, Leigh MW, Zariwala MA, Omran H. Motile ciliopathies. Nat Rev Dis Primers. 2020;6(1):77.

54. Lemaire M, Parekh RS. A perspective on inherited kidney disease: lessons for practicing nephrologists. Clin J Am Soc Nephrol. 2017;12(12):1914–6.

55. Sawyer SL, Hartley T, Dyment DA, Beaulieu CL, Schwartzentruber J, Smith A, et al. Utility of whole-exome sequencing for those near the end of the diagnostic odyssey: time to address gaps in care. Clin Genet. 2016;89:275–84.

56. Joly D, Beroud C, Grünfeld JP. Rare inherited disorders with renal involvement-approach to the patient. Kidney Int. 2015;87:901–8.

57. König J, Titieni A, Konrad M. Network for Early Onset Cystic Kidney Diseases (NEOCYST)—a comprehensive multidisciplinary approach to hereditary cystic kidney diseases in childhood. Front Pediatr. 2018;6:24.

58. Eckardt KU, et al. Autosomal dominant tubulointerstitial kidney disease: diagnosis, classification, and management—KDIGO consensus report. Kidney Int. 2015;88:676–83.

59. Goldman SH, Walker SR, Merigan TCJ, Gardner KDJ, Bull JM. Hereditary occurrence of cystic disease of the renal medulla. N Engl J Med. 1966;274:984–92.

60. Strauss MB, Sommers SC. Medullary cystic disease and familial juvenile nephronophthisis. N Engl J Med. 1967;277:863–4.

61. Devuyst O, Olinger E, Weber S, Eckardt KU, Kmoch S, Rampoldi L, Bleyer AJ. Autosomal dominant tubulointerstitial kidney disease. Nat Rev Dis Primers. 2019;5(1):60.

62. Wolf MT, Mucha BE, Attanasio M, Zalewski I, Karle SM, Neumann HP, Rahman N, Bader B, Baldamus CA, Otto E, Witzgall R, Fuchshuber A, Hildebrandt F. Mutations of the Uromodulin gene in MCKD type 2 patients cluster in exon 4, which encodes three EGF-like domains. Kidney Int. 2003;64:1580–7.

63. Bates JM, et al. Tamm-Horsfall protein knockout mice are more prone to urinary tract infection rapid communication. Kidney Int. 2004;65:791–7.

64. Gudbjartsson DF, et al. Association of variants at UMOD with chronic kidney disease and kidney stones-role of age and comorbid diseases. PLoS Genet. 2010;6:e1001039.

65. Mutig K, Kahl T, Saritas T, Godes M, Persson P, Bates J, Raffi H, Rampoldi L, Uchida S, Hille S, Dosche C, Kumar S, Castaneda-Bueno M, Gamba G, Bachmann S. Na+K+2Cl-Cotransporter (NKCC2) is regulated by Tamm-Horsfall-Protein (THP). American Society of Nephrology Annual Meeting, 2008; abstract 134.

66. Renigunta A, Renigunta V, Saritas T, Decher N, Mutig K, Waldegger S. Tamm-Horsfall glycoprotein interacts with renal outer medullary potassium channel ROMK2 and regulates its function. J Biol Chem. 2011;286:2224–35.

67. Ayasreh N, et al. Autosomal dominant tubulointerstitial kidney disease: clinical presentation of patients with ADTKD-*UMOD* and ADTKD-*MUC1*. Am J Kidney Dis. 2018;72:411–8.

68. Kirby A, Gnirke A, Jaffe DB, Barešová V, Pochet N, Blumenstiel B, Aird D, Stevens C, Robinson JT, Cabili MN, Gat-Viks I, Kelliher E, Daza R, DeFelice M, Hůlková H, Sovová J, Vylet'al P, Antignac C, Guttman M, Handsaker RE, Perrin D, Steelman S, Sigurdsson S, Scheinman SJ, Sougnez C, Cibulskis K, Parkin M, Green T, Rossin E, Zody MC, Xavier RJ, Pollak MR, Alper SL, Lindblad-Toh K, Gabriel S, Hart PS, Regev A, Nusbaum C, Kmoch S, Bleyer AJ, Lander ES, Daly MJ. Mutations causing medullary cystic kidney disease type 1 lie in a large VNTR in MUC1 missed by massively parallel sequencing. Nat Genet. 2013;45:299–303.

69. Clissold RL, Hamilton AJ, Hattersley AT, Ellard S, Bingham C. *HNF1B* associated renal and extrarenal disease—an expanding clinical spectrum. Nat Rev Nephrol. 2015;11:102–12.

70. Vlahakos DV, et al. Renin-angiotensin system stimulates erythropoietin secretion in chronic hemodialysis patients. Clin Nephrol. 1995;43:53–9.

71. Zivná M, Hůlková H, Matignon M, Hodanová K, Vylet'al P, Kalbácová M, Baresová V, Sikora J, Blazková H, Zivný J, Ivánek R, Stránecký V, Sovová J, Claes K, Lerut E, Fryns JP, Hart PS, Hart TC, Adams JN, Pawtowski A, Clemessy M, Gasc JM, Gubler MC, Antignac C, Elleder M, Kapp K, Grimbert P, Bleyer AJ, Kmoch S. Dominant renin gene mutations associated with early onset hyperuricemia, anemia and chronic kidney failure. Am J Hum Genet. 2009;85:204–13.

72. Gribouval O, et al. Mutations in genes in the renin angiotensin system are associated with autosomal recessive renal tubular dysgenesis. Nat Genet. 2005;37:964–8.

73. Bolar NA, et al. Heterozygous loss-of-function SEC61A1 mutations cause autosomaldominant tubulo-interstitial and glomerulocystic kidney disease with anemia. Am J Hum Genet. 2016;99:174–87.

74. Schubert D, et al. Plasma cell deficiency in human subjects with heterozygous mutations in Sec61 translocon alpha 1 subunit (SEC61A1). J Allergy Clin Immunol. 2018;141:1427–38.

75. Lang S, et al. An update on Sec 61 channel functions, mechanisms, and related diseases. Front Physiol. 2017;8:887.

76. Hart TC, Gorry MC, Hart PS, Woodard AS, Shihabi Z, Sandhu J, Shirts B, Xu L, Zhu H, Barmada MM, Bleyer AJ. Mutations of the UMOD gene are responsible for medullary cystic kidney disease 2 and familial juvenile hyperuricaemic nephropathy. J Med Genet. 2002;39(12):882–92.

77. Scolari F, Caridi G, Rampoldi L, Tardanico R, Izzi C, Pirulli D, Amoroso A, Casari G, Ghiggeri GM. Uromodulin storage disease: clinical aspects and mechanisms. Am J Kidney Dis. 2004;44:987–99.

78. Bollée G, Dahan K, Flamant M, Morinière V, Pawtowski A, Heidet L, Lacombe D, Devuyst O, Pirson Y, Antignac C, Knebelmann B. Phenotype and outcome in hereditary tubulointerstitial nephritis secondary to UMOD mutations. Clin J Am Soc Nephrol. 2011;6:2429–38.

79. Scolari F, Puzzer D, Amoroso A, Caridi G, Ghiggeri GM, Maiorca R, Aridon P, De Fusco M, Ballabio A, Casari G. Identification of a new locus for medullary cystic disease, on chromosome 16p12. Am J Hum Genet. 1999;64:1655–60.

80. Rezende-Lima W, Parreira KS, Garcia-Gonzalez M, Riveira E, Banet JF, Lens XM. Homozygosity for uromodulin disorders: FJHN and MCKD-type 2. Kidney Int. 2004;66:558–63.

81. Stavrou C, Koptides M, Tombazos C, Psara E, Patsias C, Zouvani I, Kyriacou K, Hildebrandt F, Christofides T, Pierides A, Deltas CC. Autosomaldominant medullary cystic kidney disease type 1: clinical and molecular findings in six large Cypriot families. Kidney Int. 2002;62:1385–94.

82. Wolf MT, Mucha BE, Hennies HC, Attanasio M, Panther F, Zalewski I, Karle SM, Otto EA, Deltas CC, Fuchshuber A, Hildebrandt F. Medullary cystic kidney disease type 1: mutational analysis in 37 genes based on haplotype sharing. Hum Genet. 2006;119:649–5.

83. Ulinski T, et al. Renal phenotypes related to hepatocyte nuclear factor1β (TCF2) mutations in a pediatric cohort. J Am Soc Nephrol. 2006;17:497–503.

84. Decramer S, et al. Anomalies of the *TCF2* gene are the main cause of fetal bilateral hyperechogenic kidneys. J Am Soc Nephrol. 2007;18:923–33.

85. Gondra L, et al. Hyperechogenic kidneys and polyhydramnios associated with *HNF1B* gene mutation. Pediatr Nephrol. 2016;31:1705–8.

86. Shuster S, et al. Prenatal detection of isolated bilateral hyperechogenic kidneys: etiologies and outcomes. Prenat Diagn. 2019;39:693–700.

87. Mitchel MW, et al. 17q12 recurrent deletion syndrome. GeneReviews. https://www.ncbi.nlm.nih.gov/books/NBK401562/. Accessed 8 December 2016.

88. Verhave JC, Bech AP, Wetzels JF, Nijenhuis T. Hepatocyte nuclear factor 1ß-associated kidney disease: more than renal cyst and diabetes. J Am Soc Nephrol. 2016;27(2):345–53.

89. Faguer S, et al. Diagnosis, management, and prognosis of *HNF1B* nephropathy in adulthood. Kidney Int. 2011;80:768–76.

90. Oram RA, et al. Mutations in the hepatocyte nuclear factor1β (*HNF1B*) gene are common with combined uterine and renal malformations but are not found with isolated uterine malformations. Am J Obstet Gynecol. 2010;203:364.e1–5.

91. MorenoDeLuca D, et al. Deletion 17q12 is a recurrent copy number variant that confers high risk of autism and schizophrenia. Am J Hum Genet. 2010;87:618–30.

92. Clissold RL, et al. Chromosome 17q12 microdeletions but not intragenic HNF1B mutations link developmental kidney disease and psychiatric disorder. Kidney Int. 2016;90:203–11.

93. Gimpel C, Avni FE, Bergmann C, Cetiner M, Habbig S, Haffner D, König J, Konrad M, Liebau MC, Pape L, Rellensmann G, Titieni A, von Kaisenberg C, Weber S, Winyard PJD, Schaefer F. Perinatal diagnosis, management and follow-up of cystic renal diseases: a clinical practice recommendation with systematic literature reviews. JAMA Pediatr. 2018;172(1):74–86.

94. Okorn C, Goertz A, Vester U, Beck BB, Bergmann C, Habbig S, König J, Konrad M, Müller D, Oh J, Ortiz-Brüchle N, Patzer L, Schild R, Seeman T, Staude H, Thumfart J, Tönshoff B, Walden U, Weber L, Zaniew M, Zappel H, Hoyer PF, Weber S. HNF1B nephropathy has a slow-progressive phenotype in childhood—with the exception of very early onset cases. Results of the German Multicenter HNF1B Childhood Registry. Pediatr Nephrol. 2019;34(6):1065–75.

95. Bleyer AJ, Hart TC, Shihabi ZAK, Robins V, Hoyer JR. Mutations in the uromodulin gene decrease urinary excretion of Tamm-Horsfall protein. Kidney Int. 2004;66:974–7.

96. Wenzel A, et al. Single molecule real time sequencing in ADTKD-*MUC1* allows complete assembly of the VNTR and exact positioning of causative mutations. Sci Rep. 2018;8:4170.

97. Ross LF, Saal HM, David KL, Anderson RR. Technical report: ethical and policy issues in genetic testing and screening of children. Genet Med. 2013;15:234–45.

98. Liu X, et al. Effects of uric acid-lowering therapy on the progression of chronic kidney disease: a systematic review and meta-analysis. Ren Fail. 2018;40:289–97.

99. Hamada T, et al. Uricosuric action of losartan via the inhibition of urate transporter 1 (URAT 1) in hypertensive patients. Am J Hypertens. 2008;21:1157–62.

Part IV

Glomerular Disorders

Hematuria and Proteinuria

12

Hui-Kim Yap and Perry Yew-Weng Lau

Introduction

The presence of blood or protein in the urine may be just a normal transient finding in children, usually accompanying a non-specific viral infection. More importantly, these findings may be an indicator of a kidney or urinary tract disorder. Macroscopic hematuria or the incidental finding of hematuria or proteinuria on urine dipstick examination is often an alarming occurrence to parents, bringing the child to medical attention. The etiology of hematuria and proteinuria includes a long list of conditions. Workup can be extensive, expensive and unnecessary as most children with isolated hematuria or isolated proteinuria do not have significant kidney disease and abnormal urine findings usually resolve on repeated testing. Conversely, persistent proteinuria or even persistent microscopic hematuria can be an indicator of significant glomerular disease, as well as associated with an increased risk for end-stage kidney disease (ESKD).

H.-K. Yap (✉)
Department of Pediatrics, National University of Singapore, Singapore, Singapore
e-mail: hui_kim_yap@nuhs.edu.sg

P. Y.-W. Lau
Khoo Teck Puat-National University Children's Medical Institute, National University Hospital, Singapore, Singapore
e-mail: perry_lau@nuhs.edu.sg

Hematuria

In a normal person, very few red blood cells are excreted into the urine. The passage of red blood cells (diameter 6–8 μm) through the glomerulus into the urinary space is mostly prevented by endothelial fenestrations (50–100 nm) of the glomerular filtration barrier. Increased passage of red blood cells into the urinary space can be due to glomerular diseases or conditions affecting the lower urinary tract. Glomerular hematuria can be due to structural modification of components of the glomerular filtration barrier (e.g. α-chain of type IV collagen in thin basement membrane disease and Alport syndrome) or increased inflammatory response leading to damage of capillary endothelium and glomerular basement membrane (e.g. in primary glomerulonephritis and autoimmune conditions).

Macroscopic hematuria is visible while microscopic hematuria is usually detected by a urine dipstick test during a routine examination or by microscopic examination of the urine sediment. As little as 1 mL of blood per liter of urine can produce a visible change in the urine color. If fresh blood is present in the urine, the urine will be pink or red. If left standing, even in the bladder, the urine will develop a hazy smoky or brown color. The brown color comes from the metheme derivative of the oxidized heme pigment. Some pigments and crystals, when present at a significant concentration, will cause color changes in

© The Author(s), under exclusive license to Springer Nature Switzerland AG 2023
F. Schaefer, L. A. Greenbaum (eds.), *Pediatric Kidney Disease*,
https://doi.org/10.1007/978-3-031-11665-0_12

Table 12.1 Causes of discoloration of urine

Dark yellow or orange urine	Normal concentrated urine Rifampicin Carotene Pyridium Warfarin
Dark brown or black urine	Bile pigments Methemoglobinemia Alanine, resorcinol Laxatives containing cascara or senna Alkaptonuria, homogentisic acid, melanin, Tyrosinosis Thymol Methyldopa metabolite Copper Phenol poisoning
Red or pink urine	Red blood cells (hematuria) Free hemoglobin (hemoglobinuria) Myoglobin (myoglobinuria) Porphyrins Urates in high concentration (may produce a pinkish tinge) Foods (e.g. beetroot, rhubarb, blackberries, red dyes) Drugs (e.g. benzene, chloroquine, desferoxamine, phenazopyridine, phenolphthalein)

the urine that can be misinterpreted as hematuria. Discoloration of urine can be due to intravascular hemolysis, rhabdomyolysis, metabolic disorders and a number of foods and drugs (Table 12.1).

Definition

The definition of hematuria is based on urine microscopic examination findings of red blood cells and it varies according to the method of quantification. The most commonly accepted upper limits of normal for urinary red blood cells are three red blood cells per high power field in fresh centrifuged urine [1]. There is some controversy as to the amount of red blood cells required for the diagnosis of microscopic hematuria. A population-based study of over 12,000 children in Texas by Dodge et al. [2] recommended five or more red blood cells per high power field in at least two of three consecutive fresh centrifuged urine obtained at least 1 week apart, as the definition of hematuria to capture children with significant disease. A study of 8954 Finnish school

children by Vehaskari et al. [3] defined hematuria as more than 5 red blood cells/0.9 mm^3 in a fresh uncentrifuged midstream urine specimen and this identified all children with kidney disease if the urine sample was positive twice in a 6-month period. A study using more stringent criteria has greater positive predictive value with regard to presence of disease, but loses some negative predictive value. Regardless of the criterion used, important cofactors to consider when a child has microscopic hematuria include the presence of proteinuria, urinary casts, hypertension, a family history of kidney disease and other clinical or laboratory findings suggestive of kidney or urinary tract disease.

Urine Dipstick

The urine dipstick utilizes the peroxidase-like activity of hemoglobin present in the urine. Hemoglobin peroxidase activity converts the chromogen tetramethyl benzidine incorporated in the dipstick into an oxidized form, resulting in a green-blue color. The test depends on the presence of free hemoglobin, which comes from hemolysis of the red blood cells in the urine. It is assumed that when there is significant hematuria, some of the red blood cells will always lyse and there will be sufficient free hemoglobin released to cause a positive test. The test is very sensitive, capable of detecting as little as 150 μg/L of free hemoglobin. As few as two to three red blood cells per high power field can make the urine dipstick positive.

It is important to follow the manufacturer's instructions of the dipstick. Delayed reading may produce false positive results. Positive results can also occur in hemoglobinuria following intravascular hemolysis or in myoglobinuria after rhabdomyolysis. Positive results can also be due to the presence of oxidizing agents in the urine such as hypochlorite (cleaning solution) and microbial peroxidases associated with microbial contamination, including urinary tract infection (UTI).

Conversely, false negative results can be due to the presence of large amounts of reducing agents such as ascorbic acid or urine with high specific gravity, in which the dipstick test is less sensitive.

Due to the very sensitive nature of the urine dipstick test, it is unwise to investigate based on a "trace" reading on the dipstick. Similarly, a child with dipstick reading of "1+" on one occasion and negative readings on subsequent dipstick testing is unlikely to benefit from further investigations. Only if the urine dipstick reading for blood is persistently greater than "trace" is further evaluation warranted. In clinical practice, it is important to confirm hematuria with urine microscopic examination. An absence of red blood cells in the urine with a positive dipstick reaction in a child with red or brown urine may suggest hemoglobinuria or myoglobinuria.

Urine Microscopy

Microscopic examination of the urine sediment is important in diagnosing and evaluating hematuria. When abundant, red blood cells are easy to identify by their characteristic biconcave disc appearance under microscopy. When scanty, red blood cells become distorted in the urine and it is difficult to differentiate them from other unidentified small objects.

Urine centrifugation is one way to solve this problem. After centrifugation and removal of supernatant, the deposit is resuspended in the remaining urine and examined under the microscope. Urine microscopic examination can have false negative results when the urine is of low specific gravity or has an alkaline pH. These conditions result in red blood cells hemolysing rapidly in standing urine, resulting in a positive urine dipstick test due to the free hemoglobin, but without the characteristic red blood cells seen by microscopy.

The morphology of the red blood cells may help identify the origin of the bleeding [4, 5]. Red blood cells from the lower urinary tract maintain their morphology whereas red blood cells from the glomeruli show great variation in shape, size and hemoglobin content due to sheering stresses on their surface in their passage from the capillary lumen through gaps in the glomerular filtra-

tion barrier into the urinary space [6]. Phase-contrast microscopy on freshly voided urine allows this differentiation. Red blood cells that are more than 90–95% isomorphic (i.e., of normal size and shape) are most commonly from the lower urinary tract. If more than 30% of dysmorphic red blood cells (blebs, budding and segmental loss of membrane with reduction in red cell volume) are present, the hematuria is more likely to be of glomerular origin [7].

The presence of casts, other cells and crystals in the urine can be helpful. Red blood cell casts are always pathological and usually suggest glomerulonephritis. Identification of red blood cell casts should be done on fresh urine or acidic urine stored at 4 °C, as red blood cell casts disintegrate readily in alkaline urine, taking on a granular appearance. Hence the finding of granular casts in association with hematuria may indicate that the blood has originated from the kidneys. The low rate of red blood cell cast identification using conventional microscopy is probably related to centrifugation of the urine specimen at a low speed of 400 g. A study using high speed centrifugation at 2000 g for microscopy was able to increase the red blood cell cast yield in the urine [8]. Hyaline casts are associated with proteinuria, and a few such casts may be found in concentrated early morning samples from healthy people. When white blood cells are also present in the urine, infection and interstitial or glomerular inflammatory disorders should be considered. Interstitial nephritis is even more likely if Wright stain of the urine shows the presence of eosinophils. Infections and poststreptococcal nephritis often have neutrophils on urinalysis. If the child has other findings suggestive of nephrolithiasis, the shape of the crystals may help to identify the chemical nature of the calculi. Calcium oxalate crystals may point to hypercalciuria.

Etiology

A practical approach is to determine whether the hematuria is of glomerular or non-glomerular origin. Non-glomerular bleeding occurs from the urinary tract, which includes the collecting sys-

Table 12.2 Causes of hematuria in children

Glomerular		Nonglomerular
Familial hematuria disorders • Thin basement membrane disease • Alport syndrome • MYH9-related disease • CFHR5 nephropathy • Giant fibronectin glomerulopathy	Glomerulonephritis • Acute post-infectious GN • Membranoproliferative GN • Membranous nephropathy • Rapidly progressive GN • Systemic lupus erythematosus • IgA nephropathy • IgA vasculitis nephritis • Polyarteritis nodosa • ANCA positive vasculitis Hemolytic uremic syndrome	Urinary tract infection Adenovirus hemorrhagic cystitis Urinary schistosomiasis Hypercalciuria Renal calculi Exercise-induced Trauma or instrumentation Chemical cystitis such as cyclophosphamide Coagulopathy Sickle cell trait Cystic kidney disease Structural abnormalities of kidney, ureter, bladder (e.g. vesicoureteric junction obstruction) Vascular malformations Nutcracker syndrome Renal vein thrombosis Tumors • Renal: Wilms tumor, renal cell carcinoma, mesoblastic nephroma • Bladder: rhabdomyosarcoma Menarche Factitious

tems, ureters, bladder and urethra. The various causes of hematuria in children are listed in Table 12.2. In children, the source of bleeding is more often from the glomeruli than from the urinary tract.

There are four different clinical presentations of hematuria:

1. Child with red or dark-colored urine
2. Child with lower urinary tract symptoms
3. Child with clinical features of acute glomerulonephritis
4. Asymptomatic child with incidental finding of microscopic hematuria on urine dipstick

These four clinical presentations will be considered separately as the approach is different in each of these scenarios, though there is an overlap in the causes.

Child with Red or Dark-Colored Urine

The first step in the evaluation is to exclude red discoloration of urine due to certain foods, drugs,

hemoglobinuria or myoglobinuria (Table 12.1). A urine microscopic examination is essential to confirm that the discoloration is due to red blood cells.

The causes of gross hematuria in children include:

1. Acute glomerulonephritis, especially if edema and hypertension are also present.
2. UTI, adenovirus hemorrhagic cystitis, schistosomiasis, urethritis, perineal irritation, urolithiasis, or hypercalciuria. These conditions are usually accompanied by voiding symptoms such as dysuria, frequency and urgency.
3. Exercise-induced hematuria
4. Trauma
5. Coagulopathy
6. Renal vein thrombosis
7. Urinary tract tumors
8. Recurrent gross hematuria which is seen in IgA nephropathy, nutcracker syndrome, Alport syndrome, CFHR5 nephropathy.

Exercise-induced hematuria is a transient hematuria that appears immediately after prolonged, vigorous exercise such as long-distance running, and usually disappears within 48 h. This is benign and results from relative higher vasoconstriction of the efferent glomerular arterioles compared with the afferent vessels, resulting in increased filtration pressure and excessive increase in red cell excretion into the urine [9].

Trauma sufficient to cause hematuria is usually associated with an obvious history such as urethral catheterization or abdominal injury. Mild trauma may cause hematuria in a patient with a previously unsuspected obstructed urinary tract, such as ureteropelvic junction stenosis.

Children with bleeding disorders such as hemophilia or thrombocytopenia commonly have microscopic hematuria, but may also develop gross hematuria following minor trauma. Sickle cell hemoglobinopathy can cause hematuria by causing infarction of the renal collecting systems [10]. Renal vein thrombosis is rare, but should be strongly considered when gross hematuria presents in nephrotic children, neonates with umbilical lines, severe dehydration, polycythemia or prothrombotic conditions.

Urinary tract tumors are rare in children. Children with Wilms tumor can have microscopic hematuria (rarely macroscopic hematuria), but are more commonly discovered following evaluation of abdominal distension or abdominal masses. Rhabdomyosarcoma of the bladder is extremely rare, and usually presents with voiding symptoms in addition to macroscopic hematuria.

The nutcracker phenomenon refers to compression of the left renal vein between the aorta and superior mesenteric artery before the left renal vein joins the inferior vena cava. This leads to left renal vein hypertension, which may result in rupture of the thin-walled vein into the renal calyceal fornix, with the clinical presentation of intermittent gross or microscopic hematuria. In addition, the increased venous pressure within the renal circulation can promote the development of varices of the renal pelvis and ureter. This phenomenon, with its associated symptoms of unilateral hematuria and left flank pain, is defined as the nutcracker syndrome. It occasionally presents as a varicocele in boys or abnormal menstruation in pubertal girls, as a result of the development of venous varicosities of the gonadal vein [11]. Orthostatic proteinuria has also been reported in nutcracker syndrome, although the exact mechanism is unknown [12]. Possible mechanisms include subtle glomerular lesions associated with hemodynamic abnormality, and an increased release in norepinephrine and angiotensin II on standing up [12]. Nutcracker syndrome appears more commonly in Asian communities. It may be one of the important causes of gross or microscopic hematuria in relatively young and previously healthy patients with a thin habitus [13].

Diagnosis of nutcracker syndrome can be made by renal ultrasound demonstrating compression of a pre-aortic left renal vein in the fork between the abdominal aorta and the proximal superior mesenteric artery, and Doppler flow scanning measuring the peak flow velocity ratio between the aorto-mesenteric portion and the hilar portion of the renal vein. The most accurate method for diagnosing the nutcracker syndrome is left renal venography, with measurement of the pressure gradient between the left renal vein and the inferior vena cava. Such invasive examination is difficult to perform in children. Magnetic resonance angiography can be used to demonstrate the dilated left renal vein after passing between the aorta and superior mesenteric artery. An alternative is multidetector computed tomography, which can detect the decrease in velocity of contrast enhancement to the parenchyma of the left kidney due to compression of left renal vein; however, the radiation risk in childhood is not negligible [14].

Controversy exists as to the treatment of nutcracker syndrome. Spontaneous resolution of hematuria in 75% of children with nutcracker syndrome followed up for 2 or more years has been reported following an increase in the body mass index (BMI) [13, 15, 16]. Surgical or radiological intervention are indicated for severe pain, significant hematuria and renal impairment, with percutaneous endovascular stent insertion being the preferred mode of therapy [17].

Children with IgA nephropathy and some of the familial hematuria syndromes (Table 12.3) can have macroscopic hematuria at the time of, or

Table 12.3 Familial hematuric disorders

Disorder	Gene(s)	Protein	Estimated risk of ESKD
X-linked Alport syndrome	*COL4A5*	α5(IV)	
Hemizygous (male)			100%
Heterozygous (female)			Up to 25%
Autosomal Alport syndrome	*COL4A3* or *COL4A4*	α3(IV) or α4(IV)	
Recessive (homozygous or compound heterozygous)			100%
Dominant			<1% if no risk factors (TBMN); ≥20% if risk factors present
Digenic Alport syndrome	*COL4A3* and *COL4A4*	α3(IV) and α4(IV)	
Mutations in trans			Up to 100%
Mutations in cis			Up to 20%
Mutations in *COL4A5* and in *COL4A3* or *COL4A4*			Up to 100% (affected males)
Autosomal dominant HANAC syndrome	*COL4A1*	α1(IV)	
Heterozygous			Unknown
Autosomal dominant MYH9 associated nephropathy	*MYH9*	Nonmuscle myosin heavy chain IIA	
Heterozygous			30%
CFHR5 nephropathy	*CFHR5*	Complement factor H-related protein 5	
Heterozygous (males)			80%
Heterozygous (females)			20%
Glomerulopathy associated with fibronectin deposition	*FN1*	Fibronectin 1	>90% between second to sixth decade

ESKD end-stage kidney disease; *TBMN* thin basement membrane nephropathy

1 or 2 days following, an upper respiratory tract infection, a phenomenon known as synpharyngitic hematuria. Some degree of accompanying proteinuria, at least at the time of intercurrent illness, is common. The urine can be normal between the bouts of gross hematuria but a considerable proportion has persistent microscopic hematuria between the attacks of gross hematuria.

Alport syndrome is a genetic disease with both gross and microscopic hematuria that is associated with high risk of progression to kidney failure before the fourth decade of life. The rate of progression to kidney failure is influenced by the type of *COL4A* mutations (*COL4A5*, *COL4A3*, *COL4A4*) affecting the α-chains of type IV collagen in the glomerular basement membrane. The inheritance pattern is most commonly X-linked, but may also be autosomal recessive or dominant. A family history of relatives with hematuria, renal failure or deafness may suggest Alport syndrome, but it must be remembered that a negative family history does not exclude Alport syndrome.

A syndrome in which hereditary angiopathy, nephropathy, aneurysms and muscle cramps (HANAC) linked to heterozygous mutations of *COL4A1* gene has been described [18]. HANAC syndrome is autosomal dominant and extremely rare. The kidney disease presents with microscopic or macroscopic hematuria. Cortical cysts and mild chronic kidney disease (CKD) have been described in adults. *COL4A1* gene mutation detection should be considered if there is hematuria in a patient with cerebral abnormalities (intracerebral aneurysm, stroke), cataracts and retinal arteriolar tortuosity.

Complement Factor H-Related 5 (CFHR5) nephropathy is endemic in the Greek Cypriot population and is extremely rare in the non-Cypriot population. It is one of the group of disorders known as C3 glomerulopathy. It is caused by a mutation of the *CFHR5* gene. Which encodes proteins that regulate the alternative complement pathway. It is characterized by low serum C3 levels but normal C4 levels, and kidney biopsy invariably shows mesangial C3 deposition. Genetic testing is required for the diagnosis.

Studies from families of Cypriot descent have shown that patients with duplication of exons two to three of the *CFHR5* gene present with hematuria, proteinuria and hypertension, with up to 50% progressing to kidney failure within 10 years of diagnosis [19].

Child with Associated Lower Urinary Tract Symptoms

Hematuria with accompanying dysuria, frequency, urgency, flank or abdominal pain may suggest a diagnosis of UTI, hypercalciuria or nephrolithiasis.

One third of UTIs have associated hematuria, though this is usually microscopic. UTIs are usually caused by bacteria, but viruses, fungi and parasites are potential etiological agents. Acute hemorrhagic cystitis is characterized by gross hematuria and symptoms of bladder inflammation. It is associated with adenovirus types 11 and 21. The macroscopic hematuria usually lasts 5 days and microscopic hematuria may persist for an additional 2–3 days [20]. Schistosomiasis is an important cause of hematuria in tropical Africa, Middle Eastern countries, Turkey, India, South-East Asia and in immigrants from these areas [21]. It is caused by swimming in lakes and ponds infested with snails infected by the flatworm *Schistosoma haematobium*. The trapped eggs of the flatworm in the bladder and lower urinary tract cause an intense granulomatous inflammatory reaction resulting in hematuria. In developing countries, tuberculosis of the urinary tract is another cause of hematuria, both microscopic and macroscopic, especially in the context of a child with prolonged ill health [22].

Nephrolithiasis is rare in children. The incidence of stone disease in children has been reported to account for between 0.13 and 0.94 cases per 1000 hospital admissions [23]. It can present with hematuria alone or hematuria with colic. Pain can be due to the presence of the stone or clots of blood passing down the ureter. An association between hematuria and hypercalciuria has been reported in children with asymptomatic macroscopic or microscopic hematuria without signs of renal stones [24]. Children with hypercalciuria can also have accompanying irritative urinary symptoms such as dysuria, frequency and urgency. These children have increased urinary excretion of calcium despite normal serum calcium levels. The urinary calcium to creatinine ratio in a single urine specimen is a useful index of calcium excretion for screening and monitoring purposes. In a large study, the 97th percentile level of urinary calcium to creatinine ratio in children eating an unrestricted diet was 0.69 mmol/mmol, whereas in infancy, it can reach as high as 2.2 mmol/mmol [25].

Child with Clinical Features of Acute Glomerulonephritis

Acute glomerulonephritis is characterized by sudden onset of macroscopic hematuria, accompanied by hypertension, oliguria, edema and varying degrees of abnormal kidney function. In children, the majority of cases of acute glomerulonephritis have a post-infectious etiology, most commonly following infection with group A β-hemolytic streptococcal infection of the throat or skin. It is important to identify acute glomerulonephritis in a child with hematuria because urgent appropriate management can prevent morbidity and mortality due to uncontrolled hypertension, fluid overload and abnormal kidney function.

Asymptomatic Child with Incidental Finding of Microscopic Hematuria on Urine Dipstick

Use of urine dipstick testing to screen for UTI in a febrile child or during routine school health examination in many countries detects asymptomatic microscopic hematuria. Mass urine screening programs of school-aged children suggest that approximately 1% will have two or more urine dipsticks positive for microscopic hematuria, but this only persists at 6 months in a third of the population [2, 3, 26]. Of those children who were subsequently referred for evaluation of persistent microscopic hematuria, a glomerular pathology was the most likely cause, occurring in between 22.2% and 52.3% based on either phase-contrast microscopy or kidney biopsy findings [27–30].

Isolated hematuria (without accompanying hypertension, significant proteinuria or abnormal kidney function) in children is traditionally regarded as benign. However, publications describing the long-term follow-up of patients who presented initially with microscopic hematuria has challenged this view. An adjusted hazard ratio of 18.5 for the development of ESKD was observed in Israeli adolescents and young adults with persistent asymptomatic isolated microscopic hematuria over a period of 22 years in a population-based retrospective cohort study [31]. A study in China involving 351 children who had undergone kidney biopsy secondary to persistent asymptomatic isolated hematuria reported increased adverse kidney events (i.e. development of proteinuria, hypertension, or abnormal kidney function) after 2–10 years of follow-up in those children with recurrent macroscopic hematuria and/or proteinuria as compared with patients with asymptomatic isolated microscopic hematuria (22.8% versus 6.0% respectively, p < 0.001) [32]. This finding suggests that microscopic hematuria, especially when accompanied by macroscopic hematuria and/or proteinuria, may be associated with unfavorable kidney outcome. While the clinical outcome for many children presenting with isolated hematuria is good, the lifetime risk of kidney disease is not insignificant and is dependent on the underlying pathology.

As microscopic hematuria and mild proteinuria may appear transiently during fever, illness or extreme exertion, it is therefore not cost-effective to subject every child to extensive investigations to elucidate the cause of microscopic hematuria. One practical approach is to repeat the urine dipstick and microscopic urinalysis twice within 2 weeks after the initial result. If the hematuria resolves, no further tests are required. If microscopic hematuria persists on at least two of the three consecutive samples, then further evaluation is required [33].

The common diagnoses in children with persistent microscopic hematuria without proteinuria are familial benign hematuria, idiopathic hypercalciuria, and IgA nephropathy. In addition, there is a group of genetically heterogenous monogenic conditions causing microscopic hematuria that may progress to ESKD, typically during adulthood. This group of familial hematuric disorders is caused by mutations in several genes (Table 12.3).

Benign familial hematuria, also known as thin basement membrane nephropathy (TBMN), is the most common cause of persistent microscopic hematuria in children, occurring in at least 1% of children worldwide [34]. It is autosomal dominant, and is frequently associated with heterozygous mutations of *COL4A3* or *COL4A4* genes. Absence of a family history does not exclude the diagnosis of TBMN because there may be a de novo mutation, the penetrance may not be complete, or family members may not be aware that they have microscopic hematuria [35]. The red blood cells in the urine are mainly dysmorphic and there may be red blood cell casts. Hearing deficits or eye abnormalities almost never occur in patients with TBMN or their family members. Universal thinning of glomerular basement membrane is seen on electron microscopy. A kidney biopsy is usually not indicated if TBMN is suspected, unless there are atypical features to suggest IgA nephropathy or Alport syndrome. The prognosis of TBMN was traditionally regarded as benign. However, it is now recognized that TBMN can be associated with an increased risk of kidney failure in adulthood, with up to 50% of patients developing various degrees of CKD after the age of 50 years [36]. TBMN is thought to be a spectrum of autosomal Alport syndrome, where the risk of progressive glomerulopathy is up to 20% in the presence of factors such as proteinuria, sensorineural deafness, family history of kidney failure and histological findings of focal segmental glomerulosclerosis, or glomerular basement membrane thickening and lamellation [37]. Hence, lifelong follow-up is recommended for children with persistent isolated microscopic hematuria due to suspected TBMN.

The better understanding of the genetic basis of diseases in recent years has prompted a better classification of familial hematuria into a number of rare glomerulopathies, such as CFHR5 nephropathy, MYH9-related disease and glomerulopathy with fibronectin deposition. The kidney outcome of these conditions is worse than was initially described for benign familial hematuria. Hence, genetic analysis in those children with family histories of hematuria and/or proteinuria or kidney failure may be considered for the early detection of these progressive, familial, hematuric disorders (Table 12.3).

One rare familial hematuric disorder is autosomal dominant MYH9-related disease, which includes Fechtner and Epstein syndromes [34, 38, 39]. Besides nephritis, these syndromes are associated with giant platelets, cytoplasmic leukocyte inclusions (Döhle-like bodies), sensorineural deafness and cataracts. The associated nephritis seen in 30–70% of patients presents initially with microscopic hematuria, with proteinuria developing as the disease progresses, and reaching ESKD in young adulthood.

Glomerulopathy with fibronectin deposition (GFND) is another rare autosomal dominant glomerulopathy characterized by microscopic hematuria, proteinuria, hypertension and massive fibronectin deposits in the mesangium and subendothelial space. GFND presents at different ages. The urinary abnormalities usually occur during the first decade of life, with progression to ESKD typically occurring in the second to sixth decade [40–42].

Clinical Approach

In approaching a child with hematuria, we should ensure that serious conditions are not missed, avoid unnecessary and expensive laboratory tests, reassure the family and provide guidelines for further studies if there is a change in the child's course. Obtaining a careful history and physical examination is the crucial first step in the evaluation.

History

It is helpful to determine the color of the urine and timing of color change related to the urinary stream. Macroscopic hematuria of glomerular origin is usually described as dark brown or cola-colored. In contrast, visible hematuria of lower urinary tract origin (bladder and urethra) is usually pink or red, there may be clots, and the blood may be only be visible at the beginning or end of the urinary stream. Hematuria at voiding onset is seen in urethral causes such as urethritis, whereas terminal hematuria is indicative of a bladder cause such as a bladder stone or tumor and schistosomiasis. Patients should be asked regarding history of recurrent gross hematuria, recent trauma or exercise, passage of urinary stones, recent or concurrent respiratory or skin infections, and intake of medications (including over-the-counter medications, calcium or vitamin D supplementation) or herbal compounds. In girls at peripubertal age, menarche as the cause of hematuria should be considered.

Associated symptoms may include fever, dysuria, urinary frequency and urgency, back pain, skin rashes, joint symptoms, and face and leg swelling. Predisposing illnesses such as sickle cell disease or trait should also be noted. The family history should search for documented hematuria, hypertension, intracerebral bleed, kidney stones, kidney failure, deafness, coagulopathy and polycystic kidney disease. In a sexually active teenager, the social history should consider any recent sexual activity and any known exposure to sexually transmitted diseases since cystitis and urethritis can present with hematuria.

Physical Examination

The presence of hypertension and edema, suggestive of acute glomerulonephritis, requires a more urgent and extensive evaluation. Associated rashes or arthritis may indicate hematuria due to systemic lupus erythematosus or nephritis due to IgA vasculitis. The presence of fever or loin pain may point to pyelonephritis. A palpable and ballotable kidney mass will require radiological investigations to exclude hydronephrosis, polycystic kidney or kidney tumor. Screening for eye and hearing abnormalities may be useful if there is a suggestive family history of familial hematuric disorders associated with progression to ESKD.

Investigations

Investigations to look for the cause of hematuria can be extensive. Tailoring the evaluation according to the type of clinical presentation reduces unnecessary laboratory and radiological investigations (Fig. 12.1). The first step is to confirm hematuria with urine microscopic examination. If the child has associated edema, hypertension, oliguria or proteinuria with hematuria, evaluation for glomerular causes such as acute glomerulonephritis or hemolytic uremic syndrome is required. If the child has associated irritative urinary symptoms, evaluation for UTI and nephrolithiasis should be considered. For children with an incidental finding of microscopic hematuria during illness or after exertion, further evaluation is required only if there is persistent microscopic hematuria on at least two of three consecutive samples. If the subsequent two urine samples do not show microscopic hematuria, the hematuria is transient and further evaluation is not required.

The next step in the evaluation of persistent hematuria is to determine the site of bleeding. Two investigations that should be done once hematuria is confirmed are urine tests for protein and urine phase contrast microscopic examination to look at the red blood cell morphology. Hematuria (gross or microscopic) associated with greater than 30% dysmorphic red blood cells, in particular acanthocytes (ring forms with vesicle-shaped protrusions) [43], and proteinuria indicate glomerular bleeding. It is important to remember that some proteinuria may also be present in non-glomerular causes of macroscopic hematuria. However, the proteinuria usually does not exceed 2+ (1 g/L) on dipstick examination if the only source of protein is from bleeding due to a non-glomerular etiology. Therefore, a child with proteinuria 2+ or more should be investigated for glomerulonephritis. Similarly, red blood cell casts, if present, are highly specific for glomerulonephritis.

A serum creatinine to estimate kidney function needs to be determined in children with glomerular pathology. If there is significant proteinuria, the serum albumin should be measured. In addition, laboratory investigations to look for the cause of glomerular disease should be performed. These investigations may include serum complements C3 and C4, anti-streptolysin O titer (ASOT) or anti-DNase B, anti-factor B antibody, anti-nuclear antibodies (ANA), anti-double-stranded DNA (dsDNA) antibody, anti-neutrophil cytoplasmic antibodies (ANCA), IgA level, hepatitis B surface antigen and viral titers if appropriate. Anti-factor B antibody levels, an autoantibody targeting factor B (a component of the alternative pathway C3 convertase), is highly specific for post-infectious glomerulonephritis [44]. Serum IgA levels are increased in 30–50% of adult patients, but in only 8–16% of children with IgA nephropathy [45]. In countries where IgA nephropathy is an important cause of glomerulonephritis, 10–35% of children undergoing kidney biopsy for isolated hematuria were found to have IgA nephropathy [45, 46].

The clinical presentation is important in deciding the type of investigations required. For example, a preceding sore throat, pyoderma or impetigo and the presence of edema, hypertension and proteinuria are suggestive of post-streptococcal glomerulonephritis. Serum ASOT, anti-DNase B and complement C3 levels would suffice in this case. If these tests are not informative, then further investigations are warranted to rule out other causes of glomerulonephritis. If a familial hematuric disorder is suspected, an audiological examination may be useful to detect high frequency sensorineural hearing deficit associated with Alport syndrome. If suspicion of X-linked Alport syndrome is high, skin biopsy with immunostaining for the α5(IV) chain can be useful. The presence of macrothrombocytopenia with or without basophilic cytoplasmic leukocyte inclusion bodies (Döhle-like bodies) suggests

12 Hematuria and Proteinuria

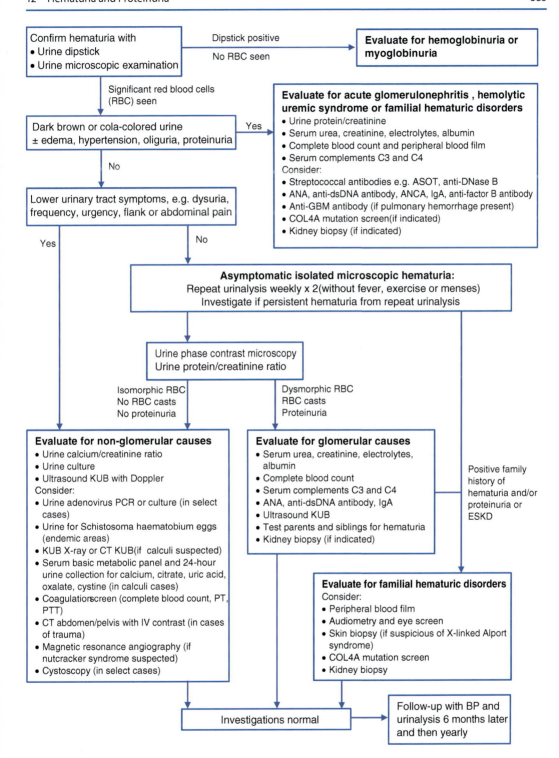

Fig. 12.1 Algorithm for investigating hematuria

MYH9-related diseases [39]. The utility of kidney ultrasonography for evaluation of the asymptomatic child with microscopic hematuria of glomerular origin remains unproven [47]. However, it may be useful to determine the size of the kidneys as a guide to chronicity in patients with evidence of progressive kidney disease, and to diagnose polycystic kidneys in the presence of a suggestive family history.

Hematuria associated with mainly isomorphic red blood cells, together with absence of red blood cell casts and proteinuria, indicate a nonglomerular cause. Urine calcium to creatinine ratio is performed to rule out hypercalciuria. In endemic areas, urine should be examined after sedimentation for *Schistosoma haematobium* eggs, especially during the day when excretion is highest. Ultrasound of the kidneys and bladder is indicated to exclude hydronephrosis, kidney calculi, tumor or cystic kidney disease. A plain abdominal x-ray may be necessary to exclude ureteric stones. If a urinary tract calculus is identified, a complete assessment of the urinary constituents associated with stone risk is needed. If the investigations reveal the presence of tumor, structural urogenital abnormality or urinary calculus, a urological referral is required. A coagulation screen may be necessary when there is a family history of bleeding diathesis. Computed tomography scan of the abdomen and pelvis may be required if there is a history of abdominal trauma followed by gross hematuria. If the nutcracker syndrome is suspected in a thin child with recurrent gross hematuria, Doppler sonography assessing the left renal vein diameter and peak velocity is a useful diagnostic tool. When Doppler renal vein ultrasonography is not diagnostic, axial imaging by computed tomography or magnetic resonance imaging may be required.

Cystoscopy may also be required in cases of children with recurrent nonglomerular macroscopic hematuria of unknown cause. Cystoscopy in children seldom reveals the cause of hematuria, but should be done when preliminary investigations have failed to find a cause, and bladder or urethral pathology is a consideration because of accompanying voiding symptoms. Vascular malformations in the bladder have been detected via cystoscopy. In the rare instance when a bladder mass is noted on ultrasound, cystoscopy is also indicated. Cystoscopy to lateralize the source of bleeding is best performed during active bleeding.

An asymptomatic child with an incidental finding of persistent microscopic hematuria often poses the greatest dilemma regarding the extent of investigations and subsequent follow-up. The most common diagnoses in children with persistent microscopic hematuria without proteinuria and hypertension are TBMN, idiopathic hypercalciuria, IgA nephropathy and Alport syndrome. It is therefore worthwhile to screen family members for microscopic hematuria. If the parents are found to have incidental asymptomatic microscopic hematuria without proteinuria and kidney failure, TBMN is the most likely cause. More extensive evaluation is then not necessary. However, it is important that these patients are followed up yearly to detect proteinuria, which is an indication of progressive kidney disease. When proteinuria is present, these patients need to undergo further evaluation, including genetic analysis for the relevant mutations associated with the familial hematuric disorders. In communities where post-infectious glomerulonephritis is common, subclinical disease is also a common cause of persistent microscopic hematuria.

Indications for Kidney Biopsy

Kidney biopsy is usually not indicated in isolated glomerular hematuria. Kidney biopsy should be considered in the following cases of hematuria associated with:

- Significant proteinuria, except in poststreptococcal glomerulonephritis
- Persistent low serum complement C3
- Unexplained azotemia
- Systemic diseases such as systemic lupus erythematosus or ANCA-associated vasculitis
- Family history of significant kidney disease suggestive of progressive forms of familial hematuric disorders including Alport syndrome

- Recurrent gross hematuria of unknown etiology where investigations are suggestive of a glomerular pathology
- Persistent glomerular hematuria where the parents are anxious about the diagnosis and prognosis.

With recent improvements in understanding the molecular genetics of the familial hematuric disorders, genetic testing, if available and affordable, can sometimes contribute useful diagnostic and prognostic information and may even obviate the need for a kidney biopsy [48].

Proteinuria

It is well-established that proteinuria is a mediator of progressive kidney insufficiency in both adults and children [49–51], as well as a risk factor for cardiovascular disease [52, 53]. Conversely, proteinuria can also be a transient finding in children, occurring during times of stress, including exercise, fever and dehydration, and does not denote kidney disease.

Renal Handling of Proteins

Plasma proteins can cross the normal glomerular filtration barrier. The ability of these proteins to cross the glomerular filtration barrier is related primarily to the molecular size and charge. The larger plasma proteins, such as globulins, are virtually excluded from the normal glomerular filtrate. Smaller proteins, mostly of low molecular weight (LMW; <40,000 Dalton), are filtered across the glomerular filtration barrier. Molecular charge plays an important role in determining glomerular permeability to macromolecules. This is due to the presence of negatively charged sialoproteins that line the surfaces of both the glomerular endothelial and epithelial cells, and glycosaminoglycans present in the glomerular basement membrane. Hence, negatively charged molecules are less able to cross the glomerulus than neutral molecules of identical size. On the other hand, positively charged molecules have enhanced clearances.

In health, albumin is the most abundant protein in serum and constitutes about 40% of the filtered urinary protein despite being anionic and molecular weight of 67,000 Dalton. The rest of the urinary proteins are immunoglobulins, peptides, enzymes, hormones and partially degraded plasma proteins. After crossing the glomerular barrier, 71% of the filtered proteins are reabsorbed by the proximal tubule, 23% by the loop of Henle and 3% by the collecting duct. The quantity of urinary proteins excreted results from a balance between the amount of these proteins filtered and the amount reabsorbed.

Under normal conditions, approximately 60% of protein in urine is filtrate of plasma protein and 40% is of kidney origin. This is a heterogeneous group of proteins, many of which are glycoproteins. Some are derived from cells lining the urinary tract and have the potential of being important diagnostic indicators. The major protein in this group is Tamm-Horsfall protein or uromodulin, which is a major constituent of urinary casts [54]. Adults excrete 30–60 mg/day. It is secreted mainly in the thick ascending limb of the loop of Henle.

Excessive urinary protein losses can be due to the following mechanisms:

- **Glomerular proteinuria:** Increased permeability of the glomerular basement membrane due to structural defects of the membrane, loss of its negative charges or damage by immune complexes or other mediators. This leads to increased filtration of macromolecules, especially albumin, across the glomerular filtration barrier
- **Tubular proteinuria:** Impaired reabsorption of normally filtered LMW proteins (e.g. α-1 microglobulin, β-2 microglobulin, retinol binding protein) by the proximal tubule
- **Secretory proteinuria:** Increased secretion of tissue proteins into the tubules, most notably Tamm-Horsfall protein in interstitial nephritis
- **Overflow proteinuria:** Marked overproduction of LMW proteins (e.g. myoglobin),

than 2200 mg/1.73 m²/day or albumin-to-creatinine ratio greater than 220 mg/mmol or 2200 mg/g [55].

With regards to using urinary albumin or protein excretion in the classification of children with CKD, variations in the definition of abnormal urinary albumin or protein excretion based on age must be taken into account. Abnormal urinary protein excretion in children should also consider the possibility of tubular versus glomerular proteinuria, depending on the underlying disease. Urinary albumin excretion rate may be normal in tubular proteinuria. Hence, in children, the quantification of total protein, as compared to the albumin only fraction, may be the preferred method of assigning risk in relation to the presence of urinary protein.

The KDIGO 2012 guidelines recommended a urinary total protein or albumin excretion rate above the normal value for age be used for children and adolescents [55]. Table 12.5 shows the categories of persistent albuminuria and proteinuria to be used in the classification of CKD. Albuminuria is classified into normal to mildly increased, moderately increased and severely increased. However, in children, urine protein-to-creatinine ratio is the preferred test, followed by albuminuria, and lastly by automated reagent strips for detection of proteinuria. This is because the vast majority of children have underlying congenital anomalies of the kidney and urinary tract, unlike in adults, where the etiology of CKD is more commonly an underlying glomerular disease such as diabetic nephropathy or hypertensive damage. The use of albumin excretion may therefore be less sensitive for diagnostic purposes in children, as those with underlying tubular conditions will tend to excrete more Tamm-Horsfall protein and other LMW proteins.

Urine Dipstick

The urine dipstick is an excellent screening test for the presence of proteinuria [64]. The dipstick is impregnated with the dye tetrabromophenol blue buffered to pH 3.5. At a constant pH, binding of protein to this dye results in the development of a blue color in proportion to the amount of protein present. If urine is protein-free, the dipstick is yellow. The color of the dipstick changes through yellow-green, to green, to a green-blue with increasing concentrations of protein. The dipstick can be read as negative, trace, 1+, 2+, 3+ and 4+, which corresponds to insignificant, less than 0.2 g/L, 0.3 g/L, 1 g/L, 3 g/L and greater than 20 g/L concentrations, respectively.

The dipstick test has a few limitations. Observer error can occur during interpretation of the color of the dipstick. False positive and false negative tests can occur. If the dipstick is kept in

Table 12.5 Categories of albuminuria in chronic kidney disease [55]

Investigation	Categories		
	Normal to mildly increased (A1)	Moderately increased (A2)	Severely increased (A3)
Albumin excretion rate (mg/1.73 m²/24 h)	<30	30–300	>300
Protein excretion rate (mg/1.73 m²/24 h)	<150	150–500	>500
Albumin:creatinine ratio (ACR)			
(g/mmol)	<0.003	0.003–0.030	>0.030
(mg/mmol)	<3	3–30	>30
(mg/g)	<30	30–300	>300
Protein:creatinine ratio (PCR)			
(g/mmol)	<0.015	0.015–0.050	>0.050
(mg/mmol)	<15	15–50	>50
(mg/g)	<150	150–500	>500
Protein reagent strip	Negative to trace	Trace to +	+ or greater

12 Hematuria and Proteinuria

the urine too long, the buffer may leach out and a false positive test may result. False positive tests for protein can also occur in the presence of gross hematuria, pyuria and bacteriuria or if the urine is contaminated with antiseptics such as chlorhexidine or benzalkonium, which are often used for skin cleansing prior to clean catch of the urine. False positive results may occur with urine specimens after the administration of radiographic contrast or with ingestion of certain medications, including penicillins, cephalosporins, tolbutamide or sulfonamides.

The result of the dipstick test can be affected by the concentration of the urine. If the urine is very dilute, the urinary protein concentration may be reduced to a level below the sensitivity of the dipstick (0.1–0.15 g/L), even in patients excreting up to 1 g of protein per day. Hence, a negative dipstick should be interpreted with caution if the urine specific gravity is less than 1.002. In contrast, if the urine specific gravity is greater than 1.025, a healthy child can register trace of protein on the dipstick, resulting in a false positive result. The dipstick test for protein can also be affected by the pH of the urine. Very alkaline urine (pH greater than 8.0) can cause a false positive result while very acid urine (pH less than 4.5) can cause a false negative result.

False negative results occur in non-albumin proteinuria. Albumin binds better to the dye than other proteins. Hence, the urine dipstick primarily detects albumin, leaving LMW proteins undetected. The dipstick results correlate better with albuminuria than with proteinuria. However, though the dipstick is more specific for albumin, it lacks the sensitivity to detect microalbuminuria associated with early glomerular injury seen in diabetic nephropathy or cardiovascular disease. A negative dipstick test for protein does not exclude the presence in the urine of low concentrations of globulins, mucoproteins or Bence-Jones protein.

Sulfosalicylic Acid Test

An alternative method to measure urine protein in patients with questionable proteinuria by dip-

Table 12.6 Sulfosalicylic acid test

Grade	Appearance	Protein concentration (g/L)
0	No turbidity	0
Trace	Slight turbidity	0.01–0.1
1+	Turbidity through which print can be read	0.15–0.3
2+	White cloud without precipitate through which heavy black lines on a white background can be seen	0.4–1
3+	White cloud with precipitate through which heavy black lines cannot be seen	1.5–3.5
4+	Flocculent precipitate	>5

stick in the office is the sulfosalicylic acid precipitation of protein in urine. This technique provides a more quantitative estimate of all the proteins present in the urine, including both albumin and the LMW proteins. This test is performed by mixing one part urine supernatant with three parts 3% sulfosalicylic acid, and the resultant turbidity is then graded, as shown in Table 12.6 [65]. As with the urine dipstick, iodinated radiocontrast agents can cause a false positive result; hence, the urine should not be tested for at least 24 h after a contrast study.

Quantification of Proteinuria: 24-h Urine Specimen Versus Spot Urine Specimen

The results obtained with urine dipstick and with quantitative 24-h protein excretion methods correlate fairly well in most situations. As mentioned earlier, the dipstick is more sensitive to albumin, whereas quantitative methods detect all proteins, including globulin and LMW protein. For example, in multiple myeloma, large amounts of protein are excreted and yet the urine dipstick for protein is negative. Hence, quantitative urinary protein measurement is necessary in this case. A more important reason why quantitative measurement of protein loss in the urine should be done is to determine whether the patient requires a more extensive evaluation. For example, many patients with a dipstick reading of 1+ protein have a normal quantitative result and additional evaluation is not indicated.

Quantification of proteinuria has traditionally demanded timed urine collection. Urinary protein excretion in adults is usually measured in a 24-h urine collection. This is more accurate than a spot urine protein analysis. However, 24-h urine collection poses logistical problems with timing and volume measurements, especially in young children who have yet to achieve continence at night. In this case, a 12-h urine collection can be done, and the protein excretion rate is then extrapolated to a 24-h value by using the appropriate correction factor.

The other method is to obtain a single voided urine sample. The concentrations of both protein and creatinine are measured in the urine sample and protein levels are expressed per unit of creatinine. The advantages of this method include not requiring timed urine samples and not having to correct for body size. The assumption is creatinine excretion is directly related to body mass and is relatively constant throughout the day. Many studies have found that the amount of protein excreted in a 24-h urine correlates extremely well with the protein-to-creatinine ratio measured in random urine samples [66, 67].

What remains debatable is whether early morning urine samples or random urine samples obtained during normal activities during the day are better indicators of kidney disease. The urine protein-to-creatinine ratio is higher in urine samples obtained in a person in an upright position than in a recumbent position, a phenomenon known as orthostatic proteinuria [59]. Studies that included subjects with normal kidney function as well as those with kidney failure have shown that urine protein-to-creatinine ratios from daytime samples correlated better with 24-h urine protein excretion values than did values from early morning samples [59]. Conversely, early morning samples had better correlation when data were evaluated from normal subjects and from those with kidney disease but normal glomerular filtration rates [68]. In subjects with kidney disease and orthostatic proteinuria, daytime urine protein-to-creatinine ratios can be misleading. Hence, in the evaluation of children with possible kidney disease, the first morning urine specimen is recommended for urine protein-to-creatinine ratio quantification to eliminate the effect of posture. In general, the 24-h urine collection for protein excretion is ideal as the initial diagnostic investigation, with the exception of children who have yet to achieve continence; whereas, the first morning spot urine protein-to-creatinine ratio is useful to monitor progress of proteinuria.

An important consideration when interpreting spot urine protein-to-creatinine ratio is a falsely elevated urine protein-to-creatinine ratio, which can occur when there is low creatinine excretion in children with very low muscle mass (e.g. neuromuscular disorders). The spot urine protein-to-creatinine ratio can be underestimated when there is a very concentrated urine sample with high creatinine level in the urine. One method to avoid overestimation or underestimation is to send spot urine sample for both protein-to-creatinine ratio as well as urinalysis, with the expectation that significant proteinuria will be present in both examinations.

The spot urine protein-to-osmolality ratio has been suggested as another convenient method for estimating urine protein excretion without a 24-h urine collection and to overcome the problem of low creatinine excretion in children with very low muscle mass. Compared to urine creatinine concentration, urine osmolality, which is a direct measure of degree of urine concentration, may thus have advantages of a methodology to standardize normal protein excretion on a random sample. Data describing the normal range of urine protein-to-osmolality ratios have been published for adults [69]. However, the results in the pediatric population differ from the adult population. In the pediatric population, urine protein-to-creatinine ratio was superior to urine protein-to-osmolality ratio for predicting abnormal amounts of proteinuria in children and adolescents [70]. Dilanthi et al. reported that urine protein-to-creatinine ratio (sensitivity 100%, specificity 94%) was more sensitive than urine protein-to-osmolality ratio (sensitivity 85.7%, specificity 100%) in detecting children with mild proteinuria [71]. Hence, using spot urine protein-to-osmolality as an alternative method to estimate 24-h urine protein excretion in children is not widely practiced. If spot urine protein-to-osmolality ratio is used, it is important to remember that high urine osmolality due to glycosuria can cause an underestimation of the protein-to-osmolality ratio. Glycosuria should be excluded prior to assessment of protein-to-osmolality ratio in a spot urine sample.

The dipstick, Multistix® PRO (Bayer, Elkhart, Ind., USA), is able to analyze concentrations of both urinary protein and creatinine semi-quantitatively in only 60 s and is commercially available. The semi-quantitative urine protein-to-creatinine ratio by Multistix® PRO correlated well with both quantitative urine protein-to-creatinine ratio and daily urinary protein excretion [72, 73], and use of the Multistix® PRO would avoid errors and difficulties associated with timed urine collection. It may become a useful tool to monitor the urinary protein excretion in children with kidney diseases in the outpatient setting.

Clinical Scenarios

Proteinuria can be symptomatic (presenting with edema) or asymptomatic, which can be intermittent or persistent.

Child with Edema

Proteinuria associated with edema can be due to nephrotic syndrome, nephritic syndrome or kidney failure. Nephrotic syndrome is defined as heavy proteinuria that is severe enough to cause hypoalbuminemia, edema and hypercholesterolemia. Nephrotic range proteinuria is defined as greater than 40 mg/m²/h or greater than 3 g/1.73 m²/day for timed urine collection, or random urine protein-to-creatinine ratio of greater than 0.22 g/mmol (220 mg/mmol or 2200 mg/g) [64]. The evaluation and management of a child presenting with nephrotic syndrome, nephritic syndrome or kidney failure is different from that of a child with intermittent or persistent proteinuria without edema. Nephrotic syndrome, nephritic syndrome and kidney failure are discussed elsewhere in the book.

Child with Intermittent Proteinuria

In intermittent proteinuria, protein is detectable in only some of the urine samples collected. This may be related to posture or occur at random.

Frequently, intermittent proteinuria is not related to posture. It may be found after exercise or in association with stress, seizures, dehydration or fever. It may occur on a random basis for which there is no obvious cause. This is also known as transient proteinuria, which is defined as proteinuria noted on 1 or 2 occasions, but not present on subsequent testing, especially when the inciting factor remits or is removed. A large proportion of healthy children may have an occasional urine sample with proteinuria. This is rarely associated with significant kidney disease.

Orthostatic (postural) proteinuria is defined as elevated protein excretion when the subject is upright, but normal protein excretion during recumbency. This occurs commonly in adolescents, with a prevalence of 2–5% [74]. The diagnosis is suggested by a normal protein-to-creatinine ratio in a first morning spot urine sample after the subject has been supine for the entire night, but an elevated protein-to-creatinine ratio after the subject has been upright for at least 4–6 h. Total urine protein excretion rarely exceeds 1 g/1.73 m²/day in orthostatic proteinuria. A study of healthy Turkish children aged 6–15 years old found that the prevalence of orthostatic proteinuria was lower than previous literature if at least three random urine samples at least 2 weeks apart were taken to exclude transient proteinuria [75]. For continuing assessment of proteinuria after the third sample, the first morning urine sample was collected. In this study, the prevalence of proteinuria was 3.7%, 1.3% and 0.94% on the first, second and third samples, respectively and the prevalence of orthostatic proteinuria was 0.65% after the first morning urine collection. This study also suggested that underweight children had a tendency for orthostatic proteinuria compared with overweight and obese children [75].

The postulated causes of orthostatic proteinuria are alterations in kidney or glomerular hemodynamics, circulating immune complexes and partial left renal vein entrapment, as may be seen in thin individuals [76]. The incidence of orthostatic proteinuria decreases with advancing age, possibly due to the gradual accumulation of retroperitoneal fat. Long-term studies where patients have been followed for up to 50 years have documented the benign nature of orthostatic proteinuria, although rare cases of glomerulosclerosis have been identified later in life in patients who were initially diagnosed to have orthostatic proteinuria [77, 78]. No treatment is required for children with orthostatic proteinuria. It has been recommended that children with orthostatic proteinuria should be followed up annually [79].

It is important to remember that patients with glomerular disease may have an orthostatic component to their proteinuria. Protein excretion in these patients is greater when they are active or upright than when they are resting. Hence, orthostatic proteinuria should not be diagnosed unless the recumbent urine sample is normal.

Child with Persistent Proteinuria

Persistent proteinuria is defined as proteinuria of 1+ or more by dipstick on multiple occasions. This should be further investigated. Subjects who have persistent proteinuria, especially if this is associated with additional evidence of kidney disease such as microscopic hematuria, are more likely to have significant pathology in the urinary tract. In the Japanese school screening study, which looked at almost five million children, the prevalence of persistent isolated proteinuria was 0.07% in the 6–11-year age group, and this rose to 0.37% in the 12–14 year age group [27].

The majority of cases of persistent proteinuria are of glomerular origin, though non-glomerular mechanisms can also cause marked proteinuria (Table 12.7).

Glomerular proteinuria may be due to the following factors:

Table 12.7 Causes of proteinuria in children

Intermittent proteinuria	Persistent proteinuria	
	Glomerular	Tubular
Non-postural	Primary glomerulopathies	Hereditary
Fever	Minimal change disease	Cystinosis
Exercise	Focal segmental glomerulosclerosis	Galactosemia
Seizures	Membranoproliferative	Tyrosinemia
Emotional stress	glomerulonephritis	Hereditary fructose intolerance
Dehydration	Membranous nephropathy	Wilson disease
No known cause	Rapidly progressive glomerulonephritis	Lowe syndrome
Postural	Congenital nephrotic syndrome	Mitochondrial cytopathies
(Orthostatic)	Secondary glomerulopathies	Dent's disease
	Post-infectious glomerulonephritis	Polycystic kidney disease
	Lupus nephritis	Acquired
	IgA nephropathy	Pyelonephritis
	IgA vasculitis nephritis	Tubulointerstitial nephritis
	Alport syndrome	Acute tubular necrosis
	Hepatitis B nephropathy	Analgesic abuse
	Hepatitis C nephropathy	Drugs such as penicillamine
	Human immunodeficiency virus (HIV) nephropathy	Heavy metal poisoning (e.g., lead, cadmium, gold, mercury)
	Amyloidosis	Vitamin D intoxication
	Hemolytic uremic syndrome	
	Diabetes mellitus	
	Hypertension	
	Hyperfiltration following nephron loss	
	Reflux nephropathy	

- Increase in glomerular permeability to plasma proteins in residual nephrons in cases where there is reduction in nephron mass. This mechanism probably explains the increased proteinuria seen in patients with reflux nephropathy, progressive kidney disease reaching end-stage and the increased proteinuria observed in kidney transplant donors [80].
- Loss of negative charge in the glomerular filtration barrier [81, 82]. This results in mostly albuminuria. There is little increase in glomerular permeability to globulins;hence, the proteinuria is highly selective. A typical example is minimal change disease.
- Direct injury to the glomerular filtration barrier. The glomerular capillary wall consists of three structural components that form the permselectivity barrier: the endothelial cells, glomerular basement membrane and podocytes. The podocyte is crucial for maintenance of the glomerular filter, and disruption of the epithelial slit diaphragm leads to proteinuria [83]. These changes have been demonstrated in patients with nephrotic syndrome irrespective of the primary disease. Such injury increases the "effective pore size" in the glomeruli, causing an increase in the permeability of the mechanical barriers to the filtration of proteins. Hence, there is an increase in filtration of albumin and also larger proteins such as globulins. The clearance of globulins is relatively high and the proteinuria is described as non-selective.
- Mutations of key podocyte genes. Mutations of genes involved in regulation of the slit diaphragm proteins and their interaction with the actin cytoskeleton also result in proteinuria.
- Changes in glomerular capillary pressure due to disease and resulting in increased filtration fraction [49, 50, 84]. Examples are increased filtration fraction in hyperreninemia and hyperfiltration in the early stages of diabetic nephropathy.

The increased filtered load of protein overwhelms the tubular reabsorptive mechanisms; hence, the excess protein appears in the urine.

Glomerular proteinuria can be classified as selective or nonselective. In selective proteinuria, there is a predominance of LMW proteins such as albumin or transferrin, as compared to higher molecular weight proteins such as IgG. The selectivity index is expressed as the clearance ratio of IgG over albumin or transferrin. An index less than 0.1 is indicative of highly selective proteinuria [85, 86], and this is seen in steroid-sensitive nephrotic syndrome and Finnish-type congenital nephrotic syndrome. More recent studies have shown that there is a significant relationship between selectivity of proteinuria and tubulointerstitial damage in kidney disease [87]. When proteinuria is highly selective, tubulointerstitial damage is less common.

Non-glomerular mechanisms include tubular proteinuria, overflow proteinuria and secretory proteinuria. Tubular proteinuria results when there is damage to the proximal convoluted tubule, which normally reabsorbs most of the filtered protein. The amount of protein in the urine due to tubular damage is usually not large and does not exceed more than 1 g/1.73 m^2/day. Glomerular and tubular proteinuria can be distinguished by protein electrophoresis of the urine. The primary protein in glomerular proteinuria is albumin, whereas in tubular proteinuria the LMW proteins migrate primarily in the α and β regions. β2-microglobulin, α1-microglobulin and retinol-binding protein are the markers commonly used for identification of tubular proteinuria [88]. Children with proximal tubulopathies such as Lowe syndrome and Dent's disease have tubular proteinuria. Albuminuria may eventually be detected in many tubulopathies as a marker of late glomerular involvement.

Overflow proteinuria results when the concentration of filterable proteins in the glomerular filtrate exceeds the maximal tubular reabsorption capability for that protein. This can occur even with normal renal function. Examples include monoclonal gammopathy of undetermined significance or multiple myeloma in adults (immunoglobulin light chains or Bence-Jones protein), hemoglobinuria, myoglobinuria, β2-microglobulinemia, myelomonocytic leukemia and even following transfusions. After multiple transfusions of either albumin or whole blood, plasma albumin concentration may increase sufficiently to cause albuminuria.

In secretory proteinuria, the increased excretion of tissue proteins into the urine may result in proteinuria. The typical example is excretion of Tamm-Horsfall protein in the neonatal period, accounting for the higher levels of protein excretion typically seen at this age. In UTIs, mild proteinuria may be detected due to irritation of the urinary tract and increased secretion of tissue proteins into the urine. Secretory proteinuria also occurs in analgesic nephropathy and inflammation of the accessory sex glands.

Clinical Approach to Proteinuria

The finding of proteinuria in a single urine specimen in children and adolescents is relatively common. In large school screening programs, the prevalence of isolated proteinuria on a single urine ranged from 1.2 to 15% [2, 28, 89]. Persistent proteinuria on repeated urine testing is much less common [75]. When proteinuria is detected, it is important to determine whether it is intermittent, especially orthostatic, or persistent. It is also important to exclude kidney failure and acute nephritic or nephrotic syndrome because these conditions demand urgent investigations and treatment.

History

It is important to ask about any recent illness. Inquire about symptoms of CKD (e.g. polyuria, nocturia, pruritus, lethargy) or glomerulonephritis (e.g. edema, hematuria, oliguria), and connective tissue disorders (e.g. rashes, joint pain). A history of recurrent UTIs may suggest reflux nephropathy. Medications that are associated with proteinuria include non-steroidal anti-inflammatory medications, antibiotics (e.g. penicillin, sulfonamides, cephalosporins, quinolones, aminoglycosides), amphotericin B, cisplatin, allopurinol, and herbal medicines. A family history of polycystic kidney disease, hematuria, pro-

teinuria, nephrotic syndrome, kidney failure or deafness should be obtained.

Physical Examination

Examination may reveal evidence of CKD such as growth failure, pallor from anemia, and rickets from metabolic bone disease. Hypertension is common in CKD. The presence of raised jugular venous pressure, hepatomegaly and edema suggest the child may be fluid overloaded due to acute nephritic syndrome or severe kidney functional impairment, and thus require urgent diuresis. Nephrotic syndrome may cause generalized edema, ascites, pleural effusion and scrotal edema. Associated signs of systemic illnesses, such as palpable purpuric rash on the lower limbs suggesting IgA vasculitis nephritis (Henoch Schönlein purpura) and joint swelling suggesting connective tissue disorders, should be sought. Palpable flank masses may suggest hydronephrosis or polycystic kidney disease.

Investigations

Isolated proteinuria is benign in the vast majority of children and can be transient and postural; hence, it is inappropriate to extensively investigate all children found to have proteinuria. A step-by-step approach is recommended to evaluate isolated proteinuria in an asymptomatic child or a child with an incidental finding of urine dipstick protein 1+ or 2+ during an acute illness. However, if the child has signs and symptoms suggestive of kidney disease, a detailed investigation should start promptly. Similarly, if the initial urine dipstick shows the presence of hematuria and proteinuria, detailed evaluation for kidney disease should be performed. Microscopic hematuria is the most common indicator of a glomerular lesion in a proteinuric patient. The existence of hematuria with proteinuria carries a more serious connotation than isolated proteinuria. Investigations including kidney biopsy of school children with persistent hematuria and proteinuria have found that 25–60% had evidence of a glomerulopathy [29, 90], especially in those with proteinuria greater than 1 g/L. [29]

The first step in the evaluation of a child with isolated proteinuria is to determine whether the proteinuria is persistent (Fig. 12.2). Most children who have proteinuria on screening urine dipstick do not have kidney disease, and the proteinuria will resolve on repeat testing [27]. If proteinuria of 1+ or more persists on two subsequent dipstick tests at weekly intervals, further investigations are required. If proteinuria is absent on subsequent testing, the initial proteinuria may be transient and related to fever, vigorous exercise or emotional stress, and no further investigations are required. The parents and patient should be reassured and, as a precaution, a urine dipstick test for protein can be repeated in 3–6 months. If proteinuria on dipstick recurs or is persistent, the next step is to quantify the amount of proteinuria.

There are two methods to quantify proteinuria, spot urine protein-to-creatinine ratio and 24-h urinary total protein collection. An early morning spot urine protein-to-creatinine ratio is recommended to exclude orthostatic proteinuria. In orthostatic proteinuria, the first morning urine sample is negative for protein and the later urine samples may contain varying concentrations of protein, whereas the 24-h urinary total protein is normal or mildly elevated. If orthostatic proteinuria is strongly suspected, one way to prove this is to provide the family with urine dipsticks. The child's urine is tested twice daily for 1 week. The family should test the first urine sample voided in the morning and the last urine sample voided in the evening before the child sleeps. It is important that the bladder is completely emptied before going to sleep, and the child remains supine in bed throughout the night so that the early morning urine sample on awakening consists of urine formed in the recumbent position. The evening urine sample consists of urine formed in the upright position. If the urine dipstick is persistently negative in the morning and positive in the evening, orthostatic proteinuria is likely. No further investigations are required, and the urine should be rechecked for proteinuria yearly as a precaution.

If spot urine protein-to-creatinine ratio is more than 0.02 g/mmol (20 mg/mmol or 0.2 mg/mg), it is advisable to confirm the presence of significant proteinuria with a 24-h urinary total protein collection. After excluding transient and orthostatic proteinuria, and if the 24-h urinary total protein is greater than 0.3 g/1.73 m^2/day, it is useful to evaluate for kidney disease. Urinary protein excretion less than 0.3 g/1.73 m ^{2}/day is associated with regression of proteinuric chronic nephropathies [91], suggesting that investigations are only necessary above this level. The suggested work-up includes the following:

Urine Examination

Microscopic examination of the fresh urine sample for blood, casts and crystals is required. A clean catch urine sample for culture may be necessary to rule out occult UTI, especially if there is a history of recurrent fevers in infancy. If a tubular disorder or interstitial nephritis is suggested from the history or urinary findings of eosinophils, measurement of the urinary excretion of β2-microglobulin, α1-microglobulin and retinol-binding protein, markers of tubular proteinuria, can be helpful. Tubular proteinuria is suspected if the urinary excretion of β2-microglobulin, α1-microglobulin and retinol-binding protein exceeds 0.04, 2.2 and 0.024 mg/mmol creatinine or 4×10^{-4}, 0.022 and 2.4×10^{-4} mg/mg creatinine, respectively [88].

Blood Examination

Assess the kidney function with serum urea, creatinine and electrolytes. Creatinine clearance or application of an estimating formula such as the revised Schwartz formula [92] gives a more accurate assessment of kidney function than serum creatinine alone. A reduction in kidney function is one of the most important indications for a kidney biopsy. Serum total protein and albumin should be checked. Most proteinuric patients do not have decreased serum levels of protein or albumin unless they have nephrotic syndrome or they have heavy proteinuria for a significant period. Hypoproteinemia may be an indication for kidney biopsy. In addition, serum cholesterol

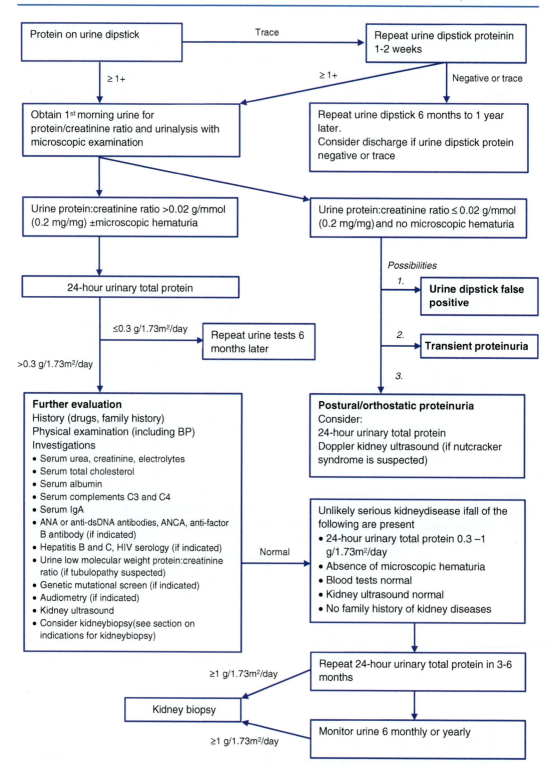

Fig. 12.2 Algorithm for investigating proteinuria

is measured as an indicator of the presence hyperlipidemia, which is suggestive of nephrotic syndrome.

Serum levels of C3 and C4 should be checked routinely as this may provide evidence of glomerulonephritis. Decreased C3 and C4 levels are seen in systemic lupus erythematosus, while decreased C3 with normal C4 levels occurs in post-infectious glomerulonephritis or C3 glomerulopathies, including membranoproliferative glomerulonephritis. Anti-factor B antibody levels, an autoantibody targeting factor B (a component of the alternative pathway C3 convertase), is highly specific for post-infectious glomerulonephritis, distinguishing it from C3 glomerulopathy [44]. ANA, anti-dsDNA antibodies, IgA levels, anti-streptolysin O titers (ASOT) or anti-DNase B titers, ANCA, hepatitis B, hepatitis C and human immunodeficiency virus (HIV) serology should be considered if the clinical setting and preliminary investigations are suggestive, as these may give a clue to the underlying etiology of the proteinuria. In addition, appropriate mutational screening should be considered if a hereditary disorder for the proteinuria or nephrotic syndrome is suspected.

Kidney Imaging

Kidney ultrasonography is done routinely in the evaluation of isolated proteinuria to identify anatomical abnormalities of the kidneys or urinary tract as these can result in reduction of nephron mass. A significant difference in the sizes of the kidneys may suggest underlying reflux nephropathy or renal dysplasia. If reflux nephropathy is suspected, a DMSA scan is useful to demonstrate the existence of renal scars. Doppler kidney ultrasonography is helpful if the patient has co-existing hypertension as proteinuria can occur in hypertensive nephropathy due to renal artery stenosis. In patients with orthostatic proteinuria, Doppler sonography of the left renal vein may be a useful screening tool to exclude the nutcracker syndrome [93].

Audiometry

Audiometry is indicated when there is a family history of nephritis, kidney failure or deafness. Deafness may be detected during later childhood in Alport syndrome, and is generally associated with progressive kidney disease.

If these urine and blood tests as well as the initial kidney ultrasound are normal, and if the proteinuria is less than 1 g/1.73 m^2/day, it is unlikely that the child has a serious kidney disease. The family should therefore be reassured that the proteinuria may disappear or it may persist without any evidence of progressive kidney failure developing. As the level of proteinuria is associated with outcome in chronic nephropathies [49, 91, 94], it is also important to emphasize to the family that follow-up urine tests are necessary. The child should be reviewed in 3–6 months. If the repeat test shows that the proteinuria is not marked (i.e., less than 1 g/1.73 m^2/day), the child's urine is then monitored twice during the subsequent year and yearly thereafter. If there is persistent significant proteinuria on follow-up, a kidney biopsy may be indicated.

Indications for Kidney Biopsy

Kidney biopsy is indicated in the following situations:

- Persistent significant proteinuria of more than 1 g/1.73 m^2/day [95] or random urine protein-to-creatinine ratio of >0.05 g/mmol (>50 mg/mmol, >0.5 g/g) [96]. The heavier the proteinuria, the more likely a tissue diagnosis will be obtained from the kidney biopsy. A study on kidney biopsies in Japanese children with asymptomatic, persistent, isolated proteinuria showed that a 41.4% probability of significant glomerular changes, such as focal segmental glomerulosclerosis, when using a urine protein-to-creatinine ratio > 50 mg/mmol (0.5 g/g) as a biopsy criterion [96]. The exception is the child with typical steroid sensitive nephrotic syndrome suggestive of minimal change disease, where kidney biopsy is not indicated at presentation.
- Proteinuria associated with urinary sediment abnormalities (e.g. hematuria). Kidney biopsy is more likely to be diagnostic when proteinuria is associated with urinary sediment abnor-

they may impair the final stages of kidney maturation, and therefore should be avoided before a corrected post-conceptual age of 44 weeks [112].

Aliskiren, the first orally active direct renin inhibitor, has shown promising results in proteinuria reduction in adult patients with CKD [113]. In a case series of four children treated with aliskiren for refractory proteinuria, three children experienced clinically significant adverse effects, including symptomatic hypotension, hyperkalemia and accelerated loss of kidney function [114]. Hence, clinicians should exercise caution when prescribing aliskiren until appropriate pediatric trials establish dosing, efficacy and safety.

Conclusion

Hematuria or proteinuria in children is frequently encountered. Many investigations have been recommended in the workup for a child presenting with hematuria or proteinuria. Many of the cases of hematuria or proteinuria are normal transient findings. Hence, a stepwise evaluation is recommended to avoid unnecessary and expensive investigations, but identify children with serious conditions. There is an increasing role of genetic testing to establish a clinical diagnosis of hereditary causes of kidney disease. Early detection and treatment of serious conditions should hopefully delay or prevent the onset of kidney functional abnormalities. Screening programs for hematuria and proteinuria may be able to identify children at an earlier stage; however, the major disadvantage is the cost effectiveness, as well as the anxiety in parents and children when the finding is spurious or transient.

References

1. Glassock R. Hematuria and pigmenturia. In: Massry SG, Glassock RJ, editors. Textbook of nephrology. Baltimore: Williams & Wilkins; 1989. p. 491–5.
2. Dodge WF, West EF, Smith EH, Bruce H 3rd. Proteinuria and hematuria in schoolchildren: epidemiology and early natural history. J Pediatr. 1976;88(2):327–47.
3. Vehaskari VM, Rapola J, Koskimies O, Savilahti E, Vilska J, Hallman N. Microscopic hematuria in school children: epidemiology and clinicopathologic evaluation. J Pediatr. 1979;95(5 Pt 1):676–84.

4. Fairley KF, Birch DF. Microscopic urinalysis in glomerulonephritis. Kidney Int Suppl. 1993;42:S9–12.
5. Pollock C, Liu PL, Györy AZ, Grigg R, Gallery ED, Caterson R, et al. Dysmorphism of urinary red blood cells—value in diagnosis. Kidney Int. 1989;36(6):1045–9.
6. Schramek P, Moritsch A, Haschkowitz H, Binder BR, Maier M. In vitro generation of dysmorphic erythrocytes. Kidney Int. 1989;36(1):72–7.
7. Shichiri M, Hosoda K, Nishio Y, Ogura M, Suenaga M, Saito H, et al. Red-cell-volume distribution curves in diagnosis of glomerular and non-glomerular haematuria. Lancet. 1988;1(8591):908–11.
8. Ito CA, Pecoits-Filho R, Bail L, Wosiack MA, Afinovicz D, Hauser AB. Comparative analysis of two methodologies for the identification of urinary red blood cell casts. J Bras Nefrol. 2011;33(4):402–7.
9. Abarbanel J, Benet AE, Lask D, Kimche D. Sports hematuria. J Urol. 1990;143(5):887–90.
10. Pham PT, Pham PC, Wilkinson AH, Lew SQ. Renal abnormalities in sickle cell disease. Kidney Int. 2000;57(1):1–8.
11. Hohenfellner M, Steinbach F, Schultz-Lampel D, Schantzen W, Walter K, Cramer BM, et al. The nutcracker syndrome: new aspects of pathophysiology, diagnosis and treatment. J Urol. 1991;146(3):685–8.
12. Mazzoni MB, Kottanatu L, Simonetti GD, Ragazzi M, Bianchetti MG, Fossali EF, et al. Renal vein obstruction and orthostatic proteinuria: a review. Nephrol Dial Transplant. 2011;26(2):562–5.
13. Okada M, Tsuzuki K, Ito S. Diagnosis of the nutcracker phenomenon using two-dimensional ultrasonography. Clin Nephrol. 1998;49(1):35–40.
14. Cho BS, Suh JS, Hahn WH, Kim SD, Lim JW. Multidetector computed tomography findings and correlations with proteinuria in nutcracker syndrome. Pediatr Nephrol. 2010;25(3):469–75.
15. Tanaka H, Waga S. Spontaneous remission of persistent severe hematuria in an adolescent with nutcracker syndrome: seven years' observation. Clin Exp Nephrol. 2004;8(1):68–70.
16. Shin JI, Park JM, Lee SM, Shin YH, Kim JH, Lee JS, et al. Factors affecting spontaneous resolution of hematuria in childhood nutcracker syndrome. Pediatr Nephrol. 2005;20(5):609–13.
17. Venkatachalam S, Bumpus K, Kapadia SR, Gray B, Lyden S, Shishehbor MH. The nutcracker syndrome. Ann Vasc Surg. 2011;25(8):1154–64.
18. Plaisier E, Gribouval O, Alamowitch S, Mougenot B, Prost C, Verpont MC, et al. COL4A1 mutations and hereditary angiopathy, nephropathy, aneurysms, and muscle cramps. N Engl J Med. 2007;357(26):2687–95.
19. Athanasiou Y, Voskarides K, Gale DP, Damianou L, Patsias C, Zavros M, et al. Familial C3 glomerulopathy associated with CFHR5 mutations: clinical characteristics of 91 patients in 16 pedigrees. Clin J Am Soc Nephrol. 2011;6(6):1436–46.
20. Mufson MA, Belshe RB, Horrigan TJ, Zollar LM. Cause of acute hemorrhagic cystitis in children. Am J Dis Child. 1973;126(5):605–9.

21. Summer AP, Stauffer W, Maroushek SR, Nevins TE. Hematuria in children due to schistosomiasis in a nonendemic setting. Clin Pediatr (Phila). 2006;45(2):177–81.
22. Altintepe L, Tonbul HZ, Ozbey I, Guney I, Odabas AR, Cetinkaya R, et al. Urinary tuberculosis: ten years' experience. Ren Fail. 2005;27(6):657–61.
23. Polinsky MS, Kaiser BA, Baluarte HJ, Gruskin AB. Renal stones and hypercalciuria. Adv Pediatr Infect Dis. 1993;40:353–84.
24. Stapleton FB, Roy S 3rd, Noe HN, Jerkins G. Hypercalciuria in children with hematuria. N Engl J Med. 1984;310(21):1345–8.
25. Shaw NJ, Wheeldon J, Brocklebank JT. Indices of intact serum parathyroid hormone and renal excretion of calcium, phosphate, and magnesium. Arch Dis Child. 1990;65(11):1208–11.
26. Kitagawa T. Lessons learned from the Japanese nephritis screening study. Pediatr Nephrol. 1988;2(2):256–63.
27. Murakami M, Yamamoto H, Ueda Y, Murakami K, Yamauchi K. Urinary screening of elementary and junior high-school children over a 13-year period in Tokyo. Pediatr Nephrol. 1991;5(1):50–3.
28. Yap HK, Quek CM, Shen Q, Joshi V, Chia KS. Role of urinary screening programmes in children in the prevention of chronic kidney disease. Ann Acad Med Singap. 2005;34(1):3–7.
29. Lin CY, Hsieh CC, Chen WP, Yang LY, Wang HH. The underlying diseases and follow-up in Taiwanese children screened by urinalysis. Pediatr Nephrol. 2001;16(3):232–7.
30. Cho BS, Kim SD, Choi YM, Kang HH. School urinalysis screening in Korea: prevalence of chronic renal disease. Pediatr Nephrol. 2001;16(12):1126–8.
31. Vivante A, Afek A, Frenkel-Nir Y, Tzur D, Farfel A, Golan E, et al. Persistent asymptomatic isolated microscopic hematuria in Israeli adolescents and young adults and risk for end-stage renal disease. JAMA. 2011;306(7):729–36.
32. Feng CY, Xia YH, Wang WJ, Xia J, Fu HD, Wang X, et al. Persistent asymptomatic isolated hematuria in children: clinical and histopathological features and prognosis. World J Pediatr. 2013;9(2):163–8.
33. Diven SC, Travis LB. A practical primary care approach to hematuria in children. Pediatr Nephrol. 2000;14(1):65–72.
34. Deltas C, Pierides A, Voskarides K. Molecular genetics of familial hematuric diseases. Nephrol Dial Transplant. 2013;28(12):2946–60.
35. Buzza M, Wilson D, Savige J. Segregation of hematuria in thin basement membrane disease with haplotypes at the loci for Alport syndrome. Kidney Int. 2001;59(5):1670–6.
36. Carasi C, Van't Hoff WG, Rees L, Risdon RA, Trompeter RS, Dillon MJ. Childhood thin GBM disease: review of 22 children with family studies and long-term follow-up. Pediatr Nephrol. 2005;20(8):1098–105.
37. Kashtan CE, Ding J, Garosi G, Heidet L, Massella L, Nakanishi K, et al. Alport syndrome: a unified classification of genetic disorders of collagen IV α345: a position paper of the Alport Syndrome Classification Working Group. Kidney Int. 2018;93(5):1045–51.
38. Seri M, Pecci A, Di Bari F, Cusano R, Savino M, Panza E, et al. MYH9-related disease: May-Hegglin anomaly, Sebastian syndrome, Fechtner syndrome, and Epstein syndrome are not distinct entities but represent a variable expression of a single illness. Medicine (Baltimore). 2003;82(3):203–15.
39. Han KH, Lee H, Kang HG, Moon KC, Lee JH, Park YS, et al. Renal manifestations of patients with MYH9-related disorders. Pediatr Nephrol. 2011;26(4):549–55.
40. Strøm EH, Banfi G, Krapf R, Abt AB, Mazzucco G, Monga G, et al. Glomerulopathy associated with predominant fibronectin deposits: a newly recognized hereditary disease. Kidney Int. 1995;48(1):163–70.
41. Castelletti F, Donadelli R, Banterla F, Hildebrandt F, Zipfel PF, Bresin E, et al. Mutations in FN1 cause glomerulopathy with fibronectin deposits. Proc Natl Acad Sci U S A. 2008;105(7):2538–43.
42. Ohtsubo H, Okada T, Nozu K, Takaoka Y, Shono A, Asanuma K, et al. Identification of mutations in FN1 leading to glomerulopathy with fibronectin deposits. Pediatr Nephrol. 2016;31(9):1459–67.
43. Köhler H, Wandel E, Brunck B. Acanthocyturia—a characteristic marker for glomerular bleeding. Kidney Int. 1991;40(1):115–20.
44. Chauvet S, Berthaud R, Devriese M, Mignotet M, Vieira Martins P, Robe-Rybkine T, et al. Anti-Factor B Antibodies and Acute Postinfectious GN in Children. J Am Soc Nephrol. 2020;31(4):829–40.
45. Yoshikawa N, Iijima K, Ito H. IgA nephropathy in children. Nephron. 1999;83(1):1–12.
46. Coppo R, Gianoglio B, Porcellini MG, Maringhini S. Frequency of renal diseases and clinical indications for renal biopsy in children (report of the Italian National Registry of Renal Biopsies in Children). Group of Renal Immunopathology of the Italian Society of Pediatric Nephrology and Group of Renal Immunopathology of the Italian Society of Nephrology. Nephrol Dial Transplant. 1998;13(2):293–7.
47. Feld LG, Meyers KE, Kaplan BS, Stapleton FB. Limited evaluation of microscopic hematuria in pediatrics. Pediatrics. 1998;102(4):E42.
48. Gale DP. How benign is hematuria? Using genetics to predict prognosis. Pediatr Nephrol. 2013;28(8):1183–93.
49. Ruggenenti P, Perna A, Mosconi L, Pisoni R, Remuzzi G. Urinary protein excretion rate is the best independent predictor of ESRF in non-diabetic proteinuric chronic nephropathies. "Gruppo Italiano di Studi Epidemiologici in Nefrologia" (GISEN). Kidney Int. 1998;53(5):1209–16.
50. Remuzzi G, Ruggenenti P, Benigni A. Understanding the nature of renal disease progression. Kidney Int. 1997;51(1):2–15.

51. Wingen AM, Fabian-Bach C, Schaefer F, Mehls O. Randomised multicentre study of a low-protein diet on the progression of chronic renal failure in children. European Study Group of Nutritional Treatment of Chronic Renal Failure in Childhood. Lancet. 1997;349(9059):1117–23.

52. Grimm RH Jr, Svendsen KH, Kasiske B, Keane WF, Wahi MM. Proteinuria is a risk factor for mortality over 10 years of follow-up. MRFIT Research Group. Multiple Risk Factor Intervention Trial. Kidney Int Suppl. 1997;63:S10–4.

53. Kannel WB, Stampfer MJ, Castelli WP, Verter J. The prognostic significance of proteinuria: the Framingham study. Am Heart J. 1984;108(5):1347–52.

54. Kumar S, Muchmore A. Tamm-Horsfall protein—uromodulin (1950-1990). Kidney Int. 1990;37(6):1395–401.

55. Chapter 1: Definition and classification of CKD. Kidney Int Suppl. 2013;3(1):19–62.

56. Rademacher ER, Sinaiko AR. Albuminuria in children. Curr Opin Nephrol Hypertens. 2009;18(3):246–51.

57. Jones CA, Francis ME, Eberhardt MS, Chavers B, Coresh J, Engelgau M, et al. Microalbuminuria in the US population: third National Health and Nutrition Examination Survey. Am J Kidney Dis. 2002;39(3):445–59.

58. Bangstad HJ, Dahl-Jørgensen K, Kjaersgaard P, Mevold K, Hanssen KF. Urinary albumin excretion rate and puberty in non-diabetic children and adolescents. Acta Paediatr. 1993;82(10):857–62.

59. Houser MT, Jahn MF, Kobayashi A, Walburn J. Assessment of urinary protein excretion in the adolescent: effect of body position and exercise. J Pediatr. 1986;109(3):556–61.

60. Amin R, Turner C, van Aken S, Bahu TK, Watts A, Lindsell DR, et al. The relationship between microalbuminuria and glomerular filtration rate in young type 1 diabetic subjects: the Oxford Regional Prospective Study. Kidney Int. 2005;68(4):1740–9.

61. Nguyen S, McCulloch C, Brakeman P, Portale A, Hsu CY. Being overweight modifies the association between cardiovascular risk factors and microalbuminuria in adolescents. Pediatrics. 2008;121(1):37–45.

62. Csernus K, Lanyi E, Erhardt E, Molnar D. Effect of childhood obesity and obesity-related cardiovascular risk factors on glomerular and tubular protein excretion. Eur J Pediatr. 2005;164(1):44–9.

63. Brem AS. Neonatal hematuria and proteinuria. Clin Perinatol. 1981;8(2):321–32.

64. Hogg RJ, Portman RJ, Milliner D, Lemley KV, Eddy A, Ingelfinger J. Evaluation and management of proteinuria and nephrotic syndrome in children: recommendations from a pediatric nephrology panel established at the National Kidney Foundation conference on proteinuria, albuminuria, risk, assessment, detection, and elimination (PARADE). Pediatrics. 2000;105(6):1242–9.

65. Rose B. Pathophysiology of renal disease. 2nd ed. New York: McGraw-Hill; 1987.

66. Elises JS, Griffiths PD, Hocking MD, Taylor CM, White RH. Simplified quantification of urinary protein excretion in children. Clin Nephrol. 1988;30(4):225–9.

67. Ginsberg JM, Chang BS, Matarese RA, Garella S. Use of single voided urine samples to estimate quantitative proteinuria. N Engl J Med. 1983;309(25):1543–6.

68. Yoshimoto M, Tsukahara H, Saito M, Hayashi S, Haruki S, Fujisawa S, et al. Evaluation of variability of proteinuria indices. Pediatr Nephrol. 1990;4(2):136–9.

69. Wilson DM, Anderson RL. Protein-osmolality ratio for the quantitative assessment of proteinuria from a random urinalysis sample. Am J Clin Pathol. 1993;100(4):419–24.

70. Morgenstern BZ, Butani L, Wollan P, Wilson DM, Larson TS. Validity of protein-osmolality versus protein-creatinine ratios in the estimation of quantitative proteinuria from random samples of urine in children. Am J Kidney Dis. 2003;41(4):760–6.

71. Hewa Warawitage Dilanthi GAMK, Subhashinie Jayasena, Dellabada Batawalage Dulani Lakmali Samaranayake, Eresha Jasinge, Vithanage Pujitha Wickramasinghe. Assessment of the validity of protein-osmolality ratio in a randomly collected urine specimen in the estimation of proteinuria in children. J Postgrad Inst Med. 2016;3(E35):1–12.

72. Kaneko K, Someya T, Nishizaki N, Shimojima T, Ohtaki R, Kaneko K. Simplified quantification of urinary protein excretion using a novel dipstick in children. Pediatr Nephrol. 2005;20(6):834–6.

73. Guy M, Newall R, Borzomato J, Kalra PA, Price C. Use of a first-line urine protein-to-creatinine ratio strip test on random urines to rule out proteinuria in patients with chronic kidney disease. Nephrol Dial Transplant. 2009;24(4):1189–93.

74. Sebestyen JF, Alon US. The teenager with asymptomatic proteinuria: think orthostatic first. Clin Pediatr (Phila). 2011;50(3):179–82.

75. Arslan Z, Koyun M, Erengin H, Akbaş H, Aksoy GK, Çomak E, et al. Orthostatic proteinuria: an overestimated phenomenon? Pediatr Nephrol. 2020;35(10):1935–40.

76. Vehaskari VM. Mechanism of orthostatic proteinuria. Pediatr Nephrol. 1990;4(4):328–30.

77. Berns JS, McDonald B, Gaudio KM, Siegel NJ. Progression of orthostatic proteinuria to focal and segmental glomerulosclerosis. Clin Pediatr (Phila). 1986;25(3):165–6.

78. Springberg PD, Garrett LE Jr, Thompson AL Jr, Collins NF, Lordon RE, Robinson RR. Fixed and reproducible orthostatic proteinuria: results of a 20-year follow-up study. Ann Intern Med. 1982;97(4):516–9.

79. Viteri B, Reid-Adam J. Hematuria and proteinuria in children. Pediatr Rev. 2018;39(12):573–87.

80. Rizvi SA, Naqvi SA, Jawad F, Ahmed E, Asghar A, Zafar MN, et al. Living kidney donor follow-up in a dedicated clinic. Transplantation. 2005;79(9):1247–51.
81. Chang RL, Deen WM, Robertson CR, Brenner BM. Permselectivity of the glomerular capillary wall: III. Restricted transport of polyanions. Kidney Int. 1975;8(4):212–8.
82. Takahashi S, Watanabe S, Wada N, Murakami H, Funaki S, Yan K, et al. Charge selective function in childhood glomerular diseases. Pediatr Res. 2006;59(2):336–40.
83. Kriz W, Kretzler M, Provoost AP, Shirato I. Stability and leakiness: opposing challenges to the glomerulus. Kidney Int. 1996;49(6):1570–4.
84. Ruggenenti P, Remuzzi G. The role of protein traffic in the progression of renal diseases. Annu Rev Med. 2000;51:315–27.
85. Joachim GR, Cameron JS, Schwartz M, Becker EL. SELECTIVITY OF PROTEIN EXCRETION IN PATIENTS WITH THE NEPHROTIC SYNDROME. J Clin Invest. 1964;43(12):2332–46.
86. Cameron JS, White RH. SELECTIVITY OF PROTEINURIA IN CHILDREN WITH THE NEPHROTIC SYNDROME. Lancet. 1965;1(7383):463–5.
87. Bazzi C, Petrini C, Rizza V, Arrigo G, D'Amico G. A modern approach to selectivity of proteinuria and tubulointerstitial damage in nephrotic syndrome. Kidney Int. 2000;58(4):1732–41.
88. Bergón E, Granados R, Fernández-Segoviano P, Miravalles E, Bergón M. Classification of renal proteinuria: a simple algorithm. Clin Chem Lab Med. 2002;40(11):1143–50.
89. Vehaskari VM, Rapola J. Isolated proteinuria: analysis of a school-age population. J Pediatr. 1982;101(5):661–8.
90. Hisano S, Ueda K. Asymptomatic haematuria and proteinuria: renal pathology and clinical outcome in 54 children. Pediatr Nephrol. 1989;3(3):229–34.
91. Ruggenenti P, Schieppati A, Remuzzi G. Progression, remission, regression of chronic renal diseases. Lancet. 2001;357(9268):1601–8.
92. Schwartz GJ, Muñoz A, Schneider MF, Mak RH, Kaskel F, Warady BA, et al. New equations to estimate GFR in children with CKD. J Am Soc Nephrol. 2009;20(3):629–37.
93. Park SJ, Lim JW, Cho BS, Yoon TY, Oh JH. Nutcracker syndrome in children with orthostatic proteinuria: diagnosis on the basis of Doppler sonography. J Ultrasound Med. 2002;21(1):39–45. quiz 6
94. Perna A, Remuzzi G. Abnormal permeability to proteins and glomerular lesions: a meta-analysis of experimental and human studies. Am J Kidney Dis. 1996;27(1):34–41.
95. Bergstein JM. A practical approach to proteinuria. Pediatr Nephrol. 1999;13(8):697–700.
96. Hama T, Nakanishi K, Shima Y, Mukaiyama H, Togawa H, Tanaka R, et al. Renal biopsy criterion in children with asymptomatic constant isolated proteinuria. Nephrol Dial Transplant. 2012;27(8):3186–90.
97. Korkmaz E, Lipska-Ziętkiewicz BS, Boyer O, Gribouval O, Fourrage C, Tabatabaei M, et al. ADCK4-associated glomerulopathy causes adolescence-onset FSGS. J Am Soc Nephrol. 2016;27(1):63–8.
98. Park E, Kang HG, Choi YH, Lee KB, Moon KC, Jeong HJ, et al. Focal segmental glomerulosclerosis and medullary nephrocalcinosis in children with ADCK4 mutations. Pediatr Nephrol. 2017;32(9):1547–54.
99. Atmaca M, Gulhan B, Korkmaz E, Inozu M, Soylemezoglu O, Candan C, et al. Follow-up results of patients with ADCK4 mutations and the efficacy of CoQ10 treatment. Pediatr Nephrol. 2017;32(8):1369–75.
100. Atmaca M, Gülhan B, Atayar E, Bayazıt AK, Candan C, Arıcı M, et al. Long-term follow-up results of patients with ADCK4 mutations who have been diagnosed in the asymptomatic period: effects of early initiation of CoQ10 supplementation. Turk J Pediatr. 2019;61(5):657–63.
101. Feng C, Wang Q, Wang J, Liu F, Shen H, Fu H, et al. Coenzyme Q10 supplementation therapy for 2 children with proteinuria renal disease and ADCK4 mutation: case reports and literature review. Medicine (Baltimore). 2017;96(47):e8880.
102. Williams JD, Coles GA. Proteinuria—a direct cause of renal morbidity? Kidney Int. 1994;45(2):443–50.
103. Kasiske BL, Lakatua JD, Ma JZ, Louis TA. A meta-analysis of the effects of dietary protein restriction on the rate of decline in renal function. Am J Kidney Dis. 1998;31(6):954–61.
104. Jureidini KF, Hogg RJ, van Renen MJ, Southwood TR, Henning PH, Cobiac L, et al. Evaluation of long-term aggressive dietary management of chronic renal failure in children. Pediatr Nephrol. 1990;4(1):1–10.
105. Uauy RD, Hogg RJ, Brewer ED, Reisch JS, Cunningham C, Holliday MA. Dietary protein and growth in infants with chronic renal insufficiency: a report from the Southwest Pediatric Nephrology Study Group and the University of California. San Francisco Pediatr Nephrol. 1994;8(1):45–50.
106. Ellis D, Vats A, Moritz ML, Reitz S, Grosso MJ, Janosky JE. Long-term antiproteinuric and renoprotective efficacy and safety of losartan in children with proteinuria. J Pediatr. 2003;143(1):89–97.
107. Wühl E, Trivelli A, Picca S, Litwin M, Peco-Antic A, Zurowska A, et al. Strict blood-pressure control and progression of renal failure in children. N Engl J Med. 2009;361(17):1639–50.
108. van den Belt SM, Heerspink HJL, Gracchi V, de Zeeuw D, Wühl E, Schaefer F. Early proteinuria lowering by angiotensin-converting enzyme inhibition predicts renal survival in children with CKD. J Am Soc Nephrol. 2018;29(8):2225–33.
109. Tabacova S. Mode of action: angiotensin-converting enzyme inhibition—developmental effects asso-

ciated with exposure to ACE inhibitors. Crit Rev Toxicol. 2005;35(8–9):747–55.

110. Lee GJ, Cohen R, Chang AC, Cleary JP. Angiotensin Converting Enzyme Inhibitor (ACEI)-induced acute renal failure in premature newborns with congenital heart disease. J Pediatr Pharmacol Ther. 2010;15(4):290–6.

111. Gantenbein MH, Bauersfeld U, Baenziger O, Frey B, Neuhaus T, Sennhauser F, et al. Side effects of angiotensin converting enzyme inhibitor (captopril) in newborns and young infants. J Perinat Med. 2008;36(5):448–52.

112. Dionne JM, Abitbol CL, Flynn JT. Hypertension in infancy: diagnosis, management and outcome. Pediatr Nephrol. 2012;27(1):17–32.

113. Persson F, Rossing P, Reinhard H, Juhl T, Stehouwer CD, Schalkwijk C, et al. Renal effects of aliskiren compared with and in combination with irbesartan in patients with type 2 diabetes, hypertension, and albuminuria. Diabetes Care. 2009;32(10):1873–9.

114. Kelland EE, McAuley LM, Filler G. Are we ready to use aliskiren in children? Pediatr Nephrol. 2011;26(3):473–7.

Steroid Sensitive Nephrotic Syndrome

13

Elisabeth M. Hodson, Deirdre Hahn,
Stephen I. Alexander, Nicole Graf,
and Hugh McCarthy

Abbreviations

APN	Arbeitsgemeinschaft für Pädiatrische Nephrologie
BMC	Bone mineral content
BMD	Bone mineral density
BMI	Body mass index
CI	Confidence intervals
CNI	Calcineurin inhibitor
DXA	Dual energy x-ray absorptiometry
ESKD	End stage kidney disease
FRNS	Frequently relapsing steroid sensitive nephrotic syndrome
FSGS	Focal and segmental glomerulosclerosis
GFR	Glomerular filtration rate
HR	Hazard ratio
ISKDC	International Study of Kidney Disease in Children
KDIGO	Kidney Disease Improving Global Outcomes
MCD	Minimal change disease
MesPGN	Mesangial proliferative glomerulonephritis
MMF	Mycophenolate mofetil
MPA	Mycophenolic acid
RCT	Randomized controlled trial
RR	Relative risk
SDNS	Steroid dependent steroid sensitive nephrotic syndrome
SDS	Standard deviation score
SIRS	Soluble immune response suppressor
SLE	Systemic lupus erythematosus
SRNS	Steroid resistant nephrotic syndrome

E. M. Hodson (✉)
Department of Nephrology and Centre for Kidney Research, The Children's Hospital at Westmead, Sydney, Australia

Sydney School of Public Health, University of Sydney, Sydney, Australia
e-mail: elisabeth.hodson@health.nsw.gov.au

D. Hahn · S. I. Alexander
Department of Nephrology and Centre for Kidney Research, The Children's Hospital at Westmead, Sydney, Australia

Discipline of Paediatrics, University of Sydney, Sydney, Australia
e-mail: deirdre.hahn@health.nsw.gov.au;
stephen.alexander@sydney.edu.au

N. Graf
Department of Histopathology, The Children's Hospital at Westmead, Sydney, Australia

Discipline of Pathology, University of Sydney, Sydney, Australia

School of Medicine, University of Western Sydney, Sydney, Australia
e-mail: nicole.graf@health.nsw.gov.au

H. McCarthy
Departments of Nephrology, Sydney Children's Hospitals Network, Sydney, Australia

School of Women's and Children's Health, University of New South Wales, Sydney, Australia
e-mail: hugh.mccarthy@health.nsw.gov.au

© The Author(s), under exclusive license to Springer Nature Switzerland AG 2023
F. Schaefer, L. A. Greenbaum (eds.), *Pediatric Kidney Disease*,
https://doi.org/10.1007/978-3-031-11665-0_13

onstrated a key role for local VEGF in maintaining glomerular endothelial integrity and again reinforced its importance though perhaps more locally in maintaining permeability [27, 28]. Soluble immune response suppressor (SIRS) was also identified as a potential protein mediating nephrotic syndrome but again the inability to characterize this protein despite many mechanistic observations led to its exclusion as the likely factor [23, 24, 29]. Other circulating factors have been proposed and the development of a functional assay of glomerular permeability by Dr. Savin in the late 1990s identified a proteinuric factor that was small, highly glycosylated, and hydrophobic [30]. This appeared to be likely to allow fractionation of nephrotic sera and identification of the factor. Other observations that protein A columns could remove the nephrotic factor post-transplant also seemed to point to identifying features [31]. More recently induction of proteinuria in rats with transfer of serum may allow models that can identify this factor as has the demonstration that overexpression of the Th2 cytokine IL-13 induces proteinuria in rats [32]. Recently podocyte-secreted angiopoietin-like-4 was found to mediate proteinuria in SSNS using overexpression in the podocyte in rat models though further confirmatory studies are awaited [33].

The central role of T cells in disease has led to a number of strategies to identify the underlying defect. The thought that the disease was caused by a low frequency pathogenic clone has given way to a view that there is a generalized alteration in the lymphocytes that is triggered in these individuals and then can be switched off by treatment. This has been studied in several ways including assessment of T cell derived cytokine responses either directly in plasma or by measurement of supernatants from activated mononuclear cells or measurement of RNA, assessment of T cell subsets by immuno-phenotyping or finally by functional assays of cell mediated immunity. More recently the identification of a role for micro-RNAs in FSGS affecting WT1 or more recently CD2AP in nephrotic syndrome suggested this may be a fruitful area of research [34, 35].

Phenotypes of Cytokine Secreting T Cells: Th1, Th2, Treg, Th17

Naïve T cells on activation become polarized into different subsets defined by their cytokine production and driven by the cytokine milieu in which they are activated. The initial division of T cells was into CD4 (originally helper) T cells, that respond to exogenous antigen presented by antigen presenting cells in the context of MHC Class II, and CD8 (originally effector) T cells that respond to internal antigens presented by all cells. CD4 T cells were further divided into Th1 and Th2 cells based on the cytokines they produced [36]. This was initially observed in mice but human Th1 cells also produce cytokines such as IFN-gamma and TNF, which are used in cell mediated immune responses. Th2 cells produce IL-4, IL-5 and IL-13 which are key to humoral immunity and are used by B cells to class switch and act as growth factors for eosinophils [37, 38]. It is now apparent that CD8 T cells can produce cytokines and can be polarized to Tc1 and Tc2 expressing similar cytokines to those in CD4 Th cell subsets [39]. The observation that allergy is more common in children with nephrotic syndrome suggested that this might be a Th2 disease [18]. A subset of T cells thought to suppress activity in other T cells was originally described as suppressor T cells and these have recently been reclassified as regulatory T cells. These are thymically derived and express regulatory cytokines such as TGF-β and IL-10 and express regulatory molecules such as CTLA-4. A key marker of these cells is the expression of the transcription factor foxp3 [40–42]. Interestingly there is now another T cell subset that is an alternative to regulatory T cells called the Th17 cell because it expresses the cytokine IL-17. Th17 cells are induced by IL-23 but can be generated by IL-6 and TGF-ß thus acting as an alternate pathway of development to regulatory T cells [42, 43]. There are now data linking Th17 cells to nephrotic syndrome and the biological effect of these cells on podocytes [44, 45].

In general, studies of cytokines have been disappointing. No clear up-regulation of Th2 type cytokines has been demonstrated. Studies of serum of patients in remission show IL-1 unchanged, IL-2 normal or undetected in four of five studies, sIL-2R increased in four of six studies, IFN-gamma normal or not detected in three and increased in two studies, IL-4 normal or decreased, IL-8 normal, increased and decreased in four studies, IL-10, IL-12 and IL-13 either normal or not detected and TNF-β normal in three of four studies [46]. Studies of culture supernatants of stimulated mononuclear cells from children with active SSNS are also highly variable though four studies suggest elevated IL-4, two studies elevated IL-12, and five studies elevated TNF-α. RNA measurements for specific cytokines in blood have been equally unrewarding as have those using intracellular cytokine staining [46]. Urinary reports are confounded by concurrent proteinuria but there has been a recent report of IL-17 increased in the urine of patients with SSNS [22, 47]. Other non-T cell inflammatory proteins associated with SSNS include neopterin which is produced by activated macrophages and is increased in SSNS [48].

Genetic Influence in the Aetiology of SSNS

Significant research effort over recent years has identified over 50 genes linked to SRNS [49] with the majority coding for proteins in the podocytes which control function and stability of the actin cytoskeleton. In stark contrast, almost no genes have been identified that have a Mendelian influence on the development of SSNS. This is despite the known ethnic variation in prevalence, familial clustering and a history of affected first degree relatives previously reported at 3% [50, 51]. Similarly to IgA Nephropathy, any genetic influence is likely mediated through complex inheritance of risk alleles in multiple genes.

Initial investigation of complex inheritance focused solely on HLA genes and identified possible association with HLA-DQ/DR. Further studies using exome wide association [52] and then genome wide association studies (GWAS) [53–56] confirmed that association across European, African, South Asian and Japanese cohorts. Through the use of HLA imputation, HLA haplotypes that confer maximum risk and also those that confer protection can be derived. Interestingly, while these were reproducible across the European and South Asian cohorts, Japanese cohorts had differing haplotypes [53–56]. The use of GWAS to study Membranous Nephropathy enabled identification of a non-HLA locus at PLA2R1 which has been incredibly informative in understanding disease pathology. In SSNS non-HLA loci have been identified (BTNL2, CALHM6/DSE, PARM1, TNFSF15 and NPHS1) but the signals are not as strong and to date are not clearly reproducible across all ethnic groups but cohort size has been relatively small [53, 55, 56]. The pathological mechanism by which an HLA haplotype may confer risk in SSNS has not yet been clearly elucidated and while it is likely to be related to the association with CD4 positive T cells, further work utilising new molecular tools may prove highly valuable [57].

Role of the Thymus

The information above, the association of nephrotic syndrome with T cell lymphomas and thymomas, the timing of thymic involution occurring around puberty at the same time as the resolution of relapses for the majority of children with uncomplicated SSNS, and the exquisite sensitivity of thymocytes to steroids all suggest a role for early T cells or other thymically derived cells in SSNS. Further evidence of early thymic emigrants in single cell analysis of CD2 positive cells from children with FSGS also supports a role for T cells, which are early emigrants from the thymus.

Role of Infection

While there has been no clear infectious agent identified as inducing nephrotic syndrome, there is an identifiable viral prodrome in around 50% of cases of relapse. Whether this merely reflects cytokine release with the initiation of nephrotic syndrome or whether this is initiation of the disease by a viral trigger is not clear. Some groups have postulated that inflammation through TLRs may upregulate CD80 on podocytes leading to activation though CD80 and nephrosis [58]. There has also been interest in CD80 as a therapeutic target in resistant nephrotic syndrome [59].

Summary

While the evidence supports a role for T cells activated to secrete a permeability factor, identifying the specific T cell changes or characterization of the factor remains a major challenge in SSNS. The clinical results with rituximab in depleting B cells, and the data on CD80 expression on podocytes raises other alternatives as potential causes of SSNS including circulating cells other than T cells and specific podocyte responses, but there are limited data so far on these pathways.

Histopathology

Steroid sensitive nephrotic syndrome comprises a spectrum of disease that includes MCD, MesPGN (also known as "diffuse mesangial hypercellularity"), IgM nephropathy and FSGS. Although these are readily distinguished on biopsy, the clinical significance of this distinction remains controversial with significant overlap in behaviour and variation in morphological diagnosis over time in a small proportion of cases. This confusion is reflected in the literature. Some studies suggest a difference in behaviour between those with and without mesangial hypercellularity in the absence of immune deposits [60]. Some studies suggest an increased risk of steroid resistance and/or development of focal sclerosing lesions with MesPGN/IgM nephropathy [61, 62] with some studies documenting transition of MCD, MesPGN and IgM nephropathy to FSGS in frequently relapsing patients over time [17, 63]. In addition some studies suggest

that the response to therapy in cases with immune deposition is "unpredictable" [64] or variable [65], and finally a number of studies have failed to find any significant difference in outcomes between these categories [66, 67]. Histological overlap also exists with MCD, MesPGN and FSGS in patients with predominant mesangial deposition of C1q (C1q nephropathy), although representing a small minority of patients with initial presentation of clinical nephrotic syndrome [68–70]. Similarly, mesangial IgA deposition in association with nephrotic syndrome has also been described in a defined subset of IgA nephropathy patients, with either MCD like changes or MesPGN on biopsy. IgA with MCD-like changes is generally responsive to steroid therapy, although with a significant rate of relapse [71]. Regardless of histopathology, children with disease resistant to steroids generally have a poorer outcome compared with those with responsive disease [72]. The ultimate prognosis for children with primary nephrotic syndrome and frequently relapsing disease associated with mesangial hypercellularity and/or positive immunofluorescence remains difficult to predict.

Minimal Change Disease (MCD)

The defining histological feature of minimal change disease (MCD) is normal appearing glomeruli on light microscopic examination (Fig. 13.1). This assumes that the specimen has an adequate sample of glomeruli, including deep glomeruli from the juxtamedullary region of the renal cortex. Glomeruli of normal young children are generally smaller compared with adults so appear relatively hypercellular. There is no significant expansion of mesangial matrix, and no increase in mesangial cellularity (either by increased numbers of mesangial cells or infiltration by inflammatory cells). The cytoplasm of the podocytes may appear to be mildly swollen or vacuolated. Glomerular capillary loops remain patent, and in many cases may appear mildly dilated. The glomerular capillary walls are thin with no evidence of basement membrane thickening. No basement membrane reduplication or

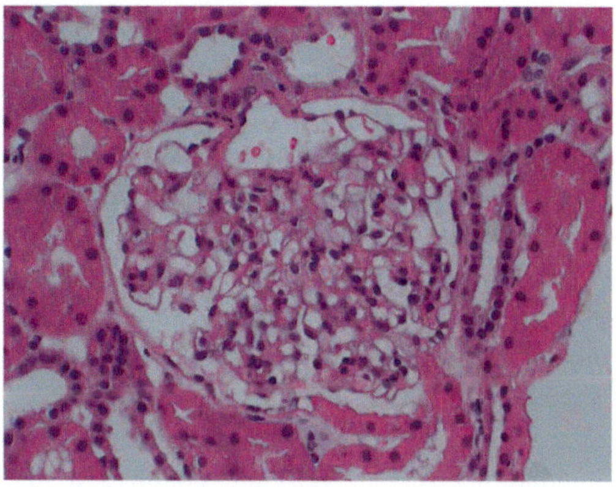

Fig. 13.1 The glomerulus appears normal to light microscopic examination, with normal mesangial matrix and cellularity. Capillary loops are dilated with normal thin capillary walls. (H&E stain, ×400)

(Courtesy Paul Kirwan, Electron Microscopy Unit, Department of Anatomical Pathology, CRGH, Concord, Sydney, Australia)

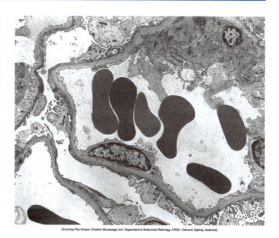

Fig. 13.2 Low power electron photomicrograph includes a capillary loop with extensive effacement of foot processes accompanied by swelling and microvillarisation of podocytes. Glomerular basement membranes are of normal appearance and no dense deposits are seen. (Courtesy of Paul Kirwan, Electron Microscopy Unit, Department of Anatomical Pathology, CRGH, Concord, Sydney, Australia)

epithelial spike formation are evident on examination of silver stained sections. The presence of an occasional glomerular "tip" lesion, defined as adhesion of the tuft to the Bowman's capsule at the site of opening of the proximal convoluted tubule, may be seen in MCD provided the glomerulus is otherwise normal in size and cellularity [73, 74]. The interstitium is normal without significant inflammation, fibrosis or tubular atrophy. Proximal tubule epithelial cells may contain hyaline droplets consistent with protein loss.

The immunofluoresence in MCD is negative. Very small amounts of IgM or C3 are considered by some to be compatible with MCD; however any significant immune reactant even in the setting of histologically normal glomeruli effectively excludes this diagnosis [64, 67, 72]. However, the clinical significance of these immune positive cases with normal histology is still controversial, and many now consider that these cases represent a spectrum of disease rather than distinct entities. Electron microscopic examination of untreated MCD shows uniform abnormality of the podocytes, with marked effacement of the foot processes over at least 50% of the glomerular capillary surface resulting in a smooth homogenous layer of epithelial cell cytoplasm which lacks the normal interdigitation. The cytoplasm of the cells may be enlarged with clear vacuoles and prominence of organelles. This is accompanied by microvillus transformation along the urinary surface of the podocytes (Fig. 13.2). The glomerular basement membrane otherwise appears normal, as do the mesangial cells and matrix. Immune deposits are absent. These changes are commonly modified with steroid treatment, and the degree of foot process effacement may be incomplete if the biopsy is taken from a partially treated patient.

Mesangial Proliferative Glomerulopathy (MesPGN)

Light microscopic examination of MesPGN shows generalized, diffuse mesangial cell hyperplasia, involving over 80% of the glomeruli. Increased numbers of mesangial cell nuclei are clearly present within mesangial matrix which is either normal or only mildly increased in amount (Fig. 13.3). There is generally no obvious lobulation of the glomerulus, and segmental sclerosis is absent. As in MCD, glomerular basement membranes remain thin and capillary loops clearly patent. By definition, spikes are not seen in silver stained sections. There is no significant intersti-

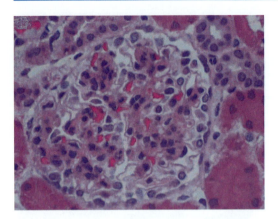

Fig. 13.3 The glomerulus shows increased numbers of mesangial cells with mildly increased matrix. The capillary loops appear normal. (H&E stain, ×400)

tial change (either tubular atrophy or fibrosis) to suggest glomerular loss. Glomerular immaturity, characterized by hypercellularity and a layer of cuboidal epithelium along the surface of the glomerular tuft, may be seen in some cases, particularly in younger children. Recent studies have suggested that these cases may have a less favourable clinical course [75].

Many cases of MesPGN show positive granular mesangial IgM ± C3 and very occasionally small amounts of C1q or IgG, although a proportion of cases have negative immunofluorescence. Some have considered these immune-positive cases as MesPGN, while others separate the positive cases into further distinct categories, most commonly IgM nephropathy. As noted earlier, these three "entities" (MCD, MesPGN, IgM Nephropathy) probably represent a spectrum rather than separate diseases. On electron microscopy there is mesangial cell hyperplasia with effacement of epithelial cell foot processes and microvillus transformation of epithelial cells. Dense deposits are not typically found, and the glomerular capillary basement membrane is normal.

IgM Nephropathy

IgM Nephropathy shows light microscopic features that may mimic those of either MCD or MesPGN. The sampled glomeruli may appear completely normal on routine stains, or may show diffuse mesangial hypercellularity. Some cases will show a combination of features, with some but not all glomeruli appearing hypercellular. As with MCD and MesPGN, segmental sclerosing lesions are not seen in an adequately sampled specimen, glomerular capillary loops remain thin walled and patent, and there is no basement membrane thickening or evidence of spike formation. Interstitial changes are absent. Granular deposits of IgM are confined to the mesangium and are generally seen in all glomeruli regardless of their histological appearance. Lesser amounts of C3 are common, and some cases may also show small amounts of C1q or IgG. In these cases, the IgM should remain as the dominant reactant. On electron microscopy there may be a mild increase in mesangial matrix. Immune deposits are often absent though some cases will show occasional small dense deposits that are located in paramesangial regions. Effacement of epithelial cell foot processes is usually seen to a varying degree, usually with microvillus transformation.

IgA Nephropathy with Nephrotic Syndrome

IgA nephropathy may present with clinical nephrotic syndrome indistinguishable from MCD in approximately 8–10% of cases. Nephrotic IgA nephropathy may show light microscopic features of MCD, MesPGN, or a focal GN (proliferative or sclerosing), however it is defined by the presence of dominant mesangial IgA deposition (frequently with some associated C3, and in approximately 50% of cases with lesser amounts of IgG and/or IgM), usually with electron microscopic evidence of immune deposits.

C1q Nephropathy

C1q nephropathy is an uncommon disorder that may also present with clinical nephrotic syndrome. Histology of these cases most commonly shows an MCD-like picture (70–75% of cases), with MesPGN (20%) and FSGS (7–13%) seen in some cases. Distinction is made with immunofluorescence finding of predominant C1q deposition in the mesangium and electron dense deposits on electron microscopic examination. Although many of these cases are clinically steroid resistant or steroid dependent, being more likely to require chronic immunosuppression and combined therapy, overall prognosis is good in particular for those with minimal changes on light microscopy. Of note, a number of studies have shown disappearance of the C1q deposits following therapy [68, 70].

Focal Segmental Glomerulosclerosis

Although FSGS more commonly results in steroid resistant disease, a proportion of cases will respond, at least initially, to steroid therapy [76, 77], and thus brief mention of the pathological features is made here. In FSGS, segmental (involving only a portion of the tuft) and focal (involving some but not all glomeruli) sclerosis of glomeruli is present. The light microscopic changes are not specific for primary idiopathic FSGS and other causes of segmental sclerosing lesions need to be excluded [78]. The sclerosed segments show collapse of the glomerular capillary with increase in matrix material though with variable patterns of glomerular involvement [79]. The uninvolved portion of the glomerular tuft should appear essentially normal. Idiopathic FSGS typically shows early preferential involvement of the deep juxtamedullary glomeruli so that adequate sampling of this region is needed to reduce the risk of missing a focal lesion. (This risk is estimated at 35% if only 10 glomeruli are examined, falling to a 12% risk if 20 glomeruli are examined [76]). Even a single segmental sclerosing lesion away from the glomerular tip is sufficient to exclude a diagnosis of MCD. Clues to the presence of possible FSGS without diagnostic sclerosing lesions include abnormal glomerular enlargement, which appears to be an early indicator of the sclerotic process, and focal interstitial fibrosis and tubular atrophy (above that expected for age), which suggest glomerular loss [76]. Typically idiopathic primary FSGS shows negative immunofluorescence though non-specific uptake of IgM may be seen, commonly within sclerosed segments. Deposits similar to that of IgM nephropathy may also be present. On electron microscopy non-sclerosed glomeruli show epithelial cell foot process fusion though this may not be complete or as widespread as in typical untreated MCD. However, this is often not helpful in making this distinction as steroid therapy may partially restore foot processes in MCD.

Clinico-pathological Correlations at Presentation of Nephrotic Syndrome

Children with MCD cannot be separated on clinical features from those with FSGS or MesPGN though children with MCD are generally younger and less likely to have haematuria, hypertension and kidney dysfunction at presentation [1]. The ISKDC found that 80% of children with MCD were aged 6 years and under compared with 50% of children with FSGS. Systolic and diastolic blood pressures were elevated at presentation in 21% and 14% of children with MCD and 49% and 33% of children with FSGS. Haematuria occurred in 23% of children with MCD and 48% of children with FSGS.

Clinical and Laboratory Features at Onset of Nephrotic Syndrome

In 30–50% cases the onset of SSNS is preceded by an upper respiratory tract infection [80, 81]. Atopy is more common in children with SSNS compared with children without SSNS [81] and more common in SSNS than SRNS [82] but an acute allergic reaction rarely precipitates a relapse. The most common initial symptom in SSNS is periorbital oedema though the significance of this finding may not be realized till the child develops generalized oedema and ascites [83]. Frequently the periorbital oedema is misdiagnosed as an allergy or as conjunctivitis particularly if the child is assessed initially in primary care rather than in emergency or paediatric care settings [84]. Symptoms may be present for longer than a year before diagnosis though 78% present within a month of the first symptom [84]. The degree of oedema is variable with some children having only mild periorbital and ankle oedema while others have pleural effusions and gross ascites with scrotal and penile oedema in boys and labial oedema in girls. The rapid formation of oedema with reduction in plasma volume may be associated with abdominal pain and malaise. Some children have serious infections at presentation including peritonitis [85]. Elevated systolic and diastolic blood pressures are present in 5–20% at presentation in children but generally hypertension does not persist [1, 80]. Urinalysis shows $\geq$3–4+ protein on urinalysis with a urine protein-creatinine ratio (uPCR) $\geq$ 200 mg/mmol ($\geq$2000 mg/g). Microscopic haematuria is present at diagnosis in 20–30% of children but rarely persists and macroscopic haematuria is rare occurring in less than 1% of children with SSNS [1, 80]. Serum albumin levels usually fall below 20 g/L and may be less than 10 g/L with a concomitant reduction in total protein levels. Kidney function is generally normal though serum creatinine may be elevated at presentation in association with intravascular volume depletion and rarely acute kidney failure. Children have elevated cholesterol and triglycerides and these continue to be abnormal while the child remains nephrotic. However it is unknown whether the intermittent lipid abnormalities seen in children with SSNS during relapses increase the risk of cardiovascular disease in adult life [86]. Serum electrolytes are usually within the normal range. Total serum calcium levels are low associated with hypoalbuminaemia but ionized calcium is usually normal. Haemoglobin and haematocrit levels may be elevated at presentation in patients with reduced plasma volumes.

Outcome of Children with SSNS

Relapse

Despite a relapsing course, the long-term prognosis for most children with SSNS is for resolution of their disease and maintenance of normal kidney function. Early follow up studies of children with SSNS and MCD [3, 5] indicated that 80–90% children relapsed one or more times. Among children who relapsed, 35–50% relapsed frequently or became steroid dependent [3, 5]. A recent retrospective observational study of 631 children diagnosed with idiopathic nephrotic syndrome (589 with SSNS) between 1993 and 2006 with a median follow up of 3.9 years (IQR 2.1–6.66 years) found that 24% children had a single episode of SSNS, 43% relapsed infrequently and 33% relapsed frequently or had SDNS [87]. In the NEPHROVIR study (a prospective population-based observational study), the 5-year relapse-free rate was 22% (36/174) [88]. The first relapse in 138 children occurred at a median of 8.3 months (IQR 3.4–11.3). Forty three children (24%) relapsed frequently and 83% of these still required treatment with prednisone and/or immunosuppressive agents at 96 months.

Although numerous predictors for a frequently relapsing or steroid dependent course have been identified, there is considerable variation in significant predictors between studies. Most studies of predictors have been retrospective studies from tertiary paediatric nephrology services. Predictors include young age at presentation [8, 88, 89], male sex [8, 89, 90], a longer time to first remission after commencing prednisone [91–95], a shorter time between first remission and first relapse [5, 94, 96], the number of relapses in the first 6 months after presentation [91, 93, 96], infection at presentation or relapse [91, 95, 96] and low birth weight [97].

Most children with SSNS cease having relapses before adulthood. The International Study of Kidney Disease in Children of 344 children with SSNS with MCD on kidney biopsy found that the proportion of children without relapses increased from 40% at 5 years to 80% at 8 years with very few children continuing to relapse at 18 years [5]. However, relapses may continue into adult life. In ten series of 705 participants with SSNS followed for 10–44 years, the proportion of people with continuing relapses varied between 9 and 50% [4, 90, 98–105]. The same series reported that the overall risk of reduced glomerular filtration rate was 0–2%. Higher numbers of relapses were reported in series with higher proportions of participants with FRNS or SDNS [4, 102]. Studies have also assessed the risk of treatment related complications in adults with childhood nephrotic syndrome. Hypertension was reported in between 0 and 32% of 569 adults (eight studies) with previous or continuing SSNS [4, 90, 100–105]. Overweight and obesity were reported in 13–46% of adults [99, 101, 102, 104, 105] though several authors pointed out that the prevalence of obesity may not differ from that in the local population [104, 105]. Short stature was reported in 2–20% of adults [99, 100, 102, 104]. Myocardial infarctions were reported in 2 of 66 participants with continuing relapses [4, 105] while a follow up study of 40 participants who had had SSNS during childhood but had no relapse for 23 years or more, identified three males who had had myocardial infarctions but all had other risk factors for cardiac disease [106]. Also the frequency of events in this group did not differ from that in the general population of the same age. No studies reported any malignancies in adults with previous nephrotic syndrome.

Kidney Function and the Development of Late Steroid Resistance

Most children with SSNS maintain normal kidney function. In a retrospective Canadian study of 78 children with SSNS followed for a median of 4.4 years (IQR 5.6), eGFR remained unchanged during follow up [107]. Development of late steroid resistance is well recognised. In European studies, most children with SSNS and biopsy proven or presumed MCD do not develop late steroid resistance and have a good prognosis for kidney function. In the ISKDC series of 334 children with SSNS and MCD, 15 (4.5%) children became transiently non-responsive to steroids but only one child (0.3%) became persistently non-responsive to therapy and developed ESKD [5]. Similarly in five series of 463 patients [4, 90, 98–100], only one patient (0.2%) developed late steroid resistance and progressed to ESKD [4]. A recent Canadian study of 589 children with initial SSNS reported that 10 (1%) children progressed to ESKD during a follow up period of up to 6.6 years [87]. Studies from the USA have identified higher risks of late steroid resistance and ESKD [108, 109]. In a retrospective analysis of 115 children with SSNS, 19 (17%) developed late steroid resistance with its development being associated with a shorter interval to first relapse and with relapse during the initial steroid therapy [109]. Although more African American children had initial steroid resistance, ethnicity did not predict for late steroid resistance [109]. A retrospective study from the USA Midwest Pediatric Nephrology Consortium investigated the outcomes in 29 children with late steroid resistance [110]. The median time to late steroid resistance was 19 months (range 2–170 months). After a mean follow up of 85 ± 47 months, 20 (70%) children were in complete or partial remission following treatment with CNI, mycophenolate mofetil (MMF) or alkylating agents. Six (21%) had persistent nephrotic range proteinuria and three (10%) had reached ESKD. Fewer African-American children responded to treatment compared with other children. These data suggest that children with late steroid resistance are more likely to respond to non-corticosteroid immunosuppressive agents and to have a better prognosis for kidney function compared with children with initial steroid resistance. Although initial steroid resistance is commonly associated with FSGS on kidney biopsy, the authors found no consistent relationship between initial or later kidney histology and late steroid resistance. Children with late steroid resistance are more likely to have recurrences of nephrotic syndrome following kidney transplantation [111]. Previous studies [112–115] have emphasized that progression to chronic kidney failure is not seen or is uncommon in children with FSGS if they continue to be steroid sensitive during follow up periods averaging about 10 years.

Other Complications of Steroid Sensitive Nephrotic Syndrome

Compared with earlier data, death is now uncommon in children with nephrotic syndrome. One study reported only one death (0.7%) associated with disease among 138 children with SSNS presenting between 1970 and 2003 [99] and no deaths were reported among 631 children presenting between 1993 and 2016 [87]. The death rate before corticosteroids and antibiotics were available was 40%, of whom half died from infection [83]. In the 1960s, 70s and 80s death rates of around 7% were reported among children with SSNS [80, 100, 116]. While upper respiratory tract infections are the most common infections, pneumonia, urinary tract infections, cellulitis, septicaemia and peritonitis are important causes of hospital admissions in children with nephrotic syndrome [117, 118]. Infections are more common in children receiving higher cumulative doses of corticosteroids and in those receiving non-corticosteroid immunosuppressive agents [119]. Routine screening for latent tuberculosis infection before treatment is indicated in areas with a high prevalence of tuberculosis but this is not cost effective in areas with a low prevalence [120]. Thromboembolism, most commonly venous, is a rare but potentially life threatening complication of SSNS though it is more common in children with congenital nephrotic syndrome or SRNS and in children aged over 12 years [121]. The majority of clinically evident venous thromboembolic episodes present in the first 3 months after nephrotic syndrome diagnosis [122]. Admissions for nephrotic syndrome complicated by acute kidney injury (AKI) increased significantly between 2000 and 2009 while admission rates for infection and thromboembolism were unchanged [117]. AKI developed in 59% of 336 children with nephrotic syndrome admitted to 27 paediatric nephrology services in USA; 237 children had SSNS. The risk of AKI was associated with infection, nephrotoxic drug exposure and duration of that exposure as well as steroid resistant disease [123]. Admissions complicated by infection, hypertension, thromboembolism and acute kidney injury result in longer hospital stays and increased costs [117, 118, 124].

Indications for Kidney Biopsy

Following the studies of the ISKDC, routine kidney biopsy at presentation and before corticosteroid administration has been abandoned. Biopsy is reserved for nephrotic children with unusual clinical and laboratory features (macroscopic haematuria, hypertension, persistent kidney insufficiency and low C3 component of complement) and for those with initial or secondary steroid resistance [125]. Rarely SSNS presents in the first year of life though more commonly nephrotic syndrome in this age group is resistant to corticosteroids and associated with monogenic podocyte disorders [126]. Where available, genetic studies should be carried out in children aged below 1 year before considering a kidney biopsy [127]. Originally biopsies at presentation were recommended for children aged above 8–10 years based on the ISKDC studies [128]. Now many paediatric nephrologists do not have a rigid upper age limit for treating children with idiopathic nephrotic syndrome without prior kidney biopsy and will give corticosteroids to children and adolescents if kidney function and complements are normal, persistent hypertension absent and microscopic haematuria transitory. This management is supported by retrospective studies of clinicopathological correlations in Indian children and adolescents, in which children without two or more abnormal clinical features generally demonstrated steroid sensitivity regardless of histology [129, 130]. However these data may not apply to African-American adolescent populations where the incidence of MCD at 20–30% [131] is much lower than the 40–50% seen in Indian or Northern European adolescents [129, 132]; kidney biopsy is recommended for children aged 12 years or above in the USA [133].

Opinions differ as to whether children with SSNS should have kidney biopsies before commencing corticosteroid sparing therapies. In some centres particularly in North America, kidney biopsies have been commonly carried out before using alternative therapy while this practice has been largely abandoned in Europe and India. Respondents to surveys in North America reported that biopsies before commencing alternative therapy provided them with prognostic information or would influence therapy with the choice of steroid sparing agent varying according to histology [134–136]. Studies from North America have demonstrated that kidney pathology (FSGS, MesPGN and IgM nephropathy) with less favourable prognoses are common in children with FRNS or SDNS [137, 138], that steroid dependent patients with MesPGN, IgM nephropathy or FSGS are more likely to have one or more relapses after cyclophosphamide therapy compared with children with MCD [63, 112] and that African American children with FSGS are more likely to progress to chronic kidney failure [139]. In contrast studies from Europe and India [113, 130, 140] have demonstrated no relationship between kidney histology and the pre-biopsy or post cyclophosphamide course even though MesPGN and FSGS are more common in selected series of children with FRNS or SDNS compared with ISKDC data. Some clinicians have argued that kidney biopsies should be obtained before commencing treatment with CNIs to provide a baseline for interstitial and tubular damage due to the underlying disease particularly in children with FSGS, where CNIs are considered the treatment of choice [134, 136]. Guidelines from KDIGO recommend that kidney biopsies are not required before commencing CNIs or other non-corticosteroid agents [125]. However kidney biopsies should be considered in children who have received prolonged treatment (2–3 years) with a CNI and are indicated in children with late resistance to corticosteroids [125, 141, 142].

Before the clinician biopsies a child with FRNS or SDNS, he or she needs to consider whether the benefits of this procedure outweigh the 1% risk of significant haemorrhage requiring blood transfusion [143, 144]. In particular, the clinician needs to know whether the kidney pathology will influence the specific therapy administered and/or whether it will provide information on the likelihood of the child progressing to ESKD. Studies show that, even if the kidney biopsy shows FSGS, the most important predictor for ESKD in idiopathic nephrotic syndrome is not the kidney pathology but the achievement and maintenance of remission following any therapy [145].

Management of Steroid Sensitive Nephrotic Syndrome

Treatment of the First Episode of Nephrotic Syndrome with Corticosteroids

Corticosteroids have been used to treat idiopathic nephrotic syndrome since the early 1950s [146]. Because of the clear net benefits of corticosteroids, no placebo-controlled trials were performed in children with nephrotic syndrome. The ISKDC agreed on a standard corticosteroid regimen for the first episode of SSNS [147] and this has provided the control group against which to test other regimens of prednisone or prednisolone therapy. At presentation children received prednisone 60 mg/m^2/day in divided doses for 4 weeks followed by 40 mg/m^2/day in divided doses on 3 consecutive days out of 7 days for 4 weeks. Subsequently a randomised controlled trial (RCT) carried out by the Arbeitsgemeinschaft für Pädiatrische Nephrologie (APN) [148] demonstrated that alternate day prednisone was more effective in maintaining remission than prednisone given on 3 consecutive days out of 7 days so alternate day prednisone dosing is generally used now in the second 4 week period. Since no significant differences in the time to remission or risk for subsequent relapse between single and divided doses of prednisone have been demonstrated [149], a single daily dose may be preferred during daily therapy to achieve greater compliance. For ease of clinical use, a dose of 2 mg/kg has commonly been substituted for

60 mg/m^2/day. Dosing per kilogram results in lower dosing for patients with weights below 30 kg [150] and two retrospective studies suggested that relative underdosing may increase the likelihood of FRNS [151, 152]. However two recent RCTs comparing dosing per kilogram with dosing by surface area in children weighing under 30 kg found no differences between dosing regimens in the time to remission and the number of relapses by 6 months with some increase in corticosteroid related adverse effects in children dosed by surface area [153, 154].

Though demonstrated to be more effective than shorter durations of treatment [155], the 8 week ISDKC/APN regimen was associated with a high relapse rate so RCTs investigated longer durations of prednisone compared with the ISKDC/APN regimen to determine if longer durations of prednisone reduced the risk of relapse and reduced the number of children, who developed FRNS or SDNS. Recently four well-designed RCTs (three placebo-controlled) involving 775 children have shown no benefit of extending the duration of treatment beyond eight (4 weeks daily and 4 weeks of alternate day prednisone) or 12 weeks (6 weeks daily and 6 weeks alternate day prednisone) on reducing the number of children with relapse or with frequent relapses (Table 13.2). Therefore children presenting with their first episode of SSNS should be

Table 13.2 Outcomes of corticosteroid treatment for initial episode of steroid sensitive nephrotic syndrome in four large well designed randomised controlled trials [150–154]

Study name	Teeninga 2013 [153]		Sinha 2014 [154]		Yoshikawa 2014 [150]		PREDNOS 2019 [151]	
Duration of treatment (months)	Three	Six	Three	Six	Two	Six	Two	Four
Number analysed	62	64	88	92	124	122	109	114
Efficacy outcomes								
Number with relapse	48	51	55	49	80	83	88	91
Number with FRNS/SDNS[a]	31	38	35	36	46	45	55	60
Median time to first relapse (months)	6 (95% CI [b] 4–8)	8 (95% CI 6–10)	6.6	9.2	8.1	8.1	2.9 (IQR [c] 2.2–4.5)	4.6 (IQR 3–6)
Number of relapses per patient	Median 2.5 (IQR = 1.0–5.0)	Median 4.0 (IQR = 1.0–6.0)	1.54 ± 1.59[d]	1.26 ± 1.58	1.25	1.33	3.61 ± 3.25	3.98 ± 3.30
Number of patients with adverse effects								
Hypertension	8	10	14	18	15	9	NR	NR
Cushingoid facies	14	21	37	37	54	61	78	83
Obesity	NR[e]	NR	5	5	20	34	NR	NR
Hirsutism	NR	NR	8	10	NR	NR	41	45
Glaucoma	0	0	NR	NR	19	13	NR	NR
Cataract	1	0	NR	NR	0	0	1	1
Adrenal insufficiency	NR	NR	NR	NR	0	1	NR	NR
Infection (episodes)	6	10	15	21	1	0	NR	NR
Hyperglycaemia	NR	NR	NR	NR	2	3	NR	NR
Glycosuria	NR	NR	NR	NR	NR	NR	14	19
Aggressive behaviour	NR	NR	4	4	NR	NR	101	94

[a] FRNS/SDNS: frequently relapsing nephrotic syndrome or steroid dependent nephrotic syndrome
[b] 95% CI: 95% confidence intervals
[c] IQR: interquartile range
[d] Standard deviation
[e] NR: not reported

treated with 8 weeks [156, 157] or 12 weeks of prednisone [158, 159]. Currently there are no adequately powered well designed RCTs comparing 8 with 12 weeks of prednisone treatment. Children under 6 years may be at higher risk of developing frequently relapsing or steroid dependent nephrotic syndrome [159]. It is uncertain whether prolonging the treatment period in young children would reduce the their risk of relapse and an RCT is underway to investigate this [160]. Meta-analyses of earlier trials had previously suggested that increasing the duration of prednisone beyond 8 to 12 weeks was associated with a reduced risk of relapse [161]. However poorly designed RCTs with inadequate allocation concealment and lack of blinding can exaggerate the efficacy of therapy [162, 163]. Therefore the 21 RCTs published between 1988 and 2018, which evaluated prednisone duration in the first episode of SSNS, were stratified in meta-analyses according to risk of bias for allocation concealment or for performance/detection bias. RCTs at low risk of bias showed no benefit of increasing the duration of prednisone while studies at high risk of bias showed a benefit of increased duration of prednisone [164].

Current international and national guidelines suggest 8–12 weeks of prednisone in the initial episode of SSNS [125, 133, 165, 166] with some guidelines including tapering of prednisone dose after 12 weeks though the recent PROPINE study found no benefit in terms of efficacy and safety of tapering prednisone dose [167]. The French protocol for the initial episode of SSNS includes the administration of three doses of intravenous methylprednisolone (1 g/1.73m^2) for those children who have not achieved remission by 30 days [165] and this protocol is used in other European centres [168]. Children who require intravenous methylprednisolone to achieve their first remission are more likely to become steroid dependent, to require ciclosporin and to develop late steroid resistance with reduced kidney function [169, 170]. Surveys of pediatric nephrologists in North America and Europe have demonstrated considerable variation among respondents in their approach to the first episode of idiopathic nephrotic syndrome [134, 136, 168, 171, 172]. A survey on SSNS management in all 12 Canadian pediatric nephrology centres indicated both within-centre and between-centre variability in prescribed doses and duration of prednisone for the first presentations and relapses of SSNS irrespective of whether or not the Centre had standard protocols [173].

Treatment of Relapsing SSNS with Corticosteroids

The ISKDC defined relapse as recurrence of proteinuria for 3 consecutive days after previously achieving remission (Table 13.1). Proteinuria may remit spontaneously in 15–30% of relapses without commencing prednisone or increasing the dose [174, 175]. Therefore it is reasonable to wait for some days of mild proteinuria ($\leq$2+ on dipstick) before commencing corticosteroids provided the child remains well and without significant oedema because spontaneous remissions may occur after several days of low grade proteinuria particularly if the child has an intercurrent viral infection. Compliance with prednisone therapy should be considered in children with multiple relapses since poor compliance could be misinterpreted as steroid dependence. If available, triamcinolone acetonide, a long acting steroid for intramuscular injection, may be used instead of oral prednisone treatment if non-compliance is suspected [176].

Paediatric nephrologists have generally treated relapses with daily prednisone (60 mg/m^2/day) till the child achieved remission and then continued alternate day therapy (40 mg/m^2) for 4 weeks or more [177]. Two observational studies and a small RCT have demonstrated that most children with relapsing SSNS achieve and maintain remission with prednisone given at a dose of 30 mg/m^2/day [178–180]. These data need confirmation in an adequately powered RCT.

In children with FRNS, observational studies have demonstrated that low-dose alternate-day prednisone (mean dose 0.48 mg/kg on alternate days) or low-dose daily prednisone (0.25 mg/kg/day) reduced the risk of relapse compared with historical controls with maintenance of growth rates [181, 182]. Guidelines recommend low-dose alternate-day prednisone in children with FRNS and SDNS [183]. However a recent RCT [184] in 61 children with FRNS or SDNS found that children receiving daily prednisone (0.2–0.3 mg/kg/day) had significantly fewer relapses than children receiving alternate day prednisone (0.5–0.7 mg/kg/day) with no increase in adverse effects. Four small RCTs have demonstrated that, in children with FRNS, increasing the frequency to daily administration at the onset of an intercurrent infection significantly reduces the risk of relapse [185–188]. However results from a large RCT with 271 children evaluated found that giving 6 days of daily low-dose prednisolone at the time of an URTI did not reduce the risk of relapse of nephrotic syndrome in children in the United Kingdom [189].

Adverse Effects of Corticosteroids

A study from the Kidney Research Network Registry [190] provides an overview of the frequency of corticosteroid adverse effects in patients with primary proteinuric kidney disease. Among a cohort of 884 patients (393 children) with primary proteinuric kidney disease, 534 received corticosteroids. At least one steroid associated adverse event was seen in 333 (62%) of those who received corticosteroids with hypertension, diabetes, overweight and obesity, infections and short stature being the most common. There was no difference in risk of steroid associated adverse effects between children and adults. The adjusted relative risk increased overall 2.5-fold for each 1 mg/kg increase in corticosteroid dose; hypertension increased 4.5-fold, obesity increased 2.9-fold and diabetes increased 1.9-fold.

Behavioural changes are common and include anxiety, depression, emotional lability, aggressive behaviour, inattention, hyperactivity and sleep disturbance [191, 192]. The adverse effects seen in the four large RCTs evaluating the initial episode of SSNS are shown in Table 13.2. Health related quality of life over time is reduced in children with nephrotic syndrome on prednisone or steroid sparing agents, compared with children not on medications [193]. In addition, nephrotic syndrome causes significant mental and economic stress on families [194].

The current practice of using alternate day rather than daily prednisone to maintain remission results from early reports that growth was less affected by alternate day prednisone. An RCT demonstrated that children given alternate day prednisone after kidney transplantation grew better than those given daily prednisone [195]. Studies of children with FRNS or SDNS, which have evaluated the adverse effects of corticosteroids on linear growth, have shown variable results. In a study of 56 children with FRNS or SDNS, children lost 0.49 ± 0.6 of height standard deviation score (SDS) during pre-pubertal growth [196]. Prednisone therapy was the only significant variable associated with the negative delta SDS. In a second study, growth rates remained normal if prednisone doses were maintained below 1.5 mg/kg on alternate days in 41 prepubertal children [197]. A third study of 64 boys found that growth rates remained stable from diagnosis for 5 years and then deteriorated [198]. In two studies final height was significantly below target in children, who required prednisone during puberty [196, 198] though partial catch up growth occurred in pubertal children permanently withdrawn from prednisone [196]. However a third study of 60 children with SSNS found that final height SDS did not differ significantly from initial height SDS (−0.60 ± 1.0 versus −0.64 ± 0.92) though the mean final height SDS differed significantly from that expected in healthy children [199].

Derangements of bone mineral metabolism may occur in patients with nephrotic syndrome and normal kidney function. Vitamin D-binding protein and 25-hydroxyvitamin D levels are reduced in nephrotic children [200] while generally levels of calcium, 1,25-dihydroxyvitamin D and parathyroid hormone levels are normal [200–202]. 25-hydroxyvitamin D levels increase in remission but remain low compared with healthy children [202] and may be associated with continuing reduction in bone mineral density [203]. Abnormalities of bone mineral metabolism are aggravated by treatment with corticosteroids. Corticosteroids reduce bone formation by inhibiting osteoblast activity and inhibiting bone matrix formation. In addition they increase bone resorption directly and by reducing calcium absorption via inhibition of Vitamin D activity with a secondary increased release of parathyroid hormone [204, 205]. Low bone area and trabecular thickness with focal areas of osteoid accumulation consistent with osteopenia and abnormal mineralisation have been found in children with steroid dependent SSNS [205]; bone formation rate correlated inversely with the daily prednisone dose. Serum osteocalcin and alkaline phosphatase levels fall during corticosteroid therapy consistent with reduced bone formation [202].

Corticosteroid therapy is associated with osteopenia (decrease in quantity of bone tissue) and osteoporosis (osteopenia with bone fragility). Trabecular bone is affected more severely than cortical bone. Dual energy x-ray absorptiometry (DXA) is widely used to assess bone mass in children with SSNS. DXA measures the mass of bone mineral per projection area (g/cm^2), which is a size dependent measure [206]. Thus results must be corrected for height in short children to prevent underestimation of bone mineral density (BMD) in comparison with age matched controls. A North American cross-sectional study of 60 children with SSNS, who had received an average of 23 g of prednisone, demonstrated that whole body bone mineral content (BMC) was increased and lumbar spine BMC was normal in children with SSNS compared with age matched local controls when adjusted for bone area, height, age, sex, pubertal stage and race [207]. Nephrotic children had significantly lower z-scores for height and higher z-scores for weight and body mass index (BMI) compared with controls. The authors concluded that corticosteroid induced increases in BMI were associated with increased whole body BMC and maintenance of BMC of spine. In contrast in 100 non obese Indian children with SSNS, who had received 5.6–18 g of prednisone, 61% had low BMD levels compared to normal values from North American controls [201]. No children developed fractures. These data indicate that differences in growth and body composition in different study populations need to be considered when interpreting studies of bone mass in children with SSNS. In a prospective Canadian study, lumbar spine BMD was studied at baseline (median 18 days from prednisone initiation), 3, 6, 9 and 12 months after the onset of nephrotic syndrome [208]. Only 51% of children were receiving prednisone by 12 months. Mean lumbar spine BMD was significantly reduced at baseline and 3 months but subsequently mean values did not differ significantly from values in healthy children. Cross sectional and longitudinal studies using peripheral quantitative computed tomography (pQCT) in children with nephrotic syndrome have confirmed differential effects of corticosteroids on cortical and trabecular bone mineral densities with evidence of reduced bone formation [209, 210].

Corticosteroid associated fractures are rare in children with SSNS unlike children with chronic inflammatory disorders such as juvenile rheumatoid arthritis. In the Canadian study, only three children (6%) of 65 children had asymptomatic vertebral fractures by 12 months after commencing prednisone [208]. Children with SSNS appear to be at a low risk of osteoporosis [206]. Bone mineral density improves in children with SSNS, who are given vitamin D and calcium supplements during prednisone therapy [211–213]. The Committee on Nutrition of the French Society of Paediatrics recommend that children with nephrotic syndrome should receive daily vitamin D supplements particularly in winter months [214].

Long term corticosteroid therapy results in suppression of the hypothalamic-pituitary-adrenal (HPA) axis in 35–60% of children with nephrotic syndrome particularly in younger children and children with FRNS or SDNS [215–218]. In the most recent study, the mean duration of prednisone in 13 children with HPA suppression was 66 months compared with 30 months in 24 children without HPA suppression with mean daily doses of 22 mg/kg and 26 mg/kg in the two groups [217]. Families with children receiving long term prednisone therapy should be educated about the possible need for hydrocortisone replacement at times of illness or stress including surgical procedures. To avoid HPA suppression, long periods of high dose prednisone therapy should be avoided by introducing non-corticosteroid sparing agents.

Corticosteroid Sparing Agents in Frequently Relapsing and Steroid Dependent SSNS

Corticosteroid sparing agents are indicated in children, who have frequent relapses despite low dose alternate day prednisone and/or who have significant adverse effects of prednisone therapy. Corticosteroid sparing agents used in children with FRNS or SDNS include alkylating agents (cyclophosphamide, chlorambucil), levamisole, calcineurin inhibitors (cyclosporin, tacrolimus), mycophenolate mofetil or mycophenolate sodium and rituximab. In addition mizoribine is used in Japan.

Alkylating Agents

Cyclophosphamide remains an important medication to treat FRNS in low and middle income countries where it is be cheaper than other non-corticosteroid immunosuppressive agents [219] while chlorambucil is less commonly used. In six RCTs combined in meta-analysis, oral cyclophosphamide 2–3 mg/kg/day for 8–12 weeks or chlorambucil 0.2 mg/kg/day administered for 8 weeks reduced the risk of relapse by 60% in frequently relapsing SSNS at 6–12 months after treatment compared with prednisone alone [220].

Two studies have shown that intravenous cyclophosphamide (500 mg/m²/dose for 6 monthly doses) was more effective than oral cyclophosphamide (2 mg/kg/day for 12 weeks) in reducing the risk for relapse at 6 months (RR 0.56; 95% CI 0.33–0.92) but not at 2 years [220–222]; in both studies the cumulative dose of cyclophosphamide was lower in the intravenously treated groups. In a systematic review of 26 observational studies of cyclophosphamide and chlorambucil usage in SSNS. relapse-free survivals after 2–5 years were 72% and 36% in children with FRNS and 40% and 24% in children with SDNS. More recent single centre studies have found similar results [223–227].

Adverse effects with alkylating agents are frequent and may be severe. A third of children will experience leucopenia so white blood counts need to be checked regularly during treatment. If leucopenia occurs, the treatment dose should be reduced or ceased temporarily to reduce the risk of infection. Latta and co-workers identified adverse effects from 38 reports involving 866 children with FRNS or SDNS, who received 906 courses of cyclophosphamide and 638 children, who received 671 courses of chlorambucil (Table 13.3) [228]. They concluded that chlorambucil in the recommended dosage was potentially more toxic than cyclophosphamide based on a higher risk of infections, malignancies and seizures so chlorambucil is rarely used now. Cyclophosphamide may reduce male fertility and cause abnormal gonadal function in men and should not be used in peripubertal male children. In SSNS there is a dose dependent relationship

Table 13.3 Adverse effects of alkylating agents in children with steroid sensitive nephrotic syndrome

Adverse effect		Cyclophosphamide		Chlorambucil	
		Total assessed	N (%) with outcome	Total assessed	N (%) with outcome
Deaths	Patients	866	7 (0.8%)	625	7 (1.1%)
Malignancies	Patients	866	2 (0.2%)	534	3 (0.6%)
Seizures	Patients	866	0 (0%)	266	9 (3.4%)
Infections	Courses	609	9 (1.5%)	552	35 (6.3%)
Haemorrhagic cystitis	Courses	762	22 (2.2%)	552	0 (0%)
Leucopenia	Courses	619	210 (32.4%)	456	151 (33%)
Thrombocytopenia	Courses	214	5 (2.1%)	408	24 (5.9%)
Hair loss	Courses	736	131 (17.8%)	237	5 (2.1%)

Reproduced with permission from Latta K, von Schnakenburg C, Ehrich JH. A meta-analysis of cytotoxic treatment for frequently relapsing nephrotic syndrome in children. Pediatric Nephrology. 16(3):271–82, 2001 [228]

between the number of patients with sperm counts below 10^6/mL and the cumulative dose of cyclophosphamide [228]. The threshold cumulative dose for safe use of cyclophosphamide remains uncertain because of individual reports of oligospermia in boys receiving less than 200 mg/kg. These data suggest that single courses of cyclophosphamide at a dose of 2 mg/kg/day should not exceed 12 weeks (cumulative dose 168 mg/kg). There are few data on gonadal toxicity with chlorambucil in SSNS. In male patients treated for lymphoma, total doses of 10–17 mg/kg led to azoospermia [229]; similar total doses are used in SSNS. Gonadal toxicity is less severe in women with most reports observing little or no toxicity with alkylating agents in SSNS [228]. The 2012 KDIGO guidelines advise that second courses of alkylating agents should not be given because of their potential long term toxicity [125].

In many countries, cyclophosphamide has been largely replaced by other non-corticosteroid medications because of its adverse effects. The main advantage of cyclophosphamide over levamisole, MMF and CNIs is that it often results in a prolonged period of remission after the medication is ceased. Rituximab also leads to a prolonged period of remission off treatment. Two recent observational studies [230, 231], which compared outcomes of children treated with cyclophosphamide with those treated with rituximab, found that 1 and 2 year relapse-free survivals were similar between treatments but adverse effects were more common with cyclophosphamide. Importantly more children treated with rituximab were able to cease steroids completely [231]. However rituximab is expensive and may not be available in resource limited countries.

Calcineurin Inhibitors

Cyclosporin has been used to treat children with frequently relapsing or steroid dependent SSNS since 1985 [232]. Two small trials enrolling 95 children demonstrated no significant difference in the risk of relapse during treatment between alkylating agents given for 6 or 8 weeks and cyclosporin given for 6 or 9 months [233–235]. However most children treated with cyclosporin relapsed when therapy was ceased so the risk of relapse with alkylating agents was lower than with cyclosporin after cyclosporin had been ceased for 12–15 months. In a prospective 2 year follow up of 44 children, in whom cyclosporin was discontinued after completion of an RCT, 37 (84%) experienced a relapse [236]. Relapses occurred in 81% (26/32), without relapse during cyclosporin therapy, and in 92% (11/12) children, who had one or more relapses during cyclosporin therapy. The probability that children would re-develop FRNS or SDNS by 2 years was 75% and 53% respectively in children with or without relapse during their previous cyclosporin therapy. Adverse effects of cyclosporin reported in four trials were common with 13% of children developing hypertension, 10% reduced kidney function, 23% gum hypertrophy and 27% hirsutism [235]. A potentially serious adverse effect of CNI is posterior reversible encephalopathy syndrome (PRES) [237]. Nephrotic syndrome per se and hypertension also are predisposing factors for PRES.

Cyclosporin (microemulsified) is usually commenced at 4–5 mg/kg/day in two divided doses with subsequent dosing altered to achieve 12 h trough whole blood levels (C_0) of 80–150 ng/mL (67–125 nmol/L) initially. In an RCT the sustained remission rate at 2 years was significantly higher in children with C_0 levels maintained between 80–100 ng/mL (50–67 nmol/L) [mean dose 4.8 mg/kg/day] compared with children treated with a fixed dose of 2.5 mg/kg/day (sustained remission rates 50% versus 15%) [238]. Hypertension and mild arteriolar hyalinosis were less common in the fixed dose group. The cyclosporin dose, required to maintain trough levels, may be reduced by one third by administering ketoconazole as a cyclosporin sparing agent with reduction in drug costs [239]. Studies in children with SSNS have demonstrated better correlations between area under the curve concentrations of cyclosporin and 2 h post dose levels (C_2) than with trough levels [240]. A Japanese RCT compared the effect of two different C_2 levels on the relapse rate in children with FRNS or SDNS [241]. Children were randomised to receive cyclosporin to achieve whole blood C_2 levels of

600–700 ng/mL (499–582 nmol/L) for 6 months followed by 450–550 ng/mL (374–457 nmol/L) for 18 months or to achieve C_2 levels of 450–550 ng/mL (374–457 nmol/L) for 6 months and then 300–400 ng/mL (250–333 nmol/L). The sustained remission rate was slightly but not significantly higher in the high C_2 level group compared with the lower C_2 level group but the relapse rate was significantly lower in the high level group; adverse effects did not differ between groups.

Tacrolimus is now the preferred CNI agent for SSNS where available largely because of the cosmetic effects of cyclosporin though it is also nephrotoxic and may be associated with diabetes mellitus. No RCTs have compared tacrolimus with cyclosporin in children with SSNS. In a prospective uncontrolled study of 74 children (50 on tacrolimus; 24 on cyclosporin), relapse frequency during 2 years follow-up did not differ significantly between treatments [242]. Nephrotoxicity defined as an increase in serum creatinine >25% above baseline was less common in tacrolimus treated children and diabetes mellitus was not reported. The starting dose of tacrolimus was 0.5–1.5 mg/kg/day in two divided doses; subsequently the dose was adjusted to 12 h trough levels of 5–12 ng/mL (6–14 nmol/L). There are also some observational data in children with SDNS suggesting that tacrolimus may be associated with less CNI nephrotoxicity than cyclosporin [243]. In a retrospective cohort study of 340 children with FRNS or SDNS examining the relative efficacy and safety of tacrolimus, MMF and levamisole as the first non-corticosteroid agent, the 30-month relapse free survival was 62% with tacrolimus, 39% with MMF and 24% with levamisole [219]. Fewer adverse effects were seen with levamisole (three reports) compared with tacrolimus (33 reports). Serious adverse effects mainly related to infection were only seen with tacrolimus.

CNI toxicity is well documented in children receiving this therapy outside the transplant setting [244] though few studies have correlated clinical toxicity with morphologic features [245, 246]. The toxic effects are essentially the same in transplant and non-transplant settings. CNI toxicity may be characterized by reduction in glomerular filtration rate with no discernible histological abnormality or by acute and chronic tubular and/or vascular changes in the kidney. Acute changes of toxic tubulopathy are classically described as "isometric" vacuolation of proximal tubular epithelial cells. However this is often a focal phenomenon and may only be seen in a small number of tubules in a biopsy sample. The vacuoles are of similar size (hence "isometric") and occur on the basis of dilatation of the smooth endoplasmic reticulum of the cells. Non-specific changes of acute tubular necrosis may be seen in some cases, with intraluminal desquamation of epithelial cells, dilatation of the tubules and regenerative nuclear changes. Acute vascular changes may result in microvascular thrombosis, endothelial and myocyte necrosis. Chronic vascular changes include nodular hyaline arteriopathy, which arises on the basis of individual myocyte necrosis of arteriolar smooth muscle, and "striped" interstitial fibrosis and tubular atrophy that reflect focal ischaemic damage. Ultimately, chronic CNI nephrotoxicity can result in glomerular changes of chronic ischaemia and/or focal and segmental glomerulosclerosis. The morphological nephrotoxic effects of tacrolimus are essentially the same as those seen with cyclosporin and include acute tubular necrosis, acute and chronic vascular changes, and interstitial fibrosis.

Cyclosporin-induced tubulointerstitial lesions on kidney biopsy are reported in 30–40% of children who have received cyclosporin for 12 months or more [247–249]. Cyclosporin associated arteriopathy is uncommon. Risk factors for fibrosis are total duration of cyclosporin therapy, having heavy proteinuria for more than 30 days during therapy [247] and higher trough cyclosporin levels [250], higher 2 h peak cyclosporin levels and concurrent use of angiotensin-converting enzyme inhibitors or angiotensin II receptor blockers [249]. Arteriopathy but not interstitial fibrosis improves after cyclosporin has been ceased for 12 months or more [251].

The duration of administration of CNIs is controversial with some authors suggesting that duration should not exceed 2 years [247]. However other authors have suggested that longer periods of CNIs may be well tolerated [252]. There are few data on kidney histology in children with SSNS who have received tacrolimus but increases in interstitial fibrosis correlated with trough tacrolimus levels [253]. These few data suggest that as with cyclosporin, the lowest possible dose of tacrolimus should be used to maintain remission.

Levamisole

Levamisole is a synthetic antihelminthic agent with immunomodulatory properties [254]. Its use in childhood nephrotic syndrome was first described by Tanphaichitr and co-workers in 1980 [255] and since then many studies have described its benefits [254]. Levamisole is usually administered in a dose of 2.5 mg/kg on alternate days. Levamisole given for 4 months to 1 year reduced the risk of relapse by 50% in comparison with prednisone alone in 6 trials (474 patients; RR 0.41, 95% CI 0.27–0.61) [220, 256–261] but was ineffective in a seventh trial, in which a lower total dose of levamisole was given [220, 262]. However several of these RCTs were at high risk of bias because of methodological problems, which may lead to an overestimation of treatment effects [163]. Recently a multicentre, double-blind RCT evaluating levamisole compared with placebo in 99 children with FRNS or SDNS confirmed the efficacy of levamisole [263]. Between 100 days and 12 months from the start of the medications, the time to relapse was significantly increased in the levamisole group compared with the placebo group (HR 0.22; 95% CI 0.11–0.43). After 12 months, 26% of levamisole treated participants remained in remission compared with 6% of placebo-treated participants. Four of 50 children treated with levamisole suffered moderate leucopenia. Adverse effects of levamisole are uncommon but include leucopenia, gastrointestinal effects and occasionally vasculitis [264, 265]. Although levamisole is a valuable corticosteroid sparing agent, it is currently unavailable in many countries.

Mycophenolate Mofetil/ Mycophenolate Sodium

Mycophenolate mofetil (MMF) and mycophenolate sodium (MPS) are converted to mycophenolic acid (MPA), which is an inhibitor of the *de novo* purine pathway with inhibitory effects on T and B lymphocyte proliferation [266]. MMF has become an important corticosteroid sparing agent in children with FRNS or SDNS and is often used as the initial non-corticosteroid immunosuppressive agent [267]. MPS is used in adults with nephrotic syndrome and minimal change disease [268] but has rarely been used in children though its efficacy can be expected to be similar to MMF [269]. Numerous observational studies have demonstrated a reduction in relapse rate during MMF treatment compared with prednisone treatment [270] though no RCT has compared MMF with prednisone alone. Its efficacy in SSNS has been evaluated in three RCTs (144 children) comparing MMF (800–1200 mg/m^2/day in two divided doses) with cyclosporin (4–5 mg/kg/day) [271, 272] and in one RCT (149 children) comparing MMF (1200 mg/m^2/day) with levamisole (2.5 mg/kg on alternate days) [273]. When combined in a meta-analysis, the relapse rate was lower with cyclosporin compared with MMF (142 children. Mean difference 0.83; 95% CI 0.33–1.33) but adverse effects of hypertension, hypertrichosis and gum hypertrophy were lower and GFR higher in MMF treated children [220]. The main adverse effects of MMF are abdominal pain, diarrhoea, anaemia, leucopenia and thrombocytopenia although MMF has been well tolerated in children with SSNS with gastrointestinal disorders reported in only 4% of 130 children in a large observational study [219]. *In utero* exposure to MMF has been associated with prenatal defects so women should be counselled that they will need to cease MMF before becoming pregnant [270].

Higher MPA exposure is required in children with nephrotic syndrome compared with levels in kidney transplant recipients [270]. Studies of therapeutic drug monitoring show that the target MPA area under the curve (AUC) needs to be above 45–50 μg h/mL to maintain remission though there is large between-patient variability [271, 274, 275]. *Post hoc* analysis of the Gellermann study revealed that the relapse rate in children with higher MPA exposure (mean MPA-AUC 74.0 mg h/mL) did not differ from that seen in cyclosporin treated children [271]. None of the RCTs reported to date have used therapeutic drug monitoring to determine the correct dose of MMF for individual patients so it remains possible that results of these RCTs would differ if drug monitoring had been included. Currently therapeutic drug monitoring of MMF in children with nephrotic syndrome is not widely available. No consistent single time point for measurement has been identified that correlates with AUC data and can be used to monitor children with FRNS or SDNS receiving MMF.

Rituximab

Rituximab is a mouse-human chimeric monoclonal antibody which binds to the CD20 antigen expressed on B cells. Treatment leads to a suppression of CD19 cells to below 1% and relapse generally occurs when levels of CD19 cells recover. Rituximab has now been evaluated in seven RCTs using one [276–278] (Fig. 13.4), two [279–281] or four doses [282] of rituximab (375 mg/m^2 per dose). In five studies including 296 children with difficult to treat SDNS, the risk for relapse was reduced by 63% at 6 months (4 studies, 239 children; RR 0.27; 95% CI 0.15–0.47) and 36% at 12 months (2 studies, 168 children; RR 0.74; 95% CI 0.58–0.94) [220]. In two studies (60 participants), which assessed RTX in children with SSNS treated with high ($\geq$0.7 mg/kg/day) or low doses ($\leq$0.4 mg/kg/day) of prednisone without other immunosuppressive agents, the risk of relapse was reduced by 94% and 74% at 6 and 12 months compared with prednisone alone [277, 278].

To gain further information about the optimum dosing regimen of rituximab, a study evaluated retrospectively the different dose regimens used in 11 tertiary centres in Asia, Europe and North America [283]. Among 511 children with complicated relapsing SSNS (defined as relapsing despite ongoing treatment with prednisone and at least one additional agent), 191 received low dose rituximab (375 mg/m^2), 208 received medium dose rituximab (750 mg/m^2) and 112 received high dose rituximab (1125–1500 mg/m^2). Fifty five percent [283] of children received concurrent immunosuppressive treatment (CNI, MMF, prednisone). Children who received low dose rituximab had shorter relapse-free periods (8.5 months) compared with those receiving medium dose (12.7 months) or high dose (14.3 months) rituximab. However when rituximab was combined with immunosuppressive therapy, relapse-free survival did not differ between different dosage groups. Two RCTs is underway to determine whether MMF compared with placebo maintains remission in children with SSNS after successful treatment with rituximab [284, 285].

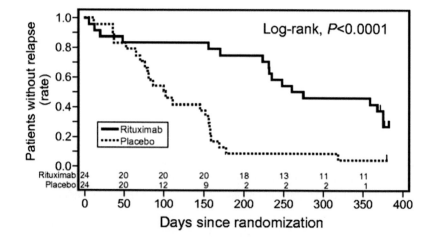

Fig. 13.4 Relapse-free survival probability in participants with relapsing nephrotic syndrome treated with rituximab. Reproduced with permission from Iijima K, Sako M, Kamei K, Nozu K. Rituximab in steroid-sensitive nephrotic syndrome: lessons from clinical trials. Pediatric Nephrology (2018) 33:1449–1455

The main adverse effects reported with rituximab have been acute episodes of bronchospasm, hypotension, fever and arthralgias occurring during or immediately after intravenous infusion. Premedication with anti-histamine and anti-pyretic agents is recommended. Adverse effects are generally mild with infusion reactions (13%) and infections (4%) being most common [283]. Mild to moderately serious infections are reported to be less commonly seen with rituximab compared with tacrolimus [280]. However rare but serious adverse effects reported in children with nephrotic syndrome treated with rituximab include fatal pulmonary fibrosis [286], *Pneumocystis jiroveci* pneumonia with respiratory failure [287, 288], bacterial pneumonia including *Pseuodomonas aeroginosa* pneumonia [289] and severe myocarditis requiring heart transplantation [290]. Though not yet reported in children with SSNS, a survey of patients with SLE treated with rituximab identified 57 patients with multifocal leucoencephalopathy caused by JC polyomavirus [291]. Fifty six children (14%) of 400 children in whom IgG levels were measured had persistent hypogammaglobulinaemia at 1 year following rituximab infusion [283]. Among 27 children who had received rituximab more than 2 years previously, most had a sustained reduction in total and switched memory B cells while 11 children had hypogammaglobulinaemia [292]. Younger patients appear to be at increased risk of hypogammaglobulinaemia [293]. More information is required to determine the longer term impact of these immunological abnormalities.

Because of the uncertainty about long term adverse effects and its cost, rituximab use was previously restricted to children with steroid and CNI dependent SSNS. However a study from the USA has demonstrated that the 1 year overall treatment costs of using rituximab compared with CNIs may not differ significantly [294]. Increasingly rituximab is being used in children with FRNS or SDNS because it can achieve long periods of remission off treatment [278] though the long term effects of prolonged B cell depression and hypogammaglobulinaema remain to be elucidated.

Choice of First Corticosteroid Sparing Agent for Children with FRNS or SDNS

RCTs to date have not provided sufficient data on the comparative efficacy and adverse effects of corticosteroid sparing agents to allow definitive recommendations on which medication should be the first agent used in FRNS or SDNS. Most international [125] and national guidelines [133, 165, 166] have not provided recommendations on which medication should be preferred as the first corticosteroid sparing agent. New guidelines from KDIGO and the International Pediatric Nephrology Association are awaited. Table 13.4 lists the advantages and disadvantages of each corticosteroid sparing medication. The choice of first agent will depend on clinician and family preferences based on an assessment of the benefits and harms as well as the cost and availability of medications.

Other Agents

In RCTs, no significant reduction in the risk of relapse has been demonstrated with azathioprine [235]. Mizoribine blocks purine biosynthesis pathways and is used in Japan for children with SSNS. In an RCT involving 197 children, who received 4 mg/kg/day of mizoribine or placebo, there was no significant difference in relapse rates and 16% of treated patients developed hyperuricaemia [295]. Recent studies suggest that some children with SSNS respond well to mizoribine and that differences in the pharmacokinetics in responders and non-reponders may explain differences in response. Mizoribine has a lower frequency of adverse effects compared with cyclophosphamide and cyclosporin so in Japan it may be used before other second line agents [296]. Two RCTs [297, 298] compared azithromycin (a macrolide antibiotic with immunomodulatory properties) and prednisone with prednisone alone and found a lower risk of relapse at 6 months in children treated with azithromycin. Adrenocorticotrophic hormone (ACTH) was widely used to try nephrotic syndrome in the 1950s but was subsequently replaced by prednisone. More recently there have been case reports of its efficacy in SSNS. However a

Table 13.4 Advantages and disadvantages of corticosteroid-sparing agents as first agent for use in frequently relapsing or steroid dependent steroid sensitive nephrotic syndrome

Medication	Advantages	Disadvantages
Cyclophosphamide	Prolonged remission off therapy Inexpensive	Less effective in SDNS Monitoring of blood count during therapy Potential serious short- and long-term adverse effects Only one course should be given
Chlorambucil	Prolonged remission off therapy Inexpensive	Less effective in SDNS Monitoring of blood count during therapy Potential serious short- and long-term adverse effects Only one course should be given
Levamisole	Prolonged remissions in some children with FRNS Generally inexpensive Few adverse effects	Continued treatment required to maintain remission Limited availability Not approved for SSNS in some countries
Mycophenolate mofetil/ Mycophenolate sodium	Prolonged remissions in some children with FRNS and SDNS Few adverse effects	Continued treatment required to maintain remission Less effective than CNIs Limited availability Expensive Risk of birth defects & pregnancy loss in first trimester of pregnancy Little data on use of mycophenolate sodium in children with SSNS
Cyclosporine	Prolonged remissions in some children with FRNS/SDNS	Continued treatment required to maintain remission Expensive Nephrotoxic Cosmetic side-effects
Tacrolimus	Prolonged remissions in some children with FRNS/SDNS	Continued treatment required to maintain remission Expensive Nephrotoxic Risk of diabetes mellitus Not approved for SSNS in some countries
Rituximab	Prolonged remissions off treatment in many children with FRNS/SDNS	Risk of prolonged B cell depression and hypogammaglobulinaemia Expensive Usually well tolerated but small risk of very serious adverse effects

FRNS frequently relapsing steroid-sensitive nephrotic syndrome; *SDNS* steroid dependent steroid-sensitive nephrotic syndrome

recent RCT found that ACTH at 80 U/1.73 m² administered twice weekly was ineffective at preventing disease relapses in children with steroid dependent SSNS [299].

Vaccinations in Children with SSNS

Physicians should encourage families to complete routine childhood vaccination programmes though the timing of administration of live vaccines (measles, mumps, rubella, varicella [MMRV]) may need to be altered if the child is receiving high dose corticosteroids or corticosteroid sparing agents. *Steptococcus pneumoniae* and *Haemophilis influenza* are important causes of invasive infections in children with SSNS. Vaccines against both organisms are included in the routine vaccination schedules of many countries. The safety and efficacy of the 13-valent pneumococcal conjugate vaccine (PCV13) and the 23-valent pneumococcal polysaccharide vaccine (PPSV23) have been demonstrated in children with SSNS [300–302]. In 42 children with nephrotic syndrome who received PCV13, serotype specific antibodies increased in all children and remained elevated for 12 months [302]. However serological responses were lower in children receiving both prednisone and non-corticosteroid immunosuppressive agents (tacrolimus, cyclosporin, MMF). Response to PPSV23 was similar in 30 nephrotic children who received PPSV23 while on prednisone 60 mg/m²/day to that seen in 13 children on low dose alternate day prednisone [300]. Similar rises in anti-pneumococcal antibody levels were detected in both groups for up to 36 months. Response was not affected by non-corticosteroid immunosuppressive agents. Relapse rates did not increase following vaccination compared with the pre-vaccination period or compared with historical controls [300]. The Centre for Disease Control and Prevention's Advisory Committee on Immunization Practices recommends that the 13-valent pneumococcal conjugate vaccine (PCV13) be given routinely to all children aged below 60 months and to children with immunocompromising conditions including nephrotic syndrome to 18 years [303]. The Committee advises that PCV13 should be administered whether or not the child has previously received PCV7 and/or PPSV23. To broaden protection against serotypes not in PCV13, PPSV23 is also recommended for all children aged 2 years and over with immuno-compromising conditions. Influenza vaccine should be given annually to children with nephrotic syndrome who are receiving corticosteroids and/or other immunosuppressive agents. Contacts of these children should also receive influenza vaccine. Hepatitis B vaccination should be administered to at risk children. Seroprotection rates were higher in SSNS than SRNS and higher in those who had received prednisone compared with those receiving prednisone with corticosteroid sparing agents [304].

Live vaccines are generally contraindicated in children on high dose prednisone or on other immunosuppressive agents. Most national recommendations on the administration of live vaccines in children do not specifically address children with SSNS. Based on a study of the South West Pediatric Nephrology Group [305], the 2012 KDIGO guidelines suggest that children not be given varicella vaccines until their prednisone dose is below 1 mg/kg/day (maximum 20 mg daily) or below 2 mg/kg on alternate days (maximum 40 mg on alternate days) and that live vaccines should not be given until children have been off cytotoxic agents for more than 3 months and off other immunosuppressive agents (CNIs, levamisole, MMF) for at least 1 month [125]. Varicella vaccination of household contacts is recommended [306]. A recent study from Japan has questioned the 2012 KDIGO guidelines [307]. The study reported no vaccine-related infections with satisfactory seroconversion rates to measles, rubella, varicella and mumps in 60 children with SSNS who were receiving immunosuppressive agent (CNI, MMF, mizoribine) with low dose prednisone when the vaccines were administered and had negative titres against one or more of these infections. Most children maintained seropositivity for these viruses at 1 year. No serious adverse reactions including vaccine-related infections were seen.

Of importance now to children with steroid sensitive nephrotic syndrome and their families is coronavirus disease 19 (COVID-19). In the United States, the Centers for Disease Control recommend COVID-19 vaccination for everyone aged 12 years and older for the prevention of COVID-19 disease [308] and their interim guidance states that immunocompromised individuals may receive COVID-19 vaccination if they have no contraindications to vaccination. There is limited information on the risk for and outcomes of COVID 19 in people with any immune related kidney disease though preliminary findings suggest that COVID 19 illnesses may be more severe than in people without such kidney disease particularly in people on high dose prednisolone [309]. The Immunonephrology Working Group of the ERA—EDTA (European Renal Association—European Dialysis and Transplant Association) recommend that all eligible people should receive vaccination against COVID-19 (except for those with known allergic reactions to any of the vaccine components) since the potential of COVID-19 vaccines to induce immunity protecting from severe COVID 19 should outweigh potential risks in most cases [310].

Conclusions

Though the long-term outlook in most children with SSNS is for resolution of nephrotic syndrome and continuing normal kidney function, approximately half of these children will suffer multiple relapses requiring corticosteroids and one or more corticosteroid sparing agents during the course of their disease and are at risk of multiple disease and treatment related complications. In summary:-

- SSNS is more common in Asian but less common in African and African-American children compared with Caucasian children.
- The aetiology and pathogenesis of SSNS remains largely uncertain.
- The outcome of SSNS is for resolution of disease and normal kidney function in the majority of patients.
- The prognosis for long-term kidney function in SSNS depends on complete remission of proteinuria rather than histology so that kidney biopsies are usually not required at presentation or before commencing corticosteroid sparing therapy in children with SSNS.
- Four large well-designed RCTs have demonstrated that there is no benefit of continuing prednisone therapy in the initial episode of SSNS beyond 2 or 3 months to reduce the risk of relapse or FRNS.
- Small studies suggest that relapses of SSNS can be treated successfully with smaller doses of prednisone (1 mg/kg/day) compared with 2 mg/kg/day but adequately powered RCTs are required to confirm this.
- RCTs and large observational studies have evaluated the relative efficacies of alkylating agents, levamisole, mycophenolate mofetil and CNIs. However these data remain insufficient to provide definitive recommendations on which corticosteroid sparing agent should be preferred as the first agent in a child with FRNS or SDNS so the choice of agent depends on patient and physician preferences based on adverse effects, availability and costs.
- In RCTs, rituximab reduces the risk of relapse compared with other therapies. However many children relapse within 6–12 months and uncertainties remain about the risk of serious adverse effects and the significance of persistent hypogammaglobulinaemia.

Further information on the underlying cause of SSNS is needed to guide therapy. New randomised controlled trials are required both to compare new therapies with existing therapies and to determine the optimal regimens for using corticosteroid therapy in SSNS. In particular further studies are required to determine the optimum dose and duration of corticosteroid therapy required in the initial episode of SSNS and in relapsing disease. Further studies on the safety of rituximab are required to determine whether it should be used ahead of other non-corticosteroid agents in children with FRNS and SDNS.

References

1. Nephrotic syndrome in children: prediction of histopathology from clinical and laboratory characteristics at time of diagnosis. A report of the International Study of Kidney Disease in Children. Kidney Int 1978;13(2):159–165.
2. The primary nephrotic syndrome in children. Identification of patients with minimal change nephrotic syndrome from initial response to prednisone. A report of the International Study of Kidney Disease in Children. J Pediatr 1981;98(4):561–564.
3. Koskimies O, Vilska J, Rapola J, Hallman N. Long-term outcome of primary nephrotic syndrome. Arch Dis Child. 1982;57(7):544–8.
4. Fakhouri F, Bocquet N, Taupin P, Presne C, Gagnadoux M-F, Landais P, et al. Steroid-sensitive nephrotic syndrome: from childhood to adulthood. Am J Kidney Dis. 2003;41(3):550–7.
5. Tarshish P, Tobin JN, Bernstein J, Edelmann CM Jr. Prognostic significance of the early course of minimal change nephrotic syndrome: report of the International Study of Kidney Disease in Children. J Am Soc Nephrol. 1997;8(5):769–76.
6. El Bakkali L, Rodrigues Pereira R, Kuik DJ, Ket JCF, van Wijk JAE. Nephrotic syndrome in The Netherlands: a population-based cohort study and a review of the literature. Pediatr Nephrol. 2011;26(8):1241–6.

7. Wong W. Idiopathic nephrotic syndrome in New Zealand children, demographic, clinical features, initial management and outcome after twelve-month follow-up: results of a three-year national surveillance study. J Paediatr Child Health. 2007;43(5):337–41.

8. Sureshkumar P, Hodson EM, Willis NS, Barzi F, Craig JC. Predictors of remission and relapse in idiopathic nephrotic syndrome: a prospective cohort study. Pediatr Nephrol. 2014;29(6):1039–46.

9. Chanchlani R, Parekh RS. Ethnic differences in childhood nephrotic syndrome. Front Pediatr. 2016;4:39.

10. Borges FF, Shiraichi L, da Silva MP, Nishimoto EI, Nogueira PC. Is focal segmental glomerulosclerosis increasing in patients with nephrotic syndrome? Pediatr Nephrol. 2007;22(9):1309–13.

11. Shalhoub RJ. Pathogenesis of lipoid nephrosis: a disorder of T-cell function. Lancet. 1974;2(7880):556–60.

12. Routledge RC, Hann IM, Jones PH. Hodgkin's disease complicated by the nephrotic syndrome. Cancer. 1976;38(4):1735–40.

13. Yum MN, Edwards JL, Kleit S. Glomerular lesions in Hodgkin disease. Arch Pathol Lab Med. 1975;99(12):645–9.

14. Keng KL, Kuipers F. Inoculation with measles virus in therapy of nephrotic syndrome. Ned Tijdschr Geneeskd. 1951;95(25):1806–14.

15. Lander HB. Effects of measles on nephrotic syndrome. AMA Am J Dis Child. 1949;78(5):813–5.

16. Rosenblum AH, Lander HB, Fisher RM. Measles in the nephrotic syndrome. J Pediatr. 1949;35(5):574–84.

17. Tejani A. Morphological transition in minimal change nephrotic syndrome. Nephron. 1985;39(3):157–9.

18. Cambon-Thomsen A, Bouissou F, Abbal M, Duprat MP, Barthe P, Calot M, et al. HLA and Bf in idiopathic nephrotic syndrome in children: differences between corticosensitive and corticoresistant forms. Pathol Biol. 1986;34(6):725–30.

19. Kobayashi T, Ogawa A, Takahashi K, Uchiyama M. HLA-DQB1 allele associates with idiopathic nephrotic syndrome in Japanese children. Acta Paediatr Jpn. 1995;37(3):293–6.

20. Lagueruela CC, Buettner TL, Cole BR, Kissane JM, Robson AM. HLA extended haplotypes in steroid-sensitive nephrotic syndrome of childhood. Kidney Int. 1990;38(1):145–50.

21. Noss G, Bachmann HJ, Olbing H. Association of minimal change nephrotic syndrome (MCNS) with HLA-B8 an B13. Clin Nephrol. 1981;15(4):172–4.

22. Brenchley PEC. Vascular permeability factors in steroid-sensitive nephrotic syndrome and focal segmental glomerulosclerosis. Nephrol Dial Transplant. 2003;18(Suppl 6):vi21–5.

23. Eddy AA, Schnaper HW. The nephrotic syndrome: from the simple to the complex. Semin Nephrol. 1998;18(3):304–16.

24. Schnaper HW, Aune TM. Identification of the lymphokine soluble immune response suppressor in urine of nephrotic children. J Clin Invest. 1985;76(1):341–9.

25. Matsumoto K, Kanmatsuse K. Elevated vascular endothelial growth factor levels in the urine of patients with minimal-change nephrotic syndrome. Clin Nephrol. 2001;55(4):269–74.

26. Webb NJ, Watson CJ, Roberts IS, Bottomley MJ, Jones CA, Lewis MA, et al. Circulating vascular endothelial growth factor is not increased during relapses of steroid-sensitive nephrotic syndrome. Kidney Int. 1999;55(3):1063–71.

27. Eremina V, Cui S, Gerber H, Ferrara N, Haigh J, Nagy A, et al. Vascular endothelial growth factor a signaling in the podocyte-endothelial compartment is required for mesangial cell migration and survival. J Am Soc Nephrol. 2006;17(3):724–35.

28. Eremina V, Sood M, Haigh J, Nagy A, Lajoie G, Ferrara N, et al. Glomerular-specific alterations of VEGF-A expression lead to distinct congenital and acquired renal diseases. J Clin Invest. 2003;111(5):707–16.

29. Schnaper HW, Aune TM. Steroid-sensitive mechanism of soluble immune response suppressor production in steroid-responsive nephrotic syndrome. J Clin Invest. 1987;79(1):257–64.

30. Savin VJ, Sharma R, Sharma M, McCarthy ET, Swan SK, Ellis E, et al. Circulating factor associated with increased glomerular permeability to albumin in recurrent focal segmental glomerulosclerosis. N Engl J Med. 1996;334(14):878–83.

31. Dantal J, Bigot E, Bogers W, Testa A, Kriaa F, Jacques Y, et al. Effect of plasma protein adsorption on protein excretion in kidney-transplant recipients with recurrent nephrotic syndrome. N Engl J Med. 1994;330(1):7–14.

32. Garin EH, Laflam PF, Muffly K. Proteinuria and fusion of podocyte foot processes in rats after infusion of cytokine from patients with idiopathic minimal lesion nephrotic syndrome. Nephron Exp Nephrol. 2006;102(3–4):e105–12.

33. Clement LC, Avila-Casado C, Mace C, Soria E, Bakker WW, Kersten S, et al. Podocyte-secreted angiopoietin-like-4 mediates proteinuria in glucocorticoid-sensitive nephrotic syndrome. Nat Med. 2011;17(1):117–22.

34. Gebeshuber CA, Kornauth C, Dong L, Sierig R, Seibler J, Reiss M, et al. Focal segmental glomerulosclerosis is induced by microRNA-193a and its downregulation of WT1. Nat Med. 2013;19(4):481–7.

35. Wang JY, Zhang DQ, Cao Q, Qiao XQ, Zhou GP. miR-939-5p decreases the enrichment of RNA polymerase II in the promoter region of CD2AP involved in nephrotic syndrome. J Cell Biochem. 2019;120:11366–74.

36. Abbas AK, Murphy KM, Sher A. Functional diversity of helper T lymphocytes. Nature. 1996;383(6603):787–93.

37. Mosmann TR, Cherwinski H, Bond MW, Giedlin MA, Coffman RL. Two types of murine helper T cell clone. I. Definition according to profiles of lym-

phokine activities and secreted proteins. J Immunol. 1986;136(7):2348–57.

38. Street NE, Mosmann TR. Functional diversity of T lymphocytes due to secretion of different cytokine patterns. FASEB J. 1991;5(2):171–7.

39. Sad S, Marcotte R, Mosmann TR. Cytokine-induced differentiation of precursor mouse CD8+ T cells into cytotoxic CD8+ T cells secreting Th1 or Th2 cytokines. Immunity. 1995;2(3):271–9.

40. Fehervari Z, Sakaguchi S. Development and function of CD25+CD4+ regulatory T cells. Curr Opin Immunol. 2004;16(2):203–8.

41. Hori S, Nomura T, Sakaguchi S. Control of regulatory T cell development by the transcription factor Foxp3. Science. 2003;299(5609):1057–61.

42. Iwakura Y, Ishigame H. The IL-23/IL-17 axis in inflammation. J Clin Invest. 2006;116(5):1218–22.

43. Weaver CT, Harrington LE, Mangan PR, Gavrieli M, Murphy KM. Th17: an effector CD4 T cell lineage with regulatory T cell ties. Immunity. 2006;24(6):677–88.

44. Motavalli R, Etemadi J, Soltani-Zangbar MS, Ardalan MR, Kahroba H, Roshangar L, et al. Altered Th17/Treg ratio as a possible mechanism in pathogenesis of idiopathic membranous nephropathy. Cytokine. 2021;141:155452.

45. May CJ, Welsh GI, Chesor M, Lait PJ, Schewitz-Bowers LP, Lee RWJ, et al. Human Th17 cells produce a soluble mediator that increases podocyte motility via signaling pathways that mimic PAR-1 activation. Am J Physiol Renal Physiol. 2019;317(4):F913–f21.

46. Araya CE, Wasserfall CH, Brusko TM, Mu W, Segal MS, Johnson RJ, et al. A case of unfulfilled expectations. Cytokines in idiopathic minimal lesion nephrotic syndrome. Pediatr Nephrol. 2006;21(5):603–10.

47. Matsumoto K, Kanmatsuse K. Increased urinary excretion of interleukin-17 in nephrotic patients. Nephron. 2002;91(2):243–9.

48. Bakr A, Rageh I, el-Azouny M, Deyab S, Lotfy H. Serum neopterin levels in children with primary nephrotic syndrome. Acta Paediatr. 2006;95(7):854–6.

49. Kopp JB, Anders HJ, Susztak K, Podesta MA, Remuzzi G, Hildebrandt F, et al. Podocytopathies. Nat Rev Dis Prim. 2020;6(1):68.

50. Dorval G, Gribouval O, Martinez-Barquero V, Machuca E, Tete MJ, Baudouin V, et al. Clinical and genetic heterogeneity in familial steroid-sensitive nephrotic syndrome. Pediatr Nephrol. 2018;33(3):473–83.

51. White RH. The familial nephrotic syndrome. I. A European survey. Clin Nephrol. 1973;1(4):215–9.

52. Gbadegesin RA, Adeyemo A, Webb NJ, Greenbaum LA, Abeyagunawardena A, Thalgahagoda S, et al. HLA-DQA1 and PLCG2 are candidate risk loci for childhood-onset steroid-sensitive nephrotic syndrome. J Am Soc Nephrol. 2015;26(7):1701–10.

53. Debiec H, Dossier C, Letouze E, Gillies CE, Vivarelli M, Putler RK, et al. Transethnic, genome-wide analysis reveals immune-related risk alleles and phenotypic correlates in pediatric steroid-sensitive nephrotic syndrome. J Am Soc Nephrol. 2018;29(7):2000–13.

54. Jia X, Horinouchi T, Hitomi Y, Shono A, Khor SS, Omae Y, et al. Strong association of the HLA-DR/DQ locus with childhood steroid-sensitive nephrotic syndrome in the Japanese population. J Am Soc Nephrol. 2018;29(8):2189–99.

55. Dufek S, Cheshire C, Levine AP, Trompeter RS, Issler N, Stubbs M, et al. Genetic identification of two novel loci associated with steroid-sensitive nephrotic syndrome. J Am Soc Nephrol. 2019;30(8):1375–84.

56. Jia X, Yamamura T, Gbadegesin R, McNulty MT, Song K, Nagano C, et al. Common risk variants in NPHS1 and TNFSF15 are associated with childhood steroid-sensitive nephrotic syndrome. Kidney Int. 2020;98(5):1308–22.

57. Stone HKPS, Eapen AA, Chen X, Harley JB, Devarajan P, Weirauch MT, Kottyan L. Comprehensive review of steroid-sensitive nephrotic syndrome genetic risk loci and transcriptional regulation as a possible mechanistic link to disease risk. Kidney Int Rep. 2020;6(1):187–95.

58. Ishimoto T, Shimada M, Gabriela G, Kosugi T, Sato W, Lee PY, et al. Toll-like receptor 3 ligand, polyIC, induces proteinuria and glomerular CD80, and increases urinary CD80 in mice. Nephrol Dial Transplant. 2013;28(6):1439–46.

59. Mundel P, Greka A. Developing therapeutic 'arrows' with the precision of William Tell: the time has come for targeted therapies in kidney disease. Curr Opin Nephrol Hypertens. 2015;24(4):388–92.

60. Murphy WM, Jukkola AF, Roy S 3rd. Nephrotic syndrome with mesangial-cell proliferation in children—a distinct entity? Am J Clin Pathol. 1979;72(1):42–7.

61. Waldherr R, Gubler MC, Levy M, Broyer M, Habib R. The significance of pure diffuse mesangial proliferation in idiopathic nephrotic syndrome. Clin Nephrol. 1978;10(5):171–9.

62. Zeis PM, Kavazarakis E, Nakopoulou L, Moustaki M, Messaritaki A, Zeis MP, et al. Glomerulopathy with mesangial IgM deposits: long-term follow up of 64 children. Pediatr Int. 2001;43(3):287–92.

63. Tejani A, Phadke K, Nicastri A, Adamson O, Chen CK, Trachtman H, et al. Efficacy of cyclophosphamide in steroid-sensitive childhood nephrotic syndrome with different morphological lesions. Nephron. 1985;41(2):170–3.

64. Kopolovic J, Shvil Y, Pomeranz A, Ron N, Rubinger D, Oren R. IgM nephropathy: morphological study related to clinical findings. Am J Nephrol. 1987;7(4):275–80.

65. Hsu HC, Chen WY, Lin GJ, Chen L, Kao SL, Huang CC, et al. Clinical and immunopathologic study of mesangial IgM nephropathy: report of 41 cases. Histopathology. 1984;8(3):435–46.

66. Habib R, Girardin E, Gagnadoux MF, Hinglais N, Levy M, Broyer M. Immunopathological findings in idiopathic nephrosis: clinical significance of

glomerular "immune deposits". Pediatr Nephrol. 1988;2(4):402–8.

67. Al-Eisa A, Carter JE, Lirenman DS, Magil AB. Childhood IgM nephropathy: comparison with minimal change disease. Nephron. 1996;72(1):37–43.

68. Fukuma Y, Hisano S, Segawa Y, Niimi K, Tsuru N, Kaku Y, et al. Clinicopathologic correlation of C1q nephropathy in children. Am J Kidney Dis. 2006;47(3):412–8.

69. Wong CS, Fink CA, Baechle J, Harris AA, Staples AO, Brandt JR. C1q nephropathy and minimal change nephrotic syndrome. Pediatr Nephrol. 2009;24(4):761–7.

70. Hisano S, Fukuma Y, Segawa Y, Niimi K, Kaku Y, Hatae K, et al. Clinicopathologic correlation and outcome of C1q nephropathy. Clin J Am Soc Nephrol. 2008;3(6):1637–43.

71. Qin J, Yang Q, Tang X, Chen W, Li Z, Mao H, et al. Clinicopathologic features and treatment response in nephrotic IgA nephropathy with minimal change disease. Clin Nephrol. 2013;79(1):37–44.

72. Myllymaki J, Saha H, Mustonen J, Helin H, Pasternack A. IgM nephropathy: clinical picture and long-term prognosis. Am J Kidney Dis. 2003;41(2):343–50.

73. Haas M, Yousefzadeh N. Glomerular tip lesion in minimal change nephropathy: a study of autopsies before 1950. Am J Kidney Dis. 2002;39(6):1168–75.

74. Howie AJ. Pathology of minimal change nephropathy and segmental sclerosing glomerular disorders. Nephrol Dial Transplant. 2003;18(Suppl 6):vi33–8.

75. Ostalska-Nowicka D, Zachwieja J, Maciejewski J, Wozniak A, Salwa-Urawska W. The prognostic value of glomerular immaturity in the nephrotic syndrome in children. Pediatr Nephrol. 2004;19(6):633–7.

76. Ichikawa I, Fogo A. Focal segmental glomerulosclerosis. Pediatr Nephrol. 1996;10(3):374–91.

77. Schnaper HW. Idiopathic focal segmental glomerulosclerosis. Semin Nephrol. 2003;23(2):183–93.

78. McAdams AJ, Valentini RP, Welch TR. The non-specificity of focal segmental glomerulosclerosis. The defining characteristics of primary focal glomerulosclerosis, mesangial proliferation, and minimal change. Medicine (Baltimore). 1997;76(1):42–52.

79. D'Agati V. Pathologic classification of focal segmental glomerulosclerosis. Semin Nephrol. 2003;23(2):117–34.

80. Habib R, Kleinknecht C. The primary nephrotic syndrome of childhood. Classification and clinicopathologic study of 406 cases. Pathol Annu. 1971;6:417–74.

81. Meadow SR, Sarsfield JK. Steroid-responsive and nephrotic syndrome and allergy: clinical studies. Arch Dis Child. 1981;56(7):509–16.

82. Salsano ME, Graziano L, Luongo I, Pilla P, Giordano M, Lama G. Atopy in childhood idiopathic nephrotic syndrome. Acta Paediatr. 2007;96(4):561–6.

83. Arneil GC. 164 children with nephrosis. Lancet. 1961;2:1103–10.

84. Hollis A, Dart A, Morgan C, Mammen C, Zappitelli M, Chanchlani R, et al. Delays in diagnosis of nephrotic syndrome in children: a survey study. Paediatr Child Health. 2019;24(4):258–62.

85. Alwadhi RK, Mathew JL, Rath B. Clinical profile of children with nephrotic syndrome not on glucorticoid therapy, but presenting with infection. J Paediatr Child Health. 2004;40(1–2):28–32.

86. Noone DG, Iijima K, Parekh R. Idiopathic nephrotic syndrome in children. [Review]. Lancet. 2018;1(10141):61–74.

87. Carter SA, Mistry S, Fitzpatrick J, Banh T, Hebert D, Langlois V, et al. Prediction of short- and long-term outcomes in childhood nephrotic syndrome. Kidney Int Rep. 2020;5(4):426–34.

88. Dossier C, Delbet JD, Boyer O, Daoud P, Mesples B, Pellegrino B, et al. Five-year outcome of children with idiopathic nephrotic syndrome: the NEPHROVIR population-based cohort study. Pediatr Nephrol. 2019;34(4):671–8.

89. Andersen RF, Thrane N, Noergaard K, Rytter L, Jespersen B, Rittig S. Early age at debut is a predictor of steroid-dependent and frequent relapsing nephrotic syndrome. Pediatr Nephrol. 2010;25(7):1299–304.

90. Lewis MA, Baildom EM, Davis N, Houston IB, Postlethwaite RJ. Nephrotic syndrome: from toddlers to twenties. Lancet. 1989;1(8632):255–9.

91. Yap HK, Han EJ, Heng CK, Gong WK. Risk factors for steroid dependency in children with idiopathic nephrotic syndrome. Pediatr Nephrol. 2001;16(12):1049–52.

92. Vivarelli M, Moscaritolo E, Tsalkidis A, Massella L, Emma F. Time for initial response to steroids is a major prognostic factor in idiopathic nephrotic syndrome. J Pediatr. 2010;156(6):965–71.

93. Fujinaga S, Hirano D, Nishizaki N. Early identification of steroid dependency in Japanese children with steroid-sensitive nephrotic syndrome undergoing short-term initial steroid therapy. Pediatr Nephrol. 2011;26(3):485–6.

94. Nakanishi K, Iijima K, Ishikura K, Hataya H, Sasaki S, Honda M, et al. Two-year outcome of the ISKDC regimen and frequently relapsing risk in children with idiopathic nephrotic syndrome. Clin J Am Soc Nephrol. 2013;8:787–96.

95. Harambat J, Godron A, Ernould S, Rigothier C, Llanas B, Leroy S. Prediction of steroid-sparing agent use in childhood idiopathic nephrotic syndrome. Pediatr Nephrol. 2013;28(4):631–8.

96. Noer MS. Predictors of relapse in steroid-sensitive nephrotic syndrome. Southeast Asian J Trop Med Public Health. 2005;36(5):1313–20.

97. Teeninga N, Schreuder MF, Bokenkamp A, Delemarre-van de Waal HA, van Wijk JAE. Influence of low birth weight on minimal change nephrotic syndrome in children, including a meta-analysis. Nephrol Dial Transplant. 2008;23(5):1615–20.

98. Lahdenkari A-T, Suvanto M, Kajantie E, Koskimies O, Kestila M, Jalanko H. Clinical features and

outcome of childhood minimal change nephrotic syndrome: is genetics involved? Pediatr Nephrol. 2005;20(8):1073–80.

99. Ruth E-M, Kemper MJ, Leumann EP, Laube GF, Neuhaus TJ. Children with steroid-sensitive nephrotic syndrome come of age: long-term outcome. J Pediatr. 2005;147(2):202–7.

100. Trompeter RS, Lloyd BW, Hicks J, White RH, Cameron JS. Long-term outcome for children with minimal-change nephrotic syndrome. Lancet. 1985;1(8425):368–70.

101. Kyrieleis HA, Levtchenko EN, Wetzels JF. Long-term outcome after cyclophosphamide treatment in children with steroid-dependent and frequently relapsing minimal change nephrotic syndrome. Am J Kidney Dis. 2007;49(5):592–7.

102. Ishikura K, Yoshikawa N, Nakazato H, Sasaki S, Nakanishi K, Matsuyama T, et al. Morbidity in children with frequently relapsing nephrosis: 10-year follow-up of a randomized controlled trial. Pediatr Nephrol. 2015;30(3):459–68.

103. Korsgaard T, Andersen RF, Joshi S, Hagstrom S, Rittig S. Childhood onset steroid-sensitive nephrotic syndrome continues into adulthood. Pediatr Nephrol. 2019;34(4):641–8.

104. Skrzypczyk P, Panczyk-Tomaszewska M, Roszkowska-Blaim M, Wawer Z, Bienias B, Zajaczkowska M, et al. Long-term outcomes in idiopathic nephrotic syndrome: from childhood to adulthood. Clin Nephrol. 2014;81(3):166–73.

105. Aydin M, Franke I, Kurylowicz L, Ganschow R, Lentze M, Born M, et al. The long-term outcome of childhood nephrotic syndrome in Germany: a cross-sectional study. Clin Exp Nephrol. 2019;23(5):676–88.

106. Lechner BL, Bockenhauer D, Iragorri S, Kennedy TL, Siegel NJ. The risk of cardiovascular disease in adults who have had childhood nephrotic syndrome. Pediatr Nephrol. 2004;19(7):744–8.

107. Alsaidi S, Wagner D, Grisaru S, Midgley J, Hamiwka L, Wade A, et al. Glomerular filtration rate trends during follow-up in children with steroid-sensitive nephrotic syndrome. Can J Kidney Health Dis. 2017;4:2054358117709496.

108. Siegel NJ, Goldberg B, Krassner LS, Hayslett JP. Long-term follow-up of children with steroid-responsive nephrotic syndrome. J Pediatr. 1972;81(2):251–8.

109. Kim JS, Bellew CA, Silverstein DM, Aviles DH, Boineau FG, Vehaskari VM. High incidence of initial and late steroid resistance in childhood nephrotic syndrome. Kidney Int. 2005;68(3):1275–81.

110. Straatmann C, Ayoob R, Gbadegesin R, Gibson K, Rheault MN, Srivastava T, et al. Treatment outcome of late steroid-resistant nephrotic syndrome: a study by the Midwest Pediatric Nephrology Consortium. Pediatr Nephrol. 2013;28(8):1235–41.

111. Ding WY, Koziell A, McCarthy HJ, Bierzynska A, Bhagavatula MK, Dudley JA, et al. Initial steroid sensitivity in children with steroid-resistant nephrotic syndrome predicts post-transplant recurrence. J Am Soc Nephrol. 2014;25(6):1342–8.

112. Berns JS, Gaudio KM, Krassner LS, Anderson FP, Durante D, McDonald BM, et al. Steroid-responsive nephrotic syndrome of childhood: a long-term study of clinical course, histopathology, efficacy of cyclophosphamide therapy, and effects on growth. Am J Kidney Dis. 1987;9(2):108–14.

113. Webb NJ, Lewis MA, Iqbal J, Smart PJ, Lendon M, Postlethwaite RJ. Childhood steroid-sensitive nephrotic syndrome: does the histology matter? Am J Kidney Dis. 1996;27(4):484–8.

114. Cattran DC, Rao P. Long-term outcome in children and adults with classic focal segmental glomerulosclerosis. Am J Kidney Dis. 1998;32(1):72–9.

115. Abrantes MM, Cardoso LSB, Lima EM, Silva JMP, Diniz JS, Bambirra EA, et al. Clinical course of 110 children and adolescents with primary focal segmental glomerulosclerosis. Pediatr Nephrol. 2006;21(4):482–9.

116. Minimal change nephrotic syndrome in children: deaths during the first 5 to 15 years' observation. Report of the International Study of Kidney Disease in Children. Pediatrics 1984;73(4):497–501.

117. Rheault MN, Wei C-C, Hains DS, Wang W, Kerlin BA, Smoyer WE. Increased frequency of acute kidney injury among children hospitalized with nephrotic syndrome. Pediatr Nephrol. 2014;29:139–47.

118. Wei C-C, Yu IW, Lin H-W, Tsai AC. Occurrence of infection among children with nephrotic syndrome during hospitalizations. Nephrology. 2012;17(8):681–8.

119. Alfakeekh K, Azar M, Sowailmi BA, Alsulaiman S, Makdob SA, Omair A, et al. Immunosuppressive burden and risk factors of infection in primary childhood nephrotic syndrome. J Infect Public Health. 2019;12(1):90–4.

120. Laskin BL, Goebel J, Starke JR, Schauer DP, Eckman MH. Cost-effectiveness of latent tuberculosis screening before steroid therapy for idiopathic nephrotic syndrome in children. Am J Kidney Dis. 2013;61(1):22–32.

121. Kerlin BA, Ayoob R, Smoyer WE. Epidemiology and pathophysiology of nephrotic syndrome-associated thromboembolic disease. Clin J Am Soc Nephrol. 2012;7(3):513–20.

122. Kerlin BA, Haworth K, Smoyer WE. Venous thromboembolism in pediatric nephrotic syndrome. Pediatr Nephrol. 2014;29(6):989–97.

123. Rheault MN, Zhang L, Selewski DT, Kallash M, Tran CL, Seamon M, et al. AKI in children hospitalized with nephrotic syndrome. Clin J Am Soc Nephrol. 2015;10(12):2110–8.

124. Gipson DS, Messer KL, Tran CL, Herreshoff EG, Samuel JP, Massengill SF, et al. Inpatient health care utilization in the United States among children, adolescents, and young adults with nephrotic syndrome. Am J Kidney Dis. 2013;61(6):910–7.

125. Kidney Disease: Improving Global Outcomes (KDIGO) Glomerulonephritis Work Group. KDIGO

125. clinical practice guideline for glomerulonephritis. Kidney Int. 2012;Supplement 2:139–274.

126. Hinkes BG, Mucha B, Vlangos CN, Gbadegesin R, Liu J, Hasselbacher K, et al. Nephrotic syndrome in the first year of life: two thirds of cases are caused by mutations in 4 genes (NPHS1, NPHS2, WT1, and LAMB2). Pediatrics. 2007;119(4):e907–19.

127. Lipska-Zietkiewicz BS, Ozaltin F, Holtta T, Bockenhauer D, Berody S, Levtchenko E, et al. Genetic aspects of congenital nephrotic syndrome: a consensus statement from the ERKNet-ESPN inherited glomerulopathy working group. Eur J Hum Genet. 2020;28(10):1368–78.

128. Broyer M, Meyrier A, Niaudet P, Habib R. Minimal changes and focal and segmental glomerulosclerosis. In: Cameron JS, Davison AM, Grunfeld J-P, Kerr D, Ritz E, editors. Oxford textbook of clinical nephrology. Oxford: Oxford University Press; 1992. p. 298–339.

129. Gulati S, Sural S, Sharma RK, Gupta A, Gupta RK. Spectrum of adolescent-onset nephrotic syndrome in Indian children. Pediatr Nephrol. 2001;16(12):1045–8.

130. Gulati S, Sharma AP, Sharma RK, Gupta A, Gupta RK. Do current recommendations for kidney biopsy in nephrotic syndrome need modifications? Pediatr Nephrol. 2002;17(6):404–8.

131. Baqi N, Singh A, Balachandra S, Ahmad H, Nicastri A, Kytinski S, et al. The paucity of minimal change disease in adolescents with primary nephrotic syndrome. Pediatr Nephrol. 1998;12(2):105–7.

132. McKinney PA, Feltbower RG, Brocklebank JT, Fitzpatrick MM. Time trends and ethnic patterns of childhood nephrotic syndrome in Yorkshire, UK. Pediatr Nephrol. 2001;16(12):1040–4.

133. Gipson DS, Massengill SF, Yao L, Nagaraj S, Smoyer WE, Mahan JD, et al. Management of childhood onset nephrotic syndrome. Pediatrics. 2009;124(2):747–57.

134. MacHardy N, Miles PV, Massengill SF, Smoyer WE, Mahan JD, Greenbaum L, et al. Management patterns of childhood-onset nephrotic syndrome. Pediatr Nephrol. 2009;24(11):2193–201.

135. Primack WA, Schulman SL, Kaplan BS. An analysis of the approach to management of childhood nephrotic syndrome by pediatric nephrologists. Am J Kidney Dis. 1994;23(4):524–7.

136. Samuel S, Morgan CJ, Bitzan N, Mammen C, Dart AB, Manns BJ, et al. Substantial practice variation exists in the management of childhood nephrotic syndrome. Pediatr Nephrol. 2013;29(12):2289–98.

137. Siegel NJ, Gaudio KM, Krassner LS, McDonald BM, Anderson FP, Kashgarian M. Steroid-dependent nephrotic syndrome in children: histopathology and relapses after cyclophosphamide treatment. Kidney Int. 1981;19(3):454–9.

138. Trachtman H, Carroll F, Phadke K, Khawar M, Nicastri A, Chen CK, et al. Paucity of minimal-change lesion in children with early frequently relapsing steroid-responsive nephrotic syndrome. Am J Nephrol. 1987;7(1):13–7.

139. Sorof JM, Hawkins EP, Brewer ED, Boydstun II, Kale AS, Powell DR. Age and ethnicity affect the risk and outcome of focal segmental glomerulosclerosis. Pediatr Nephrol. 1998;12(9):764–8.

140. Stadermann MB, Lilien MR, van de Kar NCAJ, Monnens LAH, Schroder CH. Is biopsy required prior to cyclophosphamide in steroid-sensitive nephrotic syndrome? Clin Nephrol. 2003;60(5):315–7.

141. Samuel S, Bitzan M, Zappitelli M, Dart A, Mammen C, Pinsk M, et al. Canadian Society of Nephrology Commentary on the 2012 KDIGO clinical practice guideline for glomerulonephritis: management of nephrotic syndrome in children. Am J Kidney Dis. 2014;63(3):354–62.

142. Trautmann A, Vivarelli M, Samuel S, Gipson D, Sinha A, Schaefer F, et al. IPNA clinical practice recommendations for the diagnosis and management of children with steroid-resistant nephrotic syndrome. Pediatr Nephrol. 2020;35(8):1529–61.

143. White RH, Poole C. Day care renal biopsy. Pediatr Nephrol. 1996;10(4):408–11.

144. Varnell CD Jr, Stone HK, Welge JA. Bleeding complications after pediatric kidney biopsy: a systematic review and meta-analysis. Clin J Am Soc Nephrol. 2019;1(1):57–65.

145. Gipson DS, Chin H, Presler TP, Jennette C, Ferris ME, Massengill S, et al. Differential risk of remission and ESRD in childhood FSGS. Pediatr Nephrol. 2006;21(3):344–9.

146. Arneil GC. Treatment of nephrosis with prednisolone. Lancet. 1956;270(6920):409–11.

147. Arneil GC. The nephrotic syndrome. Pediatr Clin N Am. 1971;18(2):547–59.

148. Alternate-day versus intermittent prednisone in frequently relapsing nephrotic syndrome. A report of "Arbetsgemeinschaft fur Padiatrische Nephrologie". Lancet. 1979;1(8113):401–3.

149. Ekka BK, Bagga A, Srivastava RN. Single- versus divided-dose prednisolone therapy for relapses of nephrotic syndrome. Pediatr Nephrol. 1997;11(5):597–9.

150. Feber J, Al-Matrafi J, Farhadi E, Vaillancourt R, Wolfish N. Prednisone dosing per body weight or body surface area in children with nephrotic syndrome: is it equivalent? Pediatr Nephrol. 2009;24(5):1027–31.

151. Saadeh SA, Baracco R, Jain A, Kapur G, Mattoo TK, Valentini RP. Weight or body surface area dosing of steroids in nephrotic syndrome: is there an outcome difference? Pediatr Nephrol. 2011;26(12):2167–71.

152. Hirano D, Fujimaru T. Two dosing regimens for steroid therapy in nephrotic syndrome [Letter]. Pediatr Nephrol 2013. https://doi.org/10.1007/s00467-013-2417-8.

153. Raman V, Krishnamurthy S, Harichandrakumar KT. Body weight-based prednisolone versus body surface area-based prednisolone regimen for induction of remission in children with nephrotic syndrome: a randomized, open-label, equivalence clinical trial. Pediatr Nephrol. 2016;31(4):595–604.

154. Basu B, Bhattacharyya S, Barua S, Naskar A, Roy B. Efficacy of body weight vs body surface area-based prednisolone regimen in nephrotic syndrome. Clin Exp Nephrol. 2020;24(7):622–9.

155. Short versus standard prednisone therapy for initial treatment of idiopathic nephrotic syndrome in children. Arbeitsgemeinschaft fur Padiatrische Nephrologie. Lancet 1988;1(8582):380–383.

156. Yoshikawa N, Nakanishi K, Sako M, Oba MS, Mori R, Ota E, et al. A multicenter randomized trial indicates initial prednisolone treatment for childhood nephrotic syndrome for two months is not inferior to six-month treatment. Kidney Int. 2015;87(1):225–32.

157. Webb NJA, Woolley RL, Lambe T, Frew E, Brettell EA, Barsoum EN, et al. Long term tapering versus standard prednisolone treatment for first episode of childhood nephrotic syndrome: phase III randomised controlled trial and economic evaluation. The BMJ. 2019;365 (no pagination)(l1800).

158. Teeninga N, Kist-van Holthe J, van Rijskwijk N, de Mos N, Wetzels JF, Nauta J. Extending prednisolone therapy does not reduce relapse in childhood nephrotic syndrome. J Am Soc Nephrol. 2013;24(1):149–59.

159. Sinha A, Saha A, Kumar M, Sharma S, Afzal K, Mehta A, et al. Extending initial prednisolone treatment in a randomized control trial from 3 to 6 months did not significantly influence the course of illness in children with steroid-sensitive nephrotic syndrome. Kidney Int. 2015;87(1):217–24.

160. Sinha A, Gipson D, Wong C, Massengil S, Ahmad A, Hari P, ea. 6-months versus 3-months prednisolone for initial therapy of steroid sensitive nephrotic syndrome: open label RCT [abstract no: IPN11430-80]. Pediatr Nephrol. 2019;34(10):2076.

161. Hodson EM, Willis NS, Craig JC. Corticosteroid therapy for nephrotic syndrome in children. Cochrane Database Syst Rev. 2007;(4):CD001533.

162. Moher D, Pham B, Jones A, Cook DJ, Jadad AR, Moher M, et al. Does quality of reports of randomised trials affect estimates of intervention efficacy reported in meta-analyses? Lancet. 1998;352(9128):609–13.

163. Schulz KF, Chalmers I, Hayes RJ, Altman DG. Empirical evidence of bias. Dimensions of methodological quality associated with estimates of treatment effects in controlled trials. JAMA. 1995;273(5):408–12.

164. Hahn D, Samuel SM, Willis NS, Craig JC, Hodson EM. Corticosteroid therapy for nephrotic syndrome in children. Cochrane Database Syst Rev. 2020;8:CD001533.

165. Syndrome néphrotique idiopathique de l'enfant. Haute Autorité de Santé. 2008:1–22.

166. Indian Pediatric Nephrology Group, Indian Academy of Pediatrics, Bagga A, Ali U, Banerjee S, Kanitkar M, Phadke KD, et al. Management of steroid sensitive nephrotic syndrome: revised guidelines. Indian Pediatr. 2008;45(3):203–14.

167. Gargiulo A, Massella L, Ruggiero B, Ravà L, Ciofi degli Atti M, Materassi M, et al. Results of the PROPINE randomized controlled study suggest tapering of prednisone treatment for relapses of steroid sensitive nephrotic syndrome is not necessary in children. Kidney Int. 2021;99(2):475–83.

168. Deschenes G, Vivarelli M, Peruzzi L, ESPN Working Group on Idiopathic Nephrotic syndrome. Variability of diagnostic criteria and treatment of idiopathic nephrotic syndrome across European countries. Eur J Pediatr. 2017;176(5):647–54.

169. Shenoy M, Plant ND, Lewis MA, Bradbury MG, Lennon R, Webb NJ. Intravenous methylprednisolone in idiopathic childhood nephrotic syndrome. Pediatr Nephrol. 2010;25(5):899–903.

170. Letavernier B, Letavernier E, Leroy S, Baudet-Bonneville V, Bensman A, Ulinski T. Prediction of high-degree steroid dependency in pediatric idiopathic nephrotic syndrome. Pediatr Nephrol. 2008;23(12):2221–6.

171. Lande MB, Leonard MB. Variability among pediatric nephrologists in the initial therapy of nephrotic syndrome. Pediatr Nephrol. 2000;14(8–9):766–9.

172. Pasini A, Aceto G, Ammenti A, Ardissino G, Azzolina V, Bettinelli A, et al. Best practice guidelines for idiopathic nephrotic syndrome: recommendations versus reality. Pediatr Nephrol. 2015;30(1):91–101.

173. Samuel SM, Dart A, Filler G, Bitzan M, Pinsk M, Mammen C, et al. The Canadian childhood nephrotic syndrome (CHILDNEPH) study: report on mid-study feasibility, recruitment and main measures. BMC Nephrol. 2019;20(1):159.

174. Wingen AM, Muller-Wiefel DE, Scharer K. Spontaneous remissions in frequently relapsing and steroid dependent idiopathic nephrotic syndrome. Clin Nephrol. 1985;23(1):35–40.

175. Narchi H. Nephrotic syndrome relapse: need for a better evidence based definition. Arch Dis Child. 2004;89(4):395.

176. Ulinski T, Aoun B. New treatment strategies in idiopathic nephrotic syndrome. Minerva Pediatr. 2012;64(2):135–43.

177. Anonymous. Alternate-day prednisone is more effective than intermittent prednisone in frequently relapsing nephrotic syndrome. A report of "Arbeitsgemeinschaft fur Padiatrische Nephrologie". Eur J Pediatr. 1981;135(3):229–37.

178. Choonara IA, Heney D, Meadow SR. Low dose prednisolone in nephrotic syndrome. Arch Dis Child. 1989;64(4):610–1.

179. Borovitz Y, Alfandary H, Haskin O, Levi S, Kaz S, Davidovits M, et al. Lower prednisone dosing for steroid-sensitive nephrotic syndrome relapse: a prospective randomized pilot study. Eur J Pediatr. 2020;179(2):279–83.

180. Raja K, Parikh A, Webb H, Hothi D. Use of a low-dose prednisolone regimen to treat a relapse of steroid-sensitive nephrotic syndrome in children. Pediatr Nephrol. 2017;32(1):99–105.

181. Srivastava RN, Vasudev AS, Bagga A, Sunderam KR. Long-term, low-dose prednisolone therapy in frequently relapsing nephrotic syndrome. Pediatr Nephrol. 1992;6(3):247–50.

182. Elzouki AY, Jaiswal OP. Long-term, small dose prednisone therapy in frequently relapsing nephrotic syndrome of childhood. Effect on remission, statural growth, obesity, and infection rate. Clin Pediatr (Phila). 1988;27(8):387–92.

183. Lombel RM, Gipson DS, Hodson EM. Treatment of steroid-sensitive nephrotic syndrome: new guidelines from KDIGO. Pediatr Nephrol. 2013;28(3):415–26.

184. Yadav M, Sinha A, Khandelwal P, Hari P, Bagga A. Efficacy of low-dose daily versus alternate-day prednisolone in frequently relapsing nephrotic syndrome: an open-label randomized controlled trial. Pediatr Nephrol. 2019;34(5):829–35.

185. Abeyagunawardena AS, Trompeter RS. Increasing the dose of prednisolone during viral infections reduces the risk of relapse in nephrotic syndrome: a randomised controlled trial. Arch Dis Child. 2008;93(3):226–8.

186. Gulati A, Sinha A, Sreenivas V, Math A, Hari P, Bagga A. Daily corticosteroids reduce infection-associated relapses in frequently relapsing nephrotic syndrome: a randomized controlled trial. Clin J Am Soc Nephrol. 2011;6(1):63–9.

187. Mattoo TK, Mahmoud MA. Increased maintenance corticosteroids during upper respiratory infection decrease the risk of relapse in nephrotic syndrome. Nephron. 2000;85(4):343–5.

188. Abeyagunawardena AS, Thalgahagoda RS, Dissanayake PV, Abeyagunawardena S, Illangasekera YA, Karunadasa UI, et al. Short courses of daily prednisolone during upper respiratory tract infections reduce relapse frequency in childhood nephrotic syndrome. Pediatr Nephrol. 2017;32(8):1377–82.

189. Christian M WN, Mehta S, Nafska A et al. Short course daily low-dose prednisolone at the time of upper respiratory tract infection (urti) in non-selected children with relapsing steroid sensitive nephrotic syndrome does not prevent URTI-related relapse: the Prednos 2 trial. Nephrol Dial Transplant. 2021;36(Supplement 1).

190. Oh GJ, Waldo A, Paez-Cruz F, Gipson PE, Pesenson A, Selewski DT, et al. Steroid-associated side effects in patients with primary proteinuric kidney disease. Kidney Int Rep. 2019;4(11):1608–16.

191. Mishra OP, Basu B, Upadhyay SK, Prasad R, Schaefer F. Behavioural abnormalities in children with nephrotic syndrome. Nephrol Dial Transplant. 2010;25(8):2537–41.

192. Neuhaus TJ, Langlois V, Licht C. Behavioural abnormalities in children with nephrotic syndrome—an underappreciated complication of a standard treatment? Nephrol Dial Transplant. 2010;25(8):2397–9.

193. Khullar S, Banh T, Vasilevska-Ristovska J, Chanchlani R, Brooke J, Licht CPB, et al. Impact of steroids and steroid-sparing agents on quality of life in children with nephrotic syndrome. Pediatr Nephrol. 2021;36(1):93–102.

194. Mitra S, Banerjee S. The impact of pediatric nephrotic syndrome on families. Pediatr Nephrol. 2011;26(8):1235–40.

195. Broyer M, Guest G, Gagnadoux MF. Growth rate in children receiving alternate-day corticosteroid treatment after kidney transplantation. J Pediatr. 1992;120(5):721–5.

196. Emma F, Sesto A, Rizzoni G. Long-term linear growth of children with severe steroid-responsive nephrotic syndrome. Pediatr Nephrol. 2003;18(8):783–8.

197. Simmonds J, Grundy N, Trompeter R, Tullus K. Long-term steroid treatment and growth: a study in steroid-dependent nephrotic syndrome. Arch Dis Child. 2010;95(2):146–9.

198. Leroy V, Baudouin V, Alberti C, Guest G, Niaudet P, Loirat C, et al. Growth in boys with idiopathic nephrotic syndrome on long-term cyclosporin and steroid treatment. Pediatr Nephrol. 2009;24(12):2393–400.

199. Donatti TL, Koch VH. Final height of adults with childhood-onset steroid-responsive idiopathic nephrotic syndrome. Pediatr Nephrol. 2009;24(12):2401–8.

200. Grymonprez A, Proesmans W, Van Dyck M, Jans I, Goos G, Bouillon R. Vitamin D metabolites in childhood nephrotic syndrome. Pediatr Nephrol. 1995;9(3):278–81.

201. Gulati S, Godbole M, Singh U, Gulati K, Srivastava A. Are children with idiopathic nephrotic syndrome at risk for metabolic bone disease? Am J Kidney Dis. 2003;41(6):1163–9.

202. Biyikli NK, Emre S, Sirin A, Bilge I. Biochemical bone markers in nephrotic children. Pediatr Nephrol. 2004;19(8):869–73.

203. Cetin N, Gencler A, Sivrikoz IA. Bone mineral density and vitamin D status in children with remission phase of steroid-sensitive nephrotic syndrome. Saudi J Kidney Dis Transpl. 2019;30(4):853–62.

204. Bachrach LK. Bare-bones fact—children are not small adults. N Engl J Med. 2004;351(9):924–6.

205. Freundlich M, Jofe M, Goodman WG, Salusky IB. Bone histology in steroid-treated children with non-azotemic nephrotic syndrome. Pediatr Nephrol. 2004;19(4):400–7.

206. Munns CF, Cowell CT. Prevention and treatment of osteoporosis in chronically ill children. J Musculoskelet Neuronal Interact. 2005;5(3): 262–72.

207. Leonard MB, Feldman HI, Shults J, Zemel BS, Foster BJ, Stallings VA. Long-term, high-dose glucocorticoids and bone mineral content in childhood glucocorticoid-sensitive nephrotic syndrome. N Engl J Med. 2004;351(9):868–75.

208. Phan V, Blydt-Hansen T, Feber J, Alos N, Arora S, Atkinson S, et al. Skeletal findings in the first 12 months following initiation of glucocorticoid therapy for pediatric nephrotic syndrome. Osteoporos Int. 2014;25(2):627–37.

209. Tsampalieros A, Gupta P, Denburg MR, Shults J, Zemel BS, Mostoufi-Moab S, et al. Glucocorticoid effects on changes in bone mineral density and cortical structure in childhood nephrotic syndrome. J Bone Miner Res. 2013;28(3):480–8.

210. Wetzsteon RJ, Shults J, Zemel BS, Gupta PU, Burnham JM, Herskovitz RM, et al. Divergent effects of glucocorticoids on cortical and trabecular compartment BMD in childhood nephrotic syndrome. J Bone Miner Res. 2009;24(3):503–13.

211. Gulati S, Sharma RK, Gulati K, Singh U, Srivastava A. Longitudinal follow-up of bone mineral density in children with nephrotic syndrome and the role of calcium and vitamin D supplements. Nephrol Dial Transplant. 2005;20(8):1598–603.

212. Bak M, Serdaroglu E, Guclu R. Prophylactic calcium and vitamin D treatments in steroid-treated children with nephrotic syndrome. Pediatr Nephrol. 2006;21(3):350–4.

213. Choudhary S, Agarwal I, Seshadri MS. Calcium and vitamin D for osteoprotection in children with new-onset nephrotic syndrome treated with steroids: a prospective, randomized, controlled, interventional study. Pediatr Nephrol. 2014;29(6):1025–32.

214. Vidailhet M, Mallet E, Bocquet A, Bresson JL, Briend A, Chouraqui JP, et al. Vitamin D: still a topical matter in children and adolescents. A position paper by the Committee on Nutrition of the French Society of Paediatrics. Arch Pediatr. 2012;19(3):316–28.

215. Abeyagunawardena AS, Hindmarsh P, Trompeter RS. Adrenocortical suppression increases the risk of relapse in nephrotic syndrome. Arch Dis Child. 2007;92(7):585–8.

216. Mantan M, Grover R, Kaushik S, Yadav S. Adrenocortical suppression in children with nephrotic syndrome treated with low-dose alternate day corticosteroids. Indian J Nephrol. 2018;28(3):203–8.

217. Abu Bakar K, Khalil K, Lim YN, Yap YC, Appadurai M, Sidhu S, et al. Adrenal insufficiency in children with nephrotic syndrome on corticosteroid treatment. Front Pediatr. 2020;8:164.

218. Leisti S, Vilska J, Hallman N. Adrenocortical insufficiency and relapsing in the idiopathic nephrotic syndrome of childhood. Pediatrics. 1977;60(3):334–42.

219. Basu B, Babu BG, Mahapatra TK. Long-term efficacy and safety of common steroid-sparing agents in idiopathic nephrotic children. Clin Exp Nephrol. 2017;21(1):143–51.

220. Larkins NG, Liu ID, Willis NS, Craig JC, Hodson EM. Non-corticosteroid immunosuppressive medications for steroid-sensitive nephrotic syndrome in children. Cochrane Database Syst Rev. 2020;4:CD002290.

221. Prasad N, Gulati S, Sharma RK, Singh U, Ahmed M. Pulse cyclophosphamide therapy in steroid-dependent nephrotic syndrome. Pediatr Nephrol. 2004;19(5):494–8.

222. Abeyagunawardena AS, Trompeter RS. Intravenous pulsed vs oral cyclophosphamide therapy in steroid

dependant nephrotic syndrome [abstract]. Pediatr Nephrol. 2006;21(10):1535.

223. Vester U, Kranz B, Zimmermann S, Hoyer PF. Cyclophosphamide in steroid-sensitive nephrotic syndrome: outcome and outlook. Pediatr Nephrol. 2003;18(7):661–4.

224. Zagury A, De Oliveira AL, De Moraes CAP, De Araujo Montalvao JA, Novaes RHLL, De Sa VM, et al. Long-term follow-up after cyclophosphamide therapy in steroid-dependent nephrotic syndrome. Pediatr Nephrol. 2011;26(6):915–20.

225. Azib S, Macher MA, Kwon T, Dechartres A, Alberti C, Loirat C, et al. Cyclophosphamide in steroid-dependent nephrotic syndrome. Pediatr Nephrol. 2011;26(6):927–32.

226. Cammas B, Harambat J, Bertholet-Thomas A, Bouissou F, Morin D, Guigonis V, et al. Long-term effects of cyclophosphamide therapy in steroid-dependent or frequently relapsing idiopathic nephrotic syndrome. Nephrol Dial Transplant. 2011;26(1):178–84.

227. Bajeer IA, Khatri S, Tresa V, Hashmi S, Mubarak M, Lanewala AA. Histopathological spectrum and short-term outcome of treatment with cyclophosphamide in relapsing steroid-sensitive nephrotic syndrome. J Coll Physicians Surg Pak. 2018;28(6):436–9.

228. Latta K, von Schnakenburg C, Ehrich JH. A meta-analysis of cytotoxic treatment for frequently relapsing nephrotic syndrome in children. Pediatr Nephrol. 2001;16(3):271–82.

229. Miller DG. Alkylating agents and human spermatogenesis. JAMA. 1971;217(12):1662–5.

230. Webb H, Jaureguiberry G, Dufek S, Tullus K, Bockenhauer D. Cyclophosphamide and rituximab in frequently relapsing/steroid-dependent nephrotic syndrome. Pediatr Nephrol. 2016;31(4):589–94.

231. Kari JA, Alhasan KA, Albanna AS, Safdar OY, Shalaby MA, Bockenhauer D, et al. Rituximab versus cyclophosphamide as first steroid-sparing agent in childhood frequently relapsing and steroid-dependent nephrotic syndrome. Pediatr Nephrol. 2020;35(8):1445–53.

232. Tejani A, Butt K, Khawar R, Suthabthuran M, Rosenthal CJ, Trachtman H, et al. Cyclosporine (Cy) induced remission of relapsing nephrotic syndrome (RNS) in children [Abstract]. Kidney Int. 1985;29:206.

233. Ponticelli C, Edefonti A, Ghio L, Rizzoni G, Rinaldi S, Gusmano R, et al. Cyclosporin versus cyclophosphamide for patients with steroid-dependent and frequently relapsing idiopathic nephrotic syndrome: a multicentre randomized controlled trial. Nephrol Dial Transplant. 1993;8(12):1326–32.

234. Niaudet P. Comparison of cyclosporin and chlorambucil in the treatment of steroid-dependent idiopathic nephrotic syndrome: a multicentre randomized controlled trial. The French Society of Paediatric Nephrology. Pediatr Nephrol. 1992;6(1):1–3.

235. Pravitsitthikul N, Willis NS, Hodson EM, Craig JC. Non-corticosteroid immunosuppres-

236. Ishikura K, Yoshikawa N, Nakazato H, Sasaki S, Iijima K, Nakanishi K, et al. Two-year follow-up of a prospective clinical trial of cyclosporine for frequently relapsing nephrotic syndrome in children. Clin J Am Soc Nephrol. 2012;7(10):1576–83.

237. Ishikura K, Hamasaki Y, Sakai T, Hataya H, Mak RH, Honda M. Posterior reversible encephalopathy syndrome in children with kidney diseases. Pediatr Nephrol. 2012;27(3):375–84.

238. Ishikura K, Ikeda M, Hattori S, Yoshikawa N, Sasaki S, Iijima K, et al. Effective and safe treatment with cyclosporine in nephrotic children: a prospective, randomized multicenter trial. Kidney Int. 2008;73(10):1167–73.

239. el-Husseini A, el-Basuony F, Mahmoud I, Donia A, Hassan N, Sayed-Ahmad N, et al. Co-administration of cyclosporine and ketoconazole in idiopathic childhood nephrosis. Pediatr Nephrol. 2004;19(9):976–81.

240. Filler G. How should microemulsified Cyclosporine A (Neoral) therapy in patients with nephrotic syndrome be monitored? Nephrol Dial Transplant. 2005;20(6):1032–4.

241. Iijima K, Sako M, Oba MS, Ito S, Hataya H, Tanaka R, et al. Cyclosporine C2 monitoring for the treatment of frequently relapsing nephrotic syndrome in children: a multicenter randomized phase II trial. Clin J Am Soc Nephrol. 2014;9(2):271–8.

242. Wang W, Xia Y, Mao J, Chen Y, Wang D, Shen H, et al. Treatment of tacrolimus or cyclosporine A in children with idiopathic nephrotic syndrome. Pediatr Nephrol. 2012;27(11):2073–9.

243. Delbet JD, Aoun B, Buob D, Degheili J, Brocheriou I, Ulinski T. Infrequent tacrolimus-induced nephrotoxicity in French patients with steroid-dependent nephrotic syndrome. Pediatr Nephrol. 2019;34(12):2605–8.

244. Tirelli AS, Paterlini G, Ghio L, Edefonti A, Assael BM, Bettinelli A, et al. Renal effects of cyclosporin A in children treated for idiopathic nephrotic syndrome. Acta Paediatr. 1993;82(5):463–8.

245. D'Agati VD. Morphologic features of cyclosporin nephrotoxicity. Contrib Nephrol. 1995;114:84–110.

246. Mihatsch MJ, Thiel G, Ryffel B. Morphologic diagnosis of cyclosporine nephrotoxicity. Semin Diagn Pathol. 1988;5(1):104–21.

247. Iijima K, Hamahira K, Tanaka R, Kobayashi A, Nozu K, Nakamura H, et al. Risk factors for cyclosporine-induced tubulointerstitial lesions in children with minimal change nephrotic syndrome. Kidney Int. 2002;61(5):1801–5.

248. Niaudet P, Habib R, Tete MJ, Hinglais N, Broyer M. Cyclosporin in the treatment of idiopathic nephrotic syndrome in children. Pediatr Nephrol. 1987;1(4):566–73.

249. Kengne-Wafo S, Massella L, Diomedi-Camassei F, Gianviti A, Vivarelli M, Greco M, et al. Risk factors for cyclosporin A nephrotoxicity in children with steroid-dependant nephrotic syndrome. Clin J Am Soc Nephrol. 2009;4(9):1409–16.

250. Kim JH, Park SJ, Yoon SJ, Lim BJ, Jeong HJ, Lee JS, et al. Predictive factors for ciclosporin-associated nephrotoxicity in children with minimal change nephrotic syndrome. J Clin Pathol. 2011;64(6):516–9.

251. Hamahira K, Iijima K, Tanaka R, Nakamura H, Yoshikawa N. Recovery from cyclosporine-associated arteriolopathy in childhood nephrotic syndrome. Pediatr Nephrol. 2001;16(9):723–7.

252. Kranz B, Vester U, Buscher R, Wingen A-M, Hoyer PF. Cyclosporine-A-induced nephrotoxicity in children with minimal-change nephrotic syndrome: long-term treatment up to 10 years. Pediatr Nephrol. 2008;23(4):581–6.

253. Morgan C, Sis B, Pinsk M, Yiu V. Renal interstitial fibrosis in children treated with FK506 for nephrotic syndrome. Nephrol Dial Transplant. 2011;26(9):2860–5.

254. Davin JC, Merkus MP. Levamisole in steroid-sensitive nephrotic syndrome of childhood: the lost paradise? Pediatr Nephrol. 2005;20(1):10–4.

255. Tanphaichitr P, Tanphaichitr D, Sureeratanan J, Chatasingh S. Treatment of nephrotic syndrome with levamisole. J Pediatr. 1980;96(3 Pt 1):490–3.

256. Dayal U, Dayal AK, Shastry JC, Raghupathy P. Use of levamisole in maintaining remission in steroid-sensitive nephrotic syndrome in children.[Erratum appears in Nephron 1994;67(4):507]. Nephron. 1994;66(4):408–12.

257. Levamisole for corticosteroid-dependent nephrotic syndrome in childhood. British Association for Paediatric Nephrology. Lancet. 1991;337(8757):1555–7.

258. Rashid HU, Ahmed S, Fatima N, Khanam A. Levamisole in the treatment of steroid dependent or frequently relapsing nephrotic syndrome in children. Bangladesh Renal J. 1996;15(1):6–8.

259. Abeyagunawardena AS, Trompeter RS. Efficacy of levamisole as a single agent in maintaining remission in steroid dependant nephrotic syndrome [abstract]. Pediatr Nephrol. 2006;21(10):1503.

260. Sural S, Pahari DK, Mitra K, Bhattacharya S, Mondal S, Tarapder A. Efficacy of levamisole compared to cyclophosphamide and steroid in frequently relapsing (FR) minimal change nephrotic syndrome (MCNS) [abstract]. J Am Soc Nephrol. 2001;12:126A.

261. Al-Saran K, Mirza K, Al-Ghanam G, Abdelkarim M. Experience with levamisole in frequently relapsing, steroid-dependent nephrotic syndrome. Pediatr Nephrol. 2006;21(2):201–5.

262. Weiss R. Randomized double-blind placebo controlled, multi-center trial of levamisole for children with frequently relapsing/steroid dependent

263. Gruppen MP, Bouts AH, Jansen-van der Weide MC, Merkus MP, Zurowska A, Maternik M, et al. A randomized clinical trial indicates that levamisole increases the time to relapse in children with steroid-sensitive idiopathic nephrotic syndrome. Kidney Int. 2018;93(2):510–8.

264. Palcoux JB, Niaudet P, Goumy P. Side effects of levamisole in children with nephrosis. Pediatr Nephrol. 1994;8(2):263–4.

265. Barbano G, Ginevri F, Ghiggeri GM, Gusmano R. Disseminated autoimmune disease during levamisole treatment of nephrotic syndrome. Pediatr Nephrol. 1999;13(7):602–3.

266. Bagga A, Hari P, Moudgil A, Jordan SC. Mycophenolate mofetil and prednisolone therapy in children with steroid-dependent nephrotic syndrome. Am J Kidney Dis. 2003;42(6): 1114–20.

267. Schijvens AM, van der Weerd L, van Wijk JAE, Bouts AHM, Keijzer-Veen MG, Dorresteijn EM, et al. Practice variations in the management of childhood nephrotic syndrome in the Netherlands. Eur J Pediatr. 2021;180(6):1885–94.

268. Remy P, Audard V, Natella PA, Pelle G, Dussol B, Leray-Moragues H, et al. An open-label randomized controlled trial of low-dose corticosteroid plus enteric-coated mycophenolate sodium versus standard corticosteroid treatment for minimal change nephrotic syndrome in adults (MSN Study). Kidney Int. 2018;94(6):1217–26.

269. Kapoor K, Saha A, Kaur M, Dubey NK, Upadhyay AD. Mycophenolate sodium for children with frequently relapsing or steroid dependent nephrotic syndrome. Indian Pediatr. 2017;54(10):885–6.

270. Querfeld U, Weber LT. Treatment strategies for children with steroid-dependent nephrotic syndrome: in need of controlled studies. Pediatr Nephrol. 2018;33(12):2391.

271. Gellermann J, Weber L, Pape L, Tonshoff B, Hoyer P, Querfeld U, et al. Mycophenolate mofetil versus cyclosporin A in children with frequently relapsing nephrotic syndrome. J Am Soc Nephrol. 2013;24(10):1689–97.

272. Dorresteijn EM, Kist-van Holthe JE, Levtchenko EN, Nauta J, Hop WC, van der Heijden AJ. Mycophenolate mofetil versus cyclosporine for remission maintenance in nephrotic syndrome. Pediatr Nephrol. 2008;23(11):2013–20.

273. Sinha A, Puraswani M, Kalaivani M, Goyal P, Hari P, Bagga A. Efficacy and safety of mycophenolate mofetil versus levamisole in frequently relapsing nephrotic syndrome: an open-label randomized controlled trial. Kidney Int. 2019;95(1):210–8.

274. Hackl A, Cseprekal O, Gessner M, Liebau MC, Habbig S, Ehren R, et al. Mycophenolate mofetil therapy in children with idiopathic nephrotic syndrome: does therapeutic drug monitoring make a difference? Ther Drug Monit. 2016;38(2):274–9.

275. Tellier S, Dallocchio A, Guigonis V, Saint-Marcoux F, Llanas B, Ichay L, et al. Mycophenolic acid pharmacokinetics and relapse in children with steroid-dependent idiopathic nephrotic syndrome. Clin J Am Soc Nephrol. 2016;11(10):1777–82.

276. Ravani P, Magnasco A, Edefonti A, Murer L, Rossi R, Ghio L, et al. Short-term effects of rituximab in children with steroid- and calcineurin-dependent nephrotic syndrome: a randomized controlled trial. Clin J Am Soc Nephrol. 2011;6(6):1308–15.

277. Ravani P, Rossi R, Bonanni A, Quinn RR, Sica F, Bodria M, et al. Rituximab in children with steroid-dependent nephrotic syndrome: a multicenter, open-label, noninferiority, randomized controlled trial. J Am Soc Nephrol. 2015;26(9):2259–66.

278. Ravani P, Lugani F, Pisani I, Bodria M, Piaggio G, Bartolomeo D, et al. Rituximab for very low dose steroid-dependent nephrotic syndrome in children: a randomized controlled study. Pediatr Nephrol. 2020;35(8):1437–44.

279. Boumediene A, Vachin P, Sendeyo K, Oniszczuk J, Zhang SY, Henique C, et al. NEPHRUTIX: a randomized, double-blind, placebo vs Rituximab-controlled trial assessing T-cell subset changes in Minimal Change Nephrotic Syndrome. J Autoimmun. 2018;88:91–102.

280. Basu B, Sander A, Roy B, Preussler S, Barua S, Mahapatra TKS, et al. Efficacy of rituximab vs tacrolimus in pediatric corticosteroid-dependent nephrotic syndrome a randomized clinical trial. JAMA Pediatr. 2018;172(8):757–64.

281. Ahn YH, Kim SH, Han KH, Choi HJ, Cho H, Lee JW, et al. Efficacy and safety of rituximab in childhood-onset, difficult-to-treat nephrotic syndrome: a multicenter open-label trial in Korea. Medicine. 2018;97(46):e13157.

282. Iijima K, Sako DM, Nozu K, Mori R, Tuchida N, Kamei K, et al. Rituximab for childhood-onset, complicated, frequently relapsing nephrotic syndrome or steroid-dependent nephrotic syndrome: a multicentre, double-blind, randomised, placebo-controlled trial. Lancet. 2014;384(9950):1273–81.

283. Chan EY, Webb H, Yu E, Ghiggeri GM, Kemper MJ, Ma AL, et al. Both the rituximab dose and maintenance immunosuppression in steroid-dependent/frequently-relapsing nephrotic syndrome have important effects on outcomes. Kidney Int. 2020;97(2):393–401.

284. Horinouchi T, Sako M, Nakanishi K, Ishikura K, Ito S, Nakamura H, et al. Study protocol: mycophenolate mofetil as maintenance therapy after rituximab treatment for childhood-onset, complicated, frequently-relapsing nephrotic syndrome or steroid-dependent nephrotic syndrome: a multicenter double-blind, randomized, placebo-controlled trial (JSKDC07). BMC Nephrol. 2018;19(1):302.

285. Basu B, Preussler S, Sander A, Mahapatra TKS, Schaefer F. Randomized clinical trial to compare efficacy and safety of repeated courses of rituximab to single-course rituximab followed by maintenance

285. mycophenolate-mofetil in children with steroid dependent nephrotic syndrome. BMC Nephrol. 2020;21(1):520.

286. Chaumais M-C, Garnier A, Chalard F, Peuchmaur M, Dauger S, Jacqz-Agrain E, et al. Fatal pulmonary fibrosis after rituximab administration. Pediatr Nephrol. 2009;24(9):1753–5.

287. Czarniak P, Zaluska-Lesniewska I, Zagozdzon I, Zurowska A. Difficulties in diagnosing severe *Pneumocystis jiroveci* pneumonia after rituximab therapy in steroid-dependent nephrotic syndrome. Pediatr Nephrol. 2013;29:987–8.

288. Sato M, Ito S, Ogura M, Kamei K, Miyairi I, Miyata I, et al. Atypical Pneumocystis jiroveci pneumonia with multiple nodular granulomas after rituximab for refractory nephrotic syndrome. Pediatr Nephrol. 2013;28(1):145–9.

289. Prytula A, Iijima K, Kamei K, Geary D, Gottlich E, Majeed A, et al. Rituximab in refractory nephrotic syndrome. Pediatr Nephrol. 2010;25(3):461–8.

290. Sellier-Leclerc A-L, Belli E, Guerin V, Dorfmuller P, Deschenes G. Fulminant viral myocarditis after rituximab in pediatric nephrotic syndrome. Pediatr Nephrol. 2013;28:1875–9.

291. Carson KR, Evens AM, Richey EA, Habermann TM, Focosi D, Seymour JF, et al. Progressive multifocal leukoencephalopathy after rituximab therapy in HIV-negative patients: a report of 57 cases from the Research on Adverse Drug Events and Reports project. Blood. 2009;113(20):4834–40.

292. Colucci M, Carsetti R, Serafinelli J, Rocca S, Massella L, Gargiulo A, et al. Prolonged Impairment of Immunological Memory After Anti-CD20 Treatment in Pediatric Idiopathic Nephrotic Syndrome. Front. 2019;10:1653.

293. Fujinaga S, Tomii Y. Profound effect of postrituximab mycophenolate mofetil administration for persistent hypogammaglobulinemia in young children with steroid-dependent nephrotic syndrome. Clin Exp Nephrol. 2020;24(4):386–7.

294. Iorember F, Aviles D, Kallash M, Bamgbola O. Cost analysis on the use of rituximab and calcineurin inhibitors in children and adolescents with steroid-dependent nephrotic syndrome. Pediatr Nephrol. 2018;33(2):261–7.

295. Yoshioka K, Ohashi Y, Sakai T, Ito H, Yoshikawa N, Nakamura H, et al. A multicenter trial of mizoribine compared with placebo in children with frequently relapsing nephrotic syndrome. Kidney Int. 2000;58(1):317–24.

296. Kondoh T, Ikezumi Y, Yokoi K, Nakajima Y, Matsumoto Y, Kaneko M, et al. Assessment of factors associated with mizoribine responsiveness in children with steroid-dependent nephrotic syndrome. Clin Exp Nephrol. 2019;23(9):1154–60.

297. Sawires H, Abdelaziz H, Ahmed HM, Botrous O, Agban M. Randomized controlled trial on immunomodulatory effects of azithromycin in children with steroid-dependent nephrotic syndrome. Pediatr Nephrol. 2019;34(9):1591–7.

298. Zhang B, Liu T, Wang W, Zhang X, Fan S, Liu Z, et al. A prospective randomly controlled clinical trial on azithromycin therapy for induction treatment of children with nephrotic syndrome. Eur J Pediatr. 2014;173(4):509–15.

299. Wang CS, Travers C, McCracken C, Leong T, Gbadegesin R, Quiroga A, et al. Adrenocorticotropic hormone for childhood nephrotic syndrome: the ATLANTIS randomized trial. Clin J Am Soc Nephrol. 2018;13(12):1859–65.

300. Ulinski T, Leroy S, Dubrel M, Danon S, Bensman A. High serological response to pneumococcal vaccine in nephrotic children at disease onset on high-dose prednisone. Pediatr Nephrol. 2008;23(7):1107–13.

301. Aoun B, Wannous H, Azema C, Ulinski T. Polysaccharide pneumococcal vaccination of nephrotic children at disease onset-long-term data. Pediatr Nephrol. 2010;25(9):1773–4.

302. Pittet LF, Posfay-Barbe KM, Chehade H, Rudin C, Wilhelm-Bals A, Rodriguez M, et al. Optimizing seroprotection against pneumococcus in children with nephrotic syndrome using the 13-valent pneumococcal conjugate vaccine. Vaccine. 2016;34(41):4948–54.

303. Centers for Disease Control. Use of 13-valent pneumococcal conjugate vaccine and 23-valent pneumococcal polysaccharide vaccine among children aged 6-18 years with immunocompromising conditions: recommendations of the Advisory Committee on Immunization Practices (ACIP). Morb Mortal Wkly Rep. 2013;62(25):521–4.

304. Mantan M, Pandharikar N, Yadav S, Chakravarti A, Sethi GR. Seroprotection for hepatitis B in children with nephrotic syndrome. Pediatr Nephrol. 2013;28(11):2125–30.

305. Furth SL, Arbus GS, Hogg R, Tarver J, Chan C, Fivush BA, et al. Varicella vaccination in children with nephrotic syndrome: a report of the Southwest Pediatric Nephrology Study Group. J Pediatr. 2003;142(2):145–8.

306. Australian Immunisation Handbook. 2013. http://www.health.gov.au/internet/immunise/publishing.nsf/Content/Handbook-home. Accessed 1 November 2013.

307. Kamei K, Miyairi I, Ishikura K, Ogura M, Shoji K, Funaki T, et al. Prospective study of live attenuated vaccines for patients with nephrotic syndrome receiving immunosuppressive agents. J Pediatr. 2018;196:217–22.e1.

308. Centers for Disease Control and Prevention. Interim clinical considerations for use of COVID-19 vaccines currently approved or authorized in the United States. 2021. https://www.cdc.gov/vaccines/covid-19/clinical-considerations/covid-19-vaccines-us.html. Accessed 13 September 2021.

309. Waldman M, Soler MJ, Garcia-Carro C, et al. Results from the IRoc-GN international registry of patients with COVID-19 and glomerular disease suggest close monitoring. Kidney Int. 2021;99:227–37.

310. Kronbichler A, Anders HJ, Fernandez-Juarez GM, Floege J, Goumenos D, Segelmark M, et al. Recommendations for the use of COVID-19 vaccines in patients with immune-mediated kidney diseases. Nephrol Dial Transplant. 2021;36:1160–8.

311. Consensus statement on management and audit potential for steroid responsive nephrotic syndrome. Report of a Workshop by the British Association for Paediatric Nephrology and Research Unit, Royal College of Physicians. Arch Dis Child 1994;70(2):151–7.

312. Hogg RJ, Portman RJ, Milliner D, Lemley KV, Eddy A, Ingelfinger J. Evaluation and management of proteinuria and nephrotic syndrome in children: recommendations from a pediatric nephrology panel established at the National Kidney Foundation conference on proteinuria, albuminuria, risk, assessment, detection, and elimination (PARADE). Pediatrics. 2000;105(6):1242–9.

313. Abramowicz M, Barnett HL, Edelmann CM Jr, Greifer I, Kobayashi O, Arneil GC, et al. Controlled trial of azathioprine in children with nephrotic syndrome. A report for the international study of kidney disease in children. Lancet. 1970;1(7654):959–61.

Steroid Resistant Nephrotic Syndrome

14

Rasheed Gbadegesin, Keisha Gibson, and Kimberly Reidy

Introduction

Idiopathic nephrotic syndrome is characterized by severe proteinuria, hypoalbuminemia, and/or presence of edema. Whereas approximately 85% of affected children achieve complete remission of proteinuria upon corticosteroid treatment, those who do not achieve remission are labeled as having "steroid resistant nephrotic syndrome" (SRNS). While details related to steroid sensitive forms of nephrotic syndrome are discussed in Chap. 14 of this book, our chapter will focus on the epidemiology, diagnosis, treatment and clinical outcomes of those children who fail to enter clinical remission after treatment with glucocorticoids.

R. Gbadegesin (✉)
Division of Nephrology, Department of Pediatrics, Duke University, Durham, NC, USA
e-mail: rasheed.gbadegesin@duke.edu

K. Gibson
Division of nephrology, Department of Pediatrics and Medicine, University of North Carolina, Chapel Hill, NC, USA
e-mail: keisha_gibson@med.unc.edu

K. Reidy
Division of Nephrology, Children's Hospital at Montefiore, Albert Einstein College of Medicine, Bronx, NY, USA
e-mail: KREIDY@montefiore.org

Definitions

The most important implication for a child given the label of SRNS is that he or she is at increased risk for both the development of disease complications as well as progression to chronic kidney disease (CKD) and eventually end stage kidney disease (ESKD). A major challenge of discussing the multiple issues related to children with SRNS is that its very definition has been standardized within the pediatric nephrology community only recently. In 2020, an IPNA expert committee launched a set of clinical practice recommendations for SRNS in children and in 2021, KDIGO published a clinical practice guideline for the management of glomerular diseases including a pediatric section [1, 2]. The two guidance documents provide the same uniform definitions of SRNS and its subsets:

Steroid Resistant Nephrotic Syndrome (SRNS): Children who fail to enter complete clinical remission within 4 weeks of treatment with prednisone or prednisolone at standard dose [3, 4].

It should be noted that several alternative definitions of SRNS have been used in the past, such as failure to enter remission after 6 weeks of daily oral prednisone, 4 weeks of daily followed by 4 weeks of alternate day oral prednisone, or 4 weeks of daily oral prednisone followed by three intravenous pulses of methylprednisolone [5, 6]. It is hoped that the new definition will be

© The Author(s), under exclusive license to Springer Nature Switzerland AG 2023
F. Schaefer, L. A. Greenbaum (eds.), *Pediatric Kidney Disease*,
https://doi.org/10.1007/978-3-031-11665-0_14

followed both in research settings and in routine clinical practice. This will be a prerequisite to compare the efficacy of established and novel treatments for nephrotic syndrome.

Calcineurin inhibitor responsive SRNS: Partial remission after 6 months of treatment and/or complete remission after 12 months of treatment with a CNI at adequate doses and/or levels.

Calcineurin inhibitor resistant SRNS: Absence of at least partial remission after 6 months of treatment with a CNI at adequate doses and/or levels.

Multidrug resistant SRNS: Absence of complete remission after 12 months of treatment with two mechanistically distinct steroid-sparing agents at standard doses.

Secondary SRNS: A steroid sensitive nephrotic syndrome patient at disease onset who at subsequent relapse fails to achieve remission after 4 weeks of therapy with daily prednisone or prednisolone at standard dose. Emerging data in the literature has drawn attention to this subgroup of patients with NS [7]. A unique characteristic of this group is that up to 80% of patients in this subgroup who progress to ESKD will develop recurrence of disease following kidney transplantation [8, 9].

Epidemiology

The annual incidence of nephrotic syndrome in most countries studied to date is ~1.2–17.0 new cases per 100,000 children [4, 10–14], and the prevalence is ~16 cases per 100,000 children [4]. The incidence varies widely between countries and different ethnicities [14]. In young children there is a male preponderance, with a male to female ratio of 2:1, although this gender disparity completely disappears by adolescence [11, 15–18]. Steroid resistant nephrotic syndrome (SRNS) is seen in about 15–20% of all cases of childhood nephrotic syndrome. Monogenic SRNS is responsible for 10–30% of all SRNS. The higher percentage is seen in the regions of the World here in breeding is very high and also in population where there are founder mutations. The most common causes of monogenic autosomal SRNS

are mutations in nephrin (*NPHS1*), podocin (*NPHS2*), phospholipase c epsilon 1 (*PLCE1*) and *nucleoporin* genes. Majority of all cases of autosomal dominant monogenic SRNS are due to mutations in inverted formin2 (*INF2*), transient receptor potential cation channel, subfamily C, member 6 (*TRPC6*) actinin4 alpha (*ACTN4*), and wilms tumor type 1 (*WT1*) genes.

The incidence of nephrotic syndrome has been largely unchanged over the last 35 years, but the histopathologic lesions associated with nephrotic syndrome appear to be evolving. Some reports from various countries suggest that the incidence of focal segmental glomerulosclerosis (FSGS) is increasing, even after correction for variations in renal biopsy practices, and also assuming that children who did not undergo a renal biopsy had minimal change nephrotic syndrome (MCNS) [9, 15–18].

The histologic patterns and incidence of nephrotic syndrome are also affected by **ethnicity and geographic location**. For instance, idiopathic nephrotic syndrome in the United Kingdom was found to be more common among Asian children living in the UK and Canada compared to European children [19, 20]. In contrast, in Sub-Saharan Africa, idiopathic nephrotic syndrome occurs less commonly and disease is more commonly due to infection-associated glomerular lesions [21–23]. In the US, nephrotic syndrome has a relatively higher incidence among children of various ethnic backgrounds. A review of children with nephrotic syndrome in Texas reported that the distribution of children closely resembled the ethnic composition of the surrounding community [15]. These data in conjunction with the data from African countries suggests that the interaction of environmental and genetic factors plays an important role in the pathogenesis of nephrotic syndrome. Despite this, race alone seems to have a clear correlation with the histologic lesion associated with nephrotic syndrome. Indeed, 47% of African American children with nephrotic syndrome in the above study were found to have FSGS, while only 11% of Hispanic and 18% of Caucasian children had this unfavorable pattern of injury [15]. The genetic basis for the high prevalence of

FSGS in people of African ancestry was established in 2010 when homozygous or compound heterozygous G1 and G2 genotype in the gene encoding apolipoprotein 1 (*APOL1*) were shown to confer ten times the odds of developing FSGS in African Americans [24].

The age at presentation with nephrotic syndrome also has strong correlations with the frequency of presentation, as well as the associated renal histology. The most common age for presentation with nephrotic syndrome is 2 years, and 70–80% of all cases of nephrotic syndrome develop in children <6 years of age [4, 10]. In addition, children diagnosed prior to 6 years of age comprised 80% of those with MCNS, compared to 50% of those with FSGS, and only 2.6% of those with MPGN [25]. When analyzed based on renal histology, the median age at presentation was 3 years for MCNS, 6 years for FSGS, and 10 years for MPGN [25]. Therefore, excluding presentation in the first 12 months of life, these data suggest that the likelihood of having MCNS as a cause for nephrotic syndrome decreases with increasing age, while the likelihood for having the less favorable diagnoses of FSGS or MPGN increases [25, 26].

The most common renal histologies seen in children with SRNS are FSGS, MCNS, MPGN and membranous nephropathy.

Additional variables associated with clinical steroid responsiveness include ethnicity and geographic location. While 20% of children in Western countries have steroid resistant nephrotic syndrome, studies from Africa reported steroid resistance in 50–90% of children with nephrotic syndrome, with higher proportions of children with steroid responsive disease in more affluent and diverse urban centers [23, 27–29].

Histopathological Findings

SRNS is a heterogeneous clinical condition with multiple etiologies. The histopathologic entities that may cause SRNS vary in different series depending on the age group and the population being studied. However, in different series focusing on children presenting after the first year of

Table 14.1 Pathologic findings in steroid resistant nephrotic syndrome

Histology	South-Asia[a] [25, 26] n = 326	South-Africa [28] n = 183	Poland [27] n = 34	USA[b] [9, 12] n = 253
MCD	38.4	36.1	5.9	45.4
FSGS	41.5	36.1	32.4	26.5
MESGN	14.1	8.1	55.8	10.3
MEMB	4.0	–	–	1.2
MPGN	1.0	–	5.9	7.5
Others	1.0	19.7	–	9.1

[a] Two studies one each from Pakistan and India [25, 26]
[b] Summary of two studies, some of the patients were diagnosed with frequent relapsing and steroid dependent NS [9, 12]

life, the common pathologic variants associated with SRNS include focal segmental glomerulosclerosis (FSGS), membranous glomerulopathy, membranoproliferative glomerulopathy (MPGN), and minimal change disease (MCD) [11, 15, 31–34]. The majority of cases are due to disease on the continuum between MCD and FSGS (Table 14.1). Since the MCD/FSGS spectrum represents the most common pathologic variants of SRNS, and since other chapters are devoted to each of the other histologic variants, the rest of this chapter will focus mainly on FSGS.

Focal Segmental Glomerulosclerosis (FSGS)

FSGS is a pathologic finding that is characterized by focal glomerulosclerosis or tuft collapse, segmental hyalinosis, IgM deposits on immunofluorescence staining, and podocyte foot process effacement on electron microscopy [35]. In the majority of children, it is characterized by SRNS and progression to end-stage kidney disease (ESKD) within 5–10 years of diagnosis [30]. It was first described in kidney biopsies of adults with nephrotic syndrome by Fahr in 1925, although it was Rich who later made the observation that the lesion of FSGS in children with nephrotic syndrome classically starts from the corticomedullary junction before involving other parts of the renal cortex [36, 37]. The observation of Rich is probably the explanation for why many cases of FSGS

variants is still being studied. In a cohort of adults with FSGS, it was reported that collapsing FSGS had the highest rate of renal insufficiency at presentation and worst long term outcome [45]. The most comprehensive prospective report of the clinical significance of the classification in children comes from the analysis of the kidney biopsies from the patient cohort in the NIH sponsored FSGS trial [46]. In this study FSGS NOS was the most common variant, being responsible for 68% of all cases, with collapsing, tip, perihilar and cellular variants responsible for 12%, 10%, 7% and 3%, respectively. Patients with collapsing FSGS were more likely to be black and to have nephrotic syndrome with renal impairment at presentation, compared to patients with NOS and tip variants [46]. Furthermore, globally sclerotic changes were found more commonly in the NOS variant while segmental sclerosis, tubular atrophy and interstitial fibrosis were found more commonly in collapsing FSGS [46]. At the end of 3 years follow up, 47% of patients with collapsing FSGS were in ESKD compared with 20% and 7% for the NOS and tip variants, respectively [46] (Table 14.3). These findings were confirmed in a study of 201 Japanese FSGS patients [47].

Integrated molecular and morphologic classification: Emerging data is recognizing the fact that FSGS and related morphologic descriptions such as diffuse mesangial sclerosis and minimal change disease are non-specific diagnoses but morphologic changes resulting from multiple injuries to the podocyte [48]. It is now proposed that these morphologic entities should be called **podocytopathies** [49]. The advantages of looking at FSGS and the other morphologic patterns as podocytopathies are (1) focusing on a cell that is central to pathogenesis and therefore a target for biochemical analysis and cellular therapy, (2) facilitating identification of other cellular lineage that may be working in concert with the podocyte to preserve the function and the integrity of the GFB, and (3) enabling clinical work-up focusing on identifying causes or risk factors for podocyte injury and therefore more informed prognosis and personalized therapy [48].

Pathogenesis

The hallmark of nephrotic syndrome is glomerular proteinuria [48]. While there are other causes of proteinuria, proteinuria in nephrotic syndrome results from leakage of protein through the glomerular filtration barrier (GFB). The GFB is composed of three layers: podocyte (glomerular epithelial cell), glomerular basement membrane, and fenestrated endothelium (Fig. 14.2) [24, 48–108]. Defects in any of the three layers can result in proteinuria [107, 108].

Hereditary and Monogenic Forms of SRNS

Over the past 20 years, investigations of inherited forms of nephrotic syndrome led to recognition of the importance of the podocyte in the pathogenesis of SRNS [24, 48–110]. The majority of

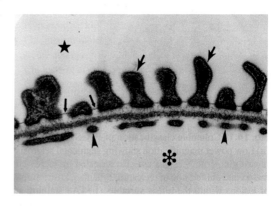

Fig. 14.2 Electron micrograph of the components of the glomerular filtration barrier. During normal glomerular filtration, plasma water is filtered from the glomerular capillary lumen (asterisk) through the fenestrated endothelial cell layer (arrowheads), then across the glomerular basement membrane (GBM) and through the slit diaphragms (small arrows) which bridge the filtration slits between adjacent podocyte foot processes (large arrows) and finally into the urinary space (star) where it enters the lumen of the proximal tubule. These podocyte foot processes are normally tall and evenly-spaced along the GBM, but during nephrotic syndrome they become spread out along the GBM, with apical displacement of the slit diaphragms. The layer of negatively-charged glycocalyx can be seen in this image as a blurry coating on the apical surfaces of the podocyte foot processes. (Adapted with permission from reference [50])

monogenic causes of SRNS affect the structure and function of the podocyte [24, 48–110]. The podocyte is a terminally differentiated epithelial cell with limited ability to regenerate [111]. The prominence of the podocyte in the pathophysiology of SRNS is highlighted by the fact that most common causes of monogenic NS are genes with preferential or selective expression in the podocyte.

In a large cohort of patients with SRNS, the top six monogenic causes of SRNS were *NPHS2* (encodes podocin), *NPHS1* (encodes nephrin), *PLCE1* (encodes phospholipase C epsilon 1), *WT-1* (encodes Wilms tumor 1), *LAMB2* (encodes laminin beta 2) and *SMARCAL* (encodes SW/SNF2 related, matrix associated, actin dependent regulator of chromatin, subfamily a-like 1) (Fig. 14.4 and Table 14.4) [112, 113]. Beyond

Table 14.4 Genetic causes of FSGS and SRNS

Gene	Protein	Mode of Inheritance
Slit diaphragm genes		
NPHS1	Nephrin	AR
NPHS2	Podocin	AR
PLCE1	Phospholipase C epsilon 1	AR
CD2AP	CD2-associated protein	AD, AR
TRPC6	Transient receptor potential channel C6	AD
CRB2	Crumbs family member 2	AR
FAT1	FAT atypical cadherin	AR
KIRREL1	kirre like nephrin family adhesion molecule 1	AR
Transcription factors and nuclear genes		
WT1	Wilm's tumor protein 1	AD
LMX1B	LIM homeobox transcription factor 1-beta	AD
SMARCL1	SMARCA-like protein	AR
NUP93	Nuclear pore complex protein 93	AR
NUP107	Nuclear pore complex protein 107	AR
NUP205	Nuclear pore complex protein 205	AR
NUP160	Nuclear pore complex protein 160	AR
NUP85	Nuclear pore complex protein 85	AR
NUP133	Nuclear pore complex protein 133	AR
XPO5	Exportin 5	AR
E2F3	E2F transcription factor	AD
NXF5	Nuclear RNA export Factor 5	X-linked recessive
PAX2	Paired box protein 2	AD
LMNA	Lamin A and C	AD
WDR73	WD repeat domain 73	AR
Cytoskeletal and membrane genes		
ACTN4	Alpha-actinin 4	AD
INF2	Inverted formin 2	AD
MYO1E	Myosin 1E	AR
MAGI2	Membrane Associated Guanylate kinase, inverted 2	AR
ANLN	Anillin actin binding protein	AD
PTPRO	Protein-tyrosine phosphatase-R O	AR
EMP2	Epithelial membrane protein 2	AR
CUBN	Cubilin	AR
PODXL	Podocalyxin	AR, AD
ARHGAP24	Rho GTPase-activating protein 24	AD
ARHGDIA	Rho GDP dissociation inhibitor alpha	AR

(continued)

Table 14.4 (continued)

Gene	Protein	Mode of Inheritance
DAAM2	Dishevelled associated activator of morphogenesis 2	AR
SYNPO	Synaptopodin	AD
SYNPO2 (Also localized to mesangial cells)	Synaptopodin 2	AR
DLC1	Deleted in liver cancer 1	AR
KANK 1/2/4	Kidney ankyrin repeat-containing protein	AR
ITSN1/2	Intersectin protein	AR
CDK20	Cyclin-dependent kinase 20	AR
NOS1AP	Nitric oxide synthase 1 adaptor protein	AR
Mitochondrial, lysosomal, metabolic, and cytosolic genes		
COQ2	Coenzyme Q2 4-hyroxybenzoate polyprenyl transferase	AR
COQ6	Coenzyme Q6 monooxygenase	AR
PDSS2	Prenyl-diphosphate synthase subunit 2	AR
ADCK4	AarF domain containing kinase 4	AR
SCARB2	Scavenger receptor class B, member 2	AR
PMM2	Phosphomannomutase 2	AR
ALG1	Asparagine-linked glycosylation 1	AR
TTC21B	Tetratricopeptide repeat protein 21B	AR
CDK20	Cyclin-dependent kinase 20	AR
CFH	Complement factor H	AR
DGKE	Diacylglycerol kinase epsilon	AR
Glomerular basement membrane genes		
LAMB2	Laminin subunit beta-2	AR
ITGB4	Integrin beta 4	AR
ITGA3	Integrin alpha 3	AR
COL4A 3/4/5	Type IV collagen alpha 3,4,5	AR, AD, X-linked
Endosomal regulator genes		
GAPVD1	GTPase Activating Protein And VPS9 Domains 1	AR
ANKFY1	Ankyrin Repeat And FYVE Domain Containing 1	AR

these top six monogenic causes of SRNS, pathogenic variants have been identified in over 60 genes in patients with SRNS (Table 14.4). Recent large cohort studies revealed that altogether 20–30% of sporadic childhood onset SRNS may be due to single gene defects [112–115]. In animal models, including transgenic mice and zebrafish, most identified single gene causes of SRNS result in podocyte dysfunction. Mechanisms of podocyte dysfunction include: (1) slit diaphragm abnormalities (*CD2AP, NPHS1, NPHS2,* and *FAT1*) (2) impaired podocyte actin cytoskeleton regulation and/or adhesion to the glomerular basement membrane (*ACTN4, ANLN, ARHGAP24, INF2, SMARCAL* and *TRPC6*); (3) defective podocyte differentiation (*PLCE1* and *WT1*), (4) mitochondrial dysfunction (*ADCK4, COQ2, COQ6, COQ8B* and

tRNA (Leu)) and (5) nuclear pore dysfunction (*NUP94, NUP107, NUP160*), Table 14.4 [48, 116–118].

Beyond the podocyte, pathogenic variants in genes encoding for key molecular components of the glomerular basement membrane are increasingly being recognized as monogenic causes of SRNS. These include *COL4A3* and *COL4A4*, which encode for type 4 collagen of the GBM, and *LAMA5* and *LAMB2*, forming laminin LM-521; α5β2γ1 that is a key component of the glomerular basement membrane. While *COL4A3* and *COL4A4* mutations typically present with the more classic phenotype of Alport syndrome (see Chap. 16), they may also phenocopy FSGS and present with SRNS [119, 120]. Further discussion of monogenic SRNS can be found in Chap. 15.

Common Gene Variants Associated with SRNS/FSGS

In addition to monogenic causes of SRNS, common variants in the gene encoding for apolipoprotein L1 (*APOL1*) are associated with FSGS [24, 122]. *APOL1* contributes to innate immunity and protection against *Trypanosoma*, the cause of African sleeping sickness. The APOL1 protein forms a channel that contributes to *Trypansomal* lysis. Two common variants (known as G1 [2 single nucleotide polymorphisms S342G and I384M] and G2 [a 6 base pair deletion (p.NYK388K] are common in people of West African descent and are associated with protection against resistant *Trypanosoma brucei rhodesiense* and *gambiense*. However, carriage of any combination of *APOL1* high risk genotype defined as homozygous or compound heterozygous G1/G2 genotypes: (G1/G1; G1/G2; or G2/G2) are associated with increased risk for kidney disease [123]. In children of African descent with SRNS, prevalence of *APOL1* high risk genotype may be as high as 40% [124, 125]. The mechanisms of *APOL1* related kidney disease continue to be a focus of ongoing investigations. The prevalence of high risk genotype is about 14% in African Americans, however less than 25% of individuals with these high risk genotypes will develop kidney disease suggesting that genetic and environmental second hits may be needed for phenotypic manifestations. Increased podocyte APOL1 expression with enhanced inflammatory signaling may be one such second hit [126, 127]. Other pathways implicated in APOL1 related kidney disease include podocyte lipid and mitochondrial dysfunction and alterations in ion channel functions [126, 128, 129]. Interestingly *APOL1* high risk genotype is also associated with increased susceptibility to infection related nephropathy, including HIV and COVID-19 nephropathy [130, 131].

Circulating Factors

Beyond genetic factors, a major mechanism of idiopathic SRNS is the presence of a circulating pathogenic factor or absence of factors that prevent proteinuria [132]. Evidence supporting the role of circulating factors includes the recurrence of FSGS post-transplant that is amenable to treatment with plasmapheresis and immunosuppression in some patients [133]. In addition, administration of plasma from FSGS patients alters glomerular and podocyte morphology *in vitro* [134]. Despite extensive efforts, a single circulating factor has not been identified to date. Several candidate factors have been proposed; one of these is sUPAR, the soluble urokinase receptor, which was shown to be elevated post FSGS recurrence and induced proteinuria in a mouse model of FSGS [135]. However, additional studies failed to confirm sUPAR as the circulating factor, although its role in disease progression remains the subject of ongoing investigations [133]. Other circulating factors that have been implicated include cardiotrophin-like cytokine factor-1 (CLCF-1), CD40 antibodies, and apolipoprotein A-Ib (ApoA-Ib) [133]. CLCF-1 is a cytokine that functions in B-cell stimulation. CD40 is a costimulatory protein expressed on immune cells. Elevated CLCF1 levels and anti-CD40 antibodies were identified in sera from patients with recurrent FSGS [136]. Application of CLCF1 or anti-CD40 antibodies to cultured podocytes induced actin cytoskeleton alterations [136]. ApoA-1 is a circulating component of the HDL complex; The ApolA-1b variant was identified by urine proteomics studies as increased in patients with recurrent FSGS [137].

Podocyte Endowment, Loss, Regeneration and Glomerulosclerosis

Glomerulosclerosis is the most common pathologic finding underlying SRNS. Regardless of the initial factor, podocyte damage and loss is key to development of the lesions of glomerulosclerosis [138]. The mechanisms by which podocyte damage evolves into the pathological appearance seen in FSGS have been studied extensively in murine models of FSGS [73]. The initial defect appears to be a reduction in podocyte number and the inability of podocytes to completely cover the glomerular tufts. The reduction in podocyte density causes the loss of separation between the glomerular tuft and Bowman's capsule, leading to the formation of synechiae or adhesions between the tuft and the Bowman's capsule [73]. The perfused capillaries lacking podocytes at the site of tuft adhesion then deliver their filtrate into the interstitium instead of Bowman's space (Fig. 14.3) [73]. This misdirected filtration through capillaries lacking podocytes leads to progression of segmental injury, tubular degeneration and interstitial fibrosis [73]. Further evidence for the role of podocytopenia in the pathogenesis of FSGS was shown using a rat model of diphtheria toxin-induced podocyte depletion in which the extent of podocyte loss is regulated [74]. In this model, mild podocyte loss resulted in hypertrophy of the remaining podocytes to cover the glomerular basement membrane. However, with moderate to severe depletion FSGS and global sclerosis developed; 30–40% of podocyte loss appear to be sufficient to drive progressive glomerulosclerosis [74].

Diagnostic Evaluation

Patient and Family History

In patients diagnosed with SRNS, the medical history should be explored for potential secondary causes of the disease such as sickle cell disease, HIV, SLE, as well as recent hepatitis B, malaria or parvovirus B19 infections. Family history should be assessed for other family members affected by nephrotic syndrome and/or chronic kidney disease, and parental consanguinity should be checked.

Clinical Assessment

The clinical evaluation of children with SRNS should include an assessment of fluid status, as well as careful exploration of extrarenal disease features such as dysmorphic features, ambiguous genitalia, skeletal, skin, ocular, hearing and neurological abnormalities. Any abnormalities should prompt further diagnostic evaluation.

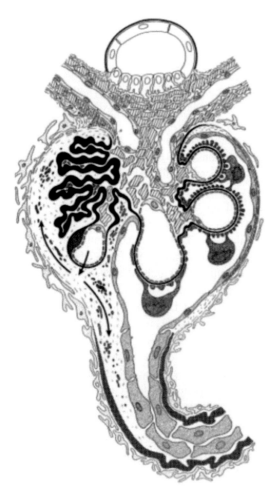

Fig. 14.3 Kriz's misdirected filtration hypothesis of evolving FSGS lesion: The glomerular basement membrane (GBM) is shown in black, podocytes are densely stippled, parietal epithelial cells are less densely stippled and interstitial as well as endothelial cells are loosely stippled, mesangial cells are hatched. The tuft adhesion contains several collapsed capillary loops. It also contains a perfused loop, which is partially hyalinized. The filtrate of this loop is delivered into a paraglomerular space that is separated from the interstitium by a layer of fibroblasts. This newly created space extends onto the outer aspect of the tubule by expanding and/or separating the tubular basement membrane from its epithelium. (Reproduced with permission from reference [73])

Laboratory Workup

Proteinuria should be quantitated by measuring the urinary protein:creatinine ratio (uPCR) in spot urine or 24-h protein excretion. Urine dipstick is not considered sufficient to make the diagnosis or monitor treatment responsiveness in

SRNS. Basic chemistries including serum creatinine, serum albumin, a complete blood count, a lipid profile and coagulation testing are important for estimating renal function, confirming the presence or absence of overt nephrosis, and evaluating the risk for disease complications.

SRNS patients require a diligent effort to rule out secondary disease processes. Tests for systemic autoimmune disorders, including antinuclear antibody (ANA), anti–double stranded DNA (anti-dsDNA) antibodies, ANCA, and complement C3 levels should be performed and testing for hepatitis B and C, HIV, malaria, parvovirus B19 and depending on geographic area and ethnicity, sickle cell disease, tuberculosis, and even syphilis may be indicated.

Genetic Testing

Genetic screening is emerging as a critically important clinical tool in the management of children with SRNS. Identification or exclusion of pathogenic gene variants potentially allows for (1) a rational approach to the use of immunosuppressive agents and avoidance of side effects; (2) selection of targeted therapies that may induce remission and/or delay progression to ESKD (e.g., COQ10 supplementation in patients with hereditary COQ10 deficiency; (3) prediction of clinical course and risk of post-transplant disease recurrence; (4) avoidance of kidney biopsy; and (5) genetic counseling and possible prenatal screening [139]. In view of these considerations, the IPNA SRNS guideline recommends genetic testing for all children as soon as the diagnosis of primary SRNS is established [1]. When considered later in the course of the disease, genetic screening is not indicated in patients who have responded to intensified immunosuppressive therapy and in patients with secondary SRNS.

Kidney Biopsy

Kidney biopsy allows the confirmation of a primary podocytopathy (MCD, FSGS, or DMS) and the exclusion of other differential diagnoses such as membranous nephropathy or MPGN. Biopsy is therefore indicated in all children with SRNS except in those with an established monogenic cause of SRNS, potentially in familial and/or syndromic cases, and in patients with known secondary SRNS due to infection or malignancy. Even in suspected or confirmed hereditary forms of SRNS, kidney biopsy may sometimes be indicated, particularly in patients with CKD stage 2 and higher, to grade the amount of tubular atrophy, interstitial fibrosis and glomerulosclerosis as prognostic markers [32, 33].

Management

The IPNA SRNS Clinical Practice Recommendation contains a refined algorithm for the management of SRNS in children (Fig. 14.4). We will describe and explain the rationale for the preferred therapeutic approaches along the lines of this recommendation.

Confirmation Period

When the diagnosis of SRNS is established after 4 weeks of standardized oral corticosteroid therapy, it is suggested to utilize a 2- to 3-week period to further confirm and elaborate the diagnosis before starting new immunosuppressive therapies other than steroids. During this period, genetic testing should be initiated and a kidney biopsy performed, oral prednisone therapy continued and/or three intravenous steroid pulses may be optionally performed. Importantly, renin-angiotensin system (RAS) blockade should be implemented by up-titrating an angiotensin converting enzyme (ACE) inhibitor or angiotensin receptor blocker (ARB) to full antiproteinuric efficacy. It is essential to measure proteinuria at the end of this period to avoid confounding the antiproteinuric effect of RAS blockade with that of any subsequent immunomodulatory therapies. If genetic screening reveals a monogenic form of SRNS, RAS blockade should be continued at the maximally effective dose, steroid therapy discontinued and no alternative immunosuppressive

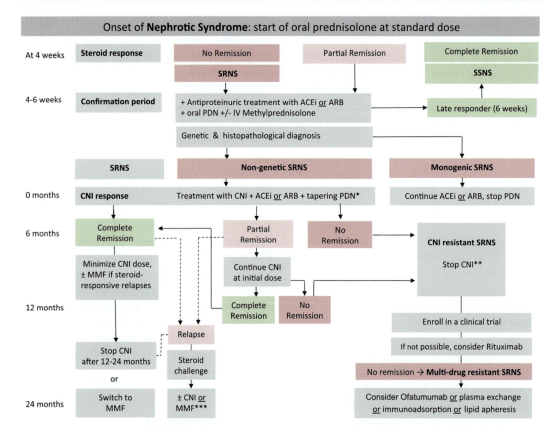

Fig. 14.4 IPNA clinical practice recommendation for management of SRNS in children (Reproduced from [1] with permission)

therapies should be started (or stopped if already started) in order to avoid a futile, potentially toxic treatment.

Therapeutic Pathway

If no genetic disorder is identified, a calcineurin inhibitor (CNI, tacrolimus or cyclosporin A) should be started, the RAS blocker continued at unchanged dose, and oral prednisone weaned over 4–5 months. The response to calcineurin inhibition should be evaluated after 6 months of treatment. If complete remission has been achieved, the patient can be classified as **CNI-responsive SRNS**. In this case, the CNI dose should be minimized and optionally supplemented by MMF. In case of persistent remission, the CNI should be stopped after 12–24 months, optionally continuing or switching to MMF monotherapy. If partial remission is achieved at 6 months, treatment should be continued for a total of 12 months. If complete remission does not occur, the CNI should be discontinued and the patient should receive the diagnosis **CNI-resistant SRNS**. In these patients, a B-cell depleting monoclonal antibody (e.g. Rituximab) can be tried. If this treatment does not yield full remission, the patient should receive the diagnosis **multidrug-resistant SRNS**. Children with CNI-resistant or multidrug-resistant SRNS are candidates for clinical trials and experimental extracorporeal rescue therapies, such as plasma exchange, immunoadsorption and lipid apheresis.

Pharmacotherapies

In the following, we describe the evidence base supporting the use of antiproteinuric and immunosuppressive pharmacotherapies in the therapeutic pathway above. It should be emphasized that due to the rarity of the disease, randomized trial evidence for any of the drugs is scarce or absent. Generally, the apparent efficacy of all of the immunosuppressive agents is lower in SRNS compared to those with frequently relapsing or steroid sensitive nephrotic syndrome [140, 141]. However, most previous treatment studies did not identify and exclude patients with genetic forms of SRNS who are highly unlikely to respond to immunosuppressive treatment. Since these cases comprise up to 30% of SRNS cases, most trial results must be considered substantially confounded. Finally, spontaneous remission of SRNS can occur and may explain some occasional responses of largely ineffective therapies.

RAS Blockade
Several controlled and non-controlled clinical studies have demonstrated the antiproteinuric efficacy of ACE inhibitors and angiotensin-receptor blockers (ARBs) in adults and children with glomerular diseases [142–148]. The antiproteinuric effects of ACEIs and ARBs are due to their ability to reduce glomerular capillary plasma flow rate, decrease transcapillary hydraulic pressure, and alter the permselectivity of the glomerular filtration barrier. On average, RAS blockers reduce proteinuria by approximately 30% in children with SRNS [149], although even complete remissions have been reported [150]. ACEIs and ARBS should be administered at the maximum approved and tolerated dosages since proteinuria reduction is dose dependent. However, the use of RAS blockers may increase the risk for AKI in patients with intravascular volume depletion [151]. Combined treatment with ACEi and ARBs is not recommended as it increases the risk for adverse events [152]. ACE inhibitor therapy may lead to a phenomenon known as 'aldosterone escape' with a long-term increase in plasma aldosterone levels. The addition of aldosterone blockade with ACE inhibition reduces urine protein excretion by 30–58% in patients with both diabetic and non-diabetic proteinuria [153]. The long-term safety of this form of combined RAS blockade remains to be elucidated.

Calcineurin Inhibition
Several randomized trials have suggested improved complete or partial remission rates in patients with SRNS when treated with cyclosporine compared with placebo, no treatment, or intravenous methylprednisolone pulses (~75% vs. 22%) [154–158].

Out of 433 children with primary SRNS in the PodoNet registry treated with CsA or Tacrolimus in the year following diagnosis, 30% achieved complete and 19% partial remission [159]. CsA and tacrolimus show similar efficacy in inducing remission [160].

In addition to immunomodulation, antiproteinuric effects of the calcineurin inhibitors may in part be mediated by hemodynamic effects that reduce renal blood flow [161]. In addition, calcineurin inhibitors may reduce proteinuria by inhibition of calcineurin-mediated degradation of synaptopodin and stabilization of the podocyte actin cytoskeleton [162, 163].

While CNIs are generally not recommended in patients with reduced eGFR due to their nephrotoxic effects, their use may be justified in SRNS patients with CKD and no other option for disease control [162]. CsA and tacrolimus have similar nephrotoxicity, but gingival hyperplasia and hypertrichosis are more prevalent with CSA and glucose intolerance occurs more frequently with tacrolimus (Table 14.5).

Mycophenolate-Mofetil (MMF)
The efficacy of MMF in inducing or maintaining remission in children with SRNS has not been demonstrated against placebo or no treatment in randomized clinical trials.

Table 14.5 Treatment options for steroid resistant nephrotic syndrome

Drug	Efficacy Evidence	Toxicity	Benefit
ACE Inhibitors/ARBs	Good	May lower eGFR Teratogenicity	Slowed progression of CKD
IV Corticosteroids	Good	Weight gain Hypertension Glucose intolerance Hyperlipidemia Striae	May ensure achieving therapeutic drug levels.
Cyclosporine	Good	Nephrotoxicity Hypertension Gingival hyperplasia	May only require low dose
Tacrolimus	Good	Nephrotoxicity Hypertension Glucose Intolerance	May only require low dose
Mycophenolate Mofetil	Mixed	GI intolerance Teratogenicity	No nephrotoxicity
Rituximab	Mixed	Infections Hypogammaglobulinemia Long-term effects unknown	May enable discontinuation of daily immunosuppressive medications

In a multicenter randomized trial of 192 children and young adults with steroid resistant FSGS, MMF in combination with dexamethasone was similarly effective as CsA (33% vs. 46%] and the rates of adverse events were similar [163]. MMF was less effective than tacrolimus in maintaining remission (45% vs. 90%) [164]. In the PodoNet registry, MMF therapy was associated with complete or partial remission in only 4 of 24 cases (17%) [159]. CNI/MMF co-treatment yielded full remission in four and partial remission in 10 of 34 patients, i.e. not different from CNI monotherapy [159].

B-Cell Depleting Agents

Rituximab is a chimeric monoclonal antibody directed against CD20. Rituximab-induced B-lymphocyte depletion may act on proteinuria in nephrotic syndrome by inducing regulatory T lymphocytes, as has been observed in patients with lupus nephritis [164]. Experimental findings suggest that Rituximab may also directly protect podocytes by stabilizing the podocyte cytoskeleton and preventing apoptosis through an interaction with the sphingomyelin phosphodiesterase acid-like 3b protein that is expressed in podocytes [165].

In a retrospective review of 33 patients with SRNS treated with two to four doses of intravenous rituximab, and followed for ≥12 months, 9 (27%) patients with SRNS showed complete remission, 7 (21%) had partial remission, and 17 (52%) had no response after 6 months of observation [166]. A similar response pattern was reported from a randomized trial in Korean children and in 66 children followed in the PodoNet registry [159, 167]. However, in an open-label, controlled trial that randomized 31 children with SRNS to either receive rituximab or continue prednisone and calcineurin inhibitors, no subjects in either arm achieved significant reduction of proteinuria. Hence, the efficacy of rituximab in the treatment of SRNS is unclear and there is a need for a randomized control trial [168].

More recently, case reports suggested that Ofatumumab (OFA), a fully humanized anti-CD20 monoclonal antibody, may be useful in inducing remission in patients with hypersensitivity reaction to rituximab or in children who are resistant to multiple immunomodulators including rituximab [169, 170]. However, a recent low-dose ofatumumab randomized placebo-controlled trial was prematurely terminated because the first 13 patients (25% of targeted enrollment) did not respond to the treatment [171]. Meanwhile, Ofatumumab has been withdrawn from the market.

Newer Therapies and Ongoing Clinical Trials

For children with CNI-resistant SRNS, consideration for entry into clinical trials evaluating novel therapies on the horizon should be strongly considered.

The FONT2 study (Novel Therapies in the Treatment of Resistant FSGS) aimed to compare novel therapies in patients with FSGS that have failed standard immunosuppressive therapies with conservative management [172]. In vitro studies have documented decreases in glomerular permeability when isolated glomeruli were incubated with galactose-containing sera [173]. The proposed mechanism suggests galactose may bind a glomerular permeability factor thus rendering it ineffective. Another proposed mechanism for proteinuria in patients with SRNS implicate Tumor Necrosis Factor-alpha (TNF-α), a pro-inflammatory cytokine that is important in the recruitment of leukocytes to the site of glomerular injury, induction of cytokines and growth factors, generation of oxygen radicals with increased glomerular endothelial cell permeability, cytotoxicity, and induction of apoptosis. In the FONT2 trial, 21 patients were randomized to one of the three study arms to receive the TNF-α antibody **adalimumab, galactose,** or standard medical therapy for 26 weeks. None of the adalimumab-treated subjects achieved the primary outcome of ≥50% reduction in proteinuria, whereas two subjects in the galactose and two in the standard medical therapy arm had a 50% reduction in proteinuria without a decline in eGFR, suggesting that some patients may benefit from treatment with oral galactose [173].

ACTH (Adrenocorticotropic Hormone) was the therapy of choice for children with nephrotic syndrome in the 1950s before corticosteroids became widely available [174, 175]. The development of an ACTH analog has made this therapy available once again as a second line agent in the treatment of SRNS. The largest published series to date by Hogan et.al reports a cumulative remission rate of 29% in 24 patients with SRNS and SDNS treated with subcutaneous ACTH [176]. In a recent systematic review that included 98 patients with FSGS, 42% achieved remission following treatment with ACTH. However, it should be noted that the population comprised frequently relapsing, steroid dependent, and steroid resistant patients [177].

Sparsentan, a dual endothelin and ARB was found to decrease proteinuria by 45% vs. 19% in a phase 2 randomized double-blind trial of those treated only with irbesartan with no differences in serious adverse events between the groups [178]. A phase-3 multicenter trial is in progress.

A small post-approval study for **low-density lipoprotein (LDL) apheresis** for children with CNI-resistant SRNS has shown increased treatment responsiveness and improved or stable eGFR over the follow-up period, it should be noted that this was not a randomized control trial [179].

Common variants in APOL1 gene termed G1 and G2 account for a significant proportion of the excess risk of progressive kidney disease in individuals of recent African ancestry with an estimated lifetime risk of kidney disease in 15% in those with a high-risk genotype [180, 181]. Novel **APOL1 inhibitors** are currently in clinical development. A Phase II trial investigating the APOL1 inhibitor VX-147 has started recruitment [182]. Antisense oligonucleotides are short, synthetic, modified chains of nucleotides that bind to the target mRNA, inducing its degradation and preventing the mRNA from being translated into a detrimental protein product. Preclinical studies with antisense oligonucleotides are showing promise as a novel therapeutic approach for APOL1 associated nephropathy [183, 184].

Treatment of Monogenic SRNS

Increased availability of genetic testing for children with SRNS has enabled the development of more personalized treatment decisions. The clinical value of genetic testing in SRNS is illustrated by our ability to make decisions on the intensity and duration of immunosuppression, as well as pre- and post-transplant management based on genomic findings [8, 9, 185, 186]. Generally, >95% of patients with monogenic SRNS will not respond to treatment with immunomodulatory agents [121, 159], and hence it is recommended to withdraw immunosuppressive therapy. RAS inhibitors should be administered at maximally effective and tolerated doses. There are anecdotal reports of individuals with mutations in *WT1, PLCE1, and MYO1E* who achieved partial or complete remission when exposed to immunosuppressive treatments, in particular calcineurin inhibitors [64, 69, 121, 187]. It is unclear if these responses, which are usually transient, are due to immunomodulatory effects or rather to their effects on stabilizing the podocyte cytoskeleton.

One of the promises of the genomic revolution is that identification of genetic causes of SRNS will lead to identification of specific and non-toxic therapeutic agents. Along this line, some monogenic causes of SRNS have given clue to novel therapeutic agents. An intriguing example is Coenzyme Q10 (CoQ10) supplementation in patients with mutations in genes encoding for components of the CoQ10 synthase complex (COQ6, COQ2, COQ8B) [67, 139, 188]. Other examples are Vitamin B12 supplementation in patients with mutations in the cubilin (CUBN) gene, and targeting of *TRPC6, TRPC5*, and RhoGTPases for potential treatment of some form of monogenic SRNS [62, 189, 190].

Long-Term Prognosis of SRNS

Most studies examining the long-term prognostic factors for kidney survival in patients with SRNS were from small cohorts, frequently single-center studies, with short term follow up, and often incomplete datasets [191, 192]. A multi-center study of 75 children with FSGS reported that within 5 years from the diagnosis of FSGS, 21% of children had developed ESKD, 23% had developed CKD, and 37% had developed persistent proteinuria, while only 11% remained in remission [30]. The most comprehensive study to date has been performed by the PodoNet consortium [159]. In this study, clinical, treatment-related, genetic, and laboratory data including kidney biopsy findings were collected from >1300 patients with SRNS with an average follow up time of about 4 years but extending up to 15 years. The overall proportion of SRNS patients with preserved kidney function was 74%, 58%, and 48% at 5, 10, and 15 years respectively. Risk factors for disease progression included lacking responsiveness to intensified immunosuppression (IIS) protocols, genetic disease, and FSGS on biopsy. Ten-year ESKD-free survival rates were 94%, 72%, and 43% in patients with complete remission, partial remission, and IIS resistance respectively (Fig. 14.5). After 15 years, kidney function was preserved in 96% of IIS-responsive, 53% of multidrug resistant and 17% of genetic SRNS patients. The histopathological findings at time of diagnosis were also predictive of outcome but less so than IIS responsiveness and genetic disease status, with 37% 15-year ESKD-free survival in patients with FSGS as compared to 79% in those with minimal change disease. The predictive value of IIS responsiveness and genetic status was independent of the histopathological diagnosis.

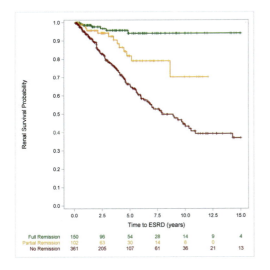
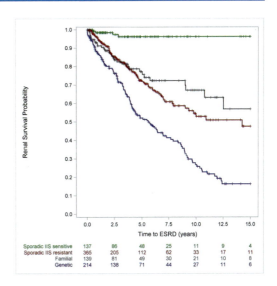

Fig. 14.5 ESKD-free survival in children with SRNS followed in PodoNet Registry. *Left panel:* Survival according to responsiveness to calcineurin inhibitor therapy (green; full remission, yellow; partial remission, red; no remission). *Right panel*: ESKD-free survival according to responsiveness to intensified immunosuppression (IIS) and genetic familial disease status (green: IIS responsive sporadic SRNS, red: multidrug resistant SRNS; grey: familial SRNS without identified genetic cause; blue: genetic SRNS). Reproduced from [159] with permission

Complications of Nephrotic Syndrome

Hyperlipidemia

Hyperlipidemia is a common clinical finding in children with nephrotic syndrome. The characteristic lipid profile includes elevations in total plasma cholesterol, very low-density lipoprotein (VLDL), and low-density lipoprotein (LDL) cholesterol, triglyceride, lipoprotein A, as well as variable alterations (more typically decreased) in high-density lipoprotein (HDL) cholesterol [193, 194]. While the hyperlipidemia in children with SSNS is often transient and usually returns to normal after remission, children with SRNS refractory to therapy often have sustained hyperlipidemia. Such chronic hyperlipidemia has been associated with an increased risk for cardiovascular complications and progressive glomerular damage in adults [195–199]. Based on this, pharmacologic treatment of hyperlipidemia in children with refractory nephrotic syndrome may both reduce the risk for cardiovascular complications later in life and reduce the risk of disease progression.

The potential usefulness of hydroxymethylglutaryl CoA (HMG CoA) reductase inhibitors (statins) in children with SRNS has been reported in a few uncontrolled trials. One study reported a 41% reduction in cholesterol and 44% reduction in triglyceride levels within 6 months of treatment [200]. A second study found significant reductions within 2–4 months in total cholesterol (40%), LDL cholesterol (44%), and triglyceride (33%) levels, but no significant changes in HDL cholesterol levels [201]. Treatment was found to be very safe in these studies, with no associated adverse clinical or laboratory events. Although the long-term safety of statins in children has not yet been established, these medications appear to be generally well tolerated in adults with nephrotic syndrome, with only minor side effects such as asymptomatic increases in liver enzymes, creatine kinase, and rarely diarrhea [202].

Thrombosis

The risk of thromboembolic events in children with nephrotic syndrome is estimated to be 1.8–5% with a higher risk reported in children with SRNS compared with those with SSNS [203, 204]. Factors contributing to an increased risk of thrombosis during nephrotic syndrome include abnormalities of the coagulation cascade, such as increased clotting factor synthesis in the liver (factors I, II, V, VII, VIII, X, and XIII) and loss of coagulation inhibitors such as anti-thrombin III in the urine. Other prothrombotic risks present in these children include increased platelet aggregability (and sometimes thrombocytosis), hyperviscosity resulting from increased fibrinogen levels, hyperlipidemia, prolonged immobilization, and the use of diuretics. In one series, the use of diuretics was the major iatrogenic risk factor for thrombosis [204].

The majority of episodes of thrombosis are venous in origin. The most common sites for thrombosis are the deep leg veins, ileofemoral veins, and the inferior vena cava. In addition, use of central venous catheters can further increase the risk of thrombosis. Renal vein thrombosis (RVT) can also occur and may manifest as gross hematuria with or without acute renal failure. Development of these features should prompt either renal Doppler ultrasonography or magnetic resonance angiography to rule out RVT. Pulmonary embolism is another important complication that may be fatal if not recognized early. Rarely, cerebral venous thrombosis, most commonly in the sagittal sinus, has also been reported [205]. In addition to imaging studies, development of thrombosis should prompt an evaluation for possible inherited hypercoagulable states.

The typical acute management of thrombosis in children with nephrotic syndrome includes initial heparin infusion or low molecular weight heparin, followed by transition to warfarin for 6 months. Children with a history of prior thrombosis and patients with severe proteinuria should also receive prophylactic anticoagulation therapy during future relapses.

Nutrition

Several recommendations supported by observational data exist regarding nutrition in pediatric patients with nephrotic syndrome. Specifically, children with nephrotic syndrome and edema should be evaluated for malabsorption and subsequent malnutrition due to bowel wall edema. In edematous patients, long-term sodium restriction is appropriate with a maximum goal of approximately 2500 mg/day. In patients with persistent hyperlipidemia due to inability to control nephrosis, a low saturated fat diet should be instituted with their HMG CoA-reductase inhibitor. Protein intake should only be supplemented at the Recommended Daily Allowance (RDA) [206]. Although it would appear intuitive that states of excess urinary protein loss should warrant increase dietary protein intake, several studies have successfully challenged this notion. In nephrotic rats, augmentation of dietary protein was found to stimulate albumin synthesis by increasing albumin mRNA content in the liver, but there was also a notable increase in glomerular permeability and subsequently increased albuminuria [207]. No change in albumin synthesis was noted with dietary protein restriction in this model or in nephrotic patients.

Immunization

Children with nephrotic syndrome are at increased risk for infections, including but not limited to streptococcus and staphylococcal species due to urinary losses of IgG, loss of factors crucial for regulation of the alternative complement pathway, and large fluid collections prone to breeding bacteria. Live-viral vaccines (rotavirus vaccine, varicella vaccine, measles, mumps, and rubella vaccine, and the live-attenuated influenza vaccine) are generally recommended to be avoided in CKD patients who are immunosuppressed and therefore should be avoided in patients that are frankly nephrotic and/or currently receiving immunosuppressive therapy. Anti-pneumococcal vaccination using the 23-valent polysaccharide vaccine (PPSV23) is recommended for children with nephrotic syndrome [208]. Due to the low immunogenicity of this vaccine in children less than 2 years of age, the 13-valent polysaccharide pneumococcal vaccine (PCV13) is recommended in this age group, followed by supplemental immunization with PPSV23 over the age of 2 years at least 8 weeks after the final dose of PCV13. A second dose of PPSV23 should be repeated in 5 years.

Kidney Transplantation

Recurrence of nephrotic syndrome may occur in up to 30% in the first kidney allograft of patients with ESKD due to FSGS and approach 100% in those who have a history of prior allograft loss due to FSGS. The risk post-transplant recurrence appears to be mainly determined by the underlying disease etiology, i.e. immune-mediated vs. genetic. Whereas patients with secondary steroid resistance have about 80% risk of recurrence, the risk appears to be close to zero in patients with genetic forms of SRNS [7–9, 139]. Hence, genetic testing should be considered mandatory in all children with SRNS considered for kidney transplantation.

In addition, young age, mesangial proliferation in the native kidneys, rapid progression to ESKD, pre-transplant bilateral nephrectomy, and white ethnicity have been associated with increased risk of recurrence post-transplant [209, 210]. The histologic variant type of FSGS does not appear to be predictive of disease recurrence. There is a higher risk of recurrence in living donor transplant pediatric recipients; however, the reduced risk of rejection and a lower immunosuppression in living-related transplants may overcome the deleterious effect of recurrent glomerulonephritis [211].

The management of recurrent FSGS disease remains controversial and results from observational reports vary. The implementation of plasma exchange is supported in part by the idea of a circulating permeability factor. Up to 70% of chil-dren with recurrent FSGS treated with repeated plasma exchanges and/or rituximab may achieve at least a partial remission.

References

1. Trautmann A, Vivarelli M, Samuel S, et al. IPNA clinical practice recommendations for the diagnosis and management of children with steroid-resistant nephrotic syndrome. Pediatr Nephrol. 2020;35(8):1529–61.
2. Kidney Disease: Improving Global Outcomes (KDIGO) Glomerular Diseases Work Group. KDIGO 2021 clinical practice guideline for the management of glomerular diseases. Kidney Int. 2021;100(4S):S1–S276.
3. ISKDC. The primary nephrotic syndrome in children. Identification of patients with minimal change nephrotic syndrome from initial response to prednisone. J Pediatr. 1981;98(4):561–4.
4. Niaudet P. Steroid-resistant idiopathic nephrotic syndrome in children. In: Avner ED, Harmon WE, Niaudet P, editors. Pediatric nephrology. Philadelphia: Lippincott Williams & Wilkins; 2004. p. 557–73.
5. International Study of Kidney Disease in Children. Primary nephrotic syndrome in children: clinical significances of histopathologic variants of minimal change. Kidney Int. 1981;20(6):765–71.
6. Niaudet P, Gagnadoux MF, Broyer M. Treatment of childhood steroid-resistant idiopathic nephrotic syndrome. Adv Nephrol Necker Hosp. 1998;28:43–61.
7. Straatmann C, Ayoob R, Gbadegesin R, et al. Treatment outcome of late steroid-resistant nephrotic syndrome: a study by the Midwest Pediatric Nephrology Consortium. Pediatr Nephrol. 2013;28(8):1235–41.
8. Ding WY, Koziell A, McCarthy HJ, et al. Initial steroid sensitivity in children with steroid-resistant nephrotic syndrome predicts post-transplant recurrence. J Am Soc Nephrol. 2014;25(6):1342–8.
9. Pelletier JH, Kumar KR, Engen R, et al. Recurrence of nephrotic syndrome following kidney transplantation is associated with initial native kidney biopsy findings. Pediatr Nephrol. 2018;33(10):1773–80.
10. Nash MA, et al. The nephrotic syndrome. In: Edelmann CMJ, editor. Pediatric kidney disease. Boston: Little, Brown, and Company; 1992. p. 1247–66.
11. Srivastava T, Simon SD, Alon US. High incidence of focal segmental glomerulosclerosis in nephrotic syndrome of childhood. Pediatr Nephrol. 1999;13(1):13–8.
12. Hogg RJ, et al. Evaluation and management of proteinuria and nephrotic syndrome in children: recommendations from a pediatric nephrology panel

established at the National Kidney Foundation Conference on Proteinuria, Albuminuria, Risk, Assessment, Detection, and Elimination (PARADE). Pediatrics. 2000;105(6):1242–9.

13. McEnery PT, Strife CF. Nephrotic syndrome in childhood. Management and treatment in patients with minimal change disease, mesangial proliferation, or focal glomerulosclerosis. Pediat Clin North Am. 1982;29(4):875–94.

14. Noone DG, Iijima K, Parekh R. Idiopathic nephrotic syndrome in children. Lancet. 2018;392(10141):61–74.

15. Bonilla-Felix M, et al. Changing patterns in the histopathology of idiopathic nephrotic syndrome in children. Kidney Int. 1999;55(5):1885–90.

16. Eddy AA, Symons JM. Nephrotic syndrome in childhood. Lancet. 2003;362(9384):629–39.

17. Filler G, et al. Is there really an increase in non-minimal change nephrotic syndrome in children? Am J Kidney Dis. 2003;42(6):1107–13.

18. Kari JA. Changing trends of histopathology in childhood nephrotic syndrome in western Saudi Arabia. Saudi Med J. 2002;23(3):317–21.

19. Sharples PM, Poulton J, White RH. Steroid responsive nephrotic syndrome is more common in Asians. Arch Dis Child. 1985;60(11):1014–7.

20. Banh TH, Hussain-Shamsy N, Patel V, Vasilevska-Ristovska J, Borges K, Sibbald C, Lipszyc D, Brooke J, Geary D, Langlois V, Reddon M, Pearl R, Levin L, Piekut M, Licht CP, Radhakrishnan S, Aitken-Menezes K, Harvey E, Hebert D, Piscione TD, Parekh RS. Ethnic differences in incidence and outcomes of childhood nephrotic syndrome. Clin J Am Soc Nephrol. 2016;11(10):1760–8.

21. Coovadia HM, Adhikari M, Morel-Maroger L. Clinico-pathological features of the nephrotic syndrome in South African children. Q J Med. 1979;48(189):77–91.

22. Hendrickse RG, et al. Quartan malarial nephrotic syndrome. Collaborative clinicopathological study in Nigerian children. Lancet. 1972;1(1761):1143–9.

23. Abdurrahman MB. Clinicopathological features of childhood nephrotic syndrome in northern Nigeria. Q J Med. 1990;75(278):563–76.

24. Genovese G, Friedman DJ, Ross MD, et al. Association of trypanolytic ApoL1 variants with kidney disease in African Americans. Science. 2010;329(5993):841–5.

25. Nephrotic syndrome in children: prediction of histopathology from clinical and laboratory characteristics at time of diagnosis. A report of the International Study of Kidney Disease in Children. Kidney Int. 1978;13:159–65.

26. Sorof JM, et al. Age and ethnicity affect the risk and outcome of focal segmental glomerulosclerosis. Pediatr Nephrol. 1998;12(9):764–8.

27. Bhimma R, Coovadia HM, Adhikari M. Nephrotic syndrome in South African children: chang-ing perspectives over 20 years. Pediatr Nephrol. 1997;11(4):429–34.

28. Doe JY, et al. Nephrotic syndrome in African children: lack of evidence for 'tropical nephrotic syndrome'? Nephrol Dial Trans. 2006;21(3):672–6.

29. Esezobor CI, Solarin AU, Gbadegesin R. Changing epidemiology of nephrotic syndrome in Nigerian children: a cross-sectional study. PLoS One. 2020;15(9):e0239300.

30. The Southwest Pediatric Nephrology Study Group. Focal segmental glomerulosclerosis in children with idiopathic nephrotic syndrome: a report of the Southwest Pediatric Nephrology Study Group. Kidney Int. 1985;27:442–9.

31. Mubarak M, Lanewala A, Kazi JI, Akhter F, Sher A, Fayyaz A, Bhatti S. Histopathological spectrum of childhood nephrotic syndrome in Pakistan. Clin Exp Nephrol. 2009;13:589–93.

32. Nammalwar BR, Vijayakumar M, Prahlad N. Experience of renal biopsy in children with nephrotic syndrome. Pediatr Nephrol. 2006;21(2):286–8.

33. Banaszak B, Banaszak P. The increasing incidence of initial steroid resistance in childhood nephrotic syndrome. Pediatr Nephrol. 2012;27(6):927–32.

34. Bhimma R, Adhikari M, Asharam K. Steroid-resistant nephrotic syndrome: the influence of race on cyclophosphamide sensitivity. Pediatr Nephrol. 2006;21(12):1847–53.

35. Churg J, Habib R, White RH. Pathology of the nephrotic syndrome in children: a report for the International Study of Kidney Disease in Children. Lancet. 1970;760:1299–302.

36. Cameron JS. Focal segmental glomerulosclerosis in adults. Nephrol Dial Transplant. 2003;18:vi45-51.

37. Rich AR. A hitherto undescribed vulnerability of the juxtamedullary glomeruli in lipoid nephrosis. Bull Johns Hopkins Hosp. 1957;100:173–86.

38. Kitiyakara C, Kopp JB, Eggers P. Trends in the epidemiology of focal segmental glomerulosclerosis. Semin Nephrol. 2003;23:172–82.

39. Kitiyakara C, Eggers P, Kopp JB. Twenty-one-year trend in ESRD due to focal segmental glomerulosclerosis in the United States. Am J Kidney Dis. 2004;44:815–25.

40. Swaminathan S, Leung N, Lager DJ, Melton LJ 3rd, Bergstralh EJ, Rohlinger A, Fervenza FC. Changing incidence of glomerular disease in Olmsted County, Minnesota: a 30-year renal biopsy study. Clin J Am Soc Nephrol. 2006;1:483–7.

41. Borges FF, Shiraichi L, da Silva MP, Nishimoto EI, Nogueira PC. Is focal segmental glomerulosclerosis increasing in patients with nephrotic syndrome? Pediatr Nephrol. 2007;22:1309–13.

42. Izzedine H, Brocheriou I, Arzouk N, et al. COVID-19-associated collapsing glomerulopathy: a report of two cases and literature review. Intern Med J. 2020;50(12):1551–8.

43. Gbadegesin RA, Winn MP, Smoyer WE. Genetic testing in nephrotic syndrome—challenges and opportunities. Nat Rev Nephrol. 2013;9:179–84.

44. D'Agati VD, Fogo AB, Bruijn JA, Jennette JC. Pathologic classification of focal segmental glomerulosclerosis: a working proposal. Am J Kidney Dis. 2004;43:368–82.

45. Stokes MB, Valeri AM, Markowitz GS, D'Agati VD. Cellular focal segmental glomerulosclerosis: clinical and pathologic features. Kidney Int. 2006;70:1783–92.

46. D'Agati VD, Alster JM, Jennette JC, Thomas DB, Pullman J, Savino DA, Cohen AH, Gipson DS, Gassman JJ, Radeva MK, Moxey-Mims MM, Friedman AL, Kaskel FJ, Trachtman H, Alpers CE, Fogo AB, Greene TH, Nast CC. Association of histologic variants in FSGS clinical trial with presenting features and outcomes. Clin J Am Soc Nephrol. 2013;8:399–406.

47. Tsuchimoto A, Matsukuma Y, Ueki K, et al. Utility of Columbia classification in focal segmental glomerulosclerosis: renal prognosis and treatment response among the pathological variants. Nephrol Dial Transplant. 2020;35(7):1219–27.

48. Kopp JB, Anders HJ, Susztak K, et al. Podocytopathies. Nat Rev Dis Primers. 2020;6(1):68. Published 2020 Aug 13.

49. Wiggins RC. The spectrum of podocytopathies: a unifying view of glomerular diseases. Kidney Int. 2007;71:1205–14.

50. Smoyer WE, Mundel P. Regulation of podocyte structure during the development of nephrotic syndrome. J Mol Med. 1998;76:172–83.

51. Partanen TA, Arola J, Saaristo A, Jussila L, Ora A, Miettinen M, Stacker SA, Achen MG, Alitalo K. VEGF-C and VEGF-D expression in neuroendocrine cells and their receptor, VEGFR-3, in fenestrated blood vessels in human tissues. FASEB J. 2000;14:2087–96.

52. Rostgaard J, Qvortrup K. Sieve plugs in fenestrae of glomerular capillaries—site of the filtration barrier? Cells Tissues Organs. 2002;170:132–8.

53. Weinbaum S, Tarbell JM, Damiano ER. The structure and function of the endothelial glycocalyx layer. Annu Rev Biomed. 2007;9:121–67.

54. Ballermann BJ, Stan RV. Resolved: capillary endothelium is a major contributor to the glomerular filtration barrier. J Am Soc Nephrol. 2007;18:2432–8.

55. Vaughan MR, Quaggin SE. How do mesangial and endothelial cells form the glomerular tuft? J Am Soc Nephrol. 2008;19:24–33.

56. Kestilä M, Lenkkeri U, Männikkö M, Lamerdin J, McCready P, Putaala H, Ruotsalainen V, Morita T, Nissinen M, Herva R, Kashtan CE, Peltonen L, Holmberg C, Olsen A. Tryggvason K (1998) Positionally cloned gene for a novel glomerular protein—nephrin—is mutated in congenital nephrotic syndrome. Mol Cell. 1998;1:575–82.

57. Shih NY, et al. Congenital nephrotic syndrome in mice lacking CD2-associated protein. Science. 1999;286(5438):312–5.

58. Boute N, Gribouval O, Roselli S, Benessy F, Lee H, Fuchshuber A, Dahan K, Gubler MC, Niaudet P, Antignac C. NPHS2, encoding the glomerular protein podocin, is mutated in autosomal recessive steroid-resistant nephrotic syndrome. Nat Genet. 2000;24:349–54.

59. Kaplan JM, et al. Mutations in ACTN4, encoding alpha-actinin-4, cause familial focal segmental glomerulosclerosis. Nat Genet. 2000;24(3):251–6.

60. Boerkoel CF, Takashima H, John J, Yan J, Stankiewicz P, Rosenbarker L, André JL, Bogdanovic R, Burguet A, Cockfield S, Cordeiro I, Fründ S, Illies F, Joseph M, Kaitila I, Lama G, Loirat C, McLeod DR, Milford DV, Petty EM, Rodrigo F, Saraiva JM, Schmidt B, Smith GC, Spranger J, Stein A, Thiele H, Tizard J, Weksberg R, Lupski JR, Stockton DW. Mutant chromatin remodeling protein SMARCAL1 causes Schimke immuno-osseous dysplasia. Nat Genet. 2002;30:215–20.

61. Zenker M, Aigner T, Wendler O, Tralau T, Müntefering H, Fenski R, Pitz S, Schumacher V, Royer-Pokora B, Wühl E, Cochat P, Bouvier R, Kraus C, Mark K, Madlon H, Dötsch J, Rascher W, Maruniak-Chudek I, Lennert T, Neumann LM, Reis A. Human laminin beta2 deficiency causes congenital nephrosis with mesangial sclerosis and distinct eye abnormalities. Hum Mol Genet. 2004;13:2625–32.

62. Winn MP, et al. A mutation in the TRPC6 cation channel causes familial focal segmental glomerulosclerosis. Science. 2005;308(5729):1801–4.

63. Niaudet P, Gubler MC. WT1 and glomerular diseases. Pediatr Nephrol. 2006;21:1653–60.

64. Hinkes B, Wiggins RC, Gbadegesin R, et al. Positional cloning uncovers mutations in plce1 responsible for a nephrotic syndrome variant that may be reversible. Nat Genet. 2006;38:1397–405.

65. Berkovic SF, et al. Array-based gene discovery with three unrelated subjects shows SCARB2/LIMP-2 deficiency causes myoclonus epilepsy and glomerulosclerosis. Am J Hum Genet. 2008;82:673–84.

66. Brown EJ, et al. Mutations in the formin gene INF2 cause focal segmental glomerulosclerosis. Nat Genet. 2010;42:72–6.

67. Heeringa SF, et al. COQ6 mutations in human patients produce nephrotic syndrome with sensorineural deafness. J Clin Invest. 2011;121:2013–24.

68. Akilesh S, et al. Arhgap24 inactivates Rac1 in mouse podocytes, and a mutant form is associated with familial focal segmental glomerulosclerosis. J Clin Invest. 2011;121:4127–37.

69. Mele C, et al. MYO1E mutations and childhood familial focal segmental glomerulosclerosis. N Engl J Med. 2011;365:295–306.

70. Ozaltin F, et al. Disruption of PTPRO causes childhood-onset nephrotic syndrome. Am J Hum Genet. 2011;89:139–47.

71. Has C, Spartà G, Kiritsi D, Weibel L, Moeller A, Vega-Warner V, Waters A, He Y, Anikster Y, Esser P, Straub BK, Hausser I, Bockenhauer D, Dekel B, Hildebrandt F, Bruckner-Tuderman L, Laube GF. Integrin α3 mutations with kidney, lung, and skin disease. N Engl J Med. 2012;366(16):1508–14.

72. Gupta IR, Baldwin C, Auguste D, Ha KC, El Andalousi J, Fahiminiya S, Bitzan M, Bernard C, Akbari MR, Narod SA, Rosenblatt DS, Majewski J, Takano T. ARHGDIA: a novel gene implicated in nephrotic syndrome. J Med Genet. 2013;50(5):330–8.

73. Kriz W. The pathogenesis of 'classic' focal segmental glomerulosclerosis-lessons from rat models. Nephrol Dial Transplant. 2003;Suppl 6:vi39-44.

74. Wharram BL, Goyal M, Wiggins JE, Sanden SK, Hussain S, Filipiak WE, Saunders TL, Dysko RC, Kohno K, Holzman LB, Wiggins RC. Podocyte depletion causes glomerulosclerosis: diphtheria toxin-induced podocyte depletion in rats expressing human diphtheria toxin receptor transgene. J Am Soc Nephrol. 2005;16:2941–52.

75. Carrie BJ, Salyer WR, Myers BD. Minimal change nephropathy: an electrochemical disorder of the glomerular membrane. Am J Med. 1981;70(2):262–8.

76. Shalhoub RJ. Pathogenesis of lipoid nephrosis: a disorder of T-cell function. Lancet. 1974;2(7880):556–60.

77. Kemper MJ, Wolf G, Muller-Wiefel DE. Transmission of glomerular permeability factor from a mother to her child. N Engl J Med. 2001;344(5):386–7.

78. Meyrier A. Mechanisms of Disease: focal segmental glomerulosclerosis. Nat Clin Pract Nephrol. 2005;1(1):44–54.

79. Sasdelli M, et al. Cell mediated immunity in idiopathic glomerulonephritis. Clin Exp Immunol. 1984;46(1):27–34.

80. Dantal J, et al. Effect of plasma protein adsorption on protein excretion in kidney-transplant recipients with recurrent nephrotic syndrome. N Engl J Med. 1994;330(1):7–14.

81. Savin VJ, et al. Circulating factor associated with increased glomerular permeability to albumin in recurrent focal segmental glomerulosclerosis. N Engl J Med. 1996;334(14):878–83.

82. Candiano G, et al. Inhibition of renal permeability towards albumin: a new function of apolipoproteins with possible pathogenetic relevance in focal glomerulosclerosis. Electrophoresis. 2001;22(9):1819–25.

83. Savin VJ, McCarthy ET, Sharma R, Charba D, Sharma M. Galactose binds to focal segmental glomerulosclerosis permeability factor and inhibits its activity. Transl Res. 2008;151(6):288–92.

84. Savin VJ, McCarthy ET, Sharma R, Reddy S, Dong J, Hess S, Kopp J. cardiotrophin-like cytokine-1: candidate for the focal segmental glomerulosclerosis permeability factor. J Am Soc Nephrol. 2008;19.

85. De Smet E, Rioux JP, Ammann H, Déziel C, Quérin S. FSGS permeability factor-associated nephrotic syndrome: remission after oral galactose therapy. Nephrol Dial Transplant. 2009;24(9):2938–40.

86. Kopač M, Meglič A, Rus RR. Partial remission of resistant nephrotic syndrome after oral galactose therapy. Ther Apher Dial. 2011;15(3):269–72.

87. Sgambat K, Banks M, Moudgil A. Effect of galactose on glomerular permeability and proteinuria in steroid-resistant nephrotic syndrome. Pediatr Nephrol. 2013;28(11):2131–5.

88. Wei C, El Hindi S, Li J, Fornoni A, Goes N, Sageshima J, Maiguel D, Karumanchi SA, Yap HK, Saleem M, Zhang Q, Nikolic B, Chaudhuri A, Daftarian P, Salido E, Torres A, Salifu M, Sarwal MM, Schaefer F, Morath C, Schwenger V, Zeier M, Gupta V, Roth D, Rastaldi MP, Burke G, Ruiz P, Reiser J. Circulating urokinase receptor as a cause of focal segmental glomerulosclerosis. Nat Med. 2011;17(8):952–60.

89. Behrendt N, Rønne E, Ploug M, Petri T, Løber D, Nielsen LS, Schleuning WD, Blasi F, Appella E, Danø K. The human receptor for urokinase plasminogen activator. NH2-terminal amino acid sequence and glycosylation variants. J Biol Chem. 1990;265(11):6453–60.

90. Sidenius N, Sier CF, Blasi F. Shedding and cleavage of the urokinase receptor (uPAR): identification and characterisation of uPAR fragments in vitro and in vivo. FEBS Lett. 2000;475(1):52–6.

91. Wei C, Trachtman H, Li J, Dong C, Friedman AL, Gassman JJ, JL MM, Radeva M, Heil KM, Trautmann A, Anarat A, Emre S, Ghiggeri GM, Ozaltin F, Haffner D, Gipson DS, Kaskel F, Fischer DC, Schaefer F, Reiser J, PodoNet and FSGS CT Study Consortia. Circulating suPAR in two cohorts of primary FSGS. J Am Soc Nephrol. 2012;23(12):2051–9.

92. Huang J, Liu G, Zhang YM, Cui Z, Wang F, Liu XJ, Chu R, Chen Y, Zhao MH. Plasma soluble urokinase receptor levels are increased but do not distinguish primary from secondary focal segmental glomerulosclerosis. Kidney Int. 2013;84(2):366–72.

93. Maas RJ, Wetzels JF, Deegens JK. Serum-soluble urokinase receptor concentration in primary FSGS. Kidney Int. 2012;81(10):1043–4.

94. Bock ME, Price HE, Gallon L, Langman CB. Serum soluble urokinase-type plasminogen activator receptor levels and idiopathic FSGS in children: a single-center report. Clin J Am Soc Nephrol. 2013;8(8):1304–11.

95. Maas RJ, Deegens JK, Wetzels JF. Serum suPAR in patients with FSGS: trash or treasure? Pediatr Nephrol. 2013;28(7):1041–8.

96. Sever S, Trachtman H, Wei C, Reiser J. Is there clinical value in measuring suPAR levels in FSGS? Clin J Am Soc Nephrol. 2013;8(8):1273–5.

97. Reiser J. Circulating permeability factor suPAR: from concept to discovery to clinic. Trans Am Clin Climatol Assoc. 2013;124:133–8.
98. Ruf RG, Lichtenberger A, Karle SM, Haas JP, Anacleto FE, Schultheiss M, Zalewski I, Imm A, Ruf EM, Mucha B, Bagga A, Neuhaus T, Fuchshuber A, Bakkaloglu A, Hildebrandt F. Arbeitsgemeinschaft Für Pädiatrische Nephrologie Study Group. Patients with mutations in NPHS2 (podocin) do not respond to standard steroid treatment of nephrotic syndrome. J Am Soc Nephrol. 2004;15:722–32.
99. Gbadegesin R, Hinkes BG, Hoskins BE, Vlangos CN, Heeringa SF, Liu J, Loirat C, Ozaltin F, Hashmi S, Ulmer F, Cleper R, Ettenger R, Antignac C, Wiggins RC, Zenker M, Hildebrandt F. Mutations in PLCE1 are a major cause of isolated diffuse mesangial sclerosis (IDMS). Nephrol Dial Transplant. 2008;23:1291–7.
100. Wing MR, Bourdon DM, Harden TK. PLC-epsilon: a shared effector protein in Ras-, Rho-, and G alpha beta gamma-mediated signaling. Mol Interv. 2003;3:273–80.
101. Boyer O, Benoit G, Gribouval O, Nevo F, Tête MJ, Dantal J, Gilbert-Dussardier B, Touchard G, Karras A, Presne C, Grunfeld JP, Legendre C, Joly D, Rieu P, Mohsin N, Hannedouche T, Moal V, Gubler MC, Broutin I, Mollet G, Antignac C. Mutations in INF2 are a major cause of autosomal dominant focal segmental glomerulosclerosis. J Am Soc Nephrol. 2011;22(2):239–45.
102. Gbadegesin RA, Lavin PJ, Hall G, Bartkowiak B, Homstad A, Jiang R, Wu G, Byrd A, Lynn K, Wolfish N, Ottati C, Stevens P, Howell D, Conlon P, Winn MP. Inverted formin 2 mutations with variable expression in patients with sporadic and hereditary focal and segmental glomerulosclerosis. Kidney Int. 2012;81(1):94–9.
103. Barua M, Brown EJ, Charoonratana VT, Genovese G, Sun H, Pollak MR. Mutations in the INF2 gene account for a significant proportion of familial but not sporadic focal and segmental glomerulosclerosis. Kidney Int. 2013;83(2):316–22.
104. Kopp JB, Smith MW, Nelson GW, Johnson RC, Freedman BI, Bowden DW, Oleksyk T, McKenzie LM, Kajiyama H, Ahuja TS, Berns JS, Briggs W, Cho ME, Dart RA, Kimmel PL, Korbet SM, Michel DM, Mokrzycki MH, Schelling JR, Simon E, Trachtman H, Vlahov D, Winkler CA. MYH9 is a major-effect risk gene for focal segmental glomerulosclerosis. Nat Genet. 2008;40:1175–84.
105. Kao WH, Klag MJ, Meoni LA, et al. Family Investigation of Nephropathy and Diabetes Research Group. MYH9 is associated with nondiabetic end-stage renal disease in African Americans. Nat Genet. 2008;40:1185–92.
106. Okamoto K, Tokunaga K, Doi K, et al. Common variation in GPC5 is associated with acquired nephrotic syndrome. Nat Genet. 2011;43:459–63.
107. Ly J, Alexander M, Quaggin SE. A podocentric view of nephrology. Curr Opin Nephrol Hypertens. 2004;13(3):299–305.
108. Miner JH. Glomerular basement membrane composition and the filtration barrier. Pediatr Nephrol. 2011;26(9):1413–7.
109. Rheault MN, Gbadegesin RA. The genetics of nephrotic syndrome. J Pediatr Genet. 2016;5(1):15–24.
110. Akchurin O, Reidy KJ. Genetic causes of proteinuria and nephrotic syndrome: impact on podocyte pathobiology. Pediatr Nephrol. 2015;30(2):221–33.
111. Shankland SJ, Pippin JW, Duffield JS. Progenitor cells and podocyte regeneration. Semin Nephrol. 2014;34(4):418–28.
112. Warejko JK, Tan W, Daga A, et al. Whole exome sequencing of patients with steroid-resistant nephrotic syndrome. Clin J Am Soc Nephrol. 2018;13(1):53–62.
113. Sadowski CE, Lovric S, Ashraf S, et al. A single-gene cause in 29.5% of cases of steroid-resistant nephrotic syndrome. J Am Soc Nephrol. 2015;26(6):1279–89.
114. Klämbt V, Mao Y, Schneider R, et al. Generation of monogenic candidate genes for human nephrotic syndrome using 3 independent approaches. Kidney Int Rep. 2020;6(2):460–71.
115. Varner JD, Chryst-Stangl M, Esezobor CI, et al. Genetic testing for steroid-resistant-nephrotic syndrome in an outbred population. Front Pediatr. 2018;6:307.
116. Feng D, Notbohm J, Benjamin A, et al. Disease-causing mutation in α-actinin-4 promotes podocyte detachment through maladaptation to periodic stretch. Proc Natl Acad Sci U S A. 2018;115(7):1517–22.
117. Gbadegesin RA, Hall G, Adeyemo A, et al. Mutations in the gene that encodes the F-actin binding protein anillin cause FSGS. J Am Soc Nephrol. 2014;25(9):1991–2002.
118. Hall G, Lane BM, Khan K, et al. The human FSGS-causing ANLN R431C mutation induces dysregulated PI3K/AKT/mTOR/Rac1 signaling in podocytes. J Am Soc Nephrol. 2018;29(8):2110–22.
119. Malone AF, Phelan PJ, Hall G, et al. Rare hereditary COL4A3/COL4A4 variants may be mistaken for familial focal segmental glomerulosclerosis. Kidney Int. 2014;86(6):1253–9.
120. Gast C, Pengelly RJ, Lyon M, et al. Collagen (COL4A) mutations are the most frequent mutations underlying adult focal segmental glomerulosclerosis. Nephrol Dial Transplant. 2016;31(6):961–70.
121. Trautmann A, Lipska-Ziętkiewicz BS, Schaefer F. Exploring the clinical and genetic spectrum of steroid resistant nephrotic syndrome: the podonet registry. Front Pediatr. 2018;6:200.
122. Kopp JB, Nelson GW, Sampath K, et al. APOL1 genetic variants in focal segmental glomerulosclerosis and HIV-associated nephropathy. J Am Soc Nephrol. 2011;22(11):2129–37.

176. Hogan J, Bomback AS, Mehta K, Canetta PA, Rao MK, Appel GB, Radhakrishnan J, Lafayette RA. Treatment of idiopathic FSGS with adrenocorticotropic hormone gel. Clin J Am Soc Nephrol. 2013;8(12):2072–81.

177. Chakraborty R, Mehta A, Nair N, et al. ACTH treatment for management of nephrotic syndrome: a systematic review and reappraisal. Int J Nephrol. 2020;2020:2597079.

178. Trachtman H, Nelson P, Adler S, et al. DUET: a phase 2 study evaluating the efficacy and safety of Sparsentan in patients with FSGS. J Am Soc Nephrol. 2018;29(11):2745–54.

179. Raina R, Krishnappa V, Sanchez-Kazi C, et al. Dextran-sulfate plasma adsorption lipoprotein apheresis in drug resistant primary focal segmental glomerulosclerosis patients: results from a prospective, multicenter, single-arm intervention study. Front Pediatr. 2019;7:454.

180. Parsa A, Kao WH, Xie D, et al. APOL1 risk variants, race, and progression of chronic kidney disease. N Engl J Med. 2013;369(23):2183–96.

181. Limou S, Nelson GW, Kopp JB, Winkler CA. APOL1 kidney risk alleles: population genetics and disease associations. Adv Chronic Kidney Dis. 2014;21(5):426–33.

182. Sabnis RW. Novel APOL1 inhibitors for treating kidney diseases. ACS Med Chem Lett. 2020;11(12):2352–3.

183. Bennett CF. Therapeutic antisense oligonucleotides are coming of age. Annu Rev Med. 2019;70:307–21.

184. Aghajan M, Booten SL, Althage M, et al. Antisense oligonucleotide treatment ameliorates IFN-γ-induced proteinuria in APOL1-transgenic mice. JCI Insight. 2019;4(12):e126124.

185. Mason AE, Sen ES, Bierzynska A, et al. Response to first course of intensified immunosuppression in genetically stratified steroid resistant nephrotic syndrome. Clin J Am Soc Nephrol. 2020;15(7):983–94.

186. Saleem MA. Molecular stratification of idiopathic nephrotic syndrome. Nat Rev Nephrol. 2019;15(12):750–65.

187. Gellermann J, Stefanidis CJ, Mitsioni A, Querfeld U. Successful treatment of steroid-resistant nephrotic syndrome associated with WT1 mutations. Pediatr Nephrol. 2010;25(7):1285–9.

188. Atmaca M, Gulhan B, Korkmaz E, et al. Follow-up results of patients with ADCK4 mutations and the efficacy of CoQ10 treatment. Pediatr Nephrol. 2017;32(8):1369–75.

189. Saleem MA, Welsh GI. Podocyte RhoGTPases: new therapeutic targets for nephrotic syndrome? F1000Res. 2019;8:F1000. Faculty Rev-1847.

190. Zhou Y, Castonguay P, Sidhom EH, et al. A small-molecule inhibitor of TRPC5 ion channels suppresses progressive kidney disease in animal models. Science. 2017;358(6368):1332–6.

191. Martinelli R, Okumura AS, Pereira LJ, Rocha H. Primary focal segmental glomerulosclerosis in children: prognostic factors. Pediatr Nephrol. 2001;16(8):658–61.

192. Gipson DS, Chin H, Presler TP, Jennette C, Ferris ME, Massengill S, Gibson K, Thomas DB. Differential risk of remission and ESRD in childhood FSGS. Pediatr Nephrol. 2006; 21:344–9.

193. Querfeld U. Should hyperlipidemia in children with the nephrotic syndrome be treated? Pediatr Nephrol. 1999;13(1):77–84.

194. Querfeld U, Lang M, Friedrich JB, Kohl B, Fiehn W, Schärer K. Lipoprotein(a) serum levels and apolipoprotein(a) phenotypes in children with chronic renal disease. Pediatr Res. 1993;34(6): 772–6.

195. Keane WF. Lipids and the kidney. Kidney Int. 1994;46(3):910–20.

196. Moorhead JF, Wheeler DC, Varghese Z. Glomerular structures and lipids in progressive renal disease. Am J Med. 1989;87(5N):12N–20N.

197. Samuelsson O, Mulec H, Knight-Gibson C, Attman PO, Kron B, Larsson R, Weiss L, Wedel H, Alaupovic P. Lipoprotein abnormalities are associated with increased rate of progression of human chronic renal insufficiency. Nephrol Dial Transplant. 1997;12(9):1908–15.

198. Taal MW. Slowing the progression of adult chronic kidney disease: therapeutic advances. Drugs. 2004;64(20):2273–89.

199. Veverka A, Jolly JL. Recent advances in the secondary prevention of coronary heart disease. Expert Rev Cardiovasc Ther. 2004;2(6):877–89.

200. Coleman JE, Watson AR. Hyperlipidaemia, diet and simvastatin therapy in steroid-resistant nephrotic syndrome of childhood. Pediatr Nephrol. 1996;10(2):171–4.

201. Sanjad SA, al-Abbad A, al-Shorafa S. Management of hyperlipidemia in children with refractory nephrotic syndrome: the effect of statin therapy. J Pediatr. 1997;130(3):470–4.

202. Olbricht CJ, Wanner C, Thiery J, Basten A. Simvastatin in nephrotic syndrome. Simvastatin in Nephrotic Syndrome Study Group. Kidney Int Suppl. 1999;71:S113–6.

203. Citak A, Emre S, Sâirin A, Bilge I, Nayir A. Hemostatic problems and thromboembolic complications in nephrotic children. Pediatr Nephrol. 2000;14(2):138–42.

204. Lilova MI, Velkovski IG, Topalov IB. Thromboembolic complications in children with nephrotic syndrome in Bulgaria (1974-1996). Pediatr Nephrol. 2000;15(1–2):74–8.

205. Gangakhedkar A, Wong W, Pitcher LA. Cerebral thrombosis in childhood nephrosis. J Paediatr Child Health. 2005;41(4):221–4.

206. Sedman A, Friedman A, Boineau F, Strife CF, Fine R. Nutritional management of the child with mild to moderate chronic renal failure. J Pediatr. 1996;129(2):s13–8.
207. Kaysen GA. Albumin metabolism in the nephrotic syndrome: the effect of dietary protein intake. Am J Kidney Dis. 1988;12(6):461–80.
208. American Academy of Pediatrics Committee on Infectious Diseases. Recommendations for the prevention of Streptococcus pneumoniae infections in infants and children: use of 13-valent pneumococcal conjugate vaccine (PCV13) and pneumococcal polysaccharide vaccine (PPSV23). Pediatrics. 2010;126(1):186–90.
209. Banfi G, Colturi C, Montagnino G, Ponticelli C. The recurrence of focal segmental glomerulosclerosis in kidney transplant patients treated with cyclosporine. Transplantation. 1990;50(4):594–6.
210. Canaud G, Dion D, Zuber J, Gubler MC, Sberro R, Thervet E, Snanoudj R, Charbit M, Salomon R, Martinez F, Legendre C, Noel LH, Niaudet P. Recurrence of nephrotic syndrome after transplantation in a mixed population of children and adults: course of glomerular lesions and value of the Columbia classification of histological variants of focal and segmental glomerulosclerosis (FSGS). Nephrol Dial Transplant. 2010;25(4):1321–8.
211. Baum MA, Stablein DM, Panzarino VM, Tejani A, Harmon WE, Alexander SR. Loss of living donor renal allograft survival advantage in children with focal segmental glomerulosclerosis. Kidney Int. 2001;59(1):328–33.

Hereditary Nephrotic Syndrome

15

Stefanie Weber

Introduction

During the past two decades defects in various genes have been associated with the development of steroid resistant nephrotic syndrome (SRNS) in children and adults. These genes encode for proteins that participate in the development and structural architecture of glomerular visceral epithelial cells (podocytes). These insights moved the podocyte with its interdigitating foot processes and slit diaphragm (SD) into the center of interest regarding the pathophysiology of proteinuria.

While light microscopy shows variable aspects ranging from minimal change nephropathy to diffuse mesangial sclerosis or focal-segmental glomerulosclerosis (Fig. 15.1a, b), all hereditary proteinuria syndromes share a common phenotype when evaluated by electron microscopy, which uniformly demonstrates the typical flattening of the foot processes and loss of the SD. With respect to the clinical course, different entities can be distinguished, especially referring to the onset of the disease and modi of inheritance. Disorders of early glomerular development most often manifest prenatally, directly after birth or in early infancy. Disorders with late-onset nephrotic syndrome typically manifest as FSGS in adolescence or adulthood, frequently following an autosomal-dominant mode of inheritance with incomplete penetrance and variable expression. In rare cases, extrarenal symptoms are associated with hereditary nephrotic syndrome, e.g., in Denys-Drash, Frasier, Schimke and Pierson syndrome as well as in mitochondrial disorders. In the following, important genes involved in hereditary nephrotic syndrome will be discussed. Given the rapid development in the field, this list is comprehensive, though may not be complete.

S. Weber (✉)
Pediatric Nephrology/Pediatrics II, University Children's Hospital Marburg, Marburg, Germany
e-mail: stefanie.weber@med.uni-marburg.de

© The Author(s), under exclusive license to Springer Nature Switzerland AG 2023
F. Schaefer, L. A. Greenbaum (eds.), *Pediatric Kidney Disease*,
https://doi.org/10.1007/978-3-031-11665-0_15

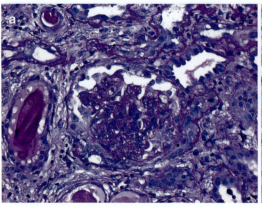 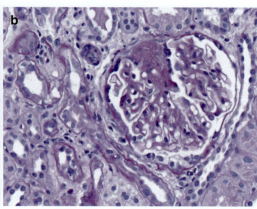

Fig. 15.1 (**a**, **b**) Kidney histology of a patient with diffuse mesangial sclerosis (**a**) and focal-segmental glomerulosclerosis (**b**), respectively. PAS staining; magnification 40×. (Courtesy of Kerstin Amann, Institute of Pathology, Department of Nephropathology, University Hospital Erlangen, Germany)

Hereditary Disorders of Early Glomerular Development

Podocytes develop from the nephrogenic blastema in a chain of events in conjunction with the development of the renal glomeruli. First, local condensation of the mesenchyme leads to the formation of the nephron anlage, i.e., the comma-shaped and the S-shaped bodies and eventually the formation of the mature glomerulus. Podocytes are the first cells that can clearly be distinguished in this process, forming a disk-like layer of epithelial cells. The subsequent differentiation to mature podocytes with interdigitating primary and secondary foot processes is associated with a general loss of the ability for further proliferation. At this stage, early cell-cell contacts (adherens junctions) have developed into a specialized structure, the SD, spanning the intercellular space. The final glomerular filtration barrier is constituted by the fenestrated endothelium, the glomerular basement membrane (GBM) and interdigitating podocytes.

A number of genes are involved in these processes (Table 15.1 and Fig. 15.2), and *WT1* is one of the major mediators of podocyte differentiation. *NPHS1* and *NPHS2* code for nephrin and podocin, respectively, two proteins that have important roles for the organization of the SD. *LAMB2* encodes laminin ß2, one component of the heterotrimeric laminins that link the podocyte to the GBM. *LMX1b* encodes the transcription factor Lmx1b that in the kidney is exclusively expressed in podocytes. It is one of the crucial genes regulating gene expression during early steps of podocyte development. Another group of genes involved in early-onset nephrotic syndrome, e.g. *PLCE1*, encoding for phospholipase C epsilon-1, are involved in podocyte signaling processes.

WT1 Gene Mutations

The *Wilms tumor* is one of the most common solid tumors of childhood, occurring in 1 of 10,000 children and accounting for 8% of childhood cancers. The Wilms' tumor suppressor gene (*WT1*) was first identified in 1990 [1]. *WT1* locates on chromosome 11p13 and encodes a zinc finger transcription factor that regulates the expression of many genes during kidney and urogenital development. Mutations in *WT1* were first identified in pediatric patients affected by Wilms'

15 Hereditary Nephrotic Syndrome

Table 15.1 Overview on important disorders causing hereditary nephrotic syndromes

	Inheritance	Locus	Gene	Protein	OMIM accession no.
Early-onset nephrotic syndrome					
Isolated DMS	AR	11p13	*WT1*	WT1	256370
Denys-Drash syndrome (typically DMS)	AD	11p13	*WT1*	WT1	194080
Congenital nephrotic syndrome/Finnish type	AR	19q13	*NPHS1*	Nephrin	602716
Recessive familial SRNS (MC/FSGS)	AR	1q25	*NPHS2*	Podocin	600995
Pierson syndrome	AR	3p21	*LAMB2*	Laminin β2	609049
Nail-patella syndrome	AD	9q34.1	*LMX1B*	LMX1B	161200
Recessive nephrotic syndrome (DMS/FSGS)	AR	10q23-q24	*NPHS3/PLCE1*	PLCE1	608414
Recessive nephrotic syndrome (FSGS)	AR	12p12.3	*PTPRO*	PTPRO	614196
Recessive congenital nephrotic syndrome (DMS)	AR	17q25.3	*ARHGDIA*	ARHGDIA	615244
Recessive childhood-onset nephrotic syndrome	AR	16p13.13	*EMP2*	EMP2	602334
NUP nephropathy	AR	multiple loci	*NUP93, NUP205, XPO5, NUP107, NUP85, NUP133, NUP160*	NUP93, NUP205, XPO5, NUP107, NUP85, NUP133, NUP160	multiple accession nos.
Late-onset nephrotic syndrome/FSGS					
Frasier syndrome (typically FSGS)	AD	11p13	*WT1*	WT1	136680
FSGS1	AD	19q13	*ACTN4*	α-Actinin 4	603278
FSGS2	AD	11q21-22	*TRPC6*	TRPC6	603965
FSGS3 (*CD2AP*-associated disease susceptibility)	AR/AD	6	*CD2AP*	CD2AP	607832
FSGS4 (*MYH9*-associated disease susceptibility)	AD	22q12.3	*MYH9/APOE1*	MYH9/APO1	612551
FSGS5	AD	14q32.33	*INF2*	INF2	613237
FSGS6	AR	15q22.2	*MYO1E*	MYO1E	614131
Mitochondrial disease					
Early-onset SRNS with variable extrarenal symptoms	AR	4q21-q22	*COQ2*	COQ2	609825
Early-onset SRNS with sensorineural deafness	AR	14q24.3	*COQ6*	Q10 mono-oxigenase 6	614647
SRNS/FSGS	AR	19q13.2	*ADCK4*	ADCK4	615573
Syndromal disease					
Schimke immuno-osseous dysplasia	AR	2q34-q36	*SMARCAL1*	SMARCAL1	242900
Galloway-Mowat Syndrome (GAMOS)	AR	15q25.2	*WDR73*	WDR73	616144
	AR	14q11.2, 20q13.12 2p13.1	*OSGEP, TP53RK, TPRKB*	OSGEP, TP53RK, TPRKB	617729 617730 617731
	X-linked	Xq28	*LAGE3*	LAGE3	301006

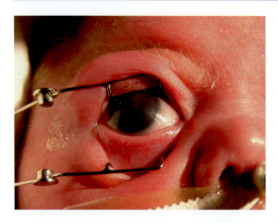

Fig. 15.2 Typical aspect of a patient with Pierson syndrome and microcoria. (Courtesy of Kveta Blahova, Pediatric Clinic, Charles University, Prague, Czech Republic)

tumor, aniridia, genitourinary malformations and mental retardation (WAGR syndrome), a contiguous gene deletion syndrome including *WT1* and *PAX6* [2]. *WT1* mutations were also identified in patients with isolated Wilms' tumor [3]. These are classically truncating mutations, associated with a complete loss-of-function of WT1. In tumor material of isolated cases both germline and somatic mutations have been detected. Familial Wilms tumor forms seem to follow a dominant pattern of inheritance, with dominant germline mutations. However, in a number of these cases the classical two-hit inactivation model, with loss of heterozygosity due to a second somatic event, has been described as the underlying cause of tumor development [4]. Alternative genes involved in familiar Wilms tumors are *CTR9*, *REST* and multiple others.

Subsequently, *WT1* mutations were also associated with Denys-Drash syndrome (DDS) [5], Frasier syndrome (FS) [6], and diffuse mesangial sclerosis (DMS) with isolated nephrotic syndrome (NS) [7]. The full picture of autosomal dominant *Denys-Drash syndrome* is characterized by early onset NS, male pseudohermaphroditism, gonadal dysgenesis and the development of Wilms tumor (in more than 90% of patients). The Wilms tumor may precede or develop after the manifestation of NS.

Of note, besides the Wilms tumor risk, individuals with 46,XY and associated disorders of sexual development (DSD) or complete gonadal dysgenesis (CGD) are at an increased risk for germ cell tumors, particularly gonadoblastoma with an observed incidence of one per 30 years at risk.

Age at onset of NS is generally within the first months of life [8]. In rare cases enlarged and hyperechogenic kidneys were already demonstrated by prenatal ultrasound [9]. Renal histology typically presents with DMS [10] and electron microscopy reveals foot process effacement. In rare cases, a histology reminiscent of MPGN may be observed. The NS is resistant to steroid treatment and renal function is deteriorating rapidly to end-stage renal disease (ESRD) already during infancy. Bilateral nephrectomy is generally advised in ESRD in order to prevent the development of Wilms tumor [11]. Recurrence of NS after kidney transplantation has not been observed so far [12].

Dominant *WT1* mutations are identified in the vast majority of DDS patients. These mutations predominantly affect exons 8 and 9 of the *WT1* gene and most of them are de novo mutations not observed in the parents. Most *WT1* mutations associated with DDS are missense mutations affecting conserved amino acids of the zinc finger domains, with p.R394W being the most frequent mutation observed. These alterations of the zinc finger structure reduce the DNA binding capacity of the *WT1* protein [13]. A heterozygous knock-in mouse model has been created for the p.R394W missense mutation, presenting with DMS and male genital anomalies [14] supporting the dominant nature of the disease.

Of note, some of the patients affected by *WT1* mutations in exons 8 and 9 do not present with the full picture of DDS but with isolated DMS or isolated (steroid-resistant) proteinuria. *WT1* analysis should therefore be performed in all children with isolated DMS and early-onset NS because of the risk of Wilms tumor development in case of a positive mutation analysis result. Close monitoring by renal ultrasound (e.g., every 6 months) is important in all children with *WT1* mutation and early-onset NS. In addition, karyotype analysis is recommended in all girls with isolated DMS to detect a possible male pseudohermaphroditism. Some patients with isolated DMS present with recessive mutations in *WT1* with both the maternal and paternal allele being affected [7].

Frasier syndrome is also characterized by a progressive glomerulopathy and male pseudohermaphroditism [15]; however, there are specific differences to DDS: the onset of proteinuria occurs later in childhood and the deterioration of renal function is slower. ESRD develops only in the second or third decade of life. As in DDS, proteinuria and NS are steroidresistant. Renal histology in FS patients typically shows focal and segmental glomerulosclerosis (FSGS) [16]; in a minority of patients only minimal change lesions are observed. In female patients, the genitourinary tract is normally developed, whereas a complete sex reversal with gonadal dysgenesis is observed in 46,XY patients. Primary amenorrhoea in conjunction with NS is a typical feature of these 46,XY patients and should prompt molecular analysis of *WT1*. While the risk to develop a Wilms tumor is low in patients with FS, gonadoblastomata, developing from gonadal dysgenesis, are frequently observed (in up to 40% of FS patients). After the diagnosis of FS, gonadectomy is highly recommended in 46,XY patients.

In 1997, it was first demonstrated that mutations in the *WT1* gene also underly the pathogenesis of FS [6]. Notably, the class of mutations in FS classically differs from DDS: whereas mutations affecting the coding sequence of exons 8 and 9 cause typical DDS, mutations associated with FS represent donor splice-site mutations located in intron 9. Similar to DDS, these mutations occur in a heterozygous state and, frequently, they are de novo mutations not observed in the parents. The donor splice-site of intron 9 plays an important role for the generation of the KTS isoform of the WT1 protein. This isoform contains three additional amino acids (lysine-threonine-serine; KTS). It has been demonstrated that the (+) KTS/(−) KTS protein dose ratio is of high relevance for WT1 action during genitourinary and kidney development. In FS patients, this ratio is markedly reduced due to the splice-site mutations [6].

Large genotype-phenotype studies confirm these associations based on the nature of the underlying mutation [17]. Still, there is some overlap and phenotypic heterogeneity in selected cases: splice-site mutations typical for FS may in some cases be found in patients with DDS [5] or isolated DMS [18], and patients with typical DDS mutations may display with isolated FSGS [19] or Wilms' tumor without NS [20]. Since the histologic findings often do not correlate with clinical findings and remarkable histopathologic heterogeneity is observed even among individuals with the same *WT1* pathogenic variant, kidney biopsy is no longer considered a first-tier diagnostic measure for patients of any age in the view of some authors. Instead, analysis of *WT1* should be included in routine genetic screening in all patients with SRNS or unexplained proteinuria. Owing to the experience of phenotypic heterogeneity, the group of clinical pictures is now entitled **WT1 disorder**s.

NPHS1 Gene Mutations Associated with Autosomal Recessive CNS of the Finnish Type (CNF)

CNS of the Finnish type is characterized by autosomal recessive inheritance and the development of proteinuria in utero [21]. The responsible gene was mapped in 1994 to chromosome 19q13 [22] and mutations in *NPHS1* have been subsequently identified in affected children [23]. *NPHS1* encodes for nephrin, a zipper-like protein of the glomerular SD. Typically, severe NS manifests before 3 months of age and renal biopsy specimens show immature glomeruli, mesangial cell hypercellularity, glomerular foot process effacement and microcystic dilatations of the proximal tubules. NS is steroid-resistant in these patients and treatment options comprise albumin infusions, pharmacological interventions with ACE inhibitors and indomethacin and ultimately unior bilateral nephrectomy [24–27].

Nephrin is exclusively expressed in podocytes, at the level of the SD once full differentiation has occurred [28]. Nephrin belongs to the immunoglobulin superfamily with a single putative transmembrane domain, a short intracellular N-terminus and long extracellular C-terminus

[23]. The extracellular C-terminus is predicted to bridge the intercellular space between the inter-digitating foot processes, rendering nephrin a key component of the SD. Nephrin strands contribute to the porous structure of the SD, forming pores of approximately 40 nm in size [29]. These pores are currently believed to be in part responsible for the size selectivity of the SD and the glomerular filtration barrier.

Apart from its role as a structural protein, nephrin also appears to participate in intracellular signaling pathways maintaining the functional integrity of the podocyte [30–32]. The SD is discussed to constitute a highly dynamic protein complex that recruits signal transduction components and initiates signaling to regulate complex biologic programs in the podocyte. A number of proteins within this signaling platform were identified to interact with nephrin, among these podocin, CD2AP and TRPC6, all of which are also associated with the development of NS when altered by gene mutations (see below). It is suggested that the plasma membrane of the filtration slit has a special lipid composition comparable to lipid rafts [33]. Lipid rafts are specialized microdomains of the plasma membrane with a unique lipid content and a concentrated assembly of signal transduction molecules [34]. It was shown that nephrin is a lipid raft-associated protein at the SD and that podocin serves to recruit nephrin into these microdomains. Disease-causing podocin mutations fail to target nephrin into rafts, altering nephrin-induced signal transduction [32]. In summary, these studies confirm the extraordinary role of SD proteins for the maintenance of the glomerular filtration barrier.

Mutations in *NPHS1* were first identified in the Finnish population, leading to the classification of "Finnish type" CNS. Two truncating mutations were found with high frequency in affected Finnish children suggesting an underlying founder effect in the Finnish population: p.L41fsX90 (Fin major, truncating the majority of the protein) and p.R1109X (Fin minor, truncating only a short C-terminal part). In subsequent studies, *NPHS1* mutations were also identified in non-Finnish patients throughout the world. The Fin major and Fin minor mutations are only rarely observed in non-Finnish patients. Several mutational hot spots were identified affecting the immunoglobulin domains of the nephrin protein [35]. The immunoglobulin domains 2, 4 and 7 appear particularly important for gene function. In addition to the high prevalence in Finland, *NPHS1* mutations are also common among Mennonites in Pennsylvania, 8% of this population is carrier of a heterozygous mutant allele [36].

Recent studies pointed out that congenital nephrotic syndrome can also be caused by recessive mutations in *NPHS2* (see below), particularly involving nonsense-, frameshift or the homozygous missense mutation p.R138Q [37–39]. In rare cases a triallelic digenic mode of inheritance was observed in patients with CNS/SRNS: in these patients, sequence variations in both *NPHS1* and *NPHS2* were identified with a total of three affected alleles (two *NPHS1* mutations and one *NPHS2* sequence variation or vice versa) [35]. It is speculated that the additional sequence variation of the second gene plays a role as a genetic modifier, possibly aggravating the clinical phenotype.

NPHS2 Gene Mutations Associated with Autosomal Recessive Steroid-Resistant Nephrotic Syndrome

The *NPHS2* gene was mapped by linkage analysis in eight families with autosomal recessive SRNS to chromosome 1q25-q31 [40] and recessive mutations in *NPHS2* were identified subsequently [41]. NS in these families was characterized by steroid-resistance, age at onset between 3 and 5 years and no recurrence of proteinuria after renal transplantation. *NPHS2* mutations have never been reported in patients with SSNS. Renal histology typically shows FSGS; however, some patients present with only minimal change lesions. In some cases, progression from minimal change lesions to FSGS has been demonstrated in repeat biopsies.

NPHS2 encodes for podocin, a 42 kD integral membrane protein expressed in both fetal and mature glomeruli [41]. By electron microscopy and immunogold labeling it was demonstrated that the site of expression is the SD of the podocytes. As both protein termini are located in the cytosol and podocin is predicted to have only one membrane domain, a hair-pin like structure of the protein was proposed. Interacting with both nephrin and CD2AP, podocin appears to link nephrin to the podocyte cytoskeleton. In patients affected by recessive mutations in *NPHS2*, SD formation is impaired and the typical foot process effacement is visible. These observations suggest that podocin has an important function for maintaining the glomerular filtration barrier. The knock-out of *Nphs2* in mice is associated with a phenotype highly reminiscent of the human disease with podocyte foot process effacement, nephrotic range proteinuria and chronic renal insufficiency [42]. As nephrin, podocin is localized in lipid rafts [33] and is important for recruiting nephrin to these microdomains of the plasma membrane [32]. Some mutations in *NPHS2* impair the ability of podocin to target nephrin to the rafts, especially the most frequent mutation identified in European patients (p. R138Q) [32].

Up to now, more than 125 pathogenic mutations have been described in *NPHS2* [43]; most mutations affect the stomatin domain located in the C-terminal part of the protein [37, 44]. Mutations in *NPHS2* were first identified in infants with SRNS and rapid progression to ESRD [41]. Subsequently, however, it became evident that defects in podocin can be responsible for SRNS manifesting at any age from birth to adulthood [45–47]. A partial genotype-phenotype correlation is apparent: while frameshift-, nonsense- and the p.R138Q mutation in homozygosity are typically associated with early-onset NS, other missense mutations (e.g., p.V180M, p. R238S) are predominantly found in patients with a later onset of SRNS [37]. A single nucleotide polymorphism in *NPHS2* (p.R229Q) has been identified to be a common cause of adulthood-onset of hereditary nephrotic syndrome when present in compound heterozygosity with specific pathogenic *NPHS2* mutations [48–50]. In the study of Machuca et al., among 119 patients diagnosed with NS presenting after 18 years of age, 18 patients were found to have one pathogenic mutation and p.R229Q, but none with two pathogenic mutations in *NPHS2* [50]. Screening for the p.R229Q variant seems therefore recommended in adolescent or adult patients. Recent data demonstrated that the pathogenicity of p. R229Q depends on the *trans*-associated mutation. It was shown that the association of *NPHS2*-p.R229Q with specific exon 7 or exon 8 mutations in *NPHS2* altered heterodimerization and mislocalisation of the encoded p.Arg229Gln podocin protein [51]. Following this study, homozygosity of *NPHS2*-p.R229Q alone is not disease causing. This observation is important as the p.R229Q variant is prevalent in heterozygous state in approximately 3% of the normal population (range 0.5–7%, depending on the genetic background) [51], resulting in a frequency of homozygous carriers of up to 1%.

Still, the p.R229Q variant is discussed to be a non-neutral PM with an enhanced frequency in FSGS patient cohorts of different ethnical origins [52]. In vitro studies have demonstrated that p.R229Q podocin shows decreased binding to its interacting protein partner nephrin [48] and in a large study of more than 1500 individuals of the general population p.R229Q was significantly associated with the prevalence of microalbuminuria, a risk factor for developing chronic renal insufficiency and cardiovascular events [53].

LAMB2 Gene Mutations Associated with Pierson Syndrome

Pierson syndrome is characterized by CNS and peculiar eye abnormalities including a typical nonreactive narrowing of the pupils (microcoria, Fig. 15.3) but also additional lens and corneal abnormalities [54]. Recessive mutations in *LAMB2* on chromosome 3p21 were identified as underlying genetic defect [55]. *LAMB2* encodes for the protein laminin β2, one component of the trimeric laminins in the kidney that crosslink the basolateral membrane of the podocyte to the GBM. Most disease-associated alleles identified in Pierson patients were truncating mutations leading to loss of laminin β2 expression in the

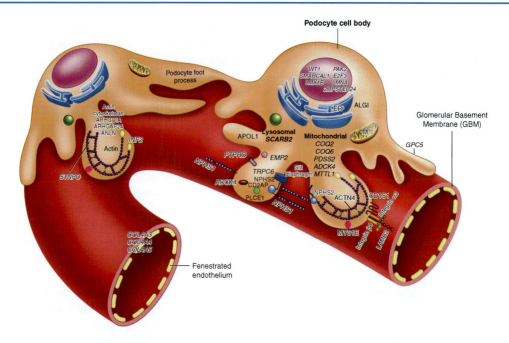

Fig. 15.3 Schema of a podocyte foot process cross-section, depicting important components involved in hereditary nephrotic syndrome

kidney [55]. Ocular laminin β2 expression in unaffected controls was strongest in the intraocular muscles, corresponding well to the characteristic hypoplasia of ciliary and pupillary muscles observed in affected patients. Subsequent genotype-phenotype studies revealed that some mutations in *LAMB2*, especially hypomorphic missense mutations, can be associated with a phenotypic spectrum that is much broader than previously anticipated including isolated CNS or CNS with minor ocular changes different from those observed in Pierson syndrome [56]. Fetal ultrasound in four consecutive fetuses of a family with Pierson syndrome and positive *LAMB2* mutation analysis consistently revealed marked hyperechogenicity of the kidneys and variable degrees of pyelectasia by 15 weeks of gestation [57]. Placentas were significantly enlarged. Hydrops fetalis due to severe hypalbuminemia demonstrated by chordocentesis occurred in one fetus and anencephaly was detected in another fetus. Development of oligohydramnios indicated a prenatal decline of renal excretory function. From these studies it can be concluded that mutational analysis in *LAMB2* should also be considered in isolated CNS if no mutations were found in *NPHS1*, *NPHS2*, or *WT1*, and in cases with prenatal onset of nephrotic disease with typical sonomorphologic findings of the kidneys and the development of oligohydramnios.

The *LAMB2* missense mutation p.C321R, for example, has been identified in congenital nephrotic syndrome with only mild extrarenal symptoms. Functional studies in cell culture and mice suggested defective intracellular trafficking of the mutant protein, associated with endoplasmatic reticulum stress [58]. Another missense mutation (p.S80R) has been identified in homozygous state a teenage girl with severe myopia since early infancy and nephrotic range proteinuria first detected at the age of 6 but normal renal function. Renal biopsy revealed mild DMS and a residual expression of laminin β2 [59].

Summarizing these reports, it becomes obvious that the phenotype associated with pathogenic *LAMB2* mutations can be very variable and that genetic testing for *LAMB2* mutations should be considered in all patients with either early-onset proteinuria or glomerular proteinuria with an abnormal ocular phenotype.

LMX1b Gene Mutations Associated with Autosomal Dominant Nail-Patella Syndrome

Nail-patella syndrome (NPS) or onychoosteodysplasia is caused by dominant mutations in the *LMX1b* gene, located on chromosome 9q34.1 and encoding the LIM-homeodomain protein Lmx1b. Lmx1b plays a central role in dorsal/ventral patterning of the vertebrate limb and targeted disruption of Lmx1b results in skeletal defects, including hypoplastic nails, absent patellae, and a unique form of renal dysplasia [60]. Prominent features of affected children are dysplasia of nails and absent or hypodysplastic patellae. In many patients, also iliac horns, dysplasia of the elbows, glaucoma and/or hearing impairment are detected. *LMX1b* is highly expressed in podocytes and patients can also present with an involvement of the kidney comprising proteinuria, nephrotic syndrome or renal insufficiency. Overall, nephropathy is reported in approximately 40% of affected patients (microalbuminuria or overt proteinuria) [61] but ESRD in less than 10% [62]. Interestingly, renal involvement appears significantly more frequent in females and in patients with a positive family history of NPS nephropathy [61]. In NPS patients with renal involvement, electron microscopy shows collagen fibril-like deposition in the GBM with typical lucent areas [63]. These characteristic ultrastructural changes can even be present in patients without apparent nephropathy [64]. Large genotype-phenotype studies demonstrated that individuals with an *LMX1B* mutation located in the homeodomain showed a significantly higher frequency of renal protein loss and higher values of proteinuria than subjects with mutations in the LIM domains [61]. Recent studies identified *LMX1B* missense mutations affecting residue p.R246 also in a subset of patients with isolated FSGS without extrarenal symptoms, expending the spectrum of FGSG-related genes to *LMX1B* [65, 66]. Insight into Lmx1b function was further obtained by the generation of *Lmx1b* knockout animals [67]. In *Lmx1b(−/−)* mice the expression of GBM collagens is reduced and podocytes have a reduced number of foot processes, are dysplastic, and lack typical SD structures. Interestingly, mRNA and protein levels for CD2AP and podocin are greatly reduced in these kidneys and several *LMX1B* binding sites were identified in the putative regulatory regions of both *CD2AP* and *NPHS2* (encoding podocin) [67]. These observations support a cooperative role for Lmx1b, CD2AP and podocin in foot process and slit diaphragm formation.

PLCE1 Gene Mutations Associated with Autosomal Recessive Nephrotic Syndrome

Following positional cloning, a gene locus for nephrotic syndrome (*NPHS3*) was mapped to chromosome 10q23-q24 and homozygous truncating mutations were identified in the gene *PLCE1*, encoding the enzyme phospholipase C-ε1 which is involved in intracellular signal transduction [68]. Onset of nephrotic syndrome was generally early in affected children and renal histology revealed DMS in most cases. In subsequent studies, mutations in *PLCE1* were identified in a relevant percentage of patients with DMS (28–33%) [69, 70] and with a lower frequency in hereditary FSGS (8%) [70]. Interestingly, two of the individuals with truncating *PLCE1* mutations entered sustained remission following steroid or cyclosporin A treatment [69]. The observation of a possible responsiveness to immunosuppression in *PLCE1* mutation carriers awaits confirmation in a larger number of affected patients.

PLCE1 is widely expressed in many tissues including also the podocytes. The knock-down of *pcle1* in zebrafish is associated with the development of podocyte foot process effacement and edematous outer appearance of the fish [68] confirming a specific role of phospholipase C epsilon-1 for the maintenance of the glomerular filtration barrier. Still, the pathogenesis of isolated podocyte damage and the development of proteinuria in patients lacking phospholipase C epsilon-1 remains to be elucidated.

PTPRO Gene Mutations Associated with Autosomal Recessive Nephrotic Syndrome

Homozygous *PTPRO* splice-site mutations were identified in two families of Turkish origin with childhood-onset nephrotic syndrome and minimal change nephropathy or FSGS on renal biopsy [71]. Nephrotic syndrome was resistant to oral prednisone therapy but a partial response to an intensified immunosuppressive regimen including pulse methylprednisolone and cyclosporin A was observed in some cases. PTPRO, identical to glomerular epithelial protein-1 (GLEPP1), is a receptor-like membrane protein tyrosine phosphatase expressed at the apical membrane of the podocyte foot processes in the kidney. Disruption of *Ptpro* in mice results in alterations of the podocyte structure and a reduction of the glomerular filtration rate indicating a role of PTPRO for proper podocyte function.

ARHGDIA Gene Mutations in Autosomal Recessive DMS

A recessive mutation in *ARHGDIA*, encoding a regulator of Rho-GTPases, was detected in two female siblings born to consanguineous parents. Both girls presented with congenital nephrotic syndrome and DMS on renal histology [72]. The homozygous 3-bp in-frame deletion mutation in *ARHGDIA* seems to be implicated in the hyperactivation of Rho-GTPases, causing a derangement of the podocyte actin cytoskeleton. *Arghdia* knock-out mice develop podocyte damage, severe proteinuria and progressive renal failure, supporting a role of human *ARHGDIA* in the pathogenesis of proteinuric disease.

EMP2 Gene Mutations Associated with Autosomal Recessive Childhood-Onset Nephrotic Syndrome

Mutations in podocyte genes have only exceptionally been identified in children with steroid-sensitive nephrotic syndrome (SSNS) [44, 73]. However, by homozygosity mapping and whole exome sequencing in 67 families biallelic mutations in *EMP2* were identified in one pair of siblings of Turkish origin, affected by frequently relapsing nephrotic syndrome with remission after cyclophosphamide treatment. In both, onset of the disease was below 3 years of age. Subsequently, more than 1600 individuals with nephrotic syndrome were screened for recessive mutations in *EMP2* and two more patients with SRNS (of Turkish and of African origin) were identified [74]. *EMP2* encodes epithelial membrane protein 2, discussed to be involved in cell proliferation and cell-cell interactions. The knock-down of *emp2* in the zebrafish resulted in pericardial effusions, consistent with a role of epithelial membrane protein 2 in keeping-up glomerular filtration [74].

NUP Nephropathy

A novel large group of genes has recently been identified to be involved in autosomal recessive steroid-resistant nephrotic syndrome leading to CKD and ESRD. These genes encode proteins of the nuclear pore complex (NPC) [75, 76]. These proteins belong to the group of nucleoporins (NUP), assembling to form NPCs, one of the largest protein complexes found in eukaryotic cells. NPCs are channels that span the nuclear envelope and allow the transport of proteins, RNAs, and ribonucleoprotein particles between the cytoplasm and nuclear interior [77]. Hitherto, mutations were reported in multiple genes encoding proteins of the NPC, including *NUP93*, *NUP205*, and *XPO5* (inner ring of the NPC) and *NUP107*, *NUP85*, *NUP133*, and *NUP160* (outer ring of the NPC) in patients with childhood-onset SRNS, accounting for approximatively 3% of cases. These human mutations seem to disturb important mechanisms of glomerulogenesis. Kidney biopsy in selected cases showed FSGS or DMS, and extrarenal symptoms identified in patients with mutations in *NUP95*, *NUP107*, and *XPO5* comprise short stature, intellectual disability, microcephaly, or dilated cardiomyopathy. However, more studies focusing on deep phenotyping will be needed to establish more reliable genotype-phenotype correlations.

Hereditary Disorders with Late-Onset Nephrotic Syndrome

Hereditary late-onset FSGS is a heterogeneous condition generally transmitted in an autosomal dominant fashion (with the exception of autosomal recessive FSGS6). Different disease loci have been mapped in affected families (FGSG1-FSGS6) and responsible genetic defects have been identified in many podocyte-associated genes, frequently involving actin cytoskeleton architecture and dynamics.

ACTN4 Gene Mutations Associated with Adulthood FSGS (FSGS1)

In 1998, a locus for autosomal dominant late-onset FSGS was mapped to chromosome 19q13 (FSGS1) [78] and mutations in *ACTN4* were identified as the underlying pathogenic cause [79]. *ACTN4* encodes for α-actinin-4, an actin-bundling protein of the cytoskeleton highly expressed in podocytes. Both a knock-down and an overexpression transgenic mouse model have been established for *Actn4*, demonstrating pro-

teinuria and podocyte alterations. It was therefore discussed that α-actinin-4 plays an important role for the cytoskeletal function of the podocyte. Young knock-out mice present with focal areas of foot process effacement and older animals with diffuse effacement and globally disrupted podocyte morphology [80]. Moreover, *Actn4* was shown to be upregulated in the kidneys of different animal models of proteinuria. Human *ACTN4* mutations were identified in three different families with FSGS [79]. The clinical course in affected family members was characterized by progressively increasing proteinuria starting in adolescence and developing into FSGS and chronic renal insufficiency later in adult life. ESRD was observed in a number of affected individuals. All *ACTN4* mutations identified so far represent non-conservative amino acid substitutions affecting the actin-binding domain of α-actinin-4. In vitro studies demonstrated that mutant α-actinin-4 binds filamentous actin more strongly than wild-type protein. Based on this observation it was proposed that dominant mutations in *ACTN4* interfere with the maintenance of podocyte architecture: a proper organisation of the cytoskeleton seems to be important for normal functioning of podocyte foot processes. Interestingly, however, not all mutation carriers of the families reported by Kaplan et al. presented with a renal phenotype. The observed incomplete penetrance suggests that additional (genetic or non-genetic) factors are involved in the pathogenesis that in conjunction with a mutation in *ACTN4* lead to the manifestation of FSGS. *ACTN4* mutations may confer *disease susceptibility*, as also discussed for mutations in *CD2AP* and *TRPC6*. However, mutations in *ACTN4* represent a rare cause of hereditary FSGS, accounting for approximately 0–4% of familial FSGS, depending on the study cohort [45, 81, 82].

TRPC6 Gene Mutations Associated with Late-Onset FSGS (FSGS2)

In 1999, a second gene locus for autosomal dominant FSGS was mapped to chromosome 11q21-q22 using a 399-member Caucasian kindred of British heritage dating back seven generations

[83]. Fourteen deceased family members had suffered from ESRD, 14 living family members were on dialysis or had undergone renal transplantation, and 3 individuals were proteinuric. Six years later, the responsible gene *TRPC6* was identified [84, 85]. *TRPC6* encodes the transient receptor potential cation channel TRPC6 that is thought to mediate capacitative calcium entry into cells. Expression analysis revealed that TRPC6 is highly expressed in the kidney and also in podocytes at the site of the SD. A dominant missense mutation was identified in the original family of Winn et al., and five additional families with mutations in *TRPC6* were characterized by Reiser et al. Two of the missense mutations in the latter study were shown to increase the current amplitudes of TRPC6, consistent with a gain-of-function effect of the mutations. Interestingly, however, both studies describe carrier individuals with a normal renal phenotype, pointing to an incomplete penetrance of the mutations. *TRPC6* mutations have been identified in very few children; early disease onset seems to be exceptional. So far, it is unknown how the dysfunction of a cation channel is related to the development of podocyte damage and loss of the glomerular filtration barrier. One hypothesis is related to the observation that MEC-2, a *C. elegans* homologue of podocin, participates in the mechanosensation of the worm. MEC-2 is physically and functionally linked to ion channels, transducing the signals of mechanosensation. Since TRPC6 interacts with podocin and nephrin at the SD, it was proposed that podocin takes part in mechanosensation processes at the glomerular filtration barrier, transducing signals to TRPC6 which in turn modulates intracellular calcium concentrations in the podocyte. Nephrin, on the other hand, is thought to stimulate different pathways of the intracellular signaling machinery. Therefore, a complex protein network involving nephrin, podocin, CD2AP and the cation channel TRPC6 is established to maintain the SD structure of the foot process. Mutations in TRPC6 likely affect this functional network by altering the intracellular calcium concentration of the podocyte.

CD2AP Gene Mutations Associated with Adulthood FSGS (FSGS3)

In 1999, FSGS3 was shown to map to chromosome 6 and reported to be caused by haploinsufficiency for *CD2AP* [86]. *CD2AP* encodes for the CD2-associated protein CD2AP, an actin-binding protein that was originally identified as a cytoplasmic ligand of the CD2 receptor on T and natural killer cells. *CD2AP* knock-out mice presented not only with impaired immune functions but also with severe NS and FSGS, accompanied by mesangial hypercellularity and extracellular matrix deposition [87]. Electron microscopy showed the typical loss of podocyte foot process integrity with process effacement and loss of the SD structure. Screening in FSGS patients led to the identification of a dominant *CD2AP* mutation (a 2-bp substitution altering the exon 7 splice acceptor site) in two adult patients with late-onset FSGS [86]. Enhanced disease susceptibility for FSGS conferred by the change in CD2AP expression was postulated as the underlying pathogenic mechanism. CD2AP interacts with nephrin and both proteins localize to lipid rafts in the plasma membrane [33], suggesting that CD2AP is required to connect nephrin (and thus the SD) to the cytoskeleton of the podocyte. An impairment of CD2AP function might be associated with enhanced cytoskeletal fragility, predisposing to podocyte damage.

Susceptibility to Genetic Locus 22q12.3 (FSGS4), Including the Genes MYH9 and APOE1

Multiple single nucleotide polymorphisms (SNP) in the gene *MYH9* were recessively associated with idiopathic and HIV-associated FSGS and hypertensive end-stage renal disease (ESRD) in African American adult patients [88]. However, subsequent genomewide analyses in large patient cohorts suggested that a positively selected risk variant could be in a larger interval containing the *APOL* genes rather than be confined to *MYH9*. Two *APOL1* risks variants for FSGS were identified to be common in African but absent in European chromosomes. As APOL1 is a serum factor that lyses trypanosomes and in vitro assays revealed that only the kidney disease-associated APOL1 variants lysed Trypanosoma brucei rhodesiense it was speculated that evolution of a critical survival factor in Africa may have contributed to the high rates of renal disease in African Americans [89].

INF2 Gene Mutations Associated with Autosomal Dominant FSGS (FSGS5) and Charcot-Marie-Tooth Disease

Mutations in *INF2*, encoding inverted formin-2, were first identified in 11 FSGS families with onset of proteinuria in adolescence or adulthood [90]. Proteinuria was typically moderate, accompanied by microscopic hematuria and hypertension in some cases. Proteinuria was progressive, often leading to ESRD. Renal biopsies showed the presence of FSGS and unusually prominent actin bundles within the foot processes, on electron microscopy. Being part of the actin cytoskeleton Inf2/inverted formin-2 interacts with actin and is involved in both polymerization and depolymerization of actin filaments. Interestingly, mutations in *INF2* were also identified in patients with dominant intermediate Charcot-Marie-Tooth (CMT) disease and FSGS-associated proteinuria [91], localizing to a distinct area of the *INF2* gene. Mutant INF2 protein was abnormally distributed in the cytoplasm and the actin cytoskeleton and microtubule network were disorganized, not only in podocytes but also in peripheral Schwann cells, leading to disturbed myelin formation and CMT.

Mutations in MYO1E in Autosomal Recessive FSGS (FSGS6)

Recessive homozygous mutations in *MYOE1*, encoding a non-muscle membrane-associated class I myosin, were reported in children and adolescent patients of consanguineous union affected by nephrotic-range proteinuria, microhematuria, hypoalbuminemia, and edema [92]. Renal biopsy demonstrated FSGS, tubular atrophy and interstitial fibrosis. *Myoe1*-knockout mice show a similar phenotype with proteinuria, hematuria and progressive renal failure, indicating a defect in the glomerular filtration barrier. Impaired intracellular trafficking of the mutant protein seems to be implicated in the pathogenesis of *MYO1E*-associated disease.

Mitochondrial Disorders Associated with Nephrotic Syndrome

Several gene mutations in different components of the coenzyme Q $_{10}$ (CoQ $_{10)}$ biosynthesis pathway have recently been identified to be involved in hereditary nephrotic syndrome, frequently associated with extrarenal symptoms. Recessive mutations in *COQ2* were first identified in 2006 in a pair of siblings with early-onset glomerular lesions, steroid resistant nephrotic syndrome and CoQ $_{10}$ deficiency [93]. The gene *COQ2* encodes for the para-hydroxybenzoate-polyprenyl transferase enzyme of the CoQ $_{10}$ synthesis pathway. An increased number of abnormal mitochondria in podocytes and other glomerular cells was demonstrated by electron microscopy. Following this initial study, more patients were identified with a similar clinical course and loss-of-function mutations in *COQ2* [94, 95]. Extrarenal symptoms of mitochondrial disease are not obligatory but developed in a subset of affected patients to a varying degree, including encephalopathy, lactacidosis, myoclonic epilepsy and hypertrophic cardiomyopathy.

Early-onset SRNS associated with sensorineural deafness has subsequently been attributed to recessive mutations in *COQ6* encoding for CoQ $_{10}$ biosynthesis monooxygenase 6 [96]. Renal histology revealed FSGS lesions in most cases with COQ6 mutation but DMS has also been observed.

Subsequently, mutations in *ADCK4 (=COQ8B)* were associated with disturbed CoQ $_{10}$ biosynthesis and identified by homozygosity mapping and whole exome sequencing in children with SRNS and school age onset of nephrotic syndrome [97]. *ADCK4/COQ8B* encodes the aarF domain containing kinase 4, a protein partially expressed in podocyte foot processes but also in podocyte mitochondria. ADCK4 colocalizes with COQ6 and COQ7. Serum CoQ $_{10}$ levels are reduced in affected patients.

Of note, *COQ2*, *COQ6* and *COQ8B* are all nuclear genes encoding mitochondrial proteins. Therefore, the inheritance of associated disorders follows the Mendelian rules of autosomal recessive disease.

These findings indicate that the podocyte reacts very sensitively to disturbances of energy supply and it can be expected that mutations in other genes encoding mitochondrial proteins will be discovered in patients with SRNS in the future.

Most importantly and in contrast to all other hereditary disorders of the podocyte, these mitochondriopathies offer for a first time a potential causal treatment option by supplementation of CoQ $_{10}$. In several patients affected by mutations in *COQ2*, *COQ6* and *COQ8B/ADCK4*, remarkable reductions of proteinuria were induced by oral medication with CoQ $_{10}$, opening a new therapeutic avenue for these patients with otherwise steroid resistant NS [96–98]. The recommended oral CoQ10 supplementation dose is 30 mg/kg/day.

Syndromal Disorders Associated with Nephrotic Syndrome

A large number of syndromes have been described on clinical grounds in patients presenting with (steroid-resistant) proteinuria in addition to various extrarenal manifestations. A genetic basis has been identified only in a minority of these syndromes. Here, we discuss two important syndromes that invariably present with SRNS, Schimke syndrome and Galloway-Mowat syndrome.

Schimke Syndrome

Schimke immuno-osseous dysplasia (SIOD) maps to chromosome 2q34–36 and is caused by

recessive mutations in the *SMARCAL1* gene [99]. *SMARCAL1* encodes the SWI/SNF-related, matrix-associated, actin-dependent regulator of chromatin subfamily a-like protein 1, a protein involved in the remodeling of chromatin to change nucleosome compaction for gene regulation, replication, recombination, and DNA repair. The clinical phenotype of Schimke immuno-osseous dysplasia is characterized by growth retardation due to spondyloepiphyseal dysplasia, a slowly progressive immune defect, cerebral infarcts, skin pigmentation, and SRNS beginning in childhood. FSGS lesions are frequently observed in kidney biopsy specimen and the majority of patients progress early to ESRD. However, disease severity and age at onset follow a continuum from early onset and severe symptoms with death early in life to later onset and mild symptoms with survival into adulthood. A considerable fraction of patients with SRNS due to SIOD is oligosymptomatic, presenting only with proteinuria and short stature [100], underpinning the role of next generation sequencing (NGS) panel sequencing including *SMARCAL1* in non-syndromic unsolved SRNS cases. Proteinuria associated with very short stature may be a reliable clue to SIOD. Genotype-phenotype studies suggest that recessive loss-of-function mutations (frameshift, stop and splice-site mutations) are generally associated with a more severe course of the disease while some missense mutations allow a retention of partial *SMARCAL1* function and thus cause milder disease [99]. This genotype-phenotype correlation is typically observed for onset of extra-renal symptoms while the renal course (median age at ESKD 8 years) seems to be independent of the mutation type [100].

Galloway-Mowat Syndrome

The Galloway-Mowat syndrome (GAMOS) is characterized by microcephaly and other brain anomalies, severe mental retardation and early-onset NS (CNS) [101]. Both FSGS and DMS were observed in kidney biopsies of affected individuals [101, 102]. An important number of

15 Hereditary Nephrotic Syndrome

patients also presents with hiatus hernia. Both males and females are affected and an occurrence in siblings of the same family has been reported. Different associated gene loci have been identified. In 2014, loss-of-function mutations in *WDR73* were described in two unrelated families [103]. In 2017, a large international consortium identified multiple mutations in KEOPS-complex genes in patients affected by autosomal recessive (*OSGEP*, *TP53RK*, *TPRKB*) or X-chromosomal linked (*LAGE3*) GAMOS [104].

Clinical Aspects

Clinical aspects of NS are discussed in all detail in former chapters. Here, we want to focus on some issues specific for genetic forms of SRNS.

Long-Term Outcome and Renal Prognosis

Large multicenter studies have provided significant data and insight into the long-term renal prognosis of hereditary forms of nephrotic syndrome. In an analysis of more than 1000 SRNS patients followed in the PodoNet Registry study the diagnosis of a genetic disease markedly impacted ESKD risk. ESKD-free survival rates were 27% and 17% in patients with a genetic diagnosis, contrasting with a favorable prognosis in children with sporadic non-genetic SRNS responsive to intensified immunosuppression, who exhibited a 15-year renal survival rate of 96% [105, 106]. Within the same study, the histopathologic diagnosis was also clearly predictive of ESKD. When adjusting for genetic status, age, proteinuria level, CKD and responsiveness to intensified immunosuppression, DMS or FSGS on biopsy implied an increased risk of progressing to ESKD [105].

Therapeutic Implications

The therapy of SRNS in general is demanding. Numerous immunosuppressive agents have shown some efficacy in a fraction of the SRNS population, including cyclosporine, mycophenolate mofetil or the anti-CD20-antibody rituximab mostly in combination with glucocorticoids. However, genetically determined forms of SRNS have mostly proven insensitive to immunosuppressive interventions, which is pathophysiologically explained by the presence of intrinsic defects in podocyte architecture and function [105, 107, 108]. A detailed review of the pertinent literature is available in the recent IPNA expert recommendations [109]. Generally, it is suggested to spare children with hereditary SRNS from immunosuppressive treatment.

Conversely, specific gene mutations have not been reported in patients with steroid sensitive NS [44], so genetic screening seems generally not indicated even in patients with reduced steroid sensitivity (such as frequent relapsers or steroid dependency). However, in former studies addressing a possible genetic basis of SSNS, associations to various gene loci and candidate genes (e.g. *CLVS1* encoding clavesin-1) have been identified [110–113].

Therefore, novel insights into the genetics and pathophysiology of SSNS can be expected.

Antiproteinuric and renoprotective pharmacological treatment with ACE inhibitors or AT1 receptor blockers (RAASi) is advised in all children with SRNS once the diagnosis is made in the maximally approved and tolerated dose in order to slow down the progression of renal insufficiency also in genetic SRNS. ACEi or ARBs should be used with caution in patients with CKD stage 4, and they should not be started or should be stopped in case of intravascular volume depletion, acute kidney injury (AKI), hyperkalemia, or frequent vomiting/diarrhea. In female adolescents, contraception should be ensured in order to avoid the teratogenic effects of RAASi [109].

Living Related Donor Transplantation

Living-related kidney transplantation is generally considered the therapy of first choice in pediatric patients with ESRD. However, in patients affected by SRNS due to germline mutations in podocyte genes several aspects need to be considered. First, it is unknown as yet how kidneys of a heterozygous donor behave and develop in a recipient with recessive SRNS: The parents of affected children with recessive SRNS carry one mutant allele each that is also present in the transplanted kidney. It could be speculated that these kidneys are more easily prone to develop proteinuria if other pro-proteinuric factors (e.g., arterial hypertension, salt-rich diet) are superposed. While animal models of SRNS do not support this hypothesis so far, comprehensive human data addressing this question are mostly lacking. Consequences for the donor should also be considered. It is as yet unknown whether the prognosis of the remaining single kidney in the heterozygous parental donor is impaired by the gene mutation. Again, the remaining heterozygous kidney might be more susceptible to proteinuric disease than single kidneys of individuals without mutations. Up to now the experience with living-related donor transplantation in hereditary SRNS is very limited and does not support a restriction in affected children. Still, careful surveillance of both donor and recipient seems advisable.

In families of patients affected by autosomal dominant late-onset SRNS, only one of the parents is carrier of the pathogenic sequence variation. Genetic testing of family members will be helpful to delineate mutation carriers in the family. If the mutation occurred as a de novo mutation in the patient, both parents are equally suitable for living donor transplantation from a genetic point of view.

Recurrence of Nephrotic Syndrome After Renal Transplantation

Many investigators have studied the pathogenesis of increased glomerular permeability and recurrence of proteinuria after transplantation in FSGS. In general, recurrence of proteinuria after renal transplantation is observed in approximately 30% of FSGS patients [108, 114]. This risk appears higher in children than in adult patients [115]. Affected patients present with proteinuria, which is often in the nephrotic range. Frequently proteinuria recurs within few days after renal transplantation. In children, the mean time to recurrent proteinuria is 14 days posttransplant [116]. Recurrence of proteinuria/FSGS following renal transplantation negatively impacts graft survival in both children and adult patients. Risk factors are an age less than 15 years, rapid progression of renal insufficiency and diffuse mesangial proliferation in the initial biopsy of the native kidney [117]. In nonhereditary FSGS/SRNS, the recurrence of proteinuria is discussed to follow a T cell dysfunction and production of proteinuric circulating factors, including soluble urokinase receptor, hemopexin, and cardiotrophin-like cytokine-1 [118, 119].

In NPHS2-associated SRNS/FSGS recurrence of post-transplant proteinuria is a rare phenomenon, observed in less than 10% of transplanted patients [37, 44, 120]. The identification of a homozygous truncating NPHS2 mutation in one patient with post-transplant NS prompted the search for anti-podocin antibodies but all results were negative excluding a de novo glomerulonephitis as underlying cause [37]. Anti-podocin antibodies were also not identifiable in a study including patients with NPHS2 missense mutations and post-transplant NS [121].

In CNF, the risk of a recurrence of proteinuria after transplantation seems to be important: it was demonstrated that especially patients affected by the Fin major mutation have a risk of approximately 25% of post-transplant NS. Subsequent studies revealed that the pathogenesis of this recurrence is related to the development of anti-nephrin antibodies directed against the wildtype nephrin protein residing in the transplanted kidney [122], analogous to the anti-GBM antibodies against type IV collagen causing post-transplant de novo glomerulonephritis in patients with Alport syndrome. Treatment options of post-transplant NS in these patients are controversially discussed due to a relative paucity of data; a subset of patients seems to respond to rituximab or cyclophosphamide [108].

Genetic Testing

Following the rapid technological development in human genetics and genome research, different approaches can be applied in order to identify gene mutations in patients with SRNS and/or FSGS. In countries where next generation sequencing (NGS) techniques are not available there may still be a rationale for conventional Sanger sequencing in patients with specific phenotypes, e.g., sequencing of *WT1* in Denys-Drash or *LAMB2* in Pierson syndrome. Sanger sequencing can also be useful in patients with congenital NS (*NPHS1*) or school-aged patients with SRNS (*NPHS2*), where the likelihood of a positive result is relatively high. In adolescents and young adults, a different screening rationale should be applied. The *NPHS2*-p.R229Q sequence variation in compound heterozygosity with specific pathogenic *NPHS2* mutations is frequently found in late-onset SRNS [45, 50, 51]. In addition, autosomal dominant disease due to mutations in *WT1*, *TRPC6*, *INF2* and *ACTN4* can be identified in adolescents and young adults, particularly in case of dominant transmission but to a minor extent also in sporadic cases [45, 123, 124].

However, panels of podocytopathy- and even more broadly kidney-disease-associated genes have been developed by many commercial and non-commercial laboratories, which now allow standardized and simultaneous sequencing of more than 50 genes in one experimental run by next NGS techniques. In addition, whole exome and whole genome sequencing (WES/WGS) are available at low costs and has been developed for many clinical diagnostic applications. Advantages of the WES approach include the identification of gene mutations in novel genes, non-coding regions (WGS), microdeletions/microduplications, copy number variations and the unraveling of gene mutations in phenotypically complex cases. Still, the interpretation of huge data sets can be challenging and necessitates biostatistical expertise. Large databases have been established offering an annotation of sequence variations in different populations. Numerous ethical issues still need to be addressed, especially with respect to the possible incidental identification of mutations in SRNS-unrelated genes with high phenotypic penetrance associated with severe disorders, e.g. different types of cancer. In these cases, genetic counseling is demanding and of high importance.

Genetic Counseling

Positive results of mutational analysis in pediatric patients with SRNS should be followed by adequate genetic counseling. This demands close collaboration between pediatric nephrologists and human geneticists. Parents of children affected by recessive disease will have a chance of 25% to give birth to another affected child. In parents of children with dominant disease, this risk amounts to 50% (with the exception of patients with de novo mutations, in these families, the risk of recurrence is very low). Parents of affected children need to be informed that treatment options are limited in hereditary SRNS and that renal function may deteriorate rapidly. Close monitoring of renal function and early treatment of complications of chronic renal insufficiency are advised. In autosomal dominant FSGS, genetic counseling might be difficult due to the fact of incomplete penetrance and variable expressivity. It seems that individual mutation carriers can be affected to a differing degree with an obvious mild phenotype in some family members and ESRD in others. Genetic counseling is not only important for the parents but also for the affected child. Children with recessive disease will transmit a heterozygous mutation to their own children in the future. As long as the other parent is not mutation carrier, all offspring will be healthy. Patients affected by dominant FSGS will transmit the pathogenic mutation in 50% of cases and offspring carrying the mutation might be affected by FSGS.

In some cases, established genotype-phenotype correlations might be helpful to estimate the risk of a more severe clinical course. In *NPHS2*-associated SRNS, for example, some mutations have been associated with early-onset and aggravated clinical course while other mutations were shown to be less pathogenic [40]. For other disease entities, the analysis of clinical symptoms of other affected family members can be of help to predict the severity of the disease: in NPS, the risk of having a child with NPS nephropathy is about 1:4 and the risk of having a child in whom renal failure will develop is about 1:10 if NPS nephropathy occurs in other family members [53]. Genetic counseling is especially important in families affected by NS with serious prognosis. In children affected by CNS with female outer appearance, mutation analysis in *WT1* is mandatory in order to rule out a risk for Wilms tumor development.

Due to the implementation of NGS techniques in the clinical routine setting, many patients are identified to carry a significant number of sequence variations of unknown relevance in different podocyte genes, not following simple Mendelian inheritance. Whether these gene variants act as modifiers, accumulate to confer a susceptibility for the development of NS or are just polymorphisms without biological function remains difficult to be designated in many cases. Genetic counseling will has to make allowance for this.

Acknowledgement I would like to thank Martin Zenker (Institute of Human Genetics, University of Erlangen-Nuremberg) for his reflections on Pierson syndrome.

References

1. Rose EA, Glaser T, Jones C, et al. Complete physical map of the WAGR region of 11p13 localizes a candidate Wilms' tumor gene. Cell. 1990;60:405–508.
2. Gessler M, Poustka A, Cavenee W, et al. Homozygous deletion in Wilms tumours of a zinc-finger gene identified by chromosome jumping. Nature. 1990;343:774–8.
3. Haber DA, Buckler AJ, Glaser T, et al. An internal deletion within an 11p13 zinc finger gene contributes to the development of Wilms' tumor. Cell. 1990;61:1257–69.
4. Schumacher V, Schneider S, Figge A, et al. Correlation of germ-line mutations and two-hit inactivation of the WT1 gene with Wilms tumors of stromal-predominant histology. Proc Natl Acad Sci U S A. 1997;94:3972–7.
5. Pelletier J, Bruening W, Kashtan CE, et al. Germline mutations in the Wilms' tumor suppressor gene are

associated with abnormal urogenital development in Denys-Drash syndrome. Cell. 1991;67(2):437–47.
6. Barbaux S, Niaudet P, Gubler MC, et al. Donor splice-site mutations in WT1 are responsible for Frasier syndrome. Nat Genet. 1997;17(4):467–70.
7. Jeanpierre C, Denamur E, Henry I, et al. Identification of constitutional WT1 mutations, in patients with isolated diffuse mesangial sclerosis, and analysis of genotype/phenotype correlations by use of a computerized mutation database. Am J Hum Genet. 1998;62(4):824–33.
8. Habib R, Gubler MC, Antignac C, et al. Diffuse mesangial sclerosis: a congenital glomerulopathy with nephrotic syndrome. Adv Nephrol Necker Hosp. 1993;22:43–57.
9. Maalouf EF, Ferguson J, van Heyningen V, et al. In utero nephropathy, Denys-Drash syndrome and Potter phenotype. Pediatr Nephrol. 1998;12(6):449–51.
10. Habib R, Loirat C, Gubler MC, et al. The nephropathy associated with male pseudohermaphroditism and Wilms' tumor (Drash syndrome): a distinctive glomerular lesion—report of 10 cases. Clin Nephrol. 1985;24(6):269–78.
11. Hu M, Zhang GY, Arbuckle S, et al. Prophylactic bilateral nephrectomies in two paediatric patients with missense mutations in the WT1 gene. Nephrol Dial Transplant. 2004;19(1):223–6.
12. Niaudet P, Gubler MC. WT1 and glomerular diseases. Pediatr Nephrol. 2006;21(11):1653–60.
13. Little M, Wells C. A clinical overview of WT1 gene mutations. Hum Mutat. 1997;9(3):209–25.
14. Gao F, Maiti S, Sun G, et al. The Wt1+/R394W mouse displays glomerulosclerosis and early-onset renal failure characteristic of human Denys-Drash syndrome. Mol Cell Biol. 2004;24(22):9899–910.
15. Frasier SD, Bashore RA, Mosier HD. Gonadoblastoma associated with pure gonadal dysgenesis in monozygous twins. J Pediatr. 1964;64:740–5.
16. Gubler MC, Yang Y, Jeanpierre C, et al. WT1, renal development, and glomerulopathies. Adv Nephrol Necker Hosp. 1999;29:299–315.
17. Lipska BS, Ranchin B, Iatropoulos P, et al. Genotype-phenotype associations in WT1 glomerulopathy. Kidney Int. 2014;85(5):1169–78.
18. Denamur E, Bocquet N, Baudouin V, et al. WT1 splice-site mutations are rarely associated with primary steroid-resistant focal and segmental glomerulosclerosis. Kidney Int. 2000;57(5):1868–72.
19. Koziell AB, Grundy R, Barratt TM, et al. Evidence for the genetic heterogeneity of nephropathic phenotypes associated with Denys-Drash and Frasier syndromes. Am J Hum Genet. 1999;64(6):1778–81.
20. Kaplinsky C, Ghahremani M, Frishberg Y, et al. Familial Wilms' tumor associated with a WT1 zinc finger mutation. Genomics. 1996;38(3):451–3.
21. Rapola J. Congenital nephrotic syndrome. Pediatr Nephrol. 1987;1(3):441–6.
22. Kestila M, Mannikko M, Holmberg C, et al. Congenital nephrotic syndrome of the Finnish type maps to

the long arm of chromosome 19. Am J Hum Genet. 1994;54:757–64.

23. Kestila M, Lenkkeri U, Mannikko M, et al. Positionally cloned gene for a novel glomerular protein—nephrin—is mutated in congenital nephrotic syndrome. Mol Cell. 1998;1(4):575–82.

24. Coulthard MG. Management of Finnish congenital nephrotic syndrome by unilateral nephrectomy. Pediatr Nephrol. 1989;3(4):451–3.

25. Holmberg C, Antikainen M, Ronnholm K, et al. Management of congenital nephrotic syndrome of the Finnish type. Pediatr Nephrol. 1995;9(1):87–93.

26. Pomeranz A, Wolach B, Bernheim J, et al. Successful treatment of Finnish congenital nephrotic syndrome with captopril and indomethacin. J Pediatr. 1995;126(1):140–2.

27. Kovacevic L, Reid CJ, Rigden SP. Management of congenital nephrotic syndrome. Pediatr Nephrol. 2003;18(5):426–30.

28. Ruotsalainen V, Ljungberg P, Wartiovaara J, et al. Nephrin is specifically located at the slit diaphragm of glomerular podocytes. Proc Natl Acad Sci U S A. 1999;96(14):7962–7.

29. Wartiovaara J, Ofverstedt LG, Khoshnoodi J, et al. Nephrin strands contribute to a porous slit diaphragm scaffold as revealed by electron tomography. J Clin Invest. 2004;114(10):1475–83.

30. Huber TB, Kottgen M, Schilling B, et al. Interaction with podocin facilitates nephrin signaling. J Biol Chem. 2001;276:41543–6.

31. Huber TB, Hartleben B, Kim J, et al. Nephrin and CD2AP associate with phosphoinositide 3-OH kinase and stimulate AKT-dependent signaling. Mol Cell Biol. 2003;23:4917–28.

32. Huber TB, Simons M, Hartleben B, et al. Molecular basis of the functional podocin-nephrin complex: mutations in the NPHS2 gene disrupt nephrin targeting to lipid raft microdomains. Hum Mol Genet. 2003;12:3397–405.

33. Schwarz K, Simons M, Reiser J, et al. Podocin, a raft-associated component of the glomerular slit diaphragm, interacts with CD2AP and nephrin. J Clin Invest. 2001;108:1621–9.

34. Simons K, Toomre D. Lipid rafts and signal transduction. Nat Rev Mol Cell Biol. 2000;1:31–9.

35. Koziell A, Grech V, Hussain S, et al. Genotype/phenotype correlations of NPHS1 and NPHS2 mutations in nephrotic syndrome advocate a functional inter-relationship in glomerular filtration. Hum Mol Genet. 2002;11(4):379–88.

36. Bolk S, Puffenberger EG, Hudson J, et al. Elevated frequency and allelic heterogeneity of congenital nephrotic syndrome, Finnish type, in the old order Mennonites. Am J Hum Genet. 1999;65(6):1785–90.

37. Weber S, Gribouval O, Esquivel EL, et al. NPHS2 mutation analysis shows genetic heterogeneity of steroid-resistant nephrotic syndrome and low post-transplant recurrence. Kidney Int. 2004;66(2):571–9.

38. Hinkes B, Vlangos C, Heeringa S, et al. Specific podocin mutations correlate with age of onset in steroid-resistant nephrotic syndrome. J Am Soc Nephrol. 2008;19(2):365–71.

39. Santín S, Tazón-Vega B, Silva I, et al. Clinical value of NPHS2 analysis in early- and adult-onset steroid-resistant nephrotic syndrome. Clin J Am Soc Nephrol. 2011;6(2):344–54.

40. Fuchshuber A, Jean G, Gribouval O, et al. Mapping a gene (SRN1) to chromosome 1q25-q31 in idiopathic nephrotic syndrome confirms a distinct entity of autosomal recessive nephrosis. Hum Molec Genet. 1995;4:2155–8.

41. Boute N, Gribouval O, Roselli S, et al. NPHS2, encoding the glomerular protein podocin, is mutated in autosomal recessive steroid-resistant nephrotic syndrome. Nat Genet. 2000;24(4):349–54.

42. Roselli S, Heidet L, Sich M, et al. Early glomerular filtration defect and severe renal disease in podocin-deficient mice. Mol Cell Biol. 2004;24:550–60.

43. Bouchireb K, Boyer O, Gribouval O, et al. NPHS2 mutations in steroid-resistant nephrotic syndrome: a mutation update and the associated phenotypic spectrum. Hum Mutat. 2014;35(2):178–86.

44. Ruf RG, Lichtenberger A, Karle SM, et al. Patients with mutations in NPHS2 (podocin) do not respond to standard steroid treatment of nephrotic syndrome. J Am Soc Nephrol. 2004;15(3):722–32.

45. Lipska BS, Iatropoulos P, Maranta R, et al. Genetic screening in adolescents with steroid-resistant nephrotic syndrome. Kidney Int. 2013;84(1): 206–13.

46. Caridi G, Bertelli R, Di Duca M, et al. Broadening the spectrum of diseases related to podocin mutations. J Am Soc Nephrol. 2003;14(5):1278–86.

47. Caridi G, Bertelli R, Scolari F, et al. Podocin mutations in sporadic focal-segmental glomerulosclerosis occurring in adulthood. Kidney Int. 2003;64(1):365.

48. Schultheiss M, Ruf RG, Mucha BE, et al. No evidence for genotype/phenotype correlation in NPHS1 and NPHS2 mutations. Pediatr Nephrol. 2004;19(12):1340–8.

49. Tsukaguchi H, Sudhakar A, Le TC, et al. NPHS2 mutations in late-onset focal segmental glomerulosclerosis: R229Q is a common disease-associated allele. J Clin Invest. 2002;110(11):1659–66.

50. Machuca E, Hummel A, Nevo F, et al. Clinical and epidemiological assessment of steroid-resistant nephrotic syndrome associated with the NPHS2 R229Q variant. Kidney Int. 2009;75(7):727–35.

51. Tory K, Menyhárd DK, Woerner S, et al. Mutation-dependent recessive inheritance of NPHS2-associated steroid-resistant nephrotic syndrome. Nat Genet. 2014;46(3):299–304. https://doi.org/10.1038/ng.2898.

52. Franceschini N, North KE, Kopp JB, et al. NPHS2 gene, nephrotic syndrome and focal segmental glomerulosclerosis: a HuGE review. Genet Med. 2006;8(2):63–75.

53. Pereira AC, Pereira AB, Mota GF, et al. NPHS2 R229Q functional variant is associated with microalbuminuria in the general population. Kidney Int. 2004;65(3):1026–30.

54. Pierson M, Cordier J, Hervouuet F, et al. An unusual congenital and familial congenital malformative combination involving the eye and the kidney. J Genet Hum. 1963;12:184–213.

55. Zenker M, Aigner T, Wendler O, et al. Human laminin beta2 deficiency causes congenital nephrosis with mesangial sclerosis and distinct eye abnormalities. Hum Mol Genet. 2004;13(21):2625–32.

56. Hasselbacher K, Wiggins RC, Matejas V, et al. Recessive missense mutations in LAMB2 expand the clinical spectrum of LAMB2-associated disorders. Kidney Int. 2006;70(6):1008–12.

57. Mrk K, Reis A, Zenker M. Prenatal findings in four consecutive pregnancies with fetal Pierson syndrome, a newly defined congenital nephrosis syndrome. Prenat Diagn. 2006;26(3):262–6.

58. Chen YM, Zhou Y, Go G, Marmerstein JT, Kikkawa Y, Miner JH. Laminin β2 gene missense mutation produces endoplasmic reticulum stress in podocytes. J Am Soc Nephrol. 2013;24(8):1223–33.

59. Lehnhardt A, Lama A, Amann K, Matejas V, Zenker M, Kemper MJ. Pierson syndromein an adolescent girl with nephrotic range proteinuria but a normal GFR. Pediatr Nephrol. 2012;27(5):865–8.

60. Chen H, Lun Y, Ovchinnikov D, et al. Limb and kidney defects in Lmx1b mutant mice suggest an involvement of LMX1B in human nail patella syndrome. Nat Genet. 1998;19(1):51–5.

61. Bongers EM, Huysmans FT, Levtchenko E, et al. Genotype-phenotype studies in nail-patella syndrome show that LMX1B mutation location is involved in the risk of developing nephropathy. Eur J Hum Genet. 2005;13(8):935–46.

62. Looij BJ Jr, te Slaa RL, Hogewind BL, et al. Genetic counselling in hereditary osteo-onychodysplasia (HOOD, nail-patella syndrome) with nephropathy. J Med Genet. 1988;25(10):682–6.

63. Browning MC, Weidner N, Lorentz WB Jr. Renal histopathology of the nail-patella syndrome in a two-year-old boy. Clin Nephrol. 1988;29(4):210–3.

64. Taguchi T, Takebayashi S, Nishimura M, et al. Nephropathy of nail-patella syndrome. Ultrastruct Pathol. 1988;12(2):175–83.

65. Boyer O, Woerner S, Yang F, et al. LMX1B mutations cause hereditary FSGS without extrarenal involvement. J Am Soc Nephrol. 2013;24(8):1216–22.

66. Isojima T, Harita Y, Furuyama M, et al. LMX1B mutation with residual transcriptional activity as a cause of isolated glomerulopathy. Nephrol Dial Transplant. 2014;29(1):81–8.

67. Miner JH, Morello R, Andrews KL, et al. Transcriptional induction of slit diaphragm genes by Lmx1b is required in podocyte differentiation. J Clin Invest. 2002;109(8):1065–72.

68. Hinkes B, Wiggins RC, Gbadegesin R, et al. Positional cloning uncovers mutations in PLCE1 responsible for a nephrotic syndrome variant that may be reversible. Nat Genet. 2006;38(12):1397–405.

69. Gbadegesin R, Hinkes BG, Hoskins BE, et al. Mutations in PLCE1 are a major cause of isolated diffuse mesangial sclerosis (IDMS). Nephrol Dial Transplant. 2008;23(4):1291–7.

70. Boyer O, Benoit G, Gribouval O, et al. Mutational analysis of the PLCE1 gene in steroid resistant nephrotic syndrome. J Med Genet. 2010;47(7):445–52.

71. Ozaltin F, Ibsirlioglu T, Taskiran EZ, et al. Disruption of PTPRO causes childhood-onset nephrotic syndrome. Am J Hum Genet. 2011;89(1):139–47.

72. Gupta IR, Baldwin C, Auguste D, et al. ARHGDIA: a novel gene implicated in nephrotic syndrome. J Med Genet. 2013;50(5):330–8.

73. Giglio S, Provenzano A, Mazzinghi B, et al. Heterogeneous genetic alterations in sporadic nephrotic syndrome associate with resistance to immunosuppression. J Am Soc Nephrol. 2014;26(1):230–6.

74. Gee HY, Ashraf S, Wan X, et al. Mutations in EMP2 cause childhood-onset nephrotic syndrome. Am J Hum Genet. 2014;94(6):884–90.

75. Braun DA, Sadowski CE, Kohl S, et al. Mutations in nuclear pore genes NUP93, NUP205 and XPO5 cause steroid-resistant nephrotic syndrome. Nat Genet. 2016;48(4):457–65.

76. Braun DA, Lovric S, Schapiro D, et al. Mutations in multiple components of the nuclear pore complex cause nephrotic syndrome. J Clin Invest. 2018;128(10):4313–28.

77. Lipska-Ziętkiewicz BS, Schaefer F. NUP nephropathy: when defective pores cause leaky glomeruli. Am J Kidney Dis. 2019;73(6):890–2.

78. Mathis BJ, Kim SH, Calabrese K, et al. A locus for inherited focal segmental glomerulosclerosis maps to chromosome 19q13. Kidney Int. 1998;53(2):282–6.

79. Kaplan JM, Kim SH, North KN, et al. Mutations in ACTN4, encoding alpha-actinin-4, cause familial focal segmental glomerulosclerosis. Nat Genet. 2000;24(3):251–6.

80. Kos CH, Le TC, Sinha S, et al. Mice deficient in alpha-actinin-4 have severe glomerular disease. J Clin Invest. 2003;111(11):1683–90.

81. Weins A, Kenlan P, Herbert S, et al. Mutational and biological analysis of alpha-actinin-4 in focal segmental glomerulosclerosis. J Am Soc Nephrol. 2005;16(12):3694–701.

82. McCarthy HJ, Bierzynska A, Wherlock M, et al. Simultaneous sequencing of 24 genes associated with steroid-resistant nephrotic syndrome. Clin J Am Soc Nephrol. 2013;8(4):637–48.

83. Winn MP, Conlon PJ, Lynn KL, et al. Linkage of a gene causing familial focal segmental glomerulosclerosis to chromosome 11 and further evidence of genetic heterogeneity. Genomics. 1999;58(2):113–20.

84. Winn MP, Conlon PJ, Lynn KL, et al. A mutation in the TRPC6 cation channel causes familial focal segmental glomerulosclerosis. Science. 2005;308(5729):1801–4.
85. Reiser J, Polu KR, Moller CC, et al. TRPC6 is a glomerular slit diaphragm-associated channel required for normal renal function. Nat Genet. 2005;37(7):739–44.
86. Kim JM, Wu H, Green G, et al. CD2-associated protein haploinsufficiency is linked to glomerular disease susceptibility. Science. 2003;300:1298–300.
87. Shih NY, Li J, Karpitskii V, et al. Congenital nephrotic syndrome in mice lacking CD2-associated protein. Science. 1999;286:312–5.
88. Kopp JB, Smith MW, Nelson GW, et al. MYH9 is a major-effect risk gene for focal segmental glomerulosclerosis. Nat Genet. 2008;40(10):1175–84.
89. Genovese G, Friedman DJ, Ross MD, et al. Association of trypanolytic ApoL1 variants with kidney disease in African Americans. Science. 2010;329(5993):841–5.
90. Brown EJ, Schlöndorff JS, Becker DJ, Tsukaguchi H, Tonna SJ, Uscinski AL, Higgs HN, Henderson JM, Pollak MR. Mutations in the formin gene INF2 cause focal segmental glomerulosclerosis. Nat Genet. 2010;42(1):72–6.
91. Boyer O, Nevo F, Plaisier E, et al. INF2 mutations in Charcot-Marie-Tooth disease with glomerulopathy. N Engl J Med. 2011;365(25):2377–88.
92. Mele C, Iatropoulos P, Donadelli R, et al. MYO1E mutations and childhood familial focal segmental glomerulosclerosis. N Engl J Med. 2011;365(4):295–306.
93. Quinzii C, Naini A, Salviati L, Trevisson E, Navas P, Dimauro S, Hirano M. A mutation in para-hydroxybenzoate-polyprenyl transferase (COQ2) causes primary coenzyme Q10 deficiency. Am J Hum Genet. 2006;78(2):345–9.
94. Diomedi-Camassei F, Di Giandomenico S, et al. COQ2 nephropathy: a newly described inherited mitochondriopathy with primary renal involvement. J Am Soc Nephrol. 2007;18(10):2773–80.
95. Scalais E, Chafai R, Van Coster R, et al. Early myoclonic epilepsy, hypertrophic cardiomyopathy and subsequently a nephrotic syndrome in a patient with CoQ10 deficiency caused by mutations in para-hydroxybenzoate-polyprenyl transferase (COQ2). Eur J Paediatr Neurol. 2013;17(6):625–30.
96. Heeringa SF, Chernin G, Chaki M, et al. COQ6 mutations in human patients produce nephrotic syndrome with sensorineural deafness. J Clin Invest. 2011;121(5):2013–24.
97. Ashraf S, Gee HY, Woerner S, et al. ADCK4 mutations promote steroid-resistant nephrotic syndrome through CoQ10 biosynthesis disruption. J Clin Invest. 2013;123(12):5179–89.
98. Montini G, Malaventura C, Salviati L. Early coenzyme Q10 supplementation in primary coenzyme Q10 deficiency. N Engl J Med. 2008;358(26):2849–50.
99. Boerkoel CF, Takashima H, John J, et al. Mutant chromatin remodeling protein SMARCAL1 causes Schimke immuno-osseous dysplasia. Nat Genet. 2002;30(2):215–20.
100. Lipska-Ziętkiewicz BS, Gellermann J, Boyer O, et al. Low renal but high extrarenal phenotype variability in Schimke immuno-osseous dysplasia. PLoS One. 2017;12(8):e0180926. https://doi.org/10.1371/journal.pone.0180926.
101. Galloway WH, Mowat AP. Congenital microcephaly with hiatus hernia and nephrotic syndrome in two sibs. J Med Genet. 1968;5(4):319–21.
102. Garty BZ, Eisenstein B, Sandbank J, et al. Microcephaly and congenital nephrotic syndrome owing to diffuse mesangial sclerosis: an autosomal recessive syndrome. J Med Genet. 1994;31(2):121–5.
103. Colin E, Huynh Cong E, Mollet G, et al. Loss-of-function mutations in WDR73 are responsible for microcephaly and steroid-resistant nephrotic syndrome: Galloway-Mowat syndrome. Am J Hum Genet. 2014;95:637–48.
104. Braun DA, Rao J, Mollet G, et al. Mutations in KEOPS-complex genes cause nephrotic syndrome with primary microcephaly. Nat Genet. 2017;49:1529–38.
105. Trautmann A, Schnaidt S, Lipska-Ziętkiewicz BS, et al. Long-term outcome of steroid-resistant nephrotic syndrome in children. J Am Soc Nephrol. 2017;28(10):3055–65.
106. Trautmann A, Lipska-Ziętkiewicz BS, Schaefer F. Exploring the clinical and genetic spectrum of steroid resistant nephrotic syndrome: the Podo-Net registry. Front Pediatr. 2018;6:200. https://doi.org/10.3389/fped.2018.00200.
107. Büscher AK, Beck BB, Melk A, et al. Rapid response to cyclosporin A and favorable renal outcome in nongenetic versus genetic steroid-resistant nephrotic syndrome. Clin J Am Soc Nephrol. 2016;11(2):245–53.
108. Trautmann A, Bodria M, Ozaltin F, et al. Spectrum of steroid-resistant and congenital nephrotic syndrome in children: the PodoNet registry cohort. Clin J Am Soc Nephrol. 2015;10:592–600.
109. Trautmann A, Vivarelli M, Samuel S, et al. IPNA clinical practice recommendations for the diagnosis and management of children with steroid-resistant nephrotic syndrome. Pediatr Nephrol. 2020;35:1529–61.
110. Gbadegesin RA, Adeyemo A, Webb NJ, et al. HLA-DQA1 and PLCG2 Are Candidate Risk Loci for Childhood-Onset Steroid-Sensitive Nephrotic Syndrome. J Am Soc Nephrol. 2015;26(7):1701–10.
111. Jia X, Horinouchi T, Hitomi Y, et al. Strong association of the HLA-DR/DQ locus with childhood steroid-sensitive nephrotic syndrome in the Japanese population. J Am Soc Nephrol. 2018;29(8):2189–99.
112. Dufek S, Cheshire C, Levine AP, et al. Genetic identification of two novel loci associated with steroid-sensitive nephrotic syndrome. J Am Soc Nephrol. 2019;30(8):1375–84.

113. Lane BM, Chryst-Stangl M, Wu G, et al. Steroid-sensitive nephrotic syndrome candidate gene CLVS1 regulates podocyte oxidative stress and endocytosis. JCI Insight. 2022;7(2):e152102. https://doi.org/10.1172/jci.insight.152102.

114. Artero M, Biava C, Amend W, et al. Recurrent focal glomerulosclerosis: natural history and response to therapy. Am J Med. 1992;92(4):375–83.

115. Senggutuvan P, Cameron JS, Hartley RB, et al. Recurrence of focal segmental glomerulosclerosis in transplanted kidneys: analysis of incidence and risk factors in 59 allografts. Pediatr Nephrol. 1990;4(1):21–8.

116. Tejani A, Stablein DH. Recurrence of focal segmental glomerulosclerosis posttransplantation: a special report of the North American Pediatric Renal Transplant Cooperative Study. J Am Soc Nephrol. 1992;2(12 Suppl):S258–63.

117. Habib R, Hebert D, Gagnadoux MF, et al. Transplantation in idiopathic nephrosis. Transplant Proc. 1982;14(3):489–95.

118. McCarthy ET, Sharma M, Savin VJ. Circulating permeability factors in idiopathic nephrotic syndrome and focal segmental glomerulosclerosis. Clin J Am Soc Nephrol. 2010;5(11):2115–21.

119. Coppo R. Different targets for treating focal segmental glomerular sclerosis. Contrib Nephrol. 2013;181:84–90.

120. Höcker B, Knüppel T, Waldherr R, et al. Recurrence of proteinuria 10 years post-transplant in NPHS2-associated focal segmental glomerulosclerosis after conversion from cyclosporin A to sirolimus. Pediatr Nephrol. 2006;21(10):1476–9.

121. Bertelli R, Ginevri F, Caridi G, et al. Recurrence of focal segmental glomerulosclerosis after renal transplantation in patients with mutations of podocin. Am J Kidney Dis. 2003;41(6):1314–21.

122. Patrakka J, Ruotsalainen V, Reponen P, et al. Recurrence of nephrotic syndrome in kidney grafts of patients with congenital nephrotic syndrome of the Finnish type: role of nephrin. Transplantation. 2002;73(3):394–403.

123. Santín S, Bullich G, Tazón-Vega B, et al. Clinical utility of genetic testing in children and adults with steroid-resistant nephrotic syndrome. Clin J Am Soc Nephrol. 2011;6(5):1139–48.

124. Büscher AK, Konrad M, Nagel M, et al. Mutations in podocyte genes are a rare cause of primary FSGS associated with ESRD in adult patients. Clin Nephrol. 2012;78(1):47–53.

Alport Syndrome and Other Type IV Collagen Disorders

16

Michelle N. Rheault and Rachel Lennon

Introduction

Several forms of familial glomerular hematuria syndromes result from genetic variants that affect type IV collagen, the major collagenous constituent of glomerular basement membranes (GBM): Alport syndrome (AS) and hereditary angiopathy with nephropathy, aneurysms and cramps (HANAC) syndrome. Persistent hematuria is a cardinal feature of each of these disorders. Variants in any of three type IV collagen genes, *COL4A3, COL4A4* or *COL4A5* can cause AS, which is characterized by progressive deterioration of kidney function with associated hearing and ocular involvement in many affected individuals. A majority of affected individuals demonstrate X-linked inheritance; however, autosomal recessive and autosomal dominant transmission is also observed. Heterozygous variants in these genes are also significant and link to a wider spectrum of kidney disease [1–3]. Variants in *COL4A3, COL4A4 or COL4A5* [4] account for about 30–50% of children with iso-

lated glomerular hematuria seen in pediatric nephrology clinics [5–8]. HANAC syndrome arises from variants in *COL4A1* [9].

Alport Syndrome

Introduction

The first description of a family with inherited hematuria appeared in 1902 in a report by Guthrie [10]. Subsequent monographs about this family by Hurst in 1923 [11] and Alport in 1927 [12] established that affected individuals in this family, particularly males, developed deafness and uremia. The advent of electron microscopy led to the discovery of unique GBM abnormalities in patients with AS [13–15], setting the stage for the histochemical [16–18] and genetic [19, 20] studies that resulted in the identification of disease causing variants in *COL4A5* [20] followed by *COL4A3* and *COL4A4* [21, 22]. AS occurs in approximately 1:50,000 live births and accounts for 1.3% and 0.4% of pediatric and adult end-stage kidney disease (ESKD) patients in the United States, respectively [23].

M. N. Rheault (✉)
Division of Pediatric Nephrology, University of Minnesota Masonic Children's Hospital, Minneapolis, MN, USA
e-mail: rheau002@umn.edu

R. Lennon
University of Manchester and Royal Manchester Children's Hospital, Manchester, UK
e-mail: Rachel.Lennon@manchester.ac.uk

© The Author(s), under exclusive license to Springer Nature Switzerland AG 2023
F. Schaefer, L. A. Greenbaum (eds.), *Pediatric Kidney Disease*,
https://doi.org/10.1007/978-3-031-11665-0_16

Etiology and Pathogenesis

Type IV Collagen Proteins, Tissue Distribution and Genes

Six chains of type IV collagen, $\alpha1(IV)$-$\alpha6(IV)$, are encoded by six genes, *COL4A1-COL4A6*. The type IV collagen genes are arranged in pairs on three chromosomes: *COL4A1-COL4A2* on chromosome 13, *COL4A3-COL4A4* on chromosome 2, and *COL4A5-COL4A6* on the X chromosome. The paired genes are arranged in a 5'-5' head-to-head fashion, separated by sequences of varying length containing regulatory elements [24, 25]. All type IV collagen chains share several basic structural features: a major collagenous domain of approximately 1400 residues containing the repetitive triplet sequence glycine (Gly)-X-Y, in which X and Y represent a variety of other amino acids; a *C*-terminal noncollagenous (NC1) domain of approximately 230 residues; and a noncollagenous *N*-terminal sequence of 15–20 residues. The collagenous domains each contain approximately 20 interruptions of the collagenous triplet sequence, while each NC1 domain contains 12 conserved cysteine residues. Type IV collagen chains self-associate to form triple helical structures or "trimers". The specificity of chain association is determined by amino acid sequences within the NC1 domains and results in only three trimeric species that are found in nature: $\alpha1_2\alpha2(IV)$, $\alpha3\alpha4\alpha5(IV)$ and $\alpha5_2\alpha6(IV)$ [26]. Unlike interstitial collagens, which lose their NC1 domains and form fibrillar networks, type IV collagen trimers form open, nonfibrillar networks through NC1-NC1 and N-terminal interactions [27].

$\alpha1_2\alpha2(IV)$ trimers are found in all basement membranes, whereas $\alpha3\alpha4\alpha5(IV)$ and $\alpha5_2\alpha6(IV)$ trimers have a more restricted distribution. In normal human kidneys, $\alpha3\alpha4\alpha5(IV)$ trimers are found in GBM, Bowman's capsules, and the basement membranes of distal tubules, while $\alpha5_2\alpha6(IV)$ trimers are detectable in Bowman's capsules, basement membranes of distal tubules and collecting ducts, but not GBM [28, 29]. $\alpha5_2\alpha6(IV)$ trimers are also present in normal epidermal basement membranes as well as some alimentary canal, ocular, and vascular basement membranes. $\alpha3\alpha4\alpha5(IV)$ trimers also occur in several basement membranes of the eye and of the cochlea [30–32].

Pathogenic variants in any of the *COL4A3*, *COL4A4*, or *COL4A5* genes will affect the formation and composition of affected basement membranes. If any of the $\alpha3(IV)$, $\alpha4(IV)$, or $\alpha5(IV)$ chains are absent due to loss of function variants (deletions, frame shift variants, premature stop codons), then the other collagen chains are degraded and no $\alpha3\alpha4\alpha5(IV)$ trimers are deposited in basement membranes [33]. In this case, the embryonic $\alpha1_2\alpha2(IV)$ network persists. Missense variants, particularly those that affect the glycine residues involved in triple helix formation, may lead to the formation of abnormally folded trimers that are either degraded or deposited into the basement membrane with formation of an abnormal type IV collagen network. Due to a greater number of disulfide bonds, the $\alpha3\alpha4\alpha5(IV)$ network is more highly cross-linked and is considered more resistant to proteases and therefore mechanical strain than the $\alpha1_2\alpha2(IV)$ network [33, 34]. In support of this network being mechanically stronger, absence of the $\alpha3\alpha4\alpha5(IV)$ network leads to increased distensibility in the lens capsule when tested in experimental models of AS [35]. Indeed, the glomerular capillary walls of AS patients may also be mechanically weak and provoke pathologic stretch-related responses in glomerular cells [36].

Genetics

AS is described in three genetic forms: X-linked (XLAS), autosomal recessive (ARAS) and autosomal dominant (ADAS), although opinions vary as to how a single gene can cause both recessive and dominant disease (Table 16.1). XLAS, caused by variants in *COL4A5*, was classically thought to account for approximately 80% of AS patients while ARAS, caused by variants in both alleles of *COL4A3* or *COL4A4*, accounted for about 15% of the AS population. Affected males with XLAS are hemizygous and carry a single abnormal *COL4A5* allele, while affected females are heterozygous with normal and abnormal alleles. Individuals with ARAS may be either homozygous, with identical variants in both

16 Alport Syndrome and Other Type IV Collagen Disorders

Table 16.1 Familial glomerular hematuria due to type IV collagen variants

	Genetic locus	Protein product	Kidney manifestations	Kidney failure	GBM ultrastructure	Extrakidney manifestations
Alport syndrome						
X-linked	COL4A5	α5(IV)	Hematuria Proteinuria Hypertension	All males, some females	Thinning (early) Lamellation (late)	Deafness Lenticonus Perimacular flecks
Autosomal recessive	COL4A3 COL4A4 (biallelic or digenic)	α3(IV) α4(IV)	Hematuria Proteinuria Hypertension	All males and females	Thinning (early) Lamellation (late)	Deafness Lenticonus Perimacular flecks
Autosomal dominant	COL4A3 COL4A4 (heterozygous)	α3(IV) α4(IV)	Hematuria Proteinuria Hypertension	Males and females (late)	Thinning (early) Lamellation (late)	Deafness
HANAC syndrome						
Autosomal dominant	COL4A1	α1(IV)	Hematuria Cysts CKD	?	Normal	Arterial aneurysms Muscle cramps

Abbreviations: *GBM* glomerular basement membrane; *CKD* chronic kidney disease

alleles of the affected gene or they may be compound heterozygotes, with different variants in the two alleles or even demonstrate digenic inheritance with one variant in *COL4A3* and the other in *COL4A4* [37, 38]. With the advent of next generation sequencing, studies are suggesting a higher percentage of patients with ADAS, up to 31% in one report [39]. ADAS is used by some clinicians to describe heterozygous variants in *COL4A3* or *COL4A4* with a progressive clinical course [40]. It is not clear why some individuals develop a progressive nephropathy while others have a slower or unremarkable clinical course; this may relate to the presence of co-segregating genetic modifiers [41].

Over 2500 pathogenic variants have been identified in the *COL4A5* gene in patients with XLAS [42]. Variants can be found along the entire 51 exons of the gene without identified hot spots. About 10–15% of *COL4A5* variants occur as spontaneous events; therefore, a family history of kidney disease is not required for a diagnosis of XLAS. A range of variants have been described: large rearrangements (~20%), small deletions and insertions (~20%), missense variants altering a glycine residue in the collagenous domain of α5(IV) (30%), other missense variants (~8%), nonsense variants (~5%) and splice-site

variants (~15%) [43]. The type of *COL4A5* variant has a significant impact on the course of XLAS in affected males [43–45]. In males with a large deletion, nonsense variant or an indel causing a reading frame shift, the risk of developing kidney failure before age 30 is 90%. In contrast, progression to kidney failure before age 30 occurs in 70% and 50% of patients with splice-site and missense variants, respectively [43]. In addition, XLAS patients with 5′ glycine missense variants demonstrate a more severe phenotype than those with 3′ glycine variants [44]. In contrast to males with XLAS, a statistical relationship between *COL4A5* genotype and kidney phenotype has not been demonstrated in females with XLAS [46].

Clinical Manifestations

Males with XLAS and ARAS inevitably develop kidney failure at a rate that is influenced by genotype [37, 43, 45]. While most females with XLAS have non-progressive or slowly progressive kidney disease, a significant minority demonstrates progression to kidney failure [47]. The course of ARAS is similar in females and males [37]. In general, patients with ADAS progress less rapidly than patients with XLAS or ARAS and are less likely to have extra-kidney manifestations [48].

Kidney Phenotype

Persistent microscopic hematuria (MH) occurs in all males with AS, regardless of genetic type, and is probably present from early infancy. Approximately 95% of heterozygous females with XLAS have persistent or intermittent MH [46], and 100% of females with ARAS have persistent MH. Gross hematuria is not unusual in boys and girls with Alport syndrome, occurring at least once in approximately 60% of affected males [43, 49].

In males with XLAS, and in males and females with ARAS, proteinuria typically becomes detectable in late childhood or early adolescence and progresses from microalbuminuria to overt proteinuria [50]. In one large cohort of females with XLAS, 75% had proteinuria, although the timing of onset was not investigated [46].

Blood pressure is typically normal in childhood but, like proteinuria, hypertension is common in adolescent males with XLAS or ARAS, and in females with ARAS. Most females with XLAS have normal blood pressure, but hypertension may develop, particularly in those with proteinuria.

All males with XLAS eventually require kidney replacement therapy, with 50% of untreated males reaching kidney failure by age 25, 80% by age 40 and 100% by age 60 [43]. The timing of kidney failure in patients with ARAS is similar to XLAS males, although ARAS patients with normal kidney function in their 30's and 40's have been reported [37]. In patients with ADAS, the age at which 50% of patients have progressed to kidney failure is approximately 50 years, or twice as long as XLAS males [48].

Females who are heterozygous for *COL4A5* variants demonstrate widely variable disease outcomes, with some women demonstrating only lifelong asymptomatic hematuria while others develop chronic progressive kidney disease including kidney failure [51]. About 12% of XLAS females reach kidney failure by age 45, 30% by age 60 and 40% by age 80 [46]. The explanation for the wide variability in outcomes for XLAS females is uncertain, but likely multifactorial. Risk factors for kidney failure in XLAS females include proteinuria and sensorineural deafness [46, 52]. X-inactivation, the process by which one X chromosome in females is silenced to adjust for gene dosage differences between males and females, may play a role in kidney disease progression in XLAS females [53, 54]. In a mouse model of female XLAS, modest skewing of X-inactivation to favor expression of the wild type $\alpha 5(IV)$ was associated with a survival advantage [55].

AS nephropathy progresses predictably through a series of clinical phases. Phase I typically lasts from birth until late childhood or early adolescence, and is characterized by isolated hematuria, with normal protein excretion and kidney function. In Phase II, microalbuminuria followed by overt proteinuria is superimposed on hematuria, but the glomerular filtration rate (GFR) remains normal. Patients in Phase III exhibit declining GFR in addition to hematuria and proteinuria, and those in Phase IV have kidney failure. These phases have histological correlates, as described in the next section. The rate of passage through these phases is primarily a function of the causative genetic variant, at least in males with XLAS. Patients with *COL4A5* variants that prevent production of any functional protein (deletions, nonsense variants) proceed through these phases more rapidly than those whose variants allow synthesis of a functional, albeit abnormal, protein (some missense variants). Females with XLAS can be viewed as passing through the same phases as males, although the rate of progression is typically slower, and the journey to kidney failure may not be completed during the individual's lifetime.

Hearing

Newborn hearing screening is normal in males with XLAS, and in males and females with ARAS, but bilateral impairment of perception of high frequency sounds frequently becomes detectable in late childhood. The hearing deficit is progressive, and extends into the range of conversational speech with advancing age. Affected individuals benefit from hearing aids since the deficit usually does not exceed 60–70 dB and speech discrimination is preserved. Sensorineural hearing loss (SNHL) is present in 50% of males with XLAS by approximately age 15, 75% by age 25, and 90% by age 40 [43]. Like the effect on kidney disease progression, missense variants in COL4A5 are associated with an attenuated risk of hearing loss. The risk of SNHL before age 30 is 60% in patients with missense variants, while the risk of SNHL before age 30 is 90% in those with other types of variants [43]. SNHL is less frequent in females with XLAS. About 10% of XLAS females have SNHL by 40 years of age, and about 20% by age 60 [46]. SNHL is also common in ARAS, with approximately 66% of individuals affected [37].

The SNHL in AS has been localized to the cochlea [56]. In control cochleae, the α3(IV), α4(IV) and α5(IV) chains are expressed in the spiral limbus, the spiral ligament, stria vascularis and in the basement membrane situated between the Organ of Corti and the basilar membrane [57–59]. However, these chains have not been detected in the cochleae of ARAS mice [58], XLAS dogs [59] or men with XLAS [32]. Examination of well-preserved cochleae from men with XLAS revealed a unique zone of separation between the organ of Corti and the underlying basilar membrane, as well as cellular infiltration of the tunnel of Corti and the spaces of Nuel [60]. These changes may be associated with abnormal tuning of basilar membrane motion and hair cell stimulation, resulting in defective hearing. An alternative hypothesis is that hearing is impaired by changes in potassium concentration in the scala media induced by abnormalities of type IV collagen in the stria vascularis [61].

Ocular Anomalies

Abnormalities of the lens and the retina are common in individuals with AS, typically becoming apparent in the second to third decade of life in XLAS males and in males and females with ARAS. The α3(IV), α4(IV) and α5(IV) chains are normal components of the anterior lens capsule and other ocular basement membranes, and variants that interfere with the formation or deposition of α3α4α5(IV) trimers prevent expression of these chains in the eye [30, 57]. Anterior lenticonus, which is considered virtually pathognomonic for AS [62], is absent at birth and manifests during the second and third decades of life in ~13–25% of affected individuals [43, 63]. In this disorder, the anterior lens capsule is markedly attenuated, especially over the central region of the lens, and exhibits focal areas of dehiscence, leading to refractive errors and, in some cases, cataracts [64, 65]. Anterior lenticonus has been described only rarely in heterozygous females with COL4A5 variants [47]. Dot-fleck retinopathy, a characteristic alteration of retinal pigmentation concentrated in the perimacular region [66], is also common in AS patients and does not appear to be associated with any abnormality in vision [43]. Recurrent corneal erosions [67, 68] and posterior polymorphous dystrophy, manifested by clear vesicles on the posterior surface of the cornea [69], have also been described in AS.

Leiomyomatosis

Several dozen families in which AS is transmitted in association with leiomyomas of the esophagus and tracheobronchial tree have been described [70]. Affected individuals carry X-chromosomal deletions that involve the COL4A5 gene and terminate within the second intron of the adjacent COL4A6 gene [71–73]. The genotype-phenotype relationship in this disorder is uncertain because deletions in this region may occur without associated leiomyomas, and conversely some families with XLAS and leiomyomas do not have deletions involving COL4A6 [74]. Those affected tend to become symptomatic in late childhood, and may exhibit dysphagia, postprandial vomiting, epigastric or retrosternal pain, recurrent bronchitis, dyspnea, cough or stridor. Females with the AS-leiomyomatosis complex may develop genital leiomyomas, with clitoral hypertrophy and variable involvement of the labia majora and uterus.

Other Findings

AS associated with mental retardation, mid-face hypoplasia and elliptocytosis has been described in association with large *COL4A5* deletions that extend beyond the 5′ terminus of the gene [75]. Early development of aortic root dilatation and aneurysms of the thoracic and abdominal aorta, as well as other arterial vessels, have been described in AS males, perhaps due to abnormalities in the α5₂α6(IV) network in arterial smooth muscle basement membranes [76].

Kidney Pathology

Children with AS typically show limited kidney parenchymal changes by light microscopy before 5 years of age. Older patients may have mesangial hypercellularity and matrix expansion. As the disease progresses, focal segmental glomerulosclerosis, tubular atrophy and interstitial fibrosis become the predominant light microscopic abnormalities. Although some patients exhibit increased numbers of immature glomeruli or interstitial foam cells, these changes are not specific for AS.

Electron microscopy is frequently diagnostic, although the expression of the pathognomonic lesion is age-dependent and, for those with XLAS, gender-dependent. In early childhood, the predominant ultrastructural lesion in males is diffuse attenuation of the GBM. The classic ultrastructural appearance is diffuse thickening of the glomerular capillary wall, accompanied by "basket-weave" transformation; intramembranous cellular components, which have been described as podocyte protrusions; scalloping of the epithelial surface of the GBM; and effacement of podocyte foot-processes (Fig. 16.1) [77]. These changes are more prevalent in affected males, typically becoming prominent in late childhood and adolescence. Affected females can display a spectrum of lesions, demonstrating predominantly normal-appearing GBM, focal GBM attenuation, diffuse GBM attenuation, focal thickening/basket-weaving, or diffuse basket-

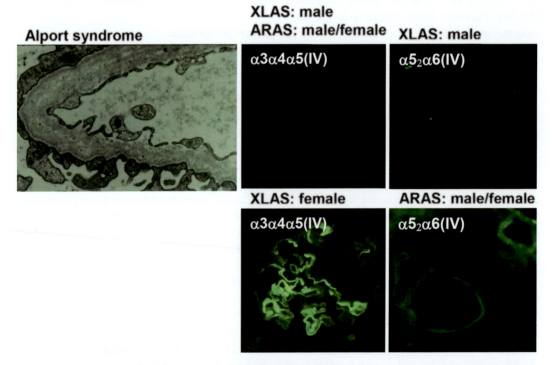

Fig. 16.1 Typical findings on electron microscopy and type IV collagen immunostaining for α5(IV) in Alport syndrome. Abbreviations: *XLAS* X-linked Alport syndrome; *ARAS* autosomal recessive Alport syndrome

weaving. The extent of the GBM lesion progresses inexorably in males, although the rate of progression may be influenced by *COL4A5* genotype. Females may have static or progressive GBM lesions. X-chromosome inactivation pattern, age and *COL4A5* genotype could all contribute to the GBM changes in affected females.

The classic GBM lesion is not found in all kindreds with AS. Adult patients who demonstrate only GBM thinning, yet have *COL4A5* variants, have been described. Although these represent a minority of Alport patients and families, they are also seen in individuals with heterozygous variants and in such patients there is an association with focal segmental glomerulosclerosis (FSGS) [1, 2]. Indeed, patients with a diagnosis of FSGS should have careful evaluation of GBM ultrastructure and, if defects are identified, genetic testing for Alport gene variants is warranted since a diagnosis of AS will enable further phenotypic evaluation in the individual as well as testing in other family members.

Routine immunofluorescence microscopy in patients with AS is normal or shows nonspecific deposition of immunoproteins. In contrast, specific immunostaining for type IV collagen α chains is frequently diagnostic, and can distinguish between XLAS and ARAS (Fig. 16.1). The utility of this approach derives from the fact that most disease-causing variants in AS alter the expression of the $\alpha3\alpha4\alpha5(IV)$ and $\alpha5_2\alpha6(IV)$ trimers in kidney basement membranes. Most *COL4A5* variants prevent expression of both trimer forms in the kidney, so that in about 80% of XLAS males immunostaining of kidney biopsy specimens for $\alpha3(IV)$, $\alpha4(IV)$ and $\alpha5(IV)$ chains is completely negative [78]. About 60–70% of XLAS females exhibit mosaic expression of these chains, while in the remainder immunostaining for these chains is normal. The biallelic variants in *COL4A3* and *COL4A4* that cause ARAS often prevent expression of $\alpha3\alpha4\alpha5(IV)$ trimers, but have no effect on expression of $\alpha5_2\alpha6(IV)$ trimers. In kidney biopsy specimens from patients with ARAS, immunostaining for $\alpha3(IV)$ and $\alpha4(IV)$ chains is negative in the GBM. However, while immunostaining of GBM for the $\alpha5(IV)$ chain is negative due to the absence of $\alpha3\alpha4\alpha5(IV)$ trimers, Bowman's capsules, distal tubular basement membranes and collecting duct basement membranes are positive for $\alpha5(IV)$ due to the unimpaired expression of $\alpha5_2\alpha6(IV)$ trimers. Heterozygous carriers of a single *COL4A3* or *COL4A4* mutation have normal kidney basement membrane immunostaining for $\alpha3(IV)$, $\alpha4(IV)$ and $\alpha5(IV)$ chains.

The $\alpha5_2\alpha6(IV)$ trimer is a normal component of the skin epidermal basement membrane (EBM). Consequently, about 80% of males with XLAS can be diagnosed by skin biopsy based on absence of $\alpha5(IV)$ expression in EBM. In 60–70% of XLAS females, there is a mosaic pattern of EBM immunostaining for $\alpha5(IV)$. EBM expression of $\alpha5(IV)$ is normal in patients with ARAS and in subjects with heterozygous variants in *COL4A3* or *COL4A4*.

Diagnosis and Differential Diagnosis

AS is one potential cause of familial and sporadic glomerular hematuria. Accurate diagnosis rests on careful clinical evaluation, a precise family history, selective application of invasive diagnostic techniques and, in appropriate patients, molecular diagnosis (Fig. 16.2).

The presence of isolated microscopic hematuria in a child with a positive family history for hematuria, an autosomal dominant pattern of inheritance, and a negative family history for kidney failure strongly suggests a diagnosis of heterozygous *COL4A3/4* variants (Fig. 16.2). Less common conditions associated with familial glomerular hematuria include the autosomal dominant *MYH9* disorders (Epstein and Fechtner syndromes), in which macrothrombocytopenia is a constant feature and familial IgA nephropathy. However, there may also be overlap with heterozygous Alport syndrome and a range of glomerular pathologies; large genetic sequencing studies will help to identify these disease group intersections.

When family history for hematuria is negative, the differential diagnosis of isolated glomerular hematuria, or hematuria associated with proteinuria includes AS, IgA nephropathy, C3

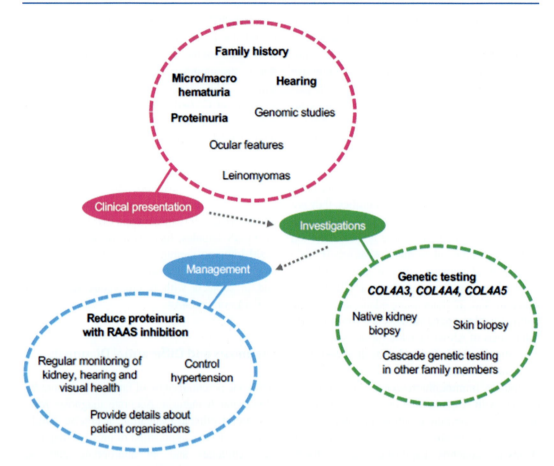

Fig. 16.2 Clinical presentation, diagnosis and management of Alport syndrome. Patients can present with a variety of clinical presentations, which should prompt investigation to confirm a diagnosis of Alport syndrome. Genetic testing for the Alport genes *COL4A3*, *COL4A4* and *COL4A5* is widely available and is the gold standard for diagnosis. Management includes the use of renin-angiotensin-aldosterone (RAAS) pathway inhibitors

glomerulopathy, membranous nephropathy, lupus nephritis, postinfectious glomerulonephritis, Henoch-Schönlein nephritis, and many other entities. Some of these conditions will be strongly suspected based on clinical findings (e.g., rash and joint complaints) while others will be suggested by laboratory findings, such as hypocomplementemia.

Formal audiometric and ophthalmological examinations should be considered as part of the diagnostic evaluation in children with persistent microscopic hematuria. Audiometry may be very helpful in children over age 6–8 years, especially boys, since high-frequency SNHL would point toward a diagnosis of AS. The presence of anterior lenticonus or the dot-fleck retinopathy may be diagnostic. However, these lesions are more prevalent in patients with advanced disease, and less likely to be present in the young patients in whom diagnostic ambiguity tends to be the greatest.

Genetic testing is the gold standard for diagnosing AS. Additional tissue studies are appropriate when clinical and pedigree information and genetic testing does not allow a diagnosis AS. Therefore, several options are available for confirming a diagnosis of AS, including genetic analysis, skin biopsy and kidney biopsy. Genetic analysis using Sanger sequencing is capable of identifying *COL4A5* variants in 80–90% of males with XLAS [79]. High variant detection rates in *COL4A3* and *COL4A4* in patients with ARAS are also possible, particularly if there is parental consanguinity. Commercial genetic testing for variants in *COL4A3, COL4A4,* and *COL4A5* is available. Next generation sequencing, which allows simultaneous analysis of *COL4A3, COL4A4* and *COL4A5,* now replaces Sanger sequencing as the preferred approach. If further investigation is required, skin biopsy is often utilized as the initial invasive diagnostic procedure in patients suspected of AS it is less invasive and expensive than a kidney biopsy. On skin biopsy, the majority of subjects with XLAS will display abnormal expression of the α5(IV) chain in EBM as described above. Normal EBM α5(IV) expression in a patient with hematuria has several possible explanations: (1) the patient has XLAS, but his or her *COL4A5* mutation allows EBM expression of α5(IV); (2) the patient has ARAS, or ADAS, in which α5(IV) expression is expected to be preserved; or (3) the patient has a disease other than AS. Kidney biopsy would then provide the opportunity to diagnose other diseases, to examine type IV collagen α chain expression in kidney basement membranes, and to evaluate GBM at the ultrastructural level.

Treatment

The goal of treatment in AS is to slow the progression of kidney disease and delay the need for dialysis or transplantation. Several therapeutic approaches have demonstrated efficacy in murine ARAS, including angiotensin blockade [80–82], inhibition of TGFβ-1 [83], chemokine receptor 1 blockade [84], administration of bone morphogenic protein-7 [85], suppression of matrix metalloproteinases [34] and bone marrow transplantation [86]. Cyclosporine therapy slowed progression of kidney disease in a canine model of AS, but human studies have demonstrated significant nephrotoxicity and adverse effects and this treatment is not recommended [87–89]. Angiotensin converting enzyme (ACE) inhibition also prolonged survival in a canine XLAS model [90]. Uncontrolled studies in human AS subjects have shown that ACE inhibition can reduce pro-

teinuria, at least transiently [91, 92]. A multicenter, randomized, double-blind study comparing losartan with placebo or amlodipine in 30 children with AS demonstrated a significant reduction in proteinuria in the losartan treated group [93]. An extension of this study showed comparable efficacy of either enalapril or losartan in reducing proteinuria in children with AS [94]. A report from the European Alport Registry, which includes 283 patients over 20 years, compared kidney outcomes in AS patients treated with ACE inhibition at various time points: at onset of microalbuminuria, at onset of proteinuria, or in chronic kidney disease (CKD) stage III-IV [95]. This retrospective review demonstrated a delay in kidney replacement therapy by 3 years in the treated CKD group and by 18 years in the treated proteinuric group [95]. These findings were confirmed in a retrospective review of kidney outcomes in men with XLAS from Japan [45]. In this study, men who received ACE inhibitors reached renal failure an average of 22 years later than those who did not receive ACE inhibitors. This beneficial effect of ACE inhibitors was also apparent in the subgroup of men with severe truncating type variants [45]. A randomized, placebo controlled trial of ramipril vs placebo in children with early Alport syndrome (microscopic hematuria alone or microalbuminuria stage) was recently reported [96]. Although not significant due to low enrollment, patients randomized to ramipril had decreased risk of progression of proteinuria and slower decline of GFR compared to patients randomized to placebo [96]. An open-label arm of this study demonstrated no safety concerns in over 200 patient years of treatment with ramipril [96].

Current clinical practice guidelines recommend treatment with an ACE inhibitor for affected males with XLAS and males and females with ARAS at the time of diagnosis if older than 12–24 months. (Table 16.2). Treatment should be started for females with XLAS and males and females with heterozygous variants in COL4A3 or COL4A4 when microalbuminuria is present [97]. Similar to other children with CKD, blood pressures

Table 16.2 Recommendations for timing of treatment with ACE inhibitors in patients with Alport syndrome

Genetic results	Indication for treatment
ARAS or male with XLAS	At time of diagnosis if age >12–24 months
XLAS female	Microalbuminuria
ADAS (heterozygous variant in COL4A3 or COL4A4)	Microalbuminuria

ARAS autosomal recessive Alport syndrome; XLAS X-linked Alport syndrome; ADAS autosomal dominant Alport syndrome

should be controlled to the 50% for age, gender, and height in children with AS in order to slow the progression of kidney disease [98].

A number of additional agents are currently in clinical development for treatment of Alport syndrome kidney disease. MicroRNAs are small, highly conserved RNAs that regulate gene expression post-transcription. One of these microRNAs, microRNA-21, is upregulated in kidneys of mice with Alport syndrome and contributes to fibrosis [99]. Treatment of Alport mice with an anti-microRNA 21 agent reduces proteinuria and kidney fibrosis and prolongs lifespan [99]. This agent is undergoing testing in a randomized phase II clinical trial in adult patients with Alport syndrome (NCT02855268). Bardoxolone is a second agent currently being tested in a randomized phase II/III clinical trial in patients with Alport syndrome (NCT03019185). Bardoxolone activates Nrf-2 and inhibits NF κB to upregulate the antioxidant response and decrease proinflammatory signaling [100]. In a clinical trial in patients with kidney disease due to type 2 diabetes, bardoxolone increased eGFR; however, the trial was halted due to increased risk of hospitalization and death from heart failure in the bardoxolone treated patients [101]. Bardoxolone treated patients also demonstrated increased proteinuria [101]. It remains controversial whether patients with Alport syndrome will have sustained benefit from treatment with bardoxolone, and long-tern studies will be required to demonstrate value in slowing progression of CKD [102].

Kidney Transplantation

In general, outcomes following kidney transplantation in patients with AS are excellent [103]. Clinicians involved in transplantation of AS patients must address two important aspects of the disease. First, the donor selection process must avoid nephrectomy in relatives at risk for ESKD. Second, post-transplant management should provide surveillance for post-transplant anti-GBM nephritis, a complication unique to AS.

Informed donor evaluation requires familiarity with the genetics of AS and the signs and symptoms of the disease. In families with XLAS, 100% of affected males and ~95% of affected females exhibit hematuria. Consequently, males who do not have hematuria are not affected, and a female without hematuria has only about a 5% risk of being affected. Given an estimated 30% risk of ESKD in women with AS [46], these women should generally be discouraged from kidney donation, even if hematuria is their only symptom. A report from Germany described five women with XLAS and one ARAS carrier who served as kidney donors [104]. One donor had proteinuria prior to transplant and all had microscopic hematuria. Three donors developed new onset hypertension and two developed new proteinuria while kidney function declined by 25–60% over 2–14 years after donation in four of the donors, highlighting the increased donor risk in this population [104].

Overt anti-GBM disease occurs in 3–5% of transplanted AS males [105]. Onset is typically within the first post-transplant year, and the disease usually results in irreversible graft failure within weeks to months of diagnosis. The risk of recurrence in subsequent allografts is high. In males with XLAS, the primary target of anti-GBM antibodies is the α5(IV) chain [106, 107]. Both males and females with ARAS can develop post-transplant anti-GBM nephritis, and in these cases the primary antibody target is the α3(IV) chain [106, 108]. The α3(IV) chain is also the target of Goodpasture autoantibodies, but the epitope identified by these antibodies differs from the α3(IV) epitope recognized by ARAS anti-GBM alloantibodies [109].

Hereditary Angiopathy with Nephropathy, Aneurysms and Cramps (HANAC Syndrome)

This autosomal dominant disorder results from variants in the *COL4A1* gene (Table 16.1) [9, 110, 111]. Complete absence of *COL4A1* is embryonic lethal in mice [112]. Missense variants that allow for expression of an abnormal α1(IV) chain lead to the development of HANAC syndrome. Kidney findings include gross and microscopic hematuria, cysts and CKD. Vascular anomalies include cerebral artery aneurysms and retinal arteriolar tortuosity. Affected individuals may have recurrent muscle cramps and elevated creatine kinase levels.

Pathology

No abnormalities of GBM ultrastructure or basement membrane expression of type IV collagen chains have been observed in kidney biopsy specimens from affected individuals with hematuria. Irregular thickening, lamellation and focal interruptions of Bowman's capsules, tubular basement membranes and interstitial capillary basement membranes have been described, as well as abnormalities of epidermal basement membranes and dermal arterial basement membranes.

Genetics

The reported variants in HANAC syndrome families affect highly conserved glycine residues in the collagenous domain of the α1(IV) chain, potentially affecting integrin binding sites. It is likely that a wider spectrum of disease will emerge in association with both *COL4A1*

and *COL4A2* variants as well as variants in other basement membrane genes as larger cohorts of patients with kidney disease phenotypes undergo whole exome and whole genome sequencing [113].

Acknowledgements The authors would like to acknowledge Dr. Clifford Kashtan for his contributions to earlier versions of this chapter.

References

1. Malone AF, Phelan PJ, Hall G, Cetincelik U, Homstad A, Alonso AS, et al. Rare hereditary COL4A3/COL4A4 variants may be mistaken for familial focal segmental glomerulosclerosis. Kidney Int. 2014;86(6):1253–9.
2. Gast C, Pengelly RJ, Lyon M, Bunyan DJ, Seaby EG, Graham N, et al. Collagen (COL4A) mutations are the most frequent mutations underlying adult focal segmental glomerulosclerosis. Nephrol Dial Transplant. 2016;31(6):961–70.
3. Li Y, Groopman EE, D'Agati V, Prakash S, Zhang J, Mizerska-Wasiak M, et al. Type IV collagen mutations in familial IgA nephropathy. Kidney Int Rep. 2020;5(7):1075–8.
4. Rana K, Wang YY, Buzza M, Tonna S, Zhang KW, Lin T, et al. The genetics of thin basement membrane nephropathy. Semin Nephrol. 2005;25:163–70.
5. Trachtman H, Weiss R, Bennett B, Griefer I. Isolated hematuria in children: indications for a renal biopsy. Kidney Int. 1984;25:94–9.
6. Schroder CH, Bontemps CM, Assmann KJM, Schuurmans-Stekhoven JH, Foidart JM, Monnens LAH, et al. Renal biopsy and family studies in 65 children with isolated hematuria. Acta Paediatr Scand. 1990;79:630–6.
7. Lang S, Stevenson B, Risdon RA. Thin basement membrane nephropathy as a cause of recurrent haematuria in childhood. Histopathology. 1990;16:331–7.
8. Piqueras AI, White RH, Raafat F, Moghal N, Milford DV. Renal biopsy diagnosis in children presenting with hematuria. Pediatr Nephrol. 1998;12:386–91.
9. Plaisier E, Gribouval O, Alamowitch S, Mougenot B, Prost C, Verpont MC, et al. COL4A1 mutations and hereditary angiopathy, nephropathy, aneurysms, and muscle cramps. N Engl J Med. 2007;357(26):2687–95.
10. Guthrie LG. "Idiopathic", or congenital, hereditary and familial hematuria. Lancet. 1902;1:1243–6.
11. Hurst AF. Hereditary familial congenital haemorrhagic nephritis occurring in sixteen individuals in three generations. Guy's Hosp Rec. 1923;3:368–70.

12. Alport AC. Hereditary familial congenital haemorrhagic nephritis. Br Med J. 1927;1:504–6.
13. Hinglais N, Grunfeld J-P, Bois LE. Characteristic ultrastructural lesion of the glomerular basement membrane in progressive hereditary nephritis (Alport's syndrome). Lab Investig. 1972;27:473–87.
14. Spear GS, Slusser RJ. Alport's syndrome: emphasizing electron microscopic studies of the glomerulus. Am J Pathol. 1972;69:213–22.
15. Churg J, Sherman RL. Pathologic characteristics of hereditary nephritis. Arch Pathol. 1973;95:374–9.
16. Olson DL, Anand SK, Landing BH, Heuser E, Grushkin CM, Lieberman E. Diagnosis of hereditary nephritis by failure of glomeruli to bind anti-glomerular basement membrane antibodies. J Pediatr. 1980;96:697–9.
17. McCoy RC, Johnson HK, Stone WJ, Wilson CB. Absence of nephritogenic GBM antigen(s) in some patients with hereditary nephritis. Kidney Int. 1982;21:642–52.
18. Kashtan C, Fish AJ, Kleppel M, Yoshioka K, Michael AF. Nephritogenic antigen determinants in epidermal and renal basement membranes of kindreds with Alport-type familial nephritis. J Clin Invest. 1986;78:1035–44.
19. Atkin CL, Hasstedt SJ, Menlove L, Cannon L, Kirschner N, Schwartz C, et al. Mapping of Alport syndrome to the long arm of the X chromosome. Am J Hum Genet. 1988;42:249–55.
20. Barker DF, Hostikka SL, Zhou J, Chow LT, Oliphant AR, Gerken SC, et al. Identification of mutations in the COL4A5 collagen gene in Alport syndrome. Science. 1990;248:1224–7.
21. Jefferson JA, Lemmink HH, Hughes AE, Hill CM, Smeets HJ, Doherty CC, et al. Autosomal dominant Alport syndrome linked to the type IV collage alpha 3 and alpha 4 genes (COL4A3 and COL4A4). Nephrol Dial Transplant. 1997;12(8):1595–9.
22. Mochizuki T, Lemmink HH, Mariyama M, Antignac C, Gubler MC, Pirson Y, et al. Identification of mutations in the alpha 3(IV) and alpha 4(IV) collagen genes in autosomal recessive Alport syndrome. Nat Genet. 1994;8(1):77–81.
23. USRDS 2013 Annual Data Report: Altas of Chronic Kidney Disease and End-Stage Renal Disease in the United States. Bethesda, MD, National Insitutes of Health NIDDK;2013.
24. Poschl E, Pollner R, Kuhn K. The genes for the alpha 1(IV) and alpha 2(IV) chains of human basement membrane collagen type IV are arranged head-to-head and separated by a bidirectional promoter of unique structure. EMBO J. 1988;7(9):2687–95.
25. Segal Y, Zhuang L, Rondeau E, Sraer JD, Zhou J. Regulation of the paired type IV collagen genes COL4A5 and COL4A6. Role of the proximal promoter region. J Biol Chem. 2001;276(15):11791–7.
26. Khoshnoodi J, Cartailler JP, Alvares K, Veis A, Hudson BG. Molecular recognition in the assembly of collagens: terminal noncollagenous domains are key recognition modules in the formation of triple helical protomers. J Biol Chem. 2006;281(50):38117–21.
27. Hudson BG. The molecular basis of Goodpasture and Alport syndromes: beacons for the discovery of the collagen IV family. J Am Soc Nephrol. 2004;15(10):2514–27.
28. Yoshioka K, Hino S, Takemura T, Maki S, Wieslander J, Takekoshi Y, et al. Type IV Collagen a5 chain: normal distribution and abnormalities in X-linked Alport syndrome revealed by monoclonal antibody. Am J Pathol. 1994;144:986–96.
29. Peissel B, Geng L, Kalluri R, Kashtan C, Rennke HG, Gallo GR, et al. Comparative distribution of the a1(IV), a5(IV) and a6(IV) collagen chains in normal human adult and fetal tissues and in kidneys from X-linked Alport syndrome patients. J Clin Invest. 1995;96:1948–57.
30. Cheong HI, Kashtan CE, Kim Y, Kleppel MM, Michael AF. Immunohistologic studies of type IV collagen in anterior lens capsules of patients with Alport syndrome. Lab Investig. 1994;70:553–7.
31. Cosgrove D, Kornak JM, Samuelson G. Expression of basement membrane type IV collagen chains during postnatal development in the murine cochlea. Hearing Res. 1996;100:21–32.
32. Zehnder AF, Adams JC, Santi PA, Kristiansen AG, Wacharasindhu C, Mann S, et al. Distribution of type IV collagen in the cochlea in Alport syndrome. Arch Otolaryngol Head Neck Surg. 2005;131:1007–13.
33. Gunwar S, Ballester F, Noelken ME, Sado Y, Ninomiya Y, Hudson BG. Glomerular basement membrane. Identification of a novel disulfide-cross-linked network of alpha3, alpha4, and alpha5 chains of type IV collagen and its implications for the pathogenesis of Alport syndrome. J Biol Chem. 1998;273(15):8767–75.
34. Zeisberg M, Khurana M, Rao VH, Cosgrove D, Rougier JP, Werner MC, et al. Stage-specific action of matrix metalloproteinases influences progressive hereditary kidney disease. PLoS Med. 2006;3(4):e100.
35. Gyoneva L, Segal Y, Dorfman KD, Barocas VH. Mechanical response of wild-type and Alport murine lens capsules during osmotic swelling. Exp Eye Res. 2013;113:87–91.
36. Meehan DT, Delimont D, Cheung L, Zallocchi M, Sansom SC, Holzclaw JD, et al. Biomechanical strain causes maladaptive gene regulation, contributing to Alport glomerular disease. Kidney Int. 2009;76(9):968–76.
37. Storey H, Savige J, Sivakumar V, Abbs S, Flinter FA. COL4A3/COL4A4 mutations and features in individuals with autosomal recessive alport syndrome. J Am Soc Nephrol. 2013;24(12):1945–54.
38. Mencarelli MA, Heidet L, Storey H, van Geel M, Knebelmann B, Fallerini C, et al. Evidence of digenic inheritance in Alport syndrome. J Med Genet. 2015;52(3):163–74.
39. Fallerini C, Dosa L, Tita R, Del Prete D, Feriozzi S, Gai G, et al. Unbiased next generation sequencing

analysis confirms the existence of autosomal dominant Alport syndrome in a relevant fraction of cases. Clin Genet. 2014;86(3):252–7.

40. Pescucci C, Mari F, Longo I, Vogiatzi P, Caselli R, Scala E, et al. Autosomal-dominant Alport syndrome: natural history of a disease due to COL4A3 or COL4A4 gene. Kidney Int. 2004; 65(5):1598–603.

41. Lemmink HH, Nillesen WN, Mochizuki T, Schroder CH, Brunner HG, van Oost BA, et al. Benign familial hematuria due to mutation of the type IV collagen alpha4 gene. J Clin Invest. 1996;98(5):1114–8.

42. Crockett DK, Pont-Kingdon G, Gedge F, Sumner K, Seamons R, Lyon E. The Alport syndrome COL4A5 variant database. Hum Mutat. 2010;31(8):E1652–7.

43. Jais JP, Knebelmann B, Giatras I, De Marchi M, Rizzoni G, Renieri A, et al. X-linked Alport syndrome: natural history in 195 families and genotype-phenotype correlations in males. J Am Soc Nephrol. 2000;11:649–57.

44. Gross O, Netzer KO, Lambrecht R, Seibold S, Weber M. Meta-analysis of genotype-phenotype correlation in X-linked Alport syndrome: impact on clnical counseling. Nephrol Dial Transpl. 2002;17:1218–27.

45. Yamamura T, Horinouchi T, Nagano C, Omori T, et al. Genotype-phenotype correlation and the influence of the genotype on response to angiotensin-targeting drugs in Japanese patients with male X-linked Alport syndrome. Kidney Int. 2020;98(6):1605–14.

46. Jais JP, Knebelmann B, Giatras I, De Marchi M, Rizzoni G, Renieri A, et al. X-linked Alport syndrome: natural history and genotype-phenotype correlations in girls and women belonging to to 195 families: a "European Community Alport Syndrome Concerted Action" study. J Am Soc Nephrol. 2003;14:2603–10.

47. Jais JP, Knebelmann B, Giatras I, De Marchi M, Rizzoni G, Renieri A, et al. X-linked Alport syndrome: natural history and genotype-phenotype correlations in girls and women belonging to 195 families: a "European Community Alport Syndrome Concerted Action" study. J Am Soc Nephrol. 2003;14(10):2603–10.

48. Marcocci E, Uliana V, Bruttini M, Artuso R, Silengo MC, Zerial M, et al. Autosomal dominant Alport syndrome: molecular analysis of the COL4A4 gene and clinical outcome. Nephrol Dial Transplant. 2009;24(5):1464–71.

49. Gubler M, Levy M, Broyer M, Naizot C, Gonzales G, Perrin D, et al. Alport's syndrome: a report of 58 cases and a review of the literature. Am J Med. 1981;70:493–505.

50. Kashtan CE, Ding J, Gregory M, Gross O, Heidet L, Knebelmann B, et al. Clinical practice recommendations for the treatment of Alport syndrome: a statement of the Alport Syndrome Research Collaborative. Pediatr Nephrol. 2013;28(1):5–11.

51. Rheault MN. Women and Alport syndrome. Pediatr Nephrol. 2012;27(1):41–6.

52. Grunfeld J-P, Noel LH, Hafez S, Droz D. Renal prognosis in women with hereditary nephritis. Clin Nephrol. 1985;23:267–71.

53. Guo C, Van Damme B, Vanrenterghem Y, Devriendt K, Cassiman JJ, Marynen P. Severe alport phenotype in a woman with two missense mutations in the same COL4A5 gene and preponderant inactivation of the X chromosome carrying the normal allele. J Clin Invest. 1995;95(4):1832–7.

54. Iijima K, Nozu K, Kamei K, Nakayama M, Ito S, Matsuoka K, et al. Severe Alport syndrome in a young woman caused by a t(X;1)(q22.3;p36.32) balanced translocation. Pediatr Nephrol. 2010;25(10):2165–70.

55. Rheault MN, Kren SM, Hartich LA, Wall M, Thomas W, Mesa HA, et al. X-inactivation modifies disease severity in female carriers of murine X-linked Alport syndrome. Nephrol Dial Transplant. 2010;25(3):764–9.

56. Wester DC, Atkin CL, Gregory MC. Alport syndrome: clinical update. J Am Acad Audiol. 1995;6:73–9.

57. Kleppel MM, Santi PA, Cameron JD, Wieslander J, Michael AF. Human tissue distribution of novel basement membrane collagen. Am J Pathol. 1989;134:813–25.

58. Cosgrove D, Samuelson G, Meehan DT, Miller C, McGee J, Walsh EJ, et al. Ultrastructural, physiological, and molecular defects in the inner ear of a gene-knockout mouse model of autosomal Alport syndrome. Hearing Res. 1998;121:84–98.

59. Harvey SJ, Mount R, Sado Y, Naito I, Ninomiya Y, Harrison R, et al. The inner ear of dogs with X-linked nephritis provides clues to the pathogenesis of hearing loss in X-linked Alport syndrome. Am J Pathol. 2001;159(3):1097–104.

60. Merchant SN, Burgess BJ, Adams JC, Kashtan CE, Gregory MC, Santi PA, et al. Temporal bone histopathology in alport syndrome. Laryngoscope. 2004;114(9):1609–18.

61. Gratton MA, Rao VH, Meehan DT, Askew C, Cosgrove D. Matrix metalloproteinase dysregulation in the stria vascularis of mice with Alport syndrome: implications for capillary basement membrane pathology. Am J Pathol. 2005;166(5):1465–74.

62. Nielsen CE. Lenticonus anterior and Alport's syndrome. Arch Ophthalmol. 1978;56:518–30.

63. Colville DJ, Savige J. Alport syndrome. A review of the ocular manifestations. Ophthalmic Genet. 1997;18(4):161–73.

64. Streeten BW, Robinson MR, Wallace R, Jones DB. Lens capsule abnormalities in Alport's syndrome. Arch Ophthalmol. 1987;105:1693–7.

65. Kato T, Watanabe Y, Nakayasu K, Kanai A, Yajima Y. The ultrastructure of the lens capsule abnormalities in Alport's syndrome. Jpn J Ophthalmol. 1998;42:401–5.

66. Perrin D, Jungers P, Grunfeld JP, Delons S, Noel LH, Zenatti C. Perimacular changes in Alport's syndrome. Clin Nephrol. 1980;13:163–7.

67. Rhys C, Snyers B, Pirson Y. Recurrent corneal erosion associated with Alport's syndrome. Kidney Int. 1997;52:208–11.
68. Burke JP, Clearkin LG, Talbot JF. Recurrent corneal epithelial erosions in Alport's syndrome. Acta Ophthalmol. 1991;69:555–7.
69. Teekhasaenee C, Nimmanit S, Wutthiphan S, Vareesangthip K, Laohapand T, Malasitr P, et al. Posterior polymorphous dystrophy and Alport syndrome. Ophthalmology. 1991;98:1207–15.
70. Antignac C, Heidet L. Mutations in Alport syndrome associated with diffuse esophageal leiomyomatosis. Contrib Nephrol. 1996;117:172–82.
71. Antignac C, Knebelmann B, Druout L, Gros F, Deschenes G, Hors-Cayla M-C, et al. Deletions in the COL4A5 collagen gene in X-linked Alport syndrome: characterization of the pathological transcripts in non-renal cells and correlation with disease expression. J Clin Invest. 1994;93:1195–207.
72. Zhou J, Mochizuki T, Smeets H, Antignac C, Laurila P, de Paepe A, et al. Deletion of the paired a5(IV) and a6(IV) collagen genes in inherited smooth muscle tumors. Science. 1993;261:1167–9.
73. Segal Y, Peissel B, Renieri A, de Marchi M, Ballabio A, Pei Y, et al. LINE-1 elements at the sites of molecular rearrangements in Alport syndrome-diffuse leiomyomatosis. Am J Hum Genet. 1999;64:62–29.
74. Sa MJ, Fieremans N, de Brouwer AP, Sousa R, et al. Deletion of the 5'exons of COL4A6 is not needed for the development of diffuse leiomyomatosis in patients with Alport syndrome. J Med Genet. 2013;50(11):745–53.
75. Jonsson JJ, Renieri A, Gallagher PG, Kashtan CE, Cherniske EM, Bruttini M, et al. Alport syndrome, mental retardation, midface hypoplasia, and elliptocytosis: a new X linked contiguous gene deletion syndrome? J Med Genet. 1998;35(4):273–8.
76. Kashtan CE, Segal Y, Flinter F, Makanjuola D, Gan JS, Watnick T. Aortic abnormalities in males with Alport syndrome. Nephrol Dial Transplant. 2010;25(11):3554–60.
77. Randles MJ, Collinson S, Starborg T, Mironov A, Krendel M, Konigshausen E, et al. Three-dimensional electron microscopy reveals the evolution of glomerular barrier injury. Sci Rep. 2016;6:35068.
78. Kashtan CE, Kleppel MM, Gubler MC. Immunohistologic findings in Alport syndrome. Contrib Nephrol. 1996;117:142–53.
79. Martin P, Heiskari N, Zhou J, Leinonen A, Tumelius T, Hertz JM, et al. High mutation detection rate in the COL4A5 collagen gene in suspected Alport syndrome using PCR and direct DNA sequencing. J Am Soc Nephrol. 1998;9:2291–301.
80. Gross O, Schulze-Lohoff E, Koepke ML, Beirowski B, Addicks K, Bloch W, et al. Antifibrotic, nephroprotective potential of ACE inhibitor vs AT1 antagonist in a murine model of renal fibrosis. Nephrol Dial Transplant. 2004;19(7):1716–23.
81. Gross O, Beirowski B, Koepke ML, Kuck J, Reiner M, Addicks K, et al. Preemptive ramipril therapy delays renal failure and reduces renal fibrosis in COL4A3-knockout mice with Alport syndrome. Kidney Int. 2003;63(2):438–46.
82. Gross O, Koepke ML, Beirowski B, Schulze-Lohoff E, Segerer S, Weber M. Nephroprotection by antifibrotic and anti-inflammatory effects of the vasopeptidase inhibitor AVE7688. Kidney Int. 2005;68:456–63.
83. Sayers R, Kalluri R, Rodgers KD, Shield CF, Meehan DT, Cosgrove D. Role for transforming growth factor-beta 1 in Alport renal disease progression. Kidney Int. 1999;56:1662–73.
84. Ninichuk V, Gross O, Reichel C, Kandoga A, Pawar RD, Ciubar R, et al. Delayed chemokine receptor 1 blockade prolongs survival in collagen 4A3-deficient miche with Alport disease. J Am Soc Nephrol. 2005;16:977–85.
85. Zeisberg M, Bottiglio C, Kumar N, Maeshima Y, Strutz F, Muller GA, et al. Bone morphogenic protein-7 inhibits progression of chronic renal fibrosis associated with two genetic mouse models. Am J Physiol Renal Physiol. 2003;285(6):F1060–7.
86. Sugimoto H, Mundel TM, Sund M, Xie L, Cosgrove D, Kalluri R. Bone-marrow-derived stem cells repair basement membrane collagen defects and reverse genetic kidney disease. Proc Natl Acad Sci U S A. 2006;103(19):7321–6.
87. Chen D, Jefferson B, Harvey SJ, Zheng K, Gartley CJ, Jacobs RM, et al. Cyclosporine a slows the progressive renal disease of alport syndrome (X-linked hereditary nephritis): results from a canine model. J Am Soc Nephrol. 2003;14(3):690–8.
88. Charbit M, Gubler MC, Dechaux M, Gagnadoux MF, Grunfeld JP, Niaudet P. Cyclosporin therapy in patients with Alport syndrome. Pediatr Nephrol. 2007;22(1):57–63.
89. Massella L, Muda AO, Legato A, Di Zazzo G, Giannakakis K, Emma F. Cyclosporine A treatment in patients with Alport syndrome: a single-center experience. Pediatr Nephrol. 2010;25(7):1269–75.
90. Grodecki KM, Gains MJ, Baumal R, Osmond DH, Cotter BV, V. E., Jacobs RM. Treatment of X-linked hereditary nephritis in Samoyed dogs with angiotensin converting enzyme inhibitor. J Comp Pathol. 1997;117:209–25.
91. Cohen EP, Lemann J. In hereditary nephritis angiotensin-converting enzyme inhibition decreases proteinuria and may slow the rate of progression. Am J Kid Dis. 1996;27:199–203.
92. Proesmans W, Van Dyck M. Enalapril in children with Alport syndrome. Pediatr Nephrol. 2004;19(3):271–5.
93. Webb NJ, Lam C, Shahinfar S, Strehlau J, Wells TG, Gleim GW, et al. Efficacy and safety of losartan in children with Alport syndrome—results from a subgroup analysis of a prospective, randomized, placebo- or amlodipine-controlled trial. Nephrol Dial Transplant. 2011;26(8):2521–6.

94. Webb NJ, Shahinfar S, Wells TG, Massaad R, Gleim GW, McCrary Sisk C, et al. Losartan and enalapril are comparable in reducing proteinuria in children with Alport syndrome. Pediatr Nephrol. 2013;28(5):737–43.

95. Gross O, Licht C, Anders HJ, Hoppe B, Beck B, Tonshoff B, et al. Early angiotensin-converting enzyme inhibition in Alport syndrome delays renal failure and improves life expectancy. Kidney Int. 2012;81(5):494–501.

96. Gross O, Tonshoff B, Weber LT, Pape L, Latta K, Fehrenbach H, et al. A multicenter, randomized, placebo-controlled, double-blind phase 3 trial with open-arm comparison indicates safety and efficacy of nephroprotective therapy with ramipril in children with Alport's syndrome. Kidney Int. 2020;97(6):1275–86.

97. Kashtan CE, Gross O. Clinical practice recommendations for the diagnosis and management of Alport syndrome in children, adolescents, and young adults-an update for 2020. Pediatr Nephrol. 2021;36(3):711–9.

98. Wuhl E, Trivelli A, Picca S, Litwin M, Peco-Antic A, Zurowska A, et al. Strict blood-pressure control and progression of renal failure in children. N Engl J Med. 2009;361(17):1639–50.

99. Gomez IG, MacKenna DA, Johnson BG, Kaimal V, Roach AM, Ren S, et al. Anti-microRNA-21 oligonucleotides prevent Alport nephropathy progression by stimulating metabolic pathways. J Clin Invest. 2015;125(1):141–56.

100. Wang YY, Yang YX, Zhe H, He ZX, Zhou SF. Bardoxolone methyl (CDDO-Me) as a therapeutic agent: an update on its pharmacokinetic and pharmacodynamic properties. Drug Des Devel Ther. 2014;8:2075–88.

101. de Zeeuw D, Akizawa T, Audhya P, Bakris GL, Chin M, Christ-Schmidt H, et al. Bardoxolone methyl in type 2 diabetes and stage 4 chronic kidney disease. N Engl J Med. 2013;369(26):2492–503.

102. Baigent C, Lennon R. Should we increase GFR with bardoxolone in alport syndrome? J Am Soc Nephrol. 2018;29(2):357–9.

103. Temme J, Kramer A, Jager KJ, Lange K, Peters F, Muller GA, et al. Outcomes of male patients with Alport syndrome undergoing renal replacement therapy. Clin J Am Soc Nephrol. 2012;7(12):1969–76.

104. Gross O, Weber M, Fries JW, Muller GA. Living donor kidney transplantation from relatives with mild urinary abnormalities in Alport syndrome: long-term risk, benefit and outcome. Nephrol Dial Transplant. 2009;24(5):1626–30.

105. Kashtan CE. Renal transplantation in patients with Alport syndrome. Pediatr Transplant. 2006;10(6):651–7.

106. Brainwood D, Kashtan C, Gubler MC, Turner AN. Targets of alloantibodies in Alport anti-glomerular basement membrane disease after renal transplantation. Kidney Int. 1998;53:762–6.

107. Dehan P, Van Den Heuvel LPWJ, Smeets HJM, Tryggvason K, Foidart J-M. Identification of post-transplant anti-a5(IV) collagen alloantibodies in X-linked Alport syndrome. Nephrol Dial Transpl. 1996;11:1983–8.

108. Kalluri R, van den Heuvel LP, Smeets HJM, Schroder CH, Lemmink HH, Boutaud A, et al. A COL4A3 gene mutation and post-transplant anti-a3(IV) collagen alloantibodies in Alport syndrome. Kidney Int. 1995;47:1199–204.

109. Wang XP, Fogo AB, Colon S, Giannico G, Abul-Ezz SR, Miner JH, et al. Distinct Epitopes for Anti-Glomerular Basement Membrane Alport Alloantibodies and Goodpasture Autoantibodies within the Noncollagenous Domain of {alpha}3(IV) Collagen: a Janus-Faced Antigen. J Am Soc Nephrol. 2005;16:3563–71.

110. Plaisier E, Chen Z, Gekeler F, Benhassine S, Dahan K, Marro B, et al. Novel COL4A1 mutations associated with HANAC syndrome: a role for the triple helical CB3[IV] domain. Am J Med Genet A. 2010;152A(10):2550–5.

111. Alamowitch S, Plaisier E, Favrole P, Prost C, Chen Z, Van Agtmael T, et al. Cerebrovascular disease related to COL4A1 mutations in HANAC syndrome. Neurology. 2009;73(22):1873–82.

112. Poschl E, Schlotzer-Schrehardt U, Brachvogel B, Saito K, Ninomiya Y, Mayer U. Collagen IV is essential for basement membrane stability but dispensable for initiation of its assembly during early development. Development. 2004;131(7):1619–28.

113. Gale DP, Oygar DD, Lin F, Oygar PD, Khan N, Connor TM, et al. A novel COL4A1 frameshift mutation in familial kidney disease: the importance of the C-terminal NC1 domain of type IV collagen. Nephrol Dial Transplant. 2016;31(11):1908–14.

IgA Nephropathy

17

Rosanna Coppo and Licia Peruzzi

Introduction

Primary IgA nephropathy (IgAN) is defined by the prevalence of immunoglobulin A over the others immunoglobulins in glomerular deposits as described by Berger et al. in 1968 [1]. IgAN is the commonest glomerular disease in children and adolescents who undergo renal biopsy because of isolated microscopic hematuria or hematuria with non-nephrotic proteinuria. After its initial identification, IgAN was considered a benign renal disease in adults and even more so in children. With longer follow-up in both age groups, a significant percentage of cases had a worsening of renal function, including the need for renal replacement therapy (RRT). The interest in IgAN in children increased with the recognition that most subjects with IgAN entering a chronic dialysis program were young adults [2], who displayed a slow renal function decline over decades (about 25% of the cases need dialysis in 20 years) [3]. It was therefore clear that the primary pathogenic events occurred in many cases in children. Hence, detecting IgAN at the beginning of its natural history in childhood may offer an important opportunity for early treatment, limiting factors favoring progression and controlling the complications, maximizing the benefits during childhood, and perhaps more importantly, for adulthood.

Epidemiology

The prevalence of IgAN in children varies in different reports, mostly due to the criteria for performing renal biopsy, ranging from routine practice after detection of urine anomalies by school screening programs to limiting renal biopsy to patients that have developed proteinuria. It is likely that cases of IgAN originating in the pediatric age group are missed because most patients are asymptomatic and do not undergo regular urine screening. IgAN is more frequently reported in Japan and Korea, where screening is routine, and IgAN is reported in 32 and 40% of renal biopsies in children [4, 5]. In contrast, the percentage of renal biopsies with IgAN in children are 20–26% in Europe [6], 17–20% in China, 14% in India, 10% in North America, 14% in South America, and 2.8% in Africa [7].

Data on incidence in children vary from 5 to 140 per million children/year [6, 8], similar to adult figures. The most recent biopsy series from global registries conclude that incidence varia-

R. Coppo
Fondazione Ricerca Molinette, Turin, Italy
e-mail: rosanna.coppo@unito.it

L. Peruzzi (✉)
Fondazione Ricerca Molinette, Turin, Italy

Pediatric Nephrology Unit, "Regina Margherita Children's Department", City of Health and Science University Hospital, Turin, Italy
e-mail: licia.peruzzi@unito.it

© The Author(s), under exclusive license to Springer Nature Switzerland AG 2023
F. Schaefer, L. A. Greenbaum (eds.), *Pediatric Kidney Disease*,
https://doi.org/10.1007/978-3-031-11665-0_17

tion is mainly due to biopsy policy and attitudes, and not secondary to true ethnic differences [9–11], although genetic studies seem to suggest a Northbound and Eastbound gradient of IgAN susceptibility [12]. Moreover, there is evidence in specific areas of China that incidence may vary based on humidity, air contaminants and other pollutants, such as polycyclic aromatic hydrocarbons [13].

Genetic Background

Familial aggregation of IgAN cases and accumulation of IgAN in certain populations suggest a complex heritable component. Familial clustering is consistent with autosomal dominant inheritance with variable penetrance of a polygenic trait, often manifesting as other autoimmune diseases. Familial cases often have a worse outcome.

Approximately 70% of IgAN subjects and 35% of their healthy relatives in different ethnic cohorts have Gd-IgA levels higher than geographically matched controls, suggesting that Gd-IgA by itself is not sufficient to induce the disease [14]. Gd-IgA has a greater specificity, sensitivity and heritability than total serum IgA [15].

Family linkage studies identified 6q22-23 as a candidate locus [16] and additional loci at 4q26-31, 17q12-22 and 2q36, but no causal underlying mutation was observed.

Next generation sequencing in the last years provided the technical tools to rapidly detect genetic variants at genome scale (whole genome sequencing) or on coding regions (whole exome sequencing), making possible large genome-wide association studies (GWAS) on multiethnic cohorts.

This powerful unbiased approach, [17, 18] supported by strict statistical methods and precise population stratification, was employed to explore disease association of common variants single nucleotide polymorphism (SNP) along the entire genome of large populations. Five large GWAS (reviewed in [17]) were carried out in populations of European and East Asian origin, evidencing strong signals in chromosome region 6p21, encoding for HLA genes involved in antigen presentation and immune response. HLA-DQA1 and DQB1 genes, which give origin to at least four HLA alleles, were associated with IgAN: DQA1*0101 and DQB1*0301 as risk alleles and DQA1*0102 and DQB1*0201 as protective [18].

A role of the non-HLA loci 1q32, encoding complement factor H (CFH), a critical inhibitor of the alternative pathway of complement, and five CFH-related (CFHR) genes [19] was identified.

The deletion in *CFHR3* and *CFHR1* genes, encoding for activators of the alternative complement pathway with a competitive effect on CFH, is associated with higher levels of CFH, lower complement activation and lower C3 deposition, with a protective effect on C3 activation in IgAN [20–22].

Other non-HLA regions associated with IgAN are 22q12, coding for several cytokines, 17p13, for TNFSF13, 8p23, for an alpha-defensin gene, 16p11, for alpha-integrins ITGAM and ITGAX, 1p13, for VAV37 and 9q34, for CARD9 [17]. In the Chinese population, other loci were found in 3q27.3, coding for ST6GAL1, in 11p11.2, for ACCS and 8q22.3, for ODF1-KLF10 [23].

Candidate genes are involved in antigen processing and presentation, innate immunity, NFkB signaling, gut mucosal immunity, IgA molecule biology and dysregulation of alternative complement pathway. Altogether these loci explain 6–8% of the risk, overlapping with other immune mediated diseases [18]. Genetic risk correlates with age at diagnosis and is associated with pathogen diversity, in particular helminths [24].

Moreover IgAN risk score varies in parallel to the geographic distribution of the disease, with a northbound and eastbound gradient, progressively increasing at growing distance from Africa and moving east [12].

Using whole exome sequencing, Zhou [25] in the Han Chinese population identified three candidate susceptibility genes in the non-HLA region (FBXL21, CCR6, and STAT3) and one in the HLA region (GABBR1), involved in modulation of IgA synthesis, response to mucosal infections and gut inflammatory response.

Pathogenesis

The development of IgAN represents the final event of a complex pathogenetic cascade, called the "four hit model", putting together the principles of an immune disease, with a genetic background and an environmental exposure. This causes inappropriate production of aberrantly glycosylated IgA1 (first hit), followed by a specific IgG response (second hit) and IgA immune-complexes circulation and glomerular deposition (third hit). The glomerular inflammatory response is elicited, with recruitment of multiple mechanisms leading to glomerular damage (fourth hit) (Fig. 17.1).

IgA is the most abundant immunoglobulin synthesized by the mucosal associated lymphoid tissue (MALT) and plays a major role for mucosal antigen defense and host commensal homeostasis.

IgA is synthetized in two subclasses, IgA1 and IgA2, which differ by an insertion of 18 amino acids in the hinge region between CH1 and CH2, which is only present in IgA1 [26] (Fig. 17.2a, b). The amino acid sequence includes three threonine and three serine residues bound to five short O-linked oligosaccharide chains. The O-glycosylation consists of a core N-acetyl galactosamine (GalNAc) which occurs alone or extended with β1,3 linked Gal or further with sialic acid in α2,3 or α2,6 linkage [27, 28]. In healthy subjects, serum IgA1 consists of a mixture of molecules with different O-glycoforms, whereas in patients with IgAN there are abnormal IgA1 O-glycoforms deficient in galactose (Gd-IgA1) with a high frequency of O-glycans

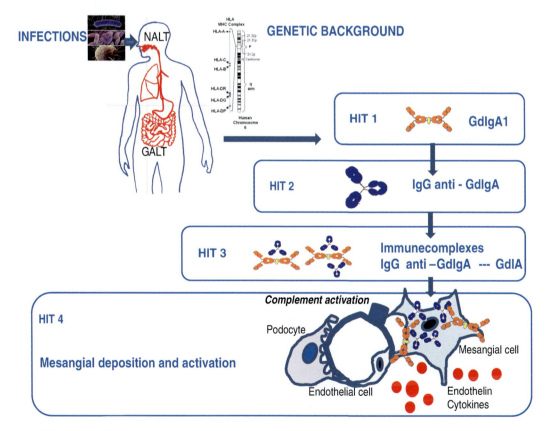

Fig. 17.1 The multihit pathogenic model

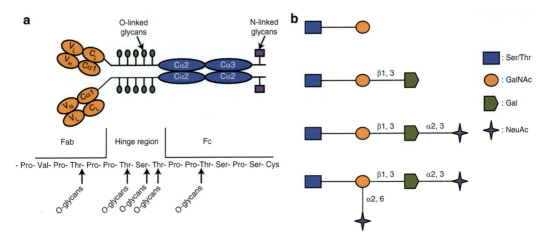

Fig. 17.2 The IgA molecule structure: (**a**) magnification of the hinge region. (**b**) Different O-glycoforms of circulating IgA1 molecules in IgAN

consisting of GalNAc alone [29–31]. Gd-IgA1 is detected in sera of up to 80% of patients with IgAN, [26, 29–33] and is prevalent in mesangial deposits of these patients [26].

The altered glycosylation of the IgA molecule confers different functional and effector mechanisms such as activation of the alternate complement pathway, Fc receptor binding, polymerization capacity and mesangial deposition due to increased affinity for matrix components. Gd-IgA1 has a hereditary component in either sporadic or familial IgAN in adults and children, [14, 15] indicated by increased plasma levels detected in healthy relatives of patients [14, 34].

Since altered glycosylation is not due to a different amino acid sequence of the hinge region [35], research efforts focused on genetically determined modifications of the B lymphocytes enzyme β 1,3-galactosyltransferase (encoded by *C1GALT1*), responsible for the terminal galactosylation of GalNAc on O-linked glycans [36] or the galactosyl transferase enzyme chaperon Cosmc (encoded by *C1GALT1C1*), but the results were not consistent with a clear genetic modification of these enzymes [34, 37].

Post-transcriptional regulation may be due to the modulatory effect of micro-RNAs, small molecules that can decrease the transcription of RNAs. Increased levels of miRNA-148b favoring the expression of the enzyme C1GALT have been detected in patients with IgAN [38].

Gd-IgA1 can circulate as monomers or participate in macromolecular self-aggregates and can elicit an IgG autoimmune response, which represents the second pathogenetic hit [29, 39]. Serum Gd-IgA1 and IgG autoantibodies have been found to correlate with disease severity and progression [40–44]. It is of interest that these IgG not only react with Gd-IgA1, but may cross-react with bacterial or viral cell-surface GalNAc-containing glycoproteins, suggesting a possible mechanism of mimicry [45]. The co-deposition of IgG in glomeruli has been demonstrated by confocal microscopy even in cases negative for routine immunofluorescence and correlates with endocapillary proliferation [46, 47].

The circulating immune-complexes (IgAIC) formed by polymeric Gd-IgA and IgG (the third hit) escape clearance by hepatic receptors and have a preferential renal deposition due to reactivity with mesangial matrix components fibronectin, laminin and collagen. The deposit on mesangial cells induces a proliferative response, matrix expansion and local inflammation [48]. IgAIC correlate with disease activity in adults and children with IgAN [40].

Macromolecular IgA also originate from interactions between human IgA1 and CD89, the soluble form of the IgA receptor [49]. The IgA1–CD89 complex binds to the transferrin 1 receptors (CD71) and transglutaminase 2 receptors (TGase2) expressed on the mesangial cell surface and increase immune deposits and inflammation [50].

The fourth pathogenic hit occurs after the renal deposition of IgAIC, Complement activation pathways are triggered and the local inflammatory process is further amplified, with release of cytokines, chemokines and inflammatory mediators acting not only on mesangial cells but also on endothelium and podocytes [51]. Mesangial cells and mesangial matrix proliferation induce a derangement of the glomerular spatial relationships, which influences podocyte behavior. Mesangial-podocyte crosstalk has been proposed as a trigger of a podocytopathy and tubulointerstitial damage, with consequent occurrence of proteinuria and disease progression [52]. In this process, activation of the RAS system also plays a crucial role [53].

The Mucosal Immunity in IgAN

The relationship between IgAN and the mucosal associated lymphoid tissue (MALT) has been considered shortly after the identification of this glomerular disease because IgA is the main product of the MALT and visible hematuria in IgAN frequently occurs during mucosal infections. About half the lymphocytes of the immune system are located in the MALT, which is at the interface with the environment [54], and thus has a major role in the defense against environmental microbes and induction of immunotolerance [55]. The principal locations of the MALT are the gut-associated lymphoid tissue (GALT) and the nasopharynx-associated lymphoid tissue (NALT), which are thought to be involved in the pathogenesis of IgAN. The GALT has up to 70% of the body's immunocytes and consists of lymphoid follicles, aggregated at the Peyer's patches, in the distal jejunum and the ileum [56]. The NALT is located in the pharynx, principally in Waldeyer's tonsillar ring, of which tonsils are the major component [57].

Peyer's patches and tonsils are the most common inductive sites where antigens prime naïve B-cells through T-cell–dependent and T-cell–independent mechanisms [58]. T cell–independent production of IgA is primarily stimulated by interleukins (IL-6 and IL-10), transforming growth factor (TGF-β), B cell activating factor (BAFF, or BLyS), and a proliferative inducing ligand (APRIL). BAFF and APRIL promote the differentiation of B cells, with class switching from IgM to IgA1 after binding to the TNF receptor homolog transmembrane activator (TACI) [59]. Activated B-cells reach the mucosal inductive sites, where they become effector cells, maturing into IgA-secreting plasma cells in the intestinal lamina propria. They produce IgA dimers, which bind a secretory component, creating secretory IgA, which is then secreted into the lumen.

The innate immune system recognizes pathogens, particularly through the activation of Toll-like receptors (TLRs), which increase IgA synthesis via promoting secretion of BAFF and enhancing lymphocytic infiltration and the expression of histocompatibility complex class II molecules on B-cells. Persistent activation of TLRs may favor increased synthesis of Gd-IgA1 in prone subjects [60].

There is a tonsil-kidney axis in IgAN. Some of the IgA eluted from renal tissue in patients with IgAN originates in tonsillar cells [61], and the number of IgA producing plasma cells in tonsils is higher in patients with IgAN than in controls [62]. These plasma cells create memory cells and may migrate to the bone marrow, where they synthesize and release Gd-IgA into the circulation. Persistent IgA deposits and hematuria were induced in mice by intranasal administration followed by systemic challenge of the respiratory Sendai virus after induction of defective mucosal tolerance [63, 64]. A microbiome study found similar tonsillar microbes in patients with IgAN and subjects with recurrent tonsillitis [65], but this observation was not confirmed [66]. Studies have shown activation of TLR9, which recognizes unmethylated DNA sequences in bacterial and viral DNA cytosine-phosphorothioate-guanine oligodeoxynucleotides (CpG ODN) in the tonsils of patients with IgAN. TLR9 expression was associated with disease activity and clinical outcome after tonsillectomy [67]. The TLR9 ligand CpG-ODN increased the expressions of APRIL, favoring the delivery of nephritogenic IgA. Human B cells infected with Epstein-Barr virus (EBV) secrete Gd-IgA1. It has recently been hypothesized that EBV infected IgA+ cells, which have homing receptors for targeting the upper respiratory tract, may be the source of galactose-deficient IgA1. Moreover, the temporal sequence of racial-specific differences in Epstein-Barr virus infection may explain the racial disparity in the prevalence of IgAN [68].

The gut-kidney axis in IgAN [69] with dysregulated GALT was postulated after the observation of the increased association of IgAN with celiac disease [70]. This hypothesis was supported by a GWAS study showing that most loci associated with IgAN are also associated with immune-mediated inflammatory bowel diseases, maintenance of the intestinal barrier and response to gut pathogens [18]. In experimental transgenic mice overexpressing BAFF and presenting with hyper-IgA, the development of IgAN is conditioned by alimentary components and intestinal microbiota [71].

The intestinal microbiota can modulate the GALT [72] and different microbiota patterns have been reported in patients with progressive IgAN [73]. Increased intestinal permeability was detected in children and adults with IgAN [74, 75], together with high levels of IgA anti-alimentary antigens [76]. Chronic enteritis, reported in China as the second most common cause of mucosal infection, present in one third of cases of IgAN, may favor increased release of bacterial lipopolysaccharide (LPS), which can interfere with the chaperone gene Cosms, leading to production of Gd-IgA1 [77]. This hypothesis is also supported by increased expression of TLR4 (LPS specific ligand) in peripheral mononuclear cells in children and adults with IgAN [78, 79].

GALT may also be triggered by abnormal response to alimentary antigens, as detected in experimental models of oral immunization in mice [80]. Mice fed a gluten-rich diet had significantly greater IgA mesangial deposits than animals fed a gluten-free diet since birth [81]. IgA anti-alimentary components and IgAIC were reduced after a gluten-free diet in subjects with IgAN [82]. The role of gliadin was confirmed in IgA1/CD89 double transgenic mice that develop spontaneous IgAN; administration of a gluten-free diet for three generations prevented IgA deposits. The same study reported high levels of anti-gliadin IgA was associated with increased proteinuria in patients with IgAN. These data suggest a role of GALT hyper-response to intestinal alimentary components or microbes in IgAN.

Complement Activation in IgAN

The presence of C3 mesangial deposits with IgA deposits has been observed since the first description of IgAN [1], but there are many recent insights into the role of complement in IgAN. The alternative pathway is the main cascade activator in IgAN and most responsible for C3 deposition, which helps to differentiate incidental IgA mesangial deposits from true IgAN. C3 deposition is found in up to 90% of biopsies, frequently in association with C4d and usually without C1q, indicating the involvement of the alternative and lectin pathways. Properdin is present in a very high percentage of biopsies (70–100%), and CFH is present with variable frequency (30–90%) [21, 83, 84]. CFHR proteins may modulate CFH activity and *CFHR1* and *CFHR3* deletions in locus 1q32 were found to limit the alternative complement pathway activation, conferring a protective effect for development of IgAN [20]. IgAN cases with significantly higher plasma levels of FHR1 were more likely to have progressive disease [20, 85], and FHR5 plasma levels directly correlated with histologic markers of kidney injury [85–88]. Increased C3 breakdown products and IgA/C3 ratio were found to be associated with worse outcomes [89, 90].

The activation of the lectin pathway is indicated by the presence of C4d without C1q, and the detection of mannose-binding lectin (Man),

though not coincident. C4d is present in the renal biopsies of most actively progressive patients with IgAN and is a significant risk predictor for children and adults [91–94]. The terminal complement products C5-C9 may play an additive inflammatory role in the pathogenesis of IgAN; they are detected in biopsies and in in vitro experimental models [95].

Systemic oxidative stress is triggered by circulating IgAIC containing Gd-IgA1 [96]. Elevated levels of advanced oxidation protein products (AOPP) have been detected in sera of patients with IgAN and found to be correlated with the amount of proteinuria and with decreased renal function during follow-up. The association of high levels of Gd-IgA1 and AOPPs represents a risk factor for progression of IgAN.

Acquired factors which modulate the immune response are likely to be activated in some patients, with increased production of IL-4 and IL-5 by Th2 lymphocytes in IgAN leading to synthesis of Gd-IgA1 which is eventually deposited in the glomeruli.

The interaction of circulating macromolecules containing Gd-IgA1 with Fcα receptors on mesangial cells results in cellular activation and phlogistic mediator synthesis, including a variety of cytokines (IL6, platelet-derived growth factor [PDGF], IL1, TNF-α, TGFβ), vasoactive factors (prostaglandins, thromboxane, leukotrienes, endothelin, PAF, NO) and chemokines (MCP-1, IL-8, MCP-1, RANTES). The influx of monocytes and lymphocytes into the mesangium is enhanced by the C3 co-deposition.

The immune activation of mesangial cells leads to cell contraction, hemodynamic modifications and activation of the RAS [53]. Angiotensin II enhances the release of cytokines and chemokines and potentiates the actions of PDGF and TGFβ as growth factors for mesangial cells, further favoring proliferation and accumulation of extracellular matrix, and ultimately promoting sclerosis. In IgAN, there is no definite evidence of altered ACE genotype frequency, though some studies reported an association of one genotype (DD) with a faster rate of progression in IgAN and a better response to ACE-I treatment [97, 98].

Proteomics identified uromodulin as a urinary marker distinguishing IgAN from healthy controls and other glomerular diseases [99].

Renal Pathology of Children with IgAN

Light Microscopy

Primary IgAN typically presents with focal or diffuse proliferation of mesangial cells and expansion of the extracellular matrix. In both adults and children, endocapillary hypercellularity or extracapillary proliferation with crescent formation can be detected in active cases, while glomerular hyalinosis and segmental or global sclerosis or tubulointerstitial fibrosis are most prominent in patients with long lasting disease. The histological features in children are usually mild or moderate, and the rapidly progressive forms with crescents involving more than 50% of glomeruli are rare. Interstitial and arteriolar changes are infrequent. The variability of pathologic features is influenced by the approach for identifying patients to receive a renal biopsy since mild lesions are common in children with asymptomatic, microscopic hematuria detected by school screening programs [4, 5].

Several authors have proposed histological classifications of IgAN based on individual lesion intensity or extension, but all had a low clinicpathological correlation [100].

The Oxford classification for IgAN is predictive of clinical outcome in children and adults with IgAN, and it is presently universally adopted [101, 102]. It consists of a combined score of four lesions (mesangial and endocapillary hypercellularity, segmental glomerulosclerosis and tubular atrophy/interstitial fibrosis), MEST, which are predictive of outcome independent of clinical assessment (Fig. 17.3a–d). The value of crescents was not found in the original cohort, but was shown in a subsequent large study of more than 3000 patients with IgAN [103], leading to the use of the combined MEST-C score in patients of any age [52, 104].

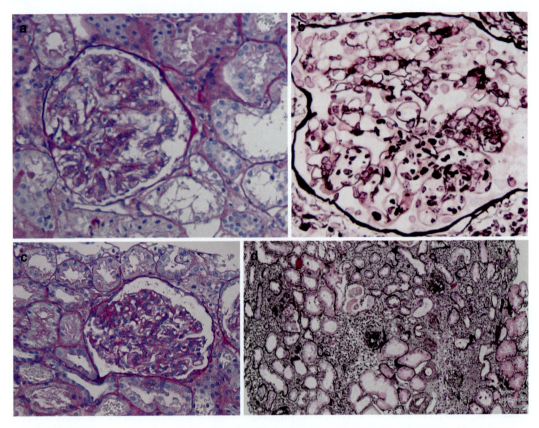

Fig. 17.3 Pathology features in IgA nephropathy. (**a**) Mesangial hypercellularity. (**b**) Endocapillary hypercellularity. (**c**) Segmental glomerulosclerosis. (**d**) Tubular atrophy/interstitial fibrosis

Although children with IgAN had more proliferative lesions and fewer chronic changes than adults, the predictive value of each lesion in the Oxford IgAN clinicopathological classification on renal survival was similar in children and adults [105].

Several validation studies have confirmed the value of the Oxford classification in children with IgAN [106–109]. The VALIGA study investigated 1147 patients with IgAN and validated the MEST score over a long-term follow-up, confirming the value of this pathology classification across the whole spectrum of IgAN, and maintaining the predictive value decades after the initial renal biopsy [110]. The search for clinical-pathological correlation and predictive value on outcome using small pediatric cohorts presents several limitations for a correct interpretation of the renal biopsy findings.

The indication to perform the renal biopsy may select cases of different severity and potential risk. Moreover, the delay from clinical onset to renal biopsy detected different lesions, with higher mesangial and endothelial hypercellularity and more frequent crescents in early renal biopsies and greater segmental sclerosis and tubulointerstitial changes in delayed biopsies. The most important feature associated with outcome, in both children and adults, is tubulointerstitial damage, a marker of irreversible changes. However, much of the interest is on the predictive value of potentially reversible pathologic features, which may support a decision to initiate therapy. This occurs with podocytopathic lesions (tip lesions and podocyte hypertrophy), which, though associated with more severe proteinuria at onset and worse outcome, improved after immunosuppressive treatment [52].

Immunofluorescence

By definition, IgA is the dominant immunoglobulin present in all glomeruli (Fig. 17.4), and it is almost exclusively polymeric IgA1 with λ light chains. C3 is detectable in up to 70% of renal biopsies with the same distribution as IgA. IgG is present in 50–70% of the renal biopsies, often as intense as IgA, a feature that explains why this disease was initially called IgA–IgG nephropathy. IgM deposits are also found, but less commonly [31–66%]. The early complement components, such as C1q and C4, are rarely detected, but when present they are invariably associated with IgG and/or IgM.

The spatial distribution of IgA and C3 in mesangial deposits, studied by confocal laser microscopy, shows IgA and C3 coated by IgA in milder cases. A stronger deposition of C3c and C4d was reported in IgAN with endocapillary proliferation and active disease [91, 92, 94]. As mentioned before, the presence of C4d deposits was found to be associated with more rapid progression of IgAN in both adults and children [111]. C4d deposits often are associated with signs of thrombotic microangiopathy, suggesting that the interaction of Gd-IgA1 with endothelial cells triggers local inflammation, and activation of the complement and coagulation pathways [112].

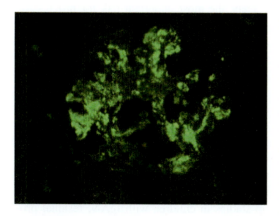

Fig. 17.4 Immunofluorescence staining with anti-IgA antibody. Mesangial distribution of IgA staining

Electron Microscopy

The most characteristic change on electron microscopy is the presence of electron-dense deposits in mesangial and para-mesangial areas.

Clinical Features

IgAN is not common in children under the age of 3 years; it is more common in adolescents [7]. In some children, the diagnosis follows an incidental finding of microscopic hematuria [113]. Asymptomatic patients may present with associated mild proteinuria (<0.5 g/day/1.73 m^2) in 3–15% of cases [114–116]. The most typical presentation of IgAN is gross hematuria coincident with upper respiratory tract infections or other mucosal inflammatory processes (in 30–40% of children). Macroscopic hematuria rarely occurs after vaccination or heavy physical exercise. The interval between the triggering event and the appearance of macroscopic hematuria is usually short (12–72 h). The macroscopic hematuria persists for few days, sometimes with flank and loin pain and fever. Some children have recurrent episodes without relevant urinary abnormalities between episodes. A transient increase in proteinuria occurs during episodes of gross hematuria. In some children, gross hematuria is associated with increased serum creatinine and hypertension [114–116], seldom with acute oliguric renal failure. In these cases, the renal biopsy shows mesangial, endocapillary and extracapillary proliferation and frequently tubular obstruction by packed red blood cells [117]. In rare cases, extensive crescentic lesions are detected [113]. Hypertension may develop during long-term follow-up or in particularly severe cases [113, 114]. An atypical presentation is nephrotic syndrome, which is reported in 7% of the cases, with podocytopathy similar to minimal change disease.

Natural History

IgAN in children is, with few exceptions, the early phase of the overall natural history of the disease. Severe clinical signs usually develop after 5–15 years, indicating the need for long follow-up, including as adults, to define the outcome of IgAN detected in childhood [118].

The natural history of IgAN varies according to the timing of performing the renal biopsy, and it differs in children diagnosed after a screening program; immediately after an onset with acute nephritic syndrome; or when there are signs of progression with decline in glomerular filtration rate (GFR). Moreover, the natural history has changed from the initial reports to the current era due to early detection and prompt therapy, including the use of RAS blockers (RASB) after diagnosis. Indeed, in the first pediatric report in 1986 of 91 French children with more than 13 years of follow-up, Levy et al. [116] reported chronic renal failure in 9%. In Finnish children, end-stage kidney disease (ESKD) from time of onset of diagnosis was found in 7% and 13% at 10 and 20 years, respectively [119]. An analysis of 500 children with IgAN in Japan showed a decrease in children reaching ESKD at 15 years from 20% to 1.2% when comparing renal biopsies before or after 1990. The European VALIGA study, over a median follow-up of 4.5 years, reported 4% of 174 children with ESKD. Since ESKD is uncommon in children, surrogate endpoints are frequently used (e.g. 50% reduction in eGFR or ESKD). In short-term follow-up studies, children seem to have a better prognosis than adults, but a 20 year survival analysis showed that IgAN in children was as progressive as in adults [115, 120]. In the long-term follow-up VALIGA study, survival to 50% reduction in eGFR or ESKD was 91% in children versus 70% in adults at 10 years and 82% in children versus 47% in adults at 20 years [110]. In a Japanese study of pediatric IgAN, patients were followed for a mean of 7 years. Clinical remission occurred in 50% and the predicted kidney survival rate was 92% at 10 years and 89% at 20 years [121]. Children with IgAN can have spontaneous remission of the urinary findings, as observed in Japanese children with IgAN and minor renal damage who did not receive medication after diagnosis [122]. Spontaneous remission could be observed after 5–8 years, but recurrences of urinary findings were detected in 20% at 5 years and in 42% at 10 years after remission. Hence, IgAN in children is a chronic disease, with phases of activity and clinical remission, rendering it difficult to provide a long-term prognosis on the basis of a short initial follow-up after renal biopsy.

Some children, usually those presenting with moderate microscopic hematuria without proteinuria and displaying the mildest lesions, do not progress to ESKD over decades of observation. In children with progressive IgAN, the clinical course is often slow and indolent. The most important factors associated with IgAN progression in adults, such as chronically reduced renal function at onset and persistent hypertension, are uncommon in children [123, 124]. The value of microscopic hematuria has been shown by some studies in adults with IgAN [125], but inter-center differences have limited the use of this urinary biomarker, so typical of IgAN, in collaborative studies.

In the VALIGA study, the clinical data, including proteinuria, blood pressure and eGFR at renal biopsy, were not significant predictors of the long-term outcome, indicating a possibility of spontaneous or drug-induced remission. Conversely, the most important risk for progression in children is the persistence of proteinuria (time-averaged) during follow-up. The threshold for time-averaged proteinuria in children is probably lower than what is accepted for adults. In adults with IgAN, only proteinuria >1 g/day is considered a significant risk for progression that deserves treatment, according to KDIGO recommendations [126]. For children, the 2021 update of KDIGO [127] suggests that those with >0.2 g/g urine protein/creatinine ratio (Up/UCr) should receive RAS inhibition. From long-term follow-up studies in children with IgAN, residual proteinuria <0.2 g/day/1.73 m^2 after treatment predicts a favorable outcome [128, 129].

In an analysis of the VALIGA cohort, only 7.5% of children with initial proteinuria >0.5 g/day/1.73 m^2 had persistent proteinuria <0.5 g/

day/1.73 m^2 at last follow-up, indicating a partial but not complete remission. The median value of proteinuria during a median 4.5 years of follow-up was 0.56 g/day/1.73 m^2, suggesting that most children with IgAN are exposed to a significant risk of progression over the following decades [106, 130].

Risk Prediction

There is a need to predict disease progression in children with IgAN to assess risk-based treatment decisions. An International IgAN Prediction Tool for adults with IgAN was recently developed to predict a 50% decline in eGFR or ESKD using clinical risk factors and MEST histology scores [131]. The variability of clinical and histological features of IgAN in children, the small number of children followed in individual centers, the short follow-up and the small number of outcome events (ESKD or 50% reduction in eGFR) represent substantial limitations for the detection of risk factors associated with progression in children. The use of the adult prediction tool was not satisfactory; hence, the global IgAN network updated the Prediction Tool for use in children using a multi-ethnic international cohort of 1060 children with IgAN followed into adulthood [132]. The Tool defined an end point of 30% reduction in eGFR or ESKD, which is considered an acceptable surrogate outcome in children with IgAN and proved to be well-calibrated. The trajectory of eGFR over time in children was different from adults: it was non-linear, with an increase in eGFR until 18 years of age followed by a linear decline similar to adults. A higher predicted risk was associated with a smaller increase in eGFR followed by a more rapid decline. This suggest that children at risk of a 30% decrease in eGFR will eventually experience a larger 50% decrease in eGFR and these two outcomes are analogous between the pediatric and adult Prediction Tools. The conclusion of this large collaborative effort was that the updated pediatric Prediction Tool could accurately predict the risk of a 30% decline in eGFR or ESKD in children with IgAN. The Prediction Tool uses a combination of commonly used clinical risk factors, and the MEST-C histology score, and is available online and in a mobile-app (www.qxmd.com/calculate-by-qxmd). The predicted risk of a 30% decline in eGFR or ESKD from the pediatric Prediction Tool at a given time horizon are similar to the predicted risks 2–3 years later of a 50% decline in eGFR or ESKD from the adult Prediction Tool.

Collectively, these results demonstrate that the Prediction Tool models are predicting clinically relevant outcomes in both children and adults and therefore can be used to identify higher-risk patients along a continuum of non-linear eGFR decline that spans the full age spectrum of patients with IgAN.

A low-risk condition according to the 2021 KDIGO recommendations, which should be the aim of treatment of children with IgAN, is persistent proteinuria <0.2 g/1.73 m^2/day and a normal GFR.

Treatment

Tonsillectomy

One of the first treatments considered for IgAN, particularly in children with recurrent gross hematuria, was tonsillectomy, which aimed to interrupt the pathogenic process initiated by an upper respiratory tract infection leading to hematuria. Tonsillectomy can eliminate a relevant source of pathogens, which multiply in tonsils, while also removing macrophages and T cells in lymphoid tonsil follicles, a potential source of aberrantly glycosylated IgA1. In children, it remains controversial whether adenotonsillectomy ultimately results in decreased serum immunoglobulins levels or, if so, whether such a decrease is associated with increased susceptibility to upper respiratory tract infections. In a randomized trial in children without IgAN [133], the IgA levels were significantly decreased after one year of follow-up; however, no relation was found between immunoglobulin levels and frequency of subsequent respiratory infections. Moreover, in children with repeated infections despite tonsillectomy, IgA levels increased again, indicating that the remaining MALT can compensate for the loss of tonsils and adenoid tissue [133]. Even though tonsillectomy can reduce the frequency of gross hematuria and produce some benefits, this intervention lacks sufficient evidence and KDIGO 2012 suggested tonsillectomy not be performed in patients with IgAN without a clinical indication beyond IgAN [134]. This is confirmed in the 2021 KDIGO [127]; however, it takes into consideration the results of tonsillectomy in two large retrospective Japanese studies which reported benefits on renal function decline after a follow-up of more than 10 years [135]. Hence, some potential benefit in Japanese patients might be considered.

Tonsillectomy has a clear indication when tonsils are a true infectious focus and in cases of recurrent tonsillitis (>3 per year). Otherwise, the efficacy of the procedure is often supported only in association with other therapy and the benefit is unclear [136]. In Europe, a VALIGA collateral study failed to show clinical benefit on outcome of a subgroup of patients who had received tonsillectomy [137].

Inhibition of the Renin-Angiotensin System

In all children with IgAN, blood pressure (BP) control should be strict. All patients should be targeted below the 90th percentile, with a target of the 50th percentile or the maximally tolerated drug dose, if proteinuria is present. This is consistent with the target recommended in adults by KDIGO [126]. The drugs of choice for BP control in IgAN are RASB, either angiotensin converting enzyme inhibitors (ACE-Is) or angiotensin receptor blockers (ARBs).

Children with IgAN and heavy proteinuria are at risk for progressive disease. RAS inhibition has a strong rationale for use in IgAN, not only because it improves two risk factors for progression (hypertension and proteinuria), but also because it can inhibit the long series of potentially negative effects caused by angiotensin II on

mesangial cells, particularly in the presence of mesangial immune deposits.

A European multicenter randomized controlled trial (RCT) included children and young patients (3–35 years old) with a constant level of proteinuria (>1 < 3.5 g/day/1.73 m^2 over the 3 months before enrolment) and normal or moderately reduced renal function. Patients were randomized to receive benazepril 0.2 mg/kg/day or placebo and the primary outcome of renal disease progression was >30% decrease in eGFR and/or worsening of proteinuria to nephrotic range. Treatment with ACE-I was an independent predictor of prognosis, while no effect on the progression of renal damage was found for gender, age, baseline GFR, systolic or diastolic blood pressure, mean arterial pressure, or proteinuria [138].

On the basis of this study, KDIGO suggested to treat children with IgAN and persistent proteinuria >0.5 and < 1 g/day/1.73 m^2 with RAS inhibition. There are no data to indicate a preference between ACE-Is or ARBs, except for fewer side effects with ARBs. No significant additional benefit was found in a RCT that investigated the addition of ARB to ACE-I in children with IgAN [139].

No RCT has addressed the effects of ACE-I in children with minimal proteinuria <0.5 g/day/1.73 m^2, but some benefits were suggested by a single-arm, collaborative, Japanese study that treated patients for 2 years [140].

Glucocorticoids

Based on the results of RCTs in adults [135, 141, 142], KDIGO in 2012 suggested that if proteinuria >1 g/day persisted unchanged after 3–6 months of RAS inhibition, glucocorticoids should be considered for treatment of IgAN in children and adults [126, 143]. In children, lower levels of persistent proteinuria (>0.5 g/day/1.73 m^2) may be considered for initiating treatment. Protocols included months regimens, using either 3 intravenous pulses of methylprednisolone (1 g) and oral prednisone (0.5 mg/kg on alternate days) [141], or oral prednisone 0.8–1 mg/kg/day for 2 months, with weaning over 6 months [142, 144]. However, subsequent RCTs in adults suggested a more cautious approach in cases with slow decline of GFR. The STOP-IgAN trial [145] did not show a superior effect of immunosuppressive therapy (monotherapy with methylprednisolone pulses for 6 months in patients with eGFR >60 ml/min; oral prednisone and cyclophosphamide followed by azathioprine in patients with lower eGFR) versus supportive care for three years. The Therapeutic Evaluation of Steroids in IgA Nephropathy Global (TESTING) study [144] compared oral methylprednisolone versus placebo. Recruitment was discontinued after 2 years because of excess serious adverse events (mostly infections, including two deaths) in patients receiving corticosteroids. The preliminary results were consistent with potential renal benefit, but early termination of the study did not allow any conclusions. These recent studies have focused attention on the potential side effects and limited benefits of corticosteroids in adults with IgAN.

In children, evidence-based reports on the effect of corticosteroids in treating IgAN are scarce [146]. Small studies in children with variable baseline data and different treatment regimens provided conflicting results [147–149]. The best results were reported in severe cases with crescentic IgAN successfully treated with pulse steroid therapy [149].

A US RCT using prednisone (60 mg/m^2 every other day for 3 months, then 40 mg/m^2 every other day for 9 months, then 30 mg/m^2 every other day for 12 month) or fish oil (4 g/day for 2 years) failed to find significant benefit of treatment [150]. However, the relatively short follow-up period, inequality of baseline proteinuria, and small numbers of patients precludes a definite conclusion.

The only RCT proving efficacy of corticosteroids in children with IgAN was performed in Japan; it enrolled children with severe mesangial proliferation. The children were randomized into two groups, with one arm (intervention) receiving prednisone, azathioprine, heparin-warfarin and dipyridamole and the other arm (control) receiving heparin-warfarin and dipyridamole.

This 2 year study reported a significant reduction in proteinuria, serum IgA concentration, mesangial deposition, and prevention of increased number of sclerosed glomeruli in the intervention arm [151]. After a follow-up of 10 years free of additional treatment, the children in the intervention arm (who had previously received the immunosuppressive combination therapy) were less likely to reach the end point of GFR <60 ml/min/1.73 m^2. In another study, a similar combination therapy produced a disappearance of IgA mesangial deposits after 2 years of treatment [152]. These reports suggest that early aggressive treatment in children with modifiable histologic risk factors for progression can in the long-term protect the kidneys from sclerosis. Side effects and limited if any benefit of prolonged anticoagulation and anti-platelet therapy suggest that they do not provide a net benefit when added to immunosuppressive therapy [153]. In adults, the addition of azathioprine to corticosteroids failed to add further benefits and caused side effects [154].

A French, uncontrolled, retrospective study [155] reported the outcome of children with severe clinical presentation and acute histologic features who received therapy with either corticosteroids (sometimes in association with cyclophosphamide) and RASB, or RASB alone. Although the two groups had different baseline proteinuria and time from onset to treatment, a large benefit of corticosteroid/immunosuppressive therapy was reported, with improvement in eGFR and decrease in proteinuria after a short follow-up of 6 months.

According to KDIGO 2021 [127], in children with proteinuria >1 g/day/1.73 m^2 and/or mesangial hypercellularity, most pediatric nephrologists will treat with glucocorticoids in addition to RAS blockade from time of diagnosis. The most common protocol is oral prednisone 1–2 mg/kg/day for 4 weeks tapered over 4–6 months. Regimens including intravenous methylprednisolone are also used. KDIGO 2021 reports that there is scarce evidence for the additional use of non-glucocorticoid immunosuppressants, but this approach may be considered in more severe cases. Children with nephrotic syndrome and histological features of minimal change disease (MCD) associated with IgAN should be treated as MCD. IgAN with rapidly progressive renal deterioration of renal function (>50% decline in eGFR in <3 months) irrespective of the percentage of glomeruli involved with crescents, may benefit from steroids and cyclophosphamide, analogous to the treatment of ANCA vasculitis [126]. Prompt use of aggressive immunosuppressive treatment, sometimes in association with plasmapheresis, has shown some benefit in slowing the progression of these difficult cases [156]. Finally, KDIGO 2021 suggests to strictly follow children with IgAN even when they enter remission, since recurrence is always possible.

New Formulations of Corticosteroids

An enteric formulation of budesonide has been developed that targets release of the drug in the distal ileum, an area within the GALT. The NEFIGAN trial compared this targeted release formulation (TRF) of budesonide with placebo in patients with persistent proteinuria despite optimized RAS blockade [157]. At 9 months, mean proteinuria decreased significantly more in TRF budesonide-treated patients than in placebo–treated patients. GFR stabilized with TRF budesonide, but decreased in the placebo arm. No increase in serious adverse events, and particularly infections, were reported in treated patients. Results from further RCT and studies in children are expected.

Mycophenolate Mofetil

The KDIGO guideline does not recommend mycophenolate mofetil in IgAN, even though some benefit in Asian adult patients have been reported [158]. A RCT that included children, young subjects and adults investigating the effects of corticosteroids, mycophenolate mofetil and fish oil was prematurely terminated for lack of benefit [159].

Cyclophosphamide

This drug, in combination with corticosteroids, was tested in adults with particularly active disease in several uncontrolled case series, and a small RCT [160] reported a protective effect of cyclophosphamide in progressive cases of adult IgAN. However, this was not confirmed by the STOP-IgAN study [145].

Rituximab

Rituximab, in a small RCT in adult patients with IgAN, had no effect on eGFR decline or remission of proteinuria [161].

Calcineurin Inhibitors

A recent meta-analysis reported limited effects of calcineurin inhibitors when used in addition to small doses of prednisone, while reporting more adverse events [162].

Future Therapies for IgAN

Hydroxychloroquine combined with RAS inhibitors significantly reduced proteinuria over 6-months in adults with IgAN [163]. Results in children are expected.

Inhibitors of endothelin-1 receptors combined with RASB are being tested in a large collaborative phase III RCT. A study in children is in preparation.

Explorative trials with Inhibitors of the BAFF-TNF receptor family (BAFF, APRIL TACI) using humanized monoclonal antibodies against these mediators are ongoing [164]. Several complement inhibitors are under investigation, including anti-C5 (eculizumab), anti-C5a receptor inhibitors (CCX168), anti-C3 (compstatin), anti-factor D (lampalizumab), and MASP-2 inhibitors (OMS721) [164, 165].

A Practical Approach to Treatment of Children with IgAN

The prospects for successful treatment of IgAN to improve long-term outcomes in children seems promising since children are more likely than adults to be treated in the early stages of the disease, when mesangial proliferative lesions/endocapillary proliferations are more prominent than sclerosis, and when proteinuria is not massive. On the other hand, we must take into consideration the toxicity and side effects of these treatments, which are particularly undesired in patients with mild disease, and the possibility of spontaneous remission in mild cases [166].

According to KDIGO 2012 and 2021 [127] recommendations, the treatment of IgAN in adults and in children is mostly driven by the level of proteinuria at renal biopsy, with advanced renal failure suggesting disease beyond "the point of no return" being the only limitation. These recommendations originate from the available evidence in the literature. However, proteinuria can be associated with active lesions, but also be the clinical manifestation of sclerotic lesions. The recent identification of pathologic features that are risk factors independent from proteinuria, blood pressure and GFR at renal biopsy, strongly suggests that there should be an integrated approach to treatment as indicated in Fig. 17.5.

For all children with IgAN, a general approach is to carefully follow BP and to target blood pressure < 50th percentile for sex and age or maximally tolerated dose using RAS inhibition if proteinuria is present.

For children with mild IgAN disease, presenting with normal GFR, urinary protein/creatinine ratio (Up/Ucr) <0.2, normal BP and with all MEST (see legend for Fig. 17.5) negative [0], watchful waiting is suggested, and prescribing a RASB if Up/Ucr exceeds 0.2 g/g.

For children with IgAN and moderate/severe IgAN (Up/Ucr >0.5), at risk of GFR decline by the prediction tool, which considers MEST scores, without severe irreversible sclerotic changes, glucocorticoids should be added to a RASB. Methylprednisolone pulses [143] or oral steroids over 6 months can be adopted.

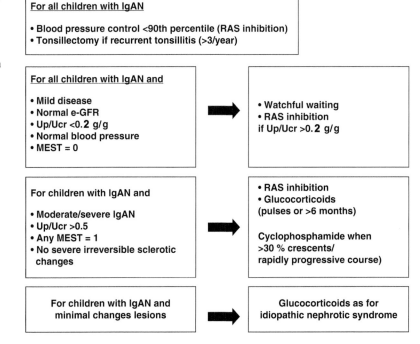

Fig. 17.5 Treatment of children with primary IgA nephropathy (IgAN). e-GFR: estimated glomerular filtration rate in children calculated with updated Schwartz formula; up/Ucr: urinary protein/creatinine ratio; normal blood pressure: <90th percentile corrected for height, sex and age; MEST: scores derived from Oxford classification of IgAN [101, 102]; M: mesangial hypercellularity; E: endocapillary hypercellularity; S: segmental sclerosis; T: tubular atrophy/interstitial fibrosis

In cases with severe endocapillary proliferation, or with crescent formation involving >30% of the glomeruli, with a rapidly progressive course, cyclophosphamide may be effective. In children with IgAN, minimal change lesions and nephrotic syndrome, a protocol similar to that recommended for idiopathic nephrotic syndrome is a suitable choice.

References

1. Berger J, Hinglais N. [Intercapillary deposits of IgA-IgG]. J Urol Nephrol (Paris). 1968;74(9):694–5.
2. Coppo R, Amore A, Hogg R, Emancipator S. Idiopathic nephropathy with IgA deposits. Pediatr Nephrol. 2000;15(1–2):139–50.
3. D'Amico G. Idiopathic IgA mesangial nephropathy. Nephron. 1985;41:1–13.
4. Sugiyama H, Yokoyama H, Sato H, Saito T, Kohda Y, Nishi S, et al. Japan Renal Biopsy Registry and Japan Kidney Disease Registry: committee report for 2009 and 2010. Clin Exp Nephrol. 2013;17(2):155–73.
5. Cho BS, Hahn WH, Il CH, Lim I, Ko CW, Kim SY, et al. A nationwide study of mass urine screening tests on Korean school children and implications for chronic kidney disease management. Clin Exp Nephrol. 2013;17(2):205–10.
6. Coppo R. Pediatric IgA nephropathy in Europe. Kidney Dis. 2019;5:182–8.
7. Coppo R, Robert T. IgA nephropathy in children and in adults: two separate entities or the same disease? J Nephrol. 2020;33:1219–29.
8. Shibano T, Takagi N, Maekawa K, Mae H, Hattori M, Takeshima Y, et al. Epidemiological survey and clinical investigation of pediatric IgA nephropathy. Clin Exp Nephrol. 2016;20(1):111–7.
9. Schena FP, IN. Epidemiology of IgA nephropathy: a global perspective. Semin Nephrol. 2018;38:435–42.
10. CM Zink SEJRUHHGJFGS. Trends of renal diseases in Germany: review of a regional renal biopsy database from 1990 to 2013. Clin Kidney J. 2019;12:795–800.
11. Su S, Yu J, Wang Y, Wang Y, Li J, Xu Z. Clinicopathologic correlations of renal biopsy findings from northeast China A 10-year retrospective study. Medicine (Baltimore). 2019;98(23):e15880.
12. Kiryluk K, Li Y, Sanna-Cherchi S, Rohanizadegan M, Suzuki H, Eitner F, et al. Geographic differences in genetic susceptibility to IgA nephropathy: GWAS replication study and geospatial risk analysis. PLoS Genet. 2012;8(6):e1002765.
13. Fan P, Song J, Chen Q, Cheng X, Liu X, Zou C, et al. The influence of environmental factors on clinical pathological changes of patients with immunoglobulin A nephropathy from different areas of China. Ren Fail. 2018;40(1):597–602.
14. Gharavi AG, Moldoveanu Z, Wyatt RJ, Barker CV, Woodford SY, Lifton RP, et al. Aberrant IgA1 glycosylation is inherited in familial and sporadic IgA nephropathy. J Am Soc Nephrol. 2008;19(5):1008–14.
15. Kiryluk K, Moldoveanu Z, Sanders JT, Eison TM, Suzuki H, Julian BA, et al. Aberrant glycosylation of IgA1 is inherited in both pediatric IgA nephropathy and Henoch-Schönlein purpura nephritis. Kidney Int. 2011;80(1):79–87.
16. Gharavi AG, Yan Y, Scolari F, Schena FP, Frasca GM, Ghiggeri GM, et al. IgA nephropathy, the most common cause of glomerulonephritis, is linked to 6q22-23. Nat Genet. 2000;26(3):354–7.
17. Neugut YD, Kiryluk K. Genetic determinants of IgA nephropathy: western perspective. Semin Nephrol. 2018;38:443–54.
18. Kiryluk K, Li Y, Scolari F, Sanna-Cherchi S, Choi M, Verbitsky M, et al. Discovery of new risk loci for IgA nephropathy implicates genes involved in immunity against intestinal pathogens. Nat Genet. 2014;46(11):1187–96.
19. Xie J, Kiryluk K, Li Y, Mladkova N, Zhu L, Hou P, et al. Fine mapping implicates a deletion of CFHR1 and CFHR3 in protection from IgA nephropathy in Han Chinese. J Am Soc Nephrol. 2016;27:3187–94.
20. Tortajada A, Gutiérrez E, Goicoechea de Jorge E, Anter J, Segarra A, Espinosa M, et al. Elevated factor H-related protein 1 and factor H pathogenic variants decrease complement regulation in IgA nephropathy. Kidney Int. 2017;92(4):953–63.
21. Tortajada A, Gutierrez E, Pickering MC, Praga Terente M, Medjeral-Thomas N. The role of complement in IgA nephropathy. Mol Immunol. 2019;114:123–32.
22. Zhu L, Zhai YL, Wang FM, Hou P, Lv JC, Xu DM, et al. Variants in complement factor H and complement factor H-related protein genes, CFHR3 and CFHR1, affect complement activation in IgA nephropathy. J Am Soc Nephrol. 2015;26(5):1195–204.
23. Li M, Foo JN, Wang JQ, Low HQ, Tang XQ, Toh KY, et al. Identification of new susceptibility loci for IgA nephropathy in Han Chinese. Nat Commun. 2015;6:7270.
24. Magistroni R, D'Agati VD, Appel GB, Kiryluk K. New developments in the genetics, pathogenesis, and therapy of IgA nephropathy. Kidney Int. 2015;88:974–89.
25. Zhou X, Tsoi LC, Hu Y, Patrick MT, He K, Berthier CC, et al. Exome chip analyses and genetic risk for IgA nephropathy among Han Chinese. Clin J Am Soc Nephrol 2021;16:CJN.06910520.
26. Hiki Y, Tanaka A, Kokubo T, Iwase H, Nishikido J, Hotta K, et al. Analyses of IgA1 hinge glycopeptides in IgA nephropathy by matrix-assisted laser desorption/ionization time-of-flight mass spectrometry. J Am Soc Nephrol. 1998;9(4):577–82.
27. Allen AC, Bailey EM, Brenchley PEC, Buck KS, Barratt J, Feehally J. Mesangial Iga1 in IgA nephrop-

athy exhibits aberrant O-glycosylation: observations in three patients. Kidney Int. 2001;60(3):969–73.

28. Novak J, Barratt J, Julian BA, Renfrow MB. Aberrant glycosylation of the IgA1 molecule in IgA nephropathy. Semin Nephrol. 2018;38:461–76.

29. Suzuki H, Moldoveanu Z, Hall S, Brown R, Julian BA, Wyatt RJ, et al. IgA nephropathy: characterization of IgG antibodies specific for galactose-deficient IgA1. Contrib Nephrol. 2007;157:129–33.

30. Mestecky J, Tomana M, Moldoveanu Z, Julian BA, Suzuki H, Matousovic K, et al. Role of aberrant glycosylation of IgA1 molecules in the pathogenesis of iga nephropathy. Kidney Blood Press Res. 2008;31:29–37.

31. Raska M, Moldoveanu Z, Suzuki H, Brown R, Kulhavy R, Andrasi J, et al. Identification and characterization of CMP-NeuAc:GalNAc-IgA1 α2,6-Sialyltransferase in IgA1-producing Cells. J Mol Biol. 2007;369(1):69–78.

32. Coppo R, Amore A, Gianoglio B, Porcellini MG, Peruzzi L, Gusmano R, et al. Macromolecular IgA and abnormal IgA reactivity in sera from children with IgA nephropathy. Clin Nephrol. 1995;43(1):1–13.

33. Allen AC, Bailey EM, Barratt J, Buck KS, Feehally J. Analysis of IgA1 O-glycans in IgA nephropathy by fluorophore-assisted carbohydrate. Electrophoresis. 1999;10(8):1763–71.

34. Sun Q, Zhang Z, Zhang H, Liu X. Aberrant IgA1 glycosylation in iga nephropathy: a systematic review. PLoS ONE 2016;11:e0166700.

35. Allen AC, Topham PS, Harper SJ, Feehally J. Leucocyte β1,3 galactosyltransferase activity in IgA nephropathy. Nephrol Dial Transplant. 1997;12(4):701–6.

36. Gale DP, Molyneux K, Wimbury D, Higgins P, Levine AP, Caplin B, et al. Galactosylation of IgA1 Is Associated with Common Variation in C1GALT1. J Am Soc Nephrol. 2017;28(7):2158–66.

37. Xing Y, Li L, Zhang Y, Wang F, He D, Liu Y, et al. C1GALT1 expression is associated with galactosylation of IgA1 in peripheral B lymphocyte in immunoglobulin a nephropathy. BMC Nephrol. 2020;21(1):18.

38. Serino G, Sallustio F, Cox SN, Pesce F, Schena FP. Abnormal miR-148b expression promotes aberrant glycosylation of IgA1 in IgA nephropathy. J Am Soc Nephrol. 2012;23(5):814–24.

39. Suzuki H, Fan R, Zhang Z, Brown R, Hall S, Julian BA, et al. Aberrantly glycosylated IgA1 in IgA nephropathy patients is recognized by IgG antibodies with restricted heterogeneity. J Clin Invest. 2009;119(6):1668–77.

40. Berthoux F, Suzuki H, Thibaudin L, Yanagawa H, Maillard N, Mariat C, et al. Autoantibodies targeting galactose-deficient IgA1 associate with progression of IgA nephropathy. J Am Soc Nephrol. 2012;23(9):1579–87.

41. Placzek WJ, Yanagawa H, Makita Y, Renfrow MB, Julian BA, Rizk DV, et al. Serum galactose-deficient-IgA1 and IgG autoantibodies correlate in patients with IgA nephropathy. PLoS One. 2018;13(1):e0190967.

42. Moldoveanu Z, Suzuki H, Reily C, Satake K, Novak L, Xu N, et al. Experimental evidence of pathogenic role of IgG autoantibodies in IgA nephropathy. J Autoimmun. 2021;118:102593.

43. Zhao N, Hou P, Lv J, Moldoveanu Z, Li Y, Kiryluk K, et al. The level of galactose-deficient IgA1 in the sera of patients with IgA nephropathy is associated with disease progression. Kidney Int. 2012;82(7):790–6.

44. Maixnerova D, Ling C, Hall S, Reily C, Brown R, Neprasova M, et al. Galactose-deficient IgA1 and the corresponding IgG autoantibodies predict IgA nephropathy progression. PLoS One. 2019;14(2):e0212254.

45. Suzuki H, Kiryluk K, Novak J, Moldoveanu Z, Herr AB, Renfrow MB, et al. The pathophysiology of IgA nephropathy. J Am Soc Nephrol. 2011;22:1795–803.

46. Rizk DV, Saha MK, Hall S, Novak L, Brown R, Huang ZQ, et al. Glomerular immunodeposits of patients with IgA nephropathy are enriched for IgG autoantibodies specific for galactose-deficient IgA1. J Am Soc Nephrol. 2019;30(10):2017–26.

47. Bellur SS, Troyanov S, Cook HT, Roberts ISD. Immunostaining findings in IgA nephropathy: correlation with histology and clinical outcome in the Oxford classification patient cohort. Nephrol Dial Transplant. 2011;26(8):2533–6.

48. Knoppova B, Reily C, Maillard N, Rizk DV, Moldoveanu Z, Mestecky J, et al. The origin and activities of IgA1-containing immune complexes in IGA nephropathy. Front Immunol. 2016;7:117.

49. Monteiro RC. Recent advances in the physiopathology of IgA nephropathy. Nephrologie et Therapeutique. 2018;14:S1–8.

50. Berthelot L, Papista C, Maciel TT, Biarnes-Pelicot M, Tissandie E, Wang PHM, et al. Transglutaminase is essential for IgA nephropathy development acting through IgA receptors. J Exp Med. 2012;209(4):793–806.

51. Lai KN, Leung JCK, Chan LYY, Saleem MA, Mathieson PW, Tam KY, et al. Podocyte injury induced by mesangial-derived cytokines in IgA nephropathy. Nephrol Dial Transplant. 2009;24(1):62–72.

52. Trimarchi H, Coppo R. Podocytopathy in the mesangial proliferative immunoglobulin A nephropathy: new insights into the mechanisms of damage and progression. Nephrol Dial Transplant. 2019;34(8):1280–5.

53. Coppo R, Amore A, Gianoglio B, Cacace G, Picciotto G, Roccatello D, et al. Angiotensin II local hyperreactivity in the progression of IgA nephropathy. Am J Kidney Dis. 1993;21(6):593–602.

54. Bienenstock KC. Characteristics and functions of mucosa-associated lymphoid tissue. In: Handbook of mucosal immunology. Part 1; 1994. p. 141–9.

55. Randall TD, Mebius RE. The development and function of mucosal lymphoid tissues: a balanc-

55. ing act with micro-organisms. Mucosal Immunol. 2014;7:455–66.
56. Cesta MF. Normal structure, function, and histology of mucosa-associated lymphoid tissue. Toxicol Pathol. 2006;34(5):599–608.
57. Harabuchi Y, Takahara M. Recent advances in the immunological understanding of association between tonsil and immunoglobulin A nephropathy as a tonsil-induced autoimmune/inflammatory syndrome. Immunity Inflammation and Disease. 2019;7:86–93.
58. Fagarasan S, Kawamoto S, Kanagawa O, Suzuki K. Adaptive immune regulation in the gut: T cell-dependent and T cell-independent IgA synthesis. Annu Rev Immunol. 2010;28:243–73.
59. Xin G, Shi W, Xu LX, Su Y, Yan LJ, Li KS. Serum BAFF is elevated in patients with IgA nephropathy and associated with clinical and histopathological features. J Nephrol. 2013;26(4):683–90.
60. Coppo R, Amore A, Peruzzi L, Vergano L, Camilla R. Innate immunity and IgA nephropathy. J Nephrol. 2010;23(6):626–32.
61. Tomino Y, Sakai H, Endoh M, Suga T, Miura M, Kaneshige H, et al. Cross-reactivity of IgA antibodies between renal mesangial areas and nuclei of tonsillar cells in patients with IgA nephropathy. Clin Exp Immunol. 1983;51(3):605–10.
62. Béné MC, Hurault de Ligny B, Kessler M, Foliguet B, Faure GC. Tonsils in IgA nephropathy. Contrib Nephrol. 1993;104:153–61.
63. Amore A, Coppo R, Nedrud JG, Sigmund N, Lamm ME, Emancipator SN. The role of nasal tolerance in a model of IgA nephropathy induced in mice by Sendai virus. Clin Immunol. 2004;113(1):101–8.
64. Gesualdo L, Lamm ME, Emancipator SN. Defective oral tolerance promotes nephritogenesis in experimental IgA nephropathy induced by oral immunization. J Immunol. 1990;145(11):3684–91.
65. Watanabe H, Goto S, Mori H, Higashi K, Hosomichi K, Aizawa N, et al. Comprehensive microbiome analysis of tonsillar crypts in IgA nephropathy. Nephrol Dial Transplant. 2017;32(12):2072–9.
66. Park JI, Kim TY, Oh B, Cho H, Kim JE, Yoo SH, et al. Comparative analysis of the tonsillar microbiota in IgA nephropathy and other glomerular diseases. Sci Rep. 2020;10(1):16206.
67. Muto M, Manfroi B, Suzuki H, Joh K, Nagai M, Wakai S, et al. Toll-like receptor 9 stimulation induces aberrant expression of a proliferation-inducing ligand by tonsillar germinal center B Cells in IgA nephropathy. J Am Soc Nephrol. 2017;28(4):1227–38.
68. Zachova K, Kosztyu P, Zadrazil J, Matousovic K, Vondrak K, Hubacek P, et al. Role of epstein-barr virus in pathogenesis and racial distribution of IgA nephropathy. Front Immunol. 2020;11:267.
69. Coppo R. The gut–kidney axis in IgA nephropathy: role of microbiota and diet on genetic predisposition. Pediatr Nephrol. 2018;33(1):53–61.
70. Collin P, Syrjanen J, Partanen J, Pasternack A, Kaukinen K, Mustonen J. Celiac disease and HLA DQ in patients with IgA nephropathy. Am J Gastroenterol. 2002;97(10):2572–6.
71. McCarthy DD, Kujawa J, Wilson C, Papandile A, Poreci U, Porfilio EA, et al. Mice overexpressing BAFF develop a commensal flora-dependent, IgA-associated nephropathy. J Clin Invest. 2011;121(10):3991–4002.
72. Bunker JJ, Bendelac A. IgA responses to microbiota. Immunity. 2018;49:211–24.
73. De Angelis M, Montemurno E, Piccolo M, Vannini L, Lauriero G, Maranzano V, et al. Microbiota and metabolome associated with Immunoglobulin A Nephropathy (IgAN). PLoS One. 2014;9(6):e99006.
74. Davin JC, Forget P, Mahieu PR. Increased intestinal permeability to (51 Cr) EDTA is correlated with IgA immune complex-plasma levels in children with IgA-associated nephropathies. Acta Paediatr Scand. 1988;77(1):118–24.
75. Rostoker G, Wirquin V, Terzidis H, Petit-Phar M, Chaumette MT, Delchier JC, et al. Mucosal immunity in primary glomerulonephritis. Nephron. 1993;63(3):286–90.
76. Coppo R, Amore A, Roccatello D, Gianoglio B, Molino A, Piccoli G, et al. IgA antibodies to dietary antigens and lectin-binding IgA in Sera From Italian, Australian, and Japanese IgA Nephropathy Patients. Am J Kidney Dis. 1991;17(4):480–7.
77. Qin W, Zhong X, Fan JM, Zhang YJ, Liu XR, Ma XY. External suppression causes the low expression of the Cosmc gene in IgA nephropathy. Nephrol Dial Transplant. 2008;23(5):1608–14.
78. Coppo R, Camilla R, Amore A, Peruzzi L, Daprà V, Loiacono E, et al. Toll-like receptor 4 expression is increased in circulating mononuclear cells of patients with immunoglobulin A nephropathy: ORIGINAL ARTICLE. Clin Exp Immunol. 2010;159(1):73–81.
79. Donadio MEL, Loiacono E, Peruzzi L, Amore A, Camilla R, Chiale F, et al. Toll-like receptors, immunoproteasome and regulatory T cells in children with Henoch-Schönlein purpura and primary IgA nephropathy. Pediatr Nephrol. 2014;29(9):1545–51.
80. Coppo R, Mazzucco G, Martina G, Roccatello D, Amore A, Novara R, et al. Gluten-induced experimental IgA glomerulopathy. Lab Investig. 1989;60(4):499–506.
81. Papista C, Lechner S, Ben Mkaddem S, Lestang MB, Abbad L, Bex-Coudrat J, et al. Gluten exacerbates IgA nephropathy in humanized mice through gliadin-CD89 interaction. Kidney Int. 2015;88(2):276–85.
82. Coppo R, Roccatello D, Amore A, Quattrocchio G, Molino A, Gianoglio B, et al. Effects of a gluten-free diet in primary IgA nephropathy. Clin Nephrol. 1990;33(2):72–86.
83. Maillard N, Wyatt RJ, Julian BA, Kiryluk K, Gharavi A, Fremeaux-Bacchi V, et al. Current understanding of the role of complement in IgA nephropathy. J Am Soc Nephrol. 2015;26(7):1503–12.

84. Daha MR, van Kooten C. Role of complement in IgA nephropathy. J Nephrol. 2016;29:1–4.
85. Medjeral-Thomas NR, Lomax-Browne HJ, Beckwith H, Willicombe M, McLean AG, Brookes P, et al. Circulating complement factor H–related proteins 1 and 5 correlate with disease activity in IgA nephropathy. Kidney Int. 2017;92(4):942–52.
86. Jia M, Zhu L, Zhai Y, Chen P, Xu B, Guo W, et al. Variation in complement factor H affects complement activation in immunoglobulin A vasculitis with nephritis. Nephrology. 2020;25(1):40–7.
87. Zhu L, Guo W-Y, Shi S-F, Liu L-J, Lv J-C, Medjeral-Thomas NR, et al. Circulating complement factor H–related protein 5 levels contribute to development and progression of IgA nephropathy. Kidney Int. 2018;94(1):150–8.
88. Guo W-Y, Sun L-J, Dong H-R, Wang G-Q, Xu X-Y, Zhao Z-R, et al. Glomerular complement factor H–related protein 5 is associated with histologic injury in immunoglobulin A nephropathy. Kidney Int Reports. 2021;6(2):404–13.
89. Wu J, Hu Z, Wang Y, Hu D, Yang Q, Li Y, et al. Severe glomerular C3 deposition indicated severe renal lesions and poor prognosis in patients with immunoglobulin A nephropathy. Histopathology. 2021;78(6):882–95.
90. Wu D, Li X, Yao X, Zhang N, Lei L, Zhang H, et al. Mesangial C3 deposition and serum C3 levels predict renal outcome in IgA nephropathy. Clin Exp Nephrol. 2021;25(6):641–51.
91. Espinosa M, Ortega R, Sanchez M, Segarra A, Salcedo MT, Gonzalez F, et al. Association of C4d deposition with clinical outcomes in IgA nephropathy. Clin J Am Soc Nephrol. 2014;9(5):897–904.
92. Nam KH, Joo YS, Lee C, Lee S, Kim J, Yun HR, et al. Predictive value of mesangial C3 and C4d deposition in IgA nephropathy. Clin Immunol. 2020;211:108331.
93. Segarra A, Romero K, Agraz I, Ramos N, Madrid A, Carnicer C, et al. Mesangial C4d deposits in early IgA nephropathy. Clin J Am Soc Nephrol. 2018;13(2):258–64.
94. Trimarchi H, Coppo R. Glomerular endothelial activation, C4d deposits and microangiopathy in immunoglobulin A nephropathy. Nephrol Dial Transplant. 36(4):581–6.
95. Stangou M, Alexopoulos E, Pantzaki A, Leonstini M, Memmos D. C5b-9 glomerular deposition and tubular $\alpha3\beta1$-integrin expression are implicated in the development of chronic lesions and predict renal function outcome in immunoglobulin a nephropathy. Scand J Urol Nephrol. 2008;42(4):373–80.
96. Camilla R, Suzuki H, Daprà V, Loiacono E, Peruzzi L, Amore A, et al. Oxidative stress and galactose-deficient IgA1 as markers of progression in IgA nephropathy. Clin J Am Soc Nephrol. 2011;6(8):1903–11.
97. Schena FP, D'Altri C, Cerullo G, Manno C, Gesualdo L. ACE gene polymorphism and IgA nephropathy: an ethnically homogeneous study and a meta-analysis. Kidney Int. 2001;60:732–40.
98. Sallustio F, Curci C, Di Leo V, Gallone A, Pesce F, Gesualdo L. A new vision of iga nephropathy: the missing link. Int J Mol Sci. 2020;21:189.
99. Graterol F, Navarro-Muñoz M, Ibernon M, López D, Troya MI, Pérez V, et al. Poor histological lesions in IgA nephropathy may be reflected in blood and urine peptide profiling. BMC Nephrol. 2013;14(1):82.
100. Haas M. Histologic subclassification of IgA nephropathy: a clinicopathologic study of 244 cases. Am J Kidney Dis. 1997;29(6):829–42.
101. Cattran DC, Coppo R, Cook HT, Feehally J, Roberts ISD, Troyanov S, et al. The Oxford classification of IgA nephropathy: rationale, clinicopathological correlations, and classification. Kidney Int. 2009;76(5):534–45.
102. Roberts ISD, Cook HT, Troyanov S, Alpers CE, Amore A, Barratt J, et al. The Oxford classification of IgA nephropathy: pathology definitions, correlations, and reproducibility. Kidney Int. 2009;76(5):546–56.
103. Haas M, Verhave JC, Liu ZH, Alpers CE, Barratt J, Becker JU, et al. A multicenter study of the predictive value of crescents in IgA nephropathy. J Am Soc Nephrol. 2017;28(2):691–701.
104. Roberts ISD. Oxford classification of immunoglobulin A nephropathy: an update. Curr Opin Nephrol Hypertens. 2013;22:281–6.
105. Coppo R, Troyanov S, Camilla R, Hogg RJ, Cattran DC, Cook HT, et al. The Oxford IgA nephropathy clinicopathological classification is valid for children as well as adults. Kidney Int. 2010;77(10):921–7.
106. Coppo R, Lofaro D, Camilla RR, Bellur S, Cattran D, Cook HT, et al. Risk factors for progression in children and young adults with IgA nephropathy: an analysis of 261 cases from the VALIGA European cohort. Pediatr Nephrol. 2017;32(1):139–50.
107. Le W, Zeng C-H, Liu Z-HZ, Liu D, Yang Q, Lin R-X, et al. Validation of the Oxford classification of IgA nephropathy for pediatric patients from China. BMC Nephrol. 2012;13(1):158.
108. Shima Y, Nakanishi K, Hama T, Mukaiyama H, Togawa H, Hashimura Y, et al. Validity of the Oxford classification of IgA nephropathy in children. Pediatr Nephrol. 2012;27(5):783–92.
109. Edström Halling S, Söderberg MP, Berg UB. Predictors of outcome in paediatric IgA nephropathy with regard to clinical and histopathological variables (Oxford classification). Nephrol Dial Transplant. 2012;27(2):715–22.
110. Coppo R, D'Arrigo G, Tripepi G, Russo ML, Roberts ISD, Bellur S, et al. Is there long-term value of pathology scoring in immunoglobulin A nephropathy? A validation study of the Oxford Classification for IgA Nephropathy (VALIGA) update. Nephrol Dial Transplant. 2020;35(6):1002–9.
111. Coppo R. Mesangial C4d deposition may predict progression of kidney disease in pediatric

111. patients with IgA nephropathy. Pediatr Nephrol. 2008;32(7):1211–20.
112. Coppo R. C4d deposits in IgA nephropathy: where does complement activation come from? Pediatr Nephrol. 2017;32:1097–101.
113. Yoshikawa N, Iijima K, Ito H. IgA nephropathy in children. Nephron. 1999;83:1–12.
114. Coppo R, Gianoglio B, Porcellini MG, Maringhini S. Frequency of renal diseases and clinical indications for renal biopsy in children (Report of the Italian National Registry of Renal Biopsies in children). Nephrol Dial Transplant. 1998;13(2):293–7.
115. Wyatt RJ, Julian BA, Bhathena DB, Mitchell BL, Holland NH, Malluche HH. IgA nephropathy: presentation, clinical course, and prognosis in children and adults. Am J Kidney Dis. 1984;4(2):192–200.
116. Lévy M, Gonzalez-Burchard G, Broyer M, Dommergues JP, Foulard M, Sorez JP, et al. Berger's disease in children: natural history and outcome. Med (United States). 1985;64(3):157–80.
117. Cambier A, Gleeson PJ, Flament H, Le Stang MB, Monteiro RC. New therapeutic perspectives for IgA nephropathy in children. Pediatr Nephrol. 2020;36(3):497–506.
118. Coppo RDG. Factors predicting progression of IgA nephropathies.itle. J Nephrol. 2005;18(5):503–12.
119. Ronkainen J, Ala-Houhala M, Autio-Harmainen H, Jahnukainen T, Koskimies O, Merenmies J, et al. Long-term outcome 19 years after childhood IgA nephritis: a retrospective cohort study. Pediatr Nephrol. 2006;21(9):1266–73.
120. Wyatt RJ, Kritchevsky SB, Woodford SY, Miller PM, Roy S, Holland NH, et al. IgA nephropathy: long-term prognosis for pediatric patients. J Pediatr. 1995;127(6):913–9.
121. Nozawa R, Suzuki J, Takahashi A, Isome M, Kawasaki Y, Suzuki S, et al. Clinicopathological features and the prognosis of IgA nephropathy in Japanese children on long-term observation. Clin Nephrol. 2005;64(3):171–9.
122. Shima Y, Nakanishi K, Hama T, Mukaiyama H, Togawa H, Sako M, et al. Spontaneous remission in children with IgA nephropathy. Pediatr Nephrol. 2013;28(1):71–6.
123. Linné T, Berg U, Bohman SO, Sigström L. Course and long-term outcome of idiopathic IgA nephropathy in children. Pediatr Nephrol. 1991;5(4):383–6.
124. Hogg RJ, Silva FG, Wyatt RJ, Reisch JS, Craig Argyle J, Savino DA. Prognostic indicators in children with IgA nephropathy—report of the Southwest Pediatric Nephrology Study Group. Pediatr Nephrol. 1994;8(1):15–20.
125. Sevillano AM, Gutiérrez E, Yuste C, Cavero T, Mérida E, Rodríguez P, et al. Remission of Hematuria Improves Renal Survival in IgA Nephropathy. J Am Soc Nephrol. 2017;28(10):3089–99.
126. Radhakrishnan J, Cattran DC. The KDIGO practice guideline on glomerulonephritis: reading between

the (guide)lines-application to the individual patient. Kidney Int. 2012;82:840–56.
127. Rovin BH, Adler SG, Barratt J, Bridoux F, Burdge KA, Chan TM, et al. KDIGO 2021 clinical practice guideline for the management of glomerular diseases. Kidney Int. 2021;100(4):S1–276.
128. Kamei K, Nakanishi K, Ito S, Saito M, Sako M, Ishikura K, et al. Long-term results of a randomized controlled trial in childhood IgA nephropathy. Clin J Am Soc Nephrol. 2011;6(6):1301–7.
129. Shima Y, Nakanishi K, Kamei K, Togawa H, Nozu K, Tanaka R, et al. Disappearance of glomerular IgA deposits in childhood IgA nephropathy showing diffuse mesangial proliferation after 2 years of combination/prednisolone therapy. Nephrol Dial Transplant. 2011;26(1):163–9.
130. Coppo R, Troyanov S, Bellur S, Cattran D, Cook HT, Feehally J, et al. Validation of the Oxford classification of IgA nephropathy in cohorts with different presentations and treatments. Kidney Int. 2014;86(4):828–36.
131. Barbour SJ, Coppo R, Zhang H, Liu ZH, Suzuki Y, Matsuzaki K, et al. Evaluating a new international risk-prediction tool in IgA nephropathy. JAMA Intern Med. 2019;179(7):942–52.
132. Barbour SJ, Coppo R, Er L, Russo ML, Liu Z-H, Ding J, et al. Updating the international IgA nephropathy prediction tool for use in children. Kidney Int. 2020;99(6):1439–50.
133. Van Den Akker EH, Sanders EAM, Van Staatj BK, Rijkers GT, Rovers MM, Hoes AW, et al. Long-term effects of pediatric adenotonsillectomy on serum immunoglobulin levels: results of a randomized controlled trial. Ann Allergy Asthma Immunol. 2006;97(2):251–6.
134. Cattran DC, Feehally J, Cook HT, Liu ZH, Fervenza FC, Mezzano SA, et al. Kidney disease: improving global outcomes (KDIGO) glomerulonephritis work group. KDIGO clinical practice guideline for glomerulonephritis. Kidney Int Suppl. 2012;2(2):139–274.
135. Floege J, Barbour SJ, Cattran DC, Hogan JJ, Nachman PH, Tang SCW, et al. Management and treatment of glomerular diseases (part 1): conclusions from a Kidney Disease: Improving Global Outcomes (KDIGO) Controversies Conference. Kidney Int. 2019;95(2):268–80.
136. Kawasaki Y, Takano K, Suyama K, Isome M, Suzuki H, Sakuma H, et al. Efficacy of tonsillectomy pulse therapy versus multiple-drug therapy for IgA nephropathy. Pediatr Nephrol. 2006;21(11):1701–6.
137. Feehally J, Coppo R, Troyanov S, Bellur SS, Cattran D, Cook T, et al. Tonsillectomy in a European Cohort of 1,147 Patients with IgA Nephropathy. Nephron. 2016;132(1):15–24.
138. Coppo R, Peruzzi L, Amore A, Piccoli A, Cochat P, Stone R, et al. IgACE: a placebo-controlled, randomized trial of angiotensin-converting enzyme inhibitors in children and young people with IgA

138. nephropathy and moderate proteinuria. J Am Soc Nephrol. 2007;18(6):1880–8.

139. Bhattacharjee R, Filler G. Additive antiproteinuric effect of ACE inhibitor and losartan in IgA nephropathy [2]. Pediatr Nephrol. 2002;17:302–4.

140. Shima Y, Nakanishi K, Sako M, Saito-Oba M, Hamasaki Y, Hataya H, et al. Lisinopril versus lisinopril and losartan for mild childhood IgA nephropathy: a randomized controlled trial (JSKDC01 study). Pediatr Nephrol. 2019;34(5):837–46.

141. Pozzi C, Bolasco PG, Fogazzi G, Andrulli S, Altieri P, Ponticelli C, et al. Corticosteroids in IgA nephropathy: a randomised controlled trial. Lancet. 1999;353(9156):883–7.

142. Manno C, Torres DD, Rossini M, Pesce F, Schena FP. Randomized controlled clinical trial of corticosteroids plus ACE-inhibitors with long-term follow-up in proteinuric IgA nephropathy. Nephrol Dial Transplant. 2009;24(12):3694–701.

143. Pozzi C, Andrulli S, Del Vecchio L, Melis P, Fogazzi GB, Altieri P, et al. Corticosteroid effectiveness in IgA nephropathy: long-term results of a randomized, controlled trial. J Am Soc Nephrol. 2004;15(1):157–63.

144. Lv J, Zhang H, Wong MG, Jardine MJ, Hladunewich M, Jha V, et al. Effect of oral methylprednisolone on clinical outcomes in patients with IgA nephropathy: the TESTING randomized clinical trial. JAMA J Am Med Assoc. 2017;318(5):432–42.

145. Rauen T, Eitner F, Fitzner C, Sommerer C, Zeier M, Otte B, et al. Intensive supportive care plus immunosuppression in IgA nephropathy. N Engl J Med. 2015;373(23):2225–36.

146. Coppo R. Pediatric IgA nephropathy: clinical and therapeutic perspectives. Semin Nephrol. 2008;28(1):18–26.

147. Waldo FB, Alexander R, Wyatt RJ, Kohaut EC. Alternate-day prednisone therapy in children with IgA-associated nephritis. Am J Kidney Dis. 1989;13(1):55–60.

148. Welch TR, Fryer C, Shely E, Witte DP, Quinlan M. Double-blind, controlled trial of short-term prednisone therapy in immunoglobulin A glomerulonephritis. J Pediatr. 1992;121(3):474–7.

149. Niaudet P, Murcia I, Beaufils H, Broyer MHR. Primary IgA nephropathies in children: prognosis and treatment. Adv Nephrol Necker Hosp. 1993;22:121–40.

150. Hogg RJ, Lee J, Nardelli N, Julian BA, Cattran D, Waldo B, et al. Clinical trial to evaluate omega-3 fatty acids and alternate day prednisone in patients with IgA nephropathy: report from the Southwest Pediatric Nephrology Study Group. Clin J Am Soc Nephrol. 2006;1(3):467–74.

151. Yoshikawa N, Ito H, Sakai T, Takekoshi Y, Honda M, Awazu M, Ito K, Iitaka K, Koitabashi Y, Yamaoka K, Nakagawa K, Nakamura H, Matsuyama S, Seino Y, Takeda N, Hattori SNM. A controlled trial of combined therapy for newly diagnosed severe childhood IgA nephropathy. The Japanese Pediatric IgA Nephropathy Treatment Study Group. J Am Soc Nephrol. 1999;10:101–9.

152. Yoshikawa N, Honda M, Iijima K, Awazu M, Hattori S, Nakanishi K, et al. Steroid treatment for severe childhood IgA nephropathy: a randomized, controlled trial. Clin J Am Soc Nephrol. 2006;1(3):511–7.

153. Shima Y, Nakanishi K, Kaku Y, Ishikura K, Hataya H, Matsuyama T, et al. Combination therapy with or without warfarin and dipyridamole for severe childhood IgA nephropathy: an RCT. Pediatr Nephrol. 2018;33(11):2103–12.

154. Pozzi C, Andrulli S, Pani A, Scaini P, Del Vecchio L, Fogazzi G, et al. Addition of azathioprine to corticosteroids does not benefit patients with IgA nephropathy. J Am Soc Nephrol. 2010;21(10):1783–90.

155. Cambier A, Rabant M, Peuchmaur M, Hertig A, Deschenes G, Couchoud C, et al. Immunosuppressive treatment in children with IgA nephropathy and the clinical value of podocytopathic features. Kidney Int Reports. 2018;3(4):916–25.

156. Shenoy M, Ognjanovic MV, Coulthard MG. Treating severe Henoch-Schönlein and IgA nephritis with plasmapheresis alone. Pediatr Nephrol. 22(8):1167–71.

157. Fellström BC, Barratt J, Cook H, Coppo R, Feehally J, de Fijter JW, et al. Targeted-release budesonide versus placebo in patients with IgA nephropathy (NEFIGAN): a double-blind, randomised, placebo-controlled phase 2b trial. Lancet. 2017;389(10084):2117–27.

158. Hou JH, Le WB, Chen N, Wang WM, Liu ZS, Liu D, et al. Mycophenolate mofetil combined with prednisone versus full-dose prednisone in IgA nephropathy with active proliferative lesions: a randomized controlled trial. Am J Kidney Dis. 2017;69(6):788–95.

159. Hogg RJ, Bay RC, Jennette JC, Sibley R, Kumar S, Fervenza FC, et al. Randomized controlled trial of mycophenolate mofetil in children, adolescents, and adults with IgA nephropathy. Am J Kidney Dis. 2015;66(5):783–91.

160. Ballardie FW, Roberts ISD. Controlled prospective trial of prednisolone and cytotoxics in progressive IgA nephropathy. J Am Soc Nephrol. 2002;13(1):142–8.

161. Lafayette RA, Canetta PA, Rovin BH, Appel GB, Novak J, Nath KA, et al. A randomized, controlled trial of rituximab in IgA nephropathy with proteinuria and renal dysfunction. J Am Soc Nephrol. 2017;28:1306–13.

162. Song YH, Cai GY, Xiao YF, Wang YP, Yuan BS, Xia YY, et al. Efficacy and safety of calcineurin inhibitor treatment for IgA nephropathy: a meta-analysis. BMC Nephrol. 2017;18(1):61.

163. Liu LJ, Yang Y-Z, Shi SF, Bao YF, Yang C, Zhu SN, et al. Effects of hydroxychloroquine on proteinuria in IgA nephropathy: a randomized controlled trial. Am J Kidney Dis. 2019;74(1):15–22.

164. Coppo R. Biomarkers and targeted new therapies for IgA nephropathy. Pediatr Nephrol. 2008;32(5):725–31.
165. Selvaskandan H, Cheung CK, Muto M, Barratt J. New strategies and perspectives on managing IgA nephropathy. Clin Exp Nephrol. 2019;23:577–88.
166. Sato M, Hotta O, Tomioka S, Horigome I, Chiba S, Miyazaki M, et al. Cohort study of advanced IgA nephropathy: efficacy and limitations of corticosteroids with tonsillectomy. Nephron Clin Pract. 2003;93(4):c137–45.

Membranous Nephropathy

18

Myda Khalid and Laurence H. Beck Jr

Incidence

Nephrotic syndrome is one of the most common kidney disorders encountered in a pediatric nephrology practice. In children, it occurs at a reported incidence of 2 per 100,000 per year and a cumulative prevalence of 16 per 100,000 children. Compared to other more commonly occurring nephrotic disorders in this population, such as minimal change disease and primary focal and segmental glomerulosclerosis, membranous nephropathy (MN) is relatively rare. Given its rarity in children, there is scant data on the true incidence, prognosis and best management practices. It is estimated that 1.5% of children with nephrotic syndrome will have membranous nephropathy based on the International Study of Kidney Disease in Children report in 1978 [1]. The incidence is higher, approaching 22%, in adolescents compared to younger children [2].

Because many children with steroid-sensitive nephrotic syndrome will never be biopsied, the relative prevalence of MN versus minimal change disease and focal segmental glomerular sclerosis is unclear. Another bias is the age range of the population. In a series from Pakistan that investigated 538 children who underwent biopsy for idiopathic nephrotic syndrome, there was a significant difference between the 3% rate of MN in children aged <13 years and the 18.5% rate found in adolescents aged 13–18 years [3]. Similar rates were found in adolescents in two different cohorts [2, 4].

MN has been reported to account for only 0.6% of pediatric chronic and end-stage kidney disease (ESKD) cases, with a median age at onset of ESKD being 16 years based on the 2007 North American Pediatric Renal Trials and Collaborative Studies report and 2012 United States Renal Data System. This is in contrast to adults, in whom MN is one of the more common forms of nephrotic syndrome and a significant contributor towards ESKD (Table 18.1).

M. Khalid (✉)
Division of Pediatric Nephrology and Hypertension,
Indiana University School of Medicine,
Indianapolis, IN, USA
e-mail: khalidm@iu.edu

L. H. Beck Jr
Section of Nephrology, Boston University School of
Medicine and Boston Medical Center,
Boston, MA, USA
e-mail: lhbeckjr@bu.edu

© The Author(s), under exclusive license to Springer Nature Switzerland AG 2023
F. Schaefer, L. A. Greenbaum (eds.), *Pediatric Kidney Disease*,
https://doi.org/10.1007/978-3-031-11665-0_18

Table 18.1 Differences between pediatric and adult membranous nephropathy

Feature	Pediatric MN	Adult MN
Disease type/subtype		
Proportion of all primary nephrotic syndrome cases that is MN	<5% (children); 5–20% (adolescents)	15–30%
MN that is primary ("idiopathic")	Minority	Majority
Proportion of primary MN that is PLA2R-associated	Less than 50% (more frequent in adolescents)	70–80%
Demographic and clinical features		
Male predominance	Variable	Yes
Full nephrotic syndrome	40–75%	75%
Microscopic hematuria	70–90% (can be macroscopic)	50%
Hypertension	<10%	30%
Thromboembolic events	<5%	10–20%
Spontaneous remission	Common	30%
Progressive renal impairment	<25%	30–40%
Pathologic features		
Mesangial deposits	Up to 50%	30%
Segmental distribution of deposits	Occasional	Very rare

MN membranous nephropathy

Etiology

The etiologies of MN have traditionally been divided into *idiopathic* (now more commonly called *primary*) and *secondary* causes. While primary MN typically reflects a kidney-specific autoimmune response, the glomerular process in secondary MN can usually be attributed to a systemic disease process, a drug or toxin, infection, or malignancy. Recent progress in the identification of target autoantigens and other specific biomarkers of MN has led the field to consider moving toward an antigen-based approach to naming the different types of MN, irrespective of primary or secondary designations [5]. However, it is still useful to subdivide MN into its autoimmune (idiopathic or primary) forms in which there is loss of tolerance to a self-antigen within the glomerulus, and secondary forms in which the antigen may be exogenous. Distinction between primary and secondary MN relies on a

systematic evaluation of historical (drugs, exposures), clinical, laboratory, and histological features, as will be discussed further later in this chapter.

Although primary autoimmune forms of MN can occur in children, there has historically been a higher frequency of secondary forms of MN when compared to adults. The main etiologies of secondary disease in the pediatric population are infections and systemic autoimmune diseases such as lupus (Table 18.2). Drugs and malignancy are less frequent causes of MN in children,

Table 18.2 Secondary causes of membranous nephropathy

A. Autoimmune diseases
1. Systemic lupus erythematosus
2. Autoimmune thyroiditis
3. Sarcoidosis
4. Sjögren syndrome
5. Rheumatoid arthritis

B. Infectious diseases
1. Hepatitis B
2. Other viruses (HIV, HCV, EBV, CMV)
3. Quartan malaria
4. Schistosomiasis
5. Filariasis
6. Congenital syphilis

C. Drugs and exposures
1. Non-steroidal anti-inflammatory agents
2. Penicillamine
3. Bucillamine
4. Mercury salts
5. Recombinant enzymes used in enzyme replacement therapy

D. Neoplastic
1. Rare associations with disparate types of malignancy

E. Other conditions
1. Familial truncating mutations in *MME* (gene for NEP)
2. Anti-cationic BSA antibodies
3. *De novo* MN after kidney transplantation
4. Immune dysregulation or deficiency syndromes (IPEX, CVID)
5. Stem cell transplantation

Abbreviations: *HIV* human immunodeficiency virus; *HCV* hepatitis C virus; *EBV* Epstein Barr virus; *CMV* cytomegalovirus; *MME* membrane metalloendopeptidase; *NEP* neutral endopeptidase; *BSA* bovine serum albumin; *IPEX* immunodysregulation, polyendocrinopathy, enteropathy, X linked; *CVID* common variable immunodeficiency

but certainly need to be considered as potentially causal when the processes are concurrent. As in adults, sarcoidosis and autoimmune thyroid disease can be linked to MN in children. Hepatitis B has historically been a major cause of secondary MN in parts of the world in which the virus is endemic [6]. Fortunately, the incidence of hepatitis B-associated MN has decreased worldwide with the introduction of vaccination programs [7–9]. Additional viral infections such as HIV, EBV, and CMV have been reported as secondary causes of childhood MN. Infections such as schistosomiasis, filariasis, malaria and congenital syphilis are also important conditions linked to development of MN in areas where these diseases are prevalent.

Dysregulation of the immune system as occurs in IPEX syndrome [10] or combined variable immunodeficiency [11] can be a cause of MN in children. Exposure of host immune system to donor antigens (or vice versa), as occurs following hematopoietic stem cell transplantation or after kidney transplantation, can lead to alloimmune forms of membranous nephropathy [12, 13].

Pathophysiology

Despite the various etiologies that can lead to the histological pattern of membranous nephropathy and its consequent clinical manifestations, much of the underlying pathophysiology is fundamentally similar. Pediatric disease has provided important conceptual information about adult disease, and vice versa.

Membranous nephropathy (also variably called membranous glomerulonephritis or glomerulopathy) is named due to a thickening of the glomerular capillary walls as visualized by light microscopy, especially with prolonged disease [14]. The thickening is a result of (1) immune complexes that deposit beneath the basal surface of the podocyte at the outer aspect of the glomerular basement membrane (GBM) and (2) the additional extracellular matrix material that is eventually secreted between and around these deposits. The subepithelial immune deposits reliably consist of several components, which aid in the pathological detection and classification of MN. The immune complexes themselves are formed by immunoglobulin (most often IgG) and a target antigen, the identities of which have been identified over the past 15 years. Components of the complement system such as C3, C4, and C5b-9, activated by these immune complexes, are also consistently found within the immune deposits. These factors are routinely identified by immunostaining of the kidney biopsy (see Pathology below). The ability to detect the specific antigen within the deposits has been an important development in both pediatric and adult MN.

The field of MN has benefited both from well-studied animal models such as Heymann nephritis as well as important insights from human disease such as the identification of a growing number of targets antigens (Fig. 18.1). The ability to detect and follow circulating antibodies against these target proteins has opened up a new era for the diagnosis and monitoring of MN from early infancy to adulthood [15, 16].

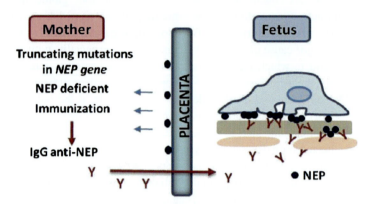
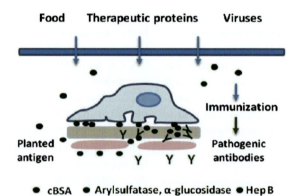
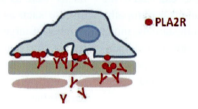

Fig. 18.1 Schematic representation of membranous nephropathy etiologies in children. (**a**) NEP-related alloimmune glomerulopathy. Neutral endopeptidase (NEP, blue dots) serves as a pathogenic antigen in the podocyte cell membrane. Antibodies to this protein originate in women who genetically lack NEP because of truncating mutations in *MME* (which encodes NEP). Immunization occurs during pregnancy when the mother's immune system is first exposed to NEP, which is strongly expressed by placental cells and by fetal cells entering the mother's blood. From about the 18th week of gestation, maternal antibodies are actively transported across the placenta to the fetus, where they bind to the NEP antigen expressed on podocytes. (**b**) Exogenous antigen-induced membranous nephropathy. Foreign, exogenous proteins commonly induce the production of antibodies. Owing to unusual physicochemical properties, these antigens can be trapped in the glomerular basement membrane where they can serve as a target for circulating antibodies, leading to the formation of in situ immune complexes. Green dots represent cationic bovine serum albumin (cBSA) from the diet, infused enzymes used in enzyme replacement therapy (arylsulfatase, α-glucosidase in this example) or hepatitis B antigens (Hep B). (**c**) PLA2R-associated primary (autoimmune) membranous nephropathy. The phospholipase A2 receptor (red dots), an integral membrane glycoprotein of podocytes, is a target antigen for circulating autoantibodies

Heymann Nephritis, the First Experimental Model of MN

An important animal model that established much of the pathophysiological paradigm for human membranous nephropathy was developed in 1959 by Walter Heymann, a pediatrician from Cleveland (Ohio, USA) and his colleagues. Lewis rats were immunized with crude extracts of rat kidney in what became known as the active Heymann nephritis model [17] and yielded a glomerular and clinical phenotype that was remarkably similar to human MN. As the experimental disease could be induced by immunizing rats with a rat proximal tubular brush border fraction, the source of the predominantly glomerular deposits was initially felt to be due to glomerular trapping of circulating immune complexes of brush border antigens and corresponding anti-brush border antibodies. Development of passive Heymann nephritis models in which the anti-brush border antibodies were first raised in rabbits or sheep and then transferred to the rats raised doubts about the importance of circulating immune complexes. Two groups, using ex vivo and isolated perfused rat kidney systems, independently demonstrated that the anti-brush border antibodies bound to an antigenic target on the podocyte (in fact, common to the podocyte and brush border) and suggested that the subepithelial deposits formed locally [18, 19].

The antigenic target common to the rat podocyte and tubular brush border was ultimately identified by Kerjaschki and Farquhar in the early 1980's as gp330 or megalin [20, 21], now known as the low-density lipoprotein receptor-related protein 2 (LRP2). Megalin was found to reside in clathrin-coated pits at the basal surface of the podocyte foot process, where it could interact with circulating anti-megalin antibodies from the capillary lumen to form immune complexes in situ. The subepithelial deposits were felt to grow in size as polyclonal anti-megalin antibodies formed highly-cross linked immune complexes with megalin that continued to be delivered to the basal surface in clathrin-coated vesicles [22]. Cleavage of the transmembrane protein megalin to release its large extracellular region into the immune complexes likely facilitated deposit formation [23].

These findings established the paradigm that a podocyte derived antigen that was expressed at the basal surface of the podocyte could react with anti-podocyte antibodies to initiate the pathologic process of MN. The search began for anti-megalin antibodies as an explanation for human MN, but it was quickly realized that human podocytes do not routinely express megalin and that other target antigens were likely the cause of human disease. Of note, anti-brush border antibodies (ABBA, now known to be anti-LRP2) are responsible for an autoimmune form of human interstitial nephritis that consistently exhibits segmental subepithelial deposits that may be due to limited megalin/LRP2 expression by aging podocytes [24].

Alloimmune Neonatal MN: Neutral Endopeptidase as the Target Antigen

The first podocyte-expressed target antigen in human MN was identified in a neonate born with MN [25] (Fig. 18.1, upper). Under the assumption that maternal antibodies might have caused this immune-complex disease in the developing fetal kidney, both maternal and infant serum was used to screen human, rat, and rabbit kidney tissue for candidate antigens. The culprit protein was identified as neutral endopeptidase (NEP) and NEP was found to co-localize with IgG and C5b-9 within the immune deposits of the infant's kidney biopsy [25, 26]. Experiments in which a pregnant rabbit was injected with IgG from the mother demonstrated that these anti-NEP antibodies were able to transfer disease [27].

NEP (which has several alternative names such as neprilysin, CD10, common acute lymphoblastic leukemia antigen or CALLA) is a product of the *MME* (membrane metalloendopeptidase) gene. It is an enzyme responsible for the degradation of biologically active peptides such as enkephalin, natriuretic peptides, endothelin, bradykinin and substance P in the vicinity of their receptors. It is present in many organs as well as granulocytes; in the kidney, NEP is detected at the podocyte surface, in the brush border and in vessel walls.

The mother of the index case of NEP-associated antenatal MN, despite having high titers of circulating anti-NEP, did not exhibit any manifestations of nephrotic syndrome herself, and it was hypothesized that she might be genetically deficient in NEP. This was confirmed at the genetic level, showing the presence of truncating mutations within the *MME* gene [26] and by the lack of reactivity of her granulocytes with a panel of anti-NEP antibodies [25]. This mother was likely alloimmunized to NEP from a prior pregnancy which was miscarried, during which NEP of paternal origin was expressed by the syncytiotrophoblastic cells of the placenta. Four additional families with maternofetal alloimmune MN were identified. All immunized mothers were NEP deficient as a result of truncating mutations in exon 7 and exon 15 of the NEP gene [26, 28].

Since the anti-NEP antibodies were of maternal origin, transferred to the fetal circulation across the placenta, it is not surprising that most of these infants exhibited rapid improvement in their renal function and proteinuria as the maternal IgG cleared from their system and the glomerular deposits were resorbed. An exception was one newborn with a long duration of kidney failure requiring dialysis. The mother in this case possessed anti-NEP with an abundance of the IgG1 subclass, in contrast to other cases in which IgG4 was predominant. In addition to possibly better activating the complement system within the glomerular deposits, this IgG1 anti-NEP was also shown to possess enzyme inhibitory function that may have had renal vascular consequences [28].

NEP-associated alloimmune antenatal MN therefore represents the first type of human MN in which an intrinsic podocyte protein was implicated as the target antigen. Furthermore, anti-NEP IgG from the mother could induce disease when transferred to a rabbit. This maternofetal incompatibility due to a maternal genetic defect leading to an alloimmune response in the fetus is rare, but could be considered in other situations in which the mother is genetically deficient in a podocyte protein normally expressed in the fetal kidney.

M-Type Phospholipase A₂ Receptor-Associated MN

As idiopathic MN in adults did not demonstrate the presence of antibodies to either megalin/LRP2 or to NEP, the search continued to identify target antigens in this disorder. A breakthrough came in 2009 with the identification of the M-type phospholipase A_2 receptor, now better known as PLA2R [29]. Sera from adult cases of MN possessed circulating IgG4 that could detect a distinct glycoprotein by immunoblotting extracts from human glomeruli. Through the use of a candidate antigen approach that was informed by a mass spectrometric analysis of human glomerular proteins immunoprecipitated with IgG from MN cases, the target antigen was ultimately identified as PLA2R [30]. Seventy to 80% of idiopathic (primary autoimmune) MN are PLA2R-associated.

Like NEP and megalin (in the rat), PLA2R is expressed as a transmembrane receptor on the podocyte surface, where circulating antibodies can target one or more epitopes in the extracellular domain (Fig. 18.1, lower). It is of interest that, like megalin, it is also delivered to and recycled from the plasma membrane in clathrin-coated vesicles. Its role within the podocyte is not clear, but it may help to internalize small secreted phospholipase A_2 enzymes that pass through the GBM. PLA2R is not expressed by podocytes in small animals and thus passive administration of human anti-PLA2R antibodies (PLA2R-ab) has not been able to transfer disease as was the case for anti-NEP alloantibodies.

The identification of PLA2R as the target antigen in the majority of adult idiopathic MN cases paved the way for a new era of diagnosis, monitoring, and understanding in MN. As the major target antigen in adult MN and after more than a decade of study, this autoantibody-target antigen system now represents the paradigm by which we understand the link between circulating antibodies and clinical manifestations of disease. We will focus on this system in the paragraphs below.

The identification of specific target antigens (like PLA2R) in MN allows for immunodetection of that antigen within immune deposits of the kidney biopsy, as well as assaying for the presence of autoantibodies to the target antigen in the circulation. Serologic assays to detect PLA2R-ab are based on ELISA using the recombinant human PLA2R protein or by immunofluorescence (IFA) of PLA2R transfected cells and are now commercially available in most countries as a clinical test. The specificity of the presence of circulating PLA2R-ab for MN is nearly 100%, especially when borderline or low-titer positive ELISA tests are confirmed by the more-sensitive IFA. Normal individuals or those with other proteinuric disease will not have PLA2R-ab. Such specificity has even led to the suggestion that a positive test for PLA2R-ab is diagnostic and may obviate the need for kidney biopsy, especially in those with normal kidney function and without other potential secondary causes of MN [31]. In situations where biopsy is difficult due to a patient already being on anticoagulation due to thromboembolic events resulting from the nephrotic state, a solitary kidney, or other relative contraindications to kidney biopsy, seropositivity for PLA2R-ab may be diagnostically sufficient to guide subsequent therapy.

A low prevalence of PLA2R-ab has been observed in forms of MN found in association with SLE, infectious disease, therapeutic drug use (especially nonsteroidal anti-inflammatory agents) or malignancy [32–35]. It is often quite difficult to assign causality of the MN to the associated condition, and in many cases a coincidental occurrence of the PLA2R-related MN and underlying disorder cannot be excluded. There may be exceptions: indeed, patients with MN associated with active sarcoidosis or replicating hepatitis B appear to have a high prevalence of PLA2R-related disease, which suggests that the immunologic setting of sarcoidosis and hepatitis B might trigger or enhance immunization against PLA2R [34, 36, 37]. Because therapeutic strategies are different for patients with idiopathic and secondary MN, discriminating between these

two groups of patients is of utmost clinical importance.

In the majority of cases of MN, a biopsy is performed, and immunodetection of the PLA2R antigen (by immunofluorescence or immunohistochemistry) within the deposits in a fine, granular peripheral capillary wall pattern can establish the type of MN as PLA2R-associated. Immunostaining for PLA2R is more sensitive for PLA2R-associated MN than are the serologic assays [38], for the reason that circulating PLA2R-ab may not be detectable or not be present due to rapid absorption in the kidney in early disease or due to the achievement of immunological remission in individuals who remain proteinuric in later disease. This test enables the retrospective diagnosis of MN in archival, paraffin-embedded biopsy specimens, which is crucial for the monitoring of patients who will benefit from a kidney graft. It should be noted that there is a small proportion of cases of biopsy-proved MN who have detectable circulating PLA2R-ab, but do not stain for PLA2R within the deposits [37, 38]. It is possible that the antigen is masked by abundant PLA2R-ab targeting multiple epitopes or by another protein that limits detection with the commonly used commercial antibodies. Further study of such cases is needed to see if the circulating PLA2R-ab correlate with disease activity (see below) or if the PLA2R-ab might be non-pathogenic and an epiphenomenon.

A fundamental observation that has revolutionized the manner in which we monitor disease activity in MN is that, as the disease resolves, circulating PLA2R-decline and disappear in a manner that precedes and predicts clinical disease activity [39]. First noted in MN patients treated with the B cell depleting agent rituximab [40], the relationship between declining autoantibody and declining proteinuria holds for all immunosuppressive agents used in the treatment of PLA2R-associated MN [41–43]. PLA2R-ab are typically present in the setting of active nephrotic syndrome, are absent at clinical remission, and return with disease relapse [44] or in the setting of recurrent PLA2R-associated MN in the kidney allograft [45, 46]. Because high titers of

PLA2R-ab tend to take longer to disappear and/or are more resistant to therapy, they are associated with a lower chance of spontaneous [47] or immunosuppressive therapy induced remission [48] and with a higher risk of deterioration of kidney function [49]. A proposal for using PLA2R-ab in clinical practice was published several years ago [50] and the main tenets were incorporated into the 2021 Kidney Disease: Improving Global Outcomes (KDIGO) guidelines for glomerulonephritis (www.kdigo.org).

Role of PLA2R-ab-Related MN in Childhood

Although the bulk of the studies investigating the utility of monitoring PLA2R-ab has been from the adult MN literature, it is likely that the same principles could be applied to pediatric MN. However, the incidence of this type of MN is clearly less in children than adults, although exact numbers are not yet known. It is exceptionally rare for a child younger than 10 years old to have PLA2R-associated MN.

With more clinical and pathological testing for PLA2R and some of the more recently described types of MN, the field is gaining an understanding of the relevance of these forms of "adult" MN within the pediatric MN population. A number of studies have assessed the prevalence of PLA2R-associated MN by immunostaining pediatric MN biopsy registries in a retrospective manner for the presence of PLA2R within immune deposits. An early study focused on 22 MN cases with no clinical evidence for secondary disease, most between the ages of 10 and 17, and identified 10 cases (45%) positive for PLA2R [51]. In contrast, the PLA2R-negative cases were more likely to have secondary features on biopsy, although no clear secondary causes emerged with 3 years of follow up. These findings suggest a more diverse and currently incompletely explained set of etiologies in pediatric MN.

International studies confirm this prevalence of PLA2R-associated MN, largely within an adolescent population. A study of adolescents (10–19 years old) with primary MN in India revealed that the majority had PLA2R staining on biopsy, circulating PLA2R-ab antibodies, or both [52]. A higher prevalence of PLA2R-associated MN in children over the age of 10 is also suggested by a report from Japan [53]. These authors found 2 cases of PLA2R-associated disease amongst 19 patients in the 10 to 15-year-old group, but no cases amongst 15 patients aged 3–9 years old. A study from China also confirms a prevalence of PLA2R-associated disease in adolescents that is similar to that found in adult primary MN and a lower rate in younger children [54]. In this cohort, the mean age of the 16 PLA2R-associated cases was 12.9 years old, while that of the PLA2R-negative cases was 6.8 years old. Nearly 82% (9/11) of MN within the older 13–17-year-old group was PLA2R-associated, whereas only 7 of 27 (25.9%) were PLA2R-associated in the 1–12-year-old group. The authors do not report the ages of these seven PLA2R-positive cases. A final case series from Japan may have identified the youngest known patient with PLA2R-associated MN. Amongst 11 pediatric (age 4–14) patients with MN, a 6 year old with 2 g/day of proteinuria was found to have PLA2R-positive granular immune deposits on biopsy; serology was not available to confirm [55].

Pregnancy and Exposure to Maternal PLA2R-ab

Although no infants have ever been shown clinically to mount an autoimmune response to PLA2R, they can rarely be exposed to maternal PLA2R-ab in utero. This scenario is theoretically similar to the cases of alloimmune fetomaternal MN with anti-NEP in which podocyte-reactive antibodies cross the placenta to cause glomerular deposits in the fetus. There are several reports of pregnancy and active PLA2R-associated MN in a 39-, 43-, 33-, and a 21-year-old mother [56–59]. In three cases, the infant was born without any evidence of proteinuria or other abnormalities. In the fourth case [58], the infant was delivered early due to worsening oligohydramnios and at birth had similar PLA2R-ab levels as the mother, but levels subsequently declined. However, with close follow-up, the infant was subsequently found to have developed proteinuria and an increased PLA2R-ab titer, which was felt to be due to ingestion/absorption of PLA2R-ab secreted in the mother's breast milk. A retrospective review of 27 women with primary MN and pregnancy showed adverse maternofetal outcomes in 10 cases [60]. Seropositivity for PLA2R-ab and the inability to achieve remission during pregnancy were risk factors for adverse events.

Additional Target Antigens Since PLA2R

Although PLA2R is the most common target antigen in primary adult MN, comprising about 80% of cases, more recent findings have implicated other target antigens or biomarkers that reveal other types of MN, some with different clinical and histologic phenotypes than the more common PLA2R-associated MN.

Thrombospondin Type-1 Domain-Containing 7A (THSD7A)

Five years after the description of the major target antigen PLA2R in adult MN, a second podocyte antigen called THSD7A was identified [61]. This protein is a well-conserved transmembrane protein that sits at the basal surface of the podocyte, directly beneath the slit diaphragms [62]. In much the same manner as the PLA2R/PLA2R-ab system, circulating antibodies to THSD7A were found in a minority of adult patients with primary MN, and appeared to correlate with disease activity [61]. THSD7A and IgG co-localized within immune deposits. Remarkably, several cases of malignancy associated MN were found to have been caused by tumor overexpression of THSD7A and regional lymph node activation of the humoral response [63, 64]. The association with malignancy may not be as common as initially reported, but is clearly greater than seen in PLA2R-associated MN [65].

THSD7A-associated MN is not common in children but can occur. The youngest patient identified with anti-THSD7A antibodies is a 4-year-old whose anti-THSD7A declined in response to treatment with rituximab [66]. A small retrospective cohort study from Germany demonstrated that 50% of their 12 pediatric MN cases had circulating antibodies to PLA2R [67], with tissue staining for PLA2R on biopsy also confirmed in two of these cases. The other six had no identifiable circulating antibodies to THSD7A, cationic bovine serum albumin (see below), or neutral endopeptidase. When Zhang and colleagues stained their 22 PLA2R-negative pediatric cases for THSD7A, none was positive [54]. It is not clear at this time what the overall prevalence of THSD7A-associated disease may be in children or adolescents.

Additional Antigens with Potential Secondary MN Associations

New findings may help to characterize cases of pediatric MN that fail to exhibit staining for PLA2R or THSD7A. Using the technique of laser capture microdissection followed by mass spectrometric analysis, Sethi and colleagues have identified a number of novel target antigens in forms of MN that were previously uncharacterized [5]. Several recent additions to the MN target antigen (or biomarker) repertoire have been identified using this methodology. NELL1 has been identified as a target of circulating antibodies in adults with MN [68]. The median age of patients diagnosed with this form of MN was nearly 67 years old, and one third of the cases were associated with underlying malignancy [69]. Several other markers or target antigens have been found that can point to underlying lupus as the etiology behind the MN. The extostosins 1 and 2 (EXT1/EXT2) are partners of a glycosyltransferase complex and seem to be a specific biomarker within deposits in a subset of secondary MN associated with lupus and other autoimmune diseases [70]. In similar manner, neural cell adhesion molecule 1 (NCAM-1) has been found as the antigen targeted by circulating antibodies and present within immune deposits in more than 6% of class V (membranous) lupus nephritis cases and in a smaller percentage of apparently primary cases. The median age for these two types of MN was in the 30's so it is possible that adolescents and young adults could develop these types of disease.

Semaphorin 3B

Another of these novel target antigens is semaphorin-3B (Sema3B), which seems to associate with a type of MN more commonly found in the pediatric population [71]. In the initial report, 73% of cases were pediatric, with a mean age of 6.9 years old, while the remainder were adults with a still younger-than-average mean age of 36.3 years old. Nearly half of the pediatric cases were under the age of 2. Unique features of this type of MN are the presence of tubular basement membrane immune deposits (exclusively found in those cases <2 years old), a predominance of the IgG1 subclass within the deposits, and a possible inherited pattern of disease in some cases [71]. In addition, although circulating anti-Sema3B antibodies could be detected in the serum, these antibodies could only recognize the recombinant human Sema3B protein under conditions in which disulfide bonds were reduced, suggesting the presence of a cryptic epitope that would not normally be available to the anti-Sema3B antibodies when the protein is in its native state. It is hoped that similar techniques as the laser capture microdissection followed by mass spectrometry method will be useful for identifying further antigens specifically in the subset of pediatric MN.

Food Antigen-Related MN

An unusual form of secondary MN in children has been described in which there are high levels of antibodies to bovine serum albumin (BSA) [72]. These four children (all younger than 5) were found to have BSA in their bloodstream that was cationic (positively charged) which is atypical for the normal protein. BSA was detected in subepithelial immune deposits only in children with both anti-BSA antibodies and high levels of circulating cationic BSA, and it colocalized with IgG, in the absence of PLA2R-ab. IgG eluted from kidney biopsy samples of children with BSA deposits belonged to IgG1 and IgG4 subclasses and specifically reacted with BSA, but not with human serum albumin.

The source of BSA in children is most likely cow's milk, and the increased permeability of the intestinal barrier in infants and young children, possibly exacerbated by episodes of gastroenteritis, is hypothesized to have allowed the entry of the whole molecule into the circulation. The precise source of the cationic form of BSA is unknown, but this modification could be due to differences in food processing (powdered infant formula) or intestinal microbiota. It is of pathophysiological and historical interest that this type of human MN seems to be equivalent to a rabbit experimental model of MN developed in the 1980's in which cationic (but not the normally anionic) BSA could induce MN [73] (Fig. 18.1, middle). These clinical findings strongly support the scenario of "planted" antigens in human disease. Based on this finding, other ingested antigenic sources or non-dietary antigens from the environment should be considered as potential targets in cases of pediatric MN in which cause remains a mystery.

Enzyme Replacement Therapy as a Cause of Alloimmune MN

The administration of recombinant enzymes or factors as replacement therapy for a genetic deficiency can lead to the development of alloantibodies. Alloantibodies may be without clinical significance or may lead to hypersensitivity reactions and decreased bioavailability and efficacy of the therapeutic proteins. They may also lead to formation of immune complexes of the replacement enzyme and alloantibody that occasionally become planted in a glomerular subepithelial location. This has occurred in a patient with mucopolysaccharidosis type VI treated with human recombinant arylsulfatase B (rhASB) [74] (Fig. 18.1, middle). The clinical circumstances in this case, particularly the resolution of proteinuria when ERT was suspended, and the finding that IgG eluted from the biopsy specimen reacted specifically with rhASB, strongly suggested that the alloimmune response to the recombinant enzyme was the cause of the disease. Other cases of nephrotic syndrome associated with MN-like subepithelial immune complexes have been induced by immune-tolerance induction regimens in which increasing doses of enzyme replacement therapy (e.g., alpha-glucosidase in Pompe disease) [75] or factors (factor IX in hemophilia B) [76] have been administered in an attempt to limit inhibitory alloantibodies.

The Case of Secondary MN

Despite our knowledge of specific proteins that comprise the immune deposits in the forms of MN described earlier in the chapter, the molecular characterization of the immune complexes in most secondary forms remains limited. Hepatitis B, hepatitis C and Helicobacter pylori antigens, tumor antigens, thyroglobulin, and DNA containing material have been detected by elution from or immunostaining of subepithelial deposits in patients with secondary MN [77, 78]. These antigens may have been trapped in the GBM owing to unusual physicochemical properties similar to what is thought to occur with cationic BSA. Alternatively, small-sized, circulating, non-precipitating IgG4 complexes containing these antigens could become deposited in the GBM as in the chronic serum sickness model, although there is no experimental evidence yet supporting this hypothesis in humans.

Genetic Factors

The finding that different forms of MN occur in different age groups may imply a complex interaction of environmental influences with an underlying genetic susceptibility. It has long been known that European Caucasians show a strong association of MN with the HLA-B8 DR3 haplotype and other HLA class II loci [79, 80]. The first genome-wide association study (GWAS) conducted, with only 556 white European adults with idiopathic MN was, sufficient to show a highly significant interaction with *HLA-DQA1* as well as *PLA2R1* [81]. The risk variants at these sites displayed an unusually strong genetic interaction such that homozygosity for the risk variants at both locations conferred an almost 80-fold increase in the risk of MN [82]. These genetic data were confirmed in ethnically distant populations from Europe [49, 83] and Asia [84–86]. Robust genetic data are lacking in children, where the prevalence of PLA2R-related MN is much lower.

Subsequent work has raised appealing suggestions as to what might underlie the robust genetic interaction between the HLA class II locus and PLA2R1 [87]. Although there was early speculation that rare single nucleotide variants leading to amino acid changes in the sequence of PLA2R might alter protein conformation, this theory was felt not to be the case as there were not specific coding variants that associated with disease [88]. A higher resolution GWAS conducted across 3782 cases of MN and over 9000 controls points to an intronic, regulatory region of *PLA2R1* that might confer increased expression of the antigen within the kidney or potentially other tissues [89]. Since the PLA2R protein is highly disulfide bonded and difficult to express in experimental settings, a genetically driven overexpression of the protein could lead to protein misfolding and presentation of aberrant protein to the immune system.

A series of studies largely from China have pointed to discrete regions within the class II MHC molecules that have been genetically linked to MN [90–92]. The most significant genetic associations can be pinpointed to variants that are predicted to alter the amino acid sequence within the binding groove of the molecule that presents peptides to the T cell receptor [89, 91, 92]. Such variants are predicted to allow PLA2R fragments to bind with potentially higher affinity to the HLA molecules encoded by the risk variants than to molecules encoded by other alleles and may therefore represent a mechanism why some genetically-predisposed individuals might more easily mount an autoimmune response to the self-protein PLA2R.

Other non-HLA alleles also predispose individuals towards the development or progression of MN such as the tumor necrosis factor (TNF) allele G308A, and polymorphisms in genes encoding IL-6, STAT4, nephrin, and plasminogen activator inhibitor type-1 (PAI1) [93]. A very large GWAS performed in MN on an international scale [89] points to two other risk loci: one in the gene for interferon response factor 4 (*IRF4*) and one within nuclear factor kappa B (*NFKB1*), suggesting that susceptibility lies in other arms of the immune regulatory system as well. Overall, these data suggest that a combination of gene variants initiates disease, and that modifier genes controlling glomerular permeability, inflammation and fibrosis might be involved in the pathogenesis of MN.

Clinical Presentation

Children with MN classically present with nephrotic syndrome or isolated sub-nephrotic proteinuria. They have hypoalbuminemia, proteinuria and may have edema on presentation. Most children have normal renal function at presentation. Microscopic hematuria is commonly seen in children, and in one study was found in 77% of children at the time of biopsy [94]. In the same pediatric cohort, eGFR at the time of biopsy was normal at 107 mL/min/1.73 m^2 [94]. The incidence of thromboembolism in children at presentation and during the course of the illness was significantly lower compared to adults [94].

It is not uncommon for children to be initially treated with oral corticosteroids for presumed minimal change disease and for MN to be discovered instead when a biopsy is performed weeks later after the patient is found to be partially responsive or non-responsive to steroids. It is also possible that there is a subset of children with MN that either spontaneously remit or respond to prednisone, who do not get biopsied.

This would be another factor limiting the determination of the true incidence of MN in children.

Distinguishing primary from secondary MN based on presentation alone is challenging. A detailed history for concomitant illnesses, recent travel and review of systems may elicit signs and symptoms of an underlying illness that would predispose a child to secondary MN. The incidence of serum PLA2R-ab and tissue PLA2R positivity at diagnosis in children has not been widely studied, with reports showing a varying degree of seropositivity, ranging from 45 to 70% [51, 95], and the specificity of these findings for primary disease is not known. Secondary etiologies of MN may present in similar fashion to primary disease, and an underlying cause is not always readily apparent. Due to the decreasing prevalence of HBV-associated MN, SLE is now the most common secondary etiology of pediatric MN. Very importantly, class V lupus nephritis can be the initial presentation of SLE in the absence of extra-renal manifestations and of serological manifestations of SLE such as hypocomplementemia or anti-double stranded DNA antibodies, which will often appear later.

Laboratory Investigations

The child or adolescent that presents with features of nephrotic syndrome should undergo standard serological workup that includes antinuclear antibodies (with anti-double stranded DNA as a confirmatory test), levels of C3 and C4, and screening tests for hepatitis B infection. Due to the possibility of finding serologically active MN, testing for PLA2R-ab should be considered in the older child or adolescent even before a biopsy diagnosis of MN is available. Specialized tests, such as anti-Sema3B, may one day be clinically available, but are currently limited to the research setting.

Children with hepatitis B-related MN show positivity of hepatitis B surface antigen (HBsAg) and usually hepatitis B surface antibody is not detected. The hepatitis B early antigen (HBeAg) can be detected in serum of 90% of patients.

Hypocomplementemia (low C3 and C4) is observed at disease onset, but levels of C3, C4 return to normal later in the disease course. Circulating immune complexes are detected in 80% of patients. Serum levels of transaminases may be elevated on presentation, which may lead the clinician to order viral hepatitis testing.

Histopathology

The glomerular features seen in membranous nephropathy are a result of the subepithelial deposits and the extra basement membrane material that is laid down surrounding them in response.

The typical *light microscopic* findings in adult MN are normal-to-enlarged glomeruli with thickened and rigid capillary walls, but without elements of proliferation. With the use of Jones' methenamine silver stain, which stains the GBM, there are spikes of new matrix between deposits in the GBM, and the deposits may be suggested by craters of absent staining (Fig. 18.2). Biopsy features in pediatric disease are similar, although mesangial deposits and a segmental distribution of the deposits seem to be more common in pediatric versus adult disease (Table 18.1). Features such as mesangial hypercellularity should prompt the clinician to look for evidence of secondary causes of disease, especially lupus.

In addition to the glomerular findings, it is important to also consider the overall health of the renal parenchyma, as prolonged glomerular disease may lead to tubulointerstitial injury. As with many glomerular diseases, the presence of glomerulosclerosis, interstitial fibrosis and tubular atrophy are signs of chronicity and tend to be associated with diminished GFR and a poorer prognosis. Intraparenchymal B cell infiltrates forming tertiary lymphoid structures have been demonstrated in human MN and other autoimmune glomuleronephritides [96, 97].

Immunofluorescence (IF) can be the most sensitive of the imaging modalities to suggest the presence of MN. In most cases of MN, there are fine granular deposits of IgG (Fig. 18.3) and C3 decorating the peripheral capillary walls in a global and diffuse distribution. The degree of complement deposition has been correlated with

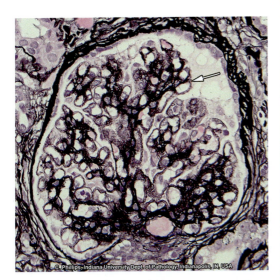

Fig. 18.2 Brightfield microscopy. Jones' silver stain of a paraffin tissue section reveals pinholes (arrow) and spikes along glomerular basement membranes (GBM) from a patient with membranous nephropathy. This GBM distortion is in response to deposition of immunoglobulin and complement (original magnification 400×). Image courtesy of Carrie L. Phillips MD, Department of Pathology, Indiana University School of Medicine

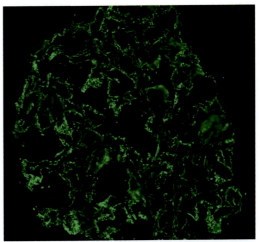

Fig. 18.3 Widefield epifluorescence microscopy. Direct immunofluorescence using fluorescein-tagged antibody to IgG shows granular deposits along glomerular capillary loops in a patient with membranous nephropathy (original magnification 400×). Image courtesy of Carrie L. Phillips MD, Department of Pathology, Indiana University School of Medicine

the rate of progression of kidney dysfunction [98]. The detection of additional immunoreactants such as C1q, IgA, and IgM can point to the presence of a secondary cause of MN. The target antigen (PLA2R, THSD7A, Sema3B) when assayed will yield a similar pattern, and co-localization studies on the same tissue section will show nearly identical patterns. Although most cases of adult MN demonstrate the global pattern in which all capillary loops exhibit immune deposits, a minority of pediatric cases will show a segmental pattern, with some loops apparently being spared from the deposits. The pathophysiological reasons behind this are currently not known.

Electron microscopy (EM) can be helpful, but it is often not needed to make the diagnosis (Fig. 18.4). EM is useful for detecting the size and distribution of deposits, and the degree of matrix reaction to the deposits. In primary disease, the deposits are largely subepithelial, while the presence of significant mesangial and/or subendothelial deposits suggests secondary etiologies of disease. The presence of tubuloreticular inclusions in endothelial cells, a sign of the interferon response, usually points to the presence of lupus or a viral infection such as HIV. Features of podocyte injury and simplification on EM are the effacement of the basal foot processes and loss of slit diaphragms, as well as the microvillous change on the apical side of the podocyte cell body.

The appearance of the electron-dense subepithelial deposits has traditionally been described as morphological stages [99]. The stages based on combination of light and electron microscopic features are as follows:

- Stage 1. Light microscopy shows normal GBM in thickness and appearance. The electron dense deposits are small and flat but discrete. The smaller deposits are often located at the site of the slit diaphragm, while larger deposits are located immediately adjacent to the effaced foot processes.
- Stage 2. Thickening of the GBM is discernible by light microscopy. The electron dense deposits are increased in number and size. These deposits are flanked by prominent spikes in almost every capillary loop.
- Stage 3. The basement membrane material (spikes) completely surrounds the deposits. These are larger and acquire intramembranous position. The capillary wall is irregular and has a moth-eaten appearance.
- Stage 4. The GBM is severely altered and irregularly thickened. The deposits are only a few in number or completely absent. The vacuolated appearance of GBM is discernible. The loss of deposits is seen as electron-lucent areas in the basement membrane.

Investigators have more recently introduced a Stage 0 in the setting of recurrent MN in the kidney allograft [100], often seen in early protocol biopsies or biopsies conducted to explore delayed graft function. In this stage, fine granular deposits of IgG can be seen by the highly sensitive IF technique, while there are no discernible electron dense deposits by EM. This stage is virtually never seen in native kidney biopsies, as there are no clinical features present at that time that would warrant a kidney biopsy.

The most common stages of deposits found in childhood MN are stages 2 and 3, which can occur in a mixed (heterogeneous) pattern. Since children with nephrotic syndrome are often tri-

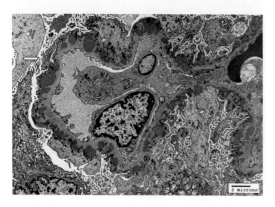

Fig. 18.4 Transmission electron microscopy. This electron micrograph shows subepithelial electron dense deposits (white arrow) along glomerular basement membranes, including some separated by spikes of extracellular matrix. Podocyte foot process effacement is extensive. Image courtesy of Carrie L Phillips MD, Department of Pathology, Indiana University School of Medicine

Specific Diagnostic Approaches

Many of the etiologies of pediatric MN are rare, and it may be difficult to rule out all potential causes. Research or clinical groups who specialize in such disorders should be contacted for further advice on testing. Much of the testing will rely on immunostaining the biopsy in a validated protocol to look for the presence of potential antigens (e.g., Sema3B, NEP, BSA) within the immune deposits. It is not expected that a renal pathologist will have the resources to look for all such antigens, and thus the availability of extra sections to send to specialized centers might be critical in making a diagnosis. Serological tests may be available for certain antigens in the future. Some specialized centers have the ability to query the proteins that accumulate over time in the deposits by means of laser capture microdissection of the glomeruli from tissue sections and then to perform mass spectrometry. This methodology is not clinically available, but may provide a diagnosis in the research setting.

Prognosis and Predictors

The course of primary MN is variable. As a general rule in adult MN, approximately one third of patients undergo spontaneous remission and maintain normal renal function with or without occasional relapses [101, 102]. Another third of patients display persistent proteinuria of variable degree, with normal or mildly impaired but stable GFR. The remaining patients develop progressive chronic kidney disease (CKD) eventually leading to ESKD. In a review of natural history studies in untreated adults with MN, 50% of these patients either died or developed ESKD within 10 years of disease onset [101].

Children seem to have a relatively better overall outcome than adults [103], with some of the more recent series reporting overall remission rates of 75% [1, 104] (Table 18.1); however, most studies still show decreased kidney function in about 20% of patients at final follow-up [1, 105]. It should be emphasized that the existing information about natural history and treatment outcomes of primary MN in children is not only uncontrolled, but there is considerable variability regarding the therapeutic protocols used and the definition of remission. Individually based decisions are therefore of paramount importance to minimize the risk of progression to renal failure.

Unfortunately, predictors of outcome are still poorly defined in children. The degree of proteinuria seems to be a valuable predictor of outcome, which is excellent in children with asymptomatic, non-nephrotic proteinuria; however, approximately 25% of those with nephrotic syndrome will develop renal failure within 1–17 years. In one cohort, all patients who developed CKD presented with nephrotic syndrome [106]. Hypertension and interstitial fibrosis on biopsy might be further predictors of adverse outcome [104, 105].

In adults, there is no difference in response to treatment between PLA2R-ab positive and PLA2R-ab negative patients, although the response rate to rituximab appears to be lower in patients with a high titer of antibodies [107]. Further studies are required to assess how the PLA2R-ab antibody titer may be of prognostic value in children.

As with adults, in children with PLA2R-related MN the quantification of PLA2R-ab antibodies will likely become an invaluable tool for the monitoring of disease immunological activity and the titration of immunosuppressive treatments. Antibodies disappear before proteinuria in patients treated with rituximab [40, 42], which leads to consideration of withdrawal of immunosuppressive treatment at the time of immunological remission before renal remission is achieved. The time-lag between immunological and renal remission most likely corresponds to the time required for restoration of the glomerular capillary wall. PLA2R-ab antibody levels at the end of therapy may also predict the subsequent course. In a series of 48 patients treated with immunosuppressive agents, 58% of antibody-negative patients were in persistent remission after 5 years compared with none of antibody-positive patients [107]. However, further prospective studies on large cohorts of patients are needed before drawing definitive conclusions and extrapolating them to children.

Treatment

The first step in the approach to treatment is ruling out secondary causes of MN including lupus, hepatitis B and C. In cases of secondary MN, treating the underlying condition results in resolution of MN. Removal of potential offending agents such as non-steroidal anti-inflammatory agents or cow's milk in infants with suspected cationic-BSA induced MN is required in these specific situations. The treatment of pediatric membranous (class V) lupus nephritis is discussed at the end of this section.

Currently, no randomized controlled trials addressing treatment of primary MN in children exist, which represents a substantial limiting factor in determining the most efficacious regimens for children with MN. Even studies predicting natural disease course are scant and limited to small cohorts. Therefore, most treatment recommendations stem from the data in adult patients. This also has its limitation given that the underlying disease mechanism in children may be different from that in adults. Serum PLA2R positivity in children appears to be lower at around 45% in children compared to 70% in adults, suggesting different pathophysiological mechanisms are often present in the pediatric population [51].

A second step in deciding on treatment course is to determine the degree of nephrosis. As with adults, it seems reasonable that children with asymptomatic, non-nephrotic presentation may be treated conservatively with angiotensin-converting enzyme (ACE) inhibitors or angiotensin receptor blockers (ARBs) for their anti-proteinuria and nephroprotective effects, along with lifestyle modifications, including a low-salt diet. This would give time for spontaneous remission to occur, which would obviate the need for immunosuppression. Therapy in children who subsequently develop or initially present with the nephrotic syndrome and nephrotic range proteinuria remains controversial. In the adults, there is a growing body of literature suggesting superiority of treatment with rituximab compared to other immunosuppressive agents. Regimens described in the pediatric and adult cohorts are discussed in detail below.

The 2021 KDIGO guidelines (www.kdigo. org) are based on evidence from adult studies and recommend conservative treatment in subjects with eGFR >60 mL/min/1.73 m^2 and proteinuria <3.5 g/day. If, however, one or more risk factors for disease progression are present then treatment with rituximab, a combination of cyclophosphamide and steroids for 6 months, or tacrolimus therapy for at least 6 months should be considered. Risk factors for disease progression include: eGFR <60 mL/min/1.73 m^2, proteinuria >4 g/day and no decrease in 6 months despite conservative therapy, high PLA2R-ab titers, significant low-molecular-weight proteinuria or life-threatening complications of nephrotic syndrome. There are no specific treatment recommendations in children, but it is noted that therapy is often initiated prior to 6 months and that rituximab and calcineurin inhibitors have been used as treatment options in children.

There is a report of the clinical characteristics and treatment response in a large, prospectively followed cohort of 48 children in India ranging from age 1 years to 20 years with primary MN [95]. The median follow-up was for 29 months and the median age was 17 years. All except one patient, who underwent a spontaneous remission, were treated with immunosuppression. The predominant treatment regimens were a minimum of 3 months with a combination of cyclophosphamide with glucocorticoids (GC; 53%), tacrolimus with GC (21%), and rituximab (15%). Response rates in the three treatment groups were similar. Remission rates were 62.2% and 70.5% at 6 and 12 months, respectively. Of note, in subjects with resistant or relapsing disease, rituximab was used as a second agent with considerable success. Serum PLA2R-ab positivity was similar to that in adult primary MN patients at 72.9% (35 subjects). In addition, the study observed a reduction in PLA2R-ab titer with disease remission/resolution [95].

Another study reported treatment patterns in a North American and European cohort of 37 children with primary MN enrolled in the Cure Glomerulopathy Network [94]. The median age was 14 years with a follow-up of 23 months. Children who had received 6 weeks or less of glucocorticoids prior to the time of the kidney biopsy were considered immunosuppression naïve and enrolled in this cohort since most children are initially treated for presumed minimal change disease without a biopsy. Twenty-three (59%) of the children were placed on immunosuppressive therapy (IST) within 6 months after biopsy, with 70% initiating IST at any time within the follow-up period. The median time to initiate IST after the diagnostic biopsy was 1.9 months. It is important to highlight that 30% of the children did not receive any IST, which is in line with some other studies. Renin-angiotensin-aldosterone system (RAAS) inhibitors were used in 73% of the children [94]. Interestingly, the first line IST treatment most commonly prescribed in children in this group were calcineurin inhibitors (46% of the 26 children that were treated). However, since this cohort included children who may have had GC prior to biopsy, it is possible that the true exposure to GC is higher if including the treatment pre-biopsy. Seven children (27%) received 30 days or more of GC as a first line single agent. Rituximab as a single agent and first line therapy was used in 4 children (11%) and mycophenolate mofetil in two children. As part of combination therapy, up to 76% of children in the treated group received GC. Seven of 26 children were transitioned to a second-line agent [94]. There were no differences observed in clinical characteristics at presentation in the group of children that were treatment with IST compared with the children who were managed with conservative therapy. This study emphasizes the variability in approach in treating children with MN, probably a result of limited evidence for a specific treatment strategy.

In an older series that predated the use of rituximab, Valentini et al. reported treatment outcomes in 12 children with biopsy proven primary MN [108]. The mean age was 11.9 years and mean follow up time was 27 months. Two patients did not receive any IST and entered spontaneous remission. The remaining ten patients were treated with oral prednisolone 2 mg/kg/day (maximum 80 mg/day) for 4–8 weeks. One patient responded to GC alone, four patients were partially-responsive, and five patients did not respond. Cyclophosphamide (2 mg/kg/day orally for 12 weeks) was used as a second line agent for the five steroid resistant patients, one partial responder, and one initially steroid-responsive subject who became steroid dependent. This treatment regimen resulted in complete remission in all but one subject who was steroid resistant [108]. There were no clinical differences at presentation in the nine children that ultimately demonstrated complete remission compared to three children that did not.

A report from India described five children with MN, ages 5–13 years. All had positive PLA2R staining of the kidney biopsy tissue and three had a positive PLA2R-ab titer at the time of biopsy [52]. These subjects had already received oral prednisolone prior to the biopsy. Two patients were treated with the modified Ponticelli protocol (pulse methylprednisolone, oral prednisone and cyclophosphamide). The remaining three were treated with tacrolimus and oral prednisone [52]. All 5 patients were in complete or partial remission by 12 months. PLA2R-ab disappeared at 6 months in one patient with complete remission and declined by 50% in another patient with a partial remission. This study suggests that in children with PLA2R-ab positivity, a response to therapy will trend with reduction in PLA2R-ab titer.

A retrospective study performed before the era of PLA2R-ab described a Korean cohort of 19 children with primary MN with a median age of onset of 11 years [1]. There were 11 children with nephrotic syndrome at presentation and eight children with proteinuria without nephrotic syndrome at presentation. In the latter group, children without nephrotic syndrome, three children did not receive any IST and entered spontaneous remission. Five children received varied regimens of corticosteroids and some also received cyclosporine. All five subjects eventually entered remission at time ranging from 1 month to 33 months after treatment. In the second group, 11 children with nephrotic syndrome, all were treated with either prednisone alone (varied regimens) or in combination with cyclosporine. Six entered remission by a median time of 12 months, but five children did not demonstrate any response to steroids or additional IS. The authors report that at last follow-up, in the 11 children with nephrotic syndrome at presentation, six had entered remission, two had persistent proteinuria with normal renal function, one patient had CKD and two patients had progressed to ESKD [1].

Current treatment recommendations are from clinical trials in the adult MN population. The GEMRITUX trial in France compared nonimmune antiproteinuric therapy (NIAT), defined as ACE inhibitor or ARB, for 6 months to the use of rituximab 375 m/m^2 given IV for two doses 1 week apart along with NIAT [109]. When this trial was initiated, there was no objective evidence of the benefits of rituximab outside of smaller pilot studies [110–112] and a large observational cohort [42, 113] in adult patients with primary MN. The patients in the GEMRITUX study were age 18 years or older, had biopsy proven primary MN and nephrotic syndrome at the time of enrollment. At 6 months, 35% of the patients receiving NIAT-rituximab combination therapy had achieved remission compared to 21% in the group receiving NIAT alone. A significant reduction in PLA2R-ab was noted in the group receiving NIAT-rituximab. By 6 months, 50% of the NIAT-rituximab group had achieved immunologic remission (disappearance of PLA2R-ab) compared to only 12% in the NIAT alone group [109]. Complication rates in the two groups were similar.

In 2019, the MENTOR trial compared the use of rituximab 1000 mg IV given in 2 doses 14 days apart, with an additional cycle at 6 months if needed, to cyclosporine taken orally at a dose of 3.5 mg/kg/day for 12 months [114]. Study subjects had 5 g/day or more of proteinuria, a GFR of 40 mL/min/1.73 m^2 or greater and had received

ACE inhibitor or ARB for at least 3 months. At one-year, complete or partial remission rates were similar: 60% in the rituximab group and 52% in the group receiving cyclosporine. However, at 24-months, complete or partial remission was more common in the rituximab group (60%) than in the cyclosporin group (20%) [114] due to a high number of relapses during cyclosporine tapering and withdrawal.

The results of the GEMRITUX and MENTOR trials support the effectiveness of rituximab in adults with primary MN. In addition, rituximab likely has a more favorable side effect profile than cytotoxic agents and glucocorticoids. The most effective dosing regimen for treating MN with rituximab is not clear. This was partially addressed by a comparison of the use of two infusions of 1 g of rituximab at a 2-week interval in 28 patients from the NICE cohort to rituximab dosed at 375 mg/m^2 given as two infusions at a 1-week interval in 27 participants from the GEMRITUX cohort [115]. Patients in both cohorts had high levels of PLA2R-ab. At 6 months, 64% of the participants from the NICE cohort were in remission compared to 30% from the GEMRITUX cohort [115]. The median time to achieve remission in the NICE cohort was 3 months and 9 months in the GEMRITUX cohort. Participants in the NICE cohort had lower levels of PLA2R-ab at 6 months compared to those in the GEMRITUX study. This suggests that a higher dose of rituximab in adults with primary MN may result in an improved response. The ideal dosing regimen in children remains unknown.

One of the main drawbacks of the use of calcineurin inhibitors such as cyclosporine and tacrolimus for treatment of MN is the high proportion of patients that experience a relapse once the medication is tapered and discontinued. The dramatic drop in the number of clinical remissions observed between 12 and 24 months in the MENTOR trial provides recent evidence of this limitation [114]. The STARMEN trial sought to reduce the rate of relapse by introducing a single dose of rituximab prior to tapering the calcineurin inhibitor [116]. In this study, 6 months of the modified Ponticelli regimen (6 months of alternating corticosteroids and cyclophosphamide) was compared to a 6 month course of tacrolimus, with 1 g rituximab given at 6 months, before a 3 month tacrolimus taper. The corticosteroid-cyclophosphamide group had a significantly higher rate of clinical remissions at 24 months (83.7% partial or complete remissions) versus the 58.1% rate in the tacrolimus-rituximab group [116]. Despite this outcome, there were fewer (12%) relapses after tapering tacrolimus than the 30–40% rate that is typically observed.

The RI-CYCLO trial was a randomized trial in adults comparing rituximab 1 g on days one and 15 to a 6 month cyclic regimen of corticosteroids alternated with cyclophosphamide every other month [117]. The cumulative dose of cyclophosphamide per patient was 180 mg/kg. Outcomes and adverse events in both groups were similar. At 12 months, 62% of the patients in the rituximab group were in complete or partial remission, and this number increased to 85% at 24 months. In comparison, 73% of patients in the cyclic treatment group were in complete or partial remission at 12 months, and by 24 months the percentage had increased to 81% [117].

Safety

The potential adverse effects of immunosuppression should be considered when deciding on treatment. Since pediatric MN may undergo spontaneous remission more often than in adults, many patients can be monitored, with the clinical course and PLA2R-ab levels in some patients determining whether the disease is likely to improve without intervention or cause long-term morbidity. For cyclophosphamide, gonadal toxicity and bone marrow suppression leading to heightened infection risk are major concerns. Peripheral blood counts should be monitored and the cytotoxic agents withheld at a total leukocyte count $<3000/mm^3$ or in the presence of an active infection. Calcineurin inhibitors have less of an infection risk, but there is a risk of nephrotoxicity with prolonged blood levels above the therapeu-

tic range. Trough blood levels be monitored regularly, and whenever there is an unexplained rise in the serum creatinine ($>20\%$) during therapy. Rituximab can be associated with infusion reactions, reactivation of latent infections, or hypogammaglobulinemia. Potential long-term adverse effects, especially in the pediatric population, are not yet known due to its relatively recent introduction for treatment of nephrotic syndrome in children.

Class V (Membranous) Lupus Nephritis

Nearly half of pediatric lupus cases will be complicated by some form of lupus nephritis, and of these, more than one quarter have class V lesions, either in isolation (16%) or in combination with other (class II, III, or IV) lesions (12%) [118]. GFR tends to be better preserved over time in patients with pure class V lesions than in patients with overlap with class III or IV, but the vast majority of pediatric lupus MN patients are treated with immunosuppressive therapy, often due to the presence of additional extrarenal features. Data from the Childhood Arthritis and Rheumatology Research Alliance, representing a majority of pediatric rheumatology centers across the United States, demonstrate that most patients with class V lupus nephritis receive hydroxychloroquine (98.7%), mycophenolate (91.9%) and daily corticosteroids (96%), with smaller proportions treated with cyclophosphamide, rituximab, calcineurin inhibitors or azathioprine [118]. As with primary MN, the majority of patients are nephrotic, and one center reported that 78% of cases received RAAS inhibitors [119]. In this single center cohort, 74% of isolated class V lupus nephritis patients achieved complete remission at 24 months, but no specific predictors of clinical outcome were found [119]. Achievement of complete remission was not rapid, and can take years. Proliferative features were present in 13% on repeat biopsy; close monitoring of renal function, proteinuria and hematuria is essential.

Conclusions

Membranous nephropathy is an uncommon cause of nephrotic syndrome in children. The diagnosis is usually established when the children are biopsied after being labeled as steroid resistant. It is imperative to evaluate the patient for secondary etiologies since these may respond to treatment of the underlying condition. The initial management of idiopathic MN should generally be conservative. Immunosuppressive therapy should be considered in those children with nephrotic-range proteinuria and/or progressive renal dysfunction. We anticipate that advances from adult disease, including the identification of new target antigens and experience using circulating autoantibodies to guide treatment decisions, will be incorporated into improved treatment and monitoring of pediatric MN.

References

1. Lee BH, Cho HY, Kang HG, et al. Idiopathic membranous nephropathy in children. Pediatr Nephrol. 2006;21(11):1707–15.
2. Moxey-Mims MM, Stapleton FB, Feld LG. Applying decision analysis to management of adolescent idiopathic nephrotic syndrome. Pediatr Nephrol. 1994;8(6):660–4.
3. Mubarak M, Kazi JI, Lanewala A, Hashmi S, Akhter F. Pathology of idiopathic nephrotic syndrome in children: are the adolescents different from young children? Nephrol Dial Transplant. 2012;27(2):722–6.
4. Hogg RJ, Silva FG, Berry PL, Wenz JE. Glomerular lesions in adolescents with gross hematuria or the nephrotic syndrome. Report of the Southwest Pediatric Nephrology Study Group. Pediatr Nephrol. 1993;7(1):27–31.
5. Sethi S. New 'Antigens' in membranous nephropathy. J Am Soc Nephrol. 2021;32(2):268–78.
6. Hsu HC, Wu CY, Lin CY, Lin GJ, Chen CH, Huang FY. Membranous nephropathy in 52 hepatitis B surface antigen (HBsAg) carrier children in Taiwan. Kidney Int. 1989;36(6):1103–7.
7. Liao MT, Chang MH, Lin FG, Tsai IJ, Chang YW, Tsau YK. Universal hepatitis B vaccination reduces childhood hepatitis B virus-associated membranous nephropathy. Pediatrics. 2011;128(3):e600–4.
8. Xu H, Sun L, Zhou LJ, Fang LJ, Sheng FY, Guo YQ. The effect of hepatitis B vaccination on the incidence of childhood HBV-associated nephritis. Pediatr Nephrol. 2003;18(12):1216–9.
9. Burnett RJ, Kramvis A, Dochez C, Meheus A. An update after 16 years of hepatitis B vaccination in South Africa. Vaccine. 2012;30(Suppl 3):C45–51.
10. Chuva T, Pfister F, Beringer O, Felgentreff K, Buttner-Herold M, Amann K. PLA2R-positive (primary) membranous nephropathy in a child with IPEX syndrome. Pediatr Nephrol. 2017;32(9):1621–4.
11. Yim HE, Yoo KH. Membranous nephropathy in a 13-year-old boy with common variable immunodeficiency. J Korean Med Sci. 2012;27(11):1436–8.
12. Brinkerhoff BT, Houghton DC, Troxell ML. Renal pathology in hematopoietic cell transplant recipients: a contemporary biopsy, nephrectomy, and autopsy series. Mod Pathol. 2016;29(6):637–52.
13. Ponticelli C, Moroni G, Glassock RJ. De novo glomerular diseases after renal transplantation. Clin J Am Soc Nephrol. 2014;9(8):1479–87.
14. Jones DB. Nephrotic glomerulonephritis. Am J Pathol. 1957;33(2):313–29.
15. Ronco P, Plaisier E, Debiec H. Advances in membranous nephropathy. J Clin Med. 2021;10(4):607.
16. Alsharhan L, Beck LH Jr. Membranous nephropathy: core curriculum 2021. Am J Kidney Dis. 2021;77(3):440–53.
17. Heymann W, Hackel DB, Harwood S, Wilson SG, Hunter JL. Production of nephrotic syndrome in rats by Freund's adjuvants and rat kidney suspensions. Proc Soc Exp Biol Med. 1959;100(4):660–4.
18. Couser WG, Steinmuller DR, Stilmant MM, Salant DJ, Lowenstein LM. Experimental glomerulonephritis in the isolated perfused rat kidney. J Clin Invest. 1978;62(6):1275–87.
19. VanDamme BJ, Fleuren GJ, Bakker WW, Vernier RL, Hoedemaeker PJ. Experimental glomerulonephritis in the rat induced by antibodies directed against tubular antigens. V. Fixed glomerular antigens in the pathogenesis of heterologous immune complex glomerulonephritis. Lab Investig. 1978;38(4):502–10.
20. Kerjaschki D, Farquhar MG. The pathogenic antigen of Heymann nephritis is a membrane glycoprotein of the renal proximal tubule brush border. Proc Natl Acad Sci U S A. 1982;79(18):5557–61.
21. Kerjaschki D, Farquhar MG. Immunocytochemical localization of the Heymann nephritis antigen (GP330) in glomerular epithelial cells of normal Lewis rats. J Exp Med. 1983;157(2):667–86.
22. Allegri L, Brianti E, Chatelet F, Manara GC, Ronco P, Verroust P. Polyvalent antigen-antibody interactions are required for the formation of electron-dense immune deposits in passive Heymann's nephritis. Am J Pathol. 1986;125(1):1–6.
23. Kerjaschki D. Pathomechanisms and molecular basis of membranous glomerulopathy. Lancet. 2004;364(9441):1194–6.
24. Larsen CP, Trivin-Avillach C, Coles P, et al. LDL receptor-related protein 2 (Megalin) as a target antigen in human kidney anti-brush border antibody disease. J Am Soc Nephrol. 2018;29(2):644–53.
25. Debiec H, Guigonis V, Mougenot B, et al. Antenatal membranous glomerulonephritis due to anti-

neutral endopeptidase antibodies. N Engl J Med. 2002;346(26):2053–60.

26. Debiec H, Nauta J, Coulet F, et al. Role of truncating mutations in MME gene in fetomaternal alloimmunisation and antenatal glomerulopathies. Lancet. 2004;364(9441):1252–9.

27. Ronco P, Debiec H. Molecular pathomechanisms of membranous nephropathy: from Heymann nephritis to alloimmunization. J Am Soc Nephrol. 2005;16(5):1205–13.

28. Vivarelli M, Emma F, Pelle T, et al. Genetic homogeneity but IgG subclass-dependent clinical variability of alloimmune membranous nephropathy with anti-neutral endopeptidase antibodies. Kidney Int. 2015;87(3):602–9.

29. Beck LH Jr, Bonegio RG, Lambeau G, et al. M-type phospholipase A2 receptor as target antigen in idiopathic membranous nephropathy. N Engl J Med. 2009;361(1):11–21.

30. Truong LD, Seshan SV. Enigma (partially) resolved: phospholipase A2 receptor is the cause of "idiopathic" membranous glomerulonephritis. Am J Physiol Renal Physiol. 2015;309(12):F1000–2.

31. Bobart SA, De Vriese AS, Pawar AS, et al. Noninvasive diagnosis of primary membranous nephropathy using phospholipase A2 receptor antibodies. Kidney Int. 2019;95(2):429–38.

32. Qin W, Beck LH Jr, Zeng C, et al. Anti-phospholipase A2 receptor antibody in membranous nephropathy. J Am Soc Nephrol. 2011;22(6):1137–43.

33. Hoxha E, Harendza S, Zahner G, et al. An immunofluorescence test for phospholipase-A2-receptor antibodies and its clinical usefulness in patients with membranous glomerulonephritis. Nephrol Dial Transplant. 2011;26(8):2526–32.

34. Knehtl M, Debiec H, Kamgang P, et al. A case of phospholipase A receptor-positive membranous nephropathy preceding sarcoid-associated granulomatous tubulointerstitial nephritis. Am J Kidney Dis. 2011;57(1):140–3.

35. Nawaz FA, Larsen CP, Troxell ML. Membranous nephropathy and nonsteroidal anti-inflammatory agents. Am J Kidney Dis. 2013;62(5):1012–7.

36. Larsen CP, Messias NC, Silva FG, Messias E, Walker PD. Determination of primary versus secondary membranous glomerulopathy utilizing phospholipase A2 receptor staining in renal biopsies. Mod Pathol. 2013;26(5):709–15.

37. Svobodova B, Honsova E, Ronco P, Tesar V, Debiec H. Kidney biopsy is a sensitive tool for retrospective diagnosis of PLA2R-related membranous nephropathy. Nephrol Dial Transplant. 2012;28(7):1839–44.

38. Debiec H, Ronco P. PLA2R autoantibodies and PLA2R glomerular deposits in membranous nephropathy. N Engl J Med. 2011;364(7):689–90.

39. Beck LH Jr, Salant DJ. Membranous nephropathy: recent travels and new roads ahead. Kidney Int. 2010;77(9):765–70.

40. Beck LH Jr, Fervenza FC, Beck DM, et al. Rituximab-induced depletion of anti-PLA2R autoantibodies predicts response in membranous nephropathy. J Am Soc Nephrol. 2011;22(8):1543–50.

41. Hoxha E, Harendza S, Pinnschmidt H, Panzer U, Stahl RA. PLA2R antibody levels and clinical outcome in patients with membranous nephropathy and non-nephrotic range proteinuria under treatment with inhibitors of the renin-angiotensin system. PLoS One. 2014;9(10):e110681.

42. Ruggenenti P, Debiec H, Ruggiero B, et al. Anti-phospholipase A2 receptor antibody titer predicts post-rituximab outcome of membranous nephropathy. J Am Soc Nephrol. 2015;26(10):2545–58.

43. Hladunewich MA, Cattran D, Beck LH, et al. A pilot study to determine the dose and effectiveness of adrenocorticotrophic hormone (H.P. Acthar(R) Gel) in nephrotic syndrome due to idiopathic membranous nephropathy. Nephrol Dial Transplant. 2014;29(8):1570–7.

44. Hofstra JM, Beck LH Jr, Beck DM, Wetzels JF, Salant DJ. Anti-phospholipase A receptor antibodies correlate with clinical status in idiopathic membranous nephropathy. Clin J Am Soc Nephrol. 2011;6(6):1286–91.

45. Debiec H, Hanoy M, Francois A, et al. Recurrent membranous nephropathy in an allograft caused by IgG3κ targeting the PLA2 receptor. J Am Soc Nephrol. 2012;23(12):1949–54.

46. Kattah A, Ayalon R, Beck LH Jr, et al. Anti-phospholipase A(2) receptor antibodies in recurrent membranous nephropathy. Am J Transplant. 2015;15(5):1349–59.

47. Hofstra JM, Debiec H, Short CD, et al. Antiphospholipase A2 receptor antibody titer and subclass in idiopathic membranous nephropathy. J Am Soc Nephrol. 2012;23(10):1735–43.

48. Hoxha E, Thiele I, Zahner G, Panzer U, Harendza S, Stahl RA. Phospholipase A2 receptor autoantibodies and clinical outcome in patients with primary membranous nephropathy. J Am Soc Nephrol. 2014;25(6):1357–66.

49. Kanigicherla D, Gummadova J, McKenzie EA, et al. Anti-PLA2R antibodies measured by ELISA predict long-term outcome in a prevalent population of patients with idiopathic membranous nephropathy. Kidney Int. 2013;83(5):940–8.

50. De Vriese AS, Glassock RJ, Nath KA, Sethi S, Fervenza FC. A proposal for a serology-based approach to membranous nephropathy. J Am Soc Nephrol. 2017;28(2):421–30.

51. Cossey LN, Walker PD, Larsen CP. Phospholipase A2 receptor staining in pediatric idiopathic membranous glomerulopathy. Pediatr Nephrol. 2013;28(12):2307–11.

52. Kumar V, Ramachandran R, Kumar A, et al. Antibodies to m-type phospholipase A2 receptor in children with idiopathic membranous nephropathy. Nephrology (Carlton). 2015;20(8):572–5.

53. Kanda S, Horita S, Yanagihara T, Shimizu A, Hattori M. M-type phospholipase A2 receptor (PLA2R) glomerular staining in pediatric idiopathic membranous nephropathy. Pediatr Nephrol. 2017;32(4):713–7.

54. Zhang D, Wu Y, Zhang C, Zhang W, Zou J, Jiang G. Compared staining of the phospholipase A2 receptor in the glomeruli of Chinese adults and children with idiopathic membranous nephropathy. Pathol Res Pract. 2019;215(5):952–6.

55. Inaguma Y, Shiratori A, Nakagawa T, et al. M-type phospholipase A2 receptor staining in children with idiopathic membranous nephropathy: PLA2R staining in children with IMN. Open Urol Nephrol J. 2019;12:27–32.

56. Al-Rabadi L, Ayalon R, Bonegio RG, et al. Pregnancy in a patient with primary membranous nephropathy and circulating anti-PLA2R antibodies: a case report. Am J Kidney Dis. 2016;67(5):775–8.

57. Uchino E, Takada D, Mogami H, Matsubara T, Tsukamoto T, Yanagita M. Membranous nephropathy associated with pregnancy: an anti-phospholipase A2 receptor antibody-positive case report. CEN Case Rep. 2018;7(1):101–6.

58. Sachdeva M, Beck LH Jr, Miller I, Bijol V, Fishbane S. Phospholipase A2 receptor antibody-positive pregnancy: a case report. Am J Kidney Dis. 2020;76(4):586–9.

59. Jankowski J, Jedynak P, Pazik J. Pregnant woman with primary membranous nephropathy—case report. Pol Merkur Lekarski. 2020;48(284):105–7.

60. Liu ZN, Cui Z, He YD, et al. Membranous nephropathy in pregnancy. Am J Nephrol. 2020;51(4):304–17.

61. Tomas NM, Beck LH Jr, Meyer-Schwesinger C, et al. Thrombospondin type-1 domain-containing 7A in idiopathic membranous nephropathy. N Engl J Med. 2014;371(24):2277–87.

62. Herwig J, Skuza S, Sachs W, et al. Thrombospondin type 1 domain-containing 7A localizes to the slit diaphragm and stabilizes membrane dynamics of fully differentiated podocytes. J Am Soc Nephrol. 2019;30(5):824–39.

63. Hoxha E, Wiech T, Stahl PR, et al. A mechanism for cancer-associated membranous nephropathy. N Engl J Med. 2016;374(20):1995–6.

64. Hoxha E, Beck LH Jr, Wiech T, et al. An indirect immunofluorescence method facilitates detection of thrombospondin type 1 domain-containing 7A-specific antibodies in membranous nephropathy. J Am Soc Nephrol. 2017;28(2):520–31.

65. Hanset N, Aydin S, Demoulin N, et al. Podocyte antigen staining to identify distinct phenotypes and outcomes in membranous nephropathy: a retrospective multicenter cohort study. Am J Kidney Dis. 2020;76(5):624–35.

66. Zaghrini C, Seitz-Polski B, Justino J, et al. Novel ELISA for thrombospondin type 1 domain-containing 7A autoantibodies in membranous nephropathy. Kidney Int. 2019;95(3):666–79.

67. Dettmar AK, Wiech T, Kemper MJ, et al. Immunohistochemical and serological characterization of membranous nephropathy in children and adolescents. Pediatr Nephrol. 2018;33(3):463–72.

68. Sethi S, Debiec H, Madden B, et al. Neural epidermal growth factor-like 1 protein (NELL-1) associated membranous nephropathy. Kidney Int. 2020;97(1):163–74.

69. Caza T, Hassen S, Dvanajscak Z, et al. NELL1 is a target antigen in malignancy-associated membranous nephropathy. Kidney Int. 2020;99(4):967–76.

70. Sethi S, Madden BJ, Debiec H, et al. Exostosin 1/ exostosin 2-associated membranous nephropathy. J Am Soc Nephrol. 2019;30(6):1123–36.

71. Sethi S, Debiec H, Madden B, et al. Semaphorin 3B-associated membranous nephropathy is a distinct type of disease predominantly present in pediatric patients. Kidney Int. 2020;98(5):1253–64.

72. Debiec H, Lefeu F, Kemper MJ, et al. Early-childhood membranous nephropathy due to cationic bovine serum albumin. N Engl J Med. 2011;364:2101–10.

73. Border WA, Ward HJ, Kamil ES, Cohen AH. Induction of membranous nephropathy in rabbits by administration of an exogenous cationic antigen. J Clin Invest. 1982;69(2):451–61.

74. Debiec H, Valayannopoulos V, Boyer O, et al. Alloimmune membranous nephropathy and recombinant aryl sulfatase replacement therapy: a need for tolerance induction therapy. J Am Soc Nephrol. 2014;25(4):675–80.

75. Hunley TE, Corzo D, Dudek M, et al. Nephrotic syndrome complicating alpha-glucosidase replacement therapy for Pompe disease. Pediatrics. 2004;114(4):e532–5.

76. Verghese P, Darrow S, Kurth MH, Reed RC, Kim Y, Kearney S. Successful management of factor IX inhibitor-associated nephrotic syndrome in a hemophilia B patient. Pediatr Nephrol. 2013;28(5):823–6.

77. Jordan SC, Buckingham B, Sakai R, Olson D. Studies of immune-complex glomerulonephritis mediated by human thyroglobulin. N Engl J Med. 1981;304(20):1212–5.

78. Takekoshi Y, Tanaka M, Miyakawa Y, Yoshizawa H, Takahashi K, Mayumi M. Free "small" and IgG-associated "large" hepatitis B e antigen in the serum and glomerular capillary walls of two patients with membranous glomerulonephritis. N Engl J Med. 1979;300(15):814–9.

79. Berthoux FC, Laurent B, le Petit JC, et al. Immunogenetics and immunopathology of human primary membranous glomerulonephritis: HLA-A, B, DR antigens; functional activity of splenic macrophage Fc-receptors and peripheral blood T-lymphocyte subpopulations. Clin Nephrol. 1984;22(1):15–20.

80. Vaughan RW, Demaine AG, Welsh KI. A DQA1 allele is strongly associated with idiopathic membranous nephropathy. Tissue Antigens. 1989;34(5):261–9.

81. Stanescu HC, Arcos-Burgos M, Medlar A, et al. Risk HLA-DQA1 and PLA(2)R1 alleles in idiopathic membranous nephropathy. N Engl J Med. 2011;364(7):616–26.

82. Kottgen A, Kiryluk K. New genetic insights into kidney physiology and disease. Nat Rev Nephrol. 2021;17(2):85–6.

83. Bullich G, Ballarin J, Oliver A, et al. HLA-DQA1 and PLA2R1 polymorphisms and risk of idiopathic membranous nephropathy. Clin J Am Soc Nephrol. 2014;9(2):335–43.

84. Liu YH, Chen CH, Chen SY, et al. Association of phospholipase A2 receptor 1 polymorphisms with idiopathic membranous nephropathy in Chinese patients in Taiwan. J Biomed Sci. 2010;17(1):81.

85. Kim S, Chin HJ, Na KY, et al. Single nucleotide polymorphisms in the phospholipase A(2) receptor gene are associated with genetic susceptibility to idiopathic membranous nephropathy. Nephron Clin Pract. 2010;117(3):c253–8.

86. Lv J, Hou W, Zhou X, et al. Interaction between PLA2R1 and HLA-DQA1 variants associates with anti-PLA2R antibodies and membranous nephropathy. J Am Soc Nephrol. 2013;24(8):1323–9.

87. Mladkova N, Kiryluk K. Genetic complexities of the HLA region and idiopathic membranous nephropathy. J Am Soc Nephrol. 2017;28(5):1331–4.

88. Coenen MJ, Hofstra JM, Debiec H, et al. Phospholipase A2 receptor (PLA2R1) sequence variants in idiopathic membranous nephropathy. J Am Soc Nephrol. 2013;24(4):677–83.

89. Xie J, Liu L, Mladkova N, et al. The genetic architecture of membranous nephropathy and its potential to improve non-invasive diagnosis. Nat Commun. 2020;11(1):1600.

90. Le WB, Shi JS, Zhang T, et al. HLA-DRB1*15:01 and HLA-DRB3*02:02 in PLA2R-related membranous nephropathy. J Am Soc Nephrol. 2017;28(5):1642–50.

91. Cui Z, Xie LJ, Chen FJ, et al. MHC class II risk alleles and amino acid residues in idiopathic membranous nephropathy. J Am Soc Nephrol. 2017;28(5):1651–64.

92. Wang HY, Cui Z, Xie LJ, et al. HLA class II alleles differing by a single amino acid associate with clinical phenotype and outcome in patients with primary membranous nephropathy. Kidney Int. 2018;94(5):974–82.

93. Ronco P, Debiec H. Pathogenesis of membranous nephropathy: recent advances and future challenges. Nat Rev Nephrol. 2012;8(4):203–13.

94. O'Shaughnessy MM, Troost JP, Bomback AS, et al. Treatment patterns among adults and children with membranous nephropathy in the cure glomerulonephropathy network (CureGN). Kidney Int Rep. 2019;4(12):1725–34.

95. Ramachandran R, Nayak S, Kumar V, et al. Primary membranous nephropathy in children and adolescents: a single-centre report from South Asia. Pediatr Nephrol. 2020;36(5):1217–26.

96. Cohen CD, Calvaresi N, Armelloni S, et al. CD20-positive infiltrates in human membranous glomerulonephritis. J Nephrol. 2005;18(3):328–33.

97. Segerer S, Schlondorff D. B cells and tertiary lymphoid organs in renal inflammation. Kidney Int. 2008;73(5):533–7.

98. Troyanov S, Roasio L, Pandes M, Herzenberg AM, Cattran DC. Renal pathology in idiopathic membranous nephropathy: a new perspective. Kidney Int. 2006;69(9):1641–8.

99. Ehrenreich T, Churg J. Pathology of membranous nephropathy. In: Sommers SC, editor. Pathology annual. New York: Appleton-Century-Crofts; 1968.

100. Rodriguez EF, Cosio FG, Nasr SH, et al. The pathology and clinical features of early recurrent membranous glomerulonephritis. Am J Transplant. 2012;12(4):1029–38.

101. Glassock RJ. Diagnosis and natural course of membranous nephropathy. Semin Nephrol. 2003;23(4):324–32.

102. Polanco N, Gutierrez E, Covarsi A, et al. Spontaneous remission of nephrotic syndrome in idiopathic membranous nephropathy. J Am Soc Nephrol. 2010;21(4):697–704.

103. Cameron JS. Membranous nephropathy in childhood and its treatment. Pediatr Nephrol. 1990;4(2):193–8.

104. Menon S, Valentini RP. Membranous nephropathy in children: clinical presentation and therapeutic approach. Pediatr Nephrol. 2010;25(8):1419–28.

105. Chen A, Frank R, Vento S, et al. Idiopathic membranous nephropathy in pediatric patients: presentation, response to therapy, and long-term outcome. BMC Nephrol. 2007;8:11.

106. Makker SP. Treatment of membranous nephropathy in children. Semin Nephrol. 2003;23(4):379–85.

107. Bech AP, Hofstra JM, Brenchley PE, Wetzels JF. Association of anti-PLA(2)R antibodies with outcomes after immunosuppressive therapy in idiopathic membranous nephropathy. Clin J Am Soc Nephrol. 2014;9(8):1386–92.

108. Valentini RP, Mattoo TK, Kapur G, Imam A. Membranous glomerulonephritis: treatment response and outcome in children. Pediatr Nephrol. 2009;24(2):301–8.

109. Dahan K, Debiec H, Plaisier E, et al. Rituximab for severe membranous nephropathy: a 6-month trial with extended follow-up. J Am Soc Nephrol. 2017;28(1):348–58.

110. Fervenza FC, Abraham RS, Erickson SB, et al. Rituximab therapy in idiopathic membranous nephropathy: a 2-year study. Clin J Am Soc Nephrol. 2010;5(12):2188–98.

111. Fervenza FC, Cosio FG, Erickson SB, et al. Rituximab treatment of idiopathic membranous nephropathy. Kidney Int. 2008;73(1):117–25.

112. Ruggenenti P, Chiurchiu C, Brusegan V, et al. Rituximab in idiopathic membranous nephropathy: a one-year prospective study. J Am Soc Nephrol. 2003;14(7):1851–7.

113. Ruggenenti P, Cravedi P, Chianca A, et al. Rituximab in idiopathic membranous nephropathy. J Am Soc Nephrol. 2012;23(8):1416–25.

114. Fervenza FC, Appel GB, Barbour SJ, et al. Rituximab or cyclosporine in the treatment of membranous nephropathy. N Engl J Med. 2019;381(1):36–46.

115. Seitz-Polski B, Dahan K, Debiec H, et al. High-dose rituximab and early remission in PLA2R1-related membranous nephropathy. Clin J Am Soc Nephrol. 2019;14(8):1173–82.
116. Fernandez-Juarez G, Rojas-Rivera J, Logt AV, et al. The STARMEN trial indicates that alternating treatment with corticosteroids and cyclophosphamide is superior to sequential treatment with tacrolimus and rituximab in primary membranous nephropathy. Kidney Int. 2020;99(4):986–98.
117. Scolari F, Delbarba E, Santoro D, et al. Rituximab or cyclophosphamide in the treatment of membranous nephropathy: the RI-CYCLO randomized trial. J Am Soc Nephrol. 2021;32(4):972–82.
118. Boneparth A, Wenderfer SE, Moorthy LN, et al. Clinical characteristics of children with membranous lupus nephritis: the Childhood Arthritis and Rheumatology Research Alliance Legacy Registry. Lupus. 2017;26(3):299–306.
119. Pereira M, Muscal E, Eldin K, et al. Clinical presentation and outcomes of childhood-onset membranous lupus nephritis. Pediatr Nephrol. 2017;32(12):2283–91.

Postinfectious and Infectious Glomerulopathies

19

Velibor Tasic and Mignon McCulloch

Introduction

It is important to utilize the correct terminology when describing the infection-related glomerulopathies. In order to better understand the pathogenesis and management of infection-related glomerulonephritis (GN), Nadasdy and Hebert suggest classification as either postinfectious GN or the GN of active infection [1]. Acute postinfectious GN (APIG) is the most common pathology in lower and middle-income countries (LMIC) and is due to a wide spectrum of infective agents. The prototypical APIG is acute poststreptococcal GN (PSGN). In APIG the infection is mild and has usually resolved spontaneously or with antibiotics at the onset of GN, 1–3 weeks later.

Conversely, in GN due to active infection the patient develops infection which does not resolve spontaneously; very often antibiotics are not administered since the infection is not recognized or not considered to be serious. Several weeks after infection begins the patient develops GN, which manifests with hematuria, proteinuria, acute nephritic syndrome or kidney failure. In contrast to postinfectious GN, where antibiotics have no effect on the course of the GN, administration of antibiotics in GN due to active infection eliminates antigen production, ultimately leading to resolution of the GN.

The clinical presentation of infection-related GN varies from subclinical disease to severe acute kidney injury, with the majority of patients having a mild clinical course. There is a growing list of organisms which may cause infection-related GN (Table 19.1).

The pathogenesis of infection-related GN is secondary to (1) formation and deposition of circulating immune-complexes in glomeruli (2) implantation of the antigen in glomerular structures, initiating immunologic reactions and formation of immune-complexes in situ or (3) modifications of native glomerular structures, which become autoantigens [2]. The end result is activation of the complement system and coagulation cascade, and production of proinflammatory cytokines, adhesion molecules and chemoattractants. This leads to proliferation of glomerular cells and infiltration with polymorphonuclear cells.

The most common histological presentation of infection-related GN is diffuse endocapillary or proliferative GN (group A Streptococcus, Streptococcus viridans, Staphylococcus aureus, Diplococcus, Brucella melitensis, measles, mumps, varicella, Cat scratch disease and others),

---

V. Tasic (✉)
University Children's Hospital, Medical School,
Skopje, North Macedonia

M. McCulloch
Paediatric Intensive Care/Nephrology, Red Cross War
Memorial Children's Hospital,
Cape Town, Western Cape, South Africa
e-mail: mignon.mcculloch@uct.ac.za

© The Author(s), under exclusive license to Springer Nature Switzerland AG 2023
F. Schaefer, L. A. Greenbaum (eds.), *Pediatric Kidney Disease*,
https://doi.org/10.1007/978-3-031-11665-0_19

Table 19.1 Etiological agents associated with infection-related glomerulonephritis

Bacterial	Viral	Fungal	Parasites
• Streptococcus group A, C, G	• Coxsackievirus	• Coccidioides immitis	• Plasmodium malariae
• Streptococcus viridans	• Echovirus	• Candida	• Plasmodium falciparum
• Staphylococcus (aureus, albus)	• Cytomegalovirus	• Histoplasma	• Schistosoma mansoni
• Pneumococcus	• Epstein Barr virus		• Leishmania
• Hemophilus	• Hepatitis B, C		• Toxoplasma gondii
• Neisseria meningitis	• HIV		• Filariasis
• Mycobacteria	• Rubella		• Trichinosis
• Salmonella typhosa	• Measles		• Trypanosomes
• Klebsiella pneumoniae	• Varicella		• Echinococcus
• E.coli	• Vaccinia		
• Yersinia enterocolitica	• Parvovirus		
• Legionella	• Influenza		
• Brucella melitensis	• Adenovirus		
• Listeria	• Rickettsial scrub typhus		
• Leptospira	• Mumps		
• Treponema pallidum	• Hantavirus		
• Corynebacterium bovis	• Rotavirus		
• Actinobacilli			
• Cat-scratch bacillus			

but it may present as focal or diffuse crescentic GN (Streptococcus, Staphylococcus aureus, varicella, Treponema pallidum). Mesangiocapillary GN is associated with hepatitis C virus and Streptococcus viridans infections. Membranous GN occurs in infections with hepatitis B virus, syphilis, filaria, schistosoma, mycobacterium, and Plasmodium falciparum. Mesangioproliferative GN (focal or diffuse) is associated with Diplococcus, salmonella, hepatitis B virus (childhood vaccination has resulted in decline in this condition), influenza virus, and adenovirus infections. Focal segmental, necrotizing and sclerosing GN is seen in bacterial endocarditis; mesangiolytic GN occurs with ECHO virus infections.

The initial infection may be mild or severe. Examples of more severe infections include pneumonia, meningitis, sepsis, endocarditis, and ventriculoatrial shunt infection [3–6]. The GN may be mild (asymptomatic proteinuria and hematuria), but patients may develop hypertension, circulatory congestion, nephrotic syndrome, and acute kidney injury. Usually there is transient hypocomplementemia.

As previously reviewed, kidney biopsy shows various glomerular lesions, of which the most common is acute endocapillary and proliferative GN, but tubulointerstitial injury also may be present [7]. Immunofluorescence (IF) studies show granular deposits of immunoglobulins and complement. Treatment of GN of active infection must include antibiotics to address the infection, with additional interventions if the infection does not respond to antibiotics alone (e.g., shunt removal, abscess drainage).

In LMIC countries, the incidence of PSGN has declined over the past 5 decades, although is still commonly seen in some countries. In contrast, Staphylococcus aureus, including methicillin-resistant strains, has increased as an etiology of GN, particularly in older adults and diabetics, who often have worse clinical features and outcomes [1, 8–10]. Kidney biopsy shows diffuse glomerular endocapillary hypercellularity with neutrophil infiltration on light microscopy; dominant IgA deposits on IF; and the presence of subepithelial humps on electron microscopy (EM). This entity was entitled IgA dominant postinfectious GN and should be differentiated from classic IgA nephropathy because of different treatment strategies. Kimata et al. [11] described the youngest patient, a 6 year old girl with methicillin-resistant Staphylococcus aureus-associated GN who initially presented with pneumonia. Vigorous antibiotic treatment resulted in resolution of the GN; in contrast, corticosteroid treatment failed.

It is believed that the outcome of infectious related GN is benign, but in the case of acute kidney injury and crescents on biopsy, corticosteroids, methylprednisolone pulses and cyclophosphamide may be benefitial [6]. The literature is sparse with studies dealing with long-term prognosis of non-streptococcal GN. In a study from Milan 50 adult patients with infection associated GN have been followed for 90 ± 78 months; at the last observation 37% had renal insufficiency or were on hemodyalisis [12]. The unfavourable outcome was due to the underlying disease and presence of interstitial infiltration on kidney biopsy.

Post-streptococcal Glomerulonephritis

PSGN is still the most common glomerulopathy in LMIC countries. The disease is characterized by the acute onset of nephritis, potentially including hematuria, edema, hypertension, oliguria and azotemia [2, 13]. It was recognized as a complication of scarlet fever in the eighteenth century. Due to improved living standards and medical care, PSGN is uncommon in western countries, mainly occurring as sporadic cases [14–16].

Epidemiology

PSGN occurs worldwide [17–22]. It is a complication of pyoderma due to hot climate and high humidity in tropical countries. Skin injuries, insect bites (such as scabies), and poor hygiene and sanitation predispose to infection with group A beta hemolytic streptococcus (GABHS) [23]. In countries with moderate and cold climates, PSGN is usually a complication of upper respiratory tract infections (pharyngitis) during the winter months. Streptococcal M types 2, 47, 49, 55, 57, 60 are associated with PSGN following pyoderma, while M types 1, 2, 3, 4, 12, 25 and 45 are

associated with PSGN following pharyngitis. While typically seasonal, isolated cases of PSGN may be seen throughout the year. In the past, epidemics of PSGN following impetigo were reported. In some areas (Trinidad, Maracaibo), epidemics occurred every 5–7 years; there is no satisfactory explanation for this phenomenon [13]. Populations at increased risk include children and soldiers, due to intimate contact, overcrowded living conditions, and poor hygiene and sanitation. The ratio male:female is up to 2:1, but when subclinical cases are included, there is no male predominance. The disease is most common in children aged 3–12 years, although PSGN has been reported in infants [24, 25]. The risk for developing PSGN after infection with a nephritogenic strain of GABHS is about 15%; for M type 49, it is 5% after pharyngeal infection and 25% after pyoderma [26]. Rarely, PSGN occurs as a complication of piercing [27] or circumcision [28]; presents in a kidney allograft [29]; or occurs secondary to immune reconstitution inflammatory syndrome in pediatric HIV infected patient [30]. Besides GABHS, streptococci from group C and G can also cause acute GN [31–33], but the concept of a common nephritogenic antigen is questionable [34].

Pathogenesis

There is clear evidence that PSGN is an immune complex disease, but the identity of the nephritogenic antigen is uncertain [35, 36]. The proposed mechanisms are;

1. Deposition of circulating immune complexes containing nephritogenic antigen in glomeruli
2. Implantation of the nephritogenic antigen into glomerular structures and in situ formation of immune complexes
3. Molecular mimicry between streptococcal antigens and glomerular antigens, which react with antibodies against streptococcal antigens
4. Direct activation of the complement system by implanted streptococcal antigens. Many proteins such as endostreptosin, preabsorbing antigen, nephritis strain–associated protein,

streptococcal pyrogenic exotoxin B (SPEB), nephritis-associated plasmin receptor (NaPlr) have been considered as potent nephritogenic antigens in PSGN [37–45].

There are several reports of infection-related GN caused by pathogens other than Streptococcus group A and C with detection of NAPlr in kidney biopsies. This lists includes Streptococcus pneumoniae, Staphylococcus aureus, Mycoplasma pneumoniae and Aggregatibacter actinomycetemcomitans [46–49].

Evidence that an antigen is nephritogenic should include identifying the antigen in kidney biopsy specimens from patients with PSGN; extracting the same antigen from streptococci obtained from PSGN patients; not identifying the antigen in streptococci cultured from patients with rheumatic fever; and demonstrating significant titer of antibodies against the nephritogenic antigen in sera from PSGN patients in the convalescent phase. Lange and his group [39, 40] considered that endostreptosin (ESS) was an ideal nephritogenic antigen because it fulfilled the these criteria. Interestingly, ESS was identified in early but not in late biopsy specimens,. In animal experiments, ESS was implanted on the glomerular basement membrane very early in the course of the disease. Late in the disease course, there was production of anti-ESS antibodies, which bound ESS and thus enabled detection of the ESS. The two main disadvantages of this theory are (1) endostreptosin is an anionic antigen and this cannot explain its implantation on the glomerular basement membrane (GBM) (2) injection of ESS has never induced histological changes and clinical features compatible with PSGN.

Vogt et al. provided evidence that cationic antigens were responsible for the immunopathogenesis of PSGN; they identified cationic antigens in 8 out of 18 biopsy specimens from PSGN patients and confirmed that streptococci cultured from PSGN patients produced cationic antigens [42]. Later this antigen was confirmed to be streptococcal pyrogenic exotoxin B (zymogen, SPEB), a plasmin binding membrane receptor. Glyceraldehyde phosphate dehydroge-

nase (GAPDH) and NAPlr/Plr are also candidate nephritogenic antigens [36, 44, 50, 51]. Both antigens induce long lasting antibody responses; antibodies against NaPlr can be detected 10 years after an acute episode. This may explain why second attacks of PSGN are rare. Nephritogenic potential is not limited to GABHS, but extends to groups C and G, with sporadic and epidemic cases of PSGN reported after infection with these streptococcal groups. The common pathway for both antigens is binding to plasmin, which activates complement, and promotes chemotaxis and degradation of GBM components. Bound plasmin can cause tissue destruction by direct action on the GBM, or by indirect activation of procollagenases and other matrix metalloproteinases. This allows circulating immune complexes to transit the damaged GBM and accumulate in the subepithelial space, seen as humps by EM.

NAPlr has been isolated from both groups A and C streptococci, and was considered as a putative antigen in the Japanese population with serum antibodies detected in 92% of convalescing PSGN patients and in 60% of patients with uncomplicated streptococcal infections [44]. Glomerular deposits and serum antibodies against these two putative antigens were examined concurrently in biopsies and sera from PSGN patients [45]. This study suggests that SPEB is the most likely major antigen involved in the pathogenesis of PSGN in patients from Latin America, US and Europe. Subsequently, a genome study of S. equi subsp. Zooepidemicus strain MGCS10565, a Lancefield group C organism that caused an epidemic of nephritis in Brazil, found that this organism lacked a gene related to SPEB and challenges the hypothesis that SPEB or antibodies reacting with it singularly cause PSGN [34].

Immune complexes deposited from the circulation or formed in situ activate the complement cascade. This leads to production of various cytokines and other cellular immune factors which initiate an inflammatory response manifested by cellular proliferation and edema of the glomerular tuft [52, 53].

In some PSGN patients, rheumatoid factor, cryoglobulins, and antineutrophil cytoplasmic antibodies (ANCA) are present [54–58]. The significance is unknown.

Pathology

The typical presentation on light microscopy is diffuse enlargement of all glomeruli due to hypercellularity (Fig. 19.1). There is swelling of the endothelial cells, which leads to the obliteration of the capillary loops. The number of mesangial cells is increased. There is recruitment of numerous inflammatory cells in the glomeruli, mainly polymorphonuclear leukocytes and monocytes; thus, this pathological picture is termed exudative proliferative GN. Polymorphonuclear leukocytes may be seen in the tubular lumen. If the mesangial proliferation is axial, then the glomerulus has a lobular appearance. Capillary walls are not thickened. Arterioles and tubules are not affected. There may be edema of the interstitium and infiltration with inflammatory cells. Rarely, proliferation of parietal cells of Bowman's capsule may result in formation of crescents; a high percentage is associated with a rapidly progressive course.

By IF, the most common finding in the acute phase is an irregular, granular capillary and mesangial staining for complement alone, or complement and immunoglobulins. During the resolving phase, there is only mesangial staining (Fig. 19.2). The predominant finding is C3 and IgG, but C4, C1q, IgM, fibrinogen and factor B may be found. Sorger et al. described three types of immune deposits in PSGN [59]. Starry sky pattern is the fine granular deposition of C3 and IgG along the capillary walls in the first week of the disease (Fig. 19.2a). Mesangial pattern is found between the fourth and sixth week after the disease onset; the only immune reactant is C3, which is found in a mesangial location (Fig. 19.2b). The garland pattern is characterized by dense, confluent deposits along the capillary loops, while mesangial and endocapillary locations are preserved (Fig. 19.2c). Subepithelial location of the deposits correlates with the humps seen on EM. The garland pattern is associated with massive proteinuria and does not correlate with the time of kidney biopsy [60]. In clinically atypical cases with acute kidney injury and nephrotic syndrome, NAPlr staining of the glomeruli is a useful tool for confirmation of the diagnosis of PSGN [61].

The typical finding on EM in the acute phase is deposits on the subepithelial side of the GBM (humps), Fig. 19.3. These deposits disappear after the sixth week of disease onset [62].

Parallel to the clinical resolution of the disease, there is marked improvement of the histological picture, with resolution of exudative and endocapillary changes; there is residual mesangial proliferation in the convalescent phase (resolving mesangioproliferative GN). Subepithelial deposits disappear or decrease in number after the sixth week; immune deposits decrease in parallel. Complete histologic resolution usually occurs by 1 year after onset.

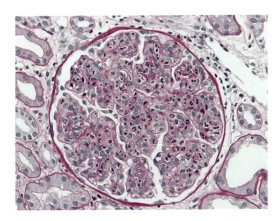

Fig. 19.1 Acute post-streptococcal glomerulonephritis, light microscopy. The glomerulus is enlarged and hypercellular; capillary loops are obliterated; and there is infiltration with polymorphonuclear leukocytes (hematoxylin and eosin, ×400). Courtesy of Prof. N. Kambham, MD, Dept. of Pathology, Stanford University

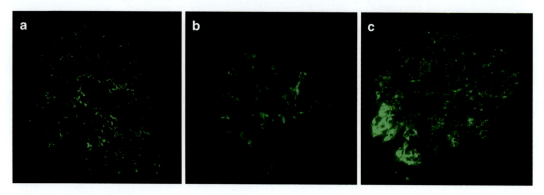

Fig. 19.2 Immunofluorescent study in acute poststreptococcal glomerulonephritis showing intensive immune deposit of C3. (**a**) Starry sky pattern (×400). (**b**) Mesangial pattern (×400). (**c**) Garland pattern (×400). Courtesy of Prof. N. Kambham, MD, Dept. of Pathology, Stanford University

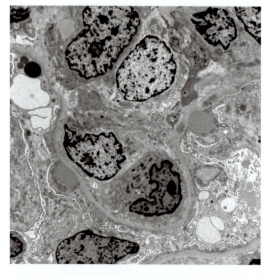

Fig. 19.3 Acute poststreptococcal glomerulonephritis, electron microscopy. Typical electron dense deposits (humps) located on the subepithelial side of the glomerular basement membrane (electron micrograph, ×8000). Courtesy of Prof. N. Kambham, MD, Dept. of Pathology, Stanford University

Clinical Features

The latent period between the upper respiratory infection (pharyngitis) or pyoderma and nephritis is usually 10–14 days or 2–4 weeks, respectively. One third of PSGN patients develop discrete microscopic hematuria and/or proteinuria in the latent period. Usually the disease has acute onset, with development of nephritic syndrome (oedema, oliguria, azotemia hematuria, hypertension). Evidence of nephritis within 2–3 days of the onset of an upper respiratory tract infection is suggestive of other etiologies such as IgA nephropathy or Alport syndrome. At the onset of the disease, non-specific symptoms may be present, such as pallor, malaise, low-grade fever, lethargy, anorexia and headache.

Gross hematuria is present in 30–70% of patients with PSGN, while microscopic hematuria is present in all patients. Microscopic examination of the urine reveals dysmorphic red blood cells and casts. The urine is described as being smoky, cola colored, tea colored or rusty. Gross hematuria may be present continuously or only a few hours during the day. Usually it resolves after 1–2 weeks and transforms into microscopic hematuria. Once gross hematuria has seemingly resolved, it may reappear after physical exercise or intercurrent infections. A few patients have minimal urinary finding (few red blood cells/per high power field), yet have a severe clinical presentation of the disease [63, 64].

Edema in PSGN results from retention of salt and water. Despite the sodium retention, the increased level of atrial natriuretic peptide in plasma of PSGN patients indicates unresponsiveness of the kidneys to its action [65]. Parents often do not appreciate the edema, but it becomes clear during the diuretic phase when there is a marked weight loss. Most children have mild morning periorbital edema; this location is due to reduced tissues resistance. There may also be pretibial edema or generalized edema (anasarca), including pleural effusions and ascites. Early salt and water restriction may prevent the consequences-circulatory congestion and hypertension.

Hypertension occurs in up to 70% of hospitalized children. Hypertension in PSGN is low renin type due to retention of water and salt, which leads to expansion of the extracellular fluid volume with consequent suppression of the renin-angiotensin-aldosterone axis. Usually it is mild and has a biphasic character. Hypertension that is severe and associated with retinal changes is suggestive of pre-existing renal disease. Normalization of the blood pressure correlates with diuresis and recovery of the kidney function. Hypertension beyond 4 weeks after disease onset may indicate rapidly progressive disease or chronic GN.

Complications

Circulatory congestion is the most common complication in hospitalized children with PSGN. If severe, it can lead to pulmonary oedema, which represents an emergency state and requires prompt and appropriate therapy. The signs and symptoms of circulatory congestions are tachycardia, dyspnoea, orthopnea, rales and cough. Sometimes clinical signs may be subtle, but a chest radiograph shows signs of congestion. Since children and young individuals have healthy cardiovascular systems, cardiac failure is rarely seen.

Posterior reversible encephalopathy syndrome (PRES), previously called hypertensive encephalopathy, is another serious complication found in 0.5–10% of hospitalized patients [13]. The most common clinical signs and symptoms are nausea, vomiting, headache, and impairment of consciousness, which varies from somnolence to coma. The children may manifest seizures, hemiparesis, amaurosis and aphasia. These symptoms are a consequence of sudden elevation of the blood pressure that impairs cerebral autoregulation leading to vasogenic edema. Electroencephalography has non-specific changes, which resolve in parallel with resolu-

tion of the neurological symptoms. Analysis of the cerebrospinal fluid may reveal the presence of protein, but no cells. On magnetic resonance imaging, there is alteration of the posterior white matter, which is termed reversible posterior leukoencephalopathy syndrome [66, 67]. The images show edematous lesions primarily involving the posterior supratentorial white matter and corticomedullary junction. Neurological complications in PSGN cannot be attributed exclusively to hypertensive encephalopathy or abnormal serum biochemistry, particularly in those patients with normal blood pressure during the incident (e.g. seizures). With advances in neuroimaging, there is evidence that some children develop cerebral vasculitis [68, 69]. This has practical implication because it may require different treatment.

PSGN may also be complicated by severe acute kidney injury. Some patients require dialysis.

Clinical Variants

Approximately 90% of patients have subclinical disease and never seek medical care due to absence of symptoms [13]. Rarely, patients may have nephrotic syndrome (0.4%) or rapidly progressive disease (0.1%). The incidence of subclinical disease (expressed as ratio subclinical: clinical disease) varies from 0.03 to 19.0 [70, 71]. This is most likely due differences in methodology and study populations, which has included epidemic contacts [26], family contacts [70, 72, 73], or patients with well-documented streptococcal infections [71, 74]. The population at risk has been tested for urinary abnormalities and hypocomplementemia once or sequentially. More frequent testing increases the likelihood of detecting abnormalities, which may be transitory and normalize within a week.

Sagel et al. followed 248 children from New York 4–6 weeks after well-documented streptococcal infections [71]. Abnormal urinalysis with hypocomplementemia was detected in 20 children, but only one had symptomatic disease. The incidence of nephritis after streptococcal infection in this report was 8.08% and the ratio subclinical/clinical nephritis 19.0. Kidney biopsy was performed in all 20 children and showed histological lesions varying from mild focal cellular proliferation to classical exudative and proliferative GN. Only one child had normal histology and lack of immune deposits. The authors concluded that only a minority of PSGN cases are detected. Yoshizawa et al. performed a similar study in Japan; 12 out of 49 patients with well-documented streptococcal infection developed subclinical nephritis (24%) and all 12 patients had abnormal kidney biopsies [74].

In a study of family contacts from Macedonia, the incidence of nephritis in parents and siblings was 0% and 9.4%, respectively [73]. It seems that parents are "protected" from developing PSGN. The ratio of subclinical/clinical nephritis in contacts was 1.28. An additional number of family contacts had glomerular type microhematuria and elevated ASO titre; thus, it is possible that they also had subclinical PSGN and that their complement levels normalized before occurrence of nephritis in the index cases. Lange et al. pointed that the finding of significant titers of endostreptosin antibodies in patients with chronic GN or on hemodialysis suggested the possibility of previous undetected subclinical PSGN [39, 75].

Nephrotic syndrome occurs in 4–25% of hospitalized children with PSGN. It usually resolves within 2–3 weeks; persistence beyond 3 weeks is associated with a poor outcome. Less than 1% of hospitalized children develop rapidly progressive disease, which is characterized by prolonged oligo-anuria, uremia, hypertension, anemia and persistent nephrotic syndrome. Crescents are present on kidney biopsy, and the percentage of crescents correlates with the severity of the disease and the outcome.

Cerebral vasculitis is an infrequent complication; cutaneous and gastrointestinal vasculitis have also been reported in PSGN patients and may mimic Henoch-Schönlein purpura [76]. PSGN is uncommonly associated with rheumatic fever [77, 78]. An unusual or atypical course of the disease is reported in patients with concurrent IgA nephropathy, diabetes mellitus, hemolytic uremic syndrome, reflux nephropathy and bilateral kidney hypoplasia [79–82]. Simultaneous occurrence of acute immune thrombocytopenia has also been reported in a few PSGNpatients [83–85]. The most likely mechanism is production of autoantibodies that cross-react against GABHS and platelets [84].

Laboratory Findings

Proteinuria and hematuria are found in almost all patients with PSGN. The presence of red blood cell casts and dysmorphic erythrocytes confirms the glomerular origin of the hematuria. In a few patients, minimal urinary findings occur despite a severe clinical presentation.

A mild dilutional anemia may be seen at the onset of the disease and is due to expansion of the extracellular fluid volume. Thrombocytopenia is extremely rare; its presence suggests the possibility of systemic lupus erythematosus or hemolytic uremic syndrome. If there is no significant impairment of glomerular filtration rate (GFR), blood chemistry is almost normal; severe reduction of renal function leads to hyperkalemia, uremia and acidosis. Hypoproteinemia, hypoalbuminemia and hyperlipidemia are evident if there is associated nephrotic syndrome.

Patients should be evaluated for evidence of previous streptococcal infection. Cultures from the throat or skin should be obtained, depending on the site of the initial infection. Antibodies against streptococcal antigens (antistreptolysin O, antihyaluronidase, anti-DNA-se B titer), or combination of antigens (streptozyme) should be measured serially during the course of the disease. Of note, in postpyodermal disease there is an insignificant rise in antistreptolysin O titres. Testing anti-zymogen titres is very sensitive and specific for diagnosing streptococcal infection in PSGN patients, but this test is not available for routine practice. A high titre of antibodies against glyceraldehydes phosphate dehydrogenase is found in PSGN patients.

There is marked depression of CH50 and C3 due to activation of the alternative pathway. In some patients, there is also depression of C2 and C4, suggesting activation of both classical and alternative pathways [86]. Usually, complement levels normalize within 6–8 weeks; persistence of hypocomplementemia beyond 3 months suggests an alternative diagnosis (membranoproliferative GN).

Complement activation was analyzed in 34 children with APIG and low C3 level at onset [87]. They demonstrated that anti-factor B (anti-FB) antibodies enhance alternative pathway convertase activity in vitro, confirming their pathogenic effect. They identified anti-FB autoantibodies in 31 of 34 (91%) children with APIG and in four of 28 (14%) children with C3 GN. Sensitivity and specificity of anti-FB antibodies for APIG diagnosis were 95% and 82%, respectively. Anti-FB antibodies were not detected in 15 patients with IgA nephropathy and 26 with lupus nephritis. During the follow-up, the anti-FB antibody levels became negative or decreased in children with APIG. The authors hypothesize that streptococcal infection may cause transient anti-FB autoantibodies, which overactivate complement with subsequent deposition of complement C3 breakdown products in the glomeruli.

Kozyro et al. tested children with PSGN for the presence of antibodies against C1q and found that 8 of 24 were positive for anti-C1q [88]. They found that anti-C1q positive children had more severe disease (hypertension, proteinuria) and unfavourable resolution of the disease.

Kidney Biopsy and Differential Diagnosis

Usually children with PSGN have a favourable disease course and outcome; thus, kidney biopsy is not necessary. In cases of severe or atypical clinical presentation or delayed recovery, then kidney biopsy is mandatory. Indications for kidney biopsy are summarized in Table 19.2.

PSGN should be differentiated from the following diseases: IgA nephritis (short latent period from infection), hereditary nephritis (family history, short latent period), MPGN (persistent hypocomplementemia and unresolving nephritic syndrome), lupus nephritis (persistent

Table 19.2 Indications for kidney biopsy

Early stage	Recovery phase
• Age <2 years • Short latent period • Anuria • Rapid progressive course • Hypertension >2 weeks • Depressed GFR >2 weeks • Normal complement levels • No elevation of antistreptococcal antibodies • Extrarenal manifestation	• Depressed GFR >4 weeks • Hypocomplementemia >12 weeks • Persistent proteinuria >6 months • Persistent microhematuria >18 months

hypocomplementemia, systemic manifestations), GN in acute and chronic infections (evidence for other non-streptococcal infection), vasculitides (polyarteritis nodosa, Henoch Schönlein purpura), haemolytic uremic syndrome (hemolysis, thrombocytopenia).

Vernon et al. described a girl who developed chronic kidney disease and persistent hypocomplementemia after streptococcal throat infection. Kidney biopsy 1 year after presentation revealed features of C3 glomerulopathy while genetic studies detected a heterozygous mutation in the complement factor H-related protein 5 gene (CFHR5) [89]. A group from the Mayo Clinic presented a series of 11 patients who had atypical postinfectious GN [90]. Kidney biopsy was performed due to persistent proteinuria, hematuria, and depressed C3. On light microscopy, there were exudative and proliferative changes; IF studies revealed dominant C3 mesangial deposits while EM revealed subepithelial humps. In 10 of 11 patients, there was an underlying defect in the alternative pathway of the complement, either autoantibodies against C3 convertase or mutations in complement regulatory genes.

Treatment

Bedrest and limited activity are indicated in the early stage of the disease, particularly if circulatory overload and hypertension are present. There is no evidence that prolonged bedrest hastens recovery.

In most cases, fluid and salt restriction are sufficient to prevent edema and hypertension. Salt intake should be limited to less than 1.0 g/day. Usually protein intake should be limited to 1.0 g/kg/day. In case of marked azotemia, calories should be provided from carbohydrates and fats. to the diet is individualized based on clinical and biochemical indices. Diuresis and body weight should be monitored every day. Loop diuretic (furosemide 1–2 mg/kg/day) is indicated if there is moderate circulatory congestion. Higher doses, up to 5 mg/kg per dose intravenously are indicated if there is pulmonary oedema, although caution is indicated if there is severe azotemia because of potential ototoxicity.

Moderate hypertension should be treated with diuretics and oral antihypertensive drugs; amlodipine is now widely used. Angiotensin converting enzyme inhibitors (ACEIs) may be effective, but there is concern for worsening hyperkalemia [91]. In a hypertensive emergency, options include intravenous labetalol (bolus or continuous infusion) and nicardipine or nitroprusside by continuous infusion. Short-acting, oral or sublingual nifedipine has been used for hypertensive emergencies without encephalopathy. However, given the occurrence of serious and fatal adverse effects in adults, it should be administered in children with great caution [92]. Amlodipine or isradipine may be safer options.

Hyperkalemia should be prevented with restricted potassium intake. If present, conservative treatment should be started immediately to prevent fatal complication. Severe hyperkalemia, azotemia, acidosis, uncontrolled hypertension, cardiovascular insufficiency and pulmonary edema are indications for urgent dialysis.

There is no clear evidence that immunosuppressive therapy has a beneficial effect in children with crescentic PSGN. In those with >30% crescents one may attempt pulse methylprednisolone 0.5–1.0 g/1.73 m² for 3–5 days. In ten children with crescentic PSGN, five were given quintuple therapy (including immunosuppressive drugs) and five were given only supportive treatment [93]. At the end of the follow-up, the outcomes were similar, though patients who received quintuple treatment had faster normalization of serum creatinine and decreased duration of hospitalization. Nevertheless, based on efficacy in other forms of rapidly progressive GN, some clinicians administer high-dose intravenous methylprednisolone for 3–5 days for severe disease based on kidney function and percentage of crescents.

Antibiotic therapy is indicated if there are still signs of streptococcal infection (pharyngitis, pyoderma) or patients have positive throat or skin culture. Oral penicillin V (or erythromycin for allergic patients) is preferred over parenteral treatment. Antibiotic treatment does not alter the course of the PSGN, but it is important to prevent spread of nephritogenic strains of GABHS. Long-term antibiotic prophylaxis is not justified since second attacks of PSGN are rare [94].

Prognosis

The prognosis of PSGN in children in the acute phase is excellent, with mortality less than 1% due to improved conservative management and availability of dialysis. There are conflicting data regarding long-term outcomes. For example, Baldwin et al. [95, 96] suggest unfavourable outcomes in many patients while Potter et al. [97] describe excellent outcomes. This is mainly due to different criteria for selection of patients for prognostic studies, excellently reviewed in detail by Cameron [98]. It is important to remember that only clinical cases (10%) are included in the analysis, while those with subclinical and mild disease may escape medical attention. Moreover, some are not referred to a nephrologist and only a small percentage have a kidney biopsy. The series describing prognosis differ in respect to following parameters: pediatric/adult, sporadic/epidemic, evidence/no evidence for previous streptococcal infection, with/without kidney biopsy, and with/without crescents on kidney biopsy.

In a study by Vogl et al. [99], 36 children and 101 adults had biopsy and serological confirmation of PSGN and had been followed for 2–13 years; none of the children reached end stage kidney disease (ESKD), but 10% had elevated serum creatinine between 1–2 mg/dL. Clark et al. provided excellent information concerning long-term outcome of PSGN in children [100]. Although their series was small, it was exclusively pediatric, with adequate documentation of streptococcal infection and initial biopsy in all children and rebiopsies in some of them. Thirty children were followed for 14.6–22 years (mean: 19 years). Urinary abnormalities were present in 20% of patients during the follow-up, but none had reduced GFR, assessed with creatinine clearance. Clark et al. questioned the role of kidney biopsy for diagnosis and follow-up of children with typical PSGN.

Baldwin et al. reported unfavourable data on long-term prognosis of PSGN [95, 96]. In their series, 37 out of 126 patients were children; 11 patients progressed to terminal uremia, nine in the first 6 months. During the follow-up of 2–15 years, proteinuria, hypertension and reduced GFR were documented in half of the patients. A total of 174 kidney biopsies were performed; in the first years after the acute episode there was a prevalence of proliferative changes, while in 2/3 of the late biopsies there were sclerosing lesions, which Baldwin considered as an indicator of chronicity. The poor outcomes may seem likely secondary to a highly selected patient population; 20% presented with nephrotic syndrome. Patients who died or rapidly progressed to uremia had crescentic nephritis at biopsy. A substantial number of patients were lost to follow-up, with selection of those who had more severe disease. Furthermore, GFR in this study was not corrected for sex, age and body surface area. The same group reported six patients with PSGN who progressed to terminal uremia 2–12 years after resolution of acute nephritis and normalization of the GFR [101]. Of note, five of six patients had nephrotic syndrome at the disease onset. Gallo et al. presented data on the morphologic alteration in kidney biopsies from patients who recovered from PSGN; they found that the incidence of glomerular and vascular sclerosis increased with time [102]. The clinical consequence of this healing process is reduced kidney functional reserve after a protein loading test [103, 104].

The two studies from Maracaibo, Venezuela also pointed to the progressive character of PSGN [105, 106]. One hundred and twenty patients (101 children) who had survived the epidemics in 1968 were evaluated between 1973–1975. Proteinuria, microhematuria, hypertension or reduced GFR were found in 36.7% of adult patients compared with 8.7% of pediatric patients. Kidney biopsies showed advanced glomerulosclerosis in all patients with abnormal findings. Mild to moderate mesangial proliferation and glomerulosclerosis were present even in those patients who had no history of any clinical abnormality.

Herrera and Rodríguez-Iturbe investigated the incidence of ESKD among Goajiros Indians, a semi-nomadic tribe that live in the northwestern part of Venezuela [107]. The incidence of ESKD was 1.7 times higher than the incidence for the country. Also, the attack rate of PSGN was double compared with the general population in the neighboring Maracaibo city. Low birth weight was common among Goajiros Indians (23% of newborns weigh less than 1000 g). The authors concluded that high attack rate of PSGN and low nephron endowment were responsible for the increased risk of ESKD in this population.

In contrast, Dodge et al. [108] and Travis et al. [109] reported excellent clinical and histological healing of the disease in their pediatric series. Dodge et al. found that the presence of proteinuria was present despite histological healing; it had an orthostatic character before definitively cleared [108]. In a study from Macedonia, 40 post-nephritic children were investigated 3 months to 10 years after the acute episode, but no increase in proteinuria was found after moderate to strenuous physical activity [110]. Perlman et al. reevaluated 61 children 10 years after the original epidemics in 1963 [111]. All children had normal GFR, 3 had proteinuria >100 mg/24, but all had normal morphology on kidney biopsy. Sixteen children had a kidney biopsy; four patients had minimal focal proliferation, but no sclerosing lesions were seen.

Three studies from Trinidad evaluated medium and long-term prognosis of PSGN. These are the largest studies, predominantly pediatric, with excellent outcomes concerning presence of urinary abnormalities, hypertension or impaired renal function [97, 112, 113]. Renal biopsy was not performed in many studies for diagnosis and follow-up of PSGN in children, but the diagnosis was based on firm clinical and serological documentation of previous streptococcal infection and transitory hypocomplementemia. Results of these studies confirmed the benign course of PSGN in children, with very low percentage having persistent urinary abnormalities, hypertension or reduced GFR [114–116]. Besides clinical healing, there was complete functional recovery in almost all patients. Drukker et al. found that natriuretic response was excellent in postnephritic children after intravenous saline loading [117].

In some indigenous communities in Australia and New Zealand, there is still high attack rate of PSGN [118, 119]. Repeated episodes of PSGN and low number of nephrons due to higher rate of prematurity contribute to higher prevalence of chronic kidney disease in the Aboriginal population [120, 121].

From analysis of multiple studies, the following risk factors for unfavourable outcome were identified: older age, high serum creatinine at presentation, nephrotic syndrome and crescents on kidney biopsy. Even after initial normalization of the kidney function, impairment of the GFR may ensue many years after disease onset; thus, children who present with crescents need indefinite follow-up [122].

Prognosis of PSGN caused by group C *Streptococcus zooepidemicus* appears less favorable. After a mean follow-up of 5.4 years after epidemics in Brazil, a relatively high percentage of patients had microalbuminuria, hypertension and reduced GFR [123]. However, it was impossible to draw conclusions for children since few were evaluated.

Shunt Nephritis

Immune complex GN associated with infection of a ventriculoatrial shunts was first reported in 1965 by Black et al. [124]. Shunt infections are common, but few patients develop GN (2%). Ventriculoperitoneal shunts are now preferred over ventriculoatrial shunts because of lower rates of complications, including shunt infections. The clinical features of shunt nephritis are variable and include proteinuria, hematuria, hypertension, nephrotic syndrome, anemia and compromised kidney function [10, 125]. Symptoms of shunt infections may be present and include fever, anemia, malaise, hepatosplenomegaly and cerebral symptoms. Colonization of the shunt may persist for months and years in otherwise asymptomatic patients. Low-grade fever may be the only sign of active shunt infection and this may result in delay of diagnosis. Staphylococcus epidermidis is the most common pathogen, occurring in 75% of shunt infections. This is a skin contaminant most likely introduced during the surgical procedure. Other isolated pathogens are S. aureus, corynebacterium, listeria, pseudomonas, Propionibacterium acnes, and Bacillus species [10, 126].

Laboratory investigations demonstrate low C3 in 90%, elevated erythrocyte sedimentation rate, cryoglobulinemia and positive blood or cerebrospinal fluid cultures. Patients with ventriculoatrial shunt with unexplained hematuria, proteinuria, or compromised kidney function should have prompt diagnostic work up for subacute shunt infection, even in the absence of fever and leukocytosis [10]. Kidney biopsy shows membranoproliferative pattern on light microscopy in the majority of patients [125]. IF studies demonstrate granular deposits of C3, IgM and IgG in subendothelial and mesangial locations. Persistent antigenemia is responsible for immune complex formation, but it is unclear whether the immune complexes are formed in the circulation or *in situ*. Their presence induces complement activation through the classical pathway, which further mediates injury to glomerular cells (through the C5–9 complex) and generates chemotactic peptides (C3a, C5a) that perpetuate local inflammation.

The prognosis of shunt nephritis is excellent, with normalization of kidney function and resolution of proteinuria, if the infected shunt is removed and appropriate antibiotic treatment is administered. Kidney function normalizes within a few weeks and hypocomplementemia also resolves [10, 125]. Delayed removal of the infected shunt may result in progressive worsening of kidney function and lead to ESKD.

Endocarditis-Associated Glomerulonephritis

Infective endocarditis (IE) is mainly a complication of congenital or rheumatic heart disease in children and still has high mortality despite appropriate antibiotic therapy. Kidney involvement occurs in about 25% of the patients with IE and manifests as kidney infarcts, GN, and interstitial nephritis [10]. The most common pathogen is Streptococcus viridians, whose indolent clinical course enables prolonged antibody response and formation of circulating immune complexes which predispose to the development of GN. Other causative pathogens include S. epidermidis, enterococcus, Hemophilus influenza, actinobacillus, chlamydia, Bartonella henselae, and Coxiella burnetti [126].

Children with acute IE) present with severe illness, including fever, anemia, heart murmur, hepatosplenomegaly, skin purpura and retinal hemorrhages (Roth spots). In contrast, those with a subacute course may have subtle symptoms that are only recognizable during the workup of the GN. GN usually ensues within 7–10 days of clinical illness. Duration of endocarditis does not increase the risk of developing GN. The clinical presentation is variable, from mild proteinuria and hematuria to a severe, rapidly progressive course. The most common presentation is acute nephritic syndrome. Laboratory investigation reveals hypocomplementemia, which correlates with the severity of kidney disease and infection. Rheumatoid factor may be positive and some patients have ANCA that react against proteinase 3.

The kidney biopsy findings are diverse; focal segmental proliferation is the most common finding, followed by diffuse endocapillary proliferation. Exudative features are similar to those seen in PSGN. Crescents and glomerular necrosis may also be present, and in some patients may affect >50% of glomeruli [6]. The tubular atrophy and fibrosis correlates with the extent of glomerular necrosis and crescents. Rarely, membranoproliferative GN resembling MPGN type I may be present and the biopsy shows diffuse mesangial and endocapillary proliferation, lobular accentuation, and GBM reduplication. During resolution of the GN, mesangial proliferation is the dominant histological pattern. IF studies show dominant deposits of C3 and less intense IgG and IgM in mesangial areas and in capillary walls. EM detects subepithelial deposits in the early phase; latter in the course of the disease they are located in subendothelial and mesangial areas.

Endocarditis-associated GN represents an immune complex disease with deposition of circulating immune complexes in the glomeruli, but also there is evidence for in situ formation of complexes. The nephritogenic bacterial antigens were identified within the affected glomeruli in S. aureus and streptococcal infections. Treatment consists of antibiotic therapy and surgery to remove valvular vegetations and eradicate the infection. Most infective and non-infective complications of IE resolve on treatment with appropriate antibiotics. In a few patients with proliferative lesions and no improvement with antibiotics, corticosteroids and cyclophosphamide may be useful [6, 127]. Patients with crescentic GN may benefit from plasmapheresis.

HIV Related Kidney Disease

The implementation of the successful prevention of mother-to-child transmission (PMTCT) program has dramatically decreased new cases of pediatric HIV infection [128, 129]. Highly active antiretroviral therapy (HAART) has significantly decreased the mortality rate in children who acquire perinatal HIV infection. However, managing and preventing contraction of HIV remains a major part of adolescent care in Africa [130]. HIV is currently the second leading cause of death among adolescents worldwide. Women aged 15–24 are the group with the highest rate of new HIV infection in sub-Saharan Africa [131].

Increased survival and complications of therapy have led to a variety of non-infectious complications in patients with HIV infection, and kidney disease is an important concern. Chronic kidney disease in children with perinatal HIV infection is the consequence of primary HIV infection, antiretroviral therapy, and other nephrotoxic drugs, including aminoglycosides. The spectrum of kidney disease includes chronic glomerular disorders, such as HIV associated nephropathy (HIVAN) and HIV immune complex kidney disease (HIVICK); the thrombotic microangiopathies (atypical haemolytic uremic syndrome and thrombotic thrombocytopenic purpura); disorders of proximal tubular function; and acute kidney injury [132].

The histology of HIVAN in children is classical FSGS, with or without mesangial hyperplasia. Other features may include microcystic tubular dilatation and interstitial inflammation. This contrasts with adults, where collapsing FSGS is the typical histological finding. Two pediatric studies have reported collapsing FSGS in 14% and 32.5% [133, 134]. This has important prognostic implications in children since collapsing FSGS has more rapid and progressive course towards ESKD compared with the classical form.

In the pathogenesis of HIVAN, the initial event is infection of the kidney epithelial cells by HIV-1, but it is still enigmatic how the virus enters the epithelial cells since podocytes and renal tubular cells do not express CD4 or other co-receptors. The injured podocytes undergo proliferation and apoptosis; then the remaining podocytes hypertrophy and leave bare segments of basement membrane that promotes the development of the sclerotic lesions that characterize HIVAN. HIV nef and tat genes are implicated for the glomerular pathology while vpr genes are

responsible for tubular lesions. Host genetic factors predispose to development of HIVAN and progression to ESKD [132]. This is supported by the observation that African-Americans have a higher incidence of HIVAN, with a rapid and unfavorable course. Polymorphisms G1 and G2 in the APOL-1 gene are highly associated with FSGS and HIVAN. These risk polymorphisms are found with increased frequencies in African populations.

HIVICK occurs as the result of deposition of circulating immune complexes in the glomeruli or their formation in situ. Immune complexes contain viral core and envelope antigens. In addition, HIV patients may have other immune complex mediated diseases (IgA nephropathy, membranous GN or membranoproliferative GN, very often associated with hepatitis A, B and C coinfection). Lupus-like GN may be also found by IF and EM studies in the absence of clinical and serological features of systemic lupus erythematosus.

In Black and Hispanic populations, FSGS with or without collapsing glomeruli and microcystic tubular dilatation are common while mesangial hyperplasia and immune complex-type disease predominates in whites. Other glomerular pathologies may be also detected in HIV infected children and adults such as postinfectious GN, minimal change disease, diabetic nephropathy, amyloidoses, and thrombotic microangiopathies.

Persistent proteinuria ($\geq$1+ on dipstick; urinary protein/creatinine ratio > 2.0 mg/mg) and microhematuria point to HIVAN [132, 135–137]. Additional suggestive features are finding of microcysts (shed epithelial cells) in the urinary sediment, highly echogenic kidneys, Black race, and nephrotic range proteinuria with or without edema or hypertension. These criteria are suggestive but not confirmatory; definitive diagnosis of HIVAN should be established by a kidney biopsy [132].

Children with perinatal HIV infection can shave tubulointerstitial nephritis, and may present with non-specific manifestations of acute kidney injury. It may be secondary to medication exposure, including non-steroidal antiinflammatory drugs, trimethoprim-sulfamethoxazole, indinavir, and ritonavir. Various electrolyte and acid-base disturbances may be found in children with perinatal HIV infections because of malnutrition, gastroenteritis, pneumonia, intracranial infections, and syndrome of inappropriate antidiuretic hormone. Antiretroviral agents such as tenofovir can cause proximal tubular dysfunction, nephrogenic diabetes insipidus, and acute kidney injury.

Children with HIVAN should be treated with HAART. If already receiving HAART, it may suggest inadequate disease control, which is supported by low CD4 counts and a high viral load. Resistance testing enables selection of the optimal HAART regimen. Since many antiretroviral drugs are excreted via the kidneys, modification of dosages based on GFR is necessary. Nephrotoxic drugs should be avoided or carefully monitored.

Although there are no controlled, randomized trials, ACEIs and angiotensin receptor blockers have been used with HAART therapy in many centers in order to decrease proteinuria. Steroids and immunosuppressive agents are not recommended for treatment of children with HIVAN [132].

Both dialysis modalities are used in HIV infected children with ESKD. Those on peritoneal dialysis have increased risk of recurrent peritonitis and worsening of malnutrition, while those on hemodialysis with central venous lines have high risk of tunnel infections and thrombosis. In the pre-HAART era, there were major concerns about transplantation in otherwise immunocompromised patients. With better control of the disease with HAART, improved prophylaxis and treatment of opportunistic infections, transplantation, as in other causes of pediatric CKD, is now the optimal treatment modality for these children. However, this requires stability on HAART with undetectable viral load for 6 months and an adequate CD4 count, and an understanding of the need for adherence to a combination of life-long HAART and immunosuppression [138].

A shortage of donor kidneys has led to adult HIV-positive kidney donors being utilized in adult HIV kidney positive transplants recipients with good success [139]. In pediatrics, this has not been described in kidney transplantation, although a successful case of living donor liver transplantation from an HIV-positive mother to her HIV-negative child has been performed as a lifesaving measure [140, 141].

Conclusion

Infectious and post-infectious GN have been important causes of pediatric kidney disease. However, there has been a decrease in these etiologies of GN due to the introduction of successful vaccines (hepatitis A and B, meningococcus, varicella and COVID-19); public health initiatives (efforts to decrease transmission of malaria and scabies); and maternal screening (HIV and syphilis).

The management of post-infectious GN focuses on addressing the clinical consequences of the GN. In contrast, eradicating the underlying infection is critical for infectious GN, although management of the GN is also important.

References

1. Nadasdy T, Hebert LA. Infection-related glomerulonephritis: understanding mechanisms. Semin Nephrol. 2011;31:369–75.
2. Sulyok E. Acute proliferative glomerulonephritis. In: Avner ED, Harmon WE, Niaudet P, editors. Pediatric nephrology. 5th ed. Philadelphia: Lippincott Williams and Wilkins; 2004. p. 601–13.
3. Forrest JW, John F, Mills LR, et al. Immune complex glomerulonephritis associated with Klebsiella pneumonia infection. Clin Nephrol. 1977;7:76–80.
4. Rainford DJ, Woodrow DF, Sloper JC, et al. Post meningococcal acute glomerulo-nephritis. Clin Nephrol. 1978;9:249–53.
5. Doregatti C, Volpi A, Torri Tarelli L, et al. Acute glomerulonephritis in human brucellosis. Nephron. 1983;41:365–6.
6. Sadikoglu B, Bilge I, Kilicaslan I, Gokce MG, Emre S, Ertugrul T. Crescentic glomerulonephritis in a child with infective endocarditis. Pediatr Nephrol. 2006;21:867–9.

7. Ferrario F, Kourilsky O, Morel-Maroger L. Acute endocapillary glomerulonephritis: a histologic and clinical comparison between patients with and without acute renal failure. Clin Nephrol. 1983;19:17–23.
8. Nasr SH, Radhakrishnan J, D'Agati VD. Bacterial infection-related glomerulonephritis in adults. Kidney Int. 2013;83:792–803.
9. Nast CC. Infection-related glomerulonephritis: changing demographics and outcomes. Adv Chronic Kidney Dis. 2012;19:68–75.
10. Kambham N. Postinfectious glomerulonephritis. Adv Anat Pathol. 2012;19:338–47.
11. Kimata T, Tsuji S, Yoshimura K, Tsukaguchi H, Kaneko K. Methicillin-resistant Staphylococcus aureus-related glomerulonephritis in a child. Pediatr Nephrol. 2012;27:2149–52.
12. Moroni G, Pozzi C, Quaglini S, et al. Long-term prognosis of diffuse proliferative glomerulonephritis associated with infection in adults. Nephrol Dial Transplant. 2002;17:1204–11.
13. Rodriguez-Iturbe B. Acute poststreptococcal glomerulonephritis. In: Schrier RW, Gottschalk CW, editors. Disease of the kidney. Boston: Little Brown; 1988. p. 1929–47.
14. Meadow SR. Poststreptococcal glomerulonephtis-A rare disease? Arch Dis Child. 1975;50:379–82.
15. Yap H, Chia K, Murugasu B, et al. Acute glomerulonephritis-changing patterns in Singapore children. Pediatr Nephrol. 1990;4:482–4.
16. Eison TM, Ault BH, Jones DP, Chesney RW, Wyatt RJ. Post-streptococcal acute glomerulonephritis in children: clinical features and pathogenesis. Pediatr Nephrol. 2011;26:165–80.
17. Knuffash FA, Sharda DC, Majeed HA. Sporadic pharyngitis-associated acute poststreptococcal glomerulonephritis. Clin Pediatr. 1986;25:181–4.
18. Sarkissian A, Papazian M, Azatian G, Arikiants N, Babloyan A, Leumann E. An epidemic of acute postinfectious glomerulonephritis in Armenia. Arch Dis Child. 1997;77:342–4.
19. Majeed HA, Khuffash FA, Sharda DC, Farwana SS, El-Sherbiny AF, Ghafour SY. Children with acute rheumatic fever and acute poststreptococcal glomerulonephritis and their families in a subtropical zone: a three-year prospective comparative epidemiological study. Int J Epidemiol. 1987;16:561–8.
20. Streeton CL, Hanna JN, Messer RD, Merianos A. An epidemic of acute post-streptococcal glomerulonephritis among aboriginal children. J Paediatr Child Health. 1995;31:245–8.
21. Leung DTY, Tseng RYM, Go SH, et al. Post-streptococcal glomerulonephritis in Hong Kong. Arch Dis Child. 1987;62:1075–6.
22. Margolis HS, Lum MKW, Bender TR, et al. Acute glomerulonephritis and streptococcal skin lesions in Eskimo children. Am J Dis Child. 1980;134:681–5.
23. Svartman M, Potter EV, Poon-King T, Earle DP. Streptococcal infection of scabetic lesions related to acute glomerulonephritis in Trinidad. J Lab Clin Med. 1973;81:182–93.

24. Li Volti S, Furnari ML, Garozzo R, et al. Acute poststreptococcal glomerulonephritis in an 8-month old girl. Pediatr Nephrol. 1993;7:737–9.
25. Kari JA, Bamagai A, Jalalah SM. Severe acute poststreptococcal glomerulonephritis in an infant. Saudi J Kidney Dis Transpl. 2013;24:546–8.
26. Anthony BF, Kaplan EL, Wannamaker LW, et al. Attack rates of acute nephritis after type 49 streptococcal infection of the skin and of the respiratory tract. J Clin Invest. 1969;48:1697–702.
27. Ahmed-Jushuf IH, Selby PL, Brownjohn AM. Acute post-streptococcal glomerulonephritis following ear piercing. Postgrad Med J. 1984;60(699):73–4.
28. Tasic V, Polenakovic M. Acute poststreptococcal glomerulonephritis following circumcision. Pediatr Nephrol. 2000;15:274–5.
29. Sorof JM, Weidner N, Potter D, Portale AA. Acute poststreptococcal glomerulonephritis in a renal allograft. Pediatr Nephrol. 1995;9:317–20.
30. Martin J, Kaul A, Schacht R. Acute poststreptococcal glomerulonephritis: a manifestation of immune reconstitution inflammatory syndrome. Pediatrics. 2012;130:e710–3.
31. Gnann JW, Gray BM, Griffin FM, Dismukes WE. Acute glomerulonephritis following group G streptococcal infection. J Infect Dis. 1987;156:411–2.
32. Barnham M, Thornton T, Lange K. Nephritis caused by streptococcus zooepidemicus (Lancefield group C). Lancet. 1983;I:945–8.
33. Francis AJ, Nimmo GR, Efstratiou A, Galanis V, Nuttall N. Investigation of milk-borne Streptococcus zooepidemicus infection associated with glomerulonephritis in Australia. J Infect. 1993;27:317–23.
34. Beres SB, Sesso R, Pinto SW, Hoe NP, Porcella SF, Deleo FR, Musser JM. Genome sequence of a Lancefield group C Streptococcus zooepidemicus strain causing epidemic nephritis: new information about an old disease. PLoS One. 2008;3:e3026.
35. Yoshizawa N. Acute glomerulonephritis. Intern Med. 2000;39:687–94.
36. Rodriguez Iturbe B. Nephritis-associated streptococcal antigens: where are we now? J Am Soc Nephrol. 2004;15:1961–2.
37. Cronin W, Deol H, Azadegan A, Lange K. Endostreptosin: isolation of the probable immunogen of acute poststreptococcal glomerulonephritis (PSGN). Clin Exp Immunol. 1989;76:198–203.
38. Cronin WJ, Lange K. Immunologic evidence for the in situ deposition of a cytoplasmatic streptococcal antigen (endostreptosin) on the glomerular basement memebrane in rats. Clin Nephrol. 1990;31:143–6.
39. Lange K, Selingson G, Cronin W. Evidence for the in situ origin of poststreptococcal glomerulonephritis: glomerular localization of endostreptosin and the clinical significance of the subsequent antibody responce. Clin Nephrol. 1983;19:3–10.
40. Lange K, Ahmed U, Kleinberger H, Treser G. A hitherto unknown streptococcal antigen and its probable relation to acute poststreptococcal glomerulonephritis. Clin Nephrol. 1976;5:207–15.

41. Rodriguez-Iturbe B, Rabideau D, Garcia R, et al. Characterization of the glomerular antibody in acute poststreptococcal glomerulonephritis. Ann Intern Med. 1980;92:478–81.
42. Vogt A, Batsford S, Rodriguez-Iturbe B, Garcia R. Cationic antigens in poststreptococcal glomerulonephritis. Clin Nephrol. 1983;20:271–9.
43. Parra G, Rodriguez-Iturbe B, Batsford S, Vogt A, Mezzano S, Olavarria F, Exeni R, Laso M, Orta N. Antibody to streptococcal zymogen in the serum of patients with acute glomerulonephritis: a multicentric study. Kidney Int. 1998;54:509–17.
44. Yoshizawa N, Yamakami K, Fujino M, Oda T, Tamura K, Matsumoto K, Sugisaki T, Boule MDP. Nephritis-associated plasmin receptor and acute glomerulonephritis: characterization of the antigen and associated immune response. J Am Soc Nephrol. 2004;15:1785–93.
45. Batsford SR, Mezzano S, Mihatsch M, Schiltz E, Rodriguez IB. Is the nephritogenic antigen in post-streptococcal glomerulonephritis pyrogenic exotoxin B (SPE B) or GAPDH? Kidney Int. 2005;68:1120–9.
46. Odaka J, Kanai T, Ito T, Saito T, Aoyagi J, Betsui H, Oda T, Ueda Y, Yamagata T. A case of postpneumococcal acute glomerulonephritis with glomerular depositions of nephritis-associated plasmin receptor. CEN Case Rep. 2015;4:112–6.
47. Uchida T, Oda T. Glomerular deposition of nephritis-associated plasmin receptor (NAPlr) and related plasmin activity: key diagnostic biomarkers of bacterial infection-related glomerulonephritis. Int J Mol Sci. 2020;21(7):2595.
48. Hirano D, Oda T, Ito A, Yamada A, Kakegawa D, Miwa S, Umeda C, Takemasa Y, Tokunaga A, Wajima T, Nakaminami H, Noguchi N, Ida H. Glyceraldehyde-3-phosphate dehydrogenase of Mycoplasma pneumoniae induces infection-related glomerulonephritis. Clin Nephrol. 2019;92(5):263–72.
49. Komaru Y, Ishioka K, Oda T, Ohtake T, Kobayashi S. Nephritis-associated plasmin receptor (NAPlr) positive glomerulonephritis caused by Aggregatibacter actinomycetemcomitans bacteremia: a case report. Clin Nephrol. 2018;90(2):155–60.
50. Oda T, Yoshizawa N, Yamakami K, Tamura K, Kuroki A, Sugisaki T, Sawanobori E, Higashida K, Ohtomo Y, Hotta O, Kumagai H, Miura S. Localization of nephritis-associated plasmin receptor in acute poststreptococcal glomerulonephritis. Hum Pathol. 2010;41:1276–85.
51. Oda T, Yoshizawa N, Yamakami K, Sakurai Y, Takechi H, Yamamoto K, Oshima N, Kumagai H. The role of nephritis-associated plasmin receptor (NAPlr) in glomerulonephritis associated with streptococcal infection. J Biomed Biotechnol. 2012;2012:417675.
52. Soto HM, Parra G, Rodriguez-Itrube B. Circulating levels of cytokines in poststreptococcal glomerulonephritis. Clin Nephrol. 1997;47:6–12.
53. Matsell DG, Wayatt RJ, Gaber LW. Terminal complement complexes in acute poststreptococcal glomerulonephritis. Pediatr Nephrol. 1994;8:671–7.
54. Garin E, Fenell R, Shulman S, et al. Clinical significance of the presence of cryoglobulins in patients with glomerulonephritis not associated with systemic disease. Clin Nephrol. 1980;13:5–11.
55. Mezzano S, Olavarria F, Ardiles L, Lopez MI. Incidence of circulating immune complexes in patients with acute poststreptococcal glomerulonephritis and in patients with streptococcal impetigo. Clin Nephrol. 1986;26:61–5.
56. Sesso RC, Ramos OL, Pereira AB. Detection of IgG-rheumatoid factor in sera of patients with acute poststreptococcal glomerulonephritis and its relationship with circulating immunocomplexes. Clin Nephrol. 1986;25:55–60.
57. Villches AR, Williams DG. Persistent anti-DNA antibodies and DNA-anti-DNA complexes in poststreptococcal glomerulonephritis. Clin Nephrol. 1984;22:97–101.
58. Ardiles LG, Valderrama G, Moya P, Mezzano SA. Incidence and studies on antigenic specificities of antineutrophil-cytoplasmic autoantibodies (ANCA) in poststreptococcal glomerulonephritis. Clin Nephrol. 1997;47:1–5.
59. Sorger K, Gessler U, Hubner FK, et al. Subtypes of acute postinfectious glomerulo-nephritis. Synopsis of clinical and pathological features. Clin Nephrol. 1982;17:114–28.
60. Sorger K, Balun J, Hubner FK, et al. The garland type of acute postinfectious glomerulonephritis: morphological characteristics and follow-up studies. Clin Nephrol. 1983;20:17–26.
61. Kokuzawa A, Morishita Y, Yoshizawa H, Iwazu K, Komada T, Akimoto T, Saito O, Oda T, Takemoto F, Ando Y, Muto S, Yumura W, Kusano E. Acute poststreptococcal glomerulonephritis with acute kidney injury in nephrotic syndrome with the glomerular deposition of nephritis-associated plasmin receptor antigen. Intern Med. 2013;52:2087–91.
62. Tornroth T. The fate of subepithelial deposits in acute poststreptococcal glomerulonephritis. Lab Investig. 1976;35:461–74.
63. Cohen JA, Levitt MF. Acute glomerulonephritis with few urinary abnormalities. Report of two cases proved by renal biopsy. New Engl. J Med. 1963;268:749–53.
64. Robson WL, Leung AK. Post-streptococcal glomerulonephritis with minimal abnormalities in the urinary sediment. J Singapore Paediatr Soc. 1992;34:232–4.
65. Ozdemir S, Saatçi U, Beşbaş N, Bakkaloglu A, Ozen S, Koray Z. Plasma atrial natriuretic peptide and endothelin levels in acute poststreptococcal glomerulonephritis. Pediatr Nephrol. 1992;6:519–22.
66. Fux CA, Bianchetti MG, Jakob SM, Remonda L. Reversible encephalopathy complicating poststreptococcal glomerulonephritis. Pediatr Infect Dis J. 2006;25:85–7.

67. Endo A, Fuchigami T, Hasegawa M, Hashimoto K, Fujita Y, Inamo Y, Mugishima H. Posterior reversible encephalopathy syndrome in childhood: report of four cases and review of the literature. Pediatr Emerg Care. 2012;28:153–7.

68. Kaplan RA, Zwick DL, Hellerstein S, et al. Cerebral vasculitis in acute poststreptococcal glomerulonephritis. Pediatr Nephrol. 1993;7:194–6.

69. Rovang RD, Zawada ET Jr, Santella RN, Jaqua RA, Boice JL, Welter RL. Cerebral vasculitis associated with acute post-streptococcal glomerulonephritis. Am J Nephrol. 1997;17:89–92.

70. Sharrett AR, Poon-King T, Potter EV, et al. Subclinical nephritis in South Trinidad. Am J Epidemiol. 1971;91:231–45.

71. Sagel I, Treser G, Ty A, et al. Occurrence and nature of glomerular lesions after group A streptococci infections in children. Ann Intern Med. 1973;79:492–9.

72. Rodriguez-Iturbe B, Rubio L, Garcia R. Attack rate of poststreptococcal glomerulonephritis in families. A prospective study. Lancet. 1981;I:401–5.

73. Tasic V, Polenakovic M. Occurrence of subclinical post-streptococcal glomerulonephritis in family contacts. J Paediatr Child Health. 2003;39:177–9.

74. Yoshizawa N, Suzuki Y, Oshima S, et al. Asymptomatic acute poststreptococcal glomerulonephritis following upper respiratory tract infections caused by Group A streptococci. Clin Nephrol. 1996;46:296–301.

75. Lange K, Azadegan AA, Seligson G, Bovie RC, Majeed H: Asymptomatic poststreptococcal glomerulonephritis in relatives of patients with symptomatic glomerulonephritis. Diagnostic value of endostreptosin antibodies. Child Nephrol Urol 1988–89;9:11–15.

76. Goodyer PR, de Chadarevian JP, Kaplan BS. Acute poststreptococcal glomerulonephritis mimicking Henoch-Schonlein purpura. J Pediatr. 1978;93:412–5.

77. Said R, Hussein M, Hassan A. Simultaneous occurrence of acute poststreptococcal glomerulonephritis and acute rheumatic fever. Am J Nephrol. 1986;6:146–8.

78. Matsell DG, Baldree LA, DiSessa TG, et al. Acute poststreptococcal glomerulonephritis and acute rheumatic fever: occurrence in the same patient. Child Nephrol Urol. 1990;10:112–4.

79. Hiki Y, Tamura K, Shigematsu H, Kobayashi Y. Superimposition of poststreptococcal acute glomerulonephritis on the course of IgA nephropathy. Nephron. 1991;57:358–64.

80. Chadaverian JP, Goodyer PR, Kaplan BS, et al. Acute glomerulonephritis and hemolytic uremic syndrome. CMA J. 1980;123:391–4.

81. Sheridan RJ, Roy S, Stapleton BF. Reflux nephropathy complicated by acute post-streptococcal glomerulonephritis. Int J Pediatr Nephrol. 1983;4:119–21.

82. Naito Yoshida Y, Hida M, Maruyama Y, Hori N, Awazu M. Poststreptococcal acute glomerulonephritis superimposed on bilateral renal hypoplasia. Clin Nephrol. 2005;63:477–80.

83. Kaplan BS, Esseltine D. Thrombocytopenia in patients with acute poststreptococcal glomerulonephritis. J Pediatr. 1978;93:974–6.

84. Tasic V, Polenakovic M. Thrombocytopenia during the course of acute poststreptococcal glomerulonephritis. Turk J Pediatr. 2003;45:148–51.

85. Guerrero AP, Musgrave JE, Lee EK. Immune globulin-responsive thrombocytopenia in acute poststreptococcal glomerulonephritis: report of a case in Hawai'i. Hawaii Med J. 2009;68:56–8.

86. Wayatt RJ, Forristal J, West CD, et al. Complement profiles in acute poststreptococcal glomerulonephritis. Pediatr Nephrol. 1988;2:219–23.

87. Chauvet S, Berthaud R, Devriese M, Mignotet M, Vieira Martins P, Robe-Rybkine T, Miteva MA, Gyulkhandanyan A, Ryckewaert A, Louillet F, Merieau E, Mestrallet G, Rousset-Rouvière C, Thervet E, Hogan J, Ulinski T, Villoutreix BO, Roumenina L, Boyer O, Frémeaux-Bacchi V. Anti-factor B antibodies and acute postinfectious GN in children. J Am Soc Nephrol. 2020;31(4):829–40.

88. Kozyro I, Perahud I, Sadallah S, Sukalo A, Titov L, Schifferli J, Trendelenburg M. Clinical value of autoantibodies against C1q in children with glomerulonephritis. Pediatrics. 2006;117:1663–8.

89. Vernon KA, Goicoechea de Jorge E, Hall AE, Fremeaux-Bacchi V, Aitman TJ, Cook HT, Hangartner R, Koziell A, Pickering MC. Acute presentation and persistent glomerulonephritis following streptococcal infection in a patient with heterozygous complement factor H-related protein 5 deficiency. Am J Kidney Dis. 2012;60:121–5.

90. Sethi S, Fervenza FC, Zhang Y, Zand L, Meyer NC, Borsa N, Nasr SH, Smith RJ. Atypical postinfectious glomerulonephritis is associated with abnormalities in the alternative pathway of complement. Kidney Int. 2013;83:293–9.

91. Parra G, Rodriguez-Iturbe B, Colina-Chourio J, Garcia R. Short term treatment with captopril in hypertension due to acute glomerulonephritis. Clin Nephrol. 1988;29:58–62.

92. Yiu V, Orrbine E, Rosychuk RJ, et al. The safety and use of short-acting nifedipine in hospitalized hypertensive children. Pediatr Nephrol. 2004;19:644–50.

93. Roy S, Murphy WM, Arant BS. Poststreptococcal crescentic glomerulonephritis in children: comparison of quintiple therapy versus supportive care. J Pediatr. 1981;98:403–10.

94. Roy S, Wall HP, Etteldorf JN. Second attacks of acute glomerulonephritis. J Pediatr. 1969;75:758–67.

95. Baldwin DS. Poststreptococcal glomerulonephritis. A progressive disease. Am J Med. 1977;62:1–11.

96. Baldwin DS, Gluck MC, Schacht RG, Gallo G. The long-term course of poststreptococcal glomerulonephritis. Ann Intern Med. 1974;80:342–58.

97. Potter E, Lipschultz SA, Abidh S, et al. Twelve to seventeen-year follow-up of patients with poststrep-

tococcal acute glomerulonephritis in Trinidad. N Engl J Med. 1982;307:725–30.

98. Cameron JS. The long-term outcome of glomerular disease. In: Schrier RW, Gottschalk CW, editors. Diseases of the kidney. Boston: Little Brown; 1988. p. 2127–89.

99. Vogl W, Renke M, Mayer-Eichberger D, et al. Long term prognosis for endocapillary glomerulonephritis of poststreptococcal type in children and adults. Nephron. 1986;44:58–65.

100. Clark G, White R, Glasgow EF, et al. Poststreptococcal glomerulonephritis in children: clinicopathological correlations and long term prognosis. Pediatr Nephrol. 1988;2:381–8.

101. Schacht RG, Gluck MC, Gallo GR, et al. Progression to uremia after remission of acute poststreptococcal glomerulonephritis. N Engl J Med. 1976;295:977–81.

102. Gallo GR, Feiner HD, Steele JM, et al. Role of intrarenal vacular sclerosis in progression of poststreptococcal glomerulonephritis. Clin Nephrol. 1980;13:49–57.

103. Rodriguez-Iturbe B, Herrera J, Garcia R. Response to acute protein load in kidney donors and in apparently normal postacute glomerulonephritis patients: evidence for glomerular hyperfiltration. Lancet. 1985;II:461–4.

104. Cleper R, Davidovitz M, Halevi R, Eisenstein B. Renal functional reserve after acute poststreptococcal glomerulonephritis. Pediatr Nephrol. 1997;11:473–6.

105. Rodriguez-Iturbe B, Garcia R, Rubio L, et al. Epidemic glomerulonephritis in Maracaibo. Evidence for progression to chronicity. Clin Nephrol. 1976;5:197–206.

106. Garcia R, Rubio L, Rodriguez-Iturbe B. Long term prognosis of epidemic poststreptococcal glomerulonephritis in Maracaibo: follow-up studies 11-12 years after the acute episode. Clin Nephrol. 1981;15:291–8.

107. Herrera J, Rodríguez-Iturbe B. End-stage renal disease and acute glomerulonephritis in Goajiro Indians. Kidney Int Suppl. 2003;83:S22–6.

108. Dodge WF, Spargo BH, Travis LB, et al. Poststreptococcal glomerulonephritis. A prospective study in children. New Engl J Med. 1971;286:273–8.

109. Travis LB, Dodge WF, Beathard GA, et al. Acute glomerulonephritis in children. A review of the natural history with emphasis on prognosis. Clin Nephrol. 1973;1:169–81.

110. Tasic V, Korneti P, Gucev Z, Korneti B. Stress tolerance test and SDS-PAGE for the analysis of urinary proteins in children and youths. Clin Chem Lab Med. 2001;39:478–3.

111. Perlman LV, Herdman RC, Kleinman H, Vernier RL. Poststreptococcal glomerulo-nephritis. A ten year follow up of an epidemics. JAMA. 1965;194:63–70.

112. Potter EV, Abidh S, Sharrett AR, et al. Clinical healing two to six years after poststreptococcal

glomerulonephritis in Trinidad. New Engl J Med. 1978;298:767–72.

113. Nissenson AR, Mayon-White R, Potter EV, et al. Continued abscence of clinical renal disease seven to twelve years after poststreptococcal acute glomerulonephritis in Trinidad. Am J Med. 1979;67:255–62.

114. Popovic-Rolovic M, Kostic M, Antic-Peco A, et al. Medium- and long-term prognosis of patients with acute postreptococcal glomerulonephritis. Nephron. 1991;58:393–9.

115. Tasic V, Polenakovic M, Kuzmanovska D, Sahpazova E, Ristoska N. Prognosis of poststreptococcal glomerulonephritis five to fifteen years after an acute episode. Pediatr Nephrol. 1998;12:C167.

116. Kasahara T, Hayakawa H, Okubo S, et al. Prognosis of acute poststreptococcal glomerulonephritis (APSGN) is excellent in children, when adequately diagnosed. Pediatr Int. 2001;43:364–7.

117. Drukker A, Pomeranz A, Reichenberg J, Mor J, Stankiewicz H. Natriuretic response to i.v. saline loading after acute poststreptococcal glomerulonephritis. Isr J Med Sci. 1986;22:779–82.

118. Marshall CS, Cheng AC, Markey PG, Towers RJ, Richardson LJ, Fagan PK, Scott L, Krause VL, Currie BJ. Acute post-streptococcal glomerulonephritis in the Northern Territory of Australia: a review of 16 years data and comparison with the literature. Am J Trop Med Hyg. 2011;85:703–10.

119. Wong W, Lennon DR, Crone S, Neutze JM, Reed PW. Prospective population-based study on the burden of disease from post-streptococcal glomerulonephritis of hospitalised children in New Zealand: epidemiology, clinical features and complications. J Paediatr Child Health. 2013;49:850–5.

120. Hoy WE, Kincaid-Smith P, Hughson MD, Fogo AB, Sinniah R, Dowling J, Samuel T, Mott SA, Douglas-Denton RN, Bertram JF. CKD in Aboriginal Australians. Am J Kidney Dis. 2010;56:983–93.

121. Hoy WE, White AV, Dowling A, Sharma SK, Bloomfield H, Tipiloura BT, Swanson CE, Mathews JD, McCredie DA. Post-streptococcal glomerulonephritis is a strong risk factor for chronic kidney disease in later life. Kidney Int. 2012;81:1026–32.

122. Tasic V, Polenakovic M, Cakalarovski K, Kuzmanovska D. Progression of crescentic poststreptococcal glomerulonephritis to terminal uremia twelve years after recovery from an acute episode (letter). Nephron. 1988;79:496.

123. Sesso R, Wyton S, Pinto L. Epidemic glomerulonephritis due to Streptococcus zooepidemicus in Nova Serrana, Brazil. Kidney Int Suppl. 2005;97:S132–6.

124. Black JA, Challacombe DN, Ockenden BG. Nephrotic syndrome associated with bacteraemia after shunt operations for hydrocephalus. Lancet. 1965;2(7419):921–4.

125. Haffner D, Schindera F, Aschoff A, Matthias S, Waldherr R, Schärer K. The clinical spectrum of shunt nephritis. Nephrol Dial Transplant. 1997;12:1143–8.

126. Kiryluk K, Preddie D, D'Agati VD, Isom R. A young man with Propionibacterium acnes-induced shunt nephritis. Kidney Int. 2008;73:1434–40.

127. Mantan M, Sethi GR, Batra VV. Post-infectious glomerulonephritis following infective endocarditis: amenable to immunosuppression. Indian J Nephrol. 2013;23:368–70.

128. Hurst SA, Appelgren KE, Kourtis AP. Prevention of mother-to-child transmission of HIV type 1: the role of neonatal and infant prophylaxis. Expert Rev Anti-Infect Ther. 2015;13(2):169–81. https://doi.org/10.1586/14787210.2015.999667.

129. Bailey H, Zash R, Rasi V, Thorne C. HIV treatment in pregnancy. Lancet HIV. 2018;5(8):e457–67. https://doi.org/10.1016/S2352-3018(18)30059-6. Epub 2018 Jun 26.

130. Davidson B, Okpechi I, McCulloch M, Wearne N. Adolescent nephrology: an emerging frontier for kidney care in sub-Saharan Africa. Nephrology (Carlton). 2017;22(12):933–9. https://doi.org/10.1111/nep.13135.

131. UNAIDS. HIV Prevention amongst Adolescent Girls and Young Women. 2016. http://www.unaids.org/sites/default/files/media_asset/UNAIDS_HIV_prevention_among_adolescent_girls_and_young_women.pdf.

132. Bhimma R, Purswani MU, Kala U. Kidney disease in children and adolescents with perinatal HIV-1 infection. J Int AIDS Soc. 2013;16:18596.

133. Ramsuran D, Bhimma R, Ramdial PK, Naicker E, Adhikari M, Deonarain J, Sing Y, Naicker T. The spectrum of HIV-related nephropathy in children. Pediatr Nephrol. 2012;27:821–7.

134. Purswani MU, Chernoff MC, Mitchell CD, Seage GR 3rd, Zilleruelo G, Abitbol C, Andiman WA, Kaiser KA, Spiegel H, Oleske JM; IMPAACT 219/219C Study Team. Chronic kidney disease associated with perinatal HIV infection in children and adolescents. Pediatr Nephrol 2012; 27: 981–989.

135. Iduoriyekemwen NJ, Sadoh WE, Sadoh AE. Prevalence of renal disease in Nigerian children infected with the human immunodeficiency virus and on highly active anti-retroviral therapy. Saudi J Kidney Dis Transpl. 2013;24:172–7.

136. Giacomet V, Erba P, Di Nello F, Coletto S, Viganò A, Zuccotti G. Proteinuria in paediatric patients with human immunodeficiency virus infection. World J Clin Cases. 2013;1:13–8.

137. Shah I, Gupta S, Shah DM, Dhabe H, Lala M. Renal manifestations of HIV infected highly active anti-retroviral therapy naive children in India. World J Pediatr. 2012;8:252–5.

138. Boyle SM, Fehr K, Deering C, Raza A, Harhay MN, Malat G, Ranganna K, Lee DH. Barriers to kidney transplant evaluation in HIV-positive patients with advanced kidney disease: a single-center study. Transpl Infect Dis. 2020;22(2):e13253. https://doi.org/10.1111/tid.13253. Epub 2020 Feb 12.

139. Muller E, Barday Z. HIV-Positive Kidney Donor Selection for HIV-Positive Transplant Recipients. J Am Soc Nephrol. 2018;29(4):1090–5. https://doi.org/10.1681/ASN.2017080853. Epub 2018 Jan 12

140. Botha J, Conradie F, Etheredge H, Fabian J, Duncan M, Haeri Mazanderani A, Paximadis M, Maher H, Britz R, Loveland J, Ströbele B, Rambarran S, Mahomed A, Terblanche A, Beretta M, Brannigan L, Pienaar M, Archibald-Durham L, Lang A, Tiemessen CT. Living donor liver transplant from an HIV-positive mother to her HIV-negative child: opening up new therapeutic options. AIDS. 2018;32(16):F13–9. https://doi.org/10.1097/QAD.0000000000002000.

141. Etheredge HR, Fabian J, Duncan M, Conradie F, Tiemessen C, Botha J. Needs must: living donor liver transplantation from an HIV-positive mother to her HIV-negative child in Johannesburg. South Africa J Med Ethics. 2019;45(5):287–90. https://doi.org/10.1136/medethics-2018-105216.

Rapidly Progressive Glomerulonephritis

20

Shina Menon and Arvind Bagga

Rapidly progressive glomerulonephritis (RPGN) is a rare syndrome in children, characterized by clinical features of glomerulonephritis (GN) and rapid loss of renal function. Histology shows crescentic extracapillary proliferation in Bowman space affecting the majority of glomeruli. This may be seen in any form of GN, including post-streptococcal GN, renal vasculitis, IgA nephropathy, systemic lupus erythematosus (SLE) and membranoproliferative GN. RPGN is a medical emergency, which if untreated rapidly progresses to irreversible loss of renal function. Prompt evaluation and specific therapy is necessary to ensure satisfactory outcome in most cases.

Definition

RPGN is a clinical syndrome characterized by an acute nephritic illness accompanied by rapid loss of renal function over days to weeks [1]. The histological correlate is the presence of crescents (crescentic GN), usually involving greater than 50% of glomeruli. The presence of crescents is a histologic marker of severe glomerular injury, which may occur in a number of conditions, including postinfectious GN, IgA nephropathy, SLE, renal vasculitis and membranoproliferative GN [1, 2]. The severity of clinical features correlates with the proportion of glomeruli that show crescents. While patients with circumferential crescents involving more than 80% of glomeruli present with more severe acute kidney injury (AKI), those with non-circumferential crescents in less than 50% of glomeruli have a relatively milder course.

Although the terms RPGN and crescentic GN are used interchangeably, similar presentation, with rapidly evolving AKI, might occur in conditions without crescents, including hemolytic uremic syndrome, diffuse proliferative GN and acute interstitial nephritis. Table 20.1 lists common conditions that present with RPGN in childhood.

S. Menon (✉)
Department of Pediatrics, University of Washington, Seattle, WA, USA

Division of Nephrology, Seattle Children's Hospital, Seattle, WA, USA
e-mail: shina.menon@seattlechildrens.org

A. Bagga
Division of Nephrology, All India Institute of Medical Sciences, New Delhi, India

© The Author(s), under exclusive license to Springer Nature Switzerland AG 2023
F. Schaefer, L. A. Greenbaum (eds.), *Pediatric Kidney Disease*,
https://doi.org/10.1007/978-3-031-11665-0_20

Table 20.1 Causes of rapidly progressive glomerulonephritis (RPGN)

Immune complex GN
Post infectious GN. Poststreptococcal nephritis, infective endocarditis, shunt nephritis, *Staphylococcus aureus* sepsis, other infections: HIV, hepatitis B and C, syphilis
Systemic disease. Systemic lupus erythematosus, IgA vasculitis, cryoglobulinemia, mixed connective tissue disorder, juvenile rheumatoid arthritis
Primary GN. IgA nephropathy, MPGN, membranous nephropathy, C1q nephropathy
Pauci-immune crescentic GN
Microscopic polyangiitis, granulomatosis with polyangiitis (Wegener granulomatosis), renal limited vasculitis, eosinophilic granulomatosis with polyangiitis (Churg-Strauss disease)
Idiopathic crescentic GN
Medications: penicillamine, hydralazine, hydrocarbons, propylthiouracil
Anti-glomerular basement membrane GN
Anti-GBM nephritis, Goodpasture syndrome, post-renal transplantation in Alport syndrome
Post-renal transplantation
Recurrence of IgA nephropathy, IgA vasculitis, MPGN, systemic lupus erythematosus
RPGN without crescents
Diffuse proliferative GN

GN glomerulonephritis; *MPGN* membranoproliferative GN; *GBM* glomerular basement membrane; *HIV* human immunodeficiency virus

Pathophysiology

Crescent formation is usually secondary to a non-specific inflammatory response to severe injury to the glomerular capillary wall. While the underlying inciting reason may differ, the final pathway is often similar.

Underlying Triggers for Crescent Formation

In immune complex crescentic GN, the underlying trigger is deposition of immune complexes in the glomerular capillary tufts. These immune complexes may be formed in the circulation or within the glomerular capillary wall.

Pauci-immune crescentic GN is associated with anti-nuclear cytoplasmic antibody (ANCA),

directed against either myeloperoxidase (MPO), proteinase 3 (PR3), or both. While the mechanisms by which ANCA arise have not been clearly elucidated, there is increasing evidence that they activate neutrophils and set off an inflammatory cascade which subsequently causes endothelial and microvascular injury, and damage to the glomerular capillary wall. Activated neutrophils result in the extrusion from the cell of neutrophil extracellular traps (NETs) containing entrapped MPO, PR3, and complement components [3, 4]. Subsequently, neutrophils undergo a form of cell death, NETosis. NETs also mediate direct injury to endothelium, transfer MPO/PR3 to vascular endothelium for antigen presentation and activate the alternate complement pathway. Involvement of the alternate complement pathway, specifically anaphylatoxin C5a and C5a receptor (CD88), has been shown in studies from an anti-MPO model in complement-deficient mice [5]. It has been proposed that there may be an amplification loop wherein activated neutrophils release properdin, activate the alternate pathway and generate C5a, resulting in additional neutrophil priming and activation. There is also emerging evidence that ANCA-negative pauci-immune GN maybe secondary to activation of the alternate and terminal pathway of complement caused by a genetic or acquired defect in the alternative pathway [6].

Finally, in anti-glomerular basement membrane (GBM) GN, there are circulating IgG antibodies directed against the non-collagenous domain of the $\alpha3$ chain of type IV collagen that is present in the GBM and alveolar basement membrane.

Pathogenesis of Crescent Formation

Crescents are defined as the presence of two or more layers of cells in Bowman space. The chief components of crescents are coagulation proteins, macrophages, T cells, fibroblasts and parietal and visceral epithelial cells [1, 7]. There is evidence that podocytes also have a role in crescent formation [8]. Perturbations of humoral immunity as well as the T helper type 1 cellular immune response contribute to the pathogenesis [1, 2]. Various pathways involving T cells, including disturbances in regulatory T cell function and stimulation of toll-like receptor 4, have been described [9, 10].

Initiation of Crescent Formation

The initial event in formation of crescents is the occurrence of a physical gap in the glomerular capillary wall and the GBM, mediated by macrophages and T lymphocytes. Breaks in the integrity of the capillary wall lead to passage of inflammatory mediators and plasma proteins into Bowman space with fibrin formation, influx of macrophages and T cells, and release of inflammatory cytokines (*e.g.,* interleukin-1 (IL-1) and tumor necrosis factor-α). Similar breaks in Bowman capsule allow cells and mediators from the interstitium to enter Bowman space and for contents of the latter to enter the interstitium, resulting in inflammation. It is proposed that podocytes, which are terminally differentiated and stationary cells, change into a migratory phenotype and contribute to crescent formation [11].

Formation

The development of a crescent results from the participation of coagulation factors and different proliferating cells, chiefly macrophages, parietal epithelial cells and interstitial fibroblasts. The presence of coagulation factors in Bowman space results in formation of a fibrin clot and recruitment of circulating macrophages. Activated neutrophils and mononuclear cells release procoagulant tissue factor, IL-1 and tumor necrosis factor-α (TNF-α), serine proteinases (elastase, PR3) and matrix metalloproteinases. The proteases cause lysis of the GBM proteins and facilitate entry of other mediators in Bowman space. Release of IL-1 and TNF-α result in expression of adhesion molecules, leading to macrophage recruitment and proliferation. Apart from macrophages, major components of the crescents are proliferating parietal and visceral epithelial cells [12].

Resolution of Crescents

The stage of inflammation is followed by development of fibrocellular and fibrous crescents. The expression of fibroblast growth factors and transforming growth factor-β is important for fibroblast proliferation and production of type I collagen, responsible for transition from cellular to fibrocellular and fibrous crescents. Transition to fibrous crescents, which occurs over days, is important since the latter is not likely to resolve following immunosuppressive therapy. The plasminogen-plasmin system is responsible for fibrinolysis and resolution of crescents.

Causes and Immunopathologic Categories

Based on pathology and immunofluorescence (IF) staining patterns, crescentic GN is classified into three categories, which reflect different mechanisms of glomerular injury [1].

1. Immune-complex GN with granular deposits of immune complexes along capillary wall and mesangium
2. Pauci-immune GN with scant or no immune deposits, and associated with systemic vasculitis
3. Anti-GBM GN with linear deposition of anti-GBM antibodies

Immune Complex Crescentic GN

These patients form a heterogeneous group in which multiple stimuli lead to proliferative GN with crescents. Immunohistology shows granular deposits of immunoglobulin and complement along capillary walls and in the mesangium. The causes include infections, systemic diseases and primary GN.

Systemic infections Poststreptococcal GN can rarely present with crescentic histology. While most patients recover completely, the presence of nephrotic range proteinuria, sustained hypertension and crescents is associated with an unsatisfactory outcome [13, 14]. Other infectious illnesses associated with crescentic GN include infective endocarditis, infected atrioventricular shunts and visceral abscesses. Crescentic GN might be associated with infection with methicillin resistant *Staphylococcus aureus,* hepatitis B and C virus, leprosy and syphilis.

Systemic immune complex disease RPGN with glomerular crescents might be seen in patients with IgA vasculitis (formerly known as Henoch Schönlein purpura) and lupus nephritis (class IV more commonly than class III).

Primary GN Patients with IgA nephropathy, immune complex mediated membranoproliferative GN (MPGN), C3 glomerulopathy (C3 GN and dense deposit disease), and membranous nephropathy may occasionally present with rapid loss of renal function and crescentic GN [13–16].

Pauci-immune Crescentic GN

This form of GN is characterized by few or no immune deposits on IF microscopy [2, 17]. This includes renal-limited vasculitis, and the renal manifestations of microscopic polyangiitis (MPA), granulomatosis with polyangiitis (GPA; formerly Wegener granulomatosis), or eosinophilic granulomatosis with polyangiitis (formerly Churg-Strauss syndrome). Most (80%) show antineutrophil cytoplasmic autoantibodies (ANCA) in blood and are collectively classified as ANCA-associated vasculitides (AAV). Some cases of ANCA positive disease might be induced by drugs, including penicillamine, propylthiouracil, minocycline and hydralazine.

In addition, approximately 10–30% of patients with pauci-immune crescentic GN are ANCA negative [18]. These patients have fewer constitutional and extrarenal symptoms than those who are ANCA-positive. Studies show differences in outcome between these groups, suggesting a different pathophysiological basis.

Anti-GBM Crescentic GN

This condition is uncommon in childhood, accounting for less than 10% of RPGN cases in children [1, 14, 19–21]. The nephritogenic autoantibody is directed against a 28 kDa monomer located on the $\alpha3$ chain of type IV collagen (Goodpasture antigen). Pulmonary involvement (Goodpasture syndrome) is uncommon. Approximately 5% of patients with Alport syndrome who receive a renal allograft develop anti-GBM autoantibodies and anti-GBM nephritis within the first year of the transplant [22]. Unlike de novo anti-GBM nephritis, pulmonary hemorrhage is not observed in post-transplant anti-GBM nephritis because the patient's lung tissue does not contain the antigen. The risk of post transplantation anti-GBM nephritis is low in subjects with normal hearing, late progression to end-stage kidney disease (ESKD), or females with X-linked Alport syndrome.

Idiopathic RPGN

This group includes patients with immune complex crescentic GN who do not fit into any identifiable category, and those with ANCA-negative pauci-immune disease. While both conditions are uncommon, the proportion varies across different regions.

Epidemiology

The incidence of RPGN in children is not known. Crescentic GN comprises about 5% of unselected renal biopsies in children. While there are no population-based studies in children, a report from Romania suggested an annual incidence of 3.3 per million adult population [23]. The 2010 NAPRTCS Annual Transplant Report shows that idiopathic crescentic GN contributes to 1.7% of all transplanted patients [24]. This figure is an underestimate since other conditions in the database, including membranoproliferative GN (2.5%), SLE (1.5%), systemic immune disorders (0.3%), GPA (0.6%), chronic GN (3.2%) and IgA

Table 20.2 Causes of crescentic glomerulonephritis in children (%)

	Mayer et al. [14] (N = 60)	Sinha et al. [20] (N = 36)	Piyaphanee et al. [11] (N = 67)	Maliakkal et al. [19] (N = 305)	Alsaad et al. [21] (N = 37)
Immune complex disease					
Unspecified	6	–	–		13.5
Systemic lupus erythematosus	17	11.1	30	21	54.1
Poststreptococcal/Post infectious GN	12	8.3	51		16.2
IgA vasculitis (Henoch-Schönlein purpura), IgA nephropathy	43	11.1	6	42	
Membranoproliferative GN		5.5			
ANCA associated Vasculitis/Pauci immune GN	17	52.7	7.5	17	8.1
Idiopathic crescentic GN		11.1	1.5	6	
Anti-glomerular basement disease	2		1.5	3	
Others	3		3		8.1

GN glomerulonephritis

nephropathy and IgA vasculitis (2.4%), might present as RPGN.

Table 20.2 outlines the underlying conditions in five series of crescentic GN reported from India [25], United States [19], Thailand [21], Germany [20] and Saudi Arabia [26]. Immune complex GN is the most common pattern of crescentic GN in children, accounting for 75–80% cases in most reports. Pauci-immune crescentic GN, while common in adults, is less frequent in children, accounting for 15–20% cases. The decline in the incidence of postinfectious GN has resulted in a change in the profile of crescentic GN.

loskeletal system (joint pain, swelling) and nervous system (seizures, altered sensorium) are common in patients with pauci-immune RPGN, with or without ANCA positivity. Relapses of systemic and renal disease occur in one-third of patients with vasculitis [2, 17]. Patients with anti-GBM antibody disease may present with hemoptysis and, less often, pulmonary hemorrhage. Similar complications are found in GPA, SLE, IgA vasculitis and severe GN with pulmonary edema. The kidney disease is most severe with anti-GBM disease, followed by pauci-immune GN and finally immune complex crescentic GN [1, 24].

Clinical Features

The spectrum of presenting features in RPGN is variable, and includes macroscopic hematuria (60–90% patients), oliguria (60–100%), hypertension (60–80%) and edema (60–90%) [14, 17]. The illness is often complicated by occurrence of severe hypertension with end organ involvement, pulmonary edema and cardiac failure. Occasionally, RPGN may have an insidious onset with initial symptoms of fatigue or edema. Nephrotic syndrome is rare and seen in patients with less severe renal insufficiency. Systemic complaints, involving the upper respiratory tract (cough, sinusitis), skin (vasculitic rash), muscu-

Investigations

Hematuria, characterized by dysmorphic red cells and red cell casts, is seen in all patients; most also have gross hematuria. A variable degree of non-selective proteinuria (2+ to 4+) is present in more than 65% of patients. Urinalysis also shows leukocyte, granular and tubular epithelial cell casts. Severe AKI is often present at diagnosis. Anemia, if present is usually mild, though may be more severe in select cases due to pulmonary hemorrhage or autoimmune hemolytic anemia in SLE; peripheral smear shows normocytic normochromic red cells. Non-specific markers of inflammation, including CRP and ESR, are elevated.

Serology

Serological investigations assist in evaluation of the cause and monitoring disease activity (Table 20.3, Fig. 20.1). Low levels of total hemolytic complement (CH50) and complement component 3 (C3) are seen in postinfectious GN and SLE. Patients with lupus may additionally show reduced levels of C1q and C4 due to activation of the classic complement pathway. Complement-mediated MPGN is usually associated with low C3; however, other complement factors may be affected depending on the site of dysregulation in the alternate pathway. Positive antistreptolysin O titers and antideoxyribonuclease B suggests streptococcal

Table 20.3 Diagnostic evaluation of patients with rapidly progressive glomerulonephritis

Complete blood counts; peripheral smear for type of anemia; reticulocyte count; erythrocyte sedimentation rate, coagulation profile
Blood levels of urea, creatinine, electrolytes, calcium, phosphate, uric acid
Urinalysis: proteinuria; microscopy for erythrocytes and leukocytes, casts
Complement levels (C3, C4, CH50); additional evaluation may be required based on biopsy findings
Antistreptolysin O, antinuclear antibody, anti-double stranded DNA antibodies; anti-extractable nuclear antibodies
Antinuclear cytoplasmic antibodies (ANCA): Indirect immunofluorescence, ELISA
Renal biopsy (light microscopy, immunofluorescence, electron microscopy)
Required in specific instances
Anti-GBM IgG antibodies
Blood levels of cryoglobulin, hepatitis B and C serology
Chest: radiograph, CT (patients with Goodpasture syndrome and vasculitides)
Sinuses: radiograph, CT (patients with granulomatosis with polyangiitis)

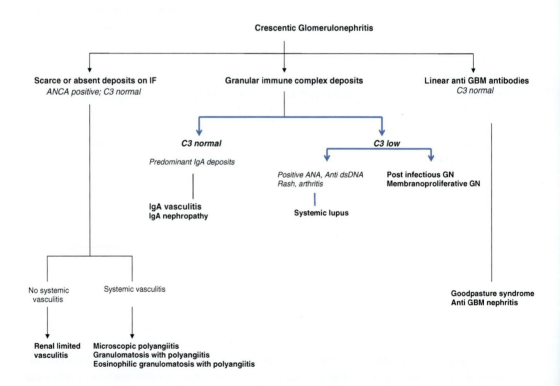

Fig. 20.1 Diagnostic evaluation of crescentic glomerulonephritis, based on renal histology and serological findings

infection in the past 3 months. Patients with SLE show antinuclear (ANA) and anti-double stranded DNA autoantibodies.

Elevated levels of ANCA suggest an underlying vasculitis, and are present in most patients with pauci-immune crescentic GN. Most ANCA have specificity for MPO or PR3. ANCA should be screened by indirect IF and positive tests confirmed by PR3-ELISA and MPO-ELISA. In patients with pauci-immune crescentic GN, negative results from IF should be tested by ELISA because 5% serum samples are positive only by the latter. GPA is associated with PR3 ANCA, which produces a cytoplasmic staining pattern on IF (c-ANCA). Renal limited vasculitis and drug induced pauci-immune crescentic GN are typically associated with MPO ANCA that shows perinuclear staining on IF (p-ANCA). Patients with MPA have equal distribution of MPO ANCA/p-ANCA and PR3 ANCA/c-ANCA. Approximately 10% of patients with GPA or MPA have negative assays for ANCA. P-ANCA autoantibodies are also found in 20–30% patients with anti-GBM GN, and occasionally in idiopathic immune complex RPGN, inflammatory bowel disease, rheumatoid arthritis and SLE [27].

Apart from diagnosis, ANCA titers have also been used for monitoring activity of systemic vasculitis. Persistent or reappearing ANCA positivity in patients in remission may be associated with disease relapse in AAV. The risk of relapse in patients who show persistently negative ANCA titers is low. An isolated rise in ANCA titers should not be used for modifying treatment in patients with systemic vasculitis [28]. The persistence or recurrence of ANCA positivity, or an increase in ANCA titers are only modestly predictive of future disease relapse and should not be used to guide treatment decisions. Such patients should be closely followed and diagnostic efforts intensified to detect and treat relapses.

Patients with AAV occasionally show autoantibodies to human lysosome-associated membrane protein-2 (hLAMP-2) [29]. These antibodies were also seen in a few patients with pauci-immune focal necrotizing crescentic GN who were negative for ANCA [30]. The hLAMP-2 autoantibodies became undetectable following initiation of immunosuppressive treatment and were detected during clinical relapse.

High titers of anti-GBM IgG antibodies, demonstrated by IF or ELISA, are seen in anti-GBM nephritis or Goodpasture syndrome and correlate with disease activity. About 5% of ANCA positive samples are also anti-GBM positive and approximately 20–30% of anti-GBM positive samples are ANCA positive. Serology for ANCA is therefore recommended in all patients with either anti-GBM antibodies in blood or linear IgG deposition along the GBM. The initial clinical outcome for these patients is similar to that of anti-GBM disease, though relapses may occur as in systemic vasculitis [1].

Renal Histology

Light Microscopy

Renal histological findings in various forms of crescentic GN are similar. A glomerular crescent is an accumulation of two or more layers of cells that partially or completely fill Bowman space. The crescent size varies from circumferential to segmental depending on the plane of the tissue section and the underlying disease. Crescents in anti-GBM nephritis or AAV are usually circumferential, while they are often segmental in immune complex GN. Interstitial changes range from acute inflammatory infiltrate to chronic interstitial scarring and tubular atrophy. Once the glomerular capillary loop is compressed by the crescent, tubules that derive their blood flow from that efferent arteriole show ischemic changes.

Crescents may be completely cellular or show variable scarring and fibrosis. Cellular crescents are characterized by proliferation of macrophages, epithelial cells and neutrophils (Fig. 20.2). Fibrocellular crescents show an admixture of collagen fibers and membrane proteins amongst the cells (Figs. 20.3 and 20.4). In fibrous crescents, the cells are replaced by collagen. Renal biopsies from patients with vasculitis show crescents in various stages of progression, indicating episodic inflammation. Early lesions have segmental fibrinoid necrosis with or without an

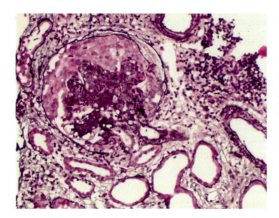

Fig. 20.2 Cellular crescent compressing the glomerular tuft. Silver methenamine stained, original magnification ×800

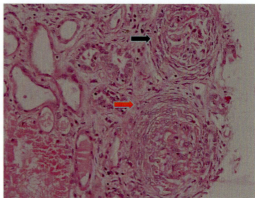

Fig. 20.4 Glomeruli showing cellular (red arrow) and fibrocellular crescents (black arrow) causing compression of underlying glomerular tuft. Note the disruption of Bowman capsule. Hematoxylin and eosin–stained, original magnification ×200

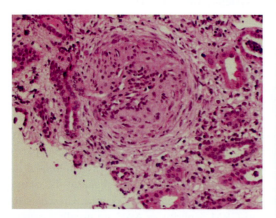

Fig. 20.3 Fibrocellular crescent with compression of glomerular tuft and partial sclerosis. There is chronic interstitial inflammation, tubular atrophy and interstitial fibrosis in surrounding area. Hematoxylin and eosin–stained, original magnification ×800

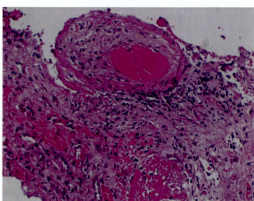

Fig. 20.5 A patient with pauci-immune crescentic glomerulonephritis. A small artery shows features of active vasculitis; its wall shows neutrophil infiltration, fibrin deposition and lumen occluded by a thrombus. The perivascular area shows interstitial hemorrhage and inflammation. Hematoxylin and eosin–stained, original magnification ×600

adjacent small crescent. Severe acute lesions show focal or diffuse necrosis in association with circumferential crescents. Features of small vessel vasculitis, affecting interlobular arteries (Fig. 20.5) and rarely angiitis involving the vasa recta might be seen.

ANCA associated GN is classified based on light microscopy findings [31]. Biopsies are categorized as focal, crescentic and sclerotic based on the predominance of normal glomeruli, cellular crescents, and globally sclerotic glomeruli, respectively. A fourth category represents a mixed or heterogeneous phenotype. Although the classification system is believed to have prognostic value for 1- and 5-year renal outcomes, and may guide therapy, it needs to be validated in children.

Immunohistology and Electron Microscopy

The presence, location and nature of immune deposits on IF and electron microscopy can help determine the underlying cause of crescentic GN. The crescents stain strongly for fibrin on IF [32]. Mesangial deposits of IgA are found in IgA nephropathy and IgA vasculitis. While IgA is dominant or co-dominant in IgA nephropathy, deposits of IgG, IgM, fibrinogen, and C3 may also be seen in the glomeruli. Postinfectious GN has granular, subepithelial deposits of IgG and C3. Full house capillary wall and mesangial deposits of granular IgG, IgA, IgM, C3, C4 and C1q are seen in SLE. Immune complex-mediated MPGN is characterized by the immunoglobulin and complement deposits, while C3 glomerulopathy is characterized by glomerular complement deposits in the absence of significant immunoglobulins. Electron microscopy usually shows subendothelial and mesangial deposits in C3 glomerulopathy and MPGN.

Anti-GBM disease is characterized by linear staining of the GBM with IgG (rarely IgM and IgA) and C3 (Fig. 20.6).

The third group of crescentic GN has few or no immune deposits by IF or electron microscopy. The majority of these patients are ANCA positive, though some may have ANCA-negative, pauci-immune crescentic GN.

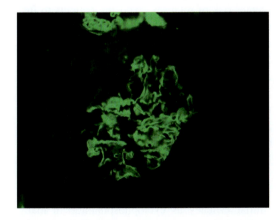

Fig. 20.6 Immunofluorescence microscopy (original magnification ×1200) in a patient with anti-glomerular basement membrane antibody-mediated crescentic glomerulonephritis showing linear deposition of IgG on the capillary wall

Evaluation and Diagnosis

It is necessary to make an accurate and rapid diagnosis in RPGN as treatment strategies vary and delay in instituting treatment increases the risk of irreversible damage. All patients should undergo a kidney biopsy promptly. While the majority have crescentic GN, the detection of thrombotic microangiopathy (affecting interlobular arteries and arterioles) or diffuse proliferative GN is not unusual. The diagnosis of the etiology of crescentic GN depends on integration of clinical data and findings on serology and renal histology (Table 20.3, Fig. 20.1).

Treatment

The heterogeneity and unsatisfactory outcome of RPGN has led to institution of multiple treatments. Evidence-based data is limited and treatment guidelines for children are based on data from case series and prospective studies in adults.

Empiric therapy with daily intravenous (IV) pulses of methylprednisolone (15–20 mg/kg, maximum 1 g) for 3 days should be initiated in patients with severe disease, particularly if kidney biopsy is likely to be delayed. This empiric initial therapy will not alter the histologic abnormalities on a kidney biopsy that is performed within a few days. Plasmapheresis can be considered in the empiric initial phase, especially if the patient presents with hemoptysis.

More specific therapy is started once the diagnosis is established. Treatment of RPGN typically comprises two phases: *induction* of remission and *maintenance* (Table 20.4). The first phase aims at control of inflammation and the associated immune response. Once remission is induced, the maintenance phase attempts to prevent further renal damage and relapses. All patients with RPGN, irrespective of the underlying diagnosis, will benefit from supportive man-

Table 20.4 Treatment of crescentic glomerulonephritis

Induction
Methylprednisolone 10–30 mg/kg (maximum 1 g) IV daily for three doses
Prednisolone 1.5–2 mg/kg/day oral for 4 weeks; taper to 0.5 mg/kg/day for 3 months; then, 0.5 mg/kg on alternate days for 3 months
[a]Cyclophosphamide 500–750 mg/m² IV every 3–4 weeks for six doses
[b]Plasma exchange (1–1.5 volume) on alternate days for 2 weeks
[c]Rituximab: 750 mg/m² (maximum 1000 mg), every 2 weeks for two doses
Maintenance
Azathioprine 1.5–2 mg/kg/day for 12–18 months
Alternate day low-dose prednisolone
Consider mycophenolate mofetil (1000–1200 mg/m²/day) if disease activity is not controlled with azathioprine or patient does not tolerate azathioprine
Rituximab can be used for maintenance, given every 6 months or when B lymphocytes reconstitute
Agents for refractory disease
Intravenous immunoglobulin, TNF-α antibody (infliximab), rituximab

[a] The dose of cyclophosphamide is increased to 750 mg/m² if there is no leukopenia before the next dose. Dose reduction is necessary in patients showing impaired renal function. Alternatively, cyclophosphamide is given orally at a dose of 2 mg/kg/day for 12 weeks

[b] Plasma exchange can be initiated early, especially if patient is dialysis-dependent at presentation or if the biopsy shows severe histological changes (>50% crescents). It is useful in anti-GBM nephritis and may be useful in ANCA-associated vasculitis. It can be considered in patients with immune complex crescentic GN if there is unsatisfactory renal recovery after steroid pulses

[c] Rituximab may be used as first line in children and adolescents with AAV, particularly PR3-AAV. It may be used as an alternative initial treatment in patients with less severe disease or in whom cyclophosphamide is contraindicated

agement, including maintenance of fluid and electrolyte balance, provision of adequate nutrition, and control of infections and hypertension. Some patients require dialysis at diagnosis or soon thereafter.

Medications

Steroids After the initial IV pulses, steroids are typically given as high-dose oral prednisone (1.5–2 mg/kg daily) for 4 weeks, with tapering to 0.5 mg/kg daily by 3 months and alternate day prednisone for 6–12 months. Based on recent studies, a reduced-dose, tapering regimen of oral glucocorticoids-could be considered for a patient with new onset or relapsing AAV [33].

Cyclophosphamide Historically, cyclophosphamide has been an important part of induction regimens. Most centers prefer the use of IV compared to oral therapy. The European Vasculitis Study Group (EUVAS) compared IV pulse cyclophosphamide (15 mg/kg every 2 weeks for 3 pulses, followed by pulses at 3-week intervals until remission, and then for another 3 months) with daily oral cyclophosphamide (2 mg/kg/day) for induction of remission [34]. They showed that the time to remission and proportion of patients in remission at 9 months was similar in both groups. The cumulative dose of cyclophosphamide in the daily oral group was twice that in the IV group (15.9 g *vs.* 8.2 g; $P < 0.001$), and the latter had a lower rate of leukopenia. A meta-analysis of nonrandomized studies showed that pulse cyclophosphamide was significantly more likely to induce remission and had a lower risk of infection and leukopenia. Pulse cyclophosphamide dosing may, however, be associated with a greater risk of relapses, exposing patients to further immunosuppression [35]. The dose of oral and IV cyclophosphamide is 2 mg/kg/day and 500–750 mg/m², respectively. The dose should be adjusted to maintain a nadir leukocyte count of 3000–4000/μL 2 weeks post-treatment. While most of the data on cyclophosphamide is from AAV or lupus nephritis, a similar regimen is recommended for crescentic IgA nephropathy or IgA vasculitis.

Rituximab B cell depletion with rituximab has similar efficacy as cyclophosphamide in many studies. It has been used successfully in patients with refractory lupus nephritis and AAV [36]. The Rituximab in ANCA-Associated Vasculitis (RAVE) trial compare rituximab with standard therapy for inducing remission in patients with AAV [37]. Patients received either rituximab (375 mg/m²/week for 4 weeks) or cyclophosphamide (2 mg/kg/day). Both groups received 1–3 pulses of methylprednisolone (1000 mg each), followed by tapering dose of prednisone. At 6 months, 64% in the rituximab group achieved remission vs. 53% in the control group. Of the subgroup that had relapsing disease, rituximab was superior to cyclophosphamide in inducing remission (67% versus 42%) at 6 months. Thus, therapy with rituximab was not inferior to treatment with cyclophosphamide for induction of remission. Patients from the RAVE study who achieved complete remission were followed through month 18 [38]. During follow-up, those treated with rituximab received no further therapy, while those treated with cyclophosphamide were converted to azathioprine. At 18 months, the proportion of patients remaining in complete remission was similar (39% rituximab vs. 33% cyclophosphamide). Interestingly, a post hoc analysis of the RAVE trial found a higher remission rate for the PR3-AAV subgroup at 6 months treated with rituximab [39]. A similar association was not seen with MPO-AAV.

The RITUXVAS study randomized patients with AAV to receive a standard steroid regimen plus either rituximab (375 mg/m²/week for 4 weeks) with two IV cyclophosphamide pulses, or IV cyclophosphamide for 3–6 months followed by azathioprine [40]. There was no significant difference in the rate of remission, severe adverse events, and death in the two groups.

Mycophenolate mofetil (MMF) MMF has been used in observational studies as part of induction therapy for vasculitis, though it may have a greater role in the maintenance phase. Results from the EUVAS MYCYC trial showed that MMF was non-inferior to cyclophosphamide for remission induction in AAV, but resulted in a higher relapse rate [41]. MMF has also been used as an alternative to azathioprine for maintenance therapy in patients with AAV. However, the IMPROVE trial (International Mycophenolate Mofetil Protocol to Reduce Outbreaks of Vasculitides) showed that relapses were significantly more common in patients receiving MMF compared to azathioprine, with no difference in severe adverse events [42]. The Kidney Disease Improving Global Outcomes (KDIGO) Clinical Practice

Guideline for Glomerulonephritis recommends using azathioprine as the first choice for maintenance therapy in ANCA vasculitis and considering MMF as an alternative in patients who are allergic to or intolerant of azathioprine [43].

Intravenous Immunoglobulin (IVIG) A number of studies have examined the efficacy of IVIG in subjects with AAV and RPGN, and reported benefit lasting for up to 3 months [44]. The exact mechanism of action is unclear with evidence for both non-specific anti-inflammatory and anti-cytokine effects and specific correction of immunoregulatory defects. In a study of AAV patients with persistent disease activity, 14/17 patients in the IVIG group had reduction in disease activity, compared to 6/17 in the placebo group [45]. The indications for initial or adjunctive treatment with IVIG is not defined.

Methotrexate The NORAM study compared the effectiveness of orally administered methotrexate and cyclophosphamide in adult patients with early systemic vasculitis and mild renal involvement [46]. Induction of remission was similar at 6 months, but relapses were more frequent after treatment withdrawal in methotrexate treated patients. Methotrexate is not recommended for patients with moderate to severe renal dysfunction.

Azathioprine Most patients with AAV need long-term maintenance immunosuppression due to the risk of relapses. Extended treatment with cyclophosphamide has been used in adults but has significant risks and is not the preferred approach for children. While azathioprine is not effective at inducing remission, it is useful for long-term prevention of relapses. The timing of the switch from cyclophosphamide to azathioprine was clarified by the CYCAZAREM trial, which compared switching from cyclophosphamide to maintenance azathioprine at 3 versus 12 months [47]. At 18 months, the two groups had similar remission rates, renal function and patient survival. There is uncertainty regarding the appropriate duration of maintenance treatment, with most patients with pauci-immune crescentic GN treated for 2 or more years.

Newer Agents

T lymphocyte depletion with Campath 1-H (alemtuzumab), an anti-CD52 monoclonal antibody, has been tried with variable success in patients with GPA and other vasculitides [48]. In a retrospective cohort study, 85% of patients with refractory AAV achieved remission after alemtuzumab, but the majority relapsed after a median of 9 months [45].

A multicenter, double-blind, placebo-controlled study evaluated belimumab for preventing relapses in patients with AAV [49]. Belimumab is a monoclonal antibody that prevents the survival of B lymphocytes by blocking the binding of soluble human B lymphocyte stimulator protein to receptors on B lymphocytes. Patients were randomized to receive azathioprine, low-dose oral steroids and either IV belimumab or placebo for maintenance of remission. The addition of belimumab did not reduce the risk of relapse.

Avacopan, which targets the complement system by blocking the C5a receptor, has been investigated as an approach to reduce corticosteroid exposure in AAV. A phase II trial showed that avacopan was well-tolerated and safe in the short-term and may be able to replace high-dose corticosteroids [50]. This was followed by a phase III randomized, controlled trial comparing avacopan with a tapering schedule of prednisone in patients with AAV concurrently treated with cyclophosphamide (followed by azathioprine) or rituximab [51]. Avacopan was noninferior to prednisone taper for the end-point of remission at week 26 and was superior to prednisone taper for sustained remission at week 52. The number of steroid-related adverse events was higher in the prednisone group than in the avacopan group.

Plasmapheresis

Plasmapheresis or plasma exchange has been used for the treatment of crescentic GN with variable success. The mechanism of action is not clear, but is believed to involve removal of pathogenic autoantibodies, complement proteins, coagulation factors and cytokines. Plasma exchange has been shown in controlled trials in adults to have therapeutic benefit in anti-GBM disease, with clearance of auto-antibodies, lower serum creatinine and improved patient and renal survival [52]. However, adults who were anuric with severe azotemia, dialysis dependent or those who had more than 85% crescents on renal biopsy had minimal benefit. The role of intensive plasma exchange versus IV methylprednisolone, in addition to oral steroids and cyclophosphamide, was examined by the MEPEX trial in patients with AAV and serum creatinine >500 μmol/L (5.65 mg/dL) at presentation [53]. Patients receiving plasma exchange were more likely to be off dialysis at 3-months (69% *vs.* 49%) and had a lower risk of ESKD at 12 months, but there were limited benefits on long-term renal function or survival. Another study showed that plasma exchange improved medium-term renal survival, even when initiated in patients with serum creatinine levels >250 μmol/L (2.85 mg/dL) [54].

More recently the PEXIVAS trial looked at initial treatment with plasma exchange vs. no plasma exchange (with either cyclophosphamide or rituximab administered to all patients) and two different regimens of oral steroids in patients with severe AAV [33]. The study failed to demonstrate that plasma exchange delayed the time to ESKD or death.

Retrospective data in children with RPGN show benefits of plasma exchange if commenced within 1 month of disease onset [55]. Anecdotal reports confirm the efficacy of plasmapheresis in patients with RPGN due to lupus, IgA vasculitis and severe proliferative GN, and in life-threatening pulmonary hemorrhage. Prospective studies in patients with pauci-immune crescentic GN suggested that kidney outcomes were better with plasma exchange and immunosuppression vs. immunosuppression alone [56]. However, a meta-analysis of renal vasculitis or idiopathic RPGN concluded that adjunctive plasma exchange did not improve renal and patient survival [57].

According to the KDIGO Guidelines, the routine use of plasma exchange is not recommended for patients presenting with a GFR <50 mL/min/1.73 m², but it can be considered in those with more severe AKI or in those with alveolar hemorrhage and hypoxemia. The dose recommended for adults is 60 mL/kg volume replacement [43]. For AAV, seven treatments over 14 days are prescribed and for patients with anti-GBM antibodies, daily exchanges are performed for 14 days or until anti-GBM antibodies are undetectable.

In our practice, we consider plasma exchange for patients with severe AKI or alveolar hemorrhage with hypoxia, and use 1–1.5 volume exchange per the schedule discussed above.

Immune Complex Crescentic GN

Therapy for immune complex crescentic GN depends on the underlying disease. The treatment of IgA nephropathy and lupus nephritis presenting with RPGN is discussed in their respective chapters. Patients with idiopathic immune complex crescentic GN should be treated similarly to those with pauci-immune crescentic GN.

Postinfectious RPGN

Poststreptococcal GN presenting with extensive crescents is rare and the benefits of intensive immunosuppressive therapy are unclear, since most patients recover spontaneously. Nevertheless, immunosuppressive therapy with corticosteroids and alkylating agents has been used in patients with renal failure and extensive glomerular crescents [58]. Despite the lack of evidence-based data, we usually treat patients with postinfectious RPGN and crescents involving 50% or more glomeruli with 3–6 IV pulses of methylprednisolone, followed by tapering doses of oral steroids for 6 months. Eradication of the infection and/or removal of infected prostheses are necessary for resolution of immune complex GN associated with active infections.

Pauci-immune Crescentic GN

Standard induction therapy is IV pulses of methylprednisolone daily for 3 days followed by oral prednisone and cyclophosphamide or rituximab. For cyclophosphamide, the choice between oral (2 mg/kg/day for 3 months) and IV (15 mg/kg every 2 weeks for three doses and then every 3 weeks for 3–6 months or 500–750 mg/m² every 2 weeks for 3–6 months) depends on institutional practice. While both oral and IV regimens are effective, IV is preferred due to the lower cumulative dose and lower risk of toxicity. After approximately 3–6 months, cyclophosphamide is replaced by a medication with a lower risk of toxicity. Rituximab, for induction is usually dosed at 750 mg/m² (maximum dose 1000 mg), with two 2 doses 14 days apart. Therapeutic plasma exchange can be added to the induction regimen for children who are dialysis dependent, those with pulmonary hemorrhage and hypoxia or not responding satisfactorily to induction treatment [33, 53].

Therapy during the maintenance phase is tapering doses of oral prednisolone and azathioprine, usually for 18–24 months. For most patients, a reduced-dose glucocorticoid tapering regimen can be used, particularly after studies like PEXIVAS showed that patients on the reduced-dose tapering regimen had similar rates of remission and fewer adverse effects compared with those on standard-dosing regimens [33].

A longer duration of therapy (3 years or more) may be needed in patients showing relapses, elevated ANCA titers and those with PR3-ANCA [2]. Approximately one-third of patients have one or more relapses, requiring reinstitution of induction therapy. Since intensive immunosuppression is associated with increased risk of infection, the use of prophylactic antimicrobials against *Pneumocystis carinii* and *Candida* may be required during induction.

For AAV, the KDIGO guidelines recommend using rituximab for children and adolescents, and for those with relapsing disease or PR3-AAV. They also suggest that for those with severe GN and creatinine >4 mg/dL, a combination of two pulses of cyclophosphamide with rituximab can be used for induction.

Anti-GBM Crescentic GN

Prompt institution of plasma exchange is necessary in these patients. Double volume exchange is done daily, and subsequently on alternate days until anti-GBM antibodies are no longer detectable (usually 2–3 weeks) [1, 59]. The patients are also treated with IV methylprednisolone (three doses of 20 mg/kg on alternate days) followed by high-dose oral prednisolone. Co-administration of cyclophosphamide (typically PO, 2 mg/kg daily for 3 months; IV may also be used) is effective in suppressing further antibody production. Pulmonary hemorrhage responds to plasma exchange and IV steroids. As anti-GBM disease does not usually have a relapsing course, long-term maintenance therapy is not required and steroids can be tapered over the next 6–9 months. Patients treated early in the course of their illness do satisfactorily. In patients who develop ESKD, transplantation should be deferred until anti-GBM antibodies are undetectable for 12 months, at which point disease recurrence is unlikely.

A proportion of patients with anti-GBM nephritis also show positive ANCA, most often p-ANCA. While the precise significance of the dual positivity is unclear, their outcome is similar to isolated anti-GBM disease. In view of a higher risk of relapses, these patients require a longer course of maintenance immunosuppressive therapy (as for ANCA-associated GN).

Outcome

The outcome for patients has improved in the last decades, such that almost 60–70% patients have normal long-term renal function. Patients with poststreptococcal crescentic GN have a better prognosis, with most showing spontaneous improvement. The prognosis is better in patients with poststreptococcal crescentic GN with sub-epithelial, rather than subendothelial or intra-membranous deposits. Outcomes in patients with pauci-immune crescentic GN, MPGN and idiopathic RPGN are less favorable than IgA vasculi-

tis or SLE. ESKD may occur on the long-term in up to 25% patients with AAV.

The outcome is determined by the severity of renal failure at presentation and promptness of intervention, renal histology and underlying diagnosis. Studies have shown that the use of plasma exchange, high percentage of normal glomeruli, and absence of glomerulosclerosis, tubular atrophy and arteriosclerosis, were associated with better renal recovery [60]. The potential for recovery correlates with the relative proportion of cellular or fibrous components in the crescents, and the extent of tubulointerstitial scarring and fibrosis.

Post-transplant Recurrence

Based on experience in adult patients, we suggest that patients with ANCA positive vasculitis should have sustained remission for 1 year before considering a transplant [61]. A positive ANCA titer at the time of transplantation does not increase the risk of allograft recurrence. Conditions associated with higher risk of histological recurrence include MPGN, IgA nephropathy, IgA vasculitis and lupus. Graft loss due recurrence is uncommon and occur in <5% of cases.

References

1. Jennette JC. Rapidly progressive crescentic glomerulonephritis. Kidney Int. 2003;63(3):1164–77.
2. Morgan MD, Harper L, Williams J, Savage C. Antineutrophil cytoplasm-associated glomerulonephritis. J Am Soc Nephrol. 2006;17(5):1224–34.
3. Kessenbrock K, Krumbholz M, Schönermarck U, Back W, Gross WL, Werb Z, et al. Netting neutrophils in autoimmune small-vessel vasculitis. Nat Med. 2009;15(6):623–5.
4. Bosch X. LAMPs and NETs in the pathogenesis of ANCA vasculitis. J Am Soc Nephrol. 2009;20(8):1654–6.
5. Xiao H, Dairaghi DJ, Powers JP, Ertl LS, Baumgart T, Wang Y, et al. C5a receptor (CD88) blockade protects against MPO-ANCA GN. J Am Soc Nephrol. 2014;25(2):225–31.
6. Sethi S, Zand L, De Vriese AS, Specks U, Vrana JA, Kanwar S, et al. Complement activation in pauci-

immune necrotizing and crescentic glomerulonephritis: results of a proteomic analysis. Nephrol Dial Transplant. 2017;32(suppl_1):i139–i45.

7. Atkins RC, Nikolic-Paterson DJ, Song Q, Lan HY. Modulators of crescentic glomerulonephritis. J Am Soc Nephrol. 1996;7(11):2271–8.

8. Thorner PS, Ho M, Eremina V, Sado Y, Quaggin S. Podocytes contribute to the formation of glomerular crescents. J Am Soc Nephrol. 2008;19(3):495–502.

9. Tipping PG, Holdsworth SR. T cells in crescentic glomerulonephritis. J Am Soc Nephrol. 2006;17(5):1253–63.

10. Paust HJ, Ostmann A, Erhardt A, Turner JE, Velden J, et al. Regulatory T cells control the Th1 immune response in murine crescentic glomerulonephritis. Kidney Int. 2011;80(2):154–64.

11. Bollée G, Flamant M, Schordan S, Fligny C, Rumpel E, Milon M, et al. Epidermal growth factor receptor promotes glomerular injury and renal failure in rapidly progressive crescentic glomerulonephritis. Nat Med. 2011;17(10):1242–50.

12. Ophascharoensuk V, Pippin JW, Gordon KL, Shankland SJ, Couser WG, Johnson RJ. Role of intrinsic renal cells versus infiltrating cells in glomerular crescent formation. Kidney Int. 1998;54(2):416–25.

13. El-Husseini AA, Sheashaa HA, Sabry AA, Moustafa FE, Sobh MA. Acute postinfectious crescentic glomerulonephritis: clinicopathologic presentation and risk factors. Int Urol Nephrol. 2005;37(3):603–9.

14. Srivastava RN, Moudgil A, Bagga A, Vasudev AS, Bhuyan UN, Sundraem KR. Crescentic glomerulonephritis in children: a review of 43 cases. Am J Nephrol. 1992;12(3):155–61.

15. Hoschek JC, Dreyer P, Dahal S, Walker PD. Rapidly progressive renal failure in childhood. Am J Kidney Dis. 2002;40(6):1342–7.

16. Bomback AS, Santoriello D, Avasare RS, Regunathan-Shenk R, Canetta PA, Ahn W, et al. C3 glomerulonephritis and dense deposit disease share a similar disease course in a large United States cohort of patients with C3 glomerulopathy. Kidney Int. 2018;93(4):977–85.

17. Hattori M, Kurayama H, Koitabashi Y, Nephrology JSP. Antineutrophil cytoplasmic autoantibody-associated glomerulonephritis in children. J Am Soc Nephrol. 2001;12(7):1493–500.

18. Chen M, Kallenberg CG, Zhao MH. ANCA-negative pauci-immune crescentic glomerulonephritis. Nat Rev Nephrol. 2009;5(6):313–8.

19. Maliakkal JG, Hicks MJ, Michael M, Selewski DT, Twombley K, Rheault MN, et al. Renal survival in children with glomerulonephritis with crescents: a pediatric nephrology research consortium cohort study. J Clin Med. 2020;9(8).

20. Mayer U, Schmitz J, Bräsen JH, Pape L. Crescentic glomerulonephritis in children. Pediatr Nephrol. 2020;35(5):829–42.

21. Piyaphanee N, Ananboontarick C, Supavekin S, Sumboonnanonda A. Renal outcome and risk factors for end-stage renal disease in pediatric rapidly progressive glomerulonephritis. Pediatr Int. 2017;59(3):334–41.

22. Kashtan CE. Renal transplantation in patients with Alport syndrome. Pediatr Transplant. 2006;10(6):651–7.

23. Covic A, Schiller A, Volovat C, Gluhovschi G, Gusbeth-Tatomir P, Petrica L, et al. Epidemiology of renal disease in Romania: a 10 year review of two regional renal biopsy databases. Nephrol Dial Transplant. 2006;21(2):419–24.

24. Studies NAPRTaC. NAPRTCS 2010 Annual Report 2010. https://web.emmes.com/study/ped/annlrept/annlrept2006.

25. Sinha A, Puri K, Hari P, Dinda AK, Bagga A. Etiology and outcome of crescentic glomerulonephritis. Indian Pediatr. 2013;50(3):283–8.

26. Alsaad K, Oudah N, Al Ameer A, Fakeeh K, Al Jomaih A, Al SA. Glomerulonephritis with crescents in children: etiology and predictors of renal outcome. ISRN Pediatr. 2011;2011:507298.

27. Bosch X, Guilabert A, Font J. Antineutrophil cytoplasmic antibodies. Lancet. 2006;368(9533):404–18.

28. Schmitt WH, van der Woude FJ. Clinical applications of antineutrophil cytoplasmic antibody testing. Curr Opin Rheumatol. 2004;16(1):9–17.

29. Kain R, Tadema H, McKinney EF, Benharkou A, Brandes R, Peschel A, et al. High prevalence of autoantibodies to hLAMP-2 in anti-neutrophil cytoplasmic antibody-associated vasculitis. J Am Soc Nephrol. 2012;23(3):556–66.

30. Peschel A, Basu N, Benharkou A, Brandes R, Brown M, Dieckmann R, et al. Autoantibodies to hLAMP-2 in ANCA-negative pauci-immune focal necrotizing GN. J Am Soc Nephrol. 2013;25(3):455–63.

31. Berden AE, Ferrario F, Hagen EC, Jayne DR, Jennette JC, Joh K, et al. Histopathologic classification of ANCA-associated glomerulonephritis. J Am Soc Nephrol. 2010;21(10):1628–36.

32. Levy J, Pusey C. Crescentic glomerulonephritis. In: Davison AMA, Cameron JS, Grunfeld J-P, Ponticelli C, Van Ypersele C, Ritz E, et al., editors. Oxford textbook of clinical nephrology. 3rd ed. Oxford: Oxford University Press; 2005.

33. Walsh M, Merkel PA, Peh CA, Szpirt WM, Puéchal X, Fujimoto S, et al. Plasma exchange and glucocorticoids in severe ANCA-associated vasculitis. N Engl J Med. 2020;382(7):622–31.

34. de Groot K, Harper L, Jayne DR, Flores Suarez LF, Gregorini G, Gross WL, et al. Pulse versus daily oral cyclophosphamide for induction of remission in antineutrophil cytoplasmic antibody-associated vasculitis: a randomized trial. Ann Intern Med. 2009;150(10):670–80.

35. de Groot K, Adu D, Savage CO, EEvs Group. The value of pulse cyclophosphamide in ANCA-associated vasculitis: meta-analysis and critical review. Nephrol Dial Transplant. 2001;16(10):2018–27.

36. Keogh KA, Ytterberg SR, Fervenza FC, Carlson KA, Schroeder DR, Specks U. Rituximab for refractory Wegener's granulomatosis: report of a prospective,

36. open-label pilot trial. Am J Respir Crit Care Med. 2006;173(2):180–7.

37. Stone JH, Merkel PA, Spiera R, Seo P, Langford CA, Hoffman GS, et al. Rituximab versus cyclophosphamide for ANCA-associated vasculitis. N Engl J Med. 2010;363(3):221–32.

38. Specks U, Merkel PA, Seo P, Spiera R, Langford CA, Hoffman GS, et al. Efficacy of remission-induction regimens for ANCA-associated vasculitis. N Engl J Med. 2013;369(5):417–27.

39. Unizony S, Villarreal M, Miloslavsky EM, Lu N, Merkel PA, Spiera R, et al. Clinical outcomes of treatment of anti-neutrophil cytoplasmic antibody (ANCA)-associated vasculitis based on ANCA type. Ann Rheum Dis. 2016;75(6):1166–9.

40. Jones RB, Tervaert JW, Hauser T, Luqmani R, Morgan MD, Peh CA, et al. Rituximab versus cyclophosphamide in ANCA-associated renal vasculitis. N Engl J Med. 2010;363(3):211–20.

41. Jones RB, Hiemstra TF, Ballarin J, Blockmans DE, Brogan P, Bruchfeld A, et al. Mycophenolate mofetil versus cyclophosphamide for remission induction in ANCA-associated vasculitis: a randomised, non-inferiority trial. Ann Rheum Dis. 2019;78(3):399–405.

42. Hiemstra TF, Walsh M, Mahr A, Savage CO, de Groot K, Harper L, et al. Mycophenolate mofetil vs azathioprine for remission maintenance in antineutrophil cytoplasmic antibody-associated vasculitis: a randomized controlled trial. JAMA. 2010;304(21):2381–8.

43. Group KDIGOGW. KDIGO clinical practice guideline for glomerulonephritis. Kidney Int. 2012;Supplement(2):139–274.

44. Ito-Ihara T, Ono T, Nogaki F, Suyama K, Tanaka M, Yonemoto S, et al. Clinical efficacy of intravenous immunoglobulin for patients with MPO-ANCA-associated rapidly progressive glomerulonephritis. Nephron Clin Pract. 2006;102(1):35–42.

45. Smith RM, Jones RB, Jayne DR. Progress in treatment of ANCA-associated vasculitis. Arthritis Res Ther. 2012;14(2):210.

46. De Groot K, Rasmussen N, Bacon PA, Tervaert JW, Feighery C, Gregorini G, et al. Randomized trial of cyclophosphamide versus methotrexate for induction of remission in early systemic antineutrophil cytoplasmic antibody-associated vasculitis. Arthritis Rheum. 2005;52(8):2461–9.

47. Jayne D, Rasmussen N, Andrassy K, Bacon P, Tervaert JW, et al. A randomized trial of maintenance therapy for vasculitis associated with antineutrophil cytoplasmic autoantibodies. N Engl J Med. 2003;349(1):36–44.

48. Jayne D. What place for the new biologics in the treatment of necrotising vasculitides. Clin Exp Rheumatol. 2006;24(2 Suppl 41):S1–5.

49. Jayne D, Blockmans D, Luqmani R, Moiseev S, Ji B, Green Y, et al. Efficacy and safety of belimumab and azathioprine for maintenance of remission in antineu-trophil cytoplasmic antibody-associated vasculitis: a randomized controlled study. Arthritis Rheumatol. 2019;71(6):952–63.

50. Jayne DRW, Bruchfeld AN, Harper L, Schaier M, Venning MC, Hamilton P, et al. Randomized trial of C5a receptor inhibitor avacopan in ANCA-associated vasculitis. J Am Soc Nephrol. 2017;28(9):2756–67.

51. Jayne DRW, Merkel PA, Schall TJ, Bekker P, Group AS. Avacopan for the treatment of ANCA-associated vasculitis. N Engl J Med. 2021;384(7):599–609.

52. Levy JB, Turner AN, Rees AJ, Pusey CD. Long-term outcome of anti-glomerular basement membrane antibody disease treated with plasma exchange and immunosuppression. Ann Intern Med. 2001;134(11):1033–42.

53. Jayne DR, Gaskin G, Rasmussen N, Abramowicz D, Ferrario F, Guillevin L, et al. Randomized trial of plasma exchange or high-dosage methylprednisolone as adjunctive therapy for severe renal vasculitis. J Am Soc Nephrol. 2007;18(7):2180–8.

54. Szpirt WM, Heaf JG, Petersen J. Plasma exchange for induction and cyclosporine A for maintenance of remission in Wegener's granulomatosis—a clinical randomized controlled trial. Nephrol Dial Transplant. 2011;26(1):206–13.

55. Gianviti A, Trompeter RS, Barratt TM, Lythgoe MF, Dillon MJ. Retrospective study of plasma exchange in patients with idiopathic rapidly progressive glomerulonephritis and vasculitis. Arch Dis Child. 1996;75(3):186–90.

56. Pusey CD, Rees AJ, Evans DJ, Peters DK, Lockwood CM. Plasma exchange in focal necrotizing glomerulonephritis without anti-GBM antibodies. Kidney Int. 1991;40(4):757–63.

57. Walsh M, Catapano F, Szpirt W, Thorlund K, Bruchfeld A, Guillevin L, et al. Plasma exchange for renal vasculitis and idiopathic rapidly progressive glomerulonephritis: a meta-analysis. Am J Kidney Dis. 2011;57(4):566–74.

58. Raff A, Hebert T, Pullman J, Coco M. Crescentic post-streptococcal glomerulonephritis with nephrotic syndrome in the adult: is aggressive therapy warranted? Clin Nephrol. 2005;63(5):375–80.

59. Jindal KK. Management of idiopathic crescentic and diffuse proliferative glomerulonephritis: evidence-based recommendations. Kidney Int Suppl. 1999;70:S33–40.

60. de Lind van Wijngaarden RA, Hauer HA, Wolterbeek R, Jayne DR, Gaskin G, Rasmussen N, et al. Chances of renal recovery for dialysis-dependent ANCA-associated glomerulonephritis. J Am Soc Nephrol. 2007;18(7):2189–97.

61. Little MA, Hassan B, Jacques S, Game D, Salisbury E, Courtney AE, et al. Renal transplantation in systemic vasculitis: when is it safe? Nephrol Dial Transplant. 2009;24(10):3219–25.

Part V

Complement Disorders

The Role of Complement in Kidney Disease

21

Michael Kirschfink and Christoph Licht

The Emerging Concept of Complement-Mediated Diseases

As a key mediator of inflammation complement also significantly contributes to tissue damage in various clinical disorders [1]. Clinical and experimental evidence underlines the prominent role of complement in the pathogenesis of numerous inflammatory diseases including immune complex and autoimmune disorders, such as systemic lupus erythematosus and autoimmune arthritis [2–4]. Complement deficiencies represent approximately 4–5% of all primary immunodeficiencies, in part closely connected with renal disorders [5].

In clinical practice, overactivation of the complement system is the cause of several inflammatory diseases and life-threatening conditions, such as adult respiratory distress syndrome (ARDS) [6], the systemic inflammatory response syndrome (SIRS), sepsis [7], and multi-organ failure after severe trauma, burns or infections [8]. Complement has also been implicated in neurodegenerative disorders, such as Alzheimer's disease, multiple sclerosis, and Guillain-Barré syndrome. In recent years complement activation has also been recognized as a major effector mechanism of ischemia/reperfusion injury [9, 10].

Over the past two decades our understanding of the role of complement in renal disorders has considerably advanced and genomic studies have revealed multiple strong associations of genetic variants of complement proteins with kidney disease [11, 12].

The inflammatory response induced by artificial surfaces in hemodialysis and other extracorporeal circuits may lead to organ dysfunction. Here, complement activation has been associated with transient neutropenia, pulmonary vascular leukostasis and occasionally even with anaphylactic shock of variable severity [13, 14].

The Complement System

With more than 50 proteins acting as components within the activation cascade and as regulators or receptors on multiple cells, complement is a vital part of the body's innate immune system which provides a highly effective means for the destruction of invading microorganisms and elimination of immune complexes [15, 16]. In addition, complement also modulates the adaptive immune response through modification of

M. Kirschfink
Insitute of Immunology, University of Heidelberg,
Heidelberg, Germany
e-mail: kirschfink@uni-hd.de

C. Licht (✉)
Division of Nephrology, The Hospital for Sick Children, Toronto, ON, Canada

Cell Biology Program, Research Institute, The Hospital for Sick Children, Toronto, ON, Canada
e-mail: christoph.licht@sickkids.ca

© The Author(s), under exclusive license to Springer Nature Switzerland AG 2023
F. Schaefer, L. A. Greenbaum (eds.), *Pediatric Kidney Disease*,
https://doi.org/10.1007/978-3-031-11665-0_21

T- and B-cell function employing specific receptors on various immune cells [17]. Moreover, a normally functioning complement system also participates in hematopoiesis, reproduction, lipid metabolism and tissue regeneration [18]. Essential intracellular immune modulatory functions of the complement system have recently been discovered promoting the survival and activation of T-lymphocytes [19].

Most complement proteins are secreted by the liver and contribute to the acute phase response. However, other tissues like the kidney also produce complement proteins to a significant amount [20]. Complement genes are distributed across different chromosomes, with 19 genes comprising three significant complement gene clusters in the human genome [21].

Complement can be activated via three pathways (Fig. 21.1), the classical, the alternative, and the lectin pathway, all of which merge in the activation of complement C3 and subsequently lead to the formation of the cytolytic membrane attack complex (MAC), C5b-9 [22, 23]. Following complement activation, the biologically active peptides (anaphylatoxins) C3a and C5a are released and elicit a number of proinflammatory effects, such as chemotaxis of leukocytes, degranulation of phagocytic cells, mast cells and basophils, smooth muscle contraction, and increase of vascular permeabiltity [24, 25]. C3a activates mesangial cells leading to proliferation and secretion of extracellular matrix [26]. It also induces in tubular epithelial cells the production of proinflammatory cytokines [27]. Upon cell activation by these complement split products the inflammatory response is further amplified by subsequent generation of toxic oxygen radicals and the induction of synthesis and release of arachidonic acid metabolites and cytokines. Consequently, an (over-)activated complement system represents a considerable risk of harming the host by directly and indirectly mediating

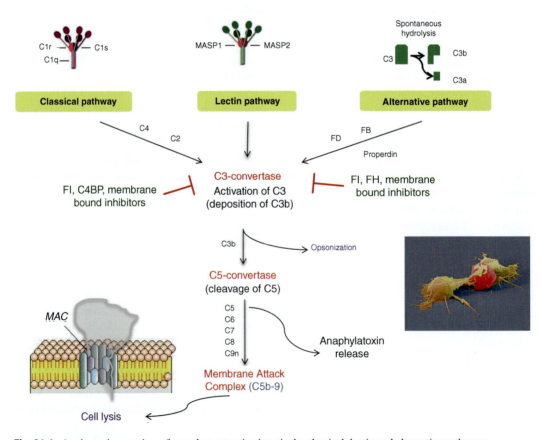

Fig. 21.1 A schematic overview of complement activation via the classical, lectin and alternative pathways

inflammatory tissue destruction [1]. Multiple interactions exist between the complement, coagulation and fibrinolytic systems altogether being of utmost importance in the pathogenesis of thrombotic microangiopathy (TMA) [28].

Under physiological conditions, activation of complement is effectively controlled by the coordinated action of soluble as well as membrane-associated regulatory proteins [29]. Soluble complement regulators, such as C1 inhibitor, C4b-binding protein (C4bp), Factors H (FH) and I (FI), clusterin and S-protein (vitronectin) restrict the action of complement in body fluids at multiple sites of the cascade (Fig. 21.1). In addition, each individual host cell is protected against the attack of homologous complement by surface proteins, such as the complement receptor 1 (CR1/CD35), the membrane cofactor protein (MCP/CD46), the glycosylphosphatidylinositol (GPI)-anchored proteins, decay-accelerating factor (DAF/CD55), and protectin (CD59) [29, 30].

Diagnosing Complement-Mediated Nephropathies

Detecting Complement Activation

In recent years, great progress has been made in complement analysis to better define disease severity, evolution and response to therapy (Tables 21.1 and 21.2) [31]. However, a comprehensive analysis going beyond C3 and C4 is still performed only in specialized laboratories (http://www.ecomplement.org/list-of-diagnostic-labs.html). The diagnostic work-up of a patient with a suspected complement-associated disease should start with the assessment of the total activity of the classical (CH50) and alternative (AH50) pathway. For rapid deficiency analysis, an ELISA has been developed that examines all three activation pathways in parallel [32]. These global tests provide information about the integrity of the entire complement cascade. A missing or

Table 21.1 Biochemical complement analysis

Functional assays	*Total complement activity (screening for complement deficiency)* • CH50 and AH50 hemolytic assays for CP and AP activity • Enzyme immunoassays (ELISA) for specific evaluation of CP, LP and AP activity using C5b-9 as readout
	Functional activity of single components • Hemolytic assays for single components (e.g. C3) using corresponding deficient sera as test system • ELISA for MBL/MASP functional activity using deposition of C4 as readout • C1 inhibitor assay (chromogenic assay or EIA) for diagnosis of HAE and acquired angioedema
Proteins	*Concentration of single components by immunoprecipitation (RID), nephelometry, ELISA* • C3 and C4 to detect "hypocomplementemia" • Follow-up of a low activity detected in total complement activity screening (any component) • C5-C9, Properdin, MBL at recurrent neisserial infections • C1 inhibitor for diagnosis of HAE and acquired angioedema
Activation products	*Concentrations of split products or protein-protein complexes by ELISA, preferentially based on antibodies to neoepitopes expressed selectively on the activation products* • Split products from components after proteolytic cleavage (e.g. C3a, C3d, C4a, C4d, C5a, Ba, Bb) • Complexes between the activated component and its inhibitor (e.g. C1rs-C1 inhibitor) • Macromolecular complexes (e.g. the AP convertase C3bBbP and the terminal sC5b-9 complex)
Autoantibodies	*Assessment of autoantibody concentrations by ELISA or functional assay* • Anti-C1q—SLE; anti-C1 inhibitor—angioedema; anti-FH—aHUS; C3 NeF/C5 NeF—MPGN, DDD/C3G
Surface proteins	*Flowcytometric quantification* • DAF/CD55 and CD59 for diagnosis of PNH

Table 21.2 Recommended complement analysis in nephropathies

Disease	Analysis
Systemic Lupus Erythematosus	CH50, C1q, C4 (C4A/B), C3, C3d or SC5b-9, anti-C1q autoantibodies
Atypical Hemolytic Uremic Syndrome	CH50, APH50, C3, C3a/C3d, SC5b-9, CFH, CFI, CFB Anti-CFH autoantibodies *C3, CFB, CFH, CFHRs, CFI, MCP/CD46, THBD/CD141 (molecular analysis)*
C3 Glomerulopathy (DDD, C3GN)	CH50, APH50, C3, C3a/C3d, SC5b-9, C3 NeF, CFH Anti-CFH autoantibodies *C3, CFB, CFH, CFHRs, CFI, MCP/CD46, THBD/CD141 (molecular analysis)*

greatly reduced activity in either test indicates primary complement deficiency affecting the classical or the alternative or both pathways but may also be due to secondary deficiency caused by increased consumption. Age- and sex-related diffrerences in the complement system should be taken into account in data interpretation [33].

Analysis of individual components and regulators provide insight in which portion of the complement cascade either a lack of function or an (over-)activation occurs. Recently, an algorithm to differentiate primary from secondary aHUS has been proposed based on the assumption that primary aHUS is caused by permanent (genetic or autoimmune) complement dysregulation as opposed to transient complement dysregulation in secondary aHUS. In brief, eculizumab treatment is proposed in TMA patients with evidence for complement activation aimimg to normalize terminal complement activity (MAC/C5b-9) in a first step. In a second step, proximal complement activity (C3 consumption; FH and FI levels) should be evaluated and eculizumab treatment should be continued in patients with proximal complement dysregulation only (primary aHUS), but not in patients with normal proximal complement activation (secondary aHUS) [34].

Analysis of the plasma concentrations of individual complement components such as C3 and C4 is still performed in many clinical laboratories. These tests, however, detect both native and activated, i.e., already "consumed" complement proteins and are strongly influenced by fluctuations in protein synthesis, in particular during the early acute-phase reaction. Modern complement analysis focuses on the quantification of complement-derived split products (e.g., C3a, C3d, C5a or Bb) and/or protein-protein complexes (e.g., sC5b-9), thereby providing comprehensive insight into the actual activation state of the complement system. The choice of the appropriate parameters allows to determine exactly which pathway is activated [35, 36]. The soluble activation product of the terminal complement cascade, sC5b-9, has received considerable attention, as unrestricted progression to its final steps has been linked to specific pathology, i.e. aHUS [37], and has recently been suggested as severity criteria in transplantation-associated thrombotic microangiopathy [38]. The therapeutic efficacy of C5 antibodies in treating aHUS patients is reflected by sC5b-9 suppression [39]. More recently, endothelial cell based ex vivo assays detecting C3 and/or C5b-9 deposition on cultured human microcvascular endothelial cells (HMEC) are offered to detect complement dysregulation in individual patients on target tissue rather than in the circulating blood [40, 41]. While not routinely available, yet, such tests add valuable insights to the complement diagnostic repertoire and have also proven to being successful in determining treatment duration [42].

Of note, complement dysregulation can be primary due to genetic (mutations in complement components and/or regulators) or autoimmune (autoantibodies) alterations, or secondary in context of underlying conditions such as infections, drugs, or mechanical stress (i.e., hypertension) of endothelail cells [43].

A recommended algorithm of complement analysis for both primary and secondary nephropathies is shown in Fig. 21.2.

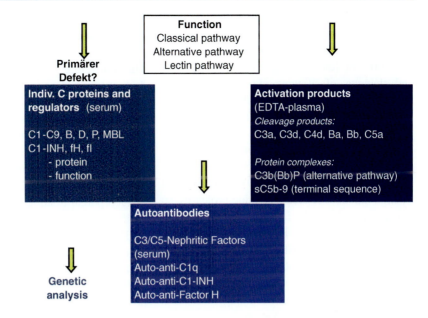

Fig. 21.2 Algorithm of complement analysis

Detecting Autoantibodies

Similar to *loss* or *gain of function* mutations in complement regulators or activating components, overactivation of complement can also be caused by autoantibodies. Autoantibodies to FH (DEAP HUS) [44], FB (DDD) [45], C1q (SLE) [46], or to C1 inhibitor (hereditary angioedema) [47] can be detected by ELISA with the respective purified complement proteins immobilized on a microtiter plate. Results from serial dilutions of patient sera or plasma should be interpreted in comparison with data from large control panels.

Nephritic factors comprise a heterogeneous group of autoantibodies against neoepitopes generated in the C3 and C5 convertases of the complement system, causing its dysregulation [48]. C3 nephritic factor (C3NeF), found in all types of MPGN [49], but especially in dense deposit disease (DDD), can be measured in a decay assay as C3NeF stabilizes the alternative pathway C3 convertase, C3bBb. In this semi-quantitative screening assay C3NeF stabilizes the C3 convertase on sheep erythrocytes, thereby causing increased complement activation and eventually hemolysis [50]. Fluid-phase conversion of C3 upon mixture of normal serum and C3Nef containing patient serum can also be visualized as emerging protein bands of C3b and C3c at lower molecular weight using an immunofixation assay [51]. Recently an ELISA for C3NeF has been reported [36]. Both C3 and C5 nephritic factors correlate with C3 consumption, while only C5 nephritic factors correlated with sC5b-9 levels [52].

Collecting Blood and Urine Samples

Proper collection of (blood and urine) samples for diagnostic analysis is essential [53]. Sample collection should aim at freezing the complement activation status of the patient at the time of blood draw. Without inhibition, physiological and pathological complement activation would continue, thereby obscuring the actual complement activation status and preventing meaningful data interpretation. Therefore, EDTA at ≥ 10 mM final concentration is used as standard anticoagulant since it blocks the *in vitro* activation of the complement system by way of its Mg^{2+} and Ca^{2+} complexing properties. Heparin and citrate are less useful [54]. Centrifuged plasma should be kept on ice or in a refrigerator if analyzed on the same day; for later processing, the sample should be aliquoted, frozen and stored at $-70\ °C$ ($-20\ °C$ for short-term [days] storage). Repeated freezing and thawing of aliquots should be avoided because of the risk of *in vitro* activation (above). If needed, frozen samples should be shipped on dry ice.

In urine, the measurement of activated complement components (such as C3) or degradation products (such as C3a or sC5b-9) can be affected by high amounts of urea and urine proteases, so that the immediate addition of protease inhibitors at sampling is required. However, as oberved by us (Kirschfink, unpublished) and shown by van der Pol et al. [55], appearance of complement activation products in proteinuria may also be the consequence of extrarenal (artificial) rather than intrarenal complement activation.

Immunohistological Diagnosis

The diagnosis of many autoimmune (or immune complex diseases) is based on the detection of immunoglobulins and complement deposition in various tissues. For immunohistochemical diagnosis, antibodies against C1q, C3b, C4b, C4d, and C5b-9 are suitable and are available for frozen and in part also for paraffin fixed tissue. Positive staining identifies a direct impact of complement in the disease process, indicates disease activity and allows for the differentiation of the complement activation pathways involved. The presence of C3b suggests ongoing inflammation, while C3d deposits in the absence of C3b point to a non-active disease process. While its specificity is debatable, for long time C4d has been accepted as biomarker of humoral renal graft rejection [56, 57]. However, more recent studies question the clinical significance of C4d in antibody-mediated rejection [58], whereas it appears as if combined C4d and C3d deposition in IgAN is associated with faster disease progression [59].

Targeting Complement in the Treatment of Kidney Disease

The unraveling of a key role for complement dysregulation in an increasing spectrum of kidney diseases provides an unprecedented treatment approach to diseases, previously only poorly managed and often progressing to ESRD and/or death [60]. Furthermore, despite significant progress in biocompatibility of hemodialysis membranes complement activation during extracorporeal treatment still remains a relevant issue [61].

The overarching principle is the restitution of proper complement control. This may be achieved by replacement of missing or defective complement factors or removal of inhibiting autoantibodies via plasma exchange (PLEX)/plasma infusion (PI). Further strategies include the replacement or supplementation of endogenous soluble complement inhibitors (such as C1-inhibitor, FH, recombinant soluble complement receptor 1 [rsCR1]), the administration of antibodies to block key proteins of the cascade reaction (e.g., C5) or to neutralize complement-derived anaphylatoxins, especially C5a (reviewed in [62–66]).

The use of C1INH (Berinert®) in patients receiving deceased donor kidney transplants with high risk for delayed graft function (DGF) may show significant improvement in outcomes post transplant [67].

Both, eculizumab and ravulizumab prevent the release of the highly potent inflammatory anaphylatoxin C5a and the assembly of the membrane attack complex C5b-9 with the advantage of leaving the activation phase of complement up to the generation of the C3 opsonins C3b and iC3b intact. Despite excellent results of treatment with eculizumab and ravulizumab in cinical trials, their is still a great uncertainty with respect the optimal treatment strategy, especially on the decision how to proceed when a patient is stable and in remission [68]. The potential risk of aHUS recurrence after discontinuation of eculizumab treatment raises the question how long eculizumab should be administered [69]. Risk factors for aHUS recurrence after eculizumab discontinuation include a positive family history of aHUS, presence of pathogenic genetic variants, and extra-renal manifestations of aHUS prior to eculizumab treatment [70]. In a recent survey, Fakhouri et al. confirmed the central role of complement mutations for aHUS recurrence but also concluded that a strategy of eculizumab discontinuation guided by the genetic diagnosis was in most patients reasonable and safe [71]. Collection of outcome data in patients with aHUS, either receiving eculizumab or other treatments, will certainly help to optimize therapy. While the treatment of aHUS with eculizumab has been highly successful in most cases [72–74], its use for other complement-mediated renal diseases is still a matter of ongoing clinical research [75, 76]. The off-label use of eculizumab in patients with C3 glomerulopathy (C3G) including dense deposit disease (DDD) and C3 glomerulonephritis (C3GN) has yielded mixed responses thus far, without uniformly countering key pathological markers (that is, proteinuria), which has prompted the evaluation of alternative therapeutics interferring with the complement cascade more proximally.

Eculizumab is currently being used in renal transplantation and has been evaluated in several clinical trials to minimize the consequences of ischemia-reoxygenation injury (IRI), prevent or treat relapsing or de novo aHUS, and to prevent and cure humoral rejection in patients at high immunological risk (i.e., DSA; ABO-incompatibility) [77, 78]. However, the C5 inhibitor appears less effective in preventing delayed graft function [78].

A second anti-C5 monoclonal antibody with increased half-life, named ravulizumab, has recently been approved by the US Food and Drug Administration for paroxysmal nocturnal haemoglobinuria (PNH) and aHUS in adults and children from 1 months of age [79]. With an extended plasma residence it only requires administration every 8 weeks instead of biweekly, an important step in improving patient management. The long-lasting anti-C5 antibody Ravulizumab has successfully been used in adult and pediatric aHUS [79, 80], and is currently being tested in clinical trials for lupus nephritis and IgA nephropathy.

Besides monitoring of eculizumab-treated patients on the basis of traditional parameters such as lactate dehydrogenase (LDH), hemoglobin (Hb), haptoglobin, platelets and serum creatinine, additional analyses of complement activation including CH50 and AH50 (reflect inhibitory efficacy), sC5b-9, C3 and C3d (indicating potential ongoing *in vivo* activation) provide valuable informations on therapeutic efficacy and may allow—together with drug monitoring—for the re-evaluation of the use and dosage of eculizumab in the heterogeneous group of complement-mediated renal diseases [68, 81].

In certain indications, broader inhibition of complement at the level of C3 may warrant investigation, leveraging clinical benefits over existing therapies, and C3-targeted therapeutics are now being evaluated in long-awaited phase II/III trials [65, 82, 83]. Specifically, alternative C3 convertase (C3bBb) inhibitors at the level of FB or C3 have successfully been tested in paroxysmal nocturnal hemoglobinuria (PNH), and are currently clinically trialed in C3 glomerulopathy (C3G).

Ongoing clinical trials are examining the efficacy of specific blockade in C3G with narsoplimab, sut-imlimab, and danicopan, all of which inhibit complement activation more proximally. Other renal diseases, such as IgA nephropathy, lupus nephritis, and membranous nephropathy are also under study with complement inhibiton. (Gavrillaki and Brodski, 2020) While broader intervention at the level of C3 or the overactive AP seems mechanistically more justified, targeted C5aR1 inhibition using the orally available drug candidate avacopan has shown early clinical promise in C3G and ANCA vasculits [84]. Moreover, an anti-MASP2 mAb is currently being evaluated in clinical trials for various nephropathies, such as IgA nephropathy, aHUS and Lupus Nephritis. Inhibitors targeting the lectin pathway, of FB, FD and C3 are currently at varying stages of clinical development [65, 85].

Summary and Perspectives

The complement system, a complex network of proteins and critical part of the innate immune response significantly contributes to the pathogenesis of inflammatory kidney diseases. A thorough understanding of the basic disease mechanism and careful follow-up are needed for optimal therapy. Comprehensive modern serological and molecular complement analysis is indispensable for correct differential diagnosis of the renal disorders.

Selective complement targeting to inhibit cascade activation can halt or even reverse renal disease. However, to delineate which pathway(s), and at what level, intervention could be effective still requires further translational and clinical research to open new avenues for successful treatment strategies for renal disease.

References

1. Ricklin D, Lambris JD. Complement in immune and inflammatory disorders: pathophysiological mechanisms. J Immunol. 2013;190:3831–8.
2. Figueroa JE, Densen P. Infectious diseases associated with complement deficiencies. Clin Microbiol Rev. 1991;4:359–95.
3. Abel G, Agnello V. Complement deficiencies: a 2004 update. In: Szebeni J, editor. The complement system Novel roles in health and disease. Boston: Kluwer Academic Publishers; 2004. p. 201–28.
4. Botto M, Kirschfink M, Macor P, Pickering MC, Wurzner R, Tedesco F. Complement in human diseases: lessons from complement deficiencies. Mol Immunol. 2009;46:2774–83.
5. Brodszki N, Frazer-Abel A, Grumach AS, Kirschfink M, Litzman J, Perez E, Seppanen MRJ, Sullivan KE, Jolles S. European Society for Immunodeficiencies (ESID) and European Reference Network on Rare Primary Immunodeficiency, Autoinflammatory and Autoimmune Diseases (ERN RITA) complement guideline: deficiencies, diagnosis, and management. J Clin Immunol. 2020;40:576–91.
6. Zilow G, Joka T, Obertacke U, Rother U, Kirschfink M. Generation of anaphylatoxin C3a in plasma and bronchoalveolar lavage fluid in trauma patients at risk for the adult respiratory distress syndrome. Crit Care Med. 1992;20:468–73.
7. Zetoune FS, Ward PA. Role of complement and histones in sepsis. Front Med (Lausanne). 2020;7:616957.
8. Rittirsch D, Redl H, Huber-Lang M. Role of complement in multiorgan failure. Clin Dev Immunol. 2012;2012:962927.
9. Farrar CA, Keogh B, McCormack W, O'Shaughnessy A, Parker A, Reilly M, Sacks SH. Inhibition of TLR2 promotes graft function in a murine model of renal transplant ischemia-reperfusion injury. FASEB J. 2012;26:799–807.
10. Farrar CA, Asgari E, Schwaeble WJ, Sacks SH. Which pathways trigger the role of complement in ischaemia/reperfusion injury? Front Immunol. 2012;3:341.
11. Willows J, Brown M, Sheerin NS. The role of complement in kidney disease. Clin Med (Lond). 2020;20:156–60.
12. Thurman JM. Complement in kidney disease: core curriculum 2015. Am J Kidney Dis. 2015;65:156–68.
13. Kirschfink M, Kovacs B, Mottaghy K. Extracorporeal circulation: in vivo and in vitro analysis of complement activation by heparin-bonded surfaces. Circ Shock. 1993;40:221–6.
14. Mollnes TE. Biocompatibility: complement as mediator of tissue damage and as indicator of incompatibility. Exp Clin Immunogenet. 1997;14:24–9.
15. Walport MJ. Complement. Second of two parts. N Engl J Med. 2001;344:1140–4.
16. Walport MJ. Complement. First of two parts. N Engl J Med. 2001;344:1058–66.
17. Carol M, Pelegri C, Castellote C, Franch A, Castell M. Immunohistochemical study of lymphoid tissues in adjuvant arthritis (AA) by image analysis; relationship with synovial lesions. Clin Exp Immunol. 2000;120:200–8.
18. Ricklin D, Hajishengallis G, Yang K, Lambris JD. Complement: a key system for immune surveillance and homeostasis. Nat Immunol. 2010;11:785–97.
19. Arbore G, Kemper C, Kolev M. Intracellular complement—the complosome—in immune cell regulation. Mol Immunol. 2017;89:2–9.
20. Zhou W, Marsh JE, Sacks SH. Intrarenal synthesis of complement. Kidney Int. 2001;59:1227–35.
21. Mayilyan KR. Complement genetics, deficiencies, and disease associations. Protein Cell. 2012;3:487–96.
22. Merle NS, Church SE, Fremeaux-Bacchi V, Roumenina LT. Complement system part I—molecular mechanisms of activation and regulation. Front Immunol. 2015;6:262.
23. Merle NS, Noe R, Halbwachs-Mecarelli L, Fremeaux-Bacchi V, Roumenina LT. Complement system part II: role in immunity. Front Immunol. 2015;6:257.
24. Klos A, Tenner AJ, Johswich KO, Ager RR, Reis ES, Kohl J. The role of the anaphylatoxins in health and disease. Mol Immunol. 2009;46:2753–66.
25. Sacks SH. Complement fragments C3a and C5a: the salt and pepper of the immune response. Eur J Immunol. 2010;40:668–70.
26. Wan JX, Fukuda N, Endo M, Tahira Y, Yao EH, Matsuda H, Ueno T, Matsumoto K. Complement

3 is involved in changing the phenotype of human glomerular mesangial cells. J Cell Physiol. 2007;213:495–501.

27. Thurman JM, Lenderink AM, Royer PA, Coleman KE, Zhou J, Lambris JD, Nemenoff RA, Quigg RJ, Holers VM. C3a is required for the production of CXC chemokines by tubular epithelial cells after renal ishemia/reperfusion. J Immunol. 2007;178:1819–28.

28. Ekdahl KN, Teramura Y, Hamad OA, Asif S, Duehrkop C, Fromell K, Gustafson E, Hong J, Kozarcanin H, Magnusson PU, Huber-Lang M, Garred P, Nilsson B. Dangerous liaisons: complement, coagulation, and kallikrein/kinin cross-talk act as a linchpin in the events leading to thromboinflammation. Immunol Rev. 2016;274:245–69.

29. Zipfel PF, Skerka C. Complement regulators and inhibitory proteins. Nat Rev Immunol. 2009;9:729–40.

30. Schmidt CQ, Lambris JD, Ricklin D. Protection of host cells by complement regulators. Immunol Rev. 2016;274:152–71.

31. Mollnes TE, Jokiranta TS, Truedsson L, Nilsson B, Rodriguez de Cordoba S, Kirschfink M. Complement analysis in the 21st century. Mol Immunol. 2007;44:3838–49.

32. Seelen MA, Roos A, Wieslander J, Mollnes TE, Sjoholm AG, Wurzner R, Loos M, Tedesco F, Sim RB, Garred P, Alexopoulos E, Turner MW, Daha MR. Functional analysis of the classical, alternative, and MBL pathways of the complement system: standardization and validation of a simple ELISA. J Immunol Methods. 2005;296:187–98.

33. Gaya da Costa M, Poppelaars F, van Kooten C, Mollnes TE, Tedesco F, Wurzner R, Trouw LA, Truedsson L, Daha MR, Roos A, Seelen MA. Age and sex-associated changes of complement activity and complement levels in a healthy caucasian population. Front Immunol. 2018;9:2664.

34. Berger BE. Atypical hemolytic uremic syndrome: a syndrome in need of clarity. Clin Kidney J. 2019;12:338–47.

35. Schroder-Braunstein J, Kirschfink M. Complement deficiencies and dysregulation: pathophysiological consequences, modern analysis, and clinical management. Mol Immunol. 2019;114:299–311.

36. Skattum L. Clinical complement analysis-an overview. Transfus Med Rev. 2019;33:207–16.

37. Noris M, Remuzzi G. Atypical hemolytic-uremic syndrome. N Engl J Med. 2009;361:1676–87.

38. Kennedy GA, Bleakley S, Butler J, Mudie K, Kearey N, Durrant S. Posttransplant thrombotic microangiopathy: sensitivity of proposed new diagnostic criteria. Transfusion. 2009;49:1884–9.

39. Legendre CM, Licht C, Muus P, Greenbaum LA, Babu S, Bedrosian C, Bingham C, Cohen DJ, Delmas Y, Douglas K, Eitner F, Feldkamp T, Fouque D, Furman RR, Gaber O, Herthelius M, Hourmant M, Karpman D, Lebranchu Y, Mariat C, Menne J, Moulin B, Nurnberger J, Ogawa M, Remuzzi G, Richard T, Sberro-Soussan R, Severino B, Sheerin NS, Trivelli A, Zimmerhackl LB, Goodship T, Loirat

C. Terminal complement inhibitor eculizumab in atypical hemolytic-uremic syndrome. N Engl J Med. 2013;368:2169–81.

40. Noris M, Galbusera M, Gastoldi S, Macor P, Banterla F, Bresin E, Tripodo C, Bettoni S, Donadelli R, Valoti E, Tedesco F, Amore A, Coppo R, Ruggenenti P, Gotti E, Remuzzi G. Dynamics of complement activation in aHUS and how to monitor eculizumab therapy. Blood. 2014;124:1715–26.

41. Galbusera M, Noris M, Gastoldi S, Bresin E, Mele C, Breno M, Cuccarolo P, Alberti M, Valoti E, Piras R, Donadelli R, Vivarelli M, Murer L, Pecoraro C, Ferrari E, Perna A, Benigni A, Portalupi V, Remuzzi G. An ex vivo test of complement activation on endothelium for individualized eculizumab therapy in hemolytic uremic syndrome. Am J Kidney Dis. 2019;74:56–72.

42. Meuleman MS, Duval A, Fremeaux-Bacchi V, Roumenina LT, Chauvet S. Ex vivo test for measuring complement attack on endothelial cells: from research to bedside. Front Immunol. 2022;13:860689.

43. Praga M, Rodriguez de Cordoba S. Secondary atypical hemolytic uremic syndromes in the era of complement blockade. Kidney Int. 2019;95:1298–300.

44. Jozsi M, Licht C, Strobel S, Zipfel SL, Richter H, Heinen S, Zipfel PF, Skerka C. Factor H autoantibodies in atypical hemolytic uremic syndrome correlate with CFHR1/CFHR3 deficiency. Blood. 2008;111:1512–4.

45. Strobel S, Zimmering M, Papp K, Prechl J, Jozsi M. Anti-factor B autoantibody in dense deposit disease. Mol Immunol. 2010;47:1476–83.

46. Mahler M, van Schaarenburg RA, Trouw LA. Anti-C1q autoantibodies, novel tests, and clinical consequences. Front Immunol. 2013;4:117.

47. Cugno M, Castelli R, Cicardi M. Angioedema due to acquired C1-inhibitor deficiency: a bridging condition between autoimmunity and lymphoproliferation. Autoimmun Rev. 2008;8:156–9.

48. Corvillo F, Okroj M, Nozal P, Melgosa M, Sanchez-Corral P, Lopez-Trascasa M. Nephritic factors: an overview of classification, diagnostic tools and clinical associations. Front Immunol. 2019;10:886.

49. Schwertz R, Rother U, Anders D, Gretz N, Scharer K, Kirschfink M. Complement analysis in children with idiopathic membranoproliferative glomerulonephritis: a long-term follow-up. Pediatr Allergy Immunol. 2001;12:166–72.

50. Rother U. A new screening test for C3 nephritis factor based on a stable cell bound convertase on sheep erythrocytes. J Immunol Methods. 1982;51:101–7.

51. Koch FJ, Jenis EH, Valeski JE. Test for C3 nephritic factor activity by immunofixation electrophoresis. Am J Clin Pathol. 1981;76:63–7.

52. Marinozzi MC, Chauvet S, Le Quintrec M, Mignotet M, Petitprez F, Legendre C, Cailliez M, Deschenes G, Fischbach M, Karras A, Nobili F, Pietrement C, Dragon-Durey MA, Fakhouri F, Roumenina LT, Fremeaux-Bacchi V. C5 nephritic factors drive the biological phenotype of C3 glomerulopathies. Kidney Int. 2017;92:1232–41.

53. Frazer-Abel A, Kirschfink M, Prohaszka Z. Expanding horizons in complement analysis and quality control. Front Immunol. 2021;12:697313.
54. Mollnes TE, Garred P, Bergseth G. Effect of time, temperature and anticoagulants on in vitro complement activation: consequences for collection and preservation of samples to be examined for complement activation. Clin Exp Immunol. 1988;73:484–8.
55. van der Pol P, de Vries DK, van Gijlswijk DJ, van Anken GE, Schlagwein N, Daha MR, Aydin Z, de Fijter JW, Schaapherder AF, van Kooten C. Pitfalls in urinary complement measurements. Transpl Immunol. 2012;27:55–8.
56. Feucht HE, Schneeberger H, Hillebrand G, Burkhardt K, Weiss M, Riethmuller G, Land W, Albert E. Capillary deposition of C4d complement fragment and early renal graft loss. Kidney Int. 1993;43:1333–8.
57. Cohen D, Colvin RB, Daha MR, Drachenberg CB, Haas M, Nickeleit V, Salmon JE, Sis B, Zhao MH, Bruijn JA, Bajema IM. Pros and cons for C4d as a biomarker. Kidney Int. 2012;81:628–39.
58. Orandi BJ, Alachkar N, Kraus ES, Naqvi F, Lonze BE, Lees L, Van Arendonk KJ, Wickliffe C, Bagnasco SM, Zachary AA, Segev DL, Montgomery RA. Presentation and outcomes of C4d-negative antibody-mediated rejection after kidney transplantation. Am J Transplant. 2016;16:213–20.
59. Faria B, Henriques C, Matos AC, Daha MR, Pestana M, Seelen M. Combined C4d and CD3 immunostaining predicts immunoglobulin (Ig)A nephropathy progression. Clin Exp Immunol. 2015;179:354–61.
60. Zipfel PF, Wiech T, Rudnick R, Afonso S, Person F, Skerka C. Complement inhibitors in clinical trials for glomerular diseases. Front Immunol. 2019;10:2166.
61. Poppelaars F, Faria B, Gaya da Costa M, Franssen CFM, van Son WJ, Berger SP, Daha MR, Seelen MA. The complement system in dialysis: a forgotten story? Front Immunol. 2018;9:71.
62. Ricklin D, Mastellos DC, Lambris JD. Therapeutic targeting of the complement system. Nat Rev Drug Discov. 2019.
63. Ricklin D, Mastellos DC, Reis ES, Lambris JD. The renaissance of complement therapeutics. Nat Rev Nephrol. 2018;14:26–47.
64. Ort M, Dingemanse J, van den Anker J, Kaufmann P. Treatment of rare inflammatory kidney diseases: drugs targeting the terminal complement pathway. Front Immunol. 2020;11:599417.
65. Mastellos DC, Ricklin D, Lambris JD. Clinical promise of next-generation complement therapeutics. Nat Rev Drug Discov. 2019;18:707–29.
66. Andrighetto S, Leventhal J, Zaza G, Cravedi P. Complement and complement targeting therapies in glomerular diseases. Int J Mol Sci. 2019;20:6336.
67. Huang E, Vo A, Choi J, Ammerman N, Lim K, Sethi S, Kim I, Kumar S, Najjar R, Peng A, Jordan SC. Three-year outcomes of a randomized, double-blind, placebo-controlled study assessing safety and efficacy of C1 esterase inhibitor for prevention of delayed graft function in deceased donor kidney transplant recipients. Clin J Am Soc Nephrol. 2020;15:109–16.
68. Wijnsma KL, Duineveld C, Wetzels JFM, van de Kar N. Eculizumab in atypical hemolytic uremic syndrome: strategies toward restrictive use. Pediatr Nephrol. 2019;34:2261–77.
69. Sahutoglu T, Basturk T, Sakaci T, Koc Y, Ahbap E, Sevinc M, Kara E, Akgol C, Caglayan FB, Unsal A, Daha MR. Can eculizumab be discontinued in aHUS? Case report and review of the literature. Medicine (Baltimore). 2016;95:e4330.
70. Ariceta G, Fakhouri F, Sartz L, Miller B, Nikolaou V, Cohen D, Siedlecki AM, Ardissino G. Eculizumab discontinuation in atypical haemolytic uraemic syndrome: TMA recurrence risk and renal outcomes. Clin Kidney J. 2021;14:2075–84.
71. Fakhouri F, Fila M, Hummel A, Ribes D, Sellier-Leclerc AL, Ville S, Pouteil-Noble C, Coindre JP, Le Quintrec M, Rondeau E, Boyer O, Provot F, Djeddi D, Hanf W, Delmas Y, Louillet F, Lahoche A, Favre G, Chatelet V, Launay EA, Presne C, Zaloszyc A, Caillard S, Bally S, Raimbourg Q, Tricot L, Mousson C, Le Thuaut A, Loirat C, Fremeaux-Bacchi V. Eculizumab discontinuation in children and adults with atypical hemolytic-uremic syndrome: a prospective multicenter study. Blood. 2021;137:2438–49.
72. Legendre CM, Licht C, Loirat C. Eculizumab in atypical hemolytic-uremic syndrome. N Engl J Med. 2013;369:1379–80.
73. Nurnberger J, Philipp T, Witzke O, Opazo Saez A, Vester U, Baba HA, Kribben A, Zimmerhackl LB, Janecke AR, Nagel M, Kirschfink M. Eculizumab for atypical hemolytic-uremic syndrome. N Engl J Med. 2009;360:542–4.
74. Gruppo RA, Rother RP. Eculizumab for congenital atypical hemolytic-uremic syndrome. N Engl J Med. 2009;360:544–6.
75. Ricklin D, Lambris JD. Progress and trends in complement therapeutics. Adv Exp Med Biol. 2013;735:1–22.
76. Emlen W, Li W, Kirschfink M. Therapeutic complement inhibition: new developments. Semin Thromb Hemost. 2010;36:660–8.
77. Grenda R, Durlik M. Eculizumab in renal transplantation: a 2017 update. Ann Transplant. 2017;22:550–4.
78. Glotz D, Russ G, Rostaing L, Legendre C, Tufveson G, Chadban S, Grinyo J, Mamode N, Rigotti P, Couzi L, Buchler M, Sandrini S, Dain B, Garfield M, Ogawa M, Richard T, Marks WH, Group CS. Safety and efficacy of eculizumab for the prevention of antibody-mediated rejection after deceased-donor kidney transplantation in patients with preformed donor-specific antibodies. Am J Transplant. 2019;19:2865–75.
79. Rondeau E, Scully M, Ariceta G, Barbour T, Cataland S, Heyne N, Miyakawa Y, Ortiz S, Swenson E, Vallee M, Yoon SS, Kavanagh D, Haller H, Studya G. The long-acting C5 inhibitor, Ravulizumab, is effective and safe in adult patients with atypical hemolytic uremic syndrome naive to complement inhibitor treatment. Kidney Int. 2020;97:1287–96.

80. Ariceta G, Dixon BP, Kim SH, Kapur G, Mauch T, Ortiz S, Vallee M, Denker AE, Kang HG, Greenbaum LA, Study G. The long-acting C5 inhibitor, ravulizumab, is effective and safe in pediatric patients with atypical hemolytic uremic syndrome naive to complement inhibitor treatment. Kidney Int. 2021;100:225–37.

81. Wehling C, Amon O, Bommer M, Hoppe B, Kentouche K, Schalk G, Weimer R, Wiesener M, Hohenstein B, Tonshoff B, Buscher R, Fehrenbach H, Gok ON, Kirschfink M. Monitoring of complement activation biomarkers and eculizumab in complement-mediated renal disorders. Clin Exp Immunol. 2017;187:304–15.

82. Smith RJH, Appel GB, Blom AM, Cook HT, D'Agati VD, Fakhouri F, Fremeaux-Bacchi V, Jozsi M, Kavanagh D, Lambris JD, Noris M, Pickering MC, Remuzzi G, de Cordoba SR, Sethi S, Van der Vlag J, Zipfel PF, Nester CM. C3 glomerulopathy—understanding a rare complement-driven renal disease. Nat Rev Nephrol. 2019;15:129–43.

83. Raina R, Vijayvargiya N, Khooblall A, Melachuri M, Deshpande S, Sharma D, Mathur K, Arora M, Sethi SK, Sandhu S. Pediatric atypical hemolytic uremic syndrome advances. Cell. 2021;10:3580.

84. Jayne DRW, Bruchfeld AN, Harper L, Schaier M, Venning MC, Hamilton P, Burst V, Grundmann F, Jadoul M, Szombati I, Tesar V, Segelmark M, Potarca A, Schall TJ, Bekker P, Group CS. Randomized trial of C5a receptor inhibitor avacopan in ANCA-associated vasculitis. J Am Soc Nephrol. 2017;28:2756–67.

85. Zelek WM, Xie L, Morgan BP, Harris CL. Compendium of current complement therapeutics. Mol Immunol. 2019;114:341–52.

Atypical Hemolytic Uremic Syndrome

22

Michal Malina ⓘ, Veronique Fremeaux-Bacchi, and Sally Johnson

Introduction

The hemolytic uremic syndrome (HUS) is a thrombotic microangiopathy (TMA) characterized by the triad of thrombocytopenia, nonimmune microangiopathic hemolytic anemia, and acute kidney injury [1]. The most frequent form of HUS in children is secondary to Shiga toxin (Stx)—producing *Escherichia coli* (STEC) and the term atypical HUS (aHUS) was initially used to designate any HUS not caused by STEC. It is now clear that within the umbrella of aHUS are a number of specific causes of HUS—for example *Streptococcus pneumoniae* infection, cobalamin C defect, Diacylglycerol kinase ε (DGKε) defect and various underlying conditions.

Atypical HUS without coexisting disease or specific infection is mostly a disease of complement alternative pathway (AP) overactivation,

due to hereditary mutations in complement genes or acquired autoantibodies against complement factor H (FH). The clinical characteristics of patients, patient outcome and genotype-phenotype correlations were described [2–7]. Therefore, the term aHUS is today preferentially used to designate HUS without coexisting disease or specific infection [5, 6, 8–11]. Plasma exchange (PE) was the mainstay of treatment for aHUS until 2009, with considerable morbidity in children [12, 13]. Since 2009, terminal complement blockade therapy by eculizumab has dramatically changed the hitherto dismal outcome of the disease [14, 15]. The aims of this chapter are to summarize the previous era of treatment, to review new knowledge in the domain of atypical HUS and to scan the horizon for future developments in the management of atypical HUS.

M. Malina (✉) · S. Johnson
National Renal Complement Therapeutics Centre and Great North Children's Hospital, Royal Victoria Infirmary, Newcastle Upon Tyne Hospitals NHS Foundation Trust, Newcastle, UK

Translation and Clinical Research Institute, Newcastle University, Tyne, UK
e-mail: michal.malina@nhs.net;
sally.johnson15@nhs.net

V. Fremeaux-Bacchi
Assistance Publique-Hôpitaux de Paris, Hôpital Européen Georges Pompidou, Laboratory of Immunology, Paris, France
e-mail: veronique.fremeaux-bacchi@aphp.fr

Definition of Atypical HUS

Atypical HUS is one of a number of causes of TMA—life or organ threatening diseases characterized by microthrombi in small blood vessels which can be classified according to etiology and/or physiopathology [16–19] (Fig. 22.1). The two most important TMAs to exclude when suspecting aHUS are thrombotic thrombocytopenic purpura (TTP) and shigatoxin associated HUS (STEC HUS). The latter is the most common TMA affecting the kidneys in children. It is caused by

---

© The Author(s), under exclusive license to Springer Nature Switzerland AG 2023
F. Schaefer, L. A. Greenbaum (eds.), *Pediatric Kidney Disease*,
https://doi.org/10.1007/978-3-031-11665-0_22

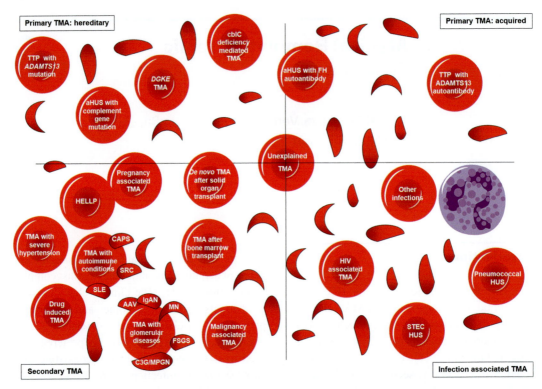

Fig. 22.1 Thrombotic microangiopathies are classified into: Inherited or acquired primary; secondary; or infection associated TMAs. Current classifications define primary TMAs as hereditary (mutations in ADAMTS13, MMACHC (cb1c deficiency), or genes encoding complement proteins) or acquired (autoantibodies to ADAMTS13, or autoantibodies to complement FH, which is associated with homozygous CFHR3/1 deletion). TMA is associated with various infections: in STEC-HUS and pneumococcal HUS, distinct mechanisms result in TMA; in other infections, the processes are not defined and in some cases the infection may trigger manifestation of a primary TMA. Secondary TMAs occur in a spectrum of conditions, and in many cases the pathogenic mechanisms are multifactorial or unknown. The classification presented here is not unequivocal: in some secondary TMAs, for example pregnancy-associated TMA or de novo TMA after transplantation, a significant proportion of individuals will have a genetic predisposition to a primary TMA. *AAV* ANCA-associated vasculitis; *ADAMTS13* a disintegrin and metalloproteinase with a thrombospondin type 1 motif, member 13; *aHUS* atypical hemolytic uremic syndrome; *C3G* C3 glomerulopathy; *CAPS* catastrophic antiphospholipid syndrome; *cblC* cobalamin C type; *DGKE* gene encoding diacylglycerol kinase ε; *FH* factor H; *HELLP* syndrome of hemolysis, elevated liver enzymes, and low platelets; *HUS* hemolytic uremic syndrome; *IgAN* IgA nephropathy; *MN* membranous nephropathy; *MPGN* membranoproliferative glomerulonephritis; *SRC* scleroderma renal crisis; *STEC* shiga toxin–producing Escherichia coli; *TMA* thrombotic microangiopathy; *TTP* thrombotic thrombocytopenic purpura. Reproduced from Brocklebank et al. [19]

intestinal infection by certain strains of E coli carrying a plasmid for producing shigatoxin, particularly serotypes O157:H7, O104:H4 and O26 and in rare cases by Shigella dysenteriae [20, 21]. This type of HUS was previously labeled as typical or D+, however this classification is now obsolete.

TTP is an important cause of TMA that must be ruled out before making a diagnosis of aHUS. It is due to a severe deficiency (<10%) in ADAMTS13 (A Disintegrin And Metalloproteinase with a ThromboSpondin type 1 motif, member 13) activity, either from a congenital absence of functional protein caused by homozygous or compound heterozygous mutations in the *ADAMTS13* gene, or due to anti-ADAMTS13 antibodies [22].

TMA can also occur secondary to a coexisting disease or condition, such as malignancy or autoimmune disease. This is more common in adults than children, with the exception of post-hematopoietic stem cell transplant (HSCT) TMA.

As the classification of TMA has evolved with increasing understanding [23], there is general agreement that the term aHUS defines patients with HUS without a coexisting disease or specific infection [5, 6, 8–11]. This chapter is focused on aHUS according to this definition.

Incidence and Prevalence of Atypical HUS

Atypical HUS, defined as indicated above, is an ultra-rare disease. In the United States, aHUS is considered to have an annual incidence rate of two new pediatric cases per million total population [24]]. An incidence of approximately 0.11 new pediatric cases per million total population per year was also observed between July 2009 and December 2010 in an exhaustive cohort of children with aHUS from France, the United Kingdom, Spain, Netherlands and Canada [13]. A recent systematic review has reported an overview of global incidence and prevalence of aHUS [25]. Eight studies were reviewed from Europe, Australia, and New Zealand [5, 26–32]. In Europe the reported incidence (all ages) ranged between 0.23 and 1.9 per million annually [5, 32]. In Australia a pediatric study reported a calculated incidence of 0.44 per million annually [28]. Studies reporting incidence for individuals under 20 years of age ranged between 0.26 and 0.75 per million annually [27, 32]. A systematic review by Yan reported that in individuals under 20 years of age, the prevalence of aHUS ranged between 2.21 and 9.4 per million people [25].

The Alternative Pathway of Complement

The alternative pathway (AP) of the complement system plays a predominant, though not exclusive role in aHUS (Fig. 22.2) [33–46]. The complement system is composed of plasma proteins that react with one another to opsonize microbes and induce a series of inflammatory responses that help the immune cells to fight infection. There is mounting evidence that complement participates not only in the defense against pathogens, but also in host homeostasis [47–52]. The complement cascade can be activated by three different pathways. While the activation of the classical and the lectin pathways occurs after binding to immune complexes or microorganisms respectively, the AP is continuously activated and generates C3b which binds indiscriminately to pathogens and host cells. On a foreign surface, C3b binds factor B (FB), which is then cleaved by Factor D to form the C3 convertase C3bBb. The C3 convertase, which is stabilized by its binding to properdin, induces exponential cleavage of C3b and the generation of C3bBbC3b complexes with C5 convertase activity. The C5 convertase cleaves C5 to generate C5a—the most potent anaphylatoxin—and C5b which initiates the formation of the membrane attack complex (MAC or C5b-9), able to lyse pathogens [52] (Fig. 22.2). The CAP amplification loop is normally strictly controlled at the surface of the host quiescent endothelium, which is protected from the local formation of the C3 convertase by complement regulatory proteins. These include regulators in serum, such as FH and Factor I (FI), as well as membrane bound CD46 (membrane cofactor protein (MCP), which cooperate locally to inactivate C3b. FH is the most important protein for the regulation of the CAP and consists of 20 short consensus repeats (SCRs) and contain two C3b-binding sites (Fig. 22.3). MCP is a widely expressed transmembrane glycoprotein that binds C3b and inhibits complement activation on host cells. The serine protease FI cleaves C3b in the presence of various cofactors including FH, complement receptor 1 (CR1, CD35) and MCP. Coagulation regulator thrombomodulin (THBD) enhances FI-mediated inactivation of C3b in the presence of FH [47, 52].

Over the past 20 years, genetic discoveries have substantially improved our understanding of the mechanisms responsible for aHUS and driven development of novel therapeutic strategies) [33–46] (Fig. 22.4). In a large genetic screen of 794 aHUS patients, rare variants in one the 5 genes (*CFH*, *C3*, *CFI*, *CFB*, or *CD46*) that encode proteins involved in the regulation of the alternative pathway of complement were identified in 41% of patients and combinations of mutations were noted

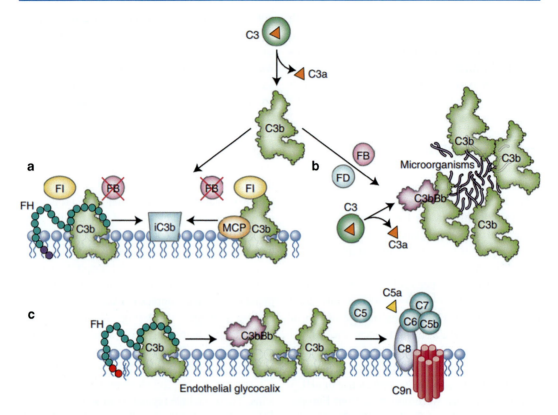

Fig. 22.2 Complement activation and its regulation. aHUS is the prototype of a disease resulting from inefficient protection of endothelial cells against complement activation. (**a**) Protection of cells surface. The AP is permanently active, with a continuous formation of small amounts of the C3 convertase C3bBb at the cell surface. To prevent unopposed complement activation resulting in cell damage, the complement system is tighly regulated. The glycocalyx is a multifunctional thick carbohydrate layer containing glycoaminoglycans (GAG) (heparin sulphate, sialic acid, polyanions) that covers all endothelial cells, in particular the glomerular endothelium in the kidney. FH binds to GAG and C3b. MCP is constitutionally anchored to endothelial membrane. Under normal conditions, the C3 convertase formation is stopped by the interaction of FH or MCP with C3b, which makes further binding of FB to C3b impossible. C3b is then cleaved by FI to iC3b, which cannot bind FB. (**b**) Activation of complement and covalent attachment of C3b to the microbial surfaces. The major function of complement is to act as a defense mechanism against microbes. Very small amounts of C3b are normally present in plasma due to low levels of spontaneous C3 cleavage but C3b can bind to bacteria. Once C3b is covalently bound to the surface of microorganisms, FB binds to it and becomes susceptible to cleavage by Factor D (FD). The resulting C3bBb complex is a C3 convertase that will continue to generate more C3b, thus amplifying C3b production. C3b attaches to bacterial surfaces for opsonization by phagocytes and simultaneous activation of the cytolytic terminal complement cascade. (**c**) In the case of aHUS, AP activation is uncontrolled and C3 convertase C3bBb and C5 convertase C3bC3bBb are formed. During complement activation, C5 is split into C5a and C5b. C5b together with complement proteins C6, C7, C8 and C9 form the C5b9 complex in sublytic quantities that activate endothelial cells to produce prothrombotic factors. *AP* alternative pathway, *C3bBb* C3 convertase; *C3bC3bBb* C5 convertase; *FB* complement factor B; *FD* complement factor D; *FH* complement factor H; *FI* complement factor I; *MCP* membrane cofactor protein (CD46)

in 3% of patients [53]. Predisposition to aHUS is inherited in an autosomal recessive or autosomal dominant manner with incomplete penetrance.

An updated database describing all rare variants identified in aHUS is available at https://www.complement-db.org [54, 55] and these genetic abnormalities are described in more detail in specific sections of this chapter. In addition, acquired autoantibodies to the FH protein (anti-FH) have been demonstrated in patients with aHUS, also described in more detail below.

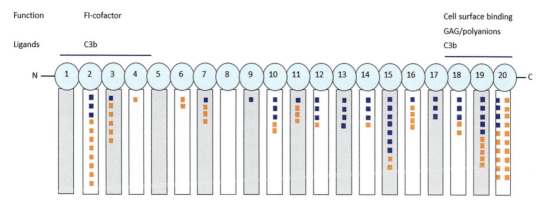

Fig. 22.3 Complement factor H. FH is a plasma protein consisting in 20 domains called short consensus repeats (SCRs) (*numbered circles*). FH has two C3b binding sites: one is localized within the N-terminal SCR 1–4, implicated in the cleavage of C3b by FI and the other in the C-terminal SCR 19–20, implicated in cell surface binding. FH regulates the formation, stability and decay of the C3 convertase C3bBb. *94 rare variants in CFH reported in the aHUS database https://www.complement-db.org are shown within columns. Blue squares indicate frameshift, deletion, nonsense and conserved cysteine affected variants (prediction of quantitative FH deficiency), orange squares indicate missense variants (with or without demonstrating functional consequences). 20% of all variants are located in the C-terminus SCR 20 and are mostly associated with normal FH plasma level. *FH* complement factor H; *FI* complement factor I; *GAG* glycoaminoglycans; *SCR* short consensus repeat

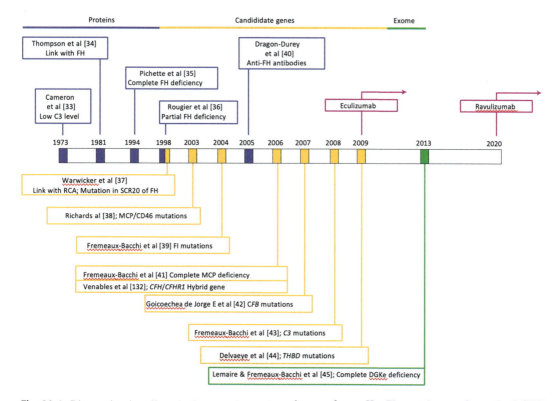

Fig. 22.4 Discoveries that allowed a better understanding of the pathophysiology of aHUS during the last decades. This led to the approval of eculizumab for the treatment of patients with aHUS, to control the overactivation of complement. *FB* complement factor B; *FH* complement factor H; *FI* complement factor I; *DGKE* diacylglycerol kinase ε; *MCP* membrane cofactor protein (CD46); *THBD* thrombomodulin; *RCA* regulators of complement activation; *CFHR* complement factor H related protein

Clinical Presentation

The majority of children with aHUS present with the complete triad of HUS; microangiopathic hemolytic anemia (with hemoglobin <10 g/dL, presence of schistocytes, high lactate dehydrogenase (LDH), decreased haptoglobin levels) thrombocytopenia with platelet count $<150 \times 10^9$/L and acute kidney injury (serum creatinine above the upper limit of normal). Approximately 60% of them require dialysis at the first episode. Severe hypertension is common. However, the complete triad may be missing at admission and a gradual onset is possible. Particularly, platelet count may be $>150 \times 10^9$/L (approximately 15% of patients) and hemoglobin may be >10 g/dL (approximately 5% of patients) [5]. Children may also have normal serum creatinine at presentation (approximately 15%) [56] and/or present with proteinuria/nephrotic syndrome/hematuria/hypertension as the only kidney manifestations. Thus, any association of two components of the triad with the third one missing can be a manifestation of HUS. While kidney biopsy is not required to establish the diagnosis when full-blown HUS is present, it is useful when hematology criteria are missing or incomplete and any time the diagnosis of HUS is uncertain, to document that the underlying histological lesion is TMA.

Age and Gender

In a cohort of French children with aHUS (66.2% of whom had a proven genetic or acquired complement abnormality), the mean age at onset was 1.5 years (0 to <15 years). 56% (50/89) of children had onset between birth and 2 years of age (28% between birth and 6 months, 28% between 6 months and 2 years) [5], similar to the proportion of 22% (10/45) of children having onset between 1 month and 1 year in another series [4] and 36.3% (53/146) less than 2 years and 19.8% (29/146) less than 1 year in another [57]. Atypical HUS in children is as frequent in females as in males (female-to-male ratio 0.9), in contrast with the female preponderance when the disease presents in adulthood (female-to-male ratio 3) [4, 5]. In a large series from the Global aHUS Registry, 387/851 (45%) of patients with aHUS presented before the age of 18 years (mean 3.8 years) and 166/387 (43%) of those with pediatric onset were female.

Age at onset in children varies according to the underlying genetic or acquired abnormality (more information about specific genetic/acquired abnormalities is given below). Onset between birth and 1 year of age has been reported in the majority of aHUS patients (37/50) reported to date with *DGKE* mutation [45, 46, 58–61] and all children with homozygous *CFH* mutation. It is also frequent in children with heterozygous *CFH* or *CFI* mutation-associated HUS. Conversely, *MCP* mutation-associated HUS in children exceptionally starts before the age of 1 year but most often between age 2 and 12 years. Anti factor H autoantibody associated HUS (anti-FH HUS) is also mostly a disease of late childhood and adolescence (onset between 5 and 12 years, mean age 7.6–9 years in five series including a total of over 500 patients with this form of aHUS [62–67]. *C3* or *CFB* mutation-associated HUS and aHUS without complement mutation or anti-FH antibodies appears to start at any age [2, 5, 25].

Family History

As indicated above, despite aHUS being a genetic disease, a family history of HUS is present in only 20–30% of patients [2, 4, 5] due to incomplete penetrance. The diagnosis of HUS may be unknown in the family and questioning should ask about cases of acute or chronic kidney failure, thrombocytopenia, anemia, hypertension, dialysis and graft failure in the pedigree as well as about consanguinity, which is significant for homozygous mutations in *CFH*, *MCP* and *DGKE*. No familial case of anti-FH antibody-associated HUS has been reported [68].

Triggering Events

Atypical HUS episodes in children are frequently triggered by intercurrent infections, whatever the genetic background. Specific reported infections include varicella [69], influenza [70, 71], Bordetella pertussis [72] and recently SarsCov2 virus [73].

Diarrhea precedes the onset of aHUS in at least one third of children and upper respiratory tract infections in at least 10% [4, 5]. This frequency of diarrhea at onset of aHUS explains why the former "post-diarrheal" or "non post-diarrheal" (or D+/D-) criterion to differentiate STEC-HUS from aHUS was frequently misleading. It is, however, often unclear whether gastrointestinal symptoms in aHUS are linked to an infectious trigger or whether they are manifestations of intestinal TMA. Rare patients (approximately 1%) have been reported in whom the first episode of aHUS was caused by STEC gastroenteritis, with the diagnosis of aHUS being retained because the patient had subsequent relapses and a familial history of aHUS (one patient with *MCP* mutation) [5], a severe course possibly favored by the genetic complement abnormality (one patient with *CFH* mutation) [74] or recurrence after kidney transplantation (two patients with *CFI* or *MCP* mutation—the latter also in the mother who donated the kidney) [75] . In a cohort of 75 patients with proven STEC HUS, four patients (5%) were found to have pathogenic variants in complement genes, including one patient with severe outcome. In aHUS secondary to anti-FH antibodies, a gastrointestinal prodrome (such as diarrhea, vomiting and/or abdominal pain) has been reported in 27.7% [65, 76, 77]. This type of aHUS is more common in the Asian subcontinent where it comprises 56% of cases compared with 10–25% of European cohorts [66, 77]. A recent study looking for gastrointestinal pathogens in aHUS secondary to anti-FH antibodies showed that twice as many patients had evidence of gastrointestinal pathogens compared with those without anti-FH (62.5% compared with 31.5%) including Clostridium difficile, Giardia intestinalis, Salmonella, Shigella, Rotavirus, Norovirus and Entamoeba histolytica. No stool was positive for Shigatoxin [78]. However, STEC has been reported as the trigger for HUS in a couple of patients with anti-FH HUS [62, 65]. Interestingly, the association of homozygous *MCP* mutation with common variable immunodeficiency has been reported [41]. Therefore, patients with homozygous *MCP* mutation should be investigated for immunodeficiency that may require immunoglobulin therapy to prevent infections—and thus decrease the frequency of HUS relapses triggered by infections.

Lastly, pregnancy is the trigger for aHUS in 20% of adult women [5] and 86% of women with pregnancy—associated HUS (mostly in the postpartum period) have a complement mutation [79]. For this reason, pregnancy-associated HUS is now classified as aHUS.

Histology of Atypical HUS

The underlying histological lesion of aHUS is TMA involving afferent arterioles and glomerular capillaries. Characteristic features during the acute phase are platelet and fibrin thrombi within glomerular capillaries and the thickening of glomerular capillary walls related to endothelial cell swelling and detachment and the accumulation of flocculent material (proteins and cellular debris) between the endothelial cells and the basement membrane, with double contour appearance. Mesangiolysis (fluffy mesangial expansion) is also common. Bloodless and ischemic glomeruli related to the narrowing or occlusion of the capillary and arteriolar lumen can be observed. Arterial changes range from endothelial swelling and intramural fibrin to fibrinoid necrosis with occlusive thrombi and fragmented red blood cells. Immunofluorescence studies for immunoglobulin G or C3 deposits are generally negative. C5b-9 staining has been reported in microangiopathy attributed to complement abnormalities and other causes, however its presence is not reliable.

Chronic lesions are characterized by mesangial sclerosis, thickening of capillary walls with sparse or diffuse double contours, ischemic changes of glomeruli and mucoid intimal hyperplasia and narrowing of the arterial lumen (onion-skinning). The time course for histological resolution of TMA is unknown and therefore it is difficult to know if presence of chronic features points to an ongoing active TMA process or to a chronic sequel [80, 81].

There is a general consensus that it is not possible to determine the etiology of TMA from histological morphology [82].

Manifestations Outside the Kidneys

Although the TMA process predominates in the kidney vasculature, other organs may be involved. The most frequent manifestation outside the kidneys during acute episodes of aHUS is brain involvement, reported in 15–20% of children with aHUS [5, 83–86]. Symptoms can be seizures, altered mental status, altered consciousness, visual problems (diplopia, sudden visual loss), paresis and coma. Computed tomography scan is useful to rule out cerebral bleeding. Magnetic resonance imaging (MRI) shows hyperdensities of variable severity and extension. Focal cerebral infarction is possible. The prognostic significance of MRI abnormalities is generally uncertain. The frequency of cardiac involvement is poorly documented, but life threatening ischemic myocardiopathy may occur, which makes sequential troponin level assay, electrocardiography and echocardiography advisable during acute episodes [86–89] . Peripheral acute ischemia leading to gangrene of fingers/hands and toes/feet [90], skin necrosis [91–93] or retinal ischemia with sudden visual loss [94] have been reported in a few patients. Manifestations outside the kidneys may also include pancreatitis (increase in pancreatic enzymes with or without clinical/radiologic signs) and/or hepatitis (increase of hepatic enzymes) (5–10% of patients) and, exceptionally, intra-alveolar hemorrhage, severe gastro-intestinal manifestations including intestinal perforation or life-threatening multiorgan failure (2–3% of patients [5, 91]. Severe gastrointestinal symptoms (abdominal pain, vomiting, diarrhea, biochemical pancreatitis and hepatitis), myocardial and neurological manifestations appear to be particularly frequent in patients with anti-FH antibodies [62, 65, 77, 84, 90].

Four children with aHUS have been reported who developed cerebral ischemic events due to stenosis of cerebral arteries after several years on dialysis [95–98]. One of them also had stenosis of coronary, pulmonary and digestive arteries [96]. These observations have suggested that local complement activation during acute episodes and/or subclinically in the long term, may lead to such macrovascular complications, independently or as aggravating factors of the vascular consequences of long-term dialysis. Prospective studies are required to document whether aHUS patients have an increased risk of cardio-or cerebro-vascular events and of arterial disease due to the local complement activation [99].

Experience of eculizumab to treat manifestations of aHUS outside the kidneys is limited to case reports. However, eculizumab was impressively effective in two children with acute distal ischemia [90] or skin necrosis and intestinal perforation [91], respectively. Eculizumab may rescue central nervous system manifestations, as suggested by nine case reports, including four in children [85, 86, 88, 100, 101]. Eculizumab also appeared life-saving in four children with myocardial involvement [86–89]. Lastly, two children who had developed cerebral artery stenosis stopped having ischemic events under eculizumab therapy, with non-progression of arterial stenosis documented in one [95, 97].

Making the Diagnosis of Atypical Hemolytic Uremic Syndrome

When the features of HUS are present (as summarized in Table 22.1), careful assessment is required to exclude possible causes before a provisional diagnosis of aHUS can be reached [102, 103] (Fig. 22.5 and Table 22.2).

Table 22.1 Investigations to support the presence of a thrombotic microangiopathy

Test to confirm a TMA	Result in aHUS	Comment
Haemoglobin	Low	
Platelet count	Low	
Blood film	Fragmented red blood cells	
Direct antiglobulin test	Negative	May be positive in pneumococcal HUS
Reticulocyte count	High	Low suggests either bone marrow problem or ESKD

Table 22.1 (continued)

Test to confirm a TMA	Result in aHUS	Comment
Lactate dehydrogenase	High	
Creatinine	High	Previous measurements are helpful to exclude CKD
Urinalysis	Blood, protein	
Kidney ultrasound scan	Normal sized or large kidneys, often echobright	Small kidneys suggest ESKD
Plasma C3	Low or normal	Not sensitive or specific for aHUS

ESKD end stage kidney disease; *CKD* chronic kidney disease

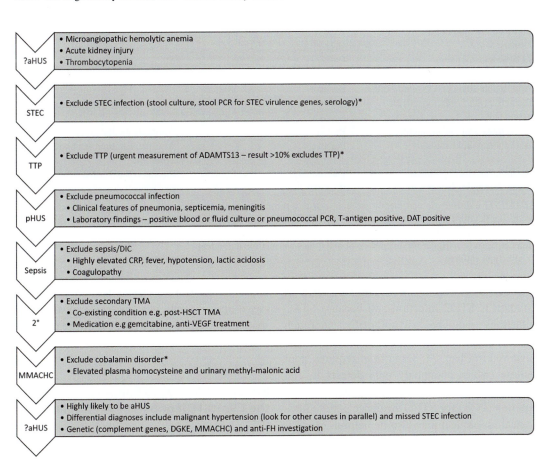

Fig. 22.5 Suggested approach to making the diagnosis of atypical HUS. When the clinical triad of microangiopathic hemolytic anemia, acute kidney injury and thrombocytopenia are present without clinical evidence of STEC infection, further evidence should be sought for STEC and pneumococcal infection. TTP should be excluded, along with secondary causes of TMA. The triad of HUS may indicate sepsis, which should be sought and excluded. Evidence for cobalamin disorder should also be sought. *these investigations may take some time to return and treatment with anti-C5 therapy should not be delayed if results are not available and the diagnosis of aHUS is strongly suspected. In practice, if an alternative diagnosis is secured after commencement of anti-C5 therapy, it can be discontinued. *STEC* shiga-toxin producing Escherichia coli; *PCR* polymerase chain reaction; *TTP* thrombotic thrombocytopenic purpura; *ADAMTS13* a disintegrin and metalloproteinase with a thrombospondin type 1 motif, member 13; *pHUS* pneumococcal haemolytic uremic syndrome; *DAT* direct antigen test; *TMA* thrombotic microangiopathy; *HSCT* hematopoietic stem cell transplant; *VEGF* vascular endothelial growth factor; *DIC* disseminated intravascular coagulation; *CRP* C-reactive protein; *DGKE* Diacylglycerol Kinase Epsilon; *MMACHC* methylmalonic aciduria and homocystinuria type C, FH factor H

Table 22.2 Investigations to rule out an alternative diagnosis

Tests for differential diagnoses	Result	Differential diagnosis
ADAMTS13 activity	<5%	TTP
Stool culture for E. coli O157	Positive	STEC HUS
Stool PCR for STEC virulence genes	Positive	STEC HUS
Serology for STEC	Positive	STEC HUS
T-antigen	Positive	Pneumococcal HUS
Pneumococcal PCR (blood/fluid)	Positive	Pneumococcal PCR
Coagulation	Prolonged PT/PTT and low fibrinogen	Sepsis/DIC
C-reactive protein	High	Sepsis/infection[a]
Plasma homocysteine	High	Cobalamin C disorder
Urinary MMA	High	Cobalamin C disorder
ECG/Echocardiogram	Evidence of left ventricular hypertrophy	Malignant hypertension
Anti-double stranded DNA antibodies	Positive	Systemic lupus erythematosus
Renal transplant—donor-specific antibodies	Positive	Antibody mediated rejection
Renal transplant—C4d staining	Positive	Antibody mediated rejection
Anti-phospholipid antibody	Positive	Anti-phospholipid antibody syndrome
Serum/urine electrophoresis[b]	Paraprotein	Plasma cell dyscrasia
Serum free light chains[b]	Positive	Plasma cell dyscrasia

ADAMTS13 a disintegrin and metalloproteinase with a thrombospondin type 1 motif, member 13; *STEC* shiga toxin producing E. coli; *PT* prothrombin time; *PTT* partial thromboplastin time; *DIC* disseminated intravascular coagulation; *MMA* methylmalonic acid
[a] Infection can be a trigger for an episode of aHUS in a susceptible individual
[b] Unlikely in children

Since the most common cause of HUS in children is STEC infection and because STEC infections may be asymptomatic, thorough microbiological assessment is required. This is reviewed in Chap. 24, but in brief requires stool culture (which commonly only detects E. coli serotype O157:H7) and stool polymerase chain reaction (PCR) for STEC virulence genes. Serological assessment may also be helpful. Medical history and physical examination usually eliminate HUS secondary to a coexisting condition—mostly HSCT- and generally suffice for the diagnosis of *Streptococcus pneumoniae*-HUS, that occurs mostly in children less than 2 years of age presenting with symptoms of invasive infection (pneumonia, meningitis, bacteremia) (see Chap. 2). Malignant hypertension can be difficult to distinguish from aHUS, and careful assessment for alternative causes of hypertension may help in this differential diagnosis. TTP must be excluded by urgent assessment of ADAMTS13 activity, since there is treatment dichotomy depending on the result. Evidence for a cobala-min C defect (raised plasma homocysteine and raised urinary methylmalonic acid) must also be sought since alternative treatment will be required [20, 102, 104–114].

Biological Assays to Support the Clinical Diagnosis of Atypical HUS

STEC infection should be ruled out as soon as possible when aHUS is suspected. Stools should be collected at admission or rectal swab performed if no stools are available, allowing stool culture and fecal PCR or immunologic assay for Stx (see Chap. 26). Negative results, mostly due to delayed stool collection or prior administration of antibiotics, are observed in at least 30% of cases classified clinically as STEC-HUS [21, 106]: in such cases, the clinical diagnosis should prevail. Congenital TTP requires urgent plasma infusion (PI) and acquired TTP requires urgent plasma exchange (PE) plus corticosteroids and rituximab. Blood samples collected before PE/PI are required for ADAMTS13 activity assays, which most commonly rely on the cleavage by plasma ADAMTS13 of the von Willebrand Factor (VWF) peptide containing the cleaving site of VWF (Fret-VWF 73). Results can be available within a few hours [115, 116]. A limitation is the interference of hyperbilirubinemia [117]. Results of commercial kits show reasonable though not full agreement (80–90% concordance) with Fret-VWF [116, 118, 119].

Lastly, assays to detect a cobalamin defect should be part of the initial biological sampling in any child suspected to have aHUS. Cobalamin defect—associated HUS, which can be rescued by hydroxocobalamine treatment, may occur in neonatal forms presenting with neurological, cardiac or multivisceral involvement, but at least as frequently in late-onset forms presenting with predominant or isolated HUS during childhood or early adulthood [110, 111, 120–122].

Complement Investigations in Patients Suspected to Have aHUS

All patients suspected of having aHUS should have blood sampling before PE/PI for measurement of C3, C4, FH, FI and FB plasma levels and screening for anti-FH antibodies. A recent publication from seven European laboratories reports the standardization of the enzyme linked immunosorbent assay technique for anti-FH antibodies [123], which could be developed in other countries. MCP surface expression on polymorphonuclear or mononuclear leucocytes is also required.

As indicated above, decreased C3 levels are observed in only 30% of children with aHUS [2, 4–6]. Therefore, a normal C3 level does not rule out the diagnosis of aHUS. Normal C4 concentration associated with decreased C3 level confirms activation of the AP as would a decreased FB concentration. As the C3 level is normal in patients with isolated MCP mutation and decreased in patients with high titer anti-FH antibodies, aHUS in a pre-adolescent or adolescent child—the age of onset in these two subgroups of complement-dependent HUS—is most likely MCP mutation-associated-HUS if C3 level is normal or anti-FH antibody-associated HUS if C3 level is low.

As indicated above, decreased FH or FI plasma levels are observed in approximately 50% and 30% of patients with mutations in *CFH* or *CFI* genes, respectively [5, 6]. Therefore, a normal FH or FI plasma level does not exclude a mutation in the corresponding gene.

Recent data suggest that levels of C5a and soluble C5b-9 (sC5b-9) are elevated during acute episodes of aHUS and may be biological markers to differentiate aHUS from TTP [124]. Increased C5a and sC5b-9 plasma levels have been confirmed in approximately half of aHUS patients during acute phases of the disease and also during remission [125]. However, a normalization of complement activation products levels after remission, including sC5b-9, has been reported by another group [126]. This, and the fact that sC5b-9 may be elevated in conditions which are not aHUS [127], means that the usefulness of these markers for routine clinical care remains to be determined.

Genetic Screening in Patients with Atypical HUS

Genetic screening results are not required for urgent therapeutic decisions but are necessary to establish whether the disease is complement-dependent or not, prognosis, risk of relapses and of progression to kidney failure, genetic counselling, decisions for complement blockade treatment duration and for kidney transplantation. The six complement genes identified as susceptibility factors for aHUS (*CFH, CFI, MCP, C3, CFB* and *THBD*) should be analysed by direct sequencing or next generation sequencing analysis. Multiplex ligation dependent probe amplification (MLPA) is required to detect hybrid *CFH* genes (5% of patients) and copy number variations in *CFH* and CFH Related (CFHR) protein genes. Because of the frequency of combined mutations indicated above, all six genes should be screened for mutations in all patients. Screening for *DGKE* mutations should be performed in children with onset of aHUS before the age of 1–2 years and maybe in older children if further reports indicate *DGKE* mutation-associated HUS may occur later in life. Sequence variants in complement genes have been identified in 5 of 13 patients with anti-FH antibody—associated HUS in one series [128], but none of 26 patients in another series [62]. Genetic analyses even when anti-FH antibodies are present may be justified. If the patient has anti-FH antibodies and a mutation, treatment should be decided according to the antibody titer and the functional consequences of the mutation [103]. Next-generation sequencing analysis allows the simultaneous study of all potentially relevant genes and should reduce the turnaround time for results and the cost of genetic analysis. Exome sequencing, which was successfully used to identify *DGKE* mutations [45], is still limited to research laboratories.

Rare Coding Variants in the CFH Gene

The role of *CFH* in aHUS was first suggested more than 40 years ago (Fig. 22.4). A decrease of plasma C3 level was first reported in 1973 in five patients with severe HUS [33] and low FH plasma levels were first reported in 1981 in a 8-month-old boy with HUS [34]. However, it is only in 1998 that Warwicker et al., by linkage analysis, could establish the link between aHUS and the Regulators of Complement Activation (RCA) region in chromosome 1q32, and the presence of mutations in *CFH*, mainly in the SCR 20, despite normal plasma levels of FH and C3 [37] .

During the last 15 years, at least 90 different rare variants of *CFH* with minor allele frequencies (MAF) <0.1% including missense or nonsense variants, short deletions or insertions, located everywhere in the gene, have been identified and referenced in the FH aHUS mutation database. The type I mutations, which induce a quantitative deficiency of the FH protein (low FH plasma levels), are located everywhere in the gene. By contrast, the mutations which induce a decreased ability of FH to bind to endothelial cells-bound C3b while plasma levels of FH are normal (namely type II mutations), are mostly located in SCR 20 (Fig. 22.3). More than 90% of reported mutations have been heterozygous and plasma C3 levels are decreased in approximately 50% of patients [2, 5, 45, 58, 65]. Less than 20 children (2–4% of reported children with aHUS), mostly from consanguineous families, carried a *CFH* homozygous variant or two heterozygous variants leading to complete FH deficiency, with permanently very low C3 levels. *CFH* pathogenic variants are the most common among aHUS patients, accounting for 20–30% of all aHUS cases in registries from the United States and Europe [1, 3–5] (Table 22.3).

The *CFH* gene is in close proximity to genes encoding for the five *CFHR* proteins that are thought to have arisen from several large genomic duplications. All *CFHRs* share a high degree of homology, which makes the region particularly prone to genomic rearrangement. The C-terminal SCR domains of CFHR1 proteins show a high level of amino acid sequence identity to the C-terminal recognition region of FH, representing the central combined cell surface anchoring- and C3b recognition region of FH. Using MLPA, genetic rearrangements between CFHR1 and FH, which result in a hybrid CFH/CFHR1 gene leading to the formation of hybrid CFH/CFHR1 protein have been reported in several unrelated aHUS patients from distinct geographic origins [129–132]. Two types of factor H/CFHR1 hybrid proteins have been described. One hybrid protein comprises the first 18 SCRs of FH linked to the C-terminal two SCRs of CFHR1. The second fusion protein has the first 19 SCRs of FH linked to SCR5 of CFHR1. Both hybrid factor H/CFHR1 proteins differ from their native C-terminal FH domain 20 by two amino acids only, at positions S1191L and V1197A [132]. They lack proper FH cell binding and protection from complement and are directly implicated in the disease pathogenesis [132].

Conversely, two types of hybrid CFHR1/CFH genes that encode a fusion protein with the first three short consensus repeats (SCRs) of FHR1 and the last two SCRs of FH or with the first four SCRs of FHR1 and the terminal SCR20 of FH have been identified in aHUS patients. Functional

22 Atypical Hemolytic Uremic Syndrome

Table 22.3 Frequency of complement and DGKE abnormalities in children and adults with atypical hemolytic uremic syndrome in four cohorts from Europe and the USA

	[2]			[5][a]			[4]	[3]
	Total	Children	Adults	Total	Children	Adults	Children	Children + adults
Number of patients	256	152	104	214	89	125	45	I44
CFH mutation, %	25.3	15.6	25	37.5	11.3	32	11	27
Homozygous	4.2	–	–	1.8	4.4	0	–	
Heterozygous	21.1	–	–	25.7	16.8	32	–	
MCP mutation, %	7	9.2	3.8	9.3	13.5	6.4	9	5
Homozygous	–	–	–	2.8	5.6	0.8	–	–
Heterozygous	–	–	–	6.5	7.8	5.6	–	–
CFI mutation, %	3.9	2.6	5.7	8.4	6.7	9.6	7	8
C3 mutation, %	4.6	3.9	5.7	8.4	7.8	8.8	9	2
CFB mutation, %	0.4	–	–	1.4	1	2.4	4	4
Anti-CFH antibodies, %	3.1	3.9	1.9	6.5	11	3.2	13	–
THBD mutation, %	5	7.8	0.9	0	0	0	0	3
Combined mutations, %	3	–	–	4.2	3.4	4.8	4	5.5
Complement-mediated HIS, %	52.3	53	43	65.7	64.7	67.2	55	46
DGKE mutation, %	–	–	–	3.2	7.9	0	–	–
No identified abnormality, %	47.7	47	57	31.1	27.4	32.8	45	54

CFB complement factor B; *CFH* complement factor H; *CFI* complement factor I; *DGKE* diacylglycerol kinase ε; *MCP* membrane cofactor protein (CD46); *THBD* thrombomodulin
% percentage of patients; – not documented
[a] DGKE mutations were identified in seven children who were previously within the group with no complement mutation identified [5]

studies revealed that the hybrid protein causes complement dysregulation at the cell surface by acting as a competitive antagonist of FH.

Rare Coding Variants in the CFI Gene

To date more than 100 *CFI* distinct rare variants have been published, located everywhere in the gene. All but one variants are heterozygous [4]. *CFI* pathogenic variants induce a default of secretion of the mutant protein (de Jong) and less frequently disrupt its cofactor activity, with altered degradation of C3b in the fluid phase and on surfaces. However, 40% of *CFI* mutations have no identified functional consequences and their link with the disease remains unclear. Plasma C3 levels are below the normal range in approximately 50% of patients with *CFI* variants and FI levels are slightly decreased in 30% [5]. *CFI* rare variants account for 4–8% of aHUS cases [5].

Rare Coding Variants in the MCP Gene

More than 100 distinct rare variants in *MCP* gene have been reported in cohorts of patients with

aHUS. Fifty percent of variants identified in MCP gene are splice site nonsense or frameshift variants. In the French aHUS cohort, one third of *MCP* mutations are homozygous and two-thirds are heterozygous [5]. Over 80% of the pathogenic variants induce a reduction in MCP expression on granulocytes. Plasma C3 level is normal in patients with isolated *MCP* mutations [5].

Rare Coding Variants in the C3 Gene

Screening the French aHUS cohort for mutations in the C3 gene led to the discovery of heterozygous pathogenic variants including a recurrent C3 variant (p.R139W) in aHUS patients. Functional studies showed that the nucleotide change induces either a defect in the ability of C3 to bind the regulatory proteins MCP and FH (indirect gain of function mutation) or an increase in the capacity of C3 to bind FB (direct gain of function mutation). In both cases, the genetic change induces enhanced C3bBb convertase formation and complement activation on cell surfaces [133]. There are now at least 90 distinct C3 mutations reported in hundreds of aHUS patients, however few functional studies have been reported. It is estimated that ~2–10% of incident aHUS patients will carry a C3 pathogenic mutation. The majority of these patients have persistently low plasma C3 levels [43].

Rare Coding Variants in the CFB Gene

Very few pathogenic variants of *CFB* with functional consequences have been identified. Therefore, *CFB* mutations account for only 1–2% of aHUS patients (Table 22.3). Functional analyses demonstrated that aHUS-associated *CFB* mutations are exclusively gain-of-function mutations that result in enhanced formation of the C3bBb convertase [134, 135]. *CFB*-mutated patients exhibit a permanent activation of the alternative pathway with very low C3.

Out of 9 *CFB* rare variants characterized using functional *in vitro* assays, only 5 revealed a gain-of-function phenotype; the other variants are classified of undetermined significance [134].

Combined Complement Gene Mutations

Only 8–10% of patients with mutations in *CFH*, *C3*, or *CFB* had combined mutations, whereas approximately 25% of patients with mutations in *MCP* or *CFI* had combined mutations [53].

Mode of Inheritance and Penetrance

Twenty to 30% of patients have a familial history of aHUS. More frequently the disease is sporadic with only one case per family. However, *de novo* mutations are exceptional [135]. Among pedigrees with familial aHUS, transmission of the disease is autosomal recessive in cases with homozygous or compound heterozygous mutations in *CFH* or *MCP*. Transmission is autosomal dominant in cases with a heterozygous mutation. Disease penetrance in family members who carry the heterozygous mutation has been evaluated to be approximately 50%, as only half of these subjects develop the disease. This may be an overestimate, due to the issue of reporting bias, since pedigrees with more that one affected individual are more likely to be studied than those with just one patient. The identified mutation therefore appears to be a risk factor for the disease rather than its direct and unique cause and aHUS has to be regarded as a complex polygenic disease which results from a combination of genetic risk factors. Homozygous haplotypes (defined by five frequent genetic variants transmitted in block) in CFH (at risk CFH tgtgt), MCP at risk (MCP ggaac) [136] and CFHR1*B allele [137] have been demonstrated to be more frequent in patients with aHUS than in controls. In addition, precipitating events or triggers appear required for the disease to manifest in patients genetically at risk.

Complement Alternative Pathway: From Gene Change to TMA Lesion

Mutations in the genes *CFH*, *MCP* and *CFI* impair the mechanisms that regulate AP activation and gain of function variants in C3 and CFB increase AP activation. Whatever the pathogenic variants identified, endothelial cells are no longer protected from complement activation [138, 139]. The increased production of MAC at the endothelial cell surface induces alterations of these cells, which become procoagulant by producing high molecular weight multimers of von Willebrand Factor, thus triggering the formation of thrombi [140–142]. In addition, complement activation at the surface of platelets triggers platelet activation and aggregation and this contributes to the formation of thrombi within the microcirculation [143]. This physiopathological model is corroborated by transgenic animal models. Mice which express a *FH* variant lacking the C-terminal 16–20 domain responsible for the interaction of FH with C3b and the endothelium develop HUS similar to the human disease [144].

Variants of Unknown Significance in Complement Genes: Disease Relevant or Benign?

Over the coming decade, the challenge will be to optimize and to implement at scale, strategies that use human genetics to further the understanding of disease, and to maximize the clinical benefit of those discoveries. The modern genetic screening test to identify genetic abnormality in aHUS patients includes next generation sequencing (NGS) with at least a panel of 5 genes (*CFH, CFI, MCP, C3* and *CFB*), Sanger sequencing and MLPA with an interpretation of the clinical consequences.

Not all detected complement gene variants have clinically relevant consequences. The standards and guidelines published in 2015 by the American College of Medical Genetics (ACMG) lay out an extensive framework of evidence for interpretation of sequence variants, including guidance for using population data and computational and predictive tools. The variants are classified along a gradient ranging from those that almost certainly have a pathogenic role to those that are very likely benign. However functional characterization of aHUS associated *FH* variants reveals limitations of routinely used variant classification methods. Access to resources that catalogue genetic variation across populations (such as gnomAD) has enabled the confident exclusion of genetic variants too common in population-level data to be plausible causes of rare diseases. As a general rule, variants with a MAF <0.1% might be considered relevant for the pathogenesis of aHUS or other complement-mediated disorders.

In 2021 this rule cannot be applied for variants in the complement genes. Genetic data are now available for >140,000 individuals from diverse populations in the Genome Aggregation Database (gnomAD). These data indicate that rare variants in the five complement genes with MAFs of <0.1% are present in 3.7% of healthy individuals and pathogenic variants can be found in 1% of samples of DNA from healthy blood donors. Only 9 out the 15 genetic changes in *CFB* identified in patients with aHUS led to functional activity changes compared to the wild-type protein [134]. Furthermore, only 29 of 79 rare variants in the *CFH* gene with a MAF <0.1% that have been identified in patients with aHUS are classified as pathogenic based upon the demonstration that they impair CFH regulatory activity [145]. The classification of complement gene variants relies on tools that help predict the potential pathogenicity of a variant [146].

In clinical practice, analysis of functional alterations in complement proteins takes into account the level of expression of the encoded protein (in plasma for CFH and CFI and at the granulocyte surface for CD46), the impact of the variant on the function of the encoded protein (assessed using *in vitro* assays and prediction of the pathogenicity of a variant based on functional domains) and *in silico* analyses. Establishing a causal relationship is difficult with the lack of experimental data. According to ACMG guidelines, more frequently the variants have only moderate evidence for pathogenicity and the variant will be classified as a variant of undetermined significance VUS). The current classification of complement gene variants is not optimal and the clinical relevance of individual variants should therefore be regularly re-evaluated.

In summary, not all detected gene variants have clinically relevant consequences. In practice, where a VUS is found in a complement gene of a patient with aHUS, it is important that other causes of a TMA are still excluded, rather than attributing causality. In addition, it is important not to screen family members for the presence of a VUS, since this could attribute risk where none exists or conversely, falsely reassure when risk still exists.

Genetic Abnormalities in Genes Not Related to Complement

Diacylglycerol Kinase ε Mutations

Diacylglycerol kinase ε (DGKε) is an intracellular lipid kinase highly expressed in glomerular capillaries, podocytes and platelets of healthy mice and humans. DGKs are enzymes that phosphorylate diacylglycerol molecules to phosphatidic acid. Using exome sequencing, deficiency in DGKε was established as a novel cause of pediatric onset aHUS in 2013 [45]. Subsequent to the first publication of 13 aHUS children from 9 kindreds, 6 new cases from 4 kindreds have been identified [58, 59], followed by a third cohort with clinical information on 15 patients based on data from the UK National Renal Complement

Therapeutics Centre including patients from UK, United Arab Emirates and New Zealand [46]. This cohort also established the presumed prevalence and incidence of DGKε-aHUS in the UK population at 0.009 per million per year, when the incidence rate of complement-mediated aHUS was 0.47 per million per year [46]. The phenotypic spectrum and outcome of *DGKE* disease was reviewed by Azukaitis et al. in a global cohort of 44 (including 10 previously unpublished) cases [60].

Transmission of *DGKε* mutations follows an autosomal recessive pattern and all patients reported to date carry homozygous or compound heterozygous nonsense, splice site or frameshift mutations. A likely explanation for the pathogenesis of *DGKε* mutations is that the loss of DGKε enhances protein kinase C activation in endothelial cells, platelets and podocytes, which may result in upregulation of prothrombic factors and platelet activation and altered podocyte function [45, 147]. However, the pathophysiological mechanisms of DGKε nephropathy have not yet been fully understood.

The aHUS relapses are clustered in early life and appear to be less prevalent later. In addition to presentation with aHUS, patients carrying *DGKε* mutations can also present with proteinuria without aHUS or steroid resistant nephrotic syndrome with MPGN pattern on biopsy. The symptoms can overlap in individuals, when in early life patients present with nephrotic range proteinuria and relapsing course of aHUS progressing further to chronic kidney disease (CKD) later in life with proteinuria, microscopic hematuria and hypertension. Neither the UK nor the global cohort found predictors that increase the risk of reaching end stage kidney disease or evidence of a significant role for complement activation on progression and relapses of *DGKε*-aHUS [46, 60]. These resolve regardless of therapy including complement blockade by eculizumab. Moreover, there were aHUS episodes or relapses during treatment with complement blocking therapy. Therefore, complement blocking therapy is probably not beneficial in this specific cohort of aHUS and patients should be managed support-

ively and in those already on eculizumab, withdrawal should be considered. DGKE nephropathy appears to take a slowly progressive course; only 20% of patients reach ESRD within 10 years of diagnosis [60]. There are no reports of DGKE nephropathy recurrence after transplantation (6 transplant cases reported as of October 2019) [46, 60]; therefore, individuals who progress to end-stage kidney disease (ESKD) should undergo kidney transplantation without the need for preemptive eculizumab [46, 60].

Cobalamin C Metabolism Defect Related HUS

A defect in the remethylation pathway caused by cobalamin C deficiency can lead to a clinical presentation very similar to HUS. It can present fulminantly in the neonatal period or later in life. The triad of HUS is also accompanied by other metabolic symptoms like delayed development and growth, seizures, hypo or hypertension and leucopenia. The inheritance is autosomal recessive, and it is usually caused by a defect in the *MMCHC* gene.

The major markers are elevated homocysteine and methylmalonic acid levels in plasma. Levels of homocysteine over 50 μM/L with normal levels of vitamin B12 and folate are pathognomonic. TMA in cobalamin C deficiency is believed to be caused by the endothelial toxicity of high plasma homocysteine levels.

Treatment is by loading dose of intramuscular vitamin B12 (hydroxycobalamin) followed by lifelong supplementation [110, 121]. Although rare, Cblc deficiency should not be missed since the prognosis of undiagnosed patients is dismal, it can easily be treated once detected. Hence, plasma homocysteine should be included in the routine diagnostic panel of aHUS.

Rare Variants in Genes with Debatable Clinical Relevance

Genetic defects in *THBD*, which encodes thrombomodulin, a protein that interconnects the coagulation cascade and complement system, have been suggested to contribute to the pathogenesis of aHUS. Few mutations in *THBD* affecting the functions of the protein have been identified to date, with a frequency varying from 0 to 5% of all aHUS cases [2, 3, 44] (Table 22.3). Burden or aggregate association tests, in which all rare variants affecting the same gene are combined into one test, are used to increase the statistical power for rare variant association. Although rare variants in *THBD* have been reported in 41 patients with aHUS, their frequency is not significantly higher in these patients than in controls the general population [148]. Therefore, the link of *THBD* with aHUS remains debatable.

The potential clinical relevance of rare variants in genes such as *PLG* (which encodes plasminogen) [149], *INF2* (which encodes inverted formin 2) [150], *VTN* (which encodes vitronectin) [148] and *CLU* (which encodes clusterin) [151] identified in patients presented with some features of HUS warrant further assessment.

Acquired Complement Abnormalities in Atypical HUS

Anti-factor H Autoantibodies

Anti-factor H (anti-FH) autoantibodies are identified in 5–11% in European aHUS cohorts and in about 20% in Asian aHUS cohorts [65, 76, 79]. Interestingly, they are identified in more than 56% cases from India [80]. A Czech cohort showed a rather outlying large proportion of anti FH antibodies in comparison to other European cohorts of aHUS at 61% which could be due to small sample size and sampling method [67].

Anti-factor H autoantibodies associated HUS (anti-FH HUS) usually manifests later than genetic types of aHUS caused by factor H mutations, usually between 5 and 15 years of age [77]. An international aHUS registry reported a median of age of 13.1 (6.1–31.3) years at presentation [81] for this group of patients. However, the youngest reported aHUS patient with anti-FH antibodies identified was younger than 1 year and the oldest reported patient was over 75 years old. Most of the published series show a slightly higher prevalence of anti-FH HUS in males.

Anti-FH antibodies bind mostly to SCR 19 and 20 of FH but also to other epitopes of FH and thus inhibit the majority of regulatory functions of FH at cell surfaces [153]. Plasma C3 level is decreased in 40–60% of patients with anti-FH antibodies during the acute phase, while FH levels are decreased in only approximately 20% of patients [62]. C3 levels are significantly lower in patients with very high anti-FH antibody titer.

Ninety percent of patients with anti-FH antibodies have a complete deficiency of *CFHR1* and *CFHR3* due to a homozygous deletion of *CFHR1-R3*, a polymorphism carried by 2–9% of European, 16% of African and ≤2% of Chinese healthy controls [128, 154]. The reason why individuals with *CFHR1-R3* deletion develop anti-FH antibodies is uncertain. The current theory linking the deletion in CFHR1 with the generation of antibodies is based upon the interaction of the FH protein that is used by pathogens for immune evasion. In individuals with *CFHR1 gene* deletion, CFHR1 protein is recognized as foreign by their immune system. When a CFHR1-deficient individual is infected by an organism that can bind CFHR1, CFHR3 and FH proteins, the FH protein is changed by the infectious organism to resemble CFHR1 and host immunity mounts a response, leading to production of anti-FH inhibiting FH, thus leading to endothelial dysfunction and symptoms of aHUS. This is corroborated by structural differences found between CFHR1 and FH [155].

Fujisawa et al. described three aHUS patients where anti-FH antibodies affected platelets directly [82]. Washed platelets aggregated more when in contact with plasma from these patients compared to plasma from healthy controls or from aHUS patients with complement genetic variants.

Anti-factor I Antibodies

Two cases of anti-FI antibody-associated HUS have been reported to date [156]. The clinical relevance of these antibodies is difficult to establish, also given their extreme rarity.

Outcome of Atypical HUS Prior to the Availability of C5 Inhibition Therapy

In the era before eculizumab became available the death rate in children with aHUS was 8% [5], 9% [4] and 14% [2] in three pediatric series at average follow-up times of 3.8, 7.5 and 3 years, respectively. Most deaths occurred in children less than 1 year of age and at first episode or during the first year after onset. Approximately 20% of children progressed to ESKD or died at first episode or within <1 month after onset, 30% within 1 year and 40% at 5 years follow-up. The most severe outcome was in children with *CFH* mutations, of whom one third progressed to ESKD or died at first episode, half at 1 year and two thirds at 5 years follow-up. The prognosis of *CFI* and *C3* mutation-associated HUS was hardly less severe than that of *CFH* mutation-associated HUS. *MCP* mutation-associated HUS in children had the best prognosis, with an ESKD risk of 25% at median follow-up of 18 years. aHUS in children with no complement mutation identified also had a relatively favorable outcome [5].

Lastly, the outcome of anti-FH antibodies associated HUS was poor when treatment was limited to PE, including death in 10% of patients, CKD in 40% and ESKD in one third at mean follow-up 39 months [62, 152]. Early treatment with a combination of PE, corticosteroids and immunosuppressants allowed a more favorable outcome, similar to that of *MCP* mutation—associated HUS [5, 64].

Less than 10% of children with *DGKE*-aHUS progress to ESKD in the first year after onset, but patients with this form of aHUS develop proteinuria and nephrotic syndrome, severe hypertension and progress to CKD stages 4–5 (eGFR 15–29 mL/min/1.73 m^2 or ESKD) between the age of 20 and 25 years [45, 46, 60].

In the pre-eculizumab era, several series suggested that approximately half of children with aHUS experienced relapses [4, 5]. Among children who had not died or reached ESKD at first episode or at 1 year follow-up, 25% had relapses during the first year and 47% after the first year.

However, a high relapse rate after the first year was mostly in patients with *DGKE* (83% during the first year, 50% up to 5 years) or *MCP* mutations (25% during the first year, 92% after the first year), while relapse rate after the first year was 20–30% in other genetic subgroups [5, 45, 46, 60]. Despite this risk of relapses in the long term, *MCP* mutation-associated HUS has the best prognosis in children, as indicated above. Last, anti-FH HUS had a relapsing course in two third of patients when untreated or treated only with PE/PI [62, 65], which was reduced to approximately 10% by early treatment combining PE + immunosuppressants + corticosteroids [5, 64].

Treatment of Atypical HUS Prior to the Availability of C5 Inhibition Therapy

Plasma Therapy

PE (or PI when PE was not possible) was first line treatment for aHUS until recent year [12] Approximately 15 case reports, mostly in children with *CFH* mutation, showed that early, intensive plasmatherapy, followed by maintenance PE/PI, could prevent relapses and preserve kidney function at follow-up up to 6 years [8, 9, 157]. However, although plasmatherapy was associated with complete or partial remission (hematologic remission with kidney sequels) in approximately 80% of aHUS episodes in children, half of them had died or reached ESKD at 3 years follow-up [2]. In addition, plasmatherapy carried significant morbidity. An audit of complications in children receiving PE for aHUS revealed 31% developed catheter-related complications (including infection, thrombosis and hemorrhage) and 11% developed plasma hypersensitivity [13]. The benefit of PE/PI is uncertain in *DGKE* mutation-associated HUS, as proteinuria, the main marker of a progressing course in *DGKE* mutation–associated HUS, persisted in 9 of the 12 patients who received plasmatherapy [45, 46, 60].

Kidney Transplantation

The risk of post-transplant recurrence of aHUS was 60% in the pre-complement blockade era [2, 104]. Forty percent of recurrences occurred during the first month after transplantation and 70% during the first year. Graft survival was 30% at 5 years follow-up in patients with recurrence, compared to 68% in those without recurrence [104]. Eighty percent of patients who had lost a prior graft from recurrence had recurrence after retransplantation. The main independent risk factor for recurrence was the presence of a complement mutation. The highest risk (approximately 80%) was in patients with *CFH* and *C3* or *CFB* gain of function mutation, the risk in patients with *CFI* mutation was approximately 50% and patients with no complement mutation identified had the lowest risk (approximately 20%) [104]. The risk of post-transplant recurrence in patients with *MCP* mutation has been shown to be low (<10%) if the mutation is isolated (the graft brings the non-mutated MCP protein), while it is approximately 30% if the *MCP* mutation is associated with a mutation in *CFH*, *CFI* or *C3* [53]. No post-transplant recurrence was observed in four patients with *DGKE* mutations [45, 46, 60]. The risk is low in anti-FH HUS if the antibody titer is low at the time of transplantation, while substantial if elevated [62, 65, 66] [128, 158]. One patient with *THBD* mutation has been reported to have had post-transplant recurrence [159].

This shows that genetic screening is necessary before listing a patient for kidney transplantation to predict the risk of post-transplant recurrence and guide decisions for the choice of the donor and the prevention of recurrence.

PE/PI for post-transplant recurrence generally failed to avoid graft loss [2, 104]. Therefore, prophylactic PE/PI was recommended [160]. The efficacy of this strategy is poorly documented. However, graft survival rate free of recurrence was significantly higher in nine patients who received prophylactic PE/PI than in 62 patients without prophylactic PE/PI [104]. Interestingly, calcineurin inhibitors (CNI) did not significantly increase the risk of recurrence in a recent series, while mTOR inhibitor use was an independent significant risk factor for recurrence, possibly related to the anti-VEGF (vascular endothelium growth factor) action of these drugs [104]. The current consensus is that aHUS is not per se a contraindication to CNI. Strict monitoring of blood levels and overdosage avoidance is recommended, while CNI-free mTOR based immunosuppressive regimens should be avoided [161].

Treatment Recommendations

During the initial manifestation of HUS, unless it is a relapse in a patient already know to carry a risk variant in genes associated to aHUS, diagnosis is challenging, and aHUS cannot be excluded purely on clinical grounds or complement markers. Children with suspected aHUS should ideally be transferred to a children's kidney center capable of kidney replacement therapy and intensive care. In contrast to adults, and because the incidence of acquired TTP in children is very low, immediate PE whilst awaiting ADAMTS13 results is not routinely recommended. Children in whom complement driven aHUS is strongly suspected or proven should receive eculizumab (see below) as first line treatment, to avoid PE and the complications of central catheters [103]. Confirmation of a complement mutation is not required for the decision of treatment initiation in such cases. As treatment delay may affect recovery of kidney function, eculizumab treatment should be initiated as soon as possible, ideally within 24–48 h of onset or admission. In addition to targeted treatment with eculizumab, symptomatic care is based on general recommendations for AKI [162] and on consensus from observational studies. The cornerstone is appropriate fluid management, kidney replacement therapy in patients with high urea or unsafe electrolyte profile and stopping of nephrotoxic drugs. Red blood cell transfusions should be given to patients who have symptoms of severe anemia or when hemoglobin falls rapidly. Platelet transfusions are not advised unless patient has a life threating bleeding or requires invasive procedure like placement of vascular catheter for adequate dialysis.

Eculizumab

Eculizumab, a monoclonal humanized anti-C5 antibody, prevents C5 cleavage and the formation of C5a and C5b-9, thus blocking the C5a pro-inflammatory and the C5b-9 pro-thrombotic consequences of complement activation. It has been the accepted treatment of paroxysmal nocturnal hemoglobinuria (PNH), another complement dependent disease, for more than 15 years [163].

The rationale for treatment with complement C5 blockade was first proposed based on first two aHUS patients treated successfully with eculizumab in 2009 [164, 165], followed by plethora of successful cases [15, 85, 87, 89–91, 166–170].

Four observational prospective single-arm non randomized multinational trials [14, 171, 172] demonstrated the efficacy of eculizumab to stop the TMA process, allowing sustained remission of aHUS with improved or preserved kidney function in the majority of patients. One of these trials [172] specifically studied eculizumab in children with aHUS. Figure 22.6 shows the remarkable efficacy of eculizumab in these patients. Data from the trials also suggested that an early switch from PE/PI to eculizumab or the use of eculizumab as first line therapy gave patients the best chance of full recovery of kidney function. Treatment was well tolerated, with no increase of adverse events over time. However, two of the 100 patients who entered these trials developed meningococcal meningitis. Eculizumab is administered by intravenous infusion according to the weight-directed dose and schedule shown in Table 22.4.

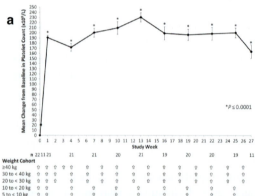

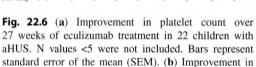

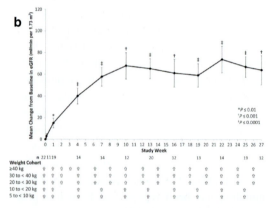

Fig. 22.6 (a) Improvement in platelet count over 27 weeks of eculizumab treatment in 22 children with aHUS. N values <5 were not included. Bars represent standard error of the mean (SEM). (b) Improvement in estimated glomerular filtration rate (eGFR) over 27 weeks of eculizumab treatment. N values <5 were not included. Bars represent SEM. Arrows denote administration of eculizumab

Table 22.4 Dosing of eculizumab based on European Medicines Agency: Summary of product characteristics Soliris, https://www.ema.europa.eu/en/documents/product-information/soliris-epar-product-information_en.pdf, February 2022

		Initial dose	Maintenance dose
Adult dosing schedule (intravenous infusion)		900 mg every week for first 4 weeks	1200 mg at week 5 then 1200 mg every 14 days
Paediatric dosing schedule according to body weight (intravenous infusion)	>40 kg	Dose as per adult schedule	Dose as per adult schedule
	30–40 kg	600 mg every week for first 2 weeks	900 mg at week 3 then 900 mg every 14 days
	20–30 kg	600 mg every week for first 2 weeks	600 mg at week 3 then 600 mg every 14 days
	10–20 kg	600 mg first week only	300 mg at week 2 then 300 mg every 14 days
	5–10 kg	300 mg first week only	300 mg at week 2 then 300 mg every 21 days

Eculizumab is currently approved by both the Food and Drug Administration and the European Medicines Agency for the treatment of atypical HUS. The cost of the drug and the presumption that patients should receive lifelong treatment played a major role in approving the cover of the costs by healthcare systems. Access and funding are achievable in USA, Australia, United Kingdom and in most states of the European Union, with exception of Bulgaria and Romania. Other countries with availability include Israel and Japan. African and Asian countries, including China and India, have no access to the drug. The availability generally corresponds to the countries' economic position (apart from New Zealand where access is very limited).

Ravulizumab

A second generation complement inhibitor, ravulizumab, has recently been developed by targeted re-engineering of eculizumab. Two structural changes were incorporated, aimed at extending the terminal half-life. The first change enhanced the dissociation rate of the mAb:C5 complex at pH 6.0, eliminating the target mediated antibody clearance. The second change enhanced the affinity of the antibody to human neonatal Fc receptor [173].

Ravulizumab has not been directly compared to eculizumab in a clinical trial. However, efficacy and safety were confirmed in a phase 3 single-arm trial in adult patients (n = 56) with aHUS naïve to complement inhibitor treatment [174]. Complete TMA response, defined as normalization of platelet count and LDH and $\geq 25\%$ improvement in serum creatinine, was achieved in 53.6% of patients in the 26 week study period. This lower response rate than reported within the eculizumab trials may have been due to broader eligibility criteria for recruitment (only 20.5% had genetic complement mutations or anti-FH identified compared with 76% in the equivalent eculizumab trial). There were no severe treatment-related events reported. Four deaths were reported, none of which were considered treatment-related by the study investigator [175].

Two trials tested the efficacy and safety of ravulizumab in children under 18 years of age with aHUS. Fourteen of 18 complement-inhibitor naïve patients with aHUS (78%), achieved complete TMA response with ravulizumab. Ten aHUS patients who were already receiving eculizumab, switched to ravulizumab for a period of 26 weeks without significant safety issues and showed unchanged kidney function and hematological remission of aHUS even after extended observation of one year. No unexpected adverse events, deaths, or meningococcal infections occurred. There were not enough data to demonstrate the effectiveness of ravulizumab in children weighing less than 10 kg [176, 177].

Taken together, these trials indicate that ravulizumab, is effective for the long-term treatment of patients with aHUS. Current evidence suggests an acceptable safety profile, although longer-term surveillance will be required. The main risk of ravulizumab treatment is similar to that of eculizumab arising from the same principle of C5 blockade. Therefore, all patients must strictly adhere to the same prevention protocols against meningococcal infection as with eculizumab. Dose and schedule information for ravulizumab are shown in Table 22.5.

There are now two licensed treatments for patients with aHUS. Clinicians and patients now have a choice between short-acting and long-acting C5 inhibition. Since the diagnosis of aHUS is complex and not all patients initiated on C5 inhibition will continue with long-term therapy, it may be an option to commence initial treatment with eculizumab, with a switch to long-acting therapy once a need for long-term treatment is established (Fig. 22.7). This approach would minimise the risk of prolonged C5 blockade for those in whom treatment is discontinued due to an alternative diagnosis (for example, a subsequent positive STEC result). However, commencing with ravulizumab at time of initial presentation is also an option.

A subcutaneous ravulizumab formulation is currently undergoing evaluation in a phase 3 trial in adult patients with PNH [177] and may be a future option also for patients with aHUS.

Table 22.5 Dosing of ravulizumab based on European Medicines Agency: Summary of product characteristics Ultomiris, https://www.ema.europa.eu/en/documents/product-information/ultomiris-epar-product-information_en.pdf, February 2022

		Initial dose	Maintenance dose
Adult dosing schedule (intravenous infusion)	≥40 to <60 kg	2400 mg loading dose followed by maintenance dose in 2 weeks	3000 mg every 8 weeks
	≥60 to <100 kg	2700 mg loading dose followed by maintenance dose in 2 weeks	3300 mg every 8 weeks
	≥100 kg	3000 mg loading dose followed by maintenance dose in 2 weeks	3600 mg every 8 weeks
Paediatric dosing schedule according to body weight (intravenous infusion)	>40 kg	Dose as per adult schedule	Dose as per adult schedule
	30–40 kg	1200 mg loading dose followed by maintenance dose in 2 weeks	2700 mg every 8 weeks
	20–30 kg	900 mg loading dose followed by maintenance dose in 2 weeks	2100 mg every 8 weeks
	10–20 kg	600 mg loading dose followed by maintenance dose in 2 weeks	600 mg every 4 weeks

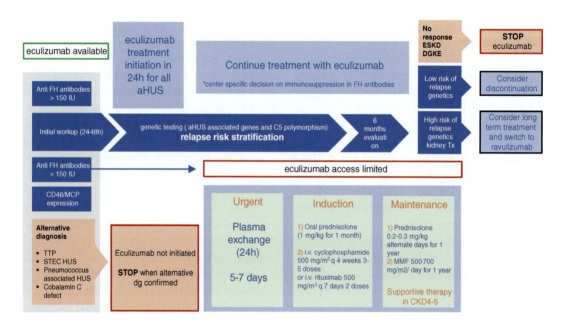

Fig. 22.7 Recommended management approach when atypical HUS is suspected

Risk of Meningococcal Infection on C5 Inhibition Therapy and Its Prevention

The host defense against *Neisseria meningitis* depends on the lytic terminal complement complex C5b-9. The incidence of meningococcal infections in patients with hereditary complete deficiency of terminal complement factors is 0.5% per year, corresponding to a 1000 to 2000-fold relative risk increase compared to the normal population [178]. Patients undergoing eculizumab or ravulizumab treatment have the same risk as these patients. Therefore, prevention of meningococcal infection is crucial, relying on vaccination and antibiotic prophylaxis. Tetravalent conjugated vaccines protect against serogroups A, C, W135 and Y. Polysaccharide vaccines against serogroup B are also available and recommended for all patients receiving eculizumab.

The frequency of invasive meningococcal infection has been approximately 0.5/100 patient years in patients with PNH treated with eculizumab, despite meningococcal vaccination (not anti-B) [179].

Two of the 100 aHUS patients treated within trial protocols and one among approximately 80 case reports developed invasive meningococcal infection despite being vaccinated [180]. The more recent analysis of eculizumab safety from the Global Atypical HUS registry showed meningococcal infection in two adult cases (0.17 per 100 patients years) and one pediatric patient (0.11 in 100 patient years) out of 1321 patients ever treated with eculizumab. Two patients recovered completely, and one case was fatal [181].

Whilst long-term antibiotic prophylaxis for patients on C5 inhibition is not mandated by the manufacturer, many clinicians add this to their patients' treatment (phenoxymethylpenicillin or erythromycin if penicillin allergic). This is strongly recommended for children and in some countries, this is obligatory [103]. Neither vaccines nor antibiotic prophylaxis guarantee full protection, hence the importance of patient and family education on signs of meningococcal infection and the provision of alert cards to be carried by the patient or their caregiver to present to their health care provider when unwell, in order to minimize delay in recognition.

Treatment of Anti-factor H Antibody Associated HUS

The first large series of patients with anti-FH HUS (treated mostly with PE without immunosuppressants) suggested that many of these patients suffer a relapsing course, leading to end stage kidney disease [62]. A much more favorable outcome, similar to that of *MCP* mutation-associated HUS, has been reported in children with this form of HUS, treated early with PE, immunosuppressants and corticosteroids [5].

The largest experience with the approach to decrease anti-FH antibodies with immunosuppressive treatment comes from India, where 55.8% of their 781 aHUS patients presented with anti-FH antibodies [66].

Combined Plasma exchange (PE) and immunosuppression improved long-term outcomes (HR 0.37; $P = 0.026$); maintenance therapy with corticosteroids and MMF reduced the relapse risk (HR 0.11; $P < 0.001$) [66].

Maintenance treatment with corticosteroids and mycophenolate mofetil (MMF) or azathioprine significantly decreased the risk of relapses, from 87% to 46% at last follow-up [64, 157].

Eculizumab was documented as an effective treatment of HUS symptoms in anti-FH HUS in several cases [88, 182].

In a cohort of 17 patients with anti-CFH antibody associated aHUS, four patients were treated with first-line eculizumab rather than PE. Patients treated with eculizumab achieved remission in 100% of cases, whereas treatment with PE and immunosuppression was associated with a poor rate of renal recovery in 7 of 11 treated. Therefore, treatment with eculizumab did not appear inferior to PE and immunosuppression [183]. This gives patients and clinicians different treatment options with different adverse effect profiles—broad immunosuppression with rituximab or cyclophosphamide, or more targeted treatment with eculizumab [103]. The National Renal Complement Therapeutics Centre in the UK recommends initial treatment with eculizumab for anti-FH HUS based upon a more favorable adverse effect profile .

Global Variations in Atypical HUS Treatment Recommendations

Eculizumab has revolutionized the management of aHUS. The current best recommendations and guidelines are challenging to implement globally, particularly in resource-limited healthcare settings due to the prohibitive cost of eculizumab and its successor ravulizumab. In response to this, the Indian Society of Pediatric Nephrology have published consensus guidelines for countries lacking access to eculizumab and complex diagnostic facilities [157].

These pragmatic guidelines are mirroring the best recommendations from the pre-eculizumab era [64]. (See also Fig. 22.7).

They recommend treating aHUS where anti-FH antibodies are not suspected with prompt initiation of PE using fresh frozen plasma (The dose is recommended as 1.5 times of the plasma volume or 60–75 mL/kg) and repeated daily until hematological remission is achieved (platelets over 100×10^9/L, schistocytes under 2% and LDH in normal range). The tapering follows after 5 days of daily PE or when remission is achieved followed by alternate days PE and 2–3 weeks of twice a week PE.

In case of positive anti-FH antibodies, additional immunosuppression is administered, starting with prednisolone 1 mg/kg daily for 4 weeks followed by alternate day dosing for another 4 weeks and tapering down for 1 year. Cyclophosphamide (500 mg/m^2 q 4 weeks, 3–5 doses) or Rituximab (500 mg/m^2 q 7 day, 2 doses) are given to further decrease the production of antibodies. Mycophenolate mofetil (500–750 mg/m2/day) or azathioprine (1–2 mg/kg/day) are used as additional long-term immunosuppression [157].

C5 Inhibition Therapy Monitoring

Data from the prospective studies show that complete complement blockade is obtained within 1 h after the first dose of eculizumab and is maintained long-term in patients receiving the recommended treatment schedule [184]. The role of assessment of complement blockade during routine use of eculizumab is uncertain. If there are features of inadequate disease control, this should be assessed. Incomplete blockade may be due to insufficient dose (especially in children with a weight just below a weight threshold requiring a higher dose) or heavy proteinuria with nephrotic syndrome (leakage of the drug in the urine). A genetic cause might also have to be considered in aHUS patients of Japanese or Asian origin with poor response to eculizumab and/or complement non-blockade, such as the C5 variant which impairs the binding of eculizumab to C5 [185]. For the long term, complement blockade assessment is mostly required in cases of apparent resistance to eculizumab, including relapse of HUS but also isolated abnormalities in platelet count, LDH and/or haptoglobin levels, appearance or increase of proteinuria or serum creatinine, especially if kidney biopsy suggests ongoing TMA.

Currently available assays of complement blockade under eculizumab are a CH50 or other hemolytic-based assays or the Wieslab Complement System [186]. Due to the site of action of eculizumab, low C3 levels as seen in some mutations are not expected to normalize under eculizumab, and this has been observed [125]. Soluble C5b-9 remains detectable or increased in aHUS patients under eculizumab and therefore cannot be recommended to monitor the efficacy of eculizumab [125, 187]. Most aHUS patients treated within the prospective trials who received the protocol schedule had suppression of CH50 activity and eculizumab trough levels ≥ 150 µg/ml [14]. However, the correlation between drug levels and complement activity in aHUS patients is not fully established and the availability of plasma eculizumab measurement is currently limited. An additional consideration is that hemolytic assay monitoring may be less accurate for ravulizumab than for eculizumab. One recent study showed that full inhibition of CH50 was not achieved despite high levels of ravulizumab present in plasma [188].

Some authors have reported using assays of hemolytic activity as a tool to lengthen the interval between doses, in an attempt to reduce cost and infusion burden [189]. This approach is not recommended by the manufacturer. It has been recommended that increasing the interval between doses should be considered only in patients who maintain CH50 activity <10% despite longer intervals or lower doses [186].

Duration of C5 Inhibition Therapy in Children with aHUS in Their Native Kidneys

Lifelong treatment with inhibition of C5 for patients with aHUS has been the accepted paradigm. However, there is no definitive evidence for persisting use. The recommendation of not stopping C5 blockade is being reconsidered for some patients with aHUS in their native kidneys based on estimating the risk of relapse by genetic testing.

Having a safe strategy for discontinuation of treatment would be beneficial not only for reducing the significant cost of the therapy but also for safety of the patients and the long-term quality of their life.

Even in the pre-eculizumab era, not all patients relapsed after successful PE. A report of 214 patients, of which 146 were treated with PE, showed that 42% of children were relapse free after 5 years of observation [5]. A Dutch cohort reported sustained remission in 25% of patients [4] and even a cohort of patients with aHUS with changes in the *CFH* gene had normalized kidney function in 22.5% [190]. Following several case reports and series of successful eculizumab discontinuation [170, 189, 191–193], more evidence to support the safety of eculizumab withdrawal appeared from larger studies. The report on this topic from the Global aHUS Registry showed that 33/151 (22%) patients experienced TMA recurrence, particularly in those with pathogenic variants in genes associated with aHUS or with a family history of aHUS. Eight percent then progressed to end-stage kidney disease and 5% required subsequent kidney transplant [194]. During an unprecedented event between 2016 and 2019 when distribution of eculizumab supply was disrupted in Brazil, the effect of discontinuation without stratifying patients based on genetic risk was demonstrated. There were 11 relapses in a cohort of 24 patients, of which 8 occurred in patients with a *CFH* gene variant [195].

A prospective, single-arm study conducted in France stopped eculizumab after at least 6 months of treatment in 55 patients of which 19 were children and showed an overall aHUS relapse rate of 23% (n = 13). Twenty-eight patients (51%) had rare variants in complement genes (*MCP* n = 12, *CFH* n = 6, *CFI* n = 6, FH antibodies, n = 4). Six out of 19 children (32%) relapsed [196]. All 13 patients who relapsed were carrying a variant in genes associated with aHUS except one that was subsequently found to have hereditary ADAMTS13 deficiency (and therefore did not have aHUS). C5 blocking therapy was restarted in all 13 patients. Eleven returned to their baseline kidney function and two remained with decreased function, one progressing to ESKD. Therefore, prompt identification of relapse in aHUS patients who stopped C5 blocking therapy seems to be crucial for preventing long term kidney damage [196].

The overall evidence suggests that patients with no mutation in known complement genes who achieve stable remission for at least 6 months are at low risk of relapse after stopping the treatment. Patients with mutations relapse at much higher rate and in this situation C5 blocking therapy must be restarted promptly to prevent loss of kidney function.

Further safety data for the withdrawal of C5 inhibition in patients with aHUS are required, particularly for patients with mutations. An ongoing trial of stopping eculizumab in patients with aHUS in UK (SETS, EudraCT Number: 2017-003916-37) [197] aims to corroborate the current evidence for safe stopping. If all evidence supports safe withdrawal of C5 inhibition in patients with aHUS, the challenge for patients and clinicians will be to implement individualized care plans to enable rapid detection of signs of relapse and facilitate immediate access to C5 inhibition when a relapse occurs. Without this in place, there is a risk that aHUS will cause ESKD.

Current evidence suggests that eculizumab can be withdrawn in a significant proportion of patients and pragmatic recommendations can be drawn from the experience and protocols used in the described trials. The prerequisite is that patient has achieved remission of HUS with no signs of TMA, normalization of platelets, LDH and stable kidney function. The duration from initiation of treatment to its discontinuation is not established, yet the arbitrary duration of 6 months chosen for the trials could be used as base recommendation. Genetic testing and testing for anti-FH antibodies could help stratifying risk of possible relapse. Patients with no mutation and no anti-FH antibodies (or low titers) are at lowest risk of relapse. Patients with variants of unknown significance and those with pathogenic variants in *CFI* and *CD46* are making a middle tier with slight risk of relapse. Patients with anti-FH antibodies in high titres, pathogenic *FH, FB* and *C3* mutations are at highest risk and the discontinuation of treatment can likely lead to relapse. Most of the relapses would occur in the first weeks after discontinuation and patients need to be reviewed frequently, ideally weekly, with testing eGFR and blood count to identify relapse quickly and restart the treatment.

Further lifelong specialist follow-up of patients who discontinued complement blocking treatment, their education and providing them with straight pathway for review and restarting treatment in case of possible relapse is essential part of the process. There is limited data on another try to stop in case of relapse and restart and it is likely these patients will need lifelong treatment, ideally with long-acting C5 complement blocker, ravulizumab.

Specific patient group are the patients after kidney transplant, where approach needs to be individualized, based on weighing the benefits of continuous or restrictive therapy.

Kidney Transplantation for aHUS Patients Today

Complement blockade therapy has transformed the approach to kidney transplantation for aHUS patients and there are international consensus guidelines regarding the use of eculizumab in this situation (KDIGO 2017). The guidelines state:

1. Kidney transplantation should be deferred until at least 6 months after the start of dialysis because limited kidney recovery may occur several months after starting eculizumab

2. The decision to use anti-complement therapy during transplantation should be based upon recurrence risk
   (a) Those with a high risk (50–100%) of recurrence include patients with previous recurrence, pathogenic mutation or gain of function mutation. They should be treated with prophylactic eculizumab to start on the day of transplantation and to continue indefinitely
   (b) Those with moderate risk of recurrence include patients with no mutation identified, isolated CFI mutations, complement gene variants of unknown significance or persistently low titer anti-FH antibodies. They can be treated with prophylactic eculizumab or PE or without preventative strategy (left to the discretion of the clinician).
   (c) Those with low recurrence risk of recurrence (<10%) include isolated *MCP* mutation or persistently negative anti-FH antibodies. These patients do not require prophylactic treatment with PE or eculizumab. NB with subsequent data, DGKE HUS can also be viewed as low recurrence risk [46].

3. Living donor transplantation can be considered, with the decision relying on a careful assessment of the risk of aHUS in the donor after kidney donation. A risk assessment for potential living related donation requires full genetic screening of the recipient and the donor, leading to the following possible outcomes:
   (a) If the mutation found in the recipient is undeniably responsible for the occurrence of HUS (e.g., *CFH* mutation in C terminus SCR 19 or 20) and is not found in the donor, the risk of HUS is low for the donor and living-related donor transplantation can proceed.
   (b) If the donor has the same mutation as the recipient, the risk of HUS is present for the donor and living-related donor transplantation should not proceed.

(c) If the role of the variant found in the recipient is uncertain (not reported in databases, unknown functional consequences) the risk of HUS is intermediate for the donor, who may share with the recipient an unknown risk factor, and living-related donor transplantation is not advised.

(d) If no mutation is identified in the recipient and the donor, the risk to the donor is not quantified. KDIGO advises that if there is no evidence of alternate complement pathway activation in the donor, donation is feasible.

In general, additional endothelial damaging factors should be avoided, such as delayed graft function (prolonged ischemia time, non-heart-beating donor), cytomegalovirus infection, high levels of CNI and the association of CNI + mTOR inhibitors and hypertension.

Prior to the availability of eculizumab, isolated liver transplantation and combined liver-kidney transplantation were recognized treatment approaches for patients with mutations in FH, C3 and FB (all synthesized in the liver). These had relatively high morbidity and mortality (for example, 20% of patients who received combined liver-kidney transplant for aHUS died) [103, 198, 199]. Eculizumab represents a safer treatment option, but liver transplantation may still have a role when eculizumab is not available [161].

Potential Future Therapies

Current therapies are limited to monoclonal antibodies against C5. Numerous drugs that inhibit complement via different targets are undergoing clinical development, some of which may be suitable for use in aHUS. OMS721 (Narsoplimab) is a monoclonal antibody targeting mannan-binding lectin associated serine protease-2, the effector enzyme of the lectin pathway of the complement system and is currently undergoing a phase 3 clinical trial in adult patients with aHUS (NCT03205995. LMP023 (Iptacopan) is an oral FB inhibitor also undergoing a phase 3 clinical trial in adult patients with aHUS (NCT04889430) [102].

Conclusion

The journey to an effective treatment for aHUS is a striking demonstration that understanding the pathophysiology of a disease opens the way to new therapies. The demonstration that aHUS was mostly a disease of complement dysregulation paralleled the development of the anti-C5 monoclonal antibody eculizumab. Prospective trials as well as off-label clinical experience confirmed the efficacy of complement blockade to prevent progression to ESKD in aHUS patients and allowed successful kidney transplantation in those on dialysis. This new era in the field of aHUS emphasizes the need for an etiology/pathophysiology-based classification of the various forms of TMAs. Hopefully, new discoveries will identify the etiology of the 30% of aHUS cases that remain unexplained today, and the aHUS denomination will then disappear.

An important current question is that of the duration of eculizumab treatment, and prospective studies are underway to define whether discontinuation can be considered, in which patients, and when. Should withdrawal be shown as feasible in some patients, this would decrease the burden and risks of continuous treatment for patients, but also the cost for health care systems.

The addition of long acting ravulizumab to the treatment armamentarium for aHUS brings choices for patients and clinicians that may improve quality of life. Over the next decade, it is possible that further agents will be shown to be effective for the treatment of aHUS. Thus, future treatment of aHUS might comprise a decision about specific treatment and mode of delivery, followed by a decision regarding continuation or discontinuation of therapy with appropriate monitoring. Such options were not imaginable by aHUS patients 20 years ago.

References

1. Nester CM, Barbour T, de Cordoba SR, et al. Atypical aHUS: state of the art. Mol Immunol. 2015;67:31–42.
2. Noris M, Caprioli J, Bresin E, et al. Relative role of genetic complement abnormalities in sporadic and familial aHUS and their impact on clinical phenotype. Clin J Am Soc Nephrol. 2010;5:1844–59.
3. Maga TK, Nishimura CJ, Weaver AE, Frees KL, Smith RJ. Mutations in alternative pathway complement proteins in American patients with atypical hemolytic uremic syndrome. Hum Mutat. 2010;31:E1445–60.
4. Geerdink LM, Westra D, van Wijk JA, et al. Atypical hemolytic uremic syndrome in children: complement mutations and clinical characteristics. Pediatr Nephrol. 2012;27:1283–91.
5. Fremeaux-Bacchi V, Fakhouri F, Garnier A, et al. Genetics and outcome of atypical hemolytic uremic syndrome: a nationwide French series comparing children and adults. Clin J Am Soc Nephrol. 2013;8:554–62.
6. Kavanagh D, Goodship TH, Richards A. Atypical hemolytic uremic syndrome. Semin Nephrol. 2013;33:508–30.
7. Rodriguez de Cordoba S, Hidalgo MS, Pinto S, Tortajada A. Genetics of atypical hemolytic uremic syndrome (aHUS). Semin Thromb Hemost. 2014;40:422–30.
8. Nester CM, Thomas CP. Atypical hemolytic uremic syndrome: what is it, how is it diagnosed, and how is it treated? Hematology Am Soc Hematol Educ Program. 2012;2012:617–25.
9. Campistol JM, Arias M, Ariceta G, et al. An update for atypical haemolytic uraemic syndrome: diagnosis and treatment. A consensus document. Nefrología (English Edition). 2015;35:421–47.
10. Scully M, Goodship T. How I treat thrombotic thrombocytopenic purpura and atypical haemolytic uraemic syndrome. Br J Haematol. 2014. https://doi.org/10.1111/bjh.12718.
11. Cataland SR, Wu HM. How I treat: the clinical differentiation and initial treatment of adult patients with atypical hemolytic uremic syndrome. Blood. 2014. https://doi.org/10.1182/blood-2013-11-516237.
12. Ariceta G, Besbas N, Johnson S, et al. Guideline for the investigation and initial therapy of diarrhea-negative hemolytic uremic syndrome. Pediatr Nephrol. 2009;24:687–96.
13. Johnson S, Stojanovic J, Ariceta G, et al. An audit analysis of a guideline for the investigation and initial therapy of diarrhea negative (atypical) hemolytic uremic syndrome. Pediatr Nephrol. 2014. https://doi.org/10.1007/s00467-014-2817-4.
14. Legendre CM, Licht C, Muus P, et al. Terminal complement inhibitor eculizumab in atypical hemolytic-uremic syndrome. N Engl J Med. 2013;368:2169–81.
15. Zuber J, Fakhouri F, Roumenina LT, Loirat C, Frémeaux-Bacchi V. Use of eculizumab for atypical haemolytic uraemic syndrome and C3 glomerulopathies. Nat Rev Nephrol. 2012;8:643–57.
16. Besbas N, Karpman D, Landau D, Loirat C, Proesmans W, Remuzzi G, Rizzoni G, Taylor CM, van de Kar N, Zimmerhackl LB. A classification of hemolytic uremic syndrome and thrombotic thrombocytopenic purpura and related disorders. Kidney Int. 2006;70:423–31.
17. Aigner C, Schmidt A, Gaggl M, Sunder-Plassmann G. An updated classification of thrombotic microangiopathies and treatment of complement gene variant-mediated thrombotic microangiopathy. Clin Kidney J. 2019;12:333–7.
18. George JN, Nester CM. Syndromes of thrombotic microangiopathy. N Engl J Med. 2014;371:654–66.
19. Brocklebank V, Wood KM, Kavanagh D. Thrombotic microangiopathy and the kidney. Clin J Am Soc Nephrol. 2018;13:300–17.
20. Joseph A, Cointe A, Mariani Kurkdjian P, Rafat C, Hertig A. Shiga toxin-associated hemolytic uremic syndrome: a narrative review. Toxins. 2020. https://doi.org/10.3390/toxins12020067.
21. Jenkins C, Byrne L, Vishram B, Sawyer C, Balasegaram S, Ahyow L, Johnson S. Shiga toxin-producing Escherichia coli haemolytic uraemic syndrome (STEC-HUS): diagnosis, surveillance and public-health management in England. J Med Microbiol. 2020;69:1034–6.
22. Coppo P, Cuker A, George JN. Thrombotic thrombocytopenic purpura: toward targeted therapy and precision medicine. Res Pract Thromb Haemost. 2019. https://doi.org/10.1002/rth2.12160.
23. Scully M, Cataland S, Coppo P, et al. Consensus on the standardization of terminology in thrombotic thrombocytopenic purpura and related thrombotic microangiopathies. J Thromb Haemost. 2017. https://doi.org/10.1111/jth.13571.
24. Constantinescu AR, Bitzan M, Weiss LS, Christen E, Kaplan BS, Cnaan A, Trachtman H. Non-enteropathic hemolytic uremic syndrome: causes and short-term course. Am J Kidney Dis. 2004. https://doi.org/10.1053/j.ajkd.2004.02.010.
25. Yan K, Desai K, Gullapalli L, Druyts E, Balijepalli C. Epidemiology of atypical hemolytic uremic syndrome: a systematic literature review. Clin Epidemiol. 2020. https://doi.org/10.2147/CLEP.S245642.
26. Bayer G, von Tokarski F, Thoreau B, et al. Etiology and outcomes of thrombotic microangiopathies. Clin J Am Soc Nephrol. 2019. CJN.11470918
27. Ardissino G, Salardi S, Colombo E, et al. Epidemiology of haemolytic uremic syndrome in children. Data from the North Italian HUS network. Eur J Pediatr. 2016. https://doi.org/10.1007/s00431-015-2642-1.
28. Durkan AM, Kim S, Craig J, Elliott E. The long-term outcomes of atypical haemolytic uraemic syndrome:

a national surveillance study. Arch Dis Child. 2016. https://doi.org/10.1136/archdischild-2015-309471.

29. Zimmerhackl LB, Besbas N, Jungraithmayr T, et al. Epidemiology, clinical presentation, and pathophysiology of atypical and recurrent hemolytic uremic syndrome. Semin Thromb Hemost. 2006. https://doi.org/10.1055/s-2006-939767.

30. Mallett A, Patel C, Salisbury A, Wang Z, Healy H, Hoy W. The prevalence and epidemiology of genetic renal disease amongst adults with chronic kidney disease in Australia. Orphanet J Rare Dis. 2014. https://doi.org/10.1186/1750-1172-9-98.

31. Jenssen GR, Hovland E, Bjerre A, Bangstad HJ, Nygard K, Vold L. Incidence and etiology of hemolytic-uremic syndrome in children in Norway, 1999-2008—a retrospective study of hospital records to assess the sensitivity of surveillance. BMC Infect Dis. 2014. https://doi.org/10.1186/1471-2334-14-265.

32. Wühl E, van Stralen KJ, Wanner C, et al. Renal replacement therapy for rare diseases affecting the kidney: an analysis of the ERA-EDTA Registry. Nephrol Dial Transplant. 2014;29(Suppl:4):iv1-8.

33. Cameron JS, Vick R. Letter: plasma-C3 in haemolytic-uraemic syndrome and thrombotic thrombocytopenic purpura. Lancet. 1973;2:975.

34. Thompson RA, Winterborn MH. Hypocomplementaemia due to a genetic deficiency of beta 1H globulin. Clin Exp Immunol. 1981;46:110–9.

35. Pichette V, Quérin S, Schürch W, Brun G, Lehner-Netsch G, Delâge JM. Familial hemolytic-uremic syndrome and homozygous factor H deficiency. Am J Kidney Dis. 1994. https://doi.org/10.1016/S0272-6386(12)81065-1.

36. Rougier N, Kazatchkine MD, Rougier JP, et al. Human complement factor H deficiency associated with hemolytic uremic syndrome. J Am Soc Nephrol. 1998. https://doi.org/10.1681/asn.v9122318.

37. Warwicker P, Goodship TH, Donne RL, Pirson Y, Nicholls A, Ward RM, Turnpenny P, Goodship JA. Genetic studies into inherited and sporadic hemolytic uremic syndrome. Kidney Int. 1998;53:836–44.

38. Richards A, Kemp EJ, Liszewski MK, et al. Mutations in human complement regulator, membrane cofactor protein (CD46), predispose to development of familial hemolytic uremic syndrome. Proc Natl Acad Sci U S A. 2003;100:12966–71.

39. Fremeaux-Bacchi V, Dragon-Durey MA, Blouin J, Vigneau C, Kuypers D, Boudailliez B, Loirat C, Rondeau E, Fridman WH. Complement factor I: a susceptibility gene for atypical haemolytic uraemic syndrome. J Med Genet. 2004;41:e84.

40. Dragon-Durey MA, Loirat C, Cloarec S, Macher MA, Blouin J, Nivet H, Weiss L, Fridman WH, Fremeaux-Bacchi V. Anti-Factor H autoantibodies associated with atypical hemolytic uremic syndrome. J Am Soc Nephrol. 2005;16:555–63.

41. Fremeaux-Bacchi V, Moulton EA, Kavanagh D, et al. Genetic and functional analyses of membrane cofactor protein (CD46) mutations in atypical hemolytic uremic syndrome. J Am Soc Nephrol. 2006;17:2017–25.

42. Goicoechea de Jorge E, Harris CL, Esparza-Gordillo J, Carreras L, Arranz EA, Garrido CA, Lopez-Trascasa M, Sanchez-Corral P, Morgan BP, Rodriguez de Cordoba S. Gain-of-function mutations in complement factor B are associated with atypical hemolytic uremic syndrome. Proc Natl Acad Sci U S A. 2007;104:240–5.

43. Frémeaux-Bacchi V, Miller EC, Liszewski MK, et al. Mutations in complement C3 predispose to development of atypical hemolytic uremic syndrome. Blood. 2008;112:4948–52.

44. Delvaeye M, Noris M, de Vriese A, et al. Thrombomodulin mutations in atypical hemolytic-uremic syndrome. N Engl J Med. 2009;361:345–57.

45. Lemaire M, Fremeaux-Bacchi V, Schaefer F, et al. Recessive mutations in DGKE cause atypical hemolytic-uremic syndrome. Nat Genet. 2013;45:531–6.

46. Brocklebank V, Kumar G, Howie AJ, et al. Long-term outcomes and response to treatment in diacylglycerol kinase epsilon nephropathy. Kidney Int. 2020. https://doi.org/10.1016/j.kint.2020.01.045.

47. Ricklin D, Hajishengallis G, Yang K, Lambris JD. Complement: a key system for immune surveillance and homeostasis. Nat Immunol. 2010;11:785–97.

48. Schmidt CQ, Lambris JD, Ricklin D. Protection of host cells by complement regulators. Immunol Rev. 2016. https://doi.org/10.1111/imr.12475.

49. Hajishengallis G, Reis ES, Mastellos DC, Ricklin D, Lambris JD. Novel mechanisms and functions of complement. Nat Immunol. 2017;18:1288–98.

50. Killick J, Morisse G, Sieger D, Astier AL. Complement as a regulator of adaptive immunity. Semin Immunopathol. 2018. https://doi.org/10.1007/s00281-017-0644-y.

51. Merle NS, Noe R, Halbwachs-Mecarelli L, Fremeaux-Bacchi V, Roumenina LT. Complement system part II: role in immunity. Front Immunol. 2015;6:257.

52. Merle NS, Church SE, Fremeaux-Bacchi V, Roumenina LT. Complement system part I—molecular mechanisms of activation and regulation. Front Immunol. 2015;6:262.

53. Bresin E, Rurali E, Caprioli J, et al. Combined complement gene mutations in atypical hemolytic uremic syndrome influence clinical phenotype. J Am Soc Nephrol. 2013;24:475–86.

54. Osborne A. Complement mutations database. https://www.complement-db.org/home.php.

55. Saunders RE, Abarrategui-Garrido C, Fremeaux-Bacchi V, et al. The interactive Factor H-atypical hemolytic uremic syndrome mutation database and website: update and integration of membrane cofac-

56. Sellier-Leclerc AL, Fremeaux-Bacchi V, Dragon-Durey MA, et al. Differential impact of complement mutations on clinical characteristics in atypical hemolytic uremic syndrome. J Am Soc Nephrol. 2007;18:2392–400.

57. Besbas N, Gulhan B, Soylemezoglu O, Ozcakar ZB, Korkmaz E, Hayran M, Ozaltin F. Turkish pediatric atypical hemolytic uremic syndrome registry: initial analysis of 146 patients. BMC Nephrol. 2017;18:6.

58. Westland R, Bodria M, Carrea A, et al. Phenotypic expansion of DGKE-associated diseases. J Am Soc Nephrol. 2014;25:1408–14.

59. Chinchilla DS, Pinto S, Hoppe B, Adragna M, Lopez L, Roldan MLJ, Peña A, Trascasa ML, Sánchez-Corral P, de Córdoba SR. Complement mutations in diacylglycerol kinase-ε–associated atypical hemolytic uremic syndrome. Clin J Am Soc Nephrol. 2014. https://doi.org/10.2215/CJN.01640214.

60. Azukaitis K, Simkova E, Abdul Majid M, et al. The phenotypic spectrum of nephropathies associated with mutations in diacylglycerol Kinase ε. J Am Soc Nephrol. 2017. https://doi.org/10.1681/ASN.2017010031.

61. Gholizad-Kolveiri S, Hooman N, Alizadeh R, Hoseini R, Otukesh H, Talebi S, Akouchekian M. Whole exome sequencing revealed a novel homozygous variant in the DGKE catalytic domain: a case report of familial hemolytic uremic syndrome. BMC Med Genet. 2020; https://doi.org/10.1186/s12881-020-01097-9.

62. Dragon-Durey MA, Sethi SK, Bagga A, et al. Clinical features of anti-factor H autoantibody-associated hemolytic uremic syndrome. J Am Soc Nephrol. 2010;21:2180–7.

63. Hofer J, Janecke AR, Zimmerhackl LB, et al. Complement factor H-related protein 1 deficiency and factor H antibodies in pediatric patients with atypical hemolytic uremic syndrome. Clin J Am Soc Nephrol. 2013;8:407–15.

64. Sinha A, Gulati A, Saini S, et al. Prompt plasma exchanges and immunosuppressive treatment improves the outcomes of anti-factor H autoantibody-associated hemolytic uremic syndrome in children. Kidney Int. 2014;85:1151–60.

65. Hofer J, Giner T, Józsi M. Complement factor h-antibody-associated hemolytic uremic syndrome: pathogenesis, clinical presentation, and treatment. Semin Thromb Hemost. 2014. https://doi.org/10.1055/s-0034-1375297.

66. Puraswani M, Khandelwal P, Saini H, et al. Clinical and immunological profile of anti-factor H antibody associated atypical hemolytic uremic syndrome: a nationwide database. Front Immunol. 2019. https://doi.org/10.3389/fimmu.2019.01282.

67. Štolbová Š, Bezdíčka M, Prohászka Z, Csuka D, Hrachovinová I, Burkert J, Šimánková N, Průhová Š, Zieg J. Molecular basis and outcomes of atypical haemolytic uraemic syndrome in Czech children. Eur J Pediatr. 2020. https://doi.org/10.1007/s00431-020-03666-9.

68. Schaefer F, Licht C, Ardissino G, Ariceta G, Kupelian V, Gasteyger C, Greenbaum LA, Ogawa M, van de Walle J, Fremeaux-Bacchi V. Manifestations of atypical haemolytic uraemic syndrome (AHUS) in children and adults: data from the global AHUS registry. Pediatr Nephrol. 2015;30:1544.

69. Condom P, Mansuy JM, Decramer S, Izopet J, Mengelle C. Atypical hemolytic uremic syndrome triggered by varicella infection. IDCases. 2017. https://doi.org/10.1016/j.idcr.2017.04.004.

70. Kobbe R, Schild R, Christner M, Oh J, Loos S, Kemper MJ. Case report—atypical hemolytic uremic syndrome triggered by influenza B. BMC Nephrol. 2017. https://doi.org/10.1186/s12882-017-0512-y.

71. van Hoeve K, Vandermeulen C, van Ranst M, Levtchenko E, van den Heuvel L, Mekahli D. Occurrence of atypical HUS associated with influenza B. Eur J Pediatr. 2017. https://doi.org/10.1007/s00431-017-2856-5.

72. Madden I, Roumenina LT, Langlois-Meurinne H, Guichoux J, Llanas B, Frémeaux-Bacchi V, Harambat J, Godron-Dubrasquet A. Hemolytic uremic syndrome associated with Bordetella pertussis infection in a 2-month-old infant carrying a pathogenic variant in complement factor H. Pediatr Nephrol. 2019. https://doi.org/10.1007/s00467-018-4174-1.

73. el Sissy C, Saldman A, Zanetta G, et al. COVID-19 as a potential trigger of complement-mediated atypical HUS. Blood. 2021. https://doi.org/10.1182/blood.2021012752.

74. Edey MM, Mead PA, Saunders RE, Strain L, Perkins SJ, Goodship THJ, Kanagasundaram NS. Association of a factor H mutation with hemolytic uremic syndrome following a diarrheal illness. Am J Kidney Dis. 2008. https://doi.org/10.1053/j.ajkd.2007.08.030.

75. Alberti M, Valoti E, Piras R, Bresin E, Galbusera M, Tripodo C, Thaiss F, Remuzzi G, Noris M. Two patients with history of STEC-HUS, posttransplant recurrence and complement gene mutations. Am J Transplant. 2013. https://doi.org/10.1111/ajt.12297.

76. Dragon-Durey MA, Blanc C, Garnier A, Hofer J, Sethi SK, Zimmerhackl LB. Anti-factor H autoantibody-associated hemolytic uremic syndrome: review of literature of the autoimmune form of HUS. Semin Thromb Hemost. 2010;36:633–40.

77. Durey MAD, Sinha A, Togarsimalemath SK, Bagga A. Anti-complement-factor H-associated glomerulopathies. Nat Rev Nephrol. 2016;12:563–78.

78. Togarsimalemath SK, Si-Mohammed A, Puraswani M, Gupta A, Vabret A, Liguori S, Mariani-Kurkdjian P, Bagga A, Dragon-Durey MA. Gastrointestinal pathogens in anti-FH antibody positive and negative Hemolytic Uremic Syndrome. Pediatr Res. 2018;84:118–24.

79. Fakhouri F, Roumenina L, Provot F, et al. Pregnancy-associated hemolytic uremic syndrome revisited in the era of complement gene mutations. J Am Soc Nephrol. 2010;21:859–67.

80. Sethi S, Fervenza FC. Pathology of renal diseases associated with dysfunction of the alternative pathway of complement: C3 glomerulopathy and atypical hemolytic uremic syndrome (aHUS). Semin Thromb Hemost. 2014. https://doi.org/10.1055/s-0034-1375701.

81. Benz K, Amann K. Pathological aspects of membranoproliferative glomerulonephritis (MPGN) and haemolytic uraemic syndrome (HUS)/thrombocyte thrombopenic purpura (TTP). Thromb Haemost. 2009. https://doi.org/10.1160/TH07-12-0761.

82. Goodship THJ, Cook HT, Fakhouri F, et al. Atypical hemolytic uremic syndrome and C3 glomerulopathy: conclusions from a "Kidney Disease: Improving Global Outcomes" (KDIGO) Controversies Conference. Kidney Int. 2017. https://doi.org/10.1016/j.kint.2016.10.005.

83. Formeck C, Swiatecka-Urban A. Extra-renal manifestations of atypical hemolytic uremic syndrome. Pediatr Nephrol. 2018. https://doi.org/10.1007/s00467-018-4039-7.

84. Hofer J, Rosales A, Fischer C, Giner T. Extra-renal manifestations of complement-mediated thrombotic microangiopathies. Front Pediatr. 2014. https://doi.org/10.3389/fped.2014.00097.

85. Gulleroglu K, Fidan K, Hancer VS, Bayrakci U, Baskin E, Soylemezoglu O. Neurologic involvement in atypical hemolytic uremic syndrome and successful treatment with eculizumab. Pediatr Nephrol. 2013;28:827–30.

86. Hu H, Nagra A, Haq MR, Gilbert RD. Eculizumab in atypical haemolytic uraemic syndrome with severe cardiac and neurological involvement. Pediatr Nephrol. 2014. https://doi.org/10.1007/s00467-013-2709-z.

87. Vilalta R, Lara E, Madrid A, Chocron S, Muñoz M, Casquero A, Nieto J. Long-term eculizumab improves clinical outcomes in atypical hemolytic uremic syndrome. Pediatr Nephrol. 2012. https://doi.org/10.1007/s00467-012-2276-8.

88. Diamante Chiodini B, Davin JC, Corazza F, Khaldi K, Dahan K, Ismaili K, Adams B. Eculizumab in anti-factor H antibodies associated with atypical hemolytic uremic syndrome. Pediatrics. 2014. https://doi.org/10.1542/peds.2013-1594.

89. Michaux K, Bacchetta J, Javouhey E, Cochat P, Frémaux-Bacchi V, Sellier-Leclerc A-L. Eculizumab in neonatal hemolytic uremic syndrome with homozygous factor H deficiency. Pediatr Nephrol. 2014;29:2415–9.

90. Malina M, Gulati A, Bagga A, Majid MA, Simkova E, Schaefer F. Peripheral gangrene in children with atypical hemolytic uremic syndrome. Pediatrics. 2013;131:e331–5.

91. Ariceta G, Arrizabalaga B, Aguirre M, Morteruel E, Lopez-Trascasa M. Eculizumab in the treatment of atypical hemolytic uremic syndrome in infants. Am J Kidney Dis. 2012. https://doi.org/10.1053/j.ajkd.2011.11.027.

92. Ardissino G, Tel F, Testa S, Marzano AV, Lazzari R, Salardi S, Edefonti A. Skin involvement in atypical hemolytic uremic syndrome. Am J Kidney Dis. 2014. https://doi.org/10.1053/j.ajkd.2013.09.020.

93. Santos C, Lopes D, Gomes A, Ventura A, Tente D, Seabra J. Cutaneous involvement in haemolytic uraemic syndrome. Clin Kidney J. 2013. https://doi.org/10.1093/ckj/sft114.

94. Larakeb A, Leroy S, Frémeaux-Bacchi V, Montchilova M, Pelosse B, Dunand O, Deschênes G, Bensman A, Ulinski T. Ocular involvement in hemolytic uremic syndrome due to factor H deficiency—are there therapeutic consequences? Pediatr Nephrol. 2007. https://doi.org/10.1007/s00467-007-0540-0.

95. Davin JC, Majoie C, Groothoff J, Gracchi V, Bouts A, Goodship TH, Loirat C. Prevention of large-vessel stenoses in atypical hemolytic uremic syndrome associated with complement dysregulation. Pediatr Nephrol. 2011;26:155–7.

96. Loirat C, Macher MA, Elmaleh-Berges M, et al. Non-atheromatous arterial stenoses in atypical haemolytic uraemic syndrome associated with complement dysregulation. Nephrol Dial Transplant. 2010;25:3421–5.

97. Békássy ZD, Kristoffersson AC, Cronqvist M, Roumenina LT, Rybkine T, Vergoz L, Hue C, Fremeaux-Bacchi V, Karpman D. Eculizumab in an anephric patient with atypical haemolytic uraemic syndrome and advanced vascular lesions. Nephrol Dial Transplant. 2013. https://doi.org/10.1093/ndt/gft340.

98. Ažukaitis K, Loirat C, Malina M, Adomaitienė I, Jankauskienė A. Macrovascular involvement in a child with atypical hemolytic uremic syndrome. Pediatr Nephrol. 2014;29:1273–7.

99. Noris M, Remuzzi G. Cardiovascular complications in atypical haemolytic uraemic syndrome. NRN. 2014:10–5.

100. Ohanian M, Cable C, Halka K. Eculizumab safely reverses neurologic impairment and eliminates need for dialysis in severe atypical hemolytic uremic syndrome. Clin Pharmacol. 2011;3:5–12.

101. Salem G, Flynn JM, Cataland SR. Profound neurological injury in a patient with atypical hemolytic uremic syndrome. Ann Hematol. 2013. https://doi.org/10.1007/s00277-012-1615-y.

102. McFarlane PA, Bitzan M, Broome C, et al. Making the correct diagnosis in thrombotic microangiopathy: a narrative review. Can J Kidney Health Dis. 2021. https://doi.org/10.1177/20543581211008707.

103. Loirat C, Fakhouri F, Ariceta G, et al. An international consensus approach to the management of atypical hemolytic uremic syndrome in children. Pediatr Nephrol. 2016. https://doi.org/10.1007/s00467-015-3076-8.

104. le Quintrec M, Zuber J, Moulin B, et al. Complement genes strongly predict recurrence and graft outcome

105. in adult renal transplant recipients with atypical hemolytic and uremic syndrome. Am J Transplant. 2013. https://doi.org/10.1111/ajt.12077.

105. Mele C, Remuzzi G, Noris M. Hemolytic uremic syndrome. Semin Immunopathol. 2014;36:399–420.

106. Espié E, Grimont F, Mariani-Kurkdjian P, et al. Surveillance of hemolytic uremic syndrome in children less than 15 years of age, a system to monitor o157 and non-o157 shiga toxin-producing escherichia coli infections in France, 1996-2006. Pediatr Infect Dis J. 2008. https://doi.org/10.1097/INF.0b013e31816a062f.

107. Loirat C, Girma JP, Desconclois C, Coppo P, Veyradier A. Thrombotic thrombocytopenic purpura related to severe ADAMTS13 deficiency in children. Pediatr Nephrol. 2009. https://doi.org/10.1007/s00467-008-0863-5.

108. Loirat C, Coppo P, Veyradier A. Thrombotic thrombocytopenic purpura in children. Curr Opin Pediatr. 2013. https://doi.org/10.1097/MOP.0b013e32835e7888.

109. Hassenpflug WA, Budde U, Schneppenheim S, Schneppenheim R. Inherited thrombotic thrombocytopenic purpura in children. Semin Thromb Hemost. 2014. https://doi.org/10.1055/s-0034-1376152.

110. Sharma AP, Greenberg CR, Prasad AN, Prasad C. Hemolytic uremic syndrome (HUS) secondary to cobalamin C (cblC) disorder. Pediatr Nephrol. 2007;22:2097–103.

111. Cornec-Le Gall E, Delmas Y, de Parscau L, Doucet L, Ogier H, Benoist JF, Fremeaux-Bacchi V, le Meur Y. Adult-onset eculizumab-resistant hemolytic uremic syndrome associated with cobalamin C deficiency. Am J Kidney Dis. 2014. https://doi.org/10.1053/j.ajkd.2013.08.031.

112. Lemoine M, François A, Grangé S, et al. Cobalamin C deficiency induces a typical histopathological pattern of renal arteriolar and glomerular thrombotic microangiopathy. Kidney Int Rep. 2018. https://doi.org/10.1016/j.ekir.2018.05.015.

113. Menni F, Testa S, Guez S, Chiarelli G, Alberti L, Esposito S. Neonatal atypical hemolytic uremic syndrome due to methylmalonic aciduria and homocystinuria. Pediatr Nephrol. 2012. https://doi.org/10.1007/s00467-012-2152-6.

114. Lawrence J, Gwee A, Quinlan C. Pneumococcal haemolytic uraemic syndrome in the postvaccine era. Arch Dis Child. 2018;103:957–61.

115. Kokame K, Nobe Y, Kokubo Y, Okayama A, Miyata T. FRETS-VWF73, a first fluorogenic substrate for ADAMTS13 assay. Br J Haematol. 2005. https://doi.org/10.1111/j.1365-2141.2005.05420.x.

116. Mackie I, Mancini I, Muia J, Kremer Hovinga J, Nair S, Machin S, Baker R. International Council for Standardization in Haematology (ICSH) recommendations for laboratory measurement of ADAMTS13. Int J Lab Hematol. 2020. https://doi.org/10.1111/ijlh.13295.

117. Meyer SC, Sulzer I, Lämmle B, Kremer Hovinga JA. Hyperbilirubinemia interferes with ADAMTS-13 activity measurement by FRETS-VWF73 assay: diagnostic relevance in patients suffering from acute thrombotic microangiopathies [4]. J Thromb Haemost. 2007. https://doi.org/10.1111/j.1538-7836.2007.02438.x.

118. Mackie I, Langley K, Chitolie A, Liesner R, Scully M, Machin S, Peyvandi F. Discrepancies between ADAMTS13 activity assays in patients with thrombotic microangiopathies. Thromb Haemost. 2013. https://doi.org/10.1160/TH12-08-0565.

119. Thouzeau S, Capdenat S, Stepanian A, Coppo P, Veyradier A. Evaluation of a commercial assay for ADAMTS13 activity measurement. Thromb Haemost. 2013. https://doi.org/10.1160/TH13-05-0393.

120. Ardissino G, Perrone M, Tel F, Testa S, Morrone A, Possenti I, Tagliaferri F, Dilena R, Menni F. Late onset cobalamin disorder and hemolytic uremic syndrome: a rare cause of nephrotic syndrome. Case Rep Pediatr. 2017. https://doi.org/10.1155/2017/2794060.

121. Topaloglu R, Inözü M, Gülhan B, Gürbüz B, Talim B, Coşkun T. Do not miss rare and treatable cause of early-onset hemolytic uremic syndrome: cobalamin C deficiency. Nephron. 2019. https://doi.org/10.1159/000497822.

122. Sloan JL, Carrillo N, Adams D. Disorders of intracellular cobalamin metabolism. In: Adam MP, Ardinger HH, Pagon RA, et al., editors. GeneReviews®; 2008.

123. Watson R, Lindner S, Bordereau P, Hunze EM, Tak F, Ngo S, Zipfel PF, Skerka C, Dragon-Durey MA, Marchbank KJ. Standardisation of the factor H autoantibody assay. Immunobiology. 2014;219:9–16.

124. Cataland SR, Holers VM, Geyer S, Yang S, Wu HM. Biomarkers of terminal complement activation confirm the diagnosis of aHUS and differentiate aHUS from TTP. Blood. 2014. https://doi.org/10.1182/blood-2013-12-547067.

125. Noris M, Galbusera M, Gastoldi S, et al. Dynamics of complement activation in aHUS and how to monitor eculizumab therapy. Blood. 2014;124:1715–26.

126. Volokhina EB, Westra D, van der Velden TJAM, van de Kar NCAJ, Mollnes TE, van den Heuvel LP. Complement activation patterns in atypical haemolytic uraemic syndrome during acute phase and in remission. Clin Exp Immunol. 2015. https://doi.org/10.1111/cei.12426.

127. Barnum SR, Bubeck D, Schein TN. Soluble membrane attack complex: biochemistry and immunobiology. Front Immunol. 2020. https://doi.org/10.3389/fimmu.2020.585108.

128. Moore I, Strain L, Pappworth I, et al. Association of factor H autoantibodies with deletions of CFHR1, CFHR3, CFHR4, and with mutations in CFH, CFI, CD46, and C3 in patients with atypical hemolytic uremic syndrome. Blood. 2010;115:379–87.

129. Venables JP, Strain L, Routledge D, et al. Atypical haemolytic uraemic syndrome associated with a hybrid complement gene. PLoS Med. 2006;3:e431.

130. Maga TK, Meyer NC, Belsha C, Nishimura CJ, Zhang Y, Smith RJ. A novel deletion in the RCA gene cluster causes atypical hemolytic uremic syndrome. Nephrol Dial Transplant. 2011;26:739–41.

131. Francis NJ, McNicholas B, Awan A, et al. A novel hybrid CFH/CFHR3 gene generated by a microhomology-mediated deletion in familial atypical hemolytic uremic syndrome. Blood. 2012:119:591–601.

132. Heinen S, Wiehl U, Lauer N, et al. Disease associated protein complement factor H related protein 1 (CFHR1) is a regulator of the human alternative complement pathway. Mol Immunol. 2008. https://doi.org/10.1016/j.molimm.2008.08.027.

133. Roumenina LT, Frimat M, Miller EC, et al. A prevalent C3 mutation in aHUS patients causes a direct C3 convertase gain of function. Blood. 2012;119:4182–91.

134. Marinozzi MC, Vergoz L, Rybkine T, et al. Complement factor b mutations in atypical hemolytic uremic syndrome-disease-relevant or benign? J Am Soc Nephrol. 2014. https://doi.org/10.1681/ASN.2013070796.

135. Roumenina LT, Jablonski M, Hue C, et al. Hyperfunctional C3 convertase leads to complement deposition on endothelial cells and contributes to atypical hemolytic uremic syndrome. Blood. 2009;114:2837–45.

136. Fremeaux-Bacchi V, Kemp EJ, Goodship JA, Dragon-Durey MA, Strain L, Loirat C, Deng HW, Goodship TH. The development of atypical haemolytic-uraemic syndrome is influenced by susceptibility factors in factor H and membrane cofactor protein: evidence from two independent cohorts. J Med Genet. 2005;42:852–6.

137. Abarrategui-Garrido C, Martínez-Barricarte R, López-Trascasa M, Rodríguez De Córdoba S, Sánchez-Corral P. Characterization of complement factor H-related (CFHR) proteins in plasma reveals novel genetic variations of CFHR1 associated with atypical hemolytic uremic syndrome. Blood. 2009. https://doi.org/10.1182/blood-2009-05-223834.

138. Meri S. Complement activation in diseases presenting with thrombotic microangiopathy. Eur J Intern Med. 2013;24:496–502.

139. Riedl M, Fakhouri F, le Quintrec M, Noone DG, Jungraithmayr TC, Fremeaux-Bacchi V, Licht C. Spectrum of complement-mediated thrombotic microangiopathies: pathogenetic insights identifying novel treatment approaches. Semin Thromb Hemost. 2014;40:444–64.

140. Turner NA, Moake J. Assembly and activation of alternative complement components on endothelial cell-anchored ultra-large von willebrand factor links complement and hemostasis-thrombosis. PLoS One. 2013; https://doi.org/10.1371/journal.pone.0059372.

141. Rayes J, Roumenina LT, Dimitrov JD, et al. The interaction between factor H and VWF increases factor H cofactor activity and regulates VWF prothrom-botic status. Blood. 2014. https://doi.org/10.1182/blood-2013-04-495853.

142. Feng S, Liang X, Cruz MA, Vu H, Zhou Z, Pemmaraju N, Dong JF, Kroll MH, Afshar-Kharghan V. The interaction between factor H and Von Willebrand factor. PLoS One. 2013. https://doi.org/10.1371/journal.pone.0073715.

143. Ståhl AL, Vaziri-Sani F, Heinen S, Kristoffersson AC, Gydell KH, Raafat R, Gutierrez A, Beringer O, Zipfel PF, Karpman D. Factor H dysfunction in patients with atypical hemolytic uremic syndrome contributes to complement deposition on platelets and their activation. Blood. 2008. https://doi.org/10.1182/blood-2007-08-106153.

144. Pickering MC, Goicoechea De Jorge E, Martinez-Barricarte R, et al. Spontaneous hemolytic uremic syndrome triggered by complement factor H lacking surface recognition domains. J Exp Med. 2007. https://doi.org/10.1084/jem.20070301.

145. Martin Merinero H, Zhang Y, Arjona E, del Angel G, Goodfellow R, Gomez-Rubio E, Ji R-R, Michelena M, Smith R, Rodríguez de Córdoba S. Functional characterization of 105 Factor H variants associated with atypical HUS: lessons for variant classification. Blood. 2021. https://doi.org/10.1182/blood.2021012037.

146. Fakhouri F, Frémeaux-Bacchi V. Thrombotic microangiopathy in aHUS and beyond: clinical clues from complement genetics. Nat Rev Nephrol. 2021. https://doi.org/10.1038/s41581-021-00424-4.

147. Quaggin SE. DGKE and atypical HUS. Nat Genet. 2013;45:475–6.

148. Bu F, Zhang Y, Wang K, et al. Genetic analysis of 400 patients refines understanding and implicates a new gene in atypical hemolytic uremic syndrome. J Am Soc Nephrol. 2018; ASN.2018070759.

149. Thergaonkar RW, Narang A, Gurjar BS, et al. Targeted exome sequencing in anti-factor H antibody negative HUS reveals multiple variations. Clin Exp Nephrol. 2018. https://doi.org/10.1007/s10157-017-1478-6.

150. Challis RC, Ring T, Xu Y, et al. Thrombotic microangiopathy in inverted formin 2-mediated renal disease. J Am Soc Nephrol. 2017. https://doi.org/10.1681/ASN.2015101189.

151. Ståhl A-L, Kristoffersson AC, Olin AI, Olsson ML, Roodhooft AM, Proesmans W, Karpman D. A novel mutation in the complement regulator clusterin in recurrent hemolytic uremic syndrome. Mol Immunol. 2009. https://doi.org/10.1016/j.molimm.2009.04.012.

152. Brocklebank V, Johnson S, Sheerin TP, et al. Factor H autoantibody is associated with atypical hemolytic uremic syndrome in children in the United Kingdom and Ireland. Kidney Int. 2017;92:1261–71.

153. Blanc C, Roumenina LT, Ashraf Y, et al. Overall neutralization of complement factor H by autoantibodies in the acute phase of the autoimmune form of atypical hemolytic uremic syndrome. J Immunol. 2012;189:3528–37.

154. Holmes LV, Strain L, Staniforth SJ, Moore I, Marchbank K, Kavanagh D, Goodship JA, Cordell HJ, Goodship THJ. Determining the population frequency of the CFHR3/CFHR1 deletion at 1q32. PLoS One. 2013. https://doi.org/10.1371/journal.pone.0060352.

155. Bhattacharjee A, Reuter S, Trojnár E, et al. The major autoantibody epitope on factor H in atypical hemolytic uremic syndrome is structurally different from its homologous site in factor H-related protein 1, supporting a novel model for induction of autoimmunity in this disease. J Biol Chem. 2015;290:9500–10.

156. Kavanagh D, Pappworth IY, Anderson H, et al. Factor i autoantibodies in patients with atypical hemolytic uremic syndrome: disease-associated or an epiphenomenon? Clin J Am Soc Nephrol. 2012;7:417–26.

157. Bagga A, Khandelwal P, Mishra K, et al. Hemolytic uremic syndrome in a developing country: consensus guidelines. Pediatr Nephrol. 2019;34:1465–82.

158. Zuber J, Quintrec ML, Krid S, et al. Eculizumab for atypical hemolytic uremic syndrome recurrence in renal transplantation. Am J Transplant. 2012. https://doi.org/10.1111/j.1600-6143.2012.04252.x.

159. Sinibaldi S, Guzzo I, Piras R, Bresin E, Emma F, dello Strologo L. Post-transplant recurrence of atypical hemolytic uremic syndrome in a patient with thrombomodulin mutation. Pediatr Transplant. 2013. https://doi.org/10.1111/petr.12151.

160. Saland JM, Ruggenenti P, Remuzzi G. Liver-kidney transplantation to cure atypical hemolytic uremic syndrome. J Am Soc Nephrol. 2009;20:940–9.

161. Zuber J, le Quintrec M, Morris H, Frémeaux-Bacchi V, Loirat C, Legendre C. Targeted strategies in the prevention and management of atypical HUS recurrence after kidney transplantation. Transplant Rev. 2013. https://doi.org/10.1016/j.trre.2013.07.003.

162. Kellum JA, Lameire N, Aspelin P, et al. Kidney disease: improving global outcomes (KDIGO) acute kidney injury work group. KDIGO clinical practice guideline for acute kidney injury. Kidney Int Suppl. 2012. https://doi.org/10.1038/kisup.2012.1.

163. Hillmen P, Hall C, Marsh JC, et al. Effect of eculizumab on hemolysis and transfusion requirements in patients with paroxysmal nocturnal hemoglobinuria. N Engl J Med. 2004;350:552–9.

164. Gruppo RA, Rother RP. Eculizumab for congenital atypical hemolytic-uremic syndrome. N Engl J Med. 2009;360:544–6.

165. Nurnberger J, Philipp T, Witzke O, et al. Eculizumab for atypical hemolytic-uremic syndrome. N Engl J Med. 2009;360:542–4.

166. Christmann M, Hansen M, Bergmann C, Schwabe D, Brand J, Schneider W. Eculizumab as first-line therapy for atypical hemolytic uremic syndrome. Pediatrics. 2014. https://doi.org/10.1542/peds.2013-1787.

167. Vaisbich MH, Henriques LDS, Watanabe A, et al. [Eculizumab for the treatment of atypical hemolytic uremic syndrome: case report and revision of the literature]. J Bras Nefrol. 2013. https://doi.org/10.5935/0101-2800.20130037.

168. Besbas N, Gulhan B, Karpman D, Topaloglu R, Duzova A, Korkmaz E, Ozaltin F. Neonatal onset atypical hemolytic uremic syndrome successfully treated with eculizumab. Pediatr Nephrol. 2013. https://doi.org/10.1007/s00467-012-2296-4.

169. Giordano M, Castellano G, Messina G, Divella C, Bellantuono R, Puteo F, Colella V, Depalo T, Gesualdo L. Preservation of renal function in atypical hemolytic uremic syndrome by eculizumab: a case report. Pediatrics. 2012. https://doi.org/10.1542/peds.2011-1685.

170. Cayci FS, Cakar N, Hancer VS, Uncu N, Acar B, Gur G. Eculizumab therapy in a child with hemolytic uremic syndrome and CFI mutation. Pediatr Nephrol. 2012. https://doi.org/10.1007/s00467-012-2283-9.

171. Licht C, Greenbaum LA, Muus P, et al. Efficacy and safety of eculizumab in atypical hemolytic uremic syndrome from 2-year extensions of phase 2 studies. Kidney Int. 2015. https://doi.org/10.1038/ki.2014.423.

172. Greenbaum LA, Fila M, Ardissino G, et al. Eculizumab is a safe and effective treatment in pediatric patients with atypical hemolytic uremic syndrome. Kidney Int. 2016;89:701–11.

173. Sheridan D, Yu ZX, Zhang Y, et al. Design and preclinical characterization of ALXN1210: a novel anti-C5 antibody with extended duration of action. PLoS One. 2018. https://doi.org/10.1371/journal.pone.0195909.

174. Rondeau E, Scully M, Ariceta G, et al. The long-acting C5 inhibitor, ravulizumab, is effective and safe in adult patients with atypical hemolytic uremic syndrome naïve to complement inhibitor treatment. Kidney Int. 2020;97:1287–96.

175. Barbour T, Scully M, Ariceta G, et al. Long-term efficacy and safety of the long-acting complement C5 inhibitor ravulizumab for the treatment of atypical hemolytic uremic syndrome in adults. Kidney Int Rep. 2021. https://doi.org/10.1016/j.ekir.2021.03.884.

176. Tanaka K, Adams B, Aris AM, Fujita N, Ogawa M, Ortiz S, Vallee M, Greenbaum LA. The long-acting C5 inhibitor, ravulizumab, is efficacious and safe in pediatric patients with atypical hemolytic uremic syndrome previously treated with eculizumab. Pediatr Nephrol. 2021;36:889–98.

177. https://www.clinicaltrialsregister.eu/ctr-search/trial/2017-002370-39/ES.

178. McNamara LA, Topaz N, Wang X, Hariri S, Fox L, MacNeil JR. High risk for invasive meningococcal disease among patients receiving eculizumab (soliris) despite receipt of meningococcal vaccine. MMWR Morb Mortal Wkly Rep. 2017;66:734–7.

179. Hillmen P, Muus P, Röth A, et al. Long-term safety and efficacy of sustained eculizumab treatment in patients with paroxysmal nocturnal haemoglobinuria. Br J Haematol. 2013. https://doi.org/10.1111/bjh.12347.

180. Struijk GH, Bouts AHM, Rijkers GT, Kuin EAC, ten Berge IJM, Bemelman FJ. Meningococcal sepsis complicating eculizumab treatment despite prior vaccination. Am J Transplant. 2013. https://doi.org/10.1111/ajt.12032.

181. Rondeau E, Cataland SR, Al-Dakkak I, Miller B, Webb NJA, Landau D. Eculizumab safety: five-year experience from the global atypical hemolytic uremic syndrome registry. Kidney Int Rep. 2019;4:1568.

182. Noone D, Waters A, Pluthero FG, Geary DF, Kirschfink M, Zipfel PF, Licht C. Successful treatment of DEAP-HUS with eculizumab. Pediatr Nephrol. 2014. https://doi.org/10.1007/s00467-013-2654-x.

183. Brocklebank V, Johnson S, Sheerin TP, et al. Factor H autoantibody associated atypical haemolytic uraemic syndrome in children in the United Kingdom and Ireland. Kidney Int. 2017;92(5):1261–71.

184. 2021. https://www.ema.europa.eu/en/medicines/human/EPAR/soliris.

185. Nishimura J, Yamamoto M, Hayashi S, et al. Genetic variants in C5 and poor response to eculizumab. N Engl J Med. 2014. https://doi.org/10.1056/nejmoa1311084.

186. Cugno M, Gualtierotti R, Possenti I, et al. Complement functional tests for monitoring eculizumab treatment in patients with atypical hemolytic uremic syndrome. J Thromb Haemost. 2014;12:1440–8.

187. Gilbert RD, Fowler DJ, Angus E, Hardy SA, Stanley L, Goodship TH. Eculizumab therapy for atypical haemolytic uraemic syndrome due to a gain-of-function mutation of complement factor B. Pediatr Nephrol. 2013;28:1315–8.

188. Willrich MAV, Ladwig PM, Martinez MA, Sridharan MR, Go RS, Murray DL. Monitoring ravulizumab effect on complement assays. J Immunol Methods. 2021;490:112944.

189. Ardissino G, Testa S, Possenti I, Tel F, Paglialonga F, Salardi S, Tedeschi S, Belingheri M, Cugno M. Discontinuation of eculizumab maintenance treatment for atypical hemolytic uremic syndrome: a report of 10 cases. Am J Kidney Dis. 2014;64:633–7.

190. Caprioli J, Noris M, Brioschi S, et al. Genetics of HUS: the impact of MCP, CFH, and IF mutations on clinical presentation, response to treatment, and outcome. Blood. 2006;108:1267–79.

191. Fakhouri F, Delmas Y, Provot F, et al. Insights from the use in clinical practice of eculizumab in adult patients with atypical hemolytic uremic syndrome affecting the native kidneys: an analysis of 19 cases. Am J Kidney Dis. 2014. https://doi.org/10.1053/j.ajkd.2013.07.011.

192. Fila M, Caillez M, Hogan J, Louillet F, Loirat C, Fremeaux Bacchi V, Fakhouri F. Outcome of 11 pediatric patients with atypical hemolytic and uremic syndrome after Eculizumab discontinuation. Pediatr Nephrol. 2016;31:233.

193. Wijnsma KL, Duineveld C, Volokhina EB, van den Heuvel LP, van de Kar NCAJ, Wetzels JFM. Safety and effectiveness of restrictive eculizumab treatment in atypical haemolytic uraemic syndrome. Nephrol Dial Transplant. 2018;33:635–45.

194. Ariceta G, Fakhouri F, Sartz L, Miller B, Nikolaou V, Cohen D, Siedlecki AM, Ardissino G. Eculizumab discontinuation in atypical haemolytic uraemic syndrome: TMA recurrence risk and renal outcomes. Clin Kidney J. 2021. https://doi.org/10.1093/ckj/sfab005.

195. Neto ME, de Moraes SL, Vasconcelos HVG, et al. Eculizumab interruption in atypical hemolytic uremic syndrome due to shortage: analysis of a Brazilian cohort. J Nephrol. 2021. https://doi.org/10.1007/s40620-020-00920-z.

196. Fakhouri F, Fila M, Hummel A, et al. Eculizumab discontinuation in children and adults with atypical hemolytic-uremic syndrome: a prospective multicenter study. Blood. 2021. https://doi.org/10.1182/blood.2020009280.

197. ISRCTN17503205. Stopping Eculizumab Treatment Safely in atypical Haemolytic Uraemic Syndrome (SETS aHUS). 2018. http://www.who.int/trialsearch/Trial2.aspx?TrialID=ISRCTN17503205.

198. Saland J. Liver-kidney transplantation to cure atypical HUS: still an option post-eculizumab? Pediatr Nephrol. 2014. https://doi.org/10.1007/s00467-013-2722-2.

199. Park SH, Kim GS. Anesthetic management of living donor liver transplantation for complement factor h deficiency hemolytic uremic syndrome: a case report. Korean J Anesthesiol. 2014. https://doi.org/10.4097/kjae.2014.66.6.481.

C3 Glomerulopathies

23

Christoph Licht, Marina Vivarelli,
Magdalena Riedl Khursigara,
and Patrick D. Walker

Introduction

Membranoproliferative glomerulonephritis (MPGN) was originally described as a pattern of glomerular injury seen in patients with Bright's Disease [1]. By mid-1970, MPGN had become a disease of children with three primary subtypes sorted by electron microscopy presenting clinically with nephrotic syndrome and hypocomplementemia [2, 3]. But over the next 40 years, as it became associated with an ever increasing variety of diseases, each with different clinical presentations and etiologies, MPGN has returned to being a pattern that only vaguely points the way to a clinicopathologic diagnosis [4].

C. Licht (✉)
Division of Nephrology, The Hospital for Sick Children, Toronto, ON, Canada

Cell Biology Program, Research Institute, The Hospital for Sick Children, Toronto, ON, Canada
e-mail: christoph.licht@sickkids.ca

M. Vivarelli
Division of Nephrology and Dialysis, Department of Pediatric Subspecialties, Bambino Gesù Pediatric Hospital – IRCCS, Rome, Italy
e-mail: marina.vivarelli@opbg.net

M. R. Khursigara
Division of Nephrology, The Hospital for Sick Children, Toronto, ON, Canada
e-mail: magdalena.riedl@sickkids.ca

P. D. Walker
Arkana Laboratories, Little Rock, AR, USA
e-mail: patrick.walker@arkanalabs.com

Due to the significantly increased understanding of the role of complement in glomerular diseases, two distinct entities have arisen from the MPGN morass, i.e. C3 Glomerulopathy (C3G) and Immune-complex mediated MPGN (Table 23.1). Glomerular diseases associated with abnormalities of the alternative pathway of complement are grouped under the term C3G [5]. There are two major subtypes, C3 glomerulonephritis (C3GN) and dense deposit disease (DDD) sorted by changes seen on electron microscopy. C3G is caused by various genetic abnormalities with or without the development of antibodies against different components of the complement pathway, so-called nephritic factors. Idiopathic MPGN also has two subtypes but these are separated by immunofluorescence findings on renal biopsy. Immune complex-mediated MPGN has dominant or co-dominant immunoglobulins with C3. There is also an immune negative variant of MPGN. The idiopathic forms of these two variants are extremely rare and a detailed search for an underlying cause is required [6]. However, otherwise idiopathic forms of MPGN may be due to abnormalities in the alternative pathway of complement, that is, C3G with immunoglobulin deposition.

© The Author(s), under exclusive license to Springer Nature Switzerland AG 2023
F. Schaefer, L. A. Greenbaum (eds.), *Pediatric Kidney Disease*,
https://doi.org/10.1007/978-3-031-11665-0_23

Table 23.1 Classification of IC-MPGN/C3G

	Characteristic findings in C3G	Characteristic findings in IC-MPGN
Light microscopy	– Membranoproliferative pattern – Mesangial glomerulopathy – Necrotizing and crescentic glomerulonephritis – Acute proliferative and exudative glomerulonephritis	– Membranoproliferative pattern – Mesangial glomerulopathy with endocapillary hypercellularity, mesangial hypercellularity and mesangial matrix expansion
Immunofluorescence microscopy	– Dominant C3 deposition along capillary loops and in mesangial areas – IgG, IgM, IgA, C1q can be present but at much lower intensity	– C3 and IgG staining (similar intensity) along capillary loops and mesangial areas
Electron microscopy	– Dense deposit disease: ribbon-like, extremely dense transformation of glomerular basement membranes – C3GN: subendothelial deposits along glomerular basement membranes and in the mesangial matrix	– Immune-complex type electron dense deposits along the subendothelial spaces and in the mesangium

Table 23.1: Overview of biopsy findings in C3G and IC-MPGN. Both entities are indistinguishable on light microscopy. IF staining will determine whether a biopsy is classified as C3G or IC-MPGN. EM can diagnose cases of DDD. C3GN and IC-MPGN are indistinguishable on EM

Histopathology of C3 Glomerulopathy

Light Microscopy (LM)

Historically, dense deposit disease and the more recently described C3 glomerulonephritis were considered to be a form of membranoproliferative glomerulonephritis (MPGN). This despite the fact that DDD and C3GN have a membranoproliferative pattern in only 25% to 30% of patients at presentation. A mesangial glomerulopathy is most common (40–50%), while necrotizing and crescentic glomerulonephritis (~10%) and acute proliferative and exudative glomerulonephritis (~10%) make up the rest (Fig. 23.1) [3, 7–9]. The name membranoproliferative glomerulonephritis describes the pathologic features found in this pattern of glomerular injury. There is new glomerular basement membrane (GBM) formation producing double contours. The proliferative component includes endocapillary and mesangial hypercellularity as well as the cellular interposition between the GBM double contours. At the time of presentation, biopsies of patients with C3G almost always have a very mild membranoproliferative pattern, particularly as opposed to patients with immune-complex mediated MPGN (see below). Mesangial glomerulopathy is limited to variable mesangial changes without GBM alterations. The changes can be so mild that the biopsy appears almost normal. In the well-developed form, there is diffuse mesangial expansion with mesangial hypercellularity. Crescentic C3G at presentation typically shows extensive cellular crescents with necrotizing areas. Where the glomerular tufts can be seen, there is usually some endocapillary and mesangial hypercellularity with neutrophilic infiltration. However, occasionally the glomerular tuft is bland, though the neutrophilic infiltration is most often still present. Acute proliferative and exudative glomerulonephritis is indistinguishable from an infection-related glomerulonephritis and most likely explains why this variant was not described in the early series [3, 10–12]. There is glomerular enlargement due to diffuse endocapillary hypercellularity with neutrophilic infiltration.

23 C3 Glomerulopathies

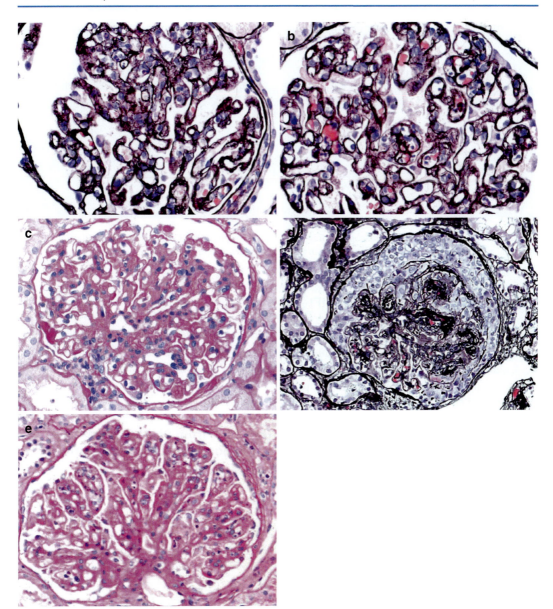

Fig. 23.1 Light microscopy findings in C3G. (**a**, **b**) Mild membranoproliferative pattern with glomerular basement membrane double contours, endocapillary and mesangial hypercellularity with mesangial matrix expansion (Jones silver stain, original magnification 600×). (**c**) Mesangiopathic glomerulopathy with mild mesangial cell and matrix increase (Periodic acid-Schiff reaction (PAS), original magnification 400×). (**d**) circumferential cellular crescent (Jones silver stain, original magnification 400×). (**e**) Acute proliferative and exudative glomerulonephritis (PAS, original magnification 400×)

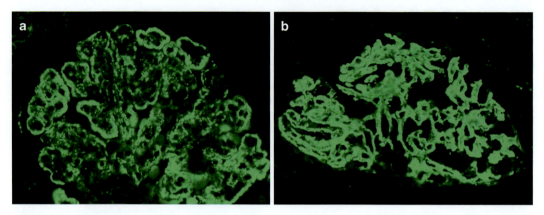

Fig. 23.2 Immunofluorescence microscopy findings in C3G. (**a**, **b**) Intense C3 staining along capillary loops and mesangial areas (fluorescein-conjugated, anti-human anti-C3c, original magnification 400×)

Immunofluorescence Microscopy (IF)

Dominant C3 deposition along capillary loops and in mesangial areas is a required feature for the diagnosis of C3G (Fig. 23.2). IgG, IgM and/or IgA are present in lower intensities in up to 36% of cases [7, 8, 13]. Surprisingly, C1q is seen in up to 30% of biopsies, again at lower intensity [7, 8]. In a large study of C3G, immunoglobulins were present in 46% of patients with C3GN and 36% with DDD [13]. Paraffin IF may reveal a dominant or co-dominant immunoglobulin [14]. The presence of immunoglobulins present on routine IF or on paraffin IF, though often found in C3G, raises the possibility of an infection-related glomerulonephritis or an autoimmune disease. Given that the latter entities are far more common than C3G, they must be ruled out before a diagnosis of C3G is made.

Electron Microscopy (EM)

C3GN is distinguished from DDD on the basis of EM (Fig. 23.3). Dense deposit disease is characterized by extremely electron dense transformation of the glomerular basement membranes with similarly dense spheroids in the mesangium. Large and equally dense sub-epithelial hump-like deposits are present in up to 50% of cases [13]. C3GN most often has electron dense deposits indistinguishable from immune-complex deposits. However, in many cases the deposits have a smudged charcoal gray appearance in the subendothelial space and in mesangial areas. Subepithelial hump-like deposits are commonly seen.

Transition from Acute Proliferative and Exudative Glomerulonephritis to C3G

There is a challenging subset of patients with C3G who initially present with an acute proliferative and exudative glomerulonephritis [15, 16]. Immunofluorescence shows C3 often with IgG in the mesangium and in a granular pattern along the capillary loops. Though this LM pattern and the finding of immunoglobulins on IF are common in C3G, these patients are thought to have an infection-related glomerulonephritis and are treated as such. The diagnosis of an infection associated GN is not surprising given that up to 40% of patients have an infection at the time of diagnosis [13]. Usually there is some renal function improvement, but continued low C3 levels and/or hematuria and proteinuria lead to a repeat biopsy and the diagnosis of C3G is made usually within months but can take several years [16–19].

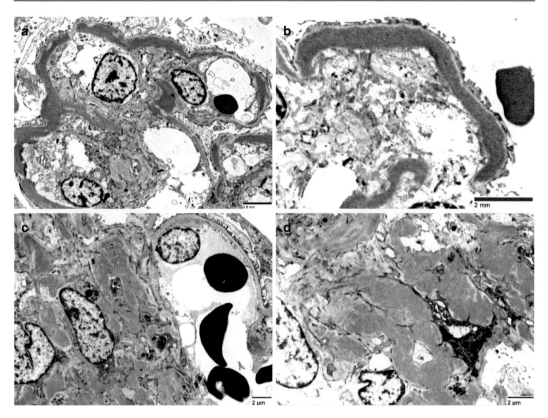

Fig. 23.3 (**a, b**) Dense deposit disease. Extremely electron dense transformation of the glomerular basement membranes forming ribbons. Similarly dense spheroids in the mesangium (**a**. unstained, original magnification 8000×; **b**. unstained, original magnification 20,000×). (**c, d**) C3GN. Smudgy gray deposits in the mesangium and in subendothelial spaces (**c**. unstained, original magnification 6000×; **d**. unstained, original magnification 8000×)

Histopathology of Immune Complex Mediated Membranoproliferative Glomerulonephritis

By definition, these patients have a membranoproliferative pattern of glomerular disease. There are glomerular basement membrane double contours with cellular interposition accompanied by endocapillary hypercellularity, mesangial hypercellularity and mesangial matrix expansion sometimes forming lobules. IF demonstrates capillary loop and mesangial deposition of C3 and immunoglobulin(s), almost always IgG with or without IgM. EM confirms the LM findings of glomerular basement membrane duplication with cells between the layers and endocapillary hypercellularity. The mesangium is expanded by cell and matrix increase. Immune-complex type electron dense deposits are found along the subendothelial spaces and in the mesangium (Fig. 23.4) [20, 21].

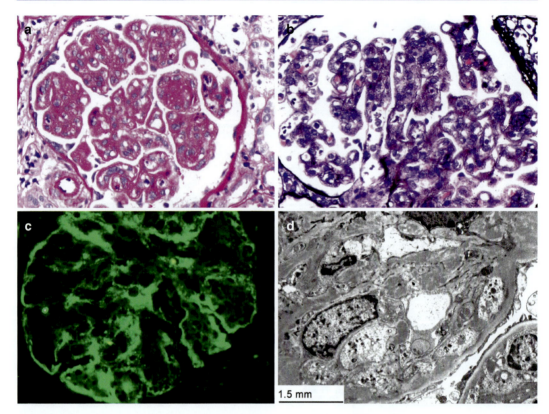

Fig. 23.4 IC-MPGN (**a**) Mesangial cell and matrix increase forming lobules. Endocapillary hypercellularity and thick glomerular basement membranes (PAS, original magnification 400x). (**b**) Endocapillary hypercellularity and mesangial cell and matrix expansion. (Jones silver, original magnification 600x). (**c**) Peripheral granular staining (fluorescein-conjugated, anti-human anti-C3c, original magnification 600x). (**d**) Mesangial and endocapillary hypercellularity. New basement membrane formation with cellular interposition. Electron dense deposits in the mesangium and in subendothelial spaces of the glomerular basement membranes (unstained, original magnification 8,000x)

Classification of C3G

The classification of C3 glomerulopathies (C3G) is based on the pattern and intensity of immunofluorescence seen on renal biopsy (Table 23.1). Prevalent Ig staining prompts the diagnosis of a *secondary* MPGN (see above), and work-up including a panel of auto-antibodies, viral serologies and, exceptionally in pediatric patients, searching for cryoglobulins and monoclonal gammopathies is warranted. However, predominant C3 staining prompts the diagnosis of a primary disease, referred to as C3 glomerulopathy (C3G). Within this category, electron microscopy assessment allows for the differentiation of patients with dense deposit disease (DDD; previously known as MPGN II), in whom dense, sausage-like very intensely osmiophilic deposits are present along the glomerular basement membrane, and patients with predominant mesangial C3 staining and possible presence of subepithelial humps as described in post-infectious mesangial glomerulonephritis. The latter group is diagnosed with MPGN I or C3 glomerulonephritis (C3GN), with MPGN I traditionally being favored in patients with membranoproliferative lesions. Of note, C3G may be familial or sporadic.

Pathogenesis

Much has been learned about C3G and MPGN by studying patients and both spontaneously occurring and genetically engineered animal models (Fig. 23.5). In summary, C3G and IC-MPGN result in principle from dysregulation of the complement alternative pathway in the fluid phase with possible terminal complement pathway (TP) activation, complement (split product) deposition in the kidney and an accompanying inflammatory response. In humans, CAP dysregulation can result from mutations in complement proteins or the presence of autoantibodies.

In animal models, Factor H (FH) deficiency resulted in C3 deposition along the GBM, terminal pathway (TP) activation followed by electron dense transformation of the GBM together with varying degrees of glomerular inflammation and structural damage, hallmark features of MPGN [22, 23]. When C5 activation was prevented by inter-crossing the Cfh−/− strain with C5-deficient mice, the abnormal glomerular C3 deposition remained unchanged but the severity of glomerulonephritis was decreased [23]. However, altering C3 convertase activation by deleting Factor B (FB) or Factor D (FD) prevented MPGN. In Cfh−/− mice that are also deficient in Factor I (FI), activated C3 remains as C3b only. Interestingly, whilst abnormal glomerular C3 developed in both strains, the C3 in the mice with combined deficiency of FH and FI was mesangial in location, whilst in the Cfh−/− strain the C3 was located along the GBM. These data indicate that during uncontrolled C3 activation the nature of the activated C3 fragment may determine the site of its glomerular deposition [24]. What those animals models have shown us is that FH is the critical regulator of glomerular C3 homeostasis, and administration of either mouse or human FH to Cfh−/− mice reduced glomerular C3 staining and increased circulating C3 levels [25]. Mutations in FH are typically associated with atypical hemolytic uremic syndrome (aHUS) indicating that defects in the CAP can give rise to at least two distinct renal phenotypes: thrombotic microangiopathy (TMA) like HUS and glomerulonephritis like C3G. The majority of aHUS-associated CFH mutations does not result in complete deficiency of FH but selectively impairs the surface C3b recognition domains of the protein. In keeping with this, mice expressing a mutant FH molecule that functionally mimicked aHUS-associated mutations known from patients developed TMA not C3G, [23] and this was dependent on C5 [26].

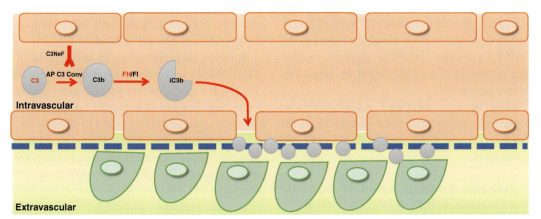

Fig. 23.5 Pathogenetic *concept* of C3G: Genetic or autoimmune factors result in fluid phase dysregulation of the complement alternative pathway at the level of the (alternative) C3 convertase. Excessive C3 activation results—in the presence of proteases (e.g. CFI) and their corresponding cofactors (e.g. CFH)—in the generation of copious amounts of C3 split products which deposit in the glomerular filter triggering local inflammatory responses

On the other hand, complement dysregulation in C3G patients may occur via different scenarios:

- Antibodies stabilizing the CAP C3 convertase and prolonging the natural decay of the CAP C3 convertase, rendering it overactive.
- Mutations or antibodies to FH or FHR that result in the absence or loss of function of FH resulting in loss of control of the CAP C3 convertase and its enhanced activity.
- Mutations in C3 or FB that result in an exceedingly stable C3 convertase with prolonged decay and enhanced function.

In all scenarios, the functional consequence is an enhanced activation rate of C3 mainly in the fluid phase. Autoantibodies associated with C3G (see below) prolong the half-life of the CAP C3 convertase, or the (CAP or CP) C5 convertase and therefore result in TP activation [27, 28].

Autoimmune Forms of C3G

Decreased serum C3 levels were long reported in patients with MPGN, which led to the hypothesis of a circulating factor leading to increased C3 cleavage [29]. When an antibody binding to a neo-epitope of the complement CAP C3 convertase (C3bBb)—delaying its natural decay and thus enhancing its function—was found, it was named C3 Nephritic Factor (C3NeF) [27, 30]. C3Nef is an autoantibody capable of binding the CAP C3 convertase, C3BbB, therefore conferring resistance to its inactivation by regulatory factors such as FH.

More recently, additional autoantibodies or nephritic factors were detected which prolong the half-life of the CAP and CP C3 and C5 convertases:

- *Antibodies that stabilize the CAP and/or CP C3 convertase:* C3NeF [31, 32], C4NeF [33, 34], Anti-Factor B antibodies [35, 36] and Anti-C3b antibodies [35];
- *Antibodies that stabilize the C5 convertase:* C4NeF [34], C5NeF [37];

- *Antibodies impairing CAP (fluid phase) regulation:* Anti-Factor H antibodies (recognizing FH N-terminus) [38–40].

C3NeF is the most prevalent antibody and was detected in 86% of DDD, 46% of C3GN, and up to 50% of patients with IC-MPGN, respectively, and is associated with decreased C3 levels [41, 42]. C3NeF might fluctuate and not correlate with disease activity and might co-exist with complement mutations [43, 44]. Therefore, a positive C3NeF still warrants comprehensive complement diagnostics. Anti-C3b and Bb antibodies, both stabilizing the CAP C3 convertase, have been reported in several patients with C3G and IC-MPGN and are associated with worse outcome if both occur at the same time [36].

Servais et al. identified mutations in complement genes in 18% of C3G patients, while the presence of circulating C3Nef was detected in 59% of cases [45]. More than half of the patients carrying complement gene mutations were also C3NeF positive. C3Nef was more frequent in patients with DDD (86%) and was associated with significantly lower levels of circulating C3. A report of 3 patients with DDD showed a correlation of moderate increases in C3Nef and slight reduction on C3 and disease recurrence post-transplant [46]. In other reports, lower circulating levels of C3 were found in patients with a membranoproliferative pattern of disease, [41] while others have reported that children have significantly lower C3 levels and more frequent C3Nef positivity compared to adults [7].

However, as reviewed by Pickering M et al. [47], C3NeF can be detected in different ways [31, 48]. It is possible that patients may be positive in some but not all available assays. C3NeF and other auto-antibodies found in MPGN were also detected in other kidney diseases, such as systemic lupus erythematosus (SLE) [49], postinfectious GN [50], and meningococcal meningitis [51]. C3Nef levels are occasionally also found in healthy individuals [52], rendering the interpretation of their pathogenic value controversial.

Therefore, the significance of C3Nef in the pathophysiology of C3G and its correlation with

Genetic Forms

Early studies found a genetic cause in approximately 18% of patients with IC-MPGN and C3G. By contrast, Bu et al., studying a larger panel of genes by next-generation sequencing (NGS), found a genetic diagnosis in up to 43% [32, 54]. Iatropoulos et al. detected mutation carriers in 17 and 18% of patients with IG-MPNG and C3G, respectively [42]. To date, mutations have been reported in the following complement genes: CFH, CFHR5, CFI, MCP, C3 and CFB and can occur in a heterozygous or homozygous fashion (Table 23.2).

Additional mutations or internal duplications in genes encoding FH related proteins (CFHR), or formation of hybrid genes, have been associated with C3G [55, 56]. In 2009 Gale et al. described 26 individuals of Cypriot ancestry with

Table 23.2 Genetic causes of IC-MPGN and C3G

Gene	Mutation/SNP	Function	Classification	References
CFH	Homo−/compound heterozygous SCRs 1–4 (regulatory domain)	Intact surface binding Reduced C3b binding Loss of FH cofactor & decay accelerating activity	C3G IC-MPGN	Licht et al. [107], Servais et al. [32], Bu et al. [54], Iatropoulos et al. [42]
CFI	Homozygous Heterozygous	Decreased FI mediated C3b degradation	C3G IC-MPGN	Servais et al. [32], Bu et al. [54], Iatropoulos et al. [42], Iatropoulos et al. (2018)
C3	Heterozygous	C3mut—resistant to cleavage by C3bBb C3mut convertase –resistant to FH inactivation C3 binding with FI or FH	C3GN IC-MPGN	Martinez-Barricarte et al. [109], Bu et al. [54], Iatropoulos et al. [42], Iatropoulos et al. (2018)
CFB	Heterozygous/ homozygous	Alters C3-FB interaction	C3G IC-MPGN	Iatropoulos et al. [42], Iatropoulos et al. (2018)
Thrombomodulin	Homozygous	Not tested	DDD	Iatropoulos et al. [42], Iatropoulos et al. (2018)
DGKE	Homozygous Heterozygous— unclear impact	Not complement mediated	MPGN	Ozaltin et al. [60], Bu et al. [54]
At risk SNPs (reviewed in Noris and Remuzzi)				
MCP/CD46	Rare SNP	Not tested	C3G IC-MPGN	Servais et al. [32]
CFH	Rare SNP e.g. Y402H (SCR 7)	Not tested	DDD	Abrera-Abeleda et al. [62]
CFHR5	Rare SNP	Not tested	DDD	Abrera-Abeleda et al. [62], Bu et al. [54]
C3	Rare SNP	Not tested	DDD	Abrera-Abeleda et al. [62]

(continued)

Table 23.2 (continued)

Gene	Mutation/SNP	Function	Classification	References
CFHR fusion proteins (reviewed in Smith et al. [83])				
CFHR3–1	CNV CFHR3–1 hybrid gene	Greater degree of FHR-mediated deregulation	C3GN	Malik et al. [55], Goicoechea de Jorge et al. [59]
CFHR2–5	CFHR2–5 hybrid gene	Stabilizes C3 convertase, reduced FH-mediated decay	DDD	
CFHR5-CFHR5	CNV Duplication in CFHR5 exons 2/3	Greater degree of FHR-mediated deregulation	C3G	Gale et al. [57], Goicoechea de Jorge et al. [59]
CFHR1-CFHR1	Internal duplication	Greater degree of FHR-mediated deregulation	C3G	
CFHR5–2	CFHR5–2 hybrid gene	Greater degree of FHR-mediated deregulation	C3GN	Smith et al. [83]
CFHR1–5	CFHR1–2 hybrid gene	Greater degree of FHR-mediated deregulation	C3G	

unexplained renal disease and a variation in CFHR5 comprising duplication in its dimerization domain, termed CFHR5 nephropathy [57]. Several more mutations and hybrid variants in CFHR genes have been detected since and are associated with C3G [58]. The role of FHR in C3G was unclear until the report, that FHR1, FHR2 and FHR5 form homo- and heterodimers amongst themselves and with FH. In the dimeric form these proteins are able to compete with FH for C3b binding and protect C3b from inactivation and the complement CAP C3 convertase from decay. This process, termed "deregulation," was increased in patients with CFHR hybrids or CFHR5 mutations [59].

Interestingly, Ozaltin et al. published several patients with MPGN with a homozygous mutation in DGKE, an intracellular lipid kinase that modulates phosphoinositol signaling in the plasma membrane [60]. DGKE mutations can also be found in thrombotic microangiopathy [61]. Bu et al. found heterozygous variants in DGKE in several patients with C3G, as well as in Thrombomodulin, Plasminogen and

ADAMTS13. The clinical relevance of these gene variants is still unclear [54].

Risk haplotypes were identified in CFH, C3 and MCP/CD46, with the CFH Y402H haplotype more frequently reported in DDD, and the MCP-652A4G polymorphism in C3G. The presence of two or more complement haplotypes increased the risk of disease [32, 62].

Clinical Presentation

MGPN, C3GN and DDD are rare diseases with an individual annual incidence estimated at 1–2 per million per total population (both pediatric and adult) [63, 64]. C3 glomerulopathies typically present with (possibly nephrotic range) proteinuria and hematuria and hypertension coupled with low circulating C3 levels [65, 66]. However, C3G has a very heterogeneous clinical presentation. This heterogeneity reflects the variety of pathogenetic mechanisms leading to a dysregulated, uncontrolled activation of the CAP.

Presentation at Onset of Disease

Age at onset is very variable, with the earliest reported case being at age 1 [67]. In the most comprehensive cohorts that include adult and pediatric patients, disease onset below age 16 years was described in 59–68% of DDD and 25–31% of C3GN patients [32, 64]. In a pediatric cohort median disease onset was approximately 10 years for both patients with IC-MPGN and C3G [68]. A slight prevalence of males (60%) was reported in some cohorts, [32, 64] but not in the cohort that included pediatric patients only [68].

Clinical symptoms are listed in Table 23.3. Data taken from the 3 cohorts indicate that patients with C3G and IC-MPGN commonly present with microscopic hematuria, significant proteinuria including nephrotic syndrome in up to 40%, hypertension and reduced renal function. Incidence of macrohematuria was reported in 10–23% [7, 64].

Disease onset is often associated with an infection as described in a report of children with DDD, in whom the appearance of renal symptoms was preceded by a respiratory infection in 57% of cases [7]. Recurrent macrohematuria during trivial infectious episodes, a clinical feature typically associated with IgA nephropathy, is not uncommon in C3G [69].

The large variation of age at presentation is probably linked to the fact that in some cases this disease has a subclinical and spontaneously remitting disease course. Hence, microhematuria and low-grade proteinuria can remain undetected for many years, leading to a delayed diagnosis when proteinuria reaches nephrotic range or when kidney failure develops. However, early onset with nephrotic proteinuria and renal failure, though less common, has been reported (patient 9 in [41]).

Worse renal function was found in pediatric patients with C3G and in adult and pediatric patients with C3GN compared to DDD. Low C3 was commonly found in patients with C3G, especially in patients with DDD and IC-MPGN. Over the course of time, C3 can normalize in some patients but might stay low in others, a persistently low C3 was more commonly found in patients with IC-MPGN [68]. C3 levels do not correlate with disease outcome [70].

Family history of glomerulonephritis must be investigated as familial forms have been described in 11% of cases [32] and genetic investigations may be channeled more effectively in these cases.

As the classification system for MPGN has recently evolved, our understanding of the differences in the clinical presentations of MPGN versus C3GN is limited. There are no unique features that clearly distinguish MPGN, DDD and C3GN on clinical grounds. An exception to this rule appears to be CFHR5 associated C3GN, which presents in childhood with persistent microscopic hematuria, synpharyngitic gross hematuria, and a strong family history of ESKD. At present this form of G3GN has been reported primarily in the Cypriot population, but also in two patients with non-Cypriot heritage [57, 71]. Patients with CFHR5 associated C3GN are also reported to have normal serum C3 concentrations.

Table 23.3 Clinical presentation of IC-MPGN and C3G

	Kirpalani (pediatric only)	Medjeral-Thomas	Servais
Number of patients	42 IC-MPGN/ 43 C3G	21 DDD/59 C3GN	29 DDD/56 C3GN
Microscopic hematuria	81/62%	76/65%	19/30%
Proteinuria	–/–	3/3 g/d	5.6/3.6 g/d
Nephrotic syndrome	22/12%	43/44%	38/27%
Hypertension	57/58%	60/39%	21/38%
Creatinine	94/168 μmmol/L	80/124 μmmol/L	–/–
eGFR (ml/min/1.73 m^2)	76/83	–/–	76/66
C3	0.26/0.39 g/L	Low 79/48%	Low 46/46%

Extra-Renal Manifestations

C3G is a complement-mediated disease, secondary to CAP dysregulation. Given that this dysregulation occurs in the fluid phase of blood, extra-renal features of disease are to be expected. In DDD, patients may develop acquired partial lipodystrophy (APL) and ocular lesions similar to soft drusen seen in age-related macular degeneration (AMD) [72].

APL—like DDD and C3GN—is associated with dysregulation of CAP on adipocytes [73] and becomes manifest in the loss of subcutaneous fat tissue, which typically occurs in the upper half of the body (starting from the face and extending to involve the neck, shoulders, arms and thorax) and precedes the onset of renal disease by several years. The median interval between the onset of APL and DDD is about eight years [74]. The majority of APL patients present with low C3 levels and, in addition, are C3NeF positive, which leads to enhanced CAP activation. MPGN was described in about 25% of patients with APL. Patients with combined disease are more likely to present with decreased C3 levels and develop APL earlier in life (about 7.7 years of age) [74].

Patients with DDD can also develop ocular lesions in the form of drusen. Drusen are retinal changes seen as crystalline yellow or white dots, which lie between the retinal pigment epithelium and Bruch's membrane [75]. Drusen can develop in the second decade of life and are responsible for visual disturbances in up to 10% of patients with DDD [72]. The drusen seen in patients with DDD are similar to those seen in age-related macular degeneration (AMD).

Diagnosis

The clinical presentations of MPGN, DDD and C3GN are extremely variable and overlap with many other glomerular diseases, ranging from subtle/subclinical to acute and severe, as exemplified in the following scenarios:

- An incidental finding on routine urinalysis of non-nephrotic proteinuria, often accompanied by microscopic hematuria.
- Macrohematuria concomitant or 2–3 weeks after an intercurrent infectious episode, most frequently of the upper respiratory tract.
- Nephrotic range proteinuria, with or without clinical signs of nephrotic syndrome and renal function impairment.
- Very rarely, an overlap with thrombotic microangiopathy.

Diagnosis of C3G is made with a renal biopsy, which includes light microscopy, immunofluorescence and electron microscopy. Extensive C3 staining allows for the diagnosis of C3GN, predominant IgG staining on the other hand is characteristic for IC-MPGN and electron dense deposits favors the diagnosis of DDD. Despite different features on biopsy, the underlying pathophysiology is similar and requires further workup for complement activation, auto-antibodies and mutations in complement genes.

Differential Diagnosis

The presentation of a nephritic/nephrotic clinical picture is compatible with a variety of diagnoses at disease onset. The clinical picture can be indistinguishable from IgA nephropathy (IgAN), particularly if circulating C3 is normal and macrohematuria in the setting of an infection is observed [69]. Familial disease does not exclude the diagnosis of C3G, particularly but not exclusively in patients of Cypriot descent [55, 57]. Renal biopsy, in particular the immunofluorescence, allows clear discrimination between C3G, in particular the familial forms, and IgAN.

In the presence of reduced levels of circulating C3, particularly in context of an infection during the preceding 2–3 weeks, the diagnosis of acute post-infectious glomerulonephritis (PIGN) is likely, but C3G is also possible though less frequent. In this case, a renal biopsy may not be definitive as the presence of "humps" in the electron microscopy is common to both, C3G and PIGN [9]. The latter presents with reduced circulating C3 levels, which typically normalize within 12 weeks from disease onset [76]. As C3 levels may be normal also in C3G and given the heterogeneity of the clinical picture of this new disease entity, we suggest that in the case of a clinical picture common to C3G and PIGN, even with normalizing C3 levels and absent proteinuria, patients be advised to perform urinalysis every 3–6 months for 2 years following resolution of the acute clinical picture and to seek medical attention if macrohematuria or significant proteinuria re-appear.

Decreased C3 and C4 are hallmark features of SLE, which can present with proteinuria, microscopic hematuria and hypertension. Low C4 was reported in a small amount of patients with C3G (5–36%) and therefore cannot be used as the differentiating factor [32, 64]. A thorough history and physical examination with attention to extrarenal disease manifestations such as arthritis, rash, neurologic, hepatic, lung or cardiac involvement combined with ANA and anti-dsDNA antibody titers, laboratory evidence of hemolysis, leukopenia, coagulopathy, or hepatitis, strongly support a diagnosis of SLE as opposed to C3G.

Laboratory Evaluation

When the diagnosis of C3G has been made by renal biopsy, analysis of the CAP is warranted:

1. Circulating complement factors including C3, C4, CFH, CFB and markers for complement pathway activation (CH50, APH50, C3d) and terminal complement activation (C5b-9).
2. Circulating autoantibodies such as C3 Nephritic Factor (C3NeF) and anti-FH autoantibodies.
3. Other antibodies that are only measured in specialized research labs can be added in spe-

cific cases: anti-CFB antibodies, C4 Nephritic Factor, C5 Nephritic Factor and anti-C3b antibodies.
4. Mutations in genes involved in the regulation of the C3 convertase such as Factor H (FH), Factor I (FI), membrane cofactor protein (MCP/CD46), C3, and Factor B (FB) and screening of the FHR locus with MLPA to detect deletions, duplications or fusion genes. Other genes associated with C3G or IC-MPGN include thrombomodulin and DGKE.
5. When family history is positive for C3G, suggesting a familial form, the FHR locus should also be screened for an internal duplication within the FHR5 gene, described mainly but not solely in individuals of Cypriot origin [57].

In patients with IC-MPGN we also recommend a detailed investigation for secondary causes as listed in Table 23.4.

Table 23.4 Causes of secondary MPGN

Immunoglobulin mediated
Infectious diseases:
Hepatitis B, C, E, EBV, HIV
Endocarditis, shunt nephritis, visceral abscess, empyema
Tuberculosis, leprosy
Brucellosis, Q Fever
Malaria, schistosomiasis
Onchocerca volvulus, Wucheria bancrofti, Loa loa infections
Systemic immune diseases:
Cryoglobulinemia
Systemic lupus erythematosus
IgA vasculitis
Sjögren's syndrome (secondary to cryoglobulinemia)
Hypocomplementemic urticarial vasculitis
Rheumatoid arthritis (Zand et al. [79])
X-linked agammaglobulinemia
Neoplasms/dysproteinemias:
Plasma cell dyscrasia
Monoclonal gammopathy of unknown significance
Fibrillary glomerulopathy
Immunotactoid glomerulonephritis

(continued)

Table 23.4 (continued)

Proliferative glomerulonephritis with monoclonal immunoglobulin deposition (Nasr et al. [7]

Proliferative glomerulonephritis with isolated light chain deposition

Membranoproliferative glomerulonephritis with masked monotypic immunoglobulin deposits

Light-chain and/or heavy-chain deposition disease

Leukemias and lymphomas (with or without cryoglobulinemia)

Bone marrow transplant

Carcinomas, Wilms' tumor, malignant melanoma

Angiofollicular lymph node hyperplasia with or without TAFRO syndrome[a]

Sinus histiocytosis with massive lymphadenopathy

Other:

Alpha-1-antitrypsin deficiency with severe liver disease

Gluten-sensitive enteropathy (celiac disease)

Immunoglobulin negative

Thrombotic microangiopathy including drug induced forms

Sickle-cell disease

Transplant glomerulopathy

POEMS syndrome[b]

[a]TAFRO = Thrombocytopenia, Anasarca, Fever, Renal dysfunction (or Reticulin myelofibrosis) and Organomegaly
[b]POEMS syndrome = Polyneuropathy, Organomegaly, Endocrinopathy, Monoclonal gammopathy and Skin changes

Outcome

Data on long-term outcomes in both native and transplant kidneys based on the new classification is limited and vary dependent on the cohort and disease onset. Medjeral-Thomas, comparing outcomes of DDD and C3GN in a cohort of 80 patients, with 50% having a pediatric onset of disease, reported progression to ESKD in 47% of DDD patients and 23% of C3GN patients with a median follow-up of 28 months. Multivariate analysis suggested crescentic changes, DDD and disease onset over 16 years of age as independent predictors for ESKD [64].

The French cohort of 134 patients reported 10-year renal survival at 63.5%, with no difference between groups (MPGN, DDD, C3GN). Median time from first observation to end-stage renal disease was about 10 years, and in the patients that underwent renal transplant, disease recurrence was observed in over half of the cases, with an additional 17% experiencing thrombotic microangiopathy (TMA) [32, 41].

A large retrospective study comprising 165 children with both IC-MPGN and C3G confirmed that children have a better outcome than adults. After a mean follow-up of 4 years kidney function was preserved, and at 10 years 80% of children analyzed did not meet the composite outcome of eGFR <30 ml/min/1.73 m^2, 50% eGFR reduction or need for kidney replacement therapy [68]. Although hypertension remained prevalent in 42.5% of the cohort at the last follow-up, and the urine protein/creatinine ratio remained elevated (mean 253.8 [range 91.9–415.7] mg/mmol).

Disease recurrence of MPGN and DDD in transplants is common (Table 23.5). Data from the ESPN/ERA-EDTA registry shows an average renal allograft loss of 32.4% at 5-years posttransplant in children [77]. Data suggesting that pediatric patients with DDD are at greater risk of graft loss from disease recurrence has also been reported in the NAPRTCS database [78]. The reason(s) for the increased risk of recurrence in children is not clear. Several limited case series confirm an increased risk of disease recurrence for C3GN and the potential negative impact on allograft survival. Disease recurrence is strongly associated with graft loss [64]. Zand et al. reported outcomes on 21 patients with C3GN, 14 (66.7%) had disease recurrence with median time to graft failure of 77 months (6.4 years) [79]. Concerning risk of relapse following renal transplantation for DDD, in one study the degree of proteinuria was strongly associated with disease recurrence, and the presence of glomerular crescents in biopsies of renal allografts had a significant negative correlation with graft survival [78].

Table 23.5 Disease recurrence post transplantation

	Medjeral-Thomas	Servais
Number of patients	7 C3GN 6 DDD	14 IC-MPGN 10 C3GN 11 DDD
MPGN	–	43%
C3G	57%	60%
DDD	100%	55%

In the familial form of C3G secondary to CFHR5 mutations described in individuals of Cypriot descent [57] prognosis differed significantly between sexes: men were by far more likely to progress to ESKD than women (78% versus 22%).

Treatment

At present, there is no treatment standard or at least a therapeutic agent of proven effectiveness in C3G available. The rarity of this disease, coupled with its protracted and variable natural history, makes clinical trials logistically challenging and the use of different end-points make uniform interpretation of results difficult [80]. However, considering that about 50% of patients proceed to ESKD and may face a high risk of disease recurrence post-renal transplant, concerted efforts to define effective treatment strategies are necessary. Several therapeutic regimens have been employed, utilizing immunosuppressive agents (glucocorticoids, mycophenolate mofetil, calcineurin inhibitors), anti-platelet agents, plasma exchange or infusion and, much more recently, complement blockers [81–83]. Renoprotective agents (such as angiotensin-converting-enzyme inhibitors, ACEi, or angiotensin II receptor antagonists, ARBs) are associated to these treatments almost invariably. As our understanding of the pathophysiology of C3G and of IC-MPGN is rapidly expanding and changing, while reviewing published cases is reasonable, its usefulness in guiding future therapeutic strategies may be limited [47].

The optimal therapeutic strategy should be driven by clinical parameters, such as the degree of proteinuria and impairment in renal function, and also by diagnostic test results (Fig. 23.6). In

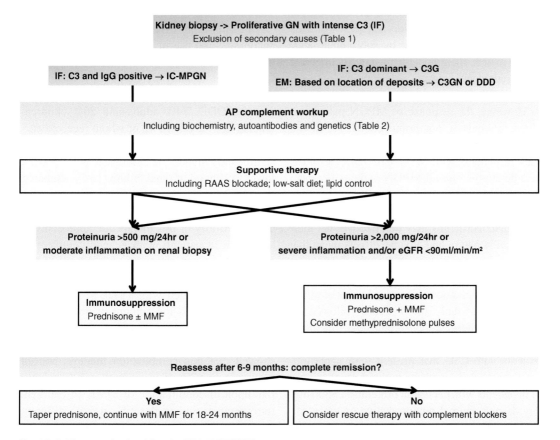

Fig. 23.6 Therapeutic algorithm for IC-MPGN/C3G

the near future, the availability of new therapeutic agents may drastically alter this strategy. Clinicians need to be aware that clinical practices in this field may evolve rapidly.

In the following paragraphs regarding treatment, for all options except eculizumab the literature cited is about different forms of IC-MPGN and C3G. Because evidence is very limited, a consensus of expert opinion currently still provides the most reasonable therapeutic approach to this disease (KDIGO) [84].

Immunosuppressive Agents

There are no published trials on the use of **prednisone** in C3G. Existing literature pertains to primary membranoproliferative glomerulonephritis of all subtypes. In children with all subtypes of primary MPGN, prednisone—specifically, long-term low-dose use of prednisone—was found to have a beneficial effect with respect to the degree of proteinuria and renal survival [85–88]. This observation was confirmed by subsequent studies, in which therapy with prolonged alternate day prednisone delayed deterioration of renal function [87, 89].

However, the response of MPGN patients to glucocorticoids is not homogenous. A MPGN subtype-specific analysis revealed a lack of efficacy in patients with MPGN II/DDD, despite a beneficial effect on all MPGN patients irrespective of the MPGN subtype [87].

Altogether, in all forms of IC-MPGN and C3G, glucocorticoids may be effective, but their nonspecific nature and adverse effects mean that a high price is paid for any beneficial effect on the renal lesion [90]. A reasonable approach based on current knowledge may be that of utilizing 60 mg/m^2 daily for 4 weeks followed by 40 mg/m^2 alternate-day prednisone for other 4 weeks then tapered for a total of 6–9 months in patients with C3G that present with nephrotic-range proteinuria, with or without renal failure, or in patients with persistent proteinuria >500 mg/day despite optimal renoprotective treatment. In children who present intense inflammation in the renal biopsy with marked endo and extracapillary proliferation, or who present an acute deterioration in renal function, intravenous methylprednisolone boluses (e.g., 1000 mg/1.73 m^2 repeated 3 times) may be added at disease presentation. If no significant reduction of proteinuria is observed, steroids should be tapered and discontinued [91]. It is important to recognize that a number of patients with C3G will not respond to this therapeutic approach [47].

Other Immunosuppressive Agents

In idiopathic MPGN patients, **MMF** was administered alone or in combination with corticosteroids, and generated encouraging results [92]. Another report of 13 adult patients with idiopathic MPGN resistant to glucocorticoid treatment (8 weeks at 1 mg/kg/day) showed that adding MMF led to significant reduction of proteinuria and increase of eGFR [93]. MMF in addition to pulse and long-term steroid treatment was also found effective in a pediatric patient [94].

In C3G, recent evidence, albeit retrospective, encourages the use of MMF. Initial findings by Rabasco et al. [95] were recently confirmed and expanded in a study by Caravaca-Fontan et al. [96] which described 97 patients (81 with C3GN, 16 with DDD, 74% adults and 26% children, median age 32 years), 42 of whom received corticosteroids plus MMF. This subgroup showed a significantly higher rate of remission (79%) and a lower likelihood of renal failure (14%) compared to patients receiving other immunosuppressive drugs, eculizumab or renoprotective treatment. The superiority of this therapeutic approach was seen both in patients with genetic complement abnormalities and in patients with autoantibodies to complement components. The only factor significantly associated with a lack of response to this approach was the amount of proteinuria at baseline. Previously, a study performed in 30 young adults [97] with a median age of 25 years showed that this combination therapy induced remission in 67% of cases with a 50% relapse rate upon discontinuation of MMF. In children, retrospective studies describe use of different immunosuppressive agents in small numbers of patients, which makes drawing meaningful conclusions difficult. Overall, similar results have been obtained [98–100]. In our experience, MMF is beneficial in patients both with IC-MPGN and with C3G with intense proteinuria. Following tapering and interruption of prednisone in 6–9 months, usually MMF monotherapy is continued for 12–18 months.

Calcineurin inhibitors (i.e. cyclosporine and tacrolimus) are also used in the treatment of MPGN. The efficacy of cyclosporin was recently tested with encouraging results in a trial involving 18 patients with refractory MPGN who also received small doses of prednisolone (0.15 mg/kg/day). Long-term proteinuria reduction with preservation of renal function was observed in 17 of the patients [101]. In two children with idiopathic MPGN with suboptimal response to a prolonged course of steroids, rapid and complete remission of the nephrotic syndrome was achieved after initiation of tacrolimus [102].

Contradictory results are published about the efficacy of cyclosporin A in the treatment of patients with MPGN II/DDD. Kiyomasu et al. report the successful treatment of a patient with MPGN II/DDD resulting in the recovery from nephrotic syndrome using a combination of alternate-day low-dose prednisone and cyclosporin [103]. The numbers of reported children in whom calcineurin inhibitors have been used are too small to draw valid conclusions. This immunosuppressive approach may reasonably be attempted, in the absence of alternatives, when MMF plus corticosteroids have failed to improve proteinuria significantly in a patient with preserved renal function.

The use of **rituximab** has been suggested in the presence of circulating C3 Nephritic Factor (C3Nef), an autoantibody that binds to C3BbB antagonizing its inactivation by circulating regulatory factors. However, to the best of our knowledge, while there are no published results showing this treatment to be effective, there are a few single case reports of its inefficacy [104, 105].

The use of **cyclophosphamide** may theoretically be considered in forms with crescentic glomerulonephritis and rapidly progressive onset, but available data is truly anecdotal.

Taken together, limited uncontrolled data suggest that especially MMF in combination with glucocorticoids may be of use in patients with C3G and intense proteinuria, while at present there is insufficient evidence to support the first-line use of calcineurin inhibitors, cyclophosphamide or rituximab in children with this disease [91].

Plasma Infusion or Plasma Exchange

As reviewed by Smith et al., [53] in FH-deficient mice with C3G, renal C3 deposition and its depletion in plasma are rapidly reversed when (either mouse or human) CFH is administered [25, 106]. These outcomes suggest that in some C3G patients with FH mutations, FH replacement therapy could restore the underlying defect and correct the disease. This has been shown in two siblings with DDD secondary to a functional FH defect in whom chronic plasma infusion prevented disease progression and development of ESKD [107, 108]. Whether administration of exogenous FH to patients without FH mutations would be therapeutically successful is not clear, but this treatment should at least in theory not be effective in patients with a known C3 mutation, in whom a C3 convertase that is resistant to regulation by FH is formed [109].

In all scenarios characterized by deficiency or functional defect of one or more complement components, replacement of this factor/these factors by either plasma infusion or plasma exchange could theoretically be effective [110].

Because of discordant reports in the literature and lack of prolonged efficacy, plasma therapy currently is used very sporadically in children with C3G and IC-MPGN. However, this therapy may be attempted, in the absence of response to immunosuppression, in rapidly progressive forms, particularly if defective FH is found.

Complement Inhibitors

The pathophysiology of C3G suggests therapeutic targeting of CAP dysregulation by complement inhibition. Based on the pathology of disease, anticomplement therapy warrants consideration. This could include (1) C3 convertase inhibition, which may have its greatest utility in limiting C3 breakdown product deposition on (glomerular) basement membranes; (2) C5 or terminal complement pathway inhibition [47]. Currently, the only commercially available options are the anti-C5 monoclonal antibodies eculizumab and its long-lasting analogue ravulizumab.

Effectiveness of anti-C5 therapy in a mouse model of DDD (*Cfh* deficient mice) [111] provided the rationale and led to the use of a humanized anti-C5 monoclonal antibody (eculizumab) in patients with different forms of C3G [104, 105, 112–115].

Eculizumab is a humanized monoclonal antibody directed against C5, which blocks C5 cleavage, preventing the release of C5a, a potent anaphylatoxin, and C5b, the initial protein of the cytotoxic membrane attack complex (MAC; C5b-9). Its use is well established for aHUS, the classic model of renal disease mediated by the CAP. In C3G, following initial encouraging single case reports and small series, [104, 112, 113, 115] two more recent larger studies have provided disappointing results.

A retrospective French study [116] evaluated 26 patients, 13 of whom pediatric, with a median treatment duration of 14 months. In this study, 6 patients (23%) had a global clinical response, 6 (23%) had a partial clinical response and 14 (54%) no response. The only prospective study that has evaluated eculizumab in IC-MPGN and C3G, the EAGLE study [117] confirmed these negative findings. It evaluated 10 patients, (6 with MPGN, 4 with C3G), all with normal renal function, severe (>3500 mg/24 h) proteinuria and highly elevated sC5b9 (>1000 ng/ml), who were treated with eculizumab for 2 sequential

48-week periods separated by one 12-week washout period. Primary outcome was change in 24-h proteinuria at 24 and 48 weeks. While terminal complement pathway inhibition was achieved in all patients, only 3/10 patients obtained partial remission of proteinuria. During the first treatment period, median proteinuria, albuminemia and lipid profile improved, but these mild benefits were lost during the washout period and never regained in 7/10 patients. More recently, two patients with a mixed aHUS/C3G phenotype benefiting from treatment for eculizumab have been described, suggesting than in patients with an endothelial CAP dysregulation as is present in aHUS, eculizumab is most likely to be beneficial [118].

However, new complement-modulating agents are now in the pipeline. Avacopan, an oral anti-C5aR inhibitor which has proven safe and effective in ANCA-associated vasculitis [119], is currently being investigated in adults and adolescents with C3G and IC-MPGN. As shown in Table 23.6, other agents which target the complement cascade upstream, at the level of the C3 convertase, are also available and studies investigating their safety and efficacy in IC-MPGN and C3G are underway or planned in the near future.

A potential benefit of complement inhibition in the treatment of complement-mediated diseases needs to be balanced against the detrimental effect of complement inhibition in situations when complement activation is required as part of the immune defense of the host, and thorough clinical trials are required before the use of these novel substances in children can be recommended.

Given the heterogeneity of potential and described mechanisms leading to CAP dysregu-

Table 23.6 Complement targeting treatment in IC-MPGN and C3G

Drug	Target	Mechanism	Clinical trial number
ACH0144471	Factor D	Prevents formation of C3 and C5 convertases	NCT03369236, NCT03459443 and NCT03124368
LNP023	Factor B	Prevents formation of C3 and C5 convertases	NCT03832114, NCT03955445
APL2	C3	Prevents formation of C3 and C5 convertases	NCT03453619
AMY101	C3	Prevents formation of C3 and C5 convertases	NCT03316521
OMS721	MASP2	Blocks initiation of lectin pathway	NCT02682407
Avacopan	C5aR1	Blocks anaphylatoxin formation (C3a, C4a and/or C5a)	NCT03301467

lation, it is most likely that no single anti-complement treatment will be universally effective. Rather, patient-tailored therapies chosen on the basis of each patient's specific alteration are the optimal therapeutic strategy. Therefore, upon diagnosis of C3G, extensive and expert assessment of the CAP in each patient is of pivotal importance and this work-up is indispensable in designing future therapeutic trials.

Renoprotective Agents

About 80% of patients are placed on ARBs or ACEi, both first line agents used to improve renal dynamics, decrease proteinuria, control blood pressure and limit glomerular leukocyte infiltration [53]. This approach, coupled with low-sodium diet and lipid-lowering agents when appropriate is recommended for all children with IC-MPGN or C3G. It can be used as exclusive treatment in two cases:

1. Non-nephrotic proteinuria with or without microhematuria and normal renal function/absence of acute renal failure. Close follow-up is needed to assess progression of disease based on renal function, proteinuria, and urine microscopy. Target proteinuria should be below 200 mg/day in children, and additional treatment should be initiated if this target is not reached within a few weeks of optimal dosing of these agents.
2. Histological evidence of advanced chronicity of the renal lesions on the biopsy. Patients with advanced chronic kidney disease (CKD), severe tubulointerstitial fibrosis (TIF), small kidney size, or other findings consistent with chronic disease sequel should—in the absence of systemic disease manifestations—not be treated with immunosuppression [91].

Treatment of Recurrence Post-Renal Transplantation

There is no proven beneficial therapy for recurrent C3G in the renal allograft following transplantation. Therapeutic approaches are similar to those used in primary disease and are therefore not discussed in detail here. Reported treatment of *recurrent idiopathic MPGN* besides conservative medications like RAAS antagonists to control proteinuria and hypertension, includes antiplatelet/anticoagulant agents [120], corticosteroids [121], cyclosporin [122], cyclophosphamide [123], and plasmapheresis [121, 124]. Reported treatment of *recurrent DDD* includes dose reduction, discontinuation or switch (cyclosporin to tacrolimus) of the calcineurin inhibitors used as part of the posttransplant immunosuppression regimen, modification of the prednisone dose (increase; switch from daily to alternate-day), pulse methylprednisolone, or plasmapheresis/plasma exchange [78, 125]. More recently, the use of terminal complement inhibition with eculizumab has been evaluated in adults with C3G post-renal transplant recurrence, once again with variable outcomes [126, 127].

Summary

In summary, the therapeutic options in C3G depend on the level of proteinuria and kidney failure and on the results of the panel of diagnostic tests performed at diagnosis. In the vast majority of patients, the empiric use of ACEi or ARBs as drugs of first choice to treat hypertension and decrease proteinuria is a common practice, which may delay the progression of renal disease [90]. Plasma therapy or, in the future, purified FH may be useful in some cases in which there is clear evidence of a FH deficiency or of the presence of anti-FH autoantibodies. There is little evidence of the effectiveness of immunosuppression, which should therefore be employed only in cases where disease is very active and proliferative with intense inflammation in the renal biopsy and nephrotic-range proteinuria.

Preliminary results on the use of complement blockers such as eculizumab are encouraging in some but not in all patients.

Lastly, improvement in renal outcome for patients with C3G largely relies on the evaluation of more targeted agents in future studies [90].

References

1. Volhard F, Fahr T. Die Brightsche Nierenkrankheit. Berlin: Springer; 1914.
2. Habib R, Kleinknecht C, Gubler MC, Maiz HB. Idiopathic membranoproliferative glomerulonephritis. In: Kincaid-Smith P, Mathew TH, Becker EL, editors. Glomerulonephritis; morphology, natural history, and treatment. 1 (part 1). New York, NY: John Wiley & Sons; 1973. p. 491–514.
3. Habib R, Gubler M-C, Loirat C, Maiz HB, Levy M. Dense deposit disease: a variant of membranoproliferative glomerulonephritis. Kidney Int. 1975;7:204–15.
4. Sethi S, Fervenza FC. Membranoproliferative glomerulonephritis— a new look at an old entity. N Engl J Med. 2012;366(12):1119–31.
5. Riedl M, Thorner P, Licht C. C3 glomerulopathy. Pediatr Nephrol. 2017;32(1):43–57.
6. Fervenza FC, Sethi S, Glassock RJ. Idiopathic membranoproliferative glomerulonephritis: does it exist? Nephrol Dial Transplant. 2012;0:1–7.
7. Nasr SH, Valeri AM, Appel GB, Sherwinter J, Stokes MB, Said SM, et al. Dense deposit disease: clinicopathologic study of 32 pediatric and adult patients. Clin J Am Soc Nephrol. 2009;4:22–32.
8. Walker PD, Ferrario F, Joh K, Bonsib SM. Dense deposit disease is not a membranoproliferative glomerulonephritis. Mod Pathol. 2007;20:605–16.
9. Sethi S, Fervenza FC, Zhang Y, Zand L, Vrana JA, Nasr SH, et al. C3 glomerulonephritis: clinicopathological findings, complement abnormalities, glomerular proteomic profile, treatment, and follow-up. Kidney Int. 2012;82(4):465–73.
10. Davis AE, Schneeberger EE, Grupe WE, McCluskey RT. Membranoproliferative glomerulonephritis (MPGN type I) and dense deposit disease (DDD) in children. Clin Nephrol. 1978;9:184–93.
11. Klein M, Poucell S, Arbus GS, McGraw M, Rance CP, Yoon S-J. Characteristics of a benign subtype of dense deposit disease: comparison with the progressive form of this disease. Clin Nephrol. 1983;20(4):163–71.
12. Hogg RJ, Silva FG, Walker PD, Cavallo T. Dense deposit disease in children: prognostic value of clinical and pathologic indicators. The Southwest Pediatric Nephrology Study Group. Am J Kidney Dis. 1985;6(3):161–9.
13. Ravindran A, Fervenza FC, Smith RJH, De Vriese AS, Sethi S. C3 glomerulopathy: ten years' experience at mayo clinic. Mayo Clin Proc. 2018;93(8):991–1008.
14. Messias NC, Walker PD, Larsen CP. Paraffin immunofluorescence in the renal pathology laboratory: more than a salvage technique. Mod Pathol. 2015;28(6):854–60.
15. Prasto J, Kaplan BS, Russo P, Chan E, Smith RJ, Meyers KE. Streptococcal infection as possible trigger for dense deposit disease (C3 glomerulopathy). Eur J Pediatr. 2014;173(6):767–72.
16. Shahidi-Asl M, Ananth M, Boineau F, Meleg-Smith S. Apparent progression of acute glomerulonephritis to dense deposit disease. Ultrastruct Pathol. 2000;24:273–7.
17. Sato H, Saito T, Seino J, Ootaka T, Kyogoku Y, Furuyama T, et al. Dense deposit disease: its possible pathogenesis suggested by an observation of a patient. Clin Nephrol. 1987;27(1):41–5.
18. Sawanobori E, Umino A, Kanai H, Matsushita K, Iwasa S, Kitamura H, et al. A prolonged course of group A streptococcus-associated nephritis: a mild case of dense deposit disease? Clin Nephrol. 2009;71(6):703–7.
19. Suzuki K, Tsugawa K, Oki E, Aita K, Endo M, Waga S, et al. Dense deposit disease presenting as endocapillary proliferative nephritis. Pediatr Int. 2009;51(5):739–41.
20. Habib R, Kleinknecht C, Gubler MC, Levy M. Idiopathic membranoproliferative glomerulonephritis in children. Report of 105 cases. Clin Nephrol. 1973;1(4):194–214.
21. Fervenza FC, Sethi S, Glassock RJ. Idiopathic membranoproliferative glomerulonephritis: does it exist? Nephrol Dial Transplant. 2012;27(12):4288–94.
22. Pickering MC, Cook HT, Warren J, Bygrave AE, Moss J, Walport MJ, et al. Uncontrolled C3 activation causes membranoproliferative glomerulonephritis in mice deficient in complement factor H. Nat Genet. 2002;31(4):424–8.
23. Pickering MC, de Jorge EG, Martinez-Barricarte R, Recalde S, Garcia-Layana A, Rose KL, et al. Spontaneous hemolytic uremic syndrome triggered by complement factor H lacking surface recognition domains. J Exp Med. 2007;204(6):1249–56.
24. Rose KL, Paixao-Cavalcante D, Fish J, Manderson AP, Malik TH, Bygrave AE, et al. Factor I is required for the development of membranoproliferative glomerulonephritis in factor H-deficient mice. J Clin Invest. 2008;118(2):608–18.
25. Fakhouri F, de Jorge EG, Brune F, Azam P, Cook HT, Pickering MC. Treatment with human complement factor H rapidly reverses renal complement deposition in factor H-deficient mice. Kidney Int. 2010;78(3):279–86.
26. de Jorge EG, Macor P, Paixao-Cavalcante D, Rose KL, Tedesco F, Cook HT, et al. The development of atypical hemolytic uremic syndrome depends on complement C5. J Am Soc Nephrol. 2011;22(1):137–45.
27. Corvillo F, Okroj M, Nozal P, Melgosa M, Sanchez-Corral P, Lopez-Trascasa M. Nephritic factors: an overview of classification, diagnostic tools and clinical associations. Front Immunol. 2019;10:886.
28. Jozsi M, Reuter S, Nozal P, Lopez-Trascasa M, Sanchez-Corral P, Prohaszka Z, et al. Autoantibodies to complement components in C3 glomerulopathy

28. and atypical hemolytic uremic syndrome. Immunol Lett. 2014;160(2):163–71.
29. Spitzer RE, Stitzel AE. On the origin and control of C3NeF. In Vivo. 1988;2(1):79–81.
30. Berthoux FC, Carpenter CB, Traeger J, Merrill JP. C3 nephritic factor and heat labile complement inactivator in chronic hypocomplementemic mesangioproliferative glomerulonephritis. [French] Le Facteur Nephritique (C3 Nephritic Factor) Et L'inactivateur Thermolabile Du Complement (Heat Labile Complement Inactivator) Dans Les Glomerulonephrites Mesangioproliferatives Hypocomplementaires Chroniques. Actualites Nephrologiques de l'Hopital Necker. 1974;1974:141–56.
31. Paixao-Cavalcante D, Lopez-Trascasa M, Skattum L, Giclas PC, Goodship TH, de Cordoba SR, et al. Sensitive and specific assays for C3 nephritic factors clarify mechanisms underlying complement dysregulation. Kidney Int. 2012;82(10):1084–92.
32. Servais A, Noel L-H, Roumenina LT, Le Quintrec M, Ngo S, Dragon-Durey M-A, et al. Acquired and genetic complement abnormalities play a critical role in dense deposit disease and other C3 glomerulopathies. Kidney Int. 2012;82(4):454–64.
33. Zhang Y, Meyer NC, Fervenza FC, Lau W, Keenan A, Cara-Fuentes G, et al. C4 nephritic factors in C3 glomerulopathy: a case series. Am J Kidney Dis. 2017;70(6):834–43.
34. Blom AM, Corvillo F, Magda M, Stasilojc G, Nozal P, Perez-Valdivia MA, et al. Testing the activity of complement convertases in serum/plasma for diagnosis of C4NeF-mediated C3 glomerulonephritis. J Clin Immunol. 2016;36(5):517–27.
35. Chen Q, Muller D, Rudolph B, Hartmann A, Kuwertz-Broking E, Wu K, et al. Combined C3b and factor B autoantibodies and MPGN type II. N Engl J Med. 2011;365(24):2340–2.
36. Strobel S, Zimmering M, Papp K, Prechl J, Jozsi M. Anti-factor B autoantibody in dense deposit disease. Mol Immunol. 2010;47(7–8):1476–83.
37. Marinozzi MC, Chauvet S, Le Quintrec M, Mignotet M, Petitprez F, Legendre C, et al. C5 nephritic factors drive the biological phenotype of C3 glomerulopathies. Kidney Int. 2017;92(5):1232–41.
38. Meri S, Koistinen V, Miettinen A, Tornroth T, Seppala IJ. Activation of the alternative pathway of complement by monoclonal lambda light chains in membranoproliferative glomerulonephritis. J Exp Med. 1992;175(4):939–50.
39. Jokiranta TS, Solomon A, Pangburn MK, Zipfel PF, Meri S. Nephritogenic lambda light chain dimer: a unique human miniautoantibody against complement factor H. J Immunol. 1999;163(8):4590–6.
40. Goodship TH, Pappworth IY, Toth T, Denton M, Houlberg K, McCormick F, et al. Factor H autoantibodies in membranoproliferative glomerulonephritis. Mol Immunol. 2012;52(3–4):200–6.

41. Servais A, Fremeaux-Bacchi V, Lequintrec M, Salomon R, Blouin J, Knebelmann B, et al. Primary glomerulonephritis with isolated C3 deposits: a new entity which shares common genetic risk factors with haemolytic uraemic syndrome. J Med Genet. 2007;44(3):193–9.
42. Iatropoulos P, Noris M, Mele C, Piras R, Valoti E, Bresin E, et al. Complement gene variants determine the risk of immunoglobulin-associated MPGN and C3 glomerulopathy and predict long-term renal outcome. Mol Immunol. 2016;71:131–42.
43. Leroy V, Fremeaux-Bacchi V, Peuchmaur M, Baudouin V, Deschenes G, Macher M-A, et al. Membranoproliferative glomerulonephritis with C3NeF and genetic complement dysregulation. Pediatr Nephrol. 2011;26(3):419–24.
44. Nicolas C, Vuiblet V, Baudouin V, Macher M-A, Vrillon I, Biebuyck-Gouge N, et al. C3 nephritic factor associated with C3 glomerulopathy in children. Pediatr Nephrol. 2014;29(1):85–94.
45. Servais A, Noel L, Fremeaux-Bacch IV, Lesavre P. C3 glomerulopathy. Contrib Nephrol. 2013;181:185–93.
46. West CD, Bissler JJ. Nephritic factor and recurrence in the renal transplant of membranoproliferative glomerulonephritis type II. Pediatr Nephrol. 2008;23(10):1867–76.
47. Pickering MC, D'Agati VD, Nester CM, Smith RJ, Haas M, Appel GB, et al. C3 glomerulopathy: consensus report. Kidney Int. 2013;84(6):1079–89.
48. Zhang Y, Meyer NC, Wang K, Nishimura C, Frees K, Jones M, et al. Causes of alternative pathway dysregulation in dense deposit disease. Clin J Am Soc Nephrol. 2012;7(2):265–74.
49. Waldo FB, Forristal J, Beischel L, West CD. A circulating inhibitor of fluid-phase amplification. C3 convertase formation in systemic lupus erythematosus. J Clin Invest. 1985;75(6):1786–95.
50. Sethi S, Fervenza FC, Zhang Y, Zand L, Meyer NC, Borsa N, et al. Atypical postinfectious glomerulonephritis is associated with abnormalities in the alternative pathway of complement. Kidney Int. 2013;83(2):293–9.
51. Lewis LA, Ram S. Meningococcal disease and the complement system. Virulence. 2014;5(1):98–126.
52. Mathieson PW, Wurzner R, Oliveria DB, Lachmann PJ, Peters DK. Complement-mediated adipocyte lysis by nephritic factor sera. J Exp Med. 1993;177(6):1827–31.
53. Smith RJ, Harris CL, Pickering MC. Dense deposit disease. Mol Immunol. 2011;48(14):1604–10.
54. Bu F, Borsa NG, Jones MB, Takanami E, Nishimura C, Hauer JJ, et al. High-throughput genetic testing for thrombotic microangiopathies and C3 glomerulopathies. J Am Soc Nephrol. 2016;27(4):1245–53.
55. Malik TH, Lavin PJ, Goicoechea de Jorge E, Vernon KA, Rose KL, Patel MP, et al. A hybrid CFHR3-1

55. gene causes familial C3 glomerulopathy. J Am Soc Nephrol. 2012;23(7):1155–60.

56. Xiao X, Pickering MC, Smith RJ. C3 glomerulopathy: the genetic and clinical findings in dense deposit disease and c3 glomerulonephritis. Semin Thromb Hemost. 2014;40(4):465–71.

57. Gale DP, de Jorge EG, Cook HT, Martinez-Barricarte R, Hadjisavvas A, McLean AG, et al. Identification of a mutation in complement factor H-related protein 5 in patients of Cypriot origin with glomerulonephritis. Lancet. 2010;376(9743):794–801.

58. Malik TH, Lavin PJ, De Jorge EG, Vernon KA, Rose KL, Patel MP, et al. A hybrid CFHR3-1 gene causes familial C3 glomerulopathy. J Am Soc Nephrol. 2012;23(7):1155–60.

59. Goicoechea de Jorge E, Caesar JJ, Malik TH, Patel M, Colledge M, Johnson S, et al. Dimerization of complement factor H-related proteins modulates complement activation in vivo. Proc Natl Acad Sci U S A. 2013;110(12):4685–90.

60. Ozaltin F, Li B, Rauhauser A, An SW, Soylemezoglu O, Gonul II, et al. DGKE variants cause a glomerular microangiopathy that mimics membranoproliferative GN. J Am Soc Nephrol. 2013;24(3):377–84.

61. Lemaire M, Fremeaux-Bacchi V, Schaefer F, Choi M, Tang WH, Le Quintrec M, et al. Recessive mutations in DGKE cause atypical hemolytic-uremic syndrome. Nat Genet. 2013;45(5):531–6.

62. Abrera-Abeleda MA, Nishimura C, Frees K, Jones M, Maga T, Katz LM, et al. Allelic variants of complement genes associated with dense deposit disease. J Am Soc Nephrol. 2011;22(8):1551–9.

63. Coppo R, Gianoglio B, Porcellini MG, Maringhini S. Frequency of renal diseases and clinical indications for renal biopsy in children (report of the Italian National Registry of Renal Biopsies in Children). Group of Renal Immunopathology of the Italian Society of Pediatric Nephrology and Group of Renal Immunopathology of the Italian Society of Nephrology. Nephrol Dial Transplant. 1998;13(2):293–7.

64. Medjeral-Thomas NR, O'Shaughnessy MM, O'Regan JA, Traynor C, Flanagan M, Wong L, et al. C3 glomerulopathy: clinicopathologic features and predictors of outcome. Clin J Am Soc Nephrol. 2014;9(1):46–53.

65. Schwertz R, Rother U, Anders D, Gretz N, Scharer K, Kirschfink M. Complement analysis in children with idiopathic membranoproliferative glomerulonephritis: a long-term follow-up. Pediatr Allergy Immunol. 2001;12(3):166–72.

66. Schwertz R, de Jong R, Gretz N, Kirschfink M, Anders D, Scharer K. Outcome of idiopathic membranoproliferative glomerulonephritis in children. Arbeitsgemeinschaft Padiatrische Nephrologie. Acta Paediatr. 1996;85(3):308–12.

67. Servais A, Noel LH, Dragon-Durey MA, Gubler MC, Remy P, Buob D, et al. Heterogeneous pattern of renal disease associated with homozygous factor H deficiency. Hum Pathol. 2011;42(9):1305–11.

68. Kirpalani A, Jawa N, Smoyer WE, Licht C, Midwest Pediatric Nephrology C. Long-term outcomes of C3 glomerulopathy and immune-complex membranoproliferative glomerulonephritis in children. Kidney Int Rep. 2020;5(12):2313–24.

69. Karumanchi SA, Thadhani R. A complement to kidney disease: CFHR5 nephropathy. Lancet. 2010;376(9743):748–50.

70. Barbour TD, Pickering MC, Terence CH. Dense deposit disease and C3 glomerulopathy. Semin Nephrol. 2013;33(6):493–507.

71. Medjeral-Thomas N, Malik TH, Patel MP, Toth T, Cook HT, Tomson C, et al. A novel CFHR5 fusion protein causes C3 glomerulopathy in a family without Cypriot ancestry. Kidney Int. 2014;85(4):933–7.

72. Appel GB, Cook HT, Hageman G, Jennette JC, Kashgarian M, Kirschfink M, et al. Membranoproliferative glomerulonephritis type II (dense deposit disease): an update. J Am Soc Nephrol. 2005;16(5):1392–403.

73. Corvillo F, Akinci B. An overview of lipodystrophy and the role of the complement system. Mol Immunol. 2019;112:223–32.

74. Misra A, Peethambaram A, Garg A. Clinical features and metabolic and autoimmune derangements in acquired partial lipodystrophy: report of 35 cases and review of the literature. Medicine (Baltimore). 2004;83(1):18–34.

75. de Jong PT. Age-related macular degeneration. N Engl J Med. 2006;355(14):1474–85.

76. Al-Ghaithi B, Chanchlani R, Riedl M, Thorner P, Licht C. C3 Glomerulopathy and post-infectious glomerulonephritis define a disease spectrum. Pediatr Nephrol. 2016;31(11):2079–86.

77. Van Stralen KJ, Verrina E, Belingheri M, Dudley J, Dusek J, Grenda R, et al. Impact of graft loss among kidney diseases with a high risk of post-transplant recurrence in the paediatric population. Nephrol Dial Transplant. 2018;33(3):542.

78. Braun MC, Stablein DM, Hamiwka LA, Bell L, Bartosh SM, Strife CF. Recurrence of membranoproliferative glomerulonephritis type II in renal allografts: the North American Pediatric Renal Transplant Cooperative Study experience. J Am Soc Nephrol. 2005;16(7):2225–33.

79. Zand L, Lorenz EC, Cosio FG, Fervenza FC, Nasr SH, Gandhi MJ, et al. Clinical findings, pathology, and outcomes of C3GN after kidney transplantation. J Am Soc Nephrol. 2014;25(5):1110–7.

80. Noris M, Remuzzi G. Translational mini-review series on complement factor H: therapies of renal diseases associated with complement factor H abnormalities: atypical haemolytic uraemic syndrome and membranoproliferative glomerulonephritis. Clin Exp Immunol. 2008;151(2):199–209.

81. Nester CM, Smith RJ. Diagnosis and treatment of C3 glomerulopathy. Clin Nephrol. 2013;80(6):395–403.

82. Nester CM, Smith RJ. Treatment options for C3 glomerulopathy. Curr Opin Nephrol Hypertens. 2013;22(2):231–7.

83. Smith RJH, Appel GB, Blom AM, Cook HT, D'Agati VD, Fakhouri F, et al. C3 glomerulopathy - understanding a rare complement-driven renal disease. Nat Rev Nephrol. 2019;15(3):129–43.

84. Goodship TH, Cook HT, Fakhouri F, Fervenza FC, Fremeaux-Bacchi V, Kavanagh D, et al. Atypical hemolytic uremic syndrome and C3 glomerulopathy: conclusions from a "Kidney Disease: Improving Global Outcomes" (KDIGO) controversies conference. Kidney Int. 2017;91(3):539–51.

85. McEnery PT. Membranoproliferative glomerulonephritis: the Cincinnati experience—cumulative renal survival from 1957 to 1989. J Pediatr. 1990;116(5):S109–14.

86. West CD. Childhood membranoproliferative glomerulonephritis: an approach to management. Kidney Int. 1986;29(5):1077–93.

87. Tarshish P, Bernstein J, Tobin JN, Edelmann CM Jr. Treatment of mesangiocapillary glomerulonephritis with alternate-day prednisone—a report of the International Study of Kidney Disease in Children. Pediatr Nephrol. 1992;6(2):123–30.

88. Ford DM, Briscoe DM, Shanley PF, Lum GM. Childhood membranoproliferative glomerulonephritis type I: limited steroid therapy. Kidney Int. 1992;41(6):1606–12.

89. Yanagihara T, Hayakawa M, Yoshida J, Tsuchiya M, Morita T, Murakami M, et al. Long-term follow-up of diffuse membranoproliferative glomerulonephritis type I. Pediatr Nephrol. 2005;20(5):585–90.

90. Alchi B, Jayne D. Membranoproliferative glomerulonephritis. Pediatr Nephrol. 2010;25(8):1409–18.

91. Beck L, Bomback AS, Choi MJ, Holzman LB, Langford C, Mariani LH, et al. KDOQI US commentary on the 2012 KDIGO clinical practice guideline for glomerulonephritis. Am J Kidney Dis. 2013;62(3):403–41.

92. Jones G, Juszczak M, Kingdon E, Harber M, Sweny P, Burns A. Treatment of idiopathic membranoproliferative glomerulonephritis with mycophenolate mofetil and steroids. Nephrol Dial Transplant. 2004;19(12):3160–4.

93. Yuan M, Zou J, Zhang X, Liu H, Teng J, Zhong Y, et al. Combination therapy with mycophenolate mofetil and prednisone in steroid-resistant idiopathic membranoproliferative glomerulonephritis. Clin Nephrol. 2010;73(5):354–9.

94. De S, Al-Nabhani D, Thorner P, Cattran D, Piscione TD, Licht C. Remission of resistant MPGN type I with mycophenolate mofetil and steroids. Pediatr Nephrol. 2009;24(3):597–600.

95. Rabasco C, Cavero T, Roman E, Rojas-Rivera J, Olea T, Espinosa M, et al. Effectiveness of mycophenolate mofetil in C3 glomerulonephritis. Kidney Int. 2015;88(5):1153–60.

96. Caravaca-Fontan F, Diaz-Encarnacion MM, Lucientes L, Cavero T, Cabello V, Ariceta G, et al. Mycophenolate MOFETIL in C3 glomerulopathy and pathogenic drivers of the disease. Clin J Am Soc Nephrol. 2020;15(9):1287–98.

97. Avasare RS, Canetta PA, Bomback AS, Marasa M, Caliskan Y, Ozluk Y, et al. Mycophenolate mofetil in combination with steroids for treatment of C3 glomerulopathy: a case series. Clin J Am Soc Nephrol. 2018;13(3):406–13.

98. Holle J, Berenberg-Gossler L, Wu K, Beringer O, Kropp F, Muller D, et al. Outcome of membranoproliferative glomerulonephritis and C3-glomerulopathy in children and adolescents. Pediatr Nephrol. 2018;33(12):2289–98.

99. Kojc N, Bahovec A, Levart TK. C3 glomerulopathy in children: Is there still a place for anti-cellular immunosuppression? Nephrology (Carlton). 2019;24(2):188–94.

100. Pinarbasi AS, Dursun I, Gokce I, Comak E, Saygili S, Bayram MT, et al. Predictors of poor kidney outcome in children with C3 glomerulopathy. Pediatr Nephrol. 2021;36(5):1195–205.

101. Bagheri N, Nemati E, Rahbar K, Nobakht A, Einollahi B, Taheri S. Cyclosporine in the treatment of membranoproliferative glomerulonephritis. Arch Iran Med. 2008;11(1):26–9.

102. Haddad M, Lau K, Butani L. Remission of membranoproliferative glomerulonephritis type I with the use of tacrolimus. Pediatr Nephrol. 2007;22(10):1787–91.

103. Kiyomasu T, Shibata M, Kurosu H, Shiraishi K, Hashimoto H, Hayashidera T, et al. Cyclosporin A treatment for membranoproliferative glomerulonephritis type II. Nephron. 2002;91(3):509–11.

104. Daina E, Noris M, Remuzzi G. Eculizumab in a patient with dense-deposit disease. N Engl J Med. 2012;366(12):1161–3.

105. McCaughan JA, O'Rourke DM, Courtney AE. Recurrent dense deposit disease after renal transplantation: an emerging role for complementary therapies. Am J Transplant. 2012;12(4):1046–51.

106. Paixao-Cavalcante D, Hanson S, Botto M, Cook HT, Pickering MC. Factor H facilitates the clearance of GBM bound iC3b by controlling C3 activation in fluid phase. Mol Immunol. 2009;46(10):1942–50.

107. Licht C, Heinen S, Jozsi M, Loschmann I, Saunders RE, Perkins SJ, et al. Deletion of Lys224 in regulatory domain 4 of Factor H reveals a novel pathomechanism for dense deposit disease (MPGN II). Kidney Int. 2006;70(1):42–50.

108. Habbig S, Kirschfink M, Zipfel PF, Hoppe B, Licht C. Long-term treatment of MPGN II tue to functional Factor H defect via FFP infusion. J Am Soc Nephrol. 2006;17(Abstracts Issue):575A.

109. Martinez-Barricarte R, Heurich M, Valdes-Canedo F, Vazquez-Martul E, Torreira E, Montes T, et al. Human C3 mutation reveals a mechanism of dense deposit disease pathogenesis and provides insights into complement activation and regulation. J Clin Invest. 2010;120(10):3702–12.

110. Licht C, Schlotzer-Schrehardt U, Kirschfink M, Zipfel PF, Hoppe B. MPGN II—genetically determined by defective complement regulation? Pediatr Nephrol. 2007;22(1):2–9.

111. Pickering MC, Warren J, Rose KL, Carlucci F, Wang Y, Walport MJ, et al. Prevention of C5 activation ameliorates spontaneous and experimental glomerulonephritis in factor H-deficient mice. Proc Natl Acad Sci U S A. 2006;103(25):9649–54.

112. Vivarelli M, Pasini A, Emma F. Eculizumab for the treatment of dense-deposit disease. N Engl J Med. 2012;366(12):1163–5.

113. Radhakrishnan S, Lunn A, Kirschfink M, Thorner P, Hebert D, Langlois V, et al. Eculizumab and refractory membranoproliferative glomerulonephritis. N Engl J Med. 2012;366(12):1165–6.

114. Gurkan S, Fyfe B, Weiss L, Xiao X, Zhang Y, Smith RJ. Eculizumab and recurrent C3 glomerulonephritis. Pediatr Nephrol. 2013;28(10): 1975–81.

115. Bomback AS, Smith RJ, Barile GR, Zhang Y, Heher EC, Herlitz L, et al. Eculizumab for dense deposit disease and C3 glomerulonephritis. Clin J Am Soc Nephrol. 2012;7(5):748–56.

116. Le Quintrec M, Lapeyraque AL, Lionet A, Sellier-Leclerc AL, Delmas Y, Baudouin V, et al. Patterns of clinical response to eculizumab in patients with C3 glomerulopathy. Am J Kidney Dis. 2018;72(1):84–92.

117. Ruggenenti P, Daina E, Gennarini A, Carrara C, Gamba S, Noris M, et al. C5 convertase blockade in membranoproliferative glomerulonephritis: a single-arm clinical trial. Am J Kidney Dis. 2019;74(2):224–38.

118. Busutti M, Diomedi-Camassei F, Donadelli R, Mele C, Emma F, Vivarelli M. Efficacy of eculizumab in coexisting complement C3 glomerulopathy and atypical hemolytic uremic syndrome. Kidney Int Rep. 2021;6(2):534–7.

119. Jayne DRW, Merkel PA, Bekker P. Avacopan for the treatment of ANCA-associated vasculitis. N Engl J Med. 2021;384(21):e81.

120. Glicklich D, Matas AJ, Sablay LB, Senitzer D, Tellis VA, Soberman R, et al. Recurrent membranoproliferative glomerulonephritis type 1 in successive renal transplants. Am J Nephrol. 1987;7(2):143–9.

121. Saxena R, Frankel WL, Sedmak DD, Falkenhain ME, Cosio FG. Recurrent type I membranoproliferative glomerulonephritis in a renal allograft: successful treatment with plasmapheresis. Am J Kidney Dis. 2000;35(4):749–52.

122. Tomlanovich S, Vincenti F, Amend W, Biava C, Melzer J, Feduska N, et al. Is cyclosporine effective in preventing recurrence of immune-mediated glomerular disease after renal transplantation? Transplant Proc. 1988;20(3 Suppl 4):285–8.

123. Lien YH, Scott K. Long-term cyclophosphamide treatment for recurrent type I membranoproliferative glomerulonephritis after transplantation. Am J Kidney Dis. 2000;35(3):539–43.

124. Muczynski KA. Plasmapheresis maintained renal function in an allograft with recurrent membranoproliferative glomerulonephritis type I. Am J Nephrol. 1995;15(5):446–9.

125. Oberkircher OR, Enama M, West JC, Campbell P, Moran J. Regression of recurrent membranoproliferative glomerulonephritis type II in a transplanted kidney after plasmapheresis therapy. Transplant Proc. 1988;20(1 Suppl 1):418–23.

126. Regunathan-Shenk R, Avasare RS, Ahn W, Canetta PA, Cohen DJ, Appel GB, et al. Kidney transplantation in C3 glomerulopathy: a case series. Am J Kidney Dis. 2019;73(3):316–23.

127. Gonzalez Suarez ML, Thongprayoon C, Hansrivijit P, Kovvuru K, Kanduri SR, Aeddula NR, et al. Treatment of C3 glomerulopathy in adult kidney transplant recipients: a systematic review. Med Sci (Basel). 2020;8(4)

Part VI

The Kidney and Systemic Disease

Postinfectious Hemolytic Uremic Syndrome

24

Martin Bitzan and Anne-Laure Lapeyraque

Abbreviations

ADAMTS13	A disintegrin and metalloprotease with a thrombospondin type 1 motif, member 13
aHUS	Atypical hemolytic uremic syndrome
AKI	Acute kidney injury
AP(C)	Alternative pathway (of complement)
C3	Complement factor 3
C4	Complement factor 4
C5	Complement factor 5
CDC	Centers for Disease Control and Prevention
CFB	Complement factor B
CFH	Complement Factor H
CKD	Chronic kidney disease
CNS	Central nervous system
CRP	C-reactive protein
CRRT	Continuous renal replacement therapy
DIC	Disseminated intravascular coagulation
EAEC	Enteroaggregative *E. coli*
eGFR	Estimated glomerular filtration rate
EHEC	Enterohemorrhagic *Escherichia coli*
eHUS	Enteropathogen (or *Escherichia coli*) induced hemolytic uremic syndrome
ELISA	Enzyme-linked immunosorbent assay
EPEC	Enteropathogenic *Escherichia coli*
ER	Endoplasmic reticulum
ESKD	End stage kidney disease
Gb3	Globotriaosylceramide
Gb4	Globotetraosylceramide
Hb	Hemoglobin
HC	Hemorrhagic colitis
HD	Hemodialysis
HUS	Hemolytic uremic syndrome
IA	Immunoabsorption
iHUS	Influenza-induced hemolytic uremic syndrome
IPD	Invasive pneumococcal disease
LDH	Lactate dehydrogenase
LPS	Lipopolysaccharide
mAb	Monoclonal antibody
MAHA	Microangiopathic hemolytic anemia
NA	Neuraminidase
NanA	Neuraminidase A

M. Bitzan (✉)
Mohammed Bin Rashid University of Medicine and Health Sciences, Kidney Center of Excellence, Al Jalila Children's Hospital, Dubai, United Arab Emirates
e-mail: martin.bitzan@mcgill.ca; martin.bitzan@ajch.ae

A.-L. Lapeyraque
Division of Nephrology, CHU Sainte-Justine, Montreal, QC, Canada
e-mail: anne.laure.lapeyraque@umontreal.ca

© The Author(s), under exclusive license to Springer Nature Switzerland AG 2023
F. Schaefer, L. A. Greenbaum (eds.), *Pediatric Kidney Disease*,
https://doi.org/10.1007/978-3-031-11665-0_24

NM	Non-motile
NSAID(s)	Non-steroidal anti-inflammatory drug(s)
OR	Odds ratio
PCR	Polymerase chain reaction
PD	Peritoneal dialysis
PE	Plasma exchange
PI	Plasma infusion
pnHUS	Pneumococcal (*Streptococcus pneumoniae*) hemolytic uremic syndrome
PRBC	Packed red blood cell(s)
RBC	Red blood cell(s)
RRT	Renal replacement therapy
SC5b-9	Serum (soluble complement factor) C5b to 9 complex (see TCC)
SD1	*Shigella dysenteriae* type 1
SLT	Shiga-like toxin
SMX/TMP	Sulfamethoxazole/trimethoprim
STEC	Shiga toxin producing *Escherichia coli*
STPB	Shiga toxin producing bacteria
Stx	Shiga toxin
TCC	Terminal complement complex
TF	Thomsen-Friedenreich (antigen)
TMA	Thrombotic microangiopathy
TTP	Thrombotic thrombocytopenic purpura
UTI	Urinary tract infection
VT	Vero(cyto)toxin
VTEC	Vero(cyto)toxin producing *Escherichia coli*

Introduction

For the purpose of this chapter, we define postinfectious hemolytic uremic syndrome (HUS) as HUS [1] caused by specific infectious organisms in patients with no identifiable HUS-associated genetic variants or autoantibodies. HUS can follow infections by Shiga toxin (Stx) producing bacteria, mainly *Escherichia coli* (STEC) and *Shigella dysenteriae* type 1, [2, 3] neuraminidase producing organisms, mainly *Streptococcus pneumoniae* and *Clostridium species* [4–7], influenza virus [8], SARS-CoV-2 [9] or HIV

[10]. Biologically diverse mechanisms affecting vascular endothelial cells, platelets and red blood cells (RBCs) have been uncovered involving Stx, neuraminidase and potentially complement that mediate thrombotic microangiopathy (TMA) [11, 12]. TMA is characterized by the simultaneous appearance of intravascular hemolysis, thrombocytopenia and acute organ injury, most commonly acute kidney injury (AKI). TMA is an umbrella term of diverse forms of HUS and thrombotic thrombocytopenic purpura (TTP). The majority of HUS episodes in children can be linked to STEC infections, depending on the geographical latitude and agricultural systems. This contrasts with HUS caused by the dysregulation of the alternative pathway of complement associated with pathogenic variants and/or autoantibodies (mainly to complement factor H), or to other genetic and metabolic causes (Box 24.1). However, HUS can arise following infection by a "specific" agent in a patient with a primary complement disorder; the "atypical" nature of such HUS is uncovered by its clinical presentation (relapsing course, recurrence after transplantation or family history) and/or genetic screening.

Box 24.1: Classification of Thrombotic Microangiopathies (TMA): HUS and TTP

1. Infection-induced HUS (caused by endothelial injury due to specific infectious agents)
   (a) Shiga toxin-producing bacteria
      (i) Shiga toxin-producing *Escherichia coli* (STEC)
      (ii) *Shigella dysenteriae* type 1
   (b) Neuraminidase-producing bacteria
      (i) *Streptococcus pneumoniae*
      (ii) *Clostridium spp.*
   (c) Influenza virus (A/H3N2, A/H1N1, B)
   (d) Severe acute respiratory syndrome corona virus-2 (SARS-CoV-2)
   (e) Human immunodeficiency virus (HIV)

2. Hereditary/genetic forms of HUS
   (a) Mutations of regulatory proteins and components of complement and coagulation pathways (soluble and membrane-bound, usually heterozygous)
   (b) Genetic abnormalities without known complement dysregulation, usually autosomal recessive (examples: methylmalonic aciduria and homocystinuria, cblC type; diacylglycerol kinase-ε)
3. Autoimmune HUS
   (a) Autoantibodies against complement regulatory proteins (example: anti-CFH antibody)
4. Thrombotic thrombocytopenic purpura (TTP)
   (a) Hereditary TTP (Upshaw Shulman Syndrome)
   (b) Autoimmune TTP (anti-ADAMS13 antibody)
5. Other forms
   (a) Endotheliotoxic therapeutics (examples: cancer drugs, anti-VEGF antibody)
   (b) NYED (not yet etiologically defined)
6. Secondary forms
   (a) SLE, anti-phospholipid syndrome, bone marrow transplantation etc.

The historical terms diarrhea-positive (D+) and diarrhea-negative (D−) HUS, introduced to distinguish STEC-induced HUS from "atypical" forms, have become obsolete. At least 1/3 of patients with complement-mediated "atypical" HUS present with diarrhea or even colitis [13, 14]. The D+/D− dichotomy also failed to differentiate postinfectious forms, such as *S. pneumoniae* HUS (pnHUS), from "atypical" HUS. An etiology-based classification and diagnosis, where possible, is essential for patient management [15].

Finally, there is emerging evidence of transient complement activation in postinfectious forms of HUS in the absence of a demonstrable genetic defect or anti-CFH autoantibodies. The precise mechanism of complement activation and its pathological significance are presently under investigation. With the evolving understanding of the complement system and of the pathogenesis of different forms of HUS, some of the descriptions and assumptions in this chapter will have to be revised in the future [8, 11, 16–19].

Shiga Toxin-Producing *Escherichia coli* HUS

History of HUS and Definitions

The term "hemolytic uremic syndrome" was first used in 1955 by the Swiss hematologist Conrad von Gasser, who described five children presenting with the triad of acute hemolytic anemia, thrombocytopenia and kidney failure [1]. It was not until 1983 when Mohamed Karmali and his group identified vero(cyto)toxin producing *Escherichia coli* as the as the cause of typical childhood HUS [2, 20]. In the same year, Allison O'Brien recognized that a toxin, produced by a newly described *E. coli* O157:H7 serovar, bore close similarity with *Shigella dysenteriae* type 1 (Shiga). Soon it became clear that verotoxin and Shiga-like toxin belong to a family of closely related bacterial protein exotoxins, subsequently name Shiga toxins (Stx), with the major subdivision Stx1 and Stx2 (and several related variants) [21]. We will use the terms STEC-HUS to describe patients with "typical" HUS, the predominant form of pediatric HUS in many countries [22].

More than 200 *E coli* serotypes have been described carrying Stx phage(s) and producing Stx, but only a limited number has been associated with human disease [23]. Shiga toxin-producing bacteria encompass STEC and *S. dysenteriae* type 1, and the occasional *Citrobacter freundii* isolates capable of Stx production [24–26].

While *E. coli* O157:H7 is responsible for the majority of sporadic hemorrhagic colitis (HC) and HUS cases and outbreaks worldwide, non-O157:H7 STEC serotypes, including *E. coli*

O111:H11/NM and O26:H11/NM have also been implicated in severe human disease [27–29]. The large-scale *E. coli* O104:H4 outbreak in Germany in 2011 [30, 31] with >850 mostly adult victims of HUS and 50 deaths represents a unique scenario where an enteroaggregative *E. coli* incorporated an *stx2* phage; this novel strain contaminated sprouts, that are usually eaten raw [31, 32].

Epidemiology of STEC Infections and STEC-HUS

The annual incidence of sporadic STEC HUS is 1–1.5 per 100,000 pediatric population (median age 2.7 years) [33, 34]. The vast majority of patients is diagnosed during the warm season. The primary reservoir is cattle and cattle manure. STEC O157:H7 can survive for months or years and multiply at low rates even under adverse conditions.

Outbreaks of STEC infections and HUS in the early 1990s were linked to the consumption of STEC O157:H7-contaminated ground beef [35, 36]. They caused widespread media attention and expensive lawsuits, and eventually resulted in improved hygiene in slaughterhouses and warnings against the consumption of undercooked meat. Consequently, the role of processed meat as the predominant outbreak vehicle diminished, and more recent epidemics were due to contaminated well water [37], aquaculture spillover [38], or agricultural produce [31, 39–42].

Non-O157:H7 STEC serotypes have been increasingly recognized as a cause of sporadic and epidemic infections and HUS. Isolation frequencies of non-O157:H7 STEC strains belonging to more than 50 *E. coli* serogroups approach or exceed those of *E. coli* O157:H7 strains in North America, Europe and elsewhere [43–47]. Transmission occurs in about equal proportions through food and person-to-person spread [48–51].

The HUS risk following STEC infection varies substantially between STEC serotypes: in pediatric populations it is between 8 and 15% for O157:H7 [52, 53], and about ten-fold lower for most non-O157:H7 serotypes [45, 54], with some notable exceptions [28, 55–59]. The global burden of STEC infections is about 2.8 million annually leading to 3890 cases of HUS, 270 cases of end-stage kidney disease (ESKD), and 230 deaths [22]. Table 24.1 summarizes large or clinically significant outbreaks of STEC infections highlighting the spectrum of involved STEC serotypes and toxins, the vehicle of transmission and calculated HUS risks.

Pathogenesis of STEC Disease and HUS

STEC display a sophisticated machinery involving bacterial and host proteins, high contagiosity and resistance to environmental factors. The central pathogenic factor leading to HC and HUS is the ability to produce Stx and to deliver it into the blood stream. STEC are not tissue invasive, and bacteremia is not a feature of STEC diarrhea or HUS.

Ingested STEC bind to epithelial cells in the terminal ileum and Payer's patches. Bacterial interaction with host cells elicits signals that enhance bacterial colonization and release of bacterium-derived pathogenic factors including lipopolysaccharide (LPS) and Stx. Tight adherence of STEC to gut epithelium facilitates toxin translocation into local microvasculature and systemic circulation without killing the epithelial cell [60, 61] (Fig. 24.1). STEC and free fecal toxin excretion often diminish when HUS becomes manifest [53, 62–64]. The concentration of measurable, circulating toxin is extremely low. This can be attributed to its avid binding to endothelial cells and transport in shed microvesicles [65, 66]. Of note, evidence of coagulation system activation and intravascular fibrin deposition can be demonstrated well before, or even in the absence of the clinical manifestation of HUS [67, 68].

Table 24.1 STEC-HUS outbreaks and epidemics

Location [year]	Vehicle	Outbreak strain (Stx type)	Cases (hospitalized)	HUS	HUS risk	Mortality	Reference
Upper Bavaria, (Germany) [Sept–Nov 1988]	?	*E. coli* O157:NM (*stx2*)	6	6 (4–17 months; dialysis 6)	100%	0/6	[362]
Lombardia, Italy [Apr–May 1992]	?	*E. coli* O111:NM (*stx1* and *stx2*)	?	9	?	1/9 (11.1%)	[363]
West Coast (USA) [Jan–Feb 1993]	Beef patties (Hamburger; errors in meat processing and cooking)	*E. coli* O157:H7 (*stx1* and *stx2*)	501 (151; 31%) Children 278	45 (37 children)	9.0% (Children 13.3%)	3/45 (6.7%) 3/501 (0.60%)	[36] See also [126, 364–366]
South Australia [Jan–Feb 1995]	Dry fermented sausage (Mettwurst)	*E. coli* O111:NM (*stx1* and *stx2*)	?	21	?	1/21 (4.8%)	[367]
Sakai (Japan) [July 1996]	Bean sprout	*E. coli* O157:H7 (*stx1* and *stx2*)	12,680 (425; 3.4%)	12	0.09%	0/12	[39, 41, 172]
Scotland (UK) [Nov–Dec 1996]	Cold cooked meat from single butcher	*E. coli* O157:H7 (*stx2*, phage type 2)	512 (120; 23.4%)	36 (Children 6)	7.0%	17/36 (47.2%) 17/512 (3.32%; all deaths >65 years)	[368–370]
Walkerton, Ont. (Canada) [May 2000]	Contaminated municipal drinking water	*E. coli* O157:H7, *Campylobacter jejuni*	Symptomatic Self-reported 2300 (65; 2.8%)	HUS 30 (Children 22)	1.3% (total)	6/30 (20%) 6/2300 (0.26%)	[371–373]
Germany [2002]	Unknown	SF (sorbitol-fermenting) EHEC O157:NM	Unknown	38	Unknown	4/38 (10.5%)	[57]
Oklahoma (USA) [August 2008]	Food (diseased food workers in restaurant)	*E. coli* O111:NM (*stx1* and *stx2*)	344 (70; 20.3%)	25	7.3%	1/25 (4.0%) 1/344 (0.29%)	[374]
Northern Germany [May–June 2011]	Fenugreek	*E. coli* O104:H4 (*stx2*; STEC/EAEC hybrid strain)	3842	855 (children 90)	22.3%	54/855 (6.3%) 54/3842 (1.41%) Pediatric HUS 1/90 (1.11%)	[31, 239, 375, 376]

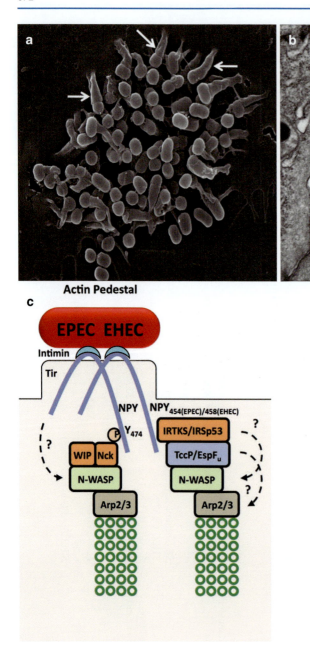

Fig. 24.1 STEC and related attaching and effacing (A/E) pathogens, such as enteropathogenic *E. coli* (EPEC), induce distinct histopathological lesions using the (bacterial) type III secretion system (T3SS) encoded by the "locus of enterocyte effacement" (LEE). (**a**) Scanning electron micrograph of pedestals induced by adherent bacteria (*arrows*). (**b**) Transmission electron micrograph showing intestinal A/E lesions (*arrow*). (**c**) Diagram depicting the actions of a subset of T3SS effectors of A/E pathogens on host cytoskeletal pathways and structures. *Green circles* represent actin filaments. (Used with permission of Jonn Wiley and Sons from Wong et al. [361])

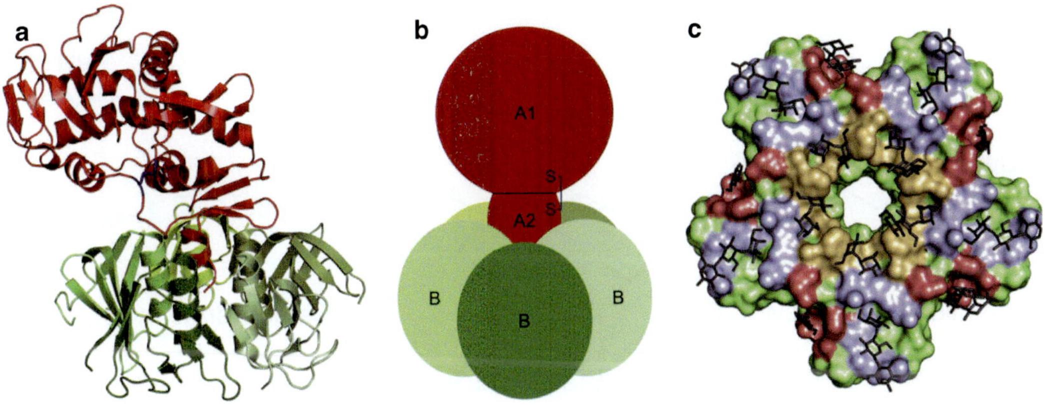

Fig. 24.2 (**a**) The structure of Shiga holotoxin as determined by X-ray crystallography. The A moiety is shown in *red*, the five B subunits in *green*, and the disulfide bridge linking the A1 and A2 fragments in *blue*. (**b**) Schematic representation of the Shiga toxin structure. (**c**) The surface of the B5 pentamer indicating the location of the 15 potential receptor binding sites, based on the structure of Shiga toxin 1. (Used with permission of Elsevier from Bergan et al. [69])

Shiga Toxin and Its Glycolipid Receptor

Shiga toxins consist of an enzymatically active 32.2 kDa A subunit and a receptor-binding B subunit, composed of 5 identical 7.7 kDa proteins (Fig. 24.2). The B subunit interacts with the terminal sugars of the glycolipid receptor, globotriaosylceramide (Gb3) [69]. Gb3 is identical with CD77 and the P^k blood group antigen [70–73] (Fig. 24.3). Although Stx1 and Stx2 display subtle differences in their affinity to Gb3, this does not readily explain why the vast majority of STEC-HUS cases are linked to Stx2 producing strains compared with Stx1 producers [74, 75].

Gb3 is the only functional receptor for Stx1 and most Stx2. Gb3 synthase knockout mice are resistant to the toxic actions of Stx [76]. Gb3 is found on microvascular endothelial cells (including glomerular and peritubular capillary endothelium), glomerular epithelial cells (podocytes), platelets and germinal center B-lymphocytes [77], and peripheral and central neurons [78, 79]. Cellular toxicity requires efficient transport of Stx to the endoplasmic reticulum and subsequent ribosomal RNA (rRNA) depurination [69, 80] (Fig. 24.4). Very few molecules are needed to paralyze the cell, making it one of the most potent known toxins. The action of Stx on the ribosome induces a ribotoxic stress response characterized by the activation of the MAP kinase pathway and apoptotic cell death [81, 82]. Evidence of apoptosis in kidney and other tissues has been demonstrated *ex vivo* in kidney biopsies from patients with STEC-HUS and in animal models of STEC infection [83–85].

Injured microvascular endothelial cells become prothrombotic. The mechanism(s) leading to intravascular hemolysis and acute thrombocytopenia are less well understood. Stx interacts with blood and plasma components and induces shedding of platelet and monocyte microparticles loaded with tissue factor and complement [86, 87] (Fig. 24.5). Biologically active microparticles and (direct) Stx-induced apoptosis of endothelial cells, including the externalization of plasma membrane phosphatidylserine [88], may provide a mechanism how microvascular thrombosis is initiated [89]. The molecular and human cellular biology of Shiga toxins has been summarized in excellent review articles [65, 90, 91].

Laboratory Diagnosis of STEC Infections

Tests must be sensitive, specific and easily accessible. Rapid microbiological diagnosis of STEC diarrhea is essential [92] and can be aided by PCR tests. The clinician should provide the labo-

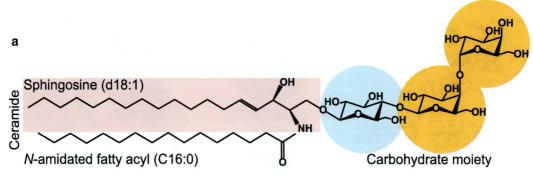

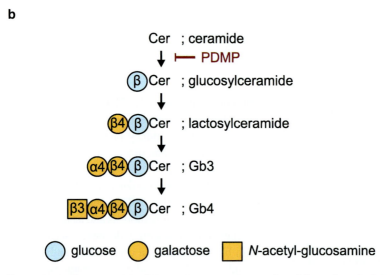

Fig. 24.3 (a) Structure of the Shiga toxin receptor Gb3. Glucose and galactose of the carbohydrate moiety are shown in *blue* and *yellow*, respectively. The ceramide moiety consists of a sphingosine backbone (in *pink*) and a variable fatty acid chain. (b) The steps in the synthesis of the globo-series of glycosphingolipids from ceramide, showing the sequential addition of carbohydrates represented by the glycan symbol system. (Used with permission of Elsevier from Bergan et al. [69])

ratory with meaningful clinical information, including the presence of painful or bloody diarrhea, or signs of HUS, and if there is a suspected outbreak. If the stool culture of an index patient is STEC negative, the pathogen may be identified in other family members [93].

An etiological diagnosis is important. It separates STEC-HUS from other HUS forms and impacts on acute treatment decisions and long-term follow-up [15, 94]. STEC detection has implications for close contacts, care facilities, restaurants/kitchens and the food industry. STEC infections are notifiable and require isolation measures to curb further transmission during an epidemic [95, 96]. In the bigger picture, bacterial isolation allows monitoring of epidemiological changes, such as the emergence of new strains and virulence traits.

Current recommendations stipulate that stools be plated simultaneously on an *E. coli* O157:H7 selective agar (or alternative bacteriological methods) and tested for the presence of Stx using a fresh stool suspension or overnight broth culture [97, 98]. Stx immunoassays or multiplex PCR

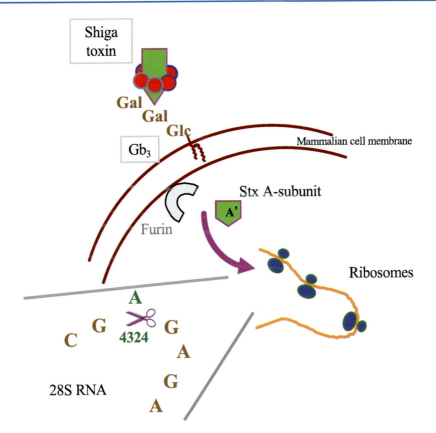

Fig. 24.4 Schematic diagram of the biological action of Stx in susceptible mammalian cells. The holotoxin binds to lipid raft-associated membrane globotriaosyl ceramide (Gb3) and enters the cell via clathrin-mediated endocytosis. A and B subunits become disengaged and the A subunit is cleaved and activated by intracellular furin. Upon "retrograde" passage through the Golgi apparatus, the A′ subunit selectively removes a specific adenine residue from the 28S RNA of the large ribosomal subunit (N-glycosidase activity). This results in (1) blockade of active (translating) ribosomes (translational inhibition), and (2) a ribotoxic cellular stress response with activation of c-jun and p38 (MAP) kinases and/or apoptotic cell death. (Used with permission of author and Elsevier from Loirat et al. [286])

alone are not sufficient for clinical samples [99]. Cell culture-based assays, although highly sensitive and specific, are not routinely performed.

Before the use of Shiga toxin assays and PCR, the isolation of non-O157:H7 STEC strains among commensal gut flora by traditional microbiological techniques was laborious, which contributed to the delayed appreciation of non-O157:H7 STEC clones as a cause of enterocolitis and HUS.

The yield of the stool diagnostic diminishes when the sample is delayed beyond 4 days after diarrhea onset [53, 63]. If stool culture or toxin assay(s) are negative, serological assays can be employed to search for elevated (or rising) IgM class antibodies to one of the more common STEC O-groups (LPS antigens) [62, 100–102]. Saliva IgA and IgM provide an alternative to serum antibodies [102, 103]. However, serodiagnostic assays are only offered in a few laboratories. Testing for Stx-specific antibodies has been used as an epidemiological tool [104, 105], but its clinical utility is limited [106].

From Colitis to HUS

The spectrum of STEC disease ranges from mild diarrhea and HC to severe HUS, and death [41, 53, 107]. The diarrhea is typically painful and

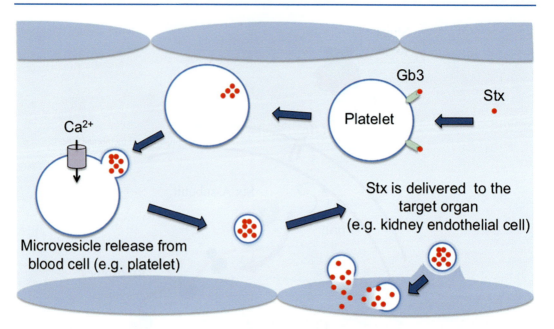

Fig. 24.5 Pathophysiological model incorporating the postulated role of microvesicles in the transfer of Shiga toxin (Stx) to target endothelium. Once in the bloodstream, Stx binds to platelets, neutrophils and red blood cells (RBC) via the toxin receptor, globotriaosylceramide (Gb3). The toxin is internalized and the activated blood cell releases microvesicles into the circulation containing the toxin. Upon reaching the target organ the microvesicles are taken up by microvascular endothelial cells, where Stx is released. In the kidney, this has been shown to occur within glomerular and peritubular capillary endothelial cells. (Used with permission from Karpman et al. [11])

frequent, with >15 small, soft or liquid stools that turn bloody by day 2 or 3 in >80% of children with STEC O157:H7 infection. The amount of visible blood varies from a few specks to frank hemorrhage. About 50% of patients develop nausea and vomiting; low-grade fever is present in one third [32, 53, 67, 92, 107]. Infections by non-O157:H7 STEC serotypes are generally milder [32, 108]. Exceptions are infections by STEC clones belonging to serogroups O26, O55, O91, O111, among others, that can be clinically indiscernible from those by classical *E. coli* O157:H7 [28, 55, 57, 109–115].

The HUS risk is greatest at the extremes of age, in children <5 years and the elderly; it decreases during childhood and adolescence, and is <0.1% in young and middle-aged adults [53, 116, 117]. Conversely, STEC colitis can lead to AKI and death without HUS, particularly in the elderly [116, 118]. Other variables impacting on the HUS risk are the STEC serotype or clone, the toxin type(s) produced, and preexisting immunity [105].

HUS starts abruptly, about 3–10 days (median 6 days) after the onset of diarrhea [53] (Fig. 24.6). Patients present from one day to the other with fatigue and pallor, become listless and may develop petechiae, often after transient clinical improvement of the colitis. Absent bowel movements during the acute phase of HUS should raise the suspicion of intussusception or ileus.

The clinical diagnosis of HUS is generally straightforward, based on the defining triad of intravascular hemolysis, thrombocytopenia and AKI. Hemolytic anemia of HUS—characterized by RBC fragmentation with schistocytes in the peripheral blood smear, with or without thrombocytopenia—is a microangiopathic hemolytic anemia (MAHA). With disease progression, serum creatinine levels rise and oligoanuria, hypertension and edema may appear, usually within 1–2 days of first HUS-related symptoms. Some patients may recover before the full picture of HUS develops. They may only demonstrate hemolytic anemia without apparent AKI, while

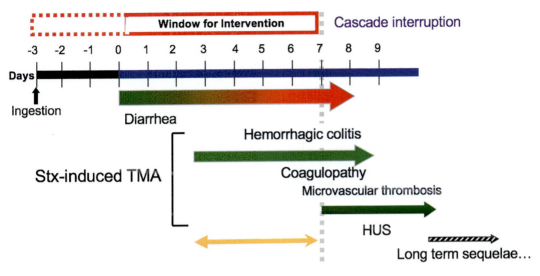

Fig. 24.6 Schematic diagram of the development of Shiga toxin-producing *E. coli* (STEC) colitis and HUS and possible window of therapeutic intervention

platelets may briefly dip within or slightly below the reference range ("partial HUS") [52, 119].

A predictive biological marker of impending HUS is the degree of systemic inflammation during the preceding colitis, particularly neutrophilia with a high-percentage shift to band forms, and a sharp rise of acute phase reactants, such as C-reactive protein or procalcitonin [41, 120–124]. Patients who progress to HUS more often have a peripheral neutrophil count above 20×10^9/L than patients without HUS [122, 125–127].

Hematologic Manifestations of STEC-HUS

Commonly, the hemoglobin level drops precipitously to <80 g/L in STEC-HUS. Hemolysis is accompanied by a rapid fall of platelet numbers, usually <50, at times $<30 \times 10^9$/L. Direct antiglobulin (Coombs) test is negative. Rising indirect bilirubin, free plasma hemoglobin and serum lactate dehydrogenase (LDH), the latter often more than five times the upper limit of normal, and haptoglobin depletion are consistent with rapid (intravascular) hemolysis. The peripheral WBC (neutrophil) count, already increased during the colitis phase, may continue to rise and, if associated with a leukemoid reaction, can herald a severe course with poor intestinal or kidney outcomes [33, 128, 129]. The severity of anemia and thrombocytopenia does not correlate with the degree of acute or chronic kidney injury.

Some authors noted an inverse relationship between Hb and disease severity [129–131]. A plausible explanation for the latter observation is the hemo concentration seen in patients with intravascular volume depletion during the first 4 days of STEC colitis [129, 132]. The recognition that hemo concentration increases the HUS risk in children with STEC diarrhea led to the development of an "HUS risk score." It is considered "high," where the sum of the concentrations of Hb plus 2x creatinine (in g/dL and mg/dL, respectively) exceeds a value of 13 [131]. The correlation between a high risk score and severe HUS/poor outcome was independently confirmed [133, 134], yet its clinical utility remains to be seen.

Thrombocytopenia and hemolysis usually resolve within 2 weeks. A rising platelet count heralds the cessation of HUS activity; platelets may transiently rebound to $>500 \times 10^9$/L. Anemia can persist for weeks after disease recovery without signs of active hemolysis.

AKI in STEC-HUS

Kidney injury in STEC-HUS ranges from microscopic hematuria and proteinuria to severe kidney failure and oligoanuria. Up to 50% of children with STEC-HUS will need acute dialysis [33, 34, 135, 136]. Arterial hypertension is common in the acute phase of HUS and may not be due to volume overload. Blood pressure instability and hypotension are not a typical feature of STEC-HUS and should raise the suspicion of sepsis. Time to recovery of kidney function ranges from a few days to weeks or even months. The risk of long-term kidney impairment (CKD, chronic hypertension, proteinuria) increases with the duration of oliguria (dialysis). A commonly cited threshold for the risk of diminished kidney recovery is anuria lasting >2–3 weeks [137, 138]. Primary ESKD is rare and should prompt investigations into a non postinfectious form of HUS [139].

Extrarenal Manifestations

There is hardly an organ system that may not be affected in STEC infection or STEC-HUS. Rare, but important extrarenal and extraintestinal manifestations are myocarditis and congestive heart failure, cardiac tamponade, pulmonary hemorrhage, pancreatitis, hepatic injury, and central nervous system (CNS) complications [140–143]. Patients with multiple organ involvement generally also have severe kidney failure and often poor outcome [141, 142, 144]. Postulated mechanisms underlying organ injury in STEC-HUS are Stx load and direct tissue toxicity, and ischemic injury [141], as evidenced by histological and autopsy findings.

Rectal prolapse and intussusception may result in transmural bowel necrosis with perforation and peritonitis [145–147]. Serum amylase and lipase activities, indicative of exocrine pancreas injury, are elevated in up to 20% of patients [145]. Transient glucose intolerance or, albeit rare, chronic insulin-dependent diabetes mellitus has been reported [146, 148–150]. Hepatomegaly and/or rising serum alanine amino transferase (ALT) are noted in up to 40% of cases. Acute myocardial insufficiency occurs in less than 1% of cases [141, 151–153]. Skeletal muscle involvement is exceedingly rare and may manifest as rhabdomyolysis [143].

Three to >41% of patients experience CNS manifestations [124, 143, 154–157]. Signs and symptoms can be vague and nonspecific and are probably underappreciated. Patients may present with irritability, lethargy or decreased level of consciousness. Brief seizures are relatively common and may reflect fluid and electrolyte imbalances and inadequate volume replacement [158]. Abnormal electroencephalograms have been reported in up to 50% of patients with HUS. Prolonged seizure activity, usually associated with acute respiratory deterioration, is an ominous sign and may indicate cerebral stroke or hemorrhage. Acute, transient or persistent isolated palsy, dysphasia, diplopia, retinal injury and cortical blindness have been noted [142, 143, 155]. Severe neurological events are associated with poor prognosis and even death [142].

Magnetic resonance imaging (MRI) of the brain is helpful in the differentiation of structural from ischemic or transient injury. In the acute phase, basal ganglia and white matter abnormalities with apparent diffusion coefficient restriction are common and reversible MRI findings [159–164] (Fig. 24.7). However, the described changes do not appear to be specific for STEC-HUS [164]. CNS lesions may be compounded by the occurrence of posterior reversible encephalopathy syndrome or hemodialysis-associated disequilibrium [164]. Peripheral nervous system involvement has been described, but pathogenesis and medical treatment of this rare complication remain unclear [165].

The *E. coli* O104:H4 HUS outbreak in Europe highlighted the occurrence of psychiatric symptoms [166, 167]. Described manifestations include cognitive impairment [168] and, in a few cases, hallucinations and affective disorders, such as severe panic attacks [166].

Histopathology of STEC-HUS

Few pathological descriptions are available from kidney biopsies of patients with acute STEC-HUS [85, 169–173]. Macroscopically, the kidneys appear swollen, with numerous petechial

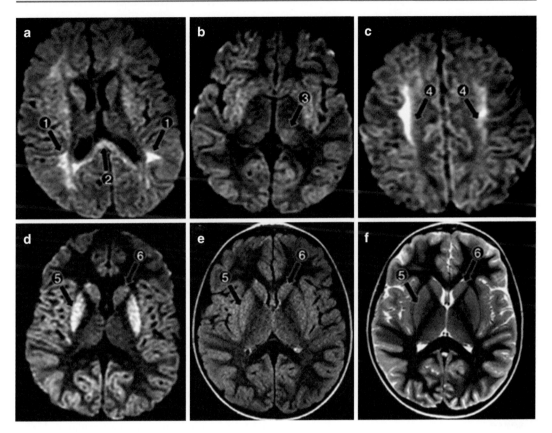

Fig. 24.7 Brain magnetic resonance imaging of patients with STEC-HUS acquired within the first 24 h after the onset of neurological symptoms. (**a–d**) Diffusion-weighted images (DWI) which demonstrate (*1*) hypersignal involving deep white matter; (*2*) corpus callosum; (*3*) thalamus; (*4*) centrum semiovale; (*5*) putamen; and (*6*) caudate nucleus. (**d–f**) Brain MRI of one of the two patients who died. (**d**) The images of this patient demonstrate deep hypersignal on DWI in putamen (*5*) and caudate nucleus (*6*), that can be detected in T2- (**e**) and fluid-attenuated inversion recovery (FLAIR) (**f**) weighted classical imaging. T2- and FLAIR-weighted images of all the surviving patients were normal (not shown). (Used with permission of John Wiley and Sons from Gitiaux et al. [164])

hemorrhages on the external surface; on section, the cortex will show areas of hemorrhage and infarction. Focal hemorrhage has also been noted in the collecting system and ureter (Chantal Bernard, unpublished communication). Prominent *light microscopic* features are the presence of fragmented RBC in *glomerular* capillary loops. Glomerular capillary and renal arteriolar microvascular thrombosis may demonstrate prominent fibrin staining. Endothelial and mesangial cell changes are also evident by *electron microscopy* (Fig. 24.8). *Immunofluorescence* is variably positive for fibrin. Immune deposits are not a feature of STEC-HUS. While glomerular histological changes dominate, the *tubulointerstitial compartment* can also be affected. In fact, all biopsies from a series of patients examined during the 2011 German HUS outbreak, including those without evidence of glomerular TMA, showed severe acute tubular injury [173].

Post-mortem studies of children with STEC-HUS [169, 170, 174] demonstrated that STEC-HUS is a systemic microangiopathy characterized by ubiquitous endothelial cell swelling and injury. There was diffuse hemorrhage with mucosal ulcerations and hemorrhage of the bowel wall as well as congestion of the serosa and extensive vascular thrombosis. The pancreas appeared enlarged and swollen, with areas of necrosis and hemorrhage (Chantal Bernard, unpublished

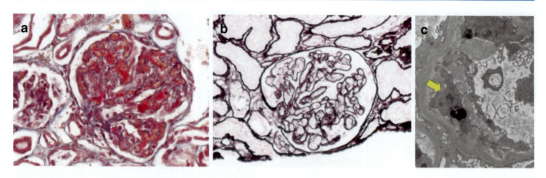

Fig. 24.8 Kidney biopsy, culture-proven STEC-HUS. (**a**) Trichrome stain of glomerulus showing fibrin and RBCs (*orange* and *red*, respectively). (**b**) Silver stain, emphasizing glomerular and tubular basement membrane structures. (**c**) Electron microscopy; a glomerular capillary is shown. *Arrow* indicates fibrin and proteinaceous material pushing toward the capillary lumen and creating the impression of double contours of the glomerular basement membrane. (Courtesy of Dr. Natacha Patey CHU Ste-Justine)

observations). CNS changes consisted of brain swelling and bilateral, symmetric necrotic lesions, mainly of the corpus striatum, and scattered necrotic lesions in the cortex and elsewhere [175].

Prevention and Treatment of STEC Disease

Preventive strategies focus on the implementation of hygienic measures. This applies to cattle farming, the management of drinking water and agricultural produce, safe practices of food preparation and consumption, and containment of the spread of the organism when cases are identified [95, 96, 176–178]. The risk of transmission is reduced by adherence to essential hygienic measures: frequent hand washing and avoiding touching the face [177, 179]. Children with proven STEC infection should only return to childcare or school 48 h after the cessation of diarrhea. Preventive measures and advice for patients and caregivers can be found in various publications [176, 177, 179].

Vaccines

Active immunization of humans, targeting the O157 LPS antigen [180, 181] and/or Stx and other bacterial antigens remains an elusive goal [182, 183]. Progress has been reported, however, in the vaccination of cattle [183, 184].

Therapeutic Interventions During STEC Colitis

Considerable work has been invested to better understand factors that facilitate the progression from colitis to HUS and to intervene at a stage where the process can be reversed, and HUS prevented or at least mitigated. Potential strategies are the elimination of STEC (or Stx) from the gut and toxin neutralization in the circulation [185–187]. None of these approaches have shown convincing results [188]. Randomized, controlled HUS prevention trials in a conventional format are extremely challenging due to the low incidence of STEC infections and the overall low risk of progression to HUS [187, 189–191].

Fluid Therapy

Volume expansion with isotonic saline administered intravenously during early STEC colitis may ameliorate the severity of HUS. In a retrospective cohort study of children with *E. coli* O157:H7 HUS [132], patients who became oligoanuric and needed dialysis had received significantly less intravenous fluid during the first 4 days of diarrhea than children who had preserved urine output and who were not dialyzed. The authors concluded that early parenteral volume expansion before the onset of HUS attenuates AKI and reduces the need for dialysis. Subsequent studies reproduced the initial findings [130, 190, 192, 193]. The "volume hypothesis" is further supported by observations linking higher Hb concentrations at presentation—as a surrogate marker of volume depletion—to severe HUS, including neurological complications [75, 131, 134, 154, 193].

The administration of isotonic solutions is not expected to affect Stx production or tissue binding, but is intended to alleviate incipient acute tubular necrosis and AKI [132, 194]. Saline infusion may also mitigate abdominal cramps caused by STEC induced ischemic colitis [193, 195]. Considering HUS rates of 8–15% in an "under 5" target population, the number needed to treat to prevent one case of HUS is about 7–12.

For practical purposes, rapid confirmation of STEC infection, mainly by PCR (ideally with a multiplex platform that allows testing for *stx1* and *stx2*, and various pathogenic bacteria and viruses in the same stool sample) and easy-to-follow protocols targeting children with bloody and non-bloody diarrhea are needed. Including non-bloody diarrhea cases is relevant, since up to 57% of STEC-HUS patients lack a history of bloody diarrhea or colitis [75, 196].

Figure 24.9 shows an abbreviated, practical algorithm to estimate the individual child's risk of HUS and initiate treatment as soon as STEC colitis is diagnosed or suspected. The risk of fluid overload and cardiopulmonary complications due to saline infusion is negligible, provided the patient is hospitalized and supervised by an experienced team [190]. Hospital admission simplifies patient monitoring. It may also mitigate parental anxiety and reduce the spread of the potentially dangerous organisms [95, 96].

Analgesia

When volume expansion with isotonic saline fails to alleviate the ischemic colitis pain, pharmacological therapy may be warranted. Acetaminophen can be tried. Morphine may be administered sparingly, although it tends to worsen post-colitis constipation or ileus. Nonsteroidal anti-inflammatory analgesic drugs

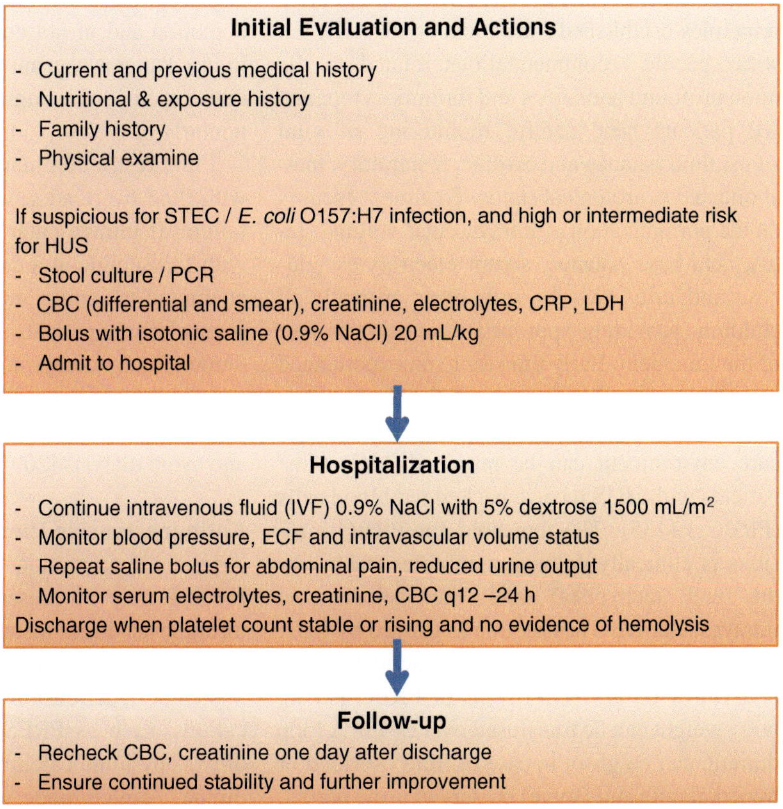

Fig. 24.9 Initial evaluation, monitoring and intervention for STEC infection. Risk of Stx HUS: Age group (>6 months) and diarrhea <4 to 7 days that is frequent, turned bloody after 2–3 days and/or is associated with abdominal cramps; recent or current hemorrhagic colitis or HUS in family or community. Rapid PCR (stool or rectal swab) or antigen assay, and culture for STEC (at least *E. coli* O157:H7), *Campylobacter*, *Salmonella*, *Shigella*, *Yersinia spp.* (Used with permission of AGA Institute from Holtz et al. [92], with modifications)

Initial Evaluation and Actions

- Current and previous medical history
- Nutritional & exposure history
- Family history
- Physical examine

If suspicious for STEC / *E. coli* O157:H7 infection, and high or intermediate risk for HUS
- Stool culture / PCR
- CBC (differential and smear), creatinine, electrolytes, CRP, LDH
- Bolus with isotonic saline (0.9% NaCl) 20 mL/kg
- Admit to hospital

Hospitalization

- Continue intravenous fluid (IVF) 0.9% NaCl with 5% dextrose 1500 mL/m^2
- Monitor blood pressure, ECF and intravascular volume status
- Repeat saline bolus for abdominal pain, reduced urine output
- Monitor serum electrolytes, creatinine, CBC q12 –24 h
Discharge when platelet count stable or rising and no evidence of hemolysis

Follow-up

- Recheck CBC, creatinine one day after discharge
- Ensure continued stability and further improvement

(NSAIDs) should not be used in patients with STEC colitis or HUS who may be intravascularly volume depleted and at risk of ischemic injury of the gut and kidneys.

Anti-Motility Drugs and Antibiotics

Antidiarrheal and antimotility agents have been associated with an increased risk of HUS and should therefore be avoided [32, 126, 154, 197–199]. The observed link between antimicrobial therapy and an increased HUS risk or fatal outcome is supported by experimental studies demonstrating that certain antibiotics stimulate Stx phage induction and toxin production [200–202]. However, the risk of HUS differs according to the class of the antibiotic and the timing of its administration [203, 204]. Evidence is emerging that rifaximin, azithromycin or fosfomycin may limit the spread of the organism and reduce the rate of complications during STEC epidemics [203–207].

Therapeutic Intervention During STEC-HUS

Symptomatic treatment of HUS follows general principles established for patients with AKI, but with specific recommendations related to the often profound hemolysis and thrombocytopenia. All patients need careful monitoring of vital signs, fluid balance and cardiac, respiratory, metabolic and neurological status. Treatment focuses on the normalization of intravascular volume status, acid-base balance, serum electrolytes, glucose and uric acid. As with other critically ill children, providing appropriate nutrition is part of the treatment. Early transfer to an experienced pediatric center is recommended, where extracorporeal purification techniques and a critical care environment can be provided 24/7. Most patients with HUS receive packed red blood cells (PRBCs) [135]. The threshold for PRBC infusions is clinically defined: symptoms (tachycardia and tachypnea) and the velocity of intravascular RBC destruction as gauged by LDH and free Hb levels in plasma. A practical cut-off is a Hb of 60 g/L. 12–15 mL of PRBC per kg body weight can be transfused over 2–4 h. A loop diuretic can be given in case of fluid overload or hyperkalemia and (some) preserved urine output.

If necessary, PRBC transfusions can be timed to coincide with dialysis sessions, particularly if hyperkalemia or volume overload are a concern. RBCs should be leucocyte and platelet depleted, as practiced in most pediatric hospitals. Peritoneal and central venous catheters can be placed safely in most children with HUS without a need for platelet transfusion [208].

AKI Management in STEC-HUS

Assessment of intravascular volume status helps guide initial treatment toward fluid replacement or restriction, and administration of diuretics or dialysis. Patients are monitored for fluid intake and changes in urine output, along with frequent measurements of blood pressure (BP) and heart rate. Weight changes correlate poorly with effective circulatory volume. Intravascular volume may be decreased due to intestinal losses and reduced oral intake during the early phase of the disease and may result in hypoperfusion of the kidneys. Third spacing, especially in the gut, and generalized edema—due to endothelial injury and capillary leak—may mask intravascular depletion and, if not corrected, worsen ischemic injury. Patients warrant diligent intravascular volume expansion to improve organ perfusion, particularly of the gut, kidneys and brain.

Fluid restriction may be necessary in patients with fluid overload secondary to oliguric kidney failure. If intravascular volume is replete, a trial with furosemide at a dose of 1–2 mg/kg may be attempted to induce diuresis and delay dialysis, particularly in patients with hyperkalemia or cardiopulmonary compromise. Aggressive challenge with high-dose loop diuretics, advocated in the past to prevent progression to oligoanuric failure and avoid dialysis [209] should be avoided.

Antihypertensive Therapy

Arterial hypertension is common in STEC-HUS. It may be caused by renal microvascular thrombosis, direct vascular endothelial cell injury or activation, and intravascular fluid overload. Systemic hypertension can lead to CNS complications, such as PRES. It is reasonable to use dihydropyridine calcium channel blockers (nifedipine, amlodipine or PO/IV nicardipine).

Treatment with renin-angiotensin system (RAS) blockers has to be balanced against concerns over impairment of kidney perfusion and hyperkalemia. However, RAS inhibition is a rationale choice for the long-term treatment of patients with HUS-induced CKD and/or chronic hypertension or proteinuria [210, 211].

Kidney Replacement Therapy

There is no evidence that early dialysis changes the evolution of acute STEC-HUS or long-term outcome. However, delaying dialysis unduly increases the risk of complications. The North American Synsorb Pk® trial protocol mandated that dialysis not be started until 72 h post diagnosis of HUS, if clinically acceptable by the responsible physician. Under these restrictive conditions, 39% of the 49 placebo-treated patients were dialyzed for a mean of 3.6 days [135]. Indications for dialysis initiation in HUS are similar to those for other causes of AKI and may evolve rapidly: severe electrolyte imbalance (hyperkalemia, hyperphosphatemia), acidosis or fluid overload refractory to medical/diuretic therapy, or symptomatic uremia.

The choice of the dialysis modality depends on clinical and practical aspects, such as availability of PD and HD and adequately trained personnel, patient size for central access creation, local preference and experience, particularly when dialyzing young children and infants. Diarrhea or colitis are not considered contraindications for peritoneal dialysis (PD) [135, 189, 212].

Continuous renal replacement therapy (CRRT) or "slow" HD offer alternatives to conventional HD in patients with severe fluid overload, cardiovascular instability, with or without sepsis, and multiorgan failure. Both are typically performed in a critical care setting. HD and CRRT can be tried with minimal or no heparin, provided there is sufficient blood flow through the circuit. Regional, citrate-based anticoagulation offers an alternative to heparin, specifically in patients with cerebral stroke or hemorrhage, or after surgery.

Some pediatric centers consider severe, life-threatening STEC-HUS an indication for plasma exchange (PE) as "rescue" therapy, especially for patients with CNS complications [189, 213]. This approach may have been influenced by the success of PE in aHUS and TTP. However, the benefit of plasma therapy (PE or plasma infusion) in STEC-HUS remains unproven [214–217]. The European Paediatric Study Group for HUS excluded STEC-HUS from PE [94]. In young children, PE requires the insertion of a large-bore central venous access (HD line), which confers additional morbidity to children not already undergoing HD [19]. The guidelines for the use of apheresis by the American Society for Apheresis (ASFA) categorized STEC-HUS as III, i.e. a disorder where the role of apheresis treatment is not established, with weak recommendation and low-quality evidence (2C) [218].

Immunoadsorption (IA) is a specialized apheresis technique for the selective removal of humoral factors such as immunoglobulins and complement from plasma via a high-affinity adsorbent column [219]. However, reports of its use for STEC-HUS is anecdotal [220–222].

Anticomplement Therapy in STEC-HUS

The role of the complement system in the pathogenesis of STEC-HUS gained traction over the past decade [223–227]. Several events stimulated scientific inquiry and clinical interest: progress in the understanding of atypical HUS caused by genetic or acquired dysregulation of the alternative pathway, availability of a potent, well-tolerated anti-C5 antibody (eculizumab), and its compassionate use during the *E. coli* O104:H4 epidemic in Northern Germany.

Increased plasma levels of complement activation products derived from factor B (CFB) and C3, and of the terminal complement complex sC5b-9 [86, 227, 228] as well as the deposition of C5b-9 in post-mortem tissue (Fig. 24.10) suggests that complement is activated in STEC-HUS. Interestingly, no correlation was found between the levels of complement products in plasma or platelet derived microparticles and the presence or absence of kidney or extrarenal complications [86, 228].

Data on the use of eculizumab in (severe) STEC-HUS have been recently summarized [229, 230]. Despite signals indicating clinical improvement,

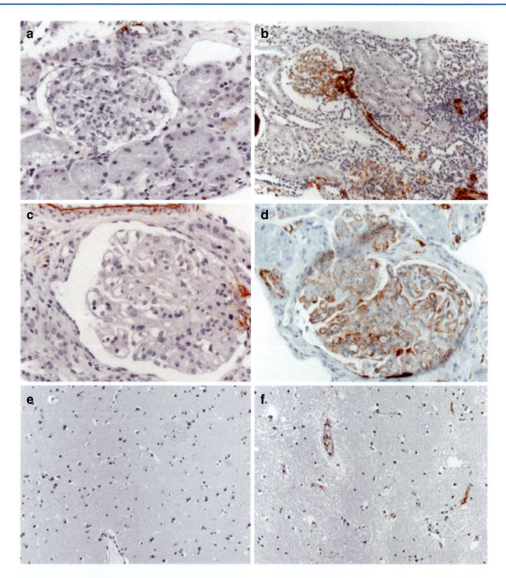

Fig. 24.10 C5b-9 (membrane attack complex, MAC) deposition in kidney and CNS sections of a child who died of STEC O157:H7 HUS. (**a**) Control (kidney). (**b**) Strong staining of kidney arteriole and glomerular capillaries with anti-MAC antibody (1:200). (**c**) Staining of afferent and efferent arterioles, minor staining within the glomerulus. (**d**) Ubiquitous glomerular capillary staining with anti- MAC antibody. (**e**) control (brain). (**f**) Staining of cerebral capillaries with anti-MAC antibody. (Courtesy of Dr. Natacha Patey CHU Ste-Justine)

mainly of neurological complications, the overall quality of evidence is low [230, 231]. It remains to be shown, if and under which conditions Stx-associated complement activation becomes deleterious and requires targeted treatment. While awaiting definitive trial results [232, 233], the off-label use of anticomplement agents in patients with STEC-HUS should be reserved for severe forms (especially in cases with CNS or cardiac involvement) and balanced against potential adverse effects and costs.

Complications and Long-Term Outcome

AKI due to STEC-HUS is frequently self-limited. Hematological improvement (decreasing LDH, increasing platelet count) generally precedes kidney recovery. Overall, the outcome of STEC-HUS has improved substantially since its first description. Reported mortality rates typically vary between <1% and 5% [234], mostly due to CNS, cardiac, or gastrointestinal complications. About 70% of patients recover completely from the acute episode [125, 129, 142, 146, 152, 153, 234–236]. Complications appear to be more frequent in adults with STEC-HUS than in children, and the lethality in the elderly population may be as high as 50% [117, 237–240].

Long-Term Outcome and Monitoring
Long-term kidney complications have been reported in 5 to 25% of patients [113, 129, 241, 242]. 15–30% of patients have proteinuria, typically mild, and 5 to 15% have arterial hypertension. CKD has been noted in approximately 10% of surviving patients and ESKD in 3% [113, 125, 138, 234, 243]. Up to one-third of children with severe HUS (defined as anuria >8 days or oliguria >15 days) developed long-term sequelae [137, 138, 244]. Yearly evaluation of kidney function, BP and urinalysis has been recommended for at least 5 years, and indefinitely for patients with decreased GFR, proteinuria and/or hypertension [113, 138, 148, 234, 243].

Up to 30% of children with CNS manifestations during HUS will develop long-term neurological sequelae [235]. There is probably underdiagnosis of subtle neurological problems such as learning and behavioral difficulties, reduced fine motor coordination, and attention deficit and hyperactivity disorder [245].

STEC-HUS and Kidney Transplantation
For the small percentage of STEC-HUS patients who progress to ESKD, kidney transplantation is the optimal therapy [113, 246]. When a genetic cause of complement dysregulation is ruled out, graft and patient survival are comparable to other kidney transplant recipients [246–250].

Shigella dysenteriae HUS

HUS due to *Shigella dysenteriae* type 1 (SD1) is rare. Yet it is the leading cause of death in outbreaks of SD1 infections [251–254]. Unlike STEC, *S. dysenteriae* is an invasive organism. It penetrates the bowel wall and enters the blood stream. Patients with SD1 infection should be treated early with appropriate antibiotics [255]. The spread of highly resistant SD1 strains is a challenge [256]. Antimicrobial treatment after the first 4 days of diarrhea has been identified as a risk factor for HUS [257].

HUS occurs four to 17 days after the onset of bloody diarrhea, and occasionally after diarrhea has improved. Shiga toxin (Stx) is involved in the pathogenesis of *S. dysenteriae* colitis and HUS. The incidence of HUS among children with SD1 dysentery is less than 0.4% (median age 3 years) [258] (Table 24.2). A high peripheral neutrophil count has been associated with the development and the severity of HUS [259, 260]. Oliguric AKI has been described in 90% of SD1-HUS cases, dialysis in 52%, and disseminated intravascular coagulation in 21% [261]. Additional complications are listed in Table 24.3.

The reported mortality of SD1-HUS is substantially higher than the mortality due to STEC-HUS. However, most of the burden of S. *dysenteriae* infections and SD1-HUS is carried by under resourced countries [255, 257, 262].

Pneumococcal (*Streptococcus pneumoniae*) HUS

Epidemiology

Invasive pneumococcal disease (IPD) may lead to HUS, referred to as pneumococcal HUS (pnHUS). It occurs in <0.7% of IPD episodes [263, 264] and affects mostly infants before the age of 2–3 years [264–266], although older children and adults are also affected [267]. The 10-year incidence is about 1.2 per 100,000 children under 15 years [268]. Indigenous populations may have a higher

Table 24.2 Pediatric *Shigella dysenteriae* type 1 (SD1) HUS [a]

Country	# of reported cases	Age in years (mean or median)	Interval between onset of diarrhea and diagnosis of HUS (days)	Case fatality rate (%)	Reference
South Africa	151	4.6	7	17	[261, 377–379]
Zimbabwe	110	1.5	11	41	[379, 380]
India	74	2.3	8	59	[381, 382]
Nepal	55	2.1	17	23	[383, 384]
Saudi Arabia	33	3.0	8	26	[385, 386]
Bangladesh	30	3.3	6	37	[259]
Kenya	21	1.6	4	52	[387]

[a] Modified from Butler [257]

Table 24.3 Organ involvement in *Shigella dysenteriae* (SD1) HUS

Organ involvement	Details	Percentage (of SD1 HUS cases)[a]
Generalized	Septicemia	18.5
	Disseminated intravascular coagulation	21.0
	Hyponatremia	69.1
	Hypoalbuminemia	82.7
Gastrointestinal	Toxic megacolon	4.9
	Gastrointestinal perforation	9.9
	Protein-losing enteropathy	32.1
	Rectal prolapse	6.2
	Hepatitis	13.6
Kidney	Oliguric AKI	90.1
	Dialysis	51.6
Central nervous system	Encephalopathy	37.0
	Convulsions	14.8
	Hemiplegia	2.3
Heart	Myocarditis	6.2
	Congestive cardiac failure	3.7
	Cardiomyopathy	3.7
	Infective endocarditis	1.2
Hematological	Leukemoid reaction	91.3

[a] Extracted from Bhimma et al. [261]. Percentages are from 81 of 107 cases of HUS, admitted between July 1994 and February 1996 in KwaZulu/Natal

disease burden than other groups [265, 268, 269]. pnHUS accounts for approximately 5% of pediatric HUS cases, and 40% of non-STEC-HUS cases [264, 270, 271]. The majority of patients presents during the winter [265, 271].

Increased vaccine coverage may have led to a decline in the incidence of pnHUS, Yet *S. pneumoniae* serotype 19A was missing in the first generation pneumococcal 7-valent conjugate vaccine (PCV7) and has emerged as the predominant isolate during the last decade [265, 266, 272–275]. It is incorporated into the present 13-valent vaccine (PCV13) [276] and the 23-valent pneumococcal polysaccharide vaccine

(PPV23). pnHUS continues to occur, e.g., due to vaccine failure and emergence of non-vaccine replacement serotypes [7, 275].

Pathogenesis

pnHUS typically develops in a patient with pneumonia or meningitis [265, 266, 274, 277, 278]. HUS has been associated with abundant *in situ* production of bacterial neuraminidase [4, 279], in particular neuraminidase A (NanA) [280]. Neuraminidases cleave terminal sialyl residues from membrane glycoproteins and glycolipids [12, 280–282]. The exposed O-glycan core is known as Thomsen-Friedenreich disaccharide (TF antigen) [283]. The TF "neo" antigen is recognized by the lectin *Arachis hypogaea*, which has been used to detect and quantify the *in vivo* effect of neuraminidase on RBCs and tissues in patients with pnHUS [4, 5, 280] (Fig. 24.11).

It was postulated that the interaction of preformed anti-TF antibodies with the exposed neoantigen induces hemolysis, platelet agglutination, microvascular thrombosis, and tissue injury [5]. However, anti-TF antibodies are generally of the IgM class and of low affinity at body temperature [284–287]. Furthermore, desialylation of RBCs is not specific for HUS: it can be found in patients with IPD without progression to HUS [288–290], and pnHUS can develop in the absence of TF antibodies [282].

Presentation of pnHUS and Clinical Course

A practical approach for diagnosing pnHUS is shown in Table 24.4. Patients with pnHUS typically present with fever and respiratory distress due to lobar pneumonia (70–80%) that is complicated in two thirds of cases by pleural effusion or empyema [265, 291]. The remaining 20–30% have pneumococcal meningitis, acute otitis media or pneumococcal sepsis. The majority (80%) is bacteremic at the time of diagnosis [292]. The interval between onset of *S. pneumoniae* infection and HUS is 1–2 weeks [289].

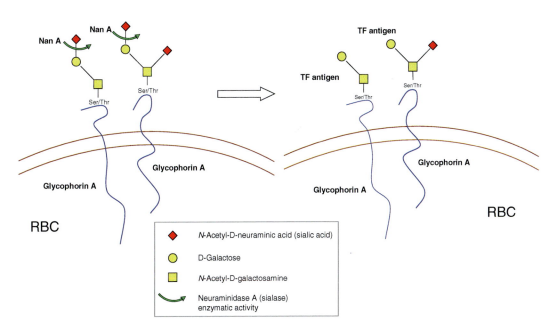

Fig. 24.11 Neuraminidase action on RBC membrane. Nan A (pneumococcal neuraminidase A) removes the terminal sialic acid. The *Arachis hypogea* lectin specifically recognizes the residual disaccharide β-D-galactose (1–3)-N-acetyl-D-galactosamine (Thomsen-Friedenreich antigen) that is O-glycosidically linked to the serine/threonine residue of glycophorin A (Used with permission of author and Elsevier from Loirat et al. [286])

The disease course can be severe or even fatal. A large proportion of patients will be admitted to the intensive care unit, of whom >50% will require mechanical ventilation and chest tube placement. About 70–85% of patients become oliguric or anuric, often with rapid clinical deterioration, and need acute dialysis [265, 291, 292]. Median time of dialysis in a large series was 10 days (range 2–240 days) [265].

In addition to microangiopathic hemolytic anemia with profound thrombocytopenia, the laboratory findings include a rapid rise of acute phase reactants (CRP, procalcitonin) [289]. The direct Coombs is positive in 58–90% of patients during the early phase of pnHUS [278, 293–295].

Patients may have DIC [278, 294, 296, 297]. *S. pneumoniae* sepsis with mild anemia, thrombocytopenia, DIC, hypotension and AKI can masquerade as HUS. Furthermore, Coombs positive hemolytic anemia may occur without thrombocytopenia and kidney injury [288, 298]. Hence, it is useful to choose a methodical approach diagnosing pnHUS [269, 274, 278] (Table 24.4).

Laboratory Studies and Biomarkers

The defining criterium is the detection of *S. pneumoniae* in a sterile fluid (blood, pleural effusion, cerebral spinal fluid, middle ear aspirate, etc.). In case of preceding antibiotic therapy, pneumococcal PCR or antigen detection should be tried.

Laboratory workup includes demonstration of TF exposure on PRBCs, a direct Coombs test and screening for DIC. It is recommended to measure C3, C4, CH50, and serum immunoglobulin levels and exclude congenital or acquired immune deficiencies that are known to predispose to invasive pneumococcal disease [299]. Serial CRP measurements are useful to confirm effective antimicrobial therapy.

No other HUS presents with a positive Coombs test or TF antigen exposure. However, the frequency of Coombs test positivity in IPD without HUS is unclear [278]. Sensitivity and specificity of TF antigen detection was reported as 86% and 57%, respectively, for pnHUS or isolated hemolytic anemia. The positive predictive value for HUS was 76%. Conversely, in

Table 24.4 Diagnostic Criteria for pnHUS[a]

pnHUS	Criteria		Details
Definite	1	Evidence of HUS	Intravascular hemolytic anemia, thrombocytopenia and acute kidney injury
	2	Evidence of invasive *S. pneumoniae* infection	Pneumococcal growth/antigen detection or positive PCR from physiologically sterile biological fluid
	3	No evidence of disseminated intravascular coagulation (DIC)	Fibrinogen consumption, prolonged prothrombin or partial thromboplastin time, and/or d-dimers *at the time of diagnosis*
Probable	1	Evidence of HUS	See above
	2	Evidence of invasive *S. pneumoniae* infection	See above
	3	a) Evidence of DIC ***and*** b) Positive Coombs test and/or evidence of TF antigen exposure	Usually cold agglutinins; TF antigen detection by *Arachis hypogaea* or specific lectin/monoclonal antibody binding [298]
Possible	1	Evidence of HUS	See above
	2	Suspected (undocumented) invasive *S. pneumoniae* infection	Negative culture/antigen detection or PCR from sterile fluid
	3	(a) No evidence of DIC, ***or*** (b) Positive Coombs test and/or TF antigen exposure	With or without evidence of DIC (see above)

Abbreviations: *TF* Thomsen-Friedenreich
[a] Modified from Copelovitch et al. [274]

children with IPD, positive and negative predictive values of TF antigen detection for pnHUS were 52 and 100% [290]. Among hospitalized patients with severe pneumococcal disease, TF antigen exposure levels peak 5–10 days after disease onset [300].

Complement and pnHUS

Informative studies on underlying complement abnormalities in pnHUS patients are scarce [287, 301, 302]. Complement consumption, primarily due to activation of the alternative pathway, is common in patients with pnHUS. Removal of sialic acids by NanA was noted to increase complement activity in whole blood, while absence of NanA blocked complement activation implying that the enzymatic removal of sialic acids can trigger pnHUS [12]. Transient CFH desialylation may play a role in disease pathogenesis [303]. While *S. pneumoniae* infection can trigger HUS in children with damaging mutations of complement regulator genes, similar to patients with "atypical" HUS, disease relapses due to *S. pneumoniae* have not been described. The emergence of specific (protective) immunity is surmised.

Treatment of pnHUS

Treatment of patients with pnHUS includes appropriate antibiotics and supportive care [278, 286]. Dialysis is required in up to 80% of patients. Previous recommendations to restrict blood transfusion to "washed" RBCs and to avoid administration of plasma which contains anti-TF antibodies [304, 305] are not based on evidence [17, 268, 278, 286, 287, 306, 307]. Indeed, plasma infusion and plasma exchange therapy have been described in pnHUS patients without apparent worsening of hemolysis or kidney function [265, 306, 308, 309].

Therapeutic complement blockade in the absence of pathogenic complement gene variants has not been systematically studied [307, 310].

Pneumococcal vaccination is an important measure for disease prevention [7].

Outcome of pnHUS

Unfavorable outcome has been noted in 20% of patients [265]. In another series, 3% of patients had died [292], 13% had neurologic sequelae, and 10% underwent kidney transplantation [292]. Important CNS complications are intracranial hemorrhage and infarction that can result in obstructive hydrocephalus [265, 268]. Waters et al. found that only 2 of 13 patients with pnHUS and meningitis had a normal neurodevelopmental outcome [265]. Pulmonary complications in addition to empyema include pneumatoceles and necrotic pneumonia [268]. Most deaths are not caused by HUS or kidney injury, but are due to meningitis and septic shock. Residual kidney dysfunction and proteinuria are expected in 20–25% [265, 311]. Kidney transplantation following pnHUS is rare, but HUS recurrence has not been reported [275, 312, 313].

Clostridium HUS

Early descriptions of HUS were traced to infections by *Clostridium perfringens*, the cause of gas gangrene, necrotizing fasciitis, and necrotizing enterocolitis [306, 314]. *C. perfringens* and other clostridial species produce neuraminidases, along with a range of other proteases and toxic enzymes [315]. A pathogenetic role of neuraminidase in clostridium HUS has been postulated [306, 314]. Newer reports have also implicated *C. difficile* in cases of HUS [316–322]. Treatment is supportive, in addition to appropriate antibiotics.

Influenza HUS

There is an established link between influenza virus infection, mostly influenza A, and HUS, but the mechanism remains speculative [8, 16].

Influenza virus shares with *S. pneumoniae* the production of neuraminidase (NA). Hemagglutinin (HA) and NA are defining and important viral pathogenicity factors in infections. NA shedding is minimal compared to *S. pneumoniae*, and it remains to be shown whether and how much it contributes to the pathogenesis HUS.

Infection of endothelial cells by influenza virus can induce apoptosis, [323] which triggers platelet adhesion directly and via extracellular matrix exposure [88, 324]. The virus also activates platelets and causes thrombin generation [325, 326]. Furthermore, influenza virus is a potent activator of complement [327–329]. Excess complement activation may lead to temporary consumption of C3 or may trigger HUS in individuals with risk variants of complement genes.

Patients with influenza HUS should be tested for plasma C3 and sC5b-9 concentrations, and ADAMTS13 activity. The presence of concomitant or complicating pneumococcal pneumonia or sepsis must be ruled out [16].

Supportive care is the main therapeutic intervention. It is unknown if the NA inhibitor oseltamivir prevents or ameliorates influenza HUS. The role of plasma therapy (PI, PLEX) or eculizumab in influenza HUS is unproven. However, recommendations for the treatment of aHUS should be followed if defective complement regulation is proven or suspected, particularly in instances of preceding HUS episode(s), a positive family history of aHUS, or recurrence of HUS after kidney transplantation [13, 94, 286].

COVID-19 and HUS

SARS-CoV-2, the virus causing COVID-19, injures the vascular endothelium, which can result in thrombotic complications [330]. SARS-CoV-2 can induce a fulminant cytokine response, including activation of the complement system and release of the chemokines C3a and C5a [331]. Multisystem inflammatory syndrome in children (MIS-C) is the most severe form of this pathologic reaction [332, 333], which may also involve the kidneys, but generally without overt TMA [334–336]. However, TMA has been observed in SARS-Cov-2 infected patients [337, 338] and after COVID-19 vaccination [339–342].

COVID-19 may cause TMA in patients without genetically determined complement abnormalities [9, 343, 344]. SARS-CoV-2 activates the alternative and lectin pathways of complement, likely via its spike surface protein [337, 345]. The pathogenic role of complement activation in COVID-19 is supported by the experimental observation that C3 deficient mice are protected against SARS-CoV-2 disease [346]. Finally, complement activation may also contribute to the hypercoagulable state in COVID-19 patients [347]. Some clinical observations, however, indicate that eculizumab may not prevent severe COVID-19 and associated endothelial cell injury [348], suggesting that blocking the terminal complement pathway is not sufficient.

HIV HUS

TMA in the context of AIDS has been variably described as HUS or TTP, and TTP has been listed as an AIDS defining condition [349, 350]. The incidence of HIV TMA has decreased since the advent of effective HIV therapies [351].

Clinical observation and animal experiments suggest that HIV can cause HUS directly [352], although the mechanism(s) remain unclear. HIV infects glomerular endothelial and mesangial cells, but not epithelial cells *in vitro* [353]. Intriguingly, a viral surface glycoprotein, pg120, binds to Gb3, the Stx receptor; this interaction has been linked to the occurrence of HIV HUS [352, 354–356]. Conversely, Gb3 has been described as natural resistance factor for the prevention of HIV infection, e.g. when given as a soluble agent [356, 357]. Kidney biopsies may show features of TMA [351, 358, 359].

Treatment of HIV TMA consists of effective antiviral therapy and supportive care, with the anecdotal use of fresh-frozen plasma infusions and plasmapheresis [351, 358–360].

References

1. Gasser C, Gautier E, Steck A, Siebenmann RE, Oechslin R. Hemolytic-uremic syndrome: bilateral necrosis of the renal cortex in acute acquired hemolytic anemia. Schweiz Med Wochenschr. 1955;85:905–9.
2. Karmali MA, Petric M, Lim C, Fleming PC, Arbus GS, Lior H. The association between idiopathic hemolytic uremic syndrome and infection by verotoxin-producing Escherichia coli. J Infect Dis. 1985;151:775–82.
3. Koster F, Levin J, Walker L, Tung KS, Gilman RH, Rahaman MM, Majid MA, Islam S, Williams RC Jr. Hemolytic-uremic syndrome after shigellosis. Relation to endotoxemia and circulating immune complexes. N Engl J Med. 1978;298:927–33.
4. Fischer K, Poschmann A, Oster H. Severe pneumonia with hemolysis caused by neuraminidase. Detection of cryptantigens by indirect immunofluorescent technic. Monatsschr Kinderheilkd. 1971;119:2–8.
5. Klein PJ, Bulla M, Newman RA, Muller P, Uhlenbruck G, Schaefer HE, Kruger G, Fisher R. Thomsen-Friedenreich antigen in haemolytic-uraemic syndrome. Lancet. 1977;2:1024–5.
6. Copelovitch L, Kaplan BS. Streptococcus pneumoniae-associated hemolytic uremic syndrome. Pediatr Nephrol. 2008;23:1951–6.
7. Agarwal HS, Latifi SQ. Streptococcus pneumoniae-associated hemolytic uremic syndrome in the era of pneumococcal vaccine. Pathogens. 2021;10(6):727.
8. Bitzan M, Zieg J. Influenza-associated thrombotic microangiopathies. Pediatr Nephrol. 2018; 33:2009–25.
9. Diorio C, McNerney KO, Lambert M, Paessler M, Anderson EM, Henrickson SE, Chase J, Liebling EJ, Burudpakdee C, Lee JH, Balamuth FB, Blatz AM, Chiotos K, Fitzgerald JC, Giglia TM, Gollomp K, Odom John AR, Jasen C, Leng T, Petrosa W, Vella LA, Witmer C, Sullivan KE, Laskin BL, Hensley SE, Bassiri H, Behrens EM, Teachey DT. Evidence of thrombotic microangiopathy in children with SARS-CoV-2 across the spectrum of clinical presentations. Blood Adv. 2020;4:6051–63.
10. Fine DM, Fogo AB, Alpers CE. Thrombotic microangiopathy and other glomerular disorders in the HIV-infected patient. Semin Nephrol. 2008;28:545–55.
11. Karpman D, Loos S, Tati R, Arvidsson I. Haemolytic uraemic syndrome. J Intern Med. 2017;281:123–48.
12. Syed S, Hakala P, Singh AK, Lapatto HAK, King SJ, Meri S, Jokiranta TS, Haapasalo K. Role of pneumococcal nana neuraminidase activity in peripheral blood. Front Cell Infect Microbiol. 2019;9:218.
13. Loirat C, Fakhouri F, Ariceta G, Besbas N, Bitzan M, Bjerre A, Coppo R, Emma F, Johnson S, Karpman D, Landau D, Langman CB, Lapeyraque AL, Licht C, Nester C, Pecoraro C, Riedl M, van de Kar NC, Van de Walle J, Vivarelli M, Fremeaux-Bacchi V, International HUS. An international consensus approach to the management of atypical hemolytic uremic syndrome in children. Pediatr Nephrol. 2016;31:15–39.
14. Schaefer F, Ardissino G, Ariceta G, Fakhouri F, Scully M, Isbel N, Lommele A, Kupelian V, Gasteyger C, Greenbaum LA, Johnson S, Ogawa M, Licht C, Vande Walle J, Fremeaux-Bacchi V, Global a HUSR. Clinical and genetic predictors of atypical hemolytic uremic syndrome phenotype and outcome. Kidney Int. 2018;94:408–18.
15. McFarlane PA, Bitzan M, Broome C, Baran D, Garland J, Girard LP, Grewal K, Lapeyraque AL, Patriquin CJ, Pavenski K, Licht C. Making the correct diagnosis in thrombotic microangiopathy: a narrative review. Can J Kidney Health Dis. 2021;8:20543581211008707.
16. Allen U, Licht C. Pandemic H1N1 influenza A infection and (atypical) HUS—more than just another trigger? Pediatr Nephrol. 2011;26:3–5.
17. Johnson S, Waters A. Is complement a culprit in infection-induced forms of haemolytic uraemic syndrome? Immunobiology. 2012;217:235–43.
18. Mele C, Remuzzi G, Noris M. Hemolytic uremic syndrome. Semin Immunopathol. 2014.
19. Johnson S, Stojanovic J, Ariceta G, Bitzan M, Besbas N, Frieling M, Karpman D, Landau D, Langman C, Licht C, Pecoraro C, Riedl M, Siomou E, van de Kar N, Walle JV, Loirat C, Taylor CM. An audit analysis of a guideline for the investigation and initial therapy of diarrhea negative (atypical) hemolytic uremic syndrome. Pediatr Nephrol. 2014;29:1967–78.
20. Karmali MA, Steele BT, Petric M, Lim C. Sporadic cases of haemolytic-uraemic syndrome associated with faecal cytotoxin and cytotoxin-producing Escherichia coli in stools. Lancet. 1983;1:619–20.
21. Scheutz F, Teel LD, Beutin L, Pierard D, Buvens G, Karch H, Mellmann A, Caprioli A, Tozzoli R, Morabito S, Strockbine NA, Melton-Celsa AR, Sanchez M, Persson S, O'Brien AD. Multicenter evaluation of a sequence-based protocol for subtyping Shiga toxins and standardizing Stx nomenclature. J Clin Microbiol. 2012;50:2951–63.
22. Majowicz SE, Scallan E, Jones-Bitton A, Sargeant JM, Stapleton J, Angulo FJ, Yeung DH, Kirk MD. Global incidence of human shiga toxin-producing escherichia coli infections and deaths: a systematic review and knowledge synthesis. Foodborne Pathog Dis. 2014;11:447–55.
23. Prager R, Fruth A, Busch U, Tietze E. Comparative analysis of virulence genes, genetic diversity, and phylogeny of Shiga toxin 2g and heat-stable enterotoxin STIa encoding Escherichia coli isolates from humans, animals, and environmental sources. Int J Med Microbiol. 2011;301:181–91.
24. Schmidt H, Montag M, Bockemuhl J, Heesemann J, Karch H. Shiga-like toxin II-related cytotoxins in Citrobacter freundii strains from humans and beef samples. Infect Immun. 1993;61:534–43.
25. Tschäpe H, Prager R, Streckel W, Fruth A, Tietze E, Bohme G. Verotoxinogenic Citrobacter freundii

25. associated with severe gastroenteritis and cases of haemolytic uraemic syndrome in a nursery school: green butter as the infection source. Epidemiol Infect. 1995;114:441–50.
26. Wickham ME, Lupp C, Mascarenhas M, Vazquez A, Coombes BK, Brown NF, Coburn BA, Deng W, Puente JL, Karmali MA, Finlay BB. Bacterial genetic determinants of non-O157 STEC outbreaks and hemolytic-uremic syndrome after infection. J Infect Dis. 2006;194:819–27.
27. Brooks JT, Sowers EG, Wells JG, Greene KD, Griffin PM, Hoekstra RM, Strockbine NA. Non-O157 Shiga toxin-producing Escherichia coli infections in the United States, 1983-2002. J Infect Dis. 2005;192:1422–9.
28. Bielaszewska M, Mellmann A, Bletz S, Zhang W, Kock R, Kossow A, Prager R, Fruth A, Orth-Holler D, Marejkova M, Morabito S, Caprioli A, Pierard D, Smith G, Jenkins C, Curova K, Karch H. Enterohemorrhagic Escherichia coli O26:H11/H-: a new virulent clone emerges in Europe. Clin Infect Dis. 2013;56:1373–81.
29. Vishram B, Jenkins C, Greig DR, Godbole G, Carroll K, Balasegaram S, Byrne L. The emerging importance of Shiga toxin-producing Escherichia coli other than serogroup O157 in England. J Med Microbiol. 2021;70
30. Bielaszewska M, Mellmann A, Zhang W, Kock R, Fruth A, Bauwens A, Peters G, Karch H. Characterisation of the Escherichia coli strain associated with an outbreak of haemolytic uraemic syndrome in Germany, 2011: a microbiological study. Lancet Infect Dis. 2011;11:671–6.
31. Buchholz U, Bernard H, Werber D, Bohmer MM, Remschmidt C, Wilking H, Delere Y, an der Heiden M, Adlhoch C, Dreesman J, Ehlers J, Ethelberg S, Faber M, Frank C, Fricke G, Greiner M, Hohle M, Ivarsson S, Jark U, Kirchner M, Koch J, Krause G, Luber P, Rosner B, Stark K, Kuhne M. German outbreak of Escherichia coli O104:H4 associated with sprouts. N Engl J Med. 2011;365:1763–70.
32. Davis TK, McKee R, Schnadower D, Tarr PI. Treatment of Shiga toxin-producing Escherichia coli infections. Infect Dis Clin N Am. 2013;27:577–97.
33. Rowe PC, Orrbine E, Wells GA, McLaine PN. Epidemiology of hemolytic-uremic syndrome in Canadian children from 1986 to 1988. The Canadian Pediatric Kidney Disease Reference Centre. J Pediatr. 1991;119:218–24.
34. McLaine PN, Rowe PC, Orrbine E. Experiences with HUS in Canada: what have we learned about childhood HUS in Canada? Kidney Int. 2009;75:S25–8.
35. Pavia AT, Nichols CR, Green DP, Tauxe RV, Mottice S, Greene KD, Wells JG, Siegler RL, Brewer ED, Hannon D, et al. Hemolytic-uremic syndrome during an outbreak of Escherichia coli O157:H7 infections in institutions for mentally retarded persons: clinical and epidemiologic observations. J Pediatr. 1990;116:544–51.
36. Bell BP, Goldoft M, Griffin PM, Davis MA, Gordon DC, Tarr PI, Bartleson CA, Lewis JH, Barrett TJ, Wells JG, et al. A multistate outbreak of Escherichia coli O157:H7-associated bloody diarrhea and hemolytic uremic syndrome from hamburgers. The Washington experience. JAMA. 1994;272:1349–53.
37. Salvadori MI, Sontrop JM, Garg AX, Moist LM, Suri RS, Clark WF. Factors that led to the Walkerton tragedy. Kidney Int Suppl. 2009;112:S33–4.
38. Kim JS, Lee MS, Kim JH. Recent updates on outbreaks of shiga toxin-producing Escherichia coli and its potential reservoirs. Front Cell Infect Microbiol. 2020;10:273.
39. Yukioka H, Kurita S. Escherichia coli O157 infection disaster in Japan, 1996. Eur J Emerg Med. 1997;4:165.
40. Ackers ML, Mahon BE, Leahy E, Goode B, Damrow T, Hayes PS, Bibb WF, Rice DH, Barrett TJ, Hutwagner L, Griffin PM, Slutsker L. An outbreak of Escherichia coli O157:H7 infections associated with leaf lettuce consumption. J Infect Dis. 1998;177:1588–93.
41. Fukushima H, Hashizume T, Morita Y, Tanaka J, Azuma K, Mizumoto Y, Kaneno M, Matsuura M, Konma K, Kitani T. Clinical experiences in Sakai City Hospital during the massive outbreak of enterohemorrhagic Escherichia coli O157 infections in Sakai City, 1996. Pediatr Int. 1999;41:213–7.
42. Marshall KE, Hexemer A, Seelman SL, Fatica MK, Blessington T, Hajmeer M, Kisselburgh H, Atkinson R, Hill K, Sharma D, Needham M, Peralta V, Higa J, Blickenstaff K, Williams IT, Jhung MA, Wise M, Gieraltowski L. Lessons learned from a decade of investigations of Shiga toxin-producing escherichia coli outbreaks linked to leafy greens, United States and Canada. Emerg Infect Dis. 2020;26:2319–28.
43. Byrne L, Vanstone GL, Perry NT, Launders N, Adak GK, Godbole G, Grant KA, Smith R, Jenkins C. Epidemiology and microbiology of Shiga toxin-producing Escherichia coli other than serogroup O157 in England, 2009-2013. J Med Microbiol. 2014;63:1181–8.
44. Luna-Gierke RE, Wymore K, Sadlowski J, Clogher P, Gierke RW, Tobin-D'Angelo M, Palmer A, Medus C, Nicholson C, McGuire S, Martin H, Garman K, Griffin PM, Mody RK. Multiple-aetiology enteric infections involving non-O157 shiga toxin-producing Escherichia coli - FoodNet, 2001-2010. Zoonoses Public Health. 2014.
45. Luna-Gierke RE, Griffin PM, Gould LH, Herman K, Bopp CA, Strockbine N, Mody RK. Outbreaks of non-O157 Shiga toxin-producing Escherichia coli infection: USA. Epidemiol Infect. 2014:1–11.
46. Hooman N, Khodadost M, Ahmadi A, Nakhaie S, Nagh Shizadian R. The Prevalence of Shiga toxin-producing Escherichia coli in patients with gastroenteritis in Iran, systematic review and meta-analysis. Iran J Kidney Dis. 2019;13:139–50.
47. Murphy V, Carroll AM, Forde K, Broni R, McNamara EB. Verocytotoxin Escherichia coli-

Associated haemolytic uraemic syndrome. Ir Med J. 2020;113:5.

48. Vasser M, Barkley J, Miller A, Gee E, Purcell K, Schroeder MN, Basler C, Neil KP. Notes from the field: multistate outbreak of Escherichia coli O26 infections linked to raw flour - United States, 2019. MMWR Morb Mortal Wkly Rep. 2021;70:600–1.

49. Spano LC, Guerrieri CG, Volpini LPB, Schuenck RP, Goulart JP, Boina E, Recco CRN, Ribeiro-Rodrigues R, Dos Santos LF, Fumian TM. EHEC O111:H8 strain and norovirus GII.4 Sydney [P16] causing an outbreak in a daycare center, Brazil, 2019. BMC Microbiol. 2021;21:95.

50. Blankenship HM, Mosci RE, Dietrich S, Burgess E, Wholehan J, McWilliams K, Pietrzen K, Benko S, Gatesy T, Rudrik JT, Soehnlen M, Manning SD. Population structure and genetic diversity of non-O157 Shiga toxin-producing Escherichia coli (STEC) clinical isolates from Michigan. Sci Rep. 2021;11:4461.

51. Butt S, Allison L, Vishram B, Greig DR, Aird H, McDonald E, Drennan G, Jenkins C, Byrne L, Licence K, Smith-Palmer A, Incident Management T. Epidemiological investigations identified an outbreak of Shiga toxin-producing Escherichia coli serotype O26:H11 associated with pre-packed sandwiches. Epidemiol Infect. 2021;149:e178.

52. Rowe PC, Orrbine E, Lior H, Wells GA, Yetisir E, Clulow M, McLaine PN. Risk of hemolytic uremic syndrome after sporadic Escherichia coli O157:H7 infection: results of a Canadian collaborative study. Investigators of the Canadian Pediatric Kidney Disease Research Center. J Pediatr. 1998;132:777–82.

53. Tarr PI, Gordon CA, Chandler WL. Shiga-toxin-producing Escherichia coli and haemolytic uraemic syndrome. Lancet. 2005;365:1073–86.

54. Preussel K, Hohle M, Stark K, Werber D. Shiga toxin-producing Escherichia coli O157 is more likely to lead to hospitalization and death than non-O157 serogroups—except O104. PLoS One. 2013;8:e78180.

55. Bielaszewska M, Kock R, Friedrich AW, von Eiff C, Zimmerhackl LB, Karch H, Mellmann A. Shiga toxin-mediated hemolytic uremic syndrome: time to change the diagnostic paradigm? PLoS One. 2007;2:e1024.

56. Feng PC, Monday SR, Lacher DW, Allison L, Siitonen A, Keys C, Eklund M, Nagano H, Karch H, Keen J, Whittam TS. Genetic diversity among clonal lineages within Escherichia coli O157:H7 stepwise evolutionary model. Emerg Infect Dis. 2007;13:1701–6.

57. Alpers K, Werber D, Frank C, Koch J, Friedrich AW, Karch H, An DERHM, Prager R, Fruth A, Bielaszewska M, Morlock G, Heissenhuber A, Diedler A, Gerber A, Ammon A. Sorbitol-fermenting enterohaemorrhagic Escherichia coli O157:H- causes another outbreak of haemolytic

uraemic syndrome in children. Epidemiol Infect. 2009;137:389–95.

58. Werber D, Bielaszewska M, Frank C, Stark K, Karch H. Watch out for the even eviler cousin-sorbitol-fermenting E coli O157. Lancet. 2011;377:298–9.

59. Chase-Topping ME, Rosser T, Allison LJ, Courcier E, Evans J, McKendrick IJ, Pearce MC, Handel I, Caprioli A, Karch H, Hanson MF, Pollock KG, Locking ME, Woolhouse ME, Matthews L, Low JC, Gally DL. Pathogenic potential to humans of bovine Escherichia coli O26, Scotland. Emerg Infect Dis. 2012;18:439–48.

60. Schuller S, Heuschkel R, Torrente F, Kaper JB, Phillips AD. Shiga toxin binding in normal and inflamed human intestinal mucosa. Microbes Infect. 2007;9:35–9.

61. Bekassy ZD, Calderon Toledo C, Leoj G, Kristoffersson A, Leopold SR, Perez MT, Karpman D. Intestinal damage in enterohemorrhagic Escherichia coli infection. Pediatr Nephrol. 2011;26:2059–71.

62. Bitzan M, Ludwig K, Klemt M, Konig H, Buren J, Muller-Wiefel DE. The role of Escherichia coli O 157 infections in the classical (enteropathic) haemolytic uraemic syndrome: results of a Central European, multicentre study. Epidemiol Infect. 1993;110:183–96.

63. Cornick NA, Jelacic S, Ciol MA, Tarr PI. Escherichia coli O157:H7 infections: discordance between filterable fecal shiga toxin and disease outcome. J Infect Dis. 2002;186:57–63.

64. Lopez EL, Contrini MM, Glatstein E, Ayala SG, Santoro R, Ezcurra G, Teplitz E, Matsumoto Y, Sato H, Sakai K, Katsuura Y, Hoshide S, Morita T, Harning R, Brookman S. An epidemiologic surveillance of Shiga-like toxin-producing Escherichia coli infection in Argentinean children: risk factors and serum Shiga-like toxin 2 values. Pediatr Infect Dis J. 2012;31:20–4.

65. Willysson A, Tontanahal A, Karpman D. Microvesicle involvement in Shiga toxin-associated infection. Toxins (Basel). 2017;9(11):376.

66. Willysson A, Stahl AL, Gillet D, Barbier J, Cintrat JC, Chambon V, Billet A, Johannes L, Karpman D. Shiga toxin uptake and sequestration in extracellular vesicles is mediated by its B-subunit. Toxins (Basel). 2020:12.

67. Chandler WL, Jelacic S, Boster DR, Ciol MA, Williams GD, Watkins SL, Igarashi T, Tarr PI. Prothrombotic coagulation abnormalities preceding the hemolytic-uremic syndrome. N Engl J Med. 2002;346:23–32.

68. Tsai HM, Chandler WL, Sarode R, Hoffman R, Jelacic S, Habeeb RL, Watkins SL, Wong CS, Williams GD, Tarr PI. von Willebrand factor and von Willebrand factor-cleaving metalloprotease activity in Escherichia coli O157:H7-associated hemolytic uremic syndrome. Pediatr Res. 2001;49:653–9.

69. Bergan J, Dyve Lingelem AB, Simm R, Skotland T, Sandvig K. Shiga toxins. Toxicon. 2012;60:1085–107.

70. Taylor CM, Milford DV, Rose PE, Roy TC, Rowe B. The expression of blood group P1 in post-enteropathic haemolytic uraemic syndrome. Pediatr Nephrol. 1990;4:59–61.

71. Armstrong GD, Fodor E, Vanmaele R. Investigation of Shiga-like toxin binding to chemically synthesized oligosaccharide sequences. J Infect Dis. 1991;164:1160–7.

72. Bitzan M, Richardson S, Huang C, Boyd B, Petric M, Karmali MA. Evidence that verotoxins (Shiga-like toxins) from Escherichia coli bind to P blood group antigens of human erythrocytes in vitro. Infect Immun. 1994;62:3337–47.

73. Cooling LL, Walker KE, Gille T, Koerner TA. Shiga toxin binds human platelets via globotriaosylceramide (Pk antigen) and a novel platelet glycosphingolipid. Infect Immun. 1998;66:4355–66.

74. Boerlin P, McEwen SA, Boerlin-Petzold F, Wilson JB, Johnson RP, Gyles CL. Associations between virulence factors of Shiga toxin-producing Escherichia coli and disease in humans. J Clin Microbiol. 1999;37:497–503.

75. Ardissino G, Vignati C, Masia C, Capone V, Colombo R, Tel F, Daprai L, Testa S, Dodaro A, Paglialonga F, Luini M, Brigotti M, Picicco D, Baldioli C, Pagani F, Ceruti R, Tommasi P, Possenti I, Cresseri D, Consonni D, Montini G, Arghittu M, ItalKid HUSN. Bloody Diarrhea and Shiga toxin-producing Escherichia coli hemolytic uremic syndrome in children: data from the ItalKid-HUS Network. J Pediatr. 2021;237(34–40):e31.

76. Okuda T, Tokuda N, Numata S, Ito M, Ohta M, Kawamura K, Wiels J, Urano T, Tajima O, Furukawa K. Targeted disruption of Gb3/CD77 synthase gene resulted in the complete deletion of globo-series glycosphingolipids and loss of sensitivity to verotoxins. J Biol Chem. 2006;281:10230–5.

77. Engedal N, Skotland T, Torgersen ML, Sandvig K. Shiga toxin and its use in targeted cancer therapy and imaging. Microb Biotechnol. 2011;4:32–46.

78. Arab S, Murakami M, Dirks P, Boyd B, Hubbard SL, Lingwood CA, Rutka JT. Verotoxins inhibit the growth of and induce apoptosis in human astrocytoma cells. J Neuro-Oncol. 1998;40:137–50.

79. Obata F, Tohyama K, Bonev AD, Kolling GL, Keepers TR, Gross LK, Nelson MT, Sato S, Obrig TG. Shiga toxin 2 affects the central nervous system through receptor globotriaosylceramide localized to neurons. J Infect Dis. 2008;198:1398–406.

80. Endo Y, Tsurugi K, Yutsudo T, Takeda Y, Ogasawara T, Igarashi K. Site of action of a Vero toxin (VT2) from Escherichia coli O157:H7 and of Shiga toxin on eukaryotic ribosomes. RNA N-glycosidase activity of the toxins. Eur J Biochem. 1988;171:45–50.

81. Jandhyala DM, Ahluwalia A, Obrig T, Thorpe CM. ZAK: a MAP3Kinase that transduces Shiga toxin- and ricin-induced proinflammatory cytokine expression. Cell Microbiol. 2008;10:1468–77.

82. Tesh VL. Activation of cell stress response pathways by Shiga toxins. Cell Microbiol. 2012;14:1–9.

83. Karpman D, Hakansson A, Perez MT, Isaksson C, Carlemalm E, Caprioli A, Svanborg C. Apoptosis of renal cortical cells in the hemolytic-uremic syndrome: in vivo and in vitro studies. Infect Immun. 1998;66:636–44.

84. Kaneko K, Kiyokawa N, Ohtomo Y, Nagaoka R, Yamashiro Y, Taguchi T, Mori T, Fujimoto J, Takeda T. Apoptosis of renal tubular cells in Shiga-toxin-mediated hemolytic uremic syndrome. Nephron. 2001;87:182–5.

85. Te Loo DM, Monnens LA, Van Den Heuvel LP, Gubler MC, Kockx MM. Detection of apoptosis in kidney biopsies of patients with d+ hemolytic uremic syndrome. Pediatr Res. 2001;49:413–6.

86. Stahl AL, Sartz L, Karpman D. Complement activation on platelet-leukocyte complexes and microparticles in enterohemorrhagic Escherichia coli-induced hemolytic uremic syndrome. Blood. 2011;117:5503–13.

87. Ge S, Hertel B, Emden SH, Beneke J, Menne J, Haller H, von Vietinghoff S. Microparticle generation and leucocyte death in Shiga toxin-mediated HUS. Nephrol Dial Transplant. 2012;27:2768–75.

88. Bombeli T, Schwartz BR, Harlan JM. Endothelial cells undergoing apoptosis become proadhesive for nonactivated platelets. Blood. 1999;93:3831–8.

89. Zoja C, Buelli S, Morigi M. Shiga toxin-associated hemolytic uremic syndrome: pathophysiology of endothelial dysfunction. Pediatr Nephrol. 2010;25:2231–40.

90. Menge C. Molecular biology of escherichia coli shiga toxins'. Effects on mammalian cells. Toxins (Basel). 2020:12.

91. Karpman D, Tontanahal A. Extracellular vesicles in renal inflammatory and infectious diseases. Free Radic Biol Med. 2021;171:42–54.

92. Holtz LR, Neill MA, Tarr PI. Acute bloody diarrhea: a medical emergency for patients of all ages. Gastroenterology. 2009;136:1887–98.

93. Luini MV, Colombo R, Dodaro A, Vignati C, Masia C, Arghittu M, Daprai L, Maisano AM, Vezzoli F, Bianchini V, Spelta C, Castiglioni B, Bertasi B, Ardissino G. Family clusters of Shiga toxin-producing Escherichia coli infection: an overlooked source of transmission. Data from the ItalKid-Hus Network. Pediatr Infect Dis J. 2021;40:1–5.

94. Ariceta G, Besbas N, Johnson S, Karpman D, Landau D, Licht C, Loirat C, Pecoraro C, Taylor CM, Van de Kar N, Vandewalle J, Zimmerhackl LB, European Paediatric Study Group for HUS. Guideline for the investigation and initial therapy of diarrhea-negative hemolytic uremic syndrome. Pediatr Nephrol. 2009;24:687–96.

95. Werber D, Mason BW, Evans MR, Salmon RL. Preventing household transmission of Shiga toxin-producing Escherichia coli O157 infection:

promptly separating siblings might be the key. Clin Infect Dis. 2008;46:1189–96.

96. Ahn CK, Klein E, Tarr PI. Isolation of patients acutely infected with Escherichia coli O157:H7: low-tech, highly effective prevention of hemolytic uremic syndrome. Clin Infect Dis. 2008;46:1197–9.

97. (CDC) CfDCaP. Laboratory-confirmed non-O157 Shiga toxin-producing Escherichia coli—Connecticut, 2000-2005. MMWR Morb Mortal Wkly Rep. 2007;56:29–31.

98. Gould LH, Bopp C, Strockbine N, Atkinson R, Baselski V, Body B, Carey R, Crandall C, Hurd S, Kaplan R, Neill M, Shea S, Somsel P, Tobin-D'Angelo M, Griffin PM, Gerner-Smidt P. Recommendations for diagnosis of shiga toxin—producing Escherichia coli infections by clinical laboratories. MMWR Recomm Rep. 2009;58:1–14.

99. Schindler EI, Sellenriek P, Storch GA, Tarr PI, Burnham CA. Shiga toxin-producing Escherichia coli: a single-center, 11-year pediatric experience. J Clin Microbiol. 2014;52:3647–53.

100. Chart H, Smith HR, Scotland SM, Rowe B, Milford DV, Taylor CM. Serological identification of Escherichia coli O157:H7 infection in haemolytic uraemic syndrome. Lancet. 1991;337:138–40.

101. Bitzan M, Moebius E, Ludwig K, Muller-Wiefel DE, Heesemann J, Karch H. High incidence of serum antibodies to Escherichia coli O157 lipopolysaccharide in children with hemolytic-uremic syndrome. J Pediatr. 1991;119:380–5.

102. Chart H, Cheasty T. Human infections with verocytotoxin-producing Escherichia coli O157--10 years of E. coli O157 serodiagnosis. J Med Microbiol. 2008;57:1389–93.

103. Ludwig K, Grabhorn E, Bitzan M, Bobrowski C, Kemper MJ, Sobottka I, Laufs R, Karch H, Muller-Wiefel DE. Saliva IgM and IgA are a sensitive indicator of the humoral immune response to Escherichia coli O157 lipopolysaccharide in children with enteropathic hemolytic uremic syndrome. Pediatr Res. 2002;52:307–13.

104. Karmali MA, Petric M, Winkler M, Bielaszewska M, Brunton J, van de Kar N, Morooka T, Nair GB, Richardson SE, Arbus GS. Enzyme-linked immunosorbent assay for detection of immunoglobulin G antibodies to Escherichia coli Vero cytotoxin 1. J Clin Microbiol. 1994;32:1457–63.

105. Karmali MA, Mascarenhas M, Petric M, Dutil L, Rahn K, Ludwig K, Arbus GS, Michel P, Sherman PM, Wilson J, Johnson R, Kaper JB. Age-specific frequencies of antibodies to Escherichia coli verocytotoxins (Shiga toxins) 1 and 2 among urban and rural populations in southern Ontario. J Infect Dis. 2003;188:1724–9.

106. Mody RK, Luna-Gierke RE, Jones TF, Comstock N, Hurd S, Scheftel J, Lathrop S, Smith G, Palmer A, Strockbine N, Talkington D, Mahon BE, Hoekstra RM, Griffin PM. Infections in pediatric postdiarrheal hemolytic uremic syndrome: factors associated with identifying shiga toxin-producing Escherichia coli. Arch Pediatr Adolesc Med. 2012:1–8.

107. Scheiring J, Andreoli SP, Zimmerhackl LB. Treatment and outcome of Shiga-toxin-associated hemolytic uremic syndrome (HUS). Pediatr Nephrol. 2008;23:1749–60.

108. Davis TK, Van De Kar N, Tarr PI. Shiga toxin/verocytotoxin-producing escherichia coli infections: practical clinical perspectives. Microbiol Spectr. 2014;2:EHEC-0025-2014.

109. Verweyen HM, Karch H, Allerberger F, Zimmerhackl LB. Enterohemorrhagic Escherichia coli (EHEC) in pediatric hemolytic-uremic syndrome: a prospective study in Germany and Austria. Infection. 1999;27:341–7.

110. Gerber A, Karch H, Allerberger F, Verweyen HM, Zimmerhackl LB. Clinical course and the role of shiga toxin-producing Escherichia coli infection in the hemolytic-uremic syndrome in pediatric patients, 1997-2000, in Germany and Austria: a prospective study. J Infect Dis. 2002;186:493–500.

111. Jelacic JK, Damrow T, Chen GS, Jelacic S, Bielaszewska M, Ciol M, Carvalho HM, Melton-Celsa AR, O'Brien AD, Tarr PI. Shiga toxin-producing Escherichia coli in Montana: bacterial genotypes and clinical profiles. J Infect Dis. 2003;188:719–29.

112. Bielaszewska M, Friedrich AW, Aldick T, Schurk-Bulgrin R, Karch H. Shiga toxin activatable by intestinal mucus in Escherichia coli isolated from humans: predictor for a severe clinical outcome. Clin Infect Dis. 2006;43:1160–7.

113. Rosales A, Hofer J, Zimmerhackl LB, Jungraithmayr TC, Riedl M, Giner T, Strasak A, Orth-Holler D, Wurzner R, Karch H, German-Austrian HUSSG. Need for long-term follow-up in enterohemorrhagic Escherichia coli-associated hemolytic uremic syndrome due to late-emerging sequelae. Clin Infect Dis. 2012;54:1413–21.

114. Gould LH, Mody RK, Ong KL, Clogher P, Cronquist AB, Garman KN, Lathrop S, Medus C, Spina NL, Webb TH, White PL, Wymore K, Gierke RE, Mahon BE, Griffin PM. Increased recognition of non-O157 Shiga toxin-producing Escherichia coli infections in the United States during 2000-2010: epidemiologic features and comparison with E. coli O157 infections. Foodborne Pathog Dis. 2013;10:453–60.

115. Sawyer C, Vishram B, Jenkins C, Jorgensen F, Byrne L, Mikhail AFW, Dallman TJ, Carroll K, Ahyow L, Vahora Q, Godbole G, Balasegaram S. Epidemiological investigation of recurrent outbreaks of haemolytic uraemic syndrome caused by Shiga toxin-producing Escherichia coli serotype O55:H7 in England, 2014-2018. Epidemiol Infect. 2021;149:e108.

116. Carter AO, Borczyk AA, Carlson JA, Harvey B, Hockin JC, Karmali MA, Krishnan C, Korn DA, Lior H. A severe outbreak of Escherichia coli O157:H7—associated hemorrhagic colitis in a nursing home. N Engl J Med. 1987;317:1496–500.

117. Dundas S, Todd WT, Stewart AI, Murdoch PS, Chaudhuri AK, Hutchinson SJ. The central Scotland Escherichia coli O157:H7 outbreak: risk factors for the hemolytic uremic syndrome and death among hospitalized patients. Clin Infect Dis. 2001;33:923–31.

118. Blanco JE, Blanco M, Alonso MP, Mora A, Dahbi G, Coira MA, Blanco J. Serotypes, virulence genes, and intimin types of Shiga toxin (verotoxin)-producing Escherichia coli isolates from human patients: prevalence in Lugo, Spain, from 1992 through 1999. J Clin Microbiol. 2004;42:311–9.

119. Lopez EL, Contrini MM, Devoto S, de Rosa MF, Grana MG, Aversa L, Gomez HF, Genero MH, Cleary TG. Incomplete hemolytic-uremic syndrome in Argentinean children with bloody diarrhea. J Pediatr. 1995;127:364–7.

120. Proulx F, Turgeon JP, Litalien C, Mariscalco MM, Robitaille P, Seidman E. Inflammatory mediators in Escherichia coli O157:H7 hemorrhagic colitis and hemolytic-uremic syndrome. Pediatr Infect Dis J. 1998;17:899–904.

121. Buteau C, Proulx F, Chaibou M, Raymond D, Clermont MJ, Mariscalco MM, Lebel MH, Seidman E. Leukocytosis in children with Escherichia coli O157:H7 enteritis developing the hemolytic-uremic syndrome. Pediatr Infect Dis J. 2000;19:642–7.

122. Ikeda M, Gunji Y, Yamasaki S, Takeda Y. Shiga toxin activates p38 MAP kinase through cellular Ca(2+) increase in Vero cells. FEBS Lett. 2000;485:94–8.

123. Decaluwe H, Harrison LM, Mariscalco MM, Gendrel D, Bohuon C, Tesh VL, Proulx F. Procalcitonin in children with Escherichia coli O157:H7 associated hemolytic uremic syndrome. Pediatr Res. 2006;59:579–83.

124. Yamamoto T, Satomura K, Okada S, Ozono K. Risk factors for neurological complications in complete hemolytic uremic syndrome caused by Escherichia coli O157. Pediatr Int. 2009;51:216–9.

125. Siegler RL. The hemolytic uremic syndrome. Pediatr Clin N Am. 1995;42:1505–29.

126. Bell BP, Griffin PM, Lozano P, Christie DL, Kobayashi JM, Tarr PI. Predictors of hemolytic uremic syndrome in children during a large outbreak of Escherichia coli O157:H7 infections. Pediatrics. 1997;100:E12.

127. Ylinen E, Salmenlinna S, Halkilahti J, Jahnukainen T, Korhonen L, Virkkala T, Rimhanen-Finne R, Nuutinen M, Kataja J, Arikoski P, Linkosalo L, Bai X, Matussek A, Jalanko H, Saxen H. Hemolytic uremic syndrome caused by Shiga toxin-producing Escherichia coli in children: incidence, risk factors, and clinical outcome. Pediatr Nephrol. 2020;35:1749–59.

128. Walters MD, Matthei IU, Kay R, Dillon MJ, Barratt TM. The polymorphonuclear leucocyte count in childhood haemolytic uraemic syndrome. Pediatr Nephrol. 1989;3:130–4.

129. Oakes RS, Siegler RL, McReynolds MA, Pysher T, Pavia AT. Predictors of fatality in postdiarrheal hemolytic uremic syndrome. Pediatrics. 2006;117:1656–62.

130. Balestracci A, Martin SM, Toledo I, Alvarado C, Wainsztein RE. Dehydration at admission increased the need for dialysis in hemolytic uremic syndrome children. Pediatr Nephrol. 2012;27:1407–10.

131. Ardissino G, Dacco V, Testa S, Civitillo CF, Tel F, Possenti I, Belingheri M, Castorina P, Bolsa-Ghiringhelli N, Tedeschi S, Paglialonga F, Salardi S, Consonni D, Zoia E, Salice P, Chidini G. Hemoconcentration: a major risk factor for neurological involvement in hemolytic uremic syndrome. Pediatr Nephrol. 2015;30:345–52.

132. Ake JA, Jelacic S, Ciol MA, Watkins SL, Murray KF, Christie DL, Klein EJ, Tarr PI. Relative nephroprotection during Escherichia coli O157:H7 infections: association with intravenous volume expansion. Pediatrics. 2005;115:e673–80.

133. Lin CY, Xie J, Freedman SB, RS MK, Schnadower D, Tarr PI, Finkelstein Y, Desai NM, Lane RD, Bergmann KR, Kaplan RL, Hariharan S, Cruz AT, Cohen DM, Dixon A, Ramgopal S, Powell EC, Kilgar J, Michelson KA, Bitzan M, Yen K, Meckler GD, Plint AC, Balamuth F, Bradin S, Gouin S, Kam AJ, Meltzer JA, Hunley TE, Avva U, Porter R, Fein DM, Louie JP, GAM T, Pediatric Emergency Research C, Pediatric Emergency Medicine Collaborative Research Committee SSG. Predicting adverse outcomes for shiga toxin-producing escherichia coli infections in emergency departments. J Pediatr. 2021;232(200–206):e204.

134. Loos S, Oh J, van de Loo L, Kemper MJ, Blohm M, Schild R. Hemoconcentration and predictors in Shiga toxin-producing E. coli-hemolytic uremic syndrome (STEC-HUS). Pediatr Nephrol. 2021;36:3777–83.

135. Trachtman H, Cnaan A, Christen E, Gibbs K, Zhao S, Acheson DW, Weiss R, Kaskel FJ, Spitzer A, Hirschman GH. Effect of an oral Shiga toxin-binding agent on diarrhea-associated hemolytic uremic syndrome in children: a randomized controlled trial. JAMA. 2003;290:1337–44.

136. Bruyand M, Mariani-Kurkdjian P, Le Hello S, King LA, Van Cauteren D, Lefevre S, Gouali M, Jourdan-da Silva N, Mailles A, Donguy MP, Loukiadis E, Sergentet-Thevenot D, Loirat C, Bonacorsi S, Weill FX, De Valk H, Reseau Francais Hospitalier de Surveillance du Shu P. Paediatric haemolytic uraemic syndrome related to Shiga toxin-producing Escherichia coli, an overview of 10 years of surveillance in France, 2007 to 2016. Euro Surveill. 2019:24.

137. Siegler RL, Milligan MK, Burningham TH, Christofferson RD, Chang SY, Jorde LB. Long-term outcome and prognostic indicators in the hemolytic-uremic syndrome. J Pediatr. 1991;118:195–200.

138. Oakes RS, Kirkhamm JK, Nelson RD, Siegler RL. Duration of oliguria and anuria as predictors of chronic renal-related sequelae in post-diarrheal hemolytic uremic syndrome. Pediatr Nephrol. 2008;23:1303–8.

139. Fakhouri F, Zuber J, Fremeaux-Bacchi V, Loirat C. Haemolytic uraemic syndrome. Lancet. 2017;390:681–96.
140. Siegler RL. Management of hemolytic-uremic syndrome. J Pediatr. 1988;112:1014–20.
141. Siegler RL. Spectrum of extrarenal involvement in postdiarrheal hemolytic-uremic syndrome. J Pediatr. 1994;125:511–8.
142. Nathanson S, Kwon T, Elmaleh M, Charbit M, Launay EA, Harambat J, Brun M, Ranchin B, Bandin F, Cloarec S, Bourdat-Michel G, Pietrement C, Champion G, Ulinski T, Deschenes G. Acute neurological involvement in diarrhea-associated hemolytic uremic syndrome. Clin J Am Soc Nephrol. 2010;5:1218–28.
143. Khalid M, Andreoli S. Extrarenal manifestations of the hemolytic uremic syndrome associated with Shiga toxin-producing Escherichia coli (STEC HUS). Pediatr Nephrol. 2019;34:2495–507.
144. Siegler RL. Hemolytic uremic syndrome in children. Curr Opin Pediatr. 1995;7:159–63.
145. de Buys Roessingh AS, de Lagausie P, Baudoin V, Loirat C, Aigrain Y. Gastrointestinal complications of post-diarrheal hemolytic uremic syndrome. Eur J Pediatr Surg. 2007;17:328–34.
146. Krogvold L, Henrichsen T, Bjerre A, Brackman D, Dollner H, Gudmundsdottir H, Syversen G, Naess PA, Bangstad HJ. Clinical aspects of a nationwide epidemic of severe haemolytic uremic syndrome (HUS) in children. Scand J Trauma Resusc Emerg Med. 2011;19:44.
147. Rahman RC, Cobenas CJ, Drut R, Amoreo OR, Ruscasso JD, Spizzirri AP, Suarez Adel C, Zalba JH, Ferrari C, Gatti MC. Hemorrhagic colitis in postdiarrheal hemolytic uremic syndrome: retrospective analysis of 54 children. Pediatr Nephrol. 2012;27:229–33.
148. Repetto HA. Long-term course and mechanisms of progression of renal disease in hemolytic uremic syndrome. Kidney Int Suppl. 2005:S102–6.
149. Suri RS, Clark WF, Barrowman N, Mahon JL, Thiessen-Philbrook HR, Rosas-Arellano MP, Zarnke K, Garland JS, Garg AX. Diabetes during diarrhea-associated hemolytic uremic syndrome: a systematic review and meta-analysis. Diabetes Care. 2005;28:2556–62.
150. Suri RS, Mahon JL, Clark WF, Moist LM, Salvadori M, Garg AX. Relationship between Escherichia coli O157:H7 and diabetes mellitus. Kidney Int Suppl. 2009:S44–6.
151. Walker AM, Benson LN, Wilson GJ, Arbus GS. Cardiomyopathy: a late complication of hemolytic uremic syndrome. Pediatr Nephrol. 1997;11:221–2.
152. Eckart P, Guillot M, Jokic M, Maragnes P, Boudailliez B, Palcoux JB, Desvignes V. Cardiac involvement during classic hemolytic uremic syndrome. Arch Pediatr. 1999;6:430–3.
153. Thayu M, Chandler WL, Jelacic S, Gordon CA, Rosenthal GL, Tarr PI. Cardiac ischemia during hemolytic uremic syndrome. Pediatr Nephrol. 2003;18:286–9.
154. Cimolai N, Morrison BJ, Carter JE. Risk factors for the central nervous system manifestations of gastroenteritis-associated hemolytic-uremic syndrome. Pediatrics. 1992;90:616–21.
155. Weissenborn K, Donnerstag F, Kielstein JT, Heeren M, Worthmann H, Hecker H, Schmitt R, Schiffer M, Pasedag T, Schuppner R, Tryc AB, Raab P, Hartmann H, Ding XQ, Hafer C, Menne J, Schmidt BM, Bultmann E, Haller H, Dengler R, Lanfermann H, Giesemann AM. Neurologic manifestations of E coli infection-induced hemolytic-uremic syndrome in adults. Neurology. 2012;79:1466–73.
156. Giordano P, Netti GS, Santangelo L, Castellano G, Carbone V, Torres DD, Martino M, Sesta M, Di Cuonzo F, Resta MC, Gaeta A, Milella L, Chironna M, Germinario C, Scavia G, Gesualdo L, Giordano M. A pediatric neurologic assessment score may drive the eculizumab-based treatment of Escherichia coli-related hemolytic uremic syndrome with neurological involvement. Pediatr Nephrol. 2019;34:517–27.
157. Costigan C, Raftery T, Carroll AG, Wildes D, Reynolds C, Cunney R, Dolan N, Drew RJ, Lynch BJ, O'Rourke DJ, Stack M, Sweeney C, Shahwan A, Twomey E, Waldron M, Riordan M, Awan A, Gorman KM. Neurological involvement in children with hemolytic uremic syndrome. Eur J Pediatr. 2022;181:501–12.
158. Milford D, Taylor CM. Hyponatraemia and haemolytic uraemic syndrome. Lancet. 1989;1:439.
159. Toldo I, Manara R, Cogo P, Sartori S, Murer L, Battistella PA, Laverda AM. Diffusion-weighted imaging findings in hemolytic uremic syndrome with central nervous system involvement. J Child Neurol. 2009;24:247–50.
160. Donnerstag F, Ding X, Pape L, Bultmann E, Lucke T, Zajaczek J, Hoy L, Das AM, Lanfermann H, Ehrich J, Hartmann H. Patterns in early diffusion-weighted MRI in children with haemolytic uraemic syndrome and CNS involvement. Eur Radiol. 2012;22:506–13.
161. Weissenborn K, Bultmann E, Donnerstag F, Giesemann AM, Gotz F, Worthmann H, Heeren M, Kielstein J, Schwarz A, Lanfermann H, Ding XQ. Quantitative MRI shows cerebral microstructural damage in hemolytic-uremic syndrome patients with severe neurological symptoms but no changes in conventional MRI. Neuroradiology. 2013;55:819–25.
162. Wengenroth M, Hoeltje J, Repenthin J, Meyer TN, Bonk F, Becker H, Faiss S, Stammel O, Urban PP, Bruening R. Central nervous system involvement in adults with epidemic hemolytic uremic syndrome. AJNR Am J Neuroradiol. 2013;34(1016–1021):S1011.
163. Meuth SG, Gobel K, Kanyshkova T, Ehling P, Ritter MA, Schwindt W, Bielaszewska M, Lebiedz P, Coulon P, Herrmann AM, Storck W, Kohmann D, Muthing J, Pavenstadt H, Kuhlmann

164. Gitiaux C, Krug P, Grevent D, Kossorotoff M, Poncet S, Eisermann M, Oualha M, Boddaert N, Salomon R, Desguerre I. Brain magnetic resonance imaging pattern and outcome in children with haemolytic-uraemic syndrome and neurological impairment treated with eculizumab. Dev Med Child Neurol. 2013;55:758–65.
165. Santangelo L, Netti GS, Torres DD, Piscopo G, Carbone V, Losito L, Milella L, Lasorella ML, Conti P, Gagliardi D, Chironna M, Spadaccino F, Bresin E, Trabacca A, Ranieri E, Giordano M. Peripheral nervous system manifestations of Shiga toxin-producing E. coli-induced haemolytic uremic syndrome in children. Ital J Pediatr. 2021;47:181.
166. Kleimann A, Toto S, Eberlein CK, Kielstein JT, Bleich S, Frieling H, Sieberer M. Psychiatric symptoms in patients with Shiga toxin-producing E. coli O104:H4 induced haemolytic-uraemic syndrome. PLoS One. 2014;9:e101839.
167. Simova O, Weineck G, Schuetze T, Wegscheider K, Panzer U, Stahl RA, Gerloff C, Magnus T. Neuropsychological outcome after complicated Shiga toxin-producing Escherichia coli infection. PLoS One. 2014;9:e103029.
168. Bauer A, Loos S, Wehrmann C, Horstmann D, Donnerstag F, Lemke J, Hillebrand G, Lobel U, Pape L, Haffner D, Bindt C, Ahlenstiel T, Melk A, Lehnhardt A, Kemper MJ, Oh J, Hartmann H. Neurological involvement in children with E. coli O104:H4-induced hemolytic uremic syndrome. Pediatr Nephrol. 2014;29:1607–15.
169. Richardson SE, Karmali MA, Becker LE, Smith CR. The histopathology of the hemolytic uremic syndrome associated with verocytotoxin-producing Escherichia coli infections. Hum Pathol. 1988;19:1102–8.
170. Gagnadoux MF, Habib R, Gubler MC, Bacri JL, Broyer M. Long-term (15-25 years) outcome of childhood hemolytic-uremic syndrome. Clin Nephrol. 1996;46:39–41.
171. Inward CD, Howie AJ, Fitzpatrick MM, Rafaat F, Milford DV, Taylor CM. Renal histopathology in fatal cases of diarrhoea-associated haemolytic uraemic syndrome. British Association for Paediatric Nephrology. Pediatr Nephrol. 1997;11:556–9.
172. Yoshioka K, Yagi K, Moriguchi N. Clinical features and treatment of children with hemolytic uremic syndrome caused by enterohemorrhagic Escherichia coli O157:H7 infection: experience of an outbreak in Sakai City, 1996. Pediatr Int. 1999;41:223–7.
173. Porubsky S, Federico G, Muthing J, Jennemann R, Gretz N, Buttner S, Obermuller N, Jung O, Hauser IA, Grone E, Geiger H, Grone HJ, Betz C. Direct acute tubular damage contributes to Shigatoxin-mediated kidney failure. J Pathol. 2014;234:120–33.
174. Burns JC, Berman ER, Fagre JL, Shikes RH, Lum GM. Pancreatic islet cell necrosis: association with hemolytic-uremic syndrome. J Pediatr. 1982;100:582–4.
175. Hrynchak M, Ang LC, Munoz DG. Bilateral striatal necrosis in hemolytic-uremic syndrome. Clin Neuropathol. 1992;11:45–8.
176. Centers for Disease Control and Prevention NCfEaZIDN (2017) Prevention.
177. Thomas DE, Elliott EJ. Interventions for preventing diarrhea-associated hemolytic uremic syndrome: systematic review. BMC Public Health. 2013;13:799.
178. Perrin F, Tenenhaus-Aziza F, Michel V, Miszczycha S, Bel N, Sanaa M. Quantitative risk assessment of haemolytic and uremic syndrome linked to O157:H7 and non-O157:H7 Shiga-toxin producing Escherichia coli strains in raw milk soft cheeses. Risk Anal. 2015;35:109–28.
179. England PH (2017) Shiga toxin-producing Escherichia coli (STEC): symptoms, how to avoid, how to treat.
180. Konadu EY, Parke JC Jr, Tran HT, Bryla DA, Robbins JB, Szu SC. Investigational vaccine for Escherichia coli O157: phase 1 study of O157 O-specific polysaccharide-Pseudomonas aeruginosa recombinant exoprotein A conjugates in adults. J Infect Dis. 1998;177:383–7.
181. Ahmed A, Li J, Shiloach Y, Robbins JB, Szu SC. Safety and immunogenicity of Escherichia coli O157 O-specific polysaccharide conjugate vaccine in 2-5-year-old children. J Infect Dis. 2006;193:515–21.
182. Goldwater PN. Treatment and prevention of enterohemorrhagic Escherichia coli infection and hemolytic uremic syndrome. Expert Rev Anti-Infect Ther. 2007;5:653–63.
183. Muhlen S, Dersch P. Treatment strategies for infections with Shiga toxin-producing Escherichia coli. Front Cell Infect Microbiol. 2020;10:169.
184. Schaut RG, Palmer MV, Boggiatto PM, Kudva IT, Loving CL, Sharma VK. Mucosal IFNgamma production and potential role in protection in Escherichia coli O157:H7 vaccinated and challenged cattle. Sci Rep. 2021;11:9769.
185. Armstrong GD, Rowe PC, Goodyer P, Orrbine E, Klassen TP, Wells G, MacKenzie A, Lior H, Blanchard C, Auclair F, et al. A phase I study of chemically synthesized verotoxin (Shiga-like toxin) Pk-trisaccharide receptors attached to chromosorb for preventing hemolytic-uremic syndrome. J Infect Dis. 1995;171:1042–5.
186. Huppertz HI, Rutkowski S, Busch DH, Eisebit R, Lissner R, Karch H. Bovine colostrum ameliorates diarrhea in infection with diarrheagenic Escherichia coli, shiga toxin-producing E. Coli, and E. coli expressing intimin and hemolysin. J Pediatr Gastroenterol Nutr. 1999;29:452–6.
187. Lopez EL, Contrini MM, Glatstein E, Gonzalez Ayala S, Santoro R, Allende D, Ezcurra G, Teplitz E,

Koyama T, Matsumoto Y, Sato H, Sakai K, Hoshide S, Komoriya K, Morita T, Harning R, Brookman S. Safety and pharmacokinetics of urtoxazumab, a humanized monoclonal antibody, against Shiga-like toxin 2 in healthy adults and in pediatric patients infected with Shiga-like toxin-producing Escherichia coli. Antimicrob Agents Chemother. 2010;54:239–43.

188. Imdad A, Mackoff SP, Urciuoli DM, Syed T, Tanner-Smith EE, Huang D, Gomez-Duarte OG. Interventions for preventing diarrhoea-associated haemolytic uraemic syndrome. Cochrane Database Syst Rev. 2021;7:CD012997.

189. Bitzan M, Schaefer F, Reymond D. Treatment of typical (enteropathic) hemolytic uremic syndrome. Semin Thromb Hemost. 2010;36:594–610.

190. Hickey CA, Beattie TJ, Cowieson J, Miyashita Y, Strife CF, Frem JC, Peterson JM, Butani L, Jones DP, Havens PL, Patel HP, Wong CS, Andreoli SP, Rothbaum RJ, Beck AM, Tarr PI. Early volume expansion during diarrhea and relative nephroprotection during subsequent hemolytic uremic syndrome. Arch Pediatr Adolesc Med. 2011;165:884–9.

191. Bitzan M, Mellmann A, Karch H, Reymond D. SHIGATEC: a phase II study evaluating Shigamabs in STEC-infected children. Zoonoses Public Health. 2012;59:18.

192. Balestracci A, Martin SM, Toledo I. Hemoconcentration in hemolytic uremic syndrome: time to review the standard case definition? Pediatr Nephrol. 2015;30:361.

193. Grisaru S, Xie J, Samuel S, Hartling L, Tarr PI, Schnadower D, Freedman SB, Alberta Provincial Pediatric Enteric Infection T. Associations between hydration status, intravenous fluid administration, and outcomes of patients infected with Shiga toxin-producing Escherichia coli: a systematic review and meta-analysis. JAMA Pediatr. 2017;171:68–76.

194. Basu RK, Zappitelli M, Brunner L, Wang Y, Wong HR, Chawla LS, Wheeler DS, Goldstein SL. Derivation and validation of the renal angina index to improve the prediction of acute kidney injury in critically ill children. Kidney Int. 2014;85:659–67.

195. Washington C, Carmichael JC. Management of ischemic colitis. Clin Colon Rectal Surg. 2012;25:228–35.

196. Loconsole D, Giordano M, Centrone F, Accogli M, Casulli D, De Robertis AL, Morea A, Quarto M, Parisi A, Scavia G, Chironna M, On Behalf Of The Bloody Diarrhea Apulia Working G. Epidemiology of Shiga toxin-producing Escherichia coli infections in Southern Italy after implementation of symptom-based surveillance of bloody diarrhea in the pediatric population. Int J Environ Res Public Health. 2020:17.

197. Cimolai N, Carter JE, Morrison BJ, Anderson JD. Risk factors for the progression of Escherichia coli O157:H7 enteritis to hemolytic-uremic syndrome. J Pediatr. 1990;116:589–92.

198. Wong CS, Jelacic S, Habeeb RL, Watkins SL, Tarr PI. The risk of the hemolytic-uremic syndrome after antibiotic treatment of Escherichia coli O157:H7 infections. N Engl J Med. 2000;342:1930–6.

199. Tarr PI, Freedman SB. Why antibiotics should not be used to treat Shiga toxin-producing Escherichia coli infections. Curr Opin Gastroenterol. 2022;38:30–8.

200. Walterspiel JN, Ashkenazi S, Morrow AL, Cleary TG. Effect of subinhibitory concentrations of antibiotics on extracellular Shiga-like toxin I. Infection. 1992;20:25–9.

201. Yoh M, Frimpong EK, Voravuthikunchai SP, Honda T. Effect of subinhibitory concentrations of antimicrobial agents (quinolones and macrolide) on the production of verotoxin by enterohemorrhagic Escherichia coli O157:H7. Can J Microbiol. 1999;45:732–9.

202. Kimmitt PT, Harwood CR, Barer MR. Toxin gene expression by shiga toxin-producing Escherichia coli: the role of antibiotics and the bacterial SOS response. Emerg Infect Dis. 2000;6:458–65.

203. Ikeda K, Ida O, Kimoto K, Takatorige T, Nakanishi N, Tatara K. Effect of early fosfomycin treatment on prevention of hemolytic uremic syndrome accompanying Escherichia coli O157:H7 infection. Clin Nephrol. 1999;52:357–62.

204. Tarr PI, Karpman D. Editorial commentary: Escherichia coli O104:H4 and hemolytic uremic syndrome: the analysis begins. Clin Infect Dis. 2012;55:760–3.

205. Safdar N, Said A, Gangnon RE, Maki DG. Risk of hemolytic uremic syndrome after antibiotic treatment of Escherichia coli O157:H7 enteritis: a meta-analysis. JAMA. 2002;288:996–1001.

206. Kakoullis L, Papachristodoulou E, Chra P, Panos G. Shiga toxin-induced haemolytic uraemic syndrome and the role of antibiotics: a global overview. J Infect. 2019;79:75–94.

207. Myojin S, Pak K, Sako M, Kobayashi T, Takahashi T, Sunagawa T, Tsuboi N, Ishikura K, Kubota M, Kubota M, Igarashi T, Morioka I, Miyairi I. Interventions for Shiga toxin-producing Escherichia coli gastroenteritis and risk of hemolytic uremic syndrome: a population-based matched case control study. PLoS One. 2022;17:e0263349.

208. Weil BR, Andreoli SP, Billmire DF. Bleeding risk for surgical dialysis procedures in children with hemolytic uremic syndrome. Pediatr Nephrol. 2010;25:1693–8.

209. Rousseau E, Blais N, O'Regan S. Decreased necessity for dialysis with loop diuretic therapy in hemolytic uremic syndrome. Clin Nephrol. 1990;34:22–5.

210. Caletti MG, Lejarraga H, Kelmansky D, Missoni M. Two different therapeutic regimes in patients with sequelae of hemolytic-uremic syndrome. Pediatr Nephrol. 2004;19:1148–52.

211. Caletti MG, Balestracci A, Missoni M, Vezzani C. Additive antiproteinuric effect of enalapril and losartan in children with hemolytic uremic syndrome. Pediatr Nephrol. 2013;28:745–50.

212. Coccia PA, Ramirez FB, Suarez ADC, Alconcher LF, Balestracci A, Garcia Chervo LA, Principi I, Vazquez A, Ratto VM, Planells MC, Montero J, Saurit M, Gutierrez M, Puga MC, Isern EM, Bettendorff MC, Boscardin MV, Bazan M, Polischuk MA, De Sarrasqueta A, Aralde A, Ripeau DB, Leroy DC, Quijada NE, Escalante RS, Giordano MI, Sanchez C, Selva VS, Caminiti A, Ojeda JM, Bonany P, Morales SE, Allende D, Arias MA, Exeni AM, Geuna JD, Arrua L. Acute peritoneal dialysis, complications and outcomes in 389 children with STEC-HUS: a multicenter experience. Pediatr Nephrol. 2021;36:1597–606.

213. Nakatani T, Tsuchida K, Yoshimura R, Sugimura K, Takemoto Y. Plasma exchange therapy for the treatment of Escherichia coli O-157 associated hemolytic uremic syndrome. Int J Mol Med. 2002;10:585–8.

214. Rizzoni G, Claris-Appiani A, Edefonti A, Facchin P, Franchini F, Gusmano R, Imbasciati E, Pavanello L, Perfumo F, Remuzzi G. Plasma infusion for hemolytic-uremic syndrome in children: results of a multicenter controlled trial. J Pediatr. 1988;112:284–90.

215. Loirat C, Sonsino E, Hinglais N, Jais JP, Landais P, Fermanian J. Treatment of the childhood haemolytic uraemic syndrome with plasma. A multicentre randomized controlled trial. The French Society of Paediatric Nephrology. Pediatr Nephrol. 1988;2:279–85.

216. Loirat C. Hemolytic uremic syndrome caused by Shiga-toxin-producing Escherichia coli. Rev Prat. 2013;63:11–6.

217. Keenswijk W, Raes A, De Clerck M, Vande Walle J. Is plasma exchange efficacious in shiga toxin-associated hemolytic uremic syndrome? a narrative review of current evidence. Ther Apher Dial. 2019;23:118–25.

218. Padmanabhan A, Connelly-Smith L, Aqui N, Balogun RA, Klingel R, Meyer E, Pham HP, Schneiderman J, Witt V, Wu Y, Zantek ND, Dunbar NM, Schwartz GEJ. Guidelines on the use of therapeutic apheresis in clinical practice - evidence-based approach from the writing committee of the american society for apheresis: the eighth special issue. J Clin Apher. 2019;34:171–354.

219. Oji S, Nomura K. Immunoadsorption in neurological disorders. Transfus Apher Sci. 2017;56:671–6.

220. Greinacher A, Friesecke S, Abel P, Dressel A, Stracke S, Fiene M, Ernst F, Selleng K, Weissenborn K, Schmidt BM, Schiffer M, Felix SB, Lerch MM, Kielstein JT, Mayerle J. Treatment of severe neurological deficits with IgG depletion through immunoadsorption in patients with Escherichia coli O104:H4-associated haemolytic uraemic syndrome: a prospective trial. Lancet. 2011;378:1166–73.

221. Combe C, Bui HN, de Precigout V, Hilbert G, Delmas Y. Immunoadsorption in patients with haemolytic uraemic syndrome. Lancet. 2012;379:517–8. author reply 518-519

222. Pietrement C, Bednarek N, Baudouin V, Fila M, Deschenes G. Immunoadsorption for paediatric post-diarrhoea haemolytic-uraemic syndrome with severe neurological involvement. Clin Kidney J. 2012;5:484–5.

223. Orth D, Khan AB, Naim A, Grif K, Brockmeyer J, Karch H, Joannidis M, Clark SJ, Day AJ, Fidanzi S, Stoiber H, Dierich MP, Zimmerhackl LB, Wurzner R. Shiga toxin activates complement and binds factor H: evidence for an active role of complement in hemolytic uremic syndrome. J Immunol. 2009;182:6394–400.

224. Orth-Holler D, Wurzner R. Role of complement in enterohemorrhagic Escherichia coli-Induced hemolytic uremic syndrome. Semin Thromb Hemost. 2014;40:503–7.

225. Arvidsson I, Stahl AL, Hedstrom MM, Kristoffersson AC, Rylander C, Westman JS, Storry JR, Olsson ML, Karpman D. Shiga toxin-induced complement-mediated hemolysis and release of complement-coated red blood cell-derived microvesicles in hemolytic uremic syndrome. J Immunol. 2015;194:2309–18.

226. Keir LS, Langman CB. Complement and the kidney in the setting of Shiga-toxin hemolytic uremic syndrome, organ transplantation, and C3 glomerulonephritis. Transfus Apher Sci. 2016;54:203–11.

227. Karpman D, Tati R. Complement contributes to the pathogenesis of Shiga toxin-associated hemolytic uremic syndrome. Kidney Int. 2016;90:726–9.

228. Thurman JM, Marians R, Emlen W, Wood S, Smith C, Akana H, Holers VM, Lesser M, Kline M, Hoffman C, Christen E, Trachtman H. Alternative pathway of complement in children with diarrhea-associated hemolytic uremic syndrome. Clin J Am Soc Nephrol. 2009.

229. Walsh PR, Johnson S. Eculizumab in the treatment of Shiga toxin haemolytic uraemic syndrome. Pediatr Nephrol. 2019;34:1485–92.

230. Mahat U, Matar RB, Rotz SJ. Use of complement monoclonal antibody eculizumab in Shiga toxin producing Escherichia coli associated hemolytic uremic syndrome: a review of current evidence. Pediatr Blood Cancer. 2019;66:e27913.

231. Monet-Didailler C, Chevallier A, Godron-Dubrasquet A, Allard L, Delmas Y, Contin-Bordes C, Brissaud O, Llanas B, Harambat J. Outcome of children with Shiga toxin-associated haemolytic uraemic syndrome treated with eculizumab: a matched cohort study. Nephrol Dial Transplant. 2020;35:2147–53.

232. Register ECT Eculizumab in Shiga-Toxin producing E. Coli Haemolytic Uraemic Syndrome (ECUSTEC): A Randomised, Double-Blind, Placebo-Controlled Trial. EudraCT Number: 2016-000997-39.

233. ClinicalTrials.gov Eculizumab in Shiga-toxin related hemolytic and uremic syndromepediatric patients - ECULISHU.

234. Spinale JM, Ruebner RL, Copelovitch L, Kaplan BS. Long-term outcomes of Shiga toxin

hemolytic uremic syndrome. Pediatr Nephrol. 2013;28:2097–105.

235. Eriksson KJ, Boyd SG, Tasker RC. Acute neurology and neurophysiology of haemolytic-uraemic syndrome. Arch Dis Child. 2001;84:434–5.

236. Garg AX, Suri RS, Barrowman N, Rehman F, Matsell D, Rosas-Arellano MP, Salvadori M, Haynes RB, Clark WF. Long-term renal prognosis of diarrhea-associated hemolytic uremic syndrome: a systematic review, meta-analysis, and meta-regression. JAMA. 2003;290:1360–70.

237. Schieppati A, Ruggenenti P, Cornejo RP, Ferrario F, Gregorini G, Zucchelli P, Rossi E, Remuzzi G. Renal function at hospital admission as a prognostic factor in adult hemolytic uremic syndrome. The Italian Registry of Haemolytic Uremic Syndrome. J Am Soc Nephrol. 1992;2:1640–4.

238. Havelaar AH, Van Duynhoven YT, Nauta MJ, Bouwknegt M, Heuvelink AE, De Wit GA, Nieuwenhuizen MG, van de Kar NC. Disease burden in The Netherlands due to infections with Shiga toxin-producing Escherichia coli O157. Epidemiol Infect. 2004;132:467–84.

239. Frank C, Faber MS, Askar M, Bernard H, Fruth A, Gilsdorf A, Hohle M, Karch H, Krause G, Prager R, Spode A, Stark K, Werber D, team HUSi. Large and ongoing outbreak of haemolytic uraemic syndrome, Germany, May 2011. Euro Surveill. 2011;16

240. Travert B, Rafat C, Mariani P, Cointe A, Dossier A, Coppo P, Joseph A. Shiga toxin-associated hemolytic uremic syndrome: specificities of adult patients and implications for critical care management. Toxins (Basel). 2021:13.

241. Siegler R, Oakes R. Hemolytic uremic syndrome; pathogenesis, treatment, and outcome. Curr Opin Pediatr. 2005;17:200–4.

242. Sharma AP, Filler G, Dwight P, Clark WF. Chronic renal disease is more prevalent in patients with hemolytic uremic syndrome who had a positive history of diarrhea. Kidney Int. 2010;78:598–604.

243. Small G, Watson AR, Evans JH, Gallagher J. Hemolytic uremic syndrome: defining the need for long-term follow-up. Clin Nephrol. 1999;52:352–6.

244. Fitzpatrick MM, Shah V, Trompeter RS, Dillon MJ, Barratt TM. Long term renal outcome of childhood haemolytic uraemic syndrome. BMJ. 1991;303:489–92.

245. Buder K, Latal B, Nef S, Neuhaus TJ, Laube GF, Sparta G. Neurodevelopmental long-term outcome in children after hemolytic uremic syndrome. Pediatr Nephrol. 2015;30:503–13.

246. Bassani CE, Ferraris J, Gianantonio CA, Ruiz S, Ramirez J. Renal transplantation in patients with classical haemolytic-uraemic syndrome. Pediatr Nephrol. 1991;5:607–11.

247. Siegler RL, Griffin PM, Barrett TJ, Strockbine NA. Recurrent hemolytic uremic syndrome secondary to Escherichia coli O157:H7 infection. Pediatrics. 1993;91:666–8.

248. Ferraris JR, Ramirez JA, Ruiz S, Caletti MG, Vallejo G, Piantanida JJ, Araujo JL, Sojo ET. Shiga toxin-associated hemolytic uremic syndrome: absence of recurrence after renal transplantation. Pediatr Nephrol. 2002;17:809–14.

249. Loirat C, Niaudet P. The risk of recurrence of hemolytic uremic syndrome after renal transplantation in children. Pediatr Nephrol. 2003;18:1095–101.

250. Alberti M, Valoti E, Piras R, Bresin E, Galbusera M, Tripodo C, Thaiss F, Remuzzi G, Noris M. Two patients with history of STEC-HUS, posttransplant recurrence and complement gene mutations. Am J Transplant. 2013;13:2201–6.

251. Ullis KC, Rosenblatt RM. Shiga bacillus dysentery complicated by bacteremia and disseminated intravascular coagulation. J Pediatr. 1973;83:90–3.

252. Chesney R. Letter: Hemolytic-uremic syndrome with shigellosis. J Pediatr. 1974;84:312–3.

253. Wimmer LE. Hemolytic-uremic syndrome with shigella antecedent. J Am Osteopath Assoc. 1974;74:139–43.

254. Raghupathy P, Date A, Shastry JC, Sudarsanam A, Jadhav M. Haemolytic-uraemic syndrome complicating shigella dystentery in south Indian children. Br Med J. 1978;1:1518–21.

255. Zaidi MB, Estrada-Garcia T. Shigella: a highly virulent and elusive pathogen. Curr Trop Med Rep. 2014;1:81–7.

256. Taneja N, Mewara A, Kumar A, Mishra A, Zaman K, Singh S, Gupta P, Mohan B. Antimicrobial resistant Shigella in North India since the turn of the 21st century. Indian J Med Microbiol. 2022;40:113–8.

257. Butler T. Haemolytic uraemic syndrome during shigellosis. Trans R Soc Trop Med Hyg. 2012;106:395–9.

258. Bennish ML, Khan WA, Begum M, Bridges EA, Ahmed S, Saha D, Salam MA, Acheson D, Ryan ET. Low risk of hemolytic uremic syndrome after early effective antimicrobial therapy for Shigella dysenteriae type 1 infection in Bangladesh. Clin Infect Dis. 2006;42:356–62.

259. Butler T, Islam MR, Azad MA, Jones PK. Risk factors for development of hemolytic uremic syndrome during shigellosis. J Pediatr. 1987;110:894–7.

260. Azim T, Islam LN, Halder RC, Hamadani J, Khanum N, Sarker MS, Salam MA, Albert MJ. Peripheral blood neutrophil responses in children with shigellosis. Clin Diagn Lab Immunol. 1995;2:616–22.

261. Bhimma R, Rollins NC, Coovadia HM, Adhikari M. Post-dysenteric hemolytic uremic syndrome in children during an epidemic of Shigella dysentery in Kwazulu/Natal. Pediatr Nephrol. 1997;11:560–4.

262. Khan WA, Griffiths JK, Bennish ML. Gastrointestinal and extra-intestinal manifestations of childhood shigellosis in a region where all four species of Shigella are endemic. PLoS One. 2013;8:e64097.

263. Cabrera GR, Fortenberry JD, Warshaw BL, Chambliss CR, Butler JC, Cooperstone BG. Hemolytic uremic syndrome associated with

317. Mbonu CC, Davison DL, El-Jazzar KM, Simon GL. Clostridium difficile colitis associated with hemolytic-uremic syndrome. Am J Kidney Dis. 2003;41:E14.
318. Keshtkar-Jahromi M, Mohebtash M. Hemolytic uremic syndrome and Clostridium difficile colitis. J Community Hosp Intern Med Perspect. 2012;2
319. Kalmanovich E, Kriger-Sharabi O, Shiloah E, Donin N, Fishelson Z, Rapoport MJ. Clostridium difficile infection and partial membrane cofactor protein (CD46) deficiency. Isr Med Assoc J. 2012;14:586–7.
320. Alvarado AS, Brodsky SV, Nadasdy T, Singh N. Hemolytic uremic syndrome associated with Clostridium difficile infection. Clin Nephrol. 2014;81:302–6.
321. Inglis JM, Barbara JA, Juneja R, Milton C, Passaris G, Li JYZ. Atypical haemolytic uraemic syndrome associated with clostridium difficile infection successfully treated with eculizumab. Case Rep Nephrol. 2018;2018:1759138.
322. Dasgupta K, Santos A, McCaul K. An unusual case of clostridium difficile colitis and hemolytic uremic syndrome in a teenager. S D Med. 2019;72:294–7.
323. Armstrong SM, Wang C, Tigdi J, Si X, Dumpit C, Charles S, Gamage A, Moraes TJ, Lee WL. Influenza infects lung microvascular endothelium leading to microvascular leak: role of apoptosis and claudin-5. PLoS One. 2012;7:e47323.
324. Armstrong SM, Darwish I, Lee WL. Endothelial activation and dysfunction in the pathogenesis of influenza A virus infection. Virulence. 2013;4:537–42.
325. Rondina MT, Brewster B, Grissom CK, Zimmerman GA, Kastendieck DH, Harris ES, Weyrich AS. In vivo platelet activation in critically ill patients with primary 2009 influenza A(H1N1). Chest. 2012;141:1490–5.
326. Boilard E, Pare G, Rousseau M, Cloutier N, Dubuc I, Levesque T, Borgeat P, Flamand L. Influenza virus H1N1 activates platelets through FcgammaRIIA signaling and thrombin generation. Blood. 2014;123:2854–63.
327. Saito D, Watanabe E, Ashida A, Kato H, Yoshida Y, Nangaku M, Ohtsuka Y, Miyata T, Hattori N, Oda S. Atypical hemolytic uremic syndrome with the p.Ile1157Thr C3 Mutation successfully treated with plasma exchange and eculizumab: a case report. Crit Care Explor. 2019;1:e0008.
328. Mittal N, Hartemayer R, Jandeska S, Giordano L. Steroid responsive atypical hemolytic uremic syndrome triggered by influenza b infection. J Pediatr Hematol Oncol. 2019;41:e63–7.
329. Sabulski A, Nehus EJ, Jodele S, Ricci K. Diagnostic considerations in H1N1 influenza-induced thrombotic microangiopathy. J Pediatr Hematol Oncol. 2022;44:e237–40.
330. Hawley HB, Chang JC. Complement-Induced Endotheliopathy-Associated Vascular Microthrombosis in Coronavirus Disease 2019. J Infect Dis. 2021;223:2198–9.

331. Chauhan AJ, Wiffen LJ, Brown TP. COVID-19: a collision of complement, coagulation and inflammatory pathways. J Thromb Haemost. 2020;18:2110–7.
332. Miller AD, Zambrano LD, Yousaf AR, Abrams JY, Meng L, Wu MJ, Melgar M, Oster ME, Godfred Cato SE, Belay ED, Campbell AP, Group M-CSA. Multisystem inflammatory syndrome in children-United States, February 2020-July 2021. Clin Infect Dis. 2021.
333. Syrimi E, Fennell E, Richter A, Vrljicak P, Stark R, Ott S, Murray PG, Al-Abadi E, Chikermane A, Dawson P, Hackett S, Jyothish D, Kanthimathinathan HK, Monaghan S, Nagakumar P, Scholefield BR, Welch S, Khan N, Faustini S, Davies K, Zelek WM, Kearns P, Taylor GS. The immune landscape of SARS-CoV-2-associated multisystem inflammatory syndrome in children (MIS-C) from acute disease to recovery. iScience. 2021;24:103215.
334. Campos YM, Drumond ALV, de Matos GM, Parreira MP, Simoes ESAC. Renal involvement in pediatric patients with COVID-19: an up-to-date. Curr Pediatr Rev. 2021.
335. Kari JA, Shalaby MA, Albanna AS, Alahmadi TS, Sukkar SA, MohamedNur HAH, AlGhamdi MS, Basri AH, Shagal RA, Alnajar A, Badawi M, Safdar OY, Zaher ZF, Temsah MH, Alhasan KA. Coronavirus disease in children: a multicentre study from the Kingdom of Saudi Arabia. J Infect Public Health. 2021;14:543–9.
336. Stewart DJ, Mudalige NL, Johnson M, Shroff R, du Pre P, Stojanovic J Acute kidney injury in paediatric inflammatory multisystem syndrome temporally associated with SARS-CoV-2 (PIMS-TS) is not associated with progression to chronic kidney disease. Arch Dis Child. 2021.
337. El Sissy C, Saldman A, Zanetta G, Martins PV, Poulain C, Cauchois R, Kaplanski G, Venetz JP, Bobot M, Dobosziewicz H, Daniel L, Koubi M, Sadallah S, Rotman S, Mousson C, Pascual M, Fremeaux-Bacchi V, Fakhouri F. COVID-19 as a potential trigger of complement-mediated atypical HUS. Blood. 2021;138:1777–82.
338. Dongre A, Jameel PZ, Deshmukh M, Bhandarkar S. Immune thrombocytopenic purpura secondary to SARS-CoV-2 infection in a child with acute lymphoblastic leukaemia: a case report and review of literature. BMJ Case Rep. 2021;14
339. Ferrer F, Roldao M, Figueiredo C, Lopes K. Atypical hemolytic uremic syndrome after ChAdOx1 nCoV-19 vaccination in a patient with homozygous CFHR3/CFHR1 gene deletion. Nephron. 2021;1–5.
340. Cugno M, Macor P, Giordano M, Manfredi M, Griffini S, Grovetti E, De Maso L, Mellone S, Valenti L, Prati D, Bonato S, Comi G, Artoni A, Meroni PL, Peyvandi F. Consumption of complement in a 26-year-old woman with severe thrombotic thrombocytopenia after ChAdOx1 nCov-19 vaccination. J Autoimmun. 2021;124:102728.
341. Lavin M, Elder PT, O'Keeffe D, Enright H, Ryan E, Kelly A, El Hassadi E, McNicholl FP, Benson G, Le

GN, Byrne M, Ryan K, O'Connell NM, O'Donnell JS. Vaccine-induced immune thrombotic thrombocytopenia (VITT) - a novel clinico-pathological entity with heterogeneous clinical presentations. Br J Haematol. 2021;195:76–84.

342. Waqar SHB, Khan AA, Memon S. Thrombotic thrombocytopenic purpura: a new menace after COVID bnt162b2 vaccine. Int J Hematol. 2021;114:626–9.

343. Gill J, Hebert CA, Colbert GB. COVID-19-associated atypical hemolytic uremic syndrome and use of Eculizumab therapy. J Nephrol. 2022;35(1):317–21.

344. Ville S, Le Bot S, Chapelet-Debout A, Blancho G, Fremeaux-Bacchi V, Deltombe C, Fakhouri F. Atypical HUS relapse triggered by COVID-19. Kidney Int. 2021;99:267–8.

345. Pfister F, Vonbrunn E, Ries T, Jack HM, Uberla K, Lochnit G, Sheriff A, Herrmann M, Buttner-Herold M, Amann K, Daniel C. Complement activation in kidneys of patients with COVID-19. Front Immunol. 2020;11:594849.

346. Yu J, Yuan X, Chen H, Chaturvedi S, Braunstein EM, Brodsky RA. Direct activation of the alternative complement pathway by SARS-CoV-2 spike proteins is blocked by factor D inhibition. Blood. 2020;136:2080–9.

347. Campbell CM, Kahwash R. Will complement inhibition be the new target in treating COVID-19-related systemic thrombosis? Circulation. 2020;141:1739–41.

348. Trimarchi H, Gianserra R, Lampo M, Monkowski M, Lodolo J. Eculizumab, SARS-CoV-2 and atypical hemolytic uremic syndrome. Clin Kidney J. 2020;13:739–41.

349. Leaf AN, Laubenstein LJ, Raphael B, Hochster H, Baez L, Karpatkin S. Thrombotic thrombocytopenic purpura associated with human immunodeficiency virus type 1 (HIV-1) infection. Ann Intern Med. 1988;109:194–7.

350. Tamkus D, Jajeh A, Osafo D, Hadad L, Bhanot B, Yogore MG 3rd. Thrombotic microangiopathy syndrome as an AIDS-defining illness: the experience of J. Stroger Hospital of Cook County. Clin Adv Hematol Oncol. 2006;4:145–9.

351. Gomes AM, Ventura A, Almeida C, Correia M, Tavares V, Mota M, Seabra J. Hemolytic uremic syndrome as a primary manifestation of acute human immunodeficiency virus infection. Clin Nephrol. 2009;71:563–6.

352. Ray PE. Shiga-like toxins and HIV-1 'go through' glycosphingolipids and lipid rafts in renal cells. Kidney Int. 2009;75:1135–7.

353. Green DF, Resnick L, Bourgoignie JJ. HIV infects glomerular endothelial and mesangial but not epithelial cells in vitro. Kidney Int. 1992;41:956–60.

354. Liu XH, Lingwood CA, Ray PE. Recruitment of renal tubular epithelial cells expressing verotoxin-1 (Stx1) receptors in HIV-1 transgenic mice with renal disease. Kidney Int. 1999;55:554–61.

355. Ray PE. Taking a hard look at the pathogenesis of childhood HIV-associated nephropathy. Pediatr Nephrol. 2009;24:2109–19.

356. Lingwood CA, Binnington B, Manis A, Branch DR. Globotriaosyl ceramide receptor function - where membrane structure and pathology intersect. FEBS Lett. 2010;584:1879–86.

357. Lund N, Branch DR, Mylvaganam M, Chark D, Ma XZ, Sakac D, Binnington B, Fantini J, Puri A, Blumenthal R, Lingwood CA. A novel soluble mimic of the glycolipid, globotriaosyl ceramide inhibits HIV infection. AIDS. 2006;20:333–43.

358. Turner ME, Kher K, Rakusan T, D'Angelo L, Kapur S, Selby D, Ray PE. A typical hemolytic uremic syndrome in human immunodeficiency virus-1-infected children. Pediatr Nephrol. 1997;11:161–3.

359. Benjamin M, Terrell DR, Vesely SK, Voskuhl GW, Dezube BJ, Kremer Hovinga JA, Lammle B, George JN. Frequency and significance of HIV infection among patients diagnosed with thrombotic thrombocytopenic purpura. Clin Infect Dis. 2009;48:1129–37.

360. Novitzky N, Thomson J, Abrahams L, du Toit C, McDonald A. Thrombotic thrombocytopenic purpura in patients with retroviral infection is highly responsive to plasma infusion therapy. Br J Haematol. 2005;128:373–9.

361. Wong AR, Pearson JS, Bright MD, Munera D, Robinson KS, Lee SF, Frankel G, Hartland EL. Enteropathogenic and enterohaemorrhagic Escherichia coli: even more subversive elements. Mol Microbiol. 2011;80:1420–38.

362. Karch H, Wiss R, Gloning H, Emmrich P, Aleksic S, Bockemuhl J. Hemolytic-uremic syndrome in infants due to verotoxin-producing Escherichia coli. Dtsch Med Wochenschr. 1990;115:489–95.

363. Caprioli A, Luzzi I, Rosmini F, Resti C, Edefonti A, Perfumo F, Farina C, Goglio A, Gianviti A, Rizzoni G. Community-wide outbreak of hemolytic-uremic syndrome associated with non-O157 verocytotoxin-producing Escherichia coli. J Infect Dis. 1994;169:208–11.

364. Shefer AM, Koo D, Werner SB, Mintz ED, Baron R, Wells JG, Barrett TJ, Ginsberg M, Bryant R, Abbott S, Griffin PM. A cluster of Escherichia coli O157:H7 infections with the hemolytic-uremic syndrome and death in California. A mandate for improved surveillance. West J Med. 1996;165:15–9.

365. Slutsker L, Ries AA, Maloney K, Wells JG, Greene KD, Griffin PM. A nationwide case-control study of Escherichia coli O157:H7 infection in the United States. J Infect Dis. 1998;177:962–6.

366. Tuttle J, Gomez T, Doyle MP, Wells JG, Zhao T, Tauxe RV, Griffin PM. Lessons from a large outbreak of Escherichia coli O157:H7 infections: insights into the infectious dose and method of widespread contamination of hamburger patties. Epidemiol Infect. 1999;122:185–92.

367. Paton AW, Ratcliff RM, Doyle RM, Seymour-Murray J, Davos D, Lanser JA, Paton JC. Molecular

microbiological investigation of an outbreak of hemolytic-uremic syndrome caused by dry fermented sausage contaminated with Shiga-like toxin-producing Escherichia coli. J Clin Microbiol. 1996;34:1622–7.

368. Dundas S, Murphy J, Soutar RL, Jones GA, Hutchinson SJ, Todd WT. Effectiveness of therapeutic plasma exchange in the 1996 Lanarkshire Escherichia coli O157:H7 outbreak. Lancet. 1999;354:1327–30.

369. Dundas S, Todd WT. Clinical presentation, complications and treatment of infection with verocytotoxin-producing Escherichia coli. Challenges for the clinician. Symp Ser Soc Appl Microbiol. 2000;29:24S–30S.

370. Cowden JM, Ahmed S, Donaghy M, Riley A. Epidemiological investigation of the central Scotland outbreak of Escherichia coli O157 infection, November to December 1996. Epidemiol Infect. 2001;126:335–41.

371. Auld H, MacIver D, Klaassen J. Heavy rainfall and waterborne disease outbreaks: the Walkerton example. J Toxicol Environ Health A. 2004;67:1879–87.

372. Garg AX, Macnab J, Clark W, Ray JG, Marshall JK, Suri RS, Devereaux PJ, Haynes B. Long-term health sequelae following E. coli and campylobacter contamination of municipal water. Population sampling and assessing non-participation biases. Can J Public Health. 2005;96:125–30.

373. Richards A. The Walkerton health study. Can Nurse. 2005;101:16–21.

374. Bradley KK, Williams JM, Burnsed LJ, Lytle MB, McDermott MD, Mody RK, Bhattarai A, Mallonee S, Piercefield EW, McDonald-Hamm CK, Smithee LK. Epidemiology of a large restaurant-associated outbreak of Shiga toxin-producing Escherichia coli O111:NM. Epidemiol Infect. 2012;140:1644–54.

375. Menne J, Nitschke M, Stingele R, Abu-Tair M, Beneke J, Bramstedt J, Bremer JP, Brunkhorst R, Busch V, Dengler R, Deuschl G, Fellermann K, Fickenscher H, Gerigk C, Goettsche A, Greeve J, Hafer C, Hagenmuller F, Haller H, Herget-Rosenthal S, Hertenstein B, Hofmann C, Lang M, Kielstein JT, Klostermeier UC, Knobloch J, Kuehbacher M, Kunzendorf U, Lehnert H, Manns MP, Menne TF, Meyer TN, Michael C, Munte T, Neumann-Grutzeck C, Nuernberger J, Pavenstaedt H, Ramazan L, Renders L, Repenthin J, Ries W, Rohr A, Rump LC, Samuelsson O, Sayk F, Schmidt BM, Schnatter S, Schocklmann H, Schreiber S, von Seydewitz CU, Steinhoff J, Stracke S, Suerbaum S, van de Loo A, Vischedyk M, Weissenborn K, Wellhoner P, Wiesner M, Zeissig S, Buning J, Schiffer M, Kuehbacher T. Validation of treatment strategies for enterohaem-

orrhagic Escherichia coli O104:H4 induced haemolytic uraemic syndrome: case-control study. BMJ. 2012;345:e4565.

376. Loos S, Ahlenstiel T, Kranz B, Staude H, Pape L, Hartel C, Vester U, Buchtala L, Benz K, Hoppe B, Beringer O, Krause M, Muller D, Pohl M, Lemke J, Hillebrand G, Kreuzer M, Konig J, Wigger M, Konrad M, Haffner D, Oh J, Kemper MJ. An outbreak of Shiga toxin-producing Escherichia coli O104:H4 hemolytic uremic syndrome in Germany: presentation and short-term outcome in children. Clin Infect Dis. 2012;55:753–9.

377. Bloom PD, MacPhail AP, Klugman K, Louw M, Raubenheimer C, Fischer C. Haemolytic-uraemic syndrome in adults with resistant Shigella dysenteriae type I. Lancet. 1994;344:206.

378. Rollins NC, Wittenberg DF, Coovadia HM, Pillay DG, Karas AJ, Sturm AW. Epidemic Shigella dysenteriae type 1 in Natal. J Trop Pediatr. 1995;41:281–4.

379. Oneko M, Nyathi MN, Doehring E. Post-dysenteric hemolytic uremic syndrome in Bulawayo, Zimbabwe. Pediatr Nephrol. 2001;16:1142–5.

380. Nathoo KJ, Sanders JA, Siziya S, Mucheche C. Haemolytic uraemic syndrome following Shigella dysenteriae type 1 outbreak in Zimbabwe: a clinical experience. Cent Afr J Med. 1995;41:267–74.

381. Srivastava RN, Moudgil A, Bagga A, Vasudev AS. Hemolytic uremic syndrome in children in northern India. Pediatr Nephrol. 1991;5:284–8.

382. Taneja N, Lyngdoh VW, Sharma M. Haemolytic uraemic syndrome due to ciprofloxacin-resistant Shigella dysenteriae serotype 1. J Med Microbiol. 2005;54:997–8.

383. Jha DK, Singh R, Raja S, Kumari N, Das BK. Clinico-laboratory profile of haemolytic uremic syndrome. Kathmandu Univ Med J (KUMJ). 2007;5:468–74.

384. Baranwal AK, Ravi R, Singh R. Diarrhea associated hemolytic uremic syndrome: a 3-year PICU experience from Nepal. Indian J Pediatr. 2009;76:1180–2.

385. Bin Saeed AA, El Bushra HE, Al-Hamdan NA. Does treatment of bloody diarrhea due to Shigella dysenteriae type 1 with ampicillin precipitate hemolytic uremic syndrome? Emerg Infect Dis. 1995;1:134–7.

386. Al-Qarawi S, Fontaine RE, Al-Qahtani MS. An outbreak of hemolytic uremic syndrome associated with antibiotic treatment of hospital inpatients for dysentery. Emerg Infect Dis. 1995;1:138–40.

387. Olotu AI, Mithwani S, Newton CR. Haemolytic uraemic syndrome in children admitted to a rural district hospital in Kenya. Trop Dr. 2008;38:165–7.

Renal Vasculitis in Children

25

Mojca Zajc Avramovič, Tadej Avčin,
and Marina Vivarelli

Abbreviations

AAGN	ANCA-associated glomerulonephritis
AAV	ANCA-associated vasculitis
ACR	American College of Rheumatology
ANA	Anti-nuclear antibody
ANCA	Antineutrophil cytoplasmic antibody
BAFF	B-cell-activating factor
BVAS	Birmingham vasculitis activity score
CHC2012	Chapel Hill Consensus Conference on the Nomenclature of Systemic Vasculitides, 2012
EGPA	Eosinophilic granuloma with polyangiitis (Churg-Strauss syndrome)
ENT	Ear, nose, and throat
ESR	Erythrocyte sedimentation rate
GBM	Glomerular basement membrane
GFR	Glomerular filtration rate
GN	Glomerulonephritis
GPA	Granulomatous polyangiitis (WG)
GWAS	Genome wide association study
HLA	Human leucocyte antigen
HUVS	Hypocomplementemic urticarial vasculitis syndrome
IgAV	IgA vasculitis
KD	Kawasaki disease
LAMP-2	Lysosome-associated membrane protein-2
MCP-1	Monocyte chemoattractant protein-1
MHC	Major histocompatibility complex
MMF	Mycophenolate mofetil
MMI	Methimazole
MPA	Microscopic polyangiitis
MPO	Myeloperoxidase
NCGN	Necrotizing crescentic glomerulonephritis
NETs	Neutrophil extracellular traps
PAN	Polyarteritis nodosa
PLEX	Plasma exchange
PR 3	Proteinase-3
PTU	Propylthiouracil
PVAS	Pediatric vasculitis activity score
pVDI	Pediatric vasculitis damage index
RCT	Randomized control trial
RLV	Renal-limited vasculitis
RPGN	Rapidly progressive glomerulonephritis
SLE	Systemic lupus erythematosus
SNP	Single nucleotide polymorphism

M. Z. Avramovič · T. Avčin
Department of Allergology, Rheumatology and Clinical Immunology, University Children's Hospital, UMC Ljubljana, Ljubljana, Slovenia

Faculty of Medicine, University of Ljubljana, Ljubljana, Slovenia
e-mail: mojca.zajc.avramovic@kclj.si; tadej.avcin@kclj.si

M. Vivarelli (✉)
Division of Nephrology, Department of Pediatric Subspecialties, Bambino Gesù Pediatric Hospital IRCCS, Rome, Italy
e-mail: marina.vivarelli@opbg.net

© The Author(s), under exclusive license to Springer Nature Switzerland AG 2023
F. Schaefer, L. A. Greenbaum (eds.), *Pediatric Kidney Disease*,
https://doi.org/10.1007/978-3-031-11665-0_25

SOV	Single-organ vasculitis
VDI	Vasculitis damage index
VVV	Variable vessel vasculitis
WG	Wegener's granulomatosis (GPA)

Introduction

Vasculitides are a wide range of disorders where the primary pathological feature is inflammation in a blood vessel wall. The clinical presentation depends on the site of involvement, vessel size, and the type and severity of pathological changes. Patients usually present with fever and constitutional symptoms, such as fatigue, weakness, weight loss, and skin lesions. Laboratory markers show inflammation, and signs of multiorgan involvement may be present at presentation. Nevertheless, the most common vasculitis in childhood, IgA vasculitis (IgAV), can present mildly, with cutaneous purpura of the lower limbs, or as a severe renal vasculitis. Vasculitis is often aggressive and can be organ- or life-threatening. Renal involvement, when present, is often rapidly progressive glomerulonephritis (RPGN) since it is extremely aggressive with severe hypertension and rapid deterioration of renal function, requiring intervention within hours of initial presentation to preserve residual kidney tissue. Classic histological features are the presence of severe inflammation with intense endocapillary and extracapillary proliferation, leading to crescents and necrosis, and in many cases (excluding IgAV and lupus nephritis) a negative (pauci-immune) immunofluorescence. Vasculitis may affect any part of the body, and patients should be treated by a multidisciplinary team including rheumatologists, nephrologists, pulmonologists, dermatologists, and neurologists. Although more common in adults, renal vasculitis occurs in childhood and may present as an isolated kidney disorder or associated with a systemic disease.

Classification of Vasculitides

Traditionally, vasculitis has been classified according to the size of the affected vasculature (Figs. 25.1 and 25.2). Large-vessel vasculitis or

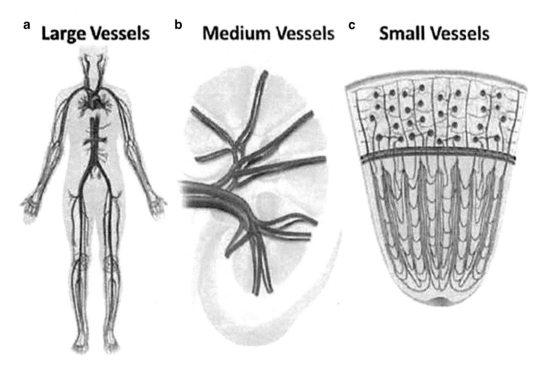

Fig. 25.1 The definition of vessel size [1]. (Reference: Jennette JC et al.:2012 Revised International Chapel Hill Consensus Conference Nomenclature of Vasculitis Arthritis & Rheumatism, 65:1–11, 2013)

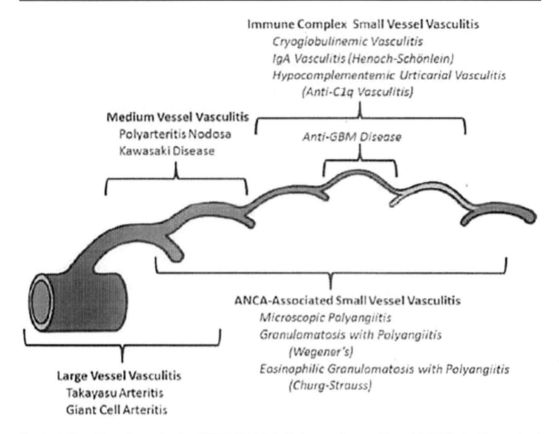

Fig. 25.2 Vasculitis and vascular size (CHCC 2012) [1]. (Reference: Jennette JC et al.:2012 Revised International Chapel Hill Consensus Conference Nomenclature of Vasculitis Arthritis & Rheumatism, 65:1–11, 2013)

arteritis affects the aorta and its major branches in diseases such as giant-cell arteritis and Takayasu arteritis, which can reduce the caliber of the abdominal aorta or of renal arteries, leading to renal ischemia and renovascular hypertension. Medium-vessel vasculitis involves medium or small arteries, leading to infarction and hemorrhage of the affected organ, and includes polyarteritis nodosa (PAN) and Kawasaki disease (KD), the only large-vessel or medium-vessel vasculitides that involves mainly infants and small children. Small-vessel vasculitides, affecting capillaries and venules, are the only forms which can by definition cause glomerulonephritis (GN). They comprise a large group of diseases; the two most common are IgAV and antineutrophil cytoplasmic antibody (ANCA)-associated vasculitis (AAV). The current nomenclature system was established at the International Chapel Hill Consensus Conference on the Nomenclature of Systemic Vasculitides in 1994 and further modified in 2012 (CHC2012), presented in Table 25.1 [1]. The most prominent modifications comprise the adoption of new names for several diseases, consistent with the trend of replacing eponyms with names that reflect the pathophysiology, the formalisation of the term AAV and categories for secondary forms of vasculitis. Monogenic forms of vasculitis, recognized more recently, were not included in the 2012 classification. The chapter includes information about rare monogenic forms of vasculitis that can affect the kidney and occur in children. The American College of Rheumatology (ACR) published a classification in 1990 of 7 vasculitides [2], which has become inadequate, and currently a joint ACR/The European Alliance of Associations for Rheumatology (EULAR) classification that will include new diagnostic criteria is being developed [3].

Kawasaki Disease

KD is an acute, self-limited vasculitis, occurring most frequently in infants and small children. Its main manifestations are fever (persisting for 5 days or more), peripheral extremity changes, a polymorphous exanthema, bilateral conjunctivitis, oral mucosal changes (e.g. red, dry, cracked lips and strawberry tongue) and non-purulent cervical lymphadenopathy [7]. It frequently affects the coronary vessels, causing aneurysms and other cardiac abnormalities; KD is one of the main causes of acquired cardiac disease in children. Renal manifestations are infrequent and their pathogenesis is unclear: pyuria, proteinuria and renal failure have been described, as well as tubulointerstitial nephritis which may be secondary to intravenous (IV) immunoglobulin, which together with aspirin is the mainstay of therapy [11].

Small-Vessel Vasculitis

The most common vasculitides affecting kidneys in children are IgAV (covered in Chap. 54) and AAV, which includes granulomatosis polyangiitis (GPA), *microscopic polyangiitis (MPA) and eosinophilic granulomatosis with polyangiitis (EGPA)*. AAV can be classified based on the autoantigen specificity. The two most recognized autoantigens are myeloperoxidase (MPO) and proteinase 3 (PR3). The categorization of a patient AAV should include both the clinicopathological phenotype and the autoantigen. The other forms of vasculitis are briefly addressed below, and the remainder of the chapter focuses on AAV.

Anti-Glomerular Basement Membrane Disease

Anti-glomerular basement membrane (GBM) disease is a rare form of small-vessel vasculitis caused by autoantibodies directed against the so-called Goodpasture antigen or non-collagenous domain 1 (NC-1), a neo-epitope of the α3 subunit of type IV collagen expressed in the GBM, where autoantibodies cause a rapidly progressive crescentic and necrotizing GN, and in pulmonary alveoli. The disease can occur in adolescents, and may be renal-limited or may, in approximately 50% of cases, involve small-vessels in the lungs as well, leading to pulmonary hemorrhage (Goodpasture syndrome). Exposure of the neo-epitope NC-1 is due to a perturbation of the structure of type IV collagen, which may be secondary to environmental exposure to reactive oxygen species (e.g. industrial hydrocarbon, cigarette smoke), systemic inflammation (e.g. AAV, which can co-exist with anti-GBM disease in approximately 25% of cases) or membranous nephropathy. Without aggressive and timely treatment, the disease is generally fulminant, and both patient and kidney survival are poor. Recommended treatment relies on the use of plasma exchange (PLEX) or immune-adsorption and immunosuppression with glucocorticoids and cyclophosphamide [12]. Treatment should be commenced without waiting for a renal biopsy when this diagnosis is suspected, and should be continued until the anti-GBM antibodies are undetectable [13].

Cryoglobulinemic Vasculitis

Cryoglobulinemic vasculitis is a rare systemic vasculitis resulting from circulating immune complex deposition in the small vessels which occurs when the temperature falls below 37° C. It has variable clinical features, including signs of hyperviscosity syndrome such as Raynaud's phenomenon, cold-induced acral ulcerations, livedo reticularis, headache and confusion, or signs of immune complex-mediated vasculitis of small vessels such as purpura, arthralgia, GN, and peripheral neuropathy. Cryoglobulinemia can result from infections (mainly hepatitis C virus and hepatitis B virus), cancer or autoimmune disease, or it can be essential. In children, essential forms predominate (72%), and renal involvement occurs, as in adults, in approximately 10% of cases [14]. Treatment is aimed at eliminating the cause, and rituximab (RTX) has been used with success. In severe forms, such as those with RPGN or symptomatic hyperviscosity, PLEX is necessary. IV immunoglobulin is contraindicated in cryoglobulinemic vasculitis as it can exacerbate immune complex precipitation, leading to multiorgan failure.

ANCA-Associated Vasculitis

Renal Pathology

The pathology of renal vasculitis is characterized by its grade of severity and anatomical location. Although there may be several stimuli that trigger vasculitis, endothelial cells are its basic target. The early pathology is an endothelitis, which is frequently seen with any endothelial injury. The more severe phenotypes are fibrinoid necrosis and occasional rupture of the corresponding vasculature, resulting in interstitial hemorrhage (Fig. 25.3a). In some cases, vasculitis is recognized by severe inflammatory infiltrates in the vascular wall; other cases show fewer inflammatory infiltrates with necrosis, such as PAN (very rare) or KD.

The key histological feature of AAV is necrotizing vasculitis, with few or no immune deposits, predominantly affecting small vessels. This can be associated with granulomatous lesions in GPA and with eosinophil-rich (and often granulomatous) inflammation in EGPA. Tissue biopsies are essential to make the diagnosis of AAV.

When renal involvement is present in patients with suspected or confirmed AAV, renal biopsy is the gold standard for diagnosis, and is an important predictor of renal outcome. ANCA-associated GN is characterized by pauci-immune immunofluorescence; necrotizing and crescentic lesions in the affected glomeruli by light microscopy; and subendothelial oedema, microthrombosis, and degranulation of neutrophils by electron microscopy [15].

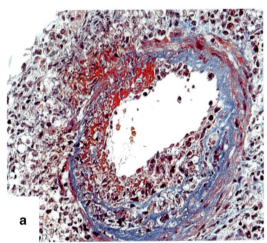

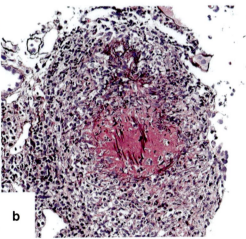

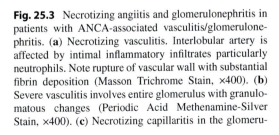

Fig. 25.3 Necrotizing angiitis and glomerulonephritis in patients with ANCA-associated vasculitis/glomerulonephritis. (**a**) Necrotizing vasculitis. Interlobular artery is affected by intimal inflammatory infiltrates particularly neutrophils. Note rupture of vascular wall with substantial fibrin deposition (Masson Trichrome Stain, ×400). (**b**) Severe vasculitis involves entire glomerulus with granulomatous changes (Periodic Acid Methenamine-Silver Stain, ×400). (**c**) Necrotizing capillaritis in the glomerulus. Note numerous neutrophils accumulation at the site of fibrinoid necrosis (Masson Trichrome Stain, ×400). (**d**) Segmental fibrinoid necrosis with nuclear fragmentation in the neutrophils (Periodic Acid Schiff Stain, ×550). (**e**) Peritubular capillaritis and interstitial inflammatory infiltrates (Masson Trichrome Stain, ×400). (**f**) Interstitial inflammatory infiltrates by electron microscopy. Note neutrophils predominant infiltration (×2000)

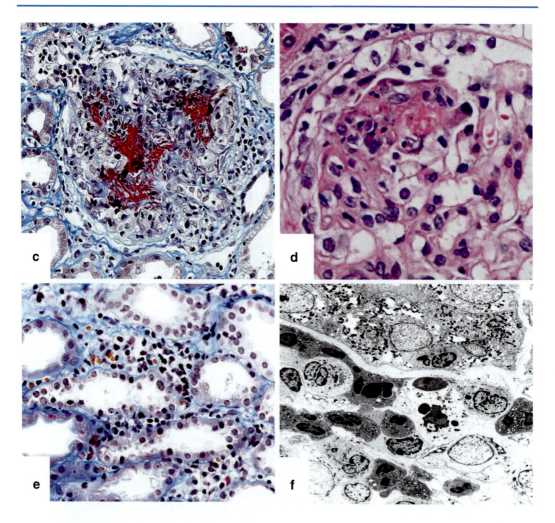

Fig. 25.3 (continued)

Light Microscopy

Renal vasculitis affects endothelial cells, causing inflammation, which manifests as endothelial cell swelling and proliferation and by inflammatory cell infiltration, in AAV mainly by neutrophils, into the subendothelial space. The typical sites of vasculitis in AAV are arterioles, glomeruli, and peritubular capillaries. In arterioles, following endothelial cell swelling, accumulation of inflammatory cells leads to intimal thickening, deposition of active coagulation product (fibrinoid necrosis), and thrombosis (Fig. 25.3a). If the lesion progresses, it leads to a defect or rupture of the vascular wall. In GPA-associated forms of AAV, angiitis can occur, targeting the glomerular hilum and resulting in the destruction of the entire glomerular structure, which is replaced by granulomatous inflammation (Fig. 25.3b). In the glomeruli, capillaritis causes necrotizing crescentic GN, which frequently progresses to glomerulosclerosis (Fig. 25.3c, d). In addition to glomerular involvement, there is also a tubulointerstitial nephritis in AAV; tubular lesions are important predictors of outcome, especially in patients treated with B-cell depleting therapy [16]. Peritubular capillaritis (Fig. 25.3e) is characterized by dilatation and adherence of inflammatory cells on the endothelium of cortical peritubular capillaries. Occasional rupture leads to interstitial hemorrhage.

GN in MPA differs from GN in GPA by the absence of granulomatous lesions and the more frequent occurrence of chronic lesions (e.g. glomerulosclerosis, fibrous crescents, interstitial fibrosis).

In 2010, an international working group of renal pathologists proposed a histopathologic classification of ANCA-associated GN that was predictive of long-term renal outcome in adult patients. Renal pathological features were divided into four categories: focal, crescentic, sclerotic, and mixed (Table 25.3). These categories predicted renal outcomes at 1 and 5 years (Fig. 25.4). Patients with focal lesions had an excellent renal outcome, whereas renal survival was poor in the sclerotic class, and severe patients also presented an increased mortality risk [17]. This classification system was confirmed in other adult cohorts [18] and in a pediatric retrospective study with biopsy-proven ANCA-associated GN (MPA and GPA) [19]. The biopsy specimens were focal in 13 patients (32.5%), crescentic in 20 (50%), mixed in 2 (5%), and sclerotic in 5 (12.5%). Mixed and crescentic were combined for analyses. This study showed rapid progression to end-stage kidney disease (ESKD) for patients in the sclerotic class, mild disease in the focal, and a slower decline over 2 years in the crescentic/mixed classes. The probability of having an estimated glomerular filtration rate (eGFR) >60 ml/min per 1.73 m^2 at 2 years was 100% for the focal, 56.5% for the crescentic/mixed, and 0% for the sclerotic biopsy categories. Renal biopsies were repeated to determine progression or because of relapses in a subset of patients. Among children with crescentic patterns who had a repeat biopsy, 80% progressed to sclerosis on a second biopsy. Among the focal group, only one child had a repeat biopsy and was reclassified as mixed. These data demonstrate a clear prognostic value of the histopathological classification and suggest for children with sclerotic class (at least 50% globally sclerotic glomeruli) that aggressive immunosuppression is unlikely to result in recovery of renal function. Therefore, it is likely that risks outweigh benefits in this setting and that when extensive sclerosis is present intense treatment should be avoided. Conversely, patients with more florid lesions require early and intensive treatment. Prospective studies are needed to achieve the objective of tailored management based on histological parameters.

Table 25.3 Classification scheme for ANCA-associated glomerulonephritis [17]

Class	Inclusion criteria[a]
Focal	≥50% normal glomeruli
Crescentic	≥50% glomeruli with crescents
Mixed	<50% normal, <50% crescentic, <50% globally sclerotic glomeruli
Sclerotic	≥50% globally sclerotic glomeruli

[a]Pauci-immune staining pattern on immunofluorescence micrography and ≥1 glomerulus with necrotizing or crescentic glomerulonephritis on light microscopy are required for inclusion in all four classes

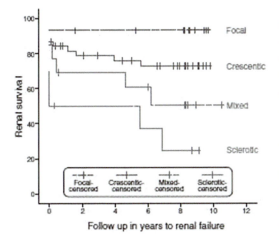

Fig. 25.4 Renal survival is depicted according to the four histological categories [17]. (Reference: Berden et al. Histological classification of ANCA-associated glomerulonephritis. JASN 21:1628–1639, 2010)

Immunofluorescence

Falk and Jennette defined "pauci-immune" as not more than 2+ staining of any immunoglobulin (on a scale of 0 to 4+) and the absence of immune-complex type electron-dense deposits by electron microscopy [20]. However, in a study of electron micrographs of 124 cases of ANCA-associated crescentic GN, 54% of the biopsies had glomerular immune-complex deposition [21], although the immunofluorescence staining was relatively weak (≤2+). Moreover, Manenti et al. evaluated 27 renal biopsies of adult patients with AAV for glomerular complement deposition by immunohistochemistry and found strong C3c staining in 11 of 27 patients (41%) and positive discrete glomerular deposition of C4d in 8 patients and of C5b-9 in 5 cases (20%), while Bb was usually negative. In this study, there was no association between tissue deposition of complement fractions and outcome [22]. In a subsequent study, patients with glomerular C3d deposition had a worse prognosis [23].

Electron Microscopy

By electron microscopy, neutrophil infiltration into the interstitium and degranulation is visible (Fig. 25.3f), together with neutrophil degranulation, subendothelial edema, and microthrombosis. Moreover, as reported above [21], in about 50% of cases immune-complex deposition was visible. These immune complexes were often few in number. Nonetheless, their presence was associated with more frequent glomerular tuft hypercellularity, greater proteinuria, and trends toward higher serum creatinine level and more widespread crescent formation compared with cases lacking deposits on electron microscopy.

Pathogenesis

The initiating events leading to AAV are multifactorial, but several risk factors and possible triggers have been recognized, including genetic factors, environmental exposures, and previous infections. The pathogenicity of ANCA plays an important role in initiating and amplifying the inflammation, and the ANCA-induced neutrophil activation is an important cause of vascular injury. The pathogenesis is presented in Fig. 25.5 [24].

Genetic Factors

Differences in the prevalence of AAV between ethnic groups, familial association studies, and genetic associations studies, including large

genome-wide association studies (GWAS) [25–28], all support the role of genetics. The strongest associations are those in the genes for human leukocyte antigen (HLA) [25–28], *SERPINA1* [25, 26, 29] and multiple genes encoding inflammatory mediators. Links with the HLA region support the central role of autoreactivity and autoimmunity in AAV. Candidate gene and GWAS studies not only indicated a highly significant association between AAV and HLA regions, but also showed genetic distinctions between different clinical phenotypes and ANCA specificity. In general, genetic associations are more closely linked with the auto-antigen specificity than with the clinical syndrome. GPA and PR3-ANCA AAV are associated with HLA-DPB1 and HLA-DPA1, while MPA and MPO-ANCA AAV are associated with HLA-DQB1 and HLA-DQA2 [25, 26, 30]. HLA-DPB1 is associated with EGPA [28]. Moreover, HLA alleles are associated with the mortality and relapse of AAV [30]. *SERPINA* codes for α1-antitrypsin, which is a major inhibitor of PR3. Involvement of the *SERPINA1* gene confirms the role of ANCA in the pathogenesis of AAV as the genetic variants may lead to decreased function α1-antitrypsin, resulting in PR3 accumulating in tissues and potentially triggering ANCA formation. Nevertheless, in a meta-analysis, not only PR3-ANCA positive patients but MPO-ANCA-positive patients and both c-ANCA and p-ANCA-positive patients are associated with *SERPINA1* [29]. One proposed hypothesis is that patients with AAV and these genetic variants have a reduced ability to inhibit PR3 released by activated neutrophils; consequently, these variants increase PR3-mediated proteolytic vessel damage. Nevertheless, the changes in *PRTN3*, which encodes PR3, were present only in PR3-ANCA-positive patients, independent of the clinical diagnosis [25, 26]. A wide range of associations in immunoregulatory genes were found, the strongest with *CTLA-4, PTPN22,* and *TLR9* [29, 30].

Environmental Factors

Infections are a known potential trigger of autoimmune disease. In AAV, more than 50% of

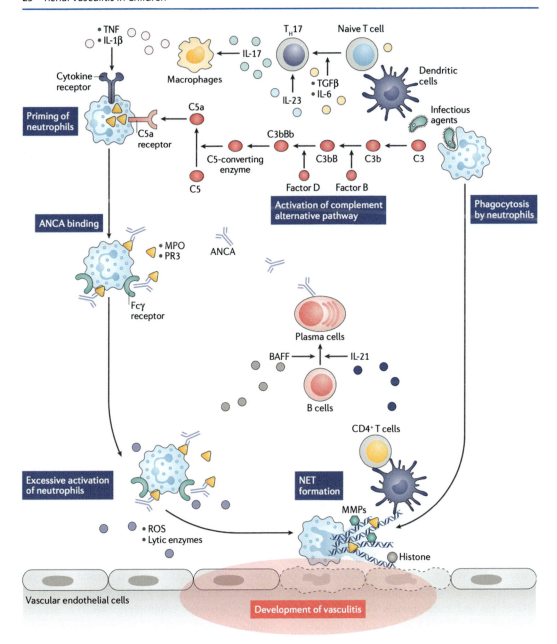

Fig. 25.5 Pathogenesis of AAV. Modified from Nature reviews Rheumatology [24]. (Reference: Nakazawa D, Masuda S, Tomaru U, Ishizu A. Pathogenesis and therapeutic interventions for ANCA-associated vasculitis. Nat Rev. Rheumatol. 2019;15(2):91–101)

patients are t nasal carriers of *Staphylococcus aureus* at the time of diagnosis, which is significantly higher than the general population. Nasal carriage of *Staphylococcus aureus* is associated with an increase risk of disease relapse [31, 32]. The underlying mechanisms is not known [32].

The human lysosome-associated membrane protein 2 (LAMP-2) epitope has complete homology with the bacterial adhesin FimH, and human LAMP-2-ANCA may cross react with this microbial protein. This supports the hypothesis of infection driven immune dysregulation in

AAV. The human antibodies directed against LAMP-2 are somewhat controversial because they have been shown in a rat model to elicit ANCA-associated GN [33], but the results were not replicated [34]. Drugs, including hydralazine, minocycline, propylthiouracil, and levamisole, may cause the development of ANCA [35, 36]. In a case series of AAV in seven children who received propylthiouracil, the most common of the recognized drugs used in childhood, the prognosis was better than non-drug induced AAV [37]. Geographic clustering, temporal clustering, seasonal variation in disease onset, and differences in urban/rural disease prevalence all suggest an environmental trigger [38]. Environmental exposure to air pollutants was investigated, with the strongest evidence for silica dust [39], which is further supported by outbreaks of AAV, mainly MPO-ANCA positive with intense pulmonary involvement, after three large earthquakes in Asia [38]. Pesticides, ultraviolet radiation, and smoking are all believed to contribute to the pathogenesis, but none is by itself sufficient to trigger the disease [38].

The Pathogenicity of ANCA

Substantial clinical and experimental data show that ANCAs are pathogenic. First, there is a strong association of the disease with ANCA, as >90% of MPA and GPA patients and >75% of EGPA patients and GN have positive ANCA. Second, there is also a partial correlation of titer with disease activity. Third, transplacental transfer of ANCA was able to induce disease in humans [40], as was the infusion of anti-MPO IgG in rat and mice models [41, 42]. Fourth, drug-induced ANCAs have a similar clinical presentation [35]. However, healthy individuals can have circulating autoantibodies against PR3 and particularly MPO, also called natural or non-pathogenic ANCAs. In comparison with ANCA from patients, the natural ANCAs have lower titers, lower avidity, less epitope specificity, and less capability to activate neutrophils [43, 44]. The transformation of natural ANCA to pathogenic is most probably an interplay between previously mentioned genetic, environmental and immunologic triggering events. The current hypothesis is that the first reaction is not against autoantigen, but against a peptide that is complementary to the autoantigen. The anti-idiotypic antibody is a response to this first immune response and it cross-reacts with the autoantigen epitopes that are complementary to the initial immunogenic peptide [45, 46]. Multiple microbial peptides are homologues of complementary PR3, including *S. aureus*.

Pathogenesis of Vascular Inflammation

Primed neutrophils, activated by ANCA, are the primary drivers of vascular inflammation in AAV. Different inflammatory signals, for example C5a, bacterial lipopolysaccharide, and TNF, can prime neutrophils to release the MPO/PR3 target autoantigens to the cell surface, where they interact with ANCA. This immune complex further activates neutrophils and causes a respiratory burst; neutrophil enzymes are degranulated; free radicals are released; and neutrophil extracellular traps (NETs) are extruded. NETs in AAV contain MPO and PR3, and further interact with ANCA. All of the above leads to injury and death of endothelial cells. Disrupted endothelium allows plasma to enter the vascular and perivascular tissue, and the following coagulation cascade results in fibroid necrosis [34, 47]. In addition, monocytes can express autoantigens (MPO and PR3) and can be activated by binding of ANCA to Fc-γ receptors (FcγRs). When activated, monocytes release proinflammatory cytokines, such as interleukin-8 (IL-8) and monocyte chemoattractant protein-1 (MCP-1). While IL-8 further activates neutrophils, MCP-1 attracts monocytes and macrophages, presumably shifting the inflammation into the next stage, from predominantly neutrophil-rich to predominantly monocyte/macrophage-rich, which includes granulomatous inflammation.

Pathogenesis of Granulomatosis

Granulomas are foci of extravascular inflammation; the exact mechanism of their formation is not known. It is believed that there is no antigen-specific response, but rather the secondary innate monocyte/macrophage response, triggered by acute vascular inflammation caused by ANCA-primed neutrophiles [47].

The Role of the Alternative Complement Pathway

The significance of the alternative complement pathway in AAV was first shown in animal studies. Ablation of C5, depletion of C3 and factor B deficiency completely inhibited disease development in a transferred anti-MPO IgG mouse model, while deficiency of classical pathway components did not prevent disease [48]. Later studies documented that the inflammatory process initiated by anti-MPO IgG is further amplified by C5aR activation on inflammatory cells, and a C5 inhibiting monoclonal antibody prevented or strongly attenuated GN development [49, 50]. The human biopsy specimens of MPO-ANCA associated GN had deposition of factor B, C3d, and the membrane attack complex (MAC) in glomeruli and small blood vessels [51]. In addition, increased levels of C3a, C5a, soluble C5b-9, and Bb were observed in the plasma of patients with active AAV, and lower levels of properdin were seen in the plasma of patients in remission. The levels of classical pathway proteins did not differ [52, 53]. Neutrophils, C5a and ANCAs create an inflammatory amplification loop, with C5a attracting and priming more neutrophils for activation by ANCAs, which causes further activation of the alternative complement pathway and consequent release of more C5a [54].

The Role of B and T Cells

The pathogenicity of ANCA, neutrophils, and complement are enabled by a defect in the regulation of the immune system. The regulatory FOXP3+ T cells are decreased and dysfunctional in AAV patients [55], even more so during active disease [56]. The subset of B cells with mostly regulatory suppressive function highly expresses CD5, and in the sera of patients with active AAV, the CD5+ B cells are reduced in number, which normalizes in remission after treatment with RTX [57, 58]. Furthermore, the sera of patients

with active AAV has elevated levels of B-cell-activating factor (BAFF), which stimulates B cells and inhibits apoptosis. The ligand for BAFF is released by activated neutrophils [59, 60]. In this way, ANCA-activated neutrophils, along with dysfunctional T- and B-cell regulation, augment the production of more ANCA.

Clinical Features

Patients typically present with non-specific systemic symptoms, such as fatigue, malaise, fever, anorexia, and weight loss. Rhinosinusitis and epistaxis can be early signs that sometimes go unnoticed, while a purpuric rash may be the first obvious reason to seek medical care. Arthralgia or overt arthritis, hematuria, hypertension, cough, diarrhea, and dyspnea can also be among the presenting features. The clinical symptoms may start suddenly or develop slowly over days or weeks.

Granulomatosis with Polyangiitis (GPA)

Upper and lower respiratory tract inflammation together with GN and positive ANCA, especially PR-3 ANCA, is typical for GPA in childhood. Granulomas are found in the tissue. The largest published cohort is the multicenter ARChiVe (A Registry for Children with Vasculitis) study, which included 183 children with GPA. A comparison of presenting features is shown in Table 25.4 [61]. Over half of the patients were female and white, while the median age at disease onset was 14 years. The median time to diagnosis was 2.1 months, but varied from 0–71 months. The most common presenting features were constitutional (88%), renal (83%), pulmonary (74%), ear, nose and throat (70%), musculoskeletal (65%), and cutaneous (47%). Renal manifestations included proteinuria (72%), hematuria (72%), decreased GFR creatinine clearance (54%), and nephrotic syndrome with edema (11%). Almost all of the patients with a biopsy had GN (94%). Thirteen percent had renal failure requiring dialysis and 7% progressed to ESKD. In the available renal biopsy specimens, pauci-immune and/or necrotizing GN was pres-

Table 25.4 Presenting features of MPA and GPA in ARChiVe study (n = 231). Adapted from Cabral et al. [61]

Clinical feature, n (%)	MPA (n = 48)	GPA (n = 183)
Constitutional/general	41 (85)	160 (88)
Malaise/fatigue	37 (77)	152 (83)
Fever	25 (52)	97 (53)
Weight Loss	15 (31)	80 (44)
Renal	36 (76)	151 (83)
Hypertension (age-adjusted)	16 (33)	39 (21)
Clinically nephrotic with edema	11 (23)	20 (11)
Renal failure requiring dialysis	12 (25)	24 (13)
End-stage renal disease	5 (10)	12 (7)
Impaired creatinine clearance or abnormal protein/creatinine ratio	28 (58)	99 (54)
Proteinuria	33 (69)	132 (72)
Hematuria >1+ or <10 hpf od red cell casts	29 (60)	132 (72)
Biopsy-proven glomerulonephritis	30 of 32 (94)	101 of 108 (94)
Pulmonary	21 (44)	136 (74)
Chronic cough	11 (23)	99 (54)
Wheeze or expiratory dyspnea	2 (4)	15 (8)
Alveolar hemorrhage/massive hemoptysis	7 (15)	76 (42)
Pleurisy	4 (8)	25 (14)
Supplemental oxygen requirement	6 (13)	40 (22)
Respiratory failure	2 (4)	22 (12)
Ear, nose, throat	0 (0)	128 (70)
Septal perforation or nasal collapse	0 (0)	15 (8)
Recurrent nasal bloody discharge/crusting/obstruction/ulcer	0 (0)	98 (53)
Chronic recurrent sinusitis	0 (0)	71 (39)
Conductive or sensorineural hearing loss	0 (0)	19 (10)
Otitis/mastoiditis	0 (0)	31 (17)
Subglottic involvement	0 (0)	19 (10)
Oral ulcers/granulomata	2 (4)	27 (15)
Eyes	15 (31)	78 (43)
Conjunctivitis	3 (6)	21 (11)
Non-specific red eye	1 (2)	19 (10)
Episcleritis	2 (4)	15 (8)
Proptosis or retro-orbital mass	0 (0)	3 (2)
Retinal exudates of hemorrhages or aneurysms or vessel thrombosis	1 (2)	0 (0)
Cutaneus	25 (52)	86 (47)
Palpable purpura/petechial rash	15 (31)	49 (27)
Gastrointestinal	28 (58)	66 (36)
Non-specific abdominal pain	18 (38)	41 (22)
Chronic nausea	16 (33)	22 (12)
Musculoskeletal	25 (52)	118 (65)
Arthralgia or confirmed arthritis	20 (42)	112 (61)
Myalgia, muscle weakness, or confirmed myositis	9 (19)	24 (14)
Nervous system	10 (21)	36 (20)
Headache	6 (13)	20 (11)
Dizziness	2 (4)	12 (7)
Cardiovascular	3 (6)	10 (5)
Venous thrombosis	0 (0)	3 (2)

ent in 80% of GPA patients [61]. In a single-center Canadian study of 25 patients with GPA, 88% had GN and 20% required dialysis at disease onset. Twenty-eight percent had elevated creatinine at disease onset and an additional 16% had an elevated creatinine during follow-up [62]. A large cohort from the PRINTO vasculitis database included 56 children with GPA. The demographic and most of the clinical data confirms results of the ARChiVe data, but patients from the PRINTO registry were younger (median 11.7 years), and had more frequent inflammation of the ears, nose, and throat (91%) and the eyes (35%) [63]. Sixty-seven percent were ANCA-PR3 positive [61, 63].

Microscopic Polyangiitis (MPA)

MPA characteristically involves small vessels of the kidneys and lungs and patients are positive for MPO-ANCA, and there are no granulomas in the pathologic specimens. The ARChiVe database included 48 pediatric MPO patients, who were significantly younger than GPA patients, with a median age at the time of diagnosis of 12 years. At presentation, the most common clinical manifestations were constitutional symptoms (85%), renal (75%), gastrointestinal (58%), musculoskeletal (52%), and cutaneous (52%). Results are shown in Table 25.4 [61]. The kidneys were more severely affected in MPA compared to GPA. The serum creatinine was moderately to severely elevated in almost half of the MPA (48%) patients. The rates of proteinuria and hematuria were 69% and 60%, similar to GPA, but almost one-quarter of patients presented with nephrotic syndrome with edema, and one-quarter of patients required dialysis. Ten percent progressed to ESKD [61]. Where renal biopsies were obtained, pauci-immune and/or necrotizing GN was seen in 78% [61]. Renal disease was a hallmark of MPA, present in 94% of MPA patients in the meta-analysis that included 130 pediatric patients [64]. The study bias was that it included studies from 1950 and MPA was previously not clearly defined. In ARChiVe, more than half of the patients had MPO-ANCA and/or p-ANCA (55%) and only 17% had PR3-ANCA and/or c-ANCA. ANCA was not present in 26% of the patients [61].

Eosinophilic Granulomatosis with Polyangiitis

EGPA is characterized by asthma or allergic rhinitis, skin disease, and vasculitis, which mostly involves small vessels and eosinophilic infiltration accompanies extravascular granulomas [65].

It is very rare in childhood, with only two out of 114 children with AAV having EGPA in the Canadian registry [66]. The largest pediatric cohorts include from 9–14 children with EGPA [67–69].

Laboratory Results

Marked elevation of inflammatory markers is typical, both erythrocyte sedimentation rate (ESR) and c-reactive protein. In half of GPA patients and one-third of MPA, total white blood cells and neutrophils are elevated. Eosinophil levels are normal for most patients with GPA and MPA. Over 80% of all patients have anemia and approximately one-third have elevated platelet counts. Von Willebrand antigen may also be elevated [61]. More than half of MPA patients and around 26% of GPA patients have MPO-ANCA and/or p-ANCA; whereas 67% of patients with GPA and 17% of patients with MPA have PR3-ANCA [61, 63]. ANCA, tested by either immunofluorescence or ELISA, was not present in 26% of MPA patients and 5% of GPA patients in ARChiVe [61, 66].

Disease Activity Assessment

Assessing disease activity and disease damage are important to help guide treatment decisions. Standardized tools are lacking in the field of childhood vasculitides. The most commonly used score in adult systemic vasculitides is the Birmingham Vasculitis Activity Score (BVAS), that was designed in 1994 [70], while the BVAS version 3 from 2009 is the most recent [71]. It is a composite score of 56 clinical features from 9 organ systems. Each feature is enumerated, according to the severity. Symptoms are categorized as new, persistent, or worsening [71]. The BVAS/WG is a disease-specific, modified version, validated for use in GPA [72]. To acknowledge the differences in childhood vasculitis, the Pediatric Vasculitis Activity Score (PVAS) was developed and validated [73]. PVAS was created by modifying BVAS. The pediatric vasculitis registry was reviewed to identify clinical features missing in the BVAS version; consequently, eight additional pediatric items were added, and others redefined, making 64 active items in nine categories. Age-specific reference ranges for blood pressure and renal function, and a pediatric definition of weight loss are incorporated. The score correlated well with physicians' global assessment, treatment decisions, and ESR [73].

Disease Damage Assessment

In 1997 the Birmingham Vasculitis Group developed and validated the Vasculitis Damage Index (VDI), a standardized tool for clinical assessment of damage in the systemic vasculitides [74]. Damage was defined as irreversible change resulting from scars. Currently, the PReS.

Childhood Arthritis and Rheumatology Research Alliance joint effort to make a pediatric version of VDI (pVDI) is underway. Vasculitis damage is defined as the presence of irreversible features present for at least 3 months since the onset of vasculitis and the pVDI contains 72

items in 10 systems [75]. Morishita et al. used pVDI to assess early outcomes in children with AAV [76].

Table 25.5 represents a roadmap of investigations suggested in all (first-line) and in certain (second-line) children with renal vasculitides [77].

Renal Transplantation

Due to the severity and rapid progression of the renal involvement in AAV, a substantial proportion of children progress to ESKD and require renal transplantation. In a recent single-center study assessing outcome of renal transplantation in these patients, seven children (3 with GPA, 4 with MPA) were described [78]. Time from diagnosis to transplant was 30 ± 12 (range, 17–48) months. Median duration of follow-up post transplantation was 27 months (range, 13–88 months). Median eGFR at last follow-up was 77 ml/min/1.73 m² (range, 7.9–83.5). One patient lost her transplant to acute cellular rejection following non-adherence to immunosuppression after

Table 25.5 Laboratory investigations in pediatric AAV. Modified from Plumb et al. [77]

First-line investigations	Second-line investigations
Hematology: Full blood count, Erythrocyte sedimentation rate, coagulation profile	Histology: renal/lung biopsy
Immunology: Lymphocyte subsets with CD19 count (pre-RTX), Immunoglobulins (Ig): IgG, IgM, IgA, IgE	Imaging: fibroendoscopy/X-ray sinuses, Chest high resolution computed tomography, MRI/MR angiography head
Biochemistry: Urea, creatinine and electrolytes, Liver function tests, Lactate dehydrogenase, Creatinine kinase, Thyroid function, Pancreatic function (amylase/lipase), Urine protein: creatinine ratio	Immunology: Anti-glomerular basement membrane antibodies, Coeliac screening
Infectious: Serology HBV, HCV, parvovirus B19, HIV, EBV, CMV, Mycoplasma, VZV and Anti-Streptolysin titre; Mantoux and/or QuantiFERON-TB testing, Blood culture, Urine microscopy and cell culture	Neurological: Nerve conduction studies
Autoantibody panel: Anti-neutrophil cytoplasmic antibodies, Antinuclear antibodies, Anti-double stranded DNA antibodies, Anti-cardiolipin and anti-phospholipid antibodies, Lupus anticoagulant	Ambulatory blood pressure monitoring; fundus oculi
Complement (C) function: C3, C4	Birmingham vasculitis activity score
Chest X-ray, Electrocardiography, Echocardiography	Renal angiography, Renal dimercaptosuccinic acid (DMSA) scan

Monogenic Forms of Renal Vasculitis

Recently, monogenic forms of autoinflammatory diseases have been identified that present predominantly with features of systemic vasculitis in childhood. Their discovery has shed light on new pathophysiological pathways which may allow innovative management, both in terms of monitoring biomarkers of disease activity and in terms of targeted therapeutic approaches [79].

Type I Interferonopathies

Type I interferons (IFNs) are regulatory proteins involved in immune response against viral infections. Their activation is induced by recognition of foreign nucleic acids and is tightly regulated by a complex network of pathways that involve both the innate and adaptive immune system. Type I interferonopathies are a group of rare monogenic disorders associated with constitutive overproduction of type I IFNs and provide unique insights into the mechanisms of differentiating self nucleic acids from non-self nucleic acids [80]. There is a marked overlap of clinical features across different type I interferonopathies, particularly the involvement of the central nervous system and skin as well as lung inflammation in certain genotypes. The clinical expression of type I interferonopathies may be influenced by differential exposure to environmental) triggers such as infection [81, 82].

Stimulator of interferon genes -associated vasculopathy with onset in infancy.

Stimulator of interferon genes (STING)-associated vasculopathy with onset in infancy (SAVI) is a type I interferonopathy caused by a gain-of-function mutation in the transmembrane protein 173 gene (*TMEM173*) [83]. *TMEM173* encodes STING, which is a transmembrane protein localized in the endoplasmic reticulum and functions in the transduction of a type I IFN response to different) types of cytosolic DNA. In patients with SAVI, constitutively activated STING leads to increased transcription of the type I IFN gene *IFNB1* and production of IFN-β, which further up-regulates the transcription of IFN-response genes.

SAVI is clinically characterized by neonatal-onset systemic inflammation, a severe cutaneous vasculopathy and major interstitial lung disease [83]. Over-expression of STING induces endothelial cell activation resulting in a severe inflammatory vaso-occlusive process leading to tissue loss on hands and feet at an early age. Renal involvement in SAVI is rare and usually mild, with microscopic hematuria and mild proteinuria associated) with hypertension [84]. One patient with SAVI developed kidney involvement with apolipoprotein L1 (APOL1)-associated collapsing glomerulopathy suggesting the role of IFN pathways in the pathogenesis of APOL1-associated nephropathy [85]. Systemic inflammation in patients with SAVI is refractory to conventional immunosuppressive medications, but treatment with JAK inhibitors (tofacitinib, ruxolitinib and baricitinib) could suppress the expression of STING-induced IFN-response genes and lead to clinical improvement.

Coatomer Associated Protein Subunit Alpha Gene Syndrome

Coatomer associated protein subunit alpha gene (COPA) syndrome is an autosomal dominant syndrome caused by mutations in the coatomer associated protein subunit alpha (COPα) gene (*COPA*) [86]. It is characterized by interstitial lung disease, inflammatory arthritis and kidney disease in childhood. COPα is part of the coatomer protein complex I involved in retrograde movement of vesicles from the Golgi apparatus to the endoplasmic reticulum (ER). Mutations in COPA lead to defective intracellular transport, resulting in immune dysregulation that can promote both autoinflammation and autoimmunity. Immunologically, COPA syndrome is associated with autoantibodies, significant skewing of CD4 T cells toward a T helper type 17 (Th17) phenotype implicated in autoimmunity, and proinflammatory cytokine expression such as IL-1β, IL-6 and IL-23. Patients with COPA syndrome have a strong upregulation of type I IFN-stimulated genes similar to patients with SAVI [87, 88].

Renal disease was reported in 45% of patients with COPA syndrome and typically presents as GN with proteinuria and decreased renal function [88, 89]. Kidney biopsy findings were heterogeneous, including crescentic GN and focal mesangial hypercellularity with immune complex deposition ranging from isolated IgA deposits to a "full house" immunofluorescence (IgM, IgG and C1q) resembling lupus nephritis. Increased type I IFN signaling suggests that JAK inhibitors as a possible treatment for COPA syndrome [87, 88].

Deficiency of Adenosine Deaminase 2

Deficiency of adenosine deaminase type 2 (DADA2) is a monogenic vasculitis syndrome caused by loss-of-function mutations in the adenosine deaminase type 2 (*ADA2*) gene, and clinically presents as an inflammatory vasculopathy [90, 91]. *ADA2* is a highly polymorphic gene, and more than 60 disease-causing mutations have been described, mostly missense variants.

Adenosine deaminase proteins regulate purine metabolism, and in the absence of ADA1 toxic deoxyadenosine nucleotides accumulate in lymphocytes leading to the severe combined immunodeficiency. ADA2, in addition to its deaminase activity, functions as a growth factor for endothelial cells and is involved in leukocyte development and differentiation. ADA2 appears to be critical for the maintenance of vascular integrity and in cross-talk between macrophages and pericytes. Increased production of proinflammatory cytokines was found in skin biopsies and blood samples from patients with DADA2 [92].

The disease has a highly variable clinical presentation, with 77% of patients presenting before the age of 10 years. A characteristic clinical feature is an inflammatory vasculopathy of small- and medium-sized arteries, with manifestations ranging from livedo reticularis to PAN and life-threatening ischemic or hemorrhagic stroke. Patients with DADA2 usually present with fever,

increased acute phase reactants and a vasculitic skin rash such as livedo reticularis, nodules, purpura, skin ulcers and digital gangrene. Vasculitis in DADA2 can affect other organs, including intestine, liver and kidney. The most common renal manifestations in patients with DADA2 are arterial hypertension, renovascular aneurysms, renal artery stenosis and kidney inflammation with dense lymphocytic infiltration and glomerular scarring [91, 93].

Genetic testing for DADA2 and measurement of ADA2 enzymatic activity should be considered for patients with early-onset PAN-like systemic vasculitis, refractory PAN and familial vasculitis. The mainstay of treatment for DADA2 is anti-TNF-α biologic drugs, which are effective in reducing fever episodes, vasculitic disease activity and preventing ischemic strokes, but are not effective for the immunodeficiency [94, 95].

Hypocomplementemic Urticarial Vasculitis Syndrome

Hypocomplementemic urticarial vasculitis syndrome (HUVS), or McDuffie syndrome, is a small vessel vasculitis associated with urticaria, hypocomplementemia (both C3 and C4) and anti-C1q circulating antibodies [96]. It affects the skin, joints, eyes, lungs and kidneys. Diagnostic criteria have been formulated [97] and diagnosis requires the presence of chronic urticarial exanthema and hypocomplementemia plus at least two minor diagnostic criteria (leukocytoclastic vasculitis, arthralgia/arthritis, GN, uveitis/episcleritis/conjunctivitis, abdominal pain, positive anti-C1q antibodies) and exclusion of autoimmune disease (systemic lupus erythematosus [SLE], Sjögren syndrome, cryoglobulinemia). It affects predominantly females with an 8:1 ratio, typically in the fifth decade of life. In a recent review of 60 cases described in the literature [98], renal involvement was identified in 14–50% of cases of HUVS. The most frequent presenting symptoms were hematuria and proteinuria (70% of patients). One third of patients with renal involvement had reduced kidney function at presentation (eGFR below 60 ml/min/1.73 m²). The most frequent glomerular pattern of injury was membranoproliferative GN (35%), followed by mesangioproliferative (21%) and membranous (19%) GN. Crescents were found in 23% of cases and were associated with a more severe presentation, as expected. By immunofluorescence, positivity for IgG, IgM, C1q and C3 was found in the mesangium and along the glomerular capillary walls, indicating immune-complex deposition. This finding, together with the observation that 50–55% of patients with HUVS have a positive ANA, indicates that this disease has similarities to SLE. Indeed, in about 50% of patients disease progression, if not prevented, leads to the development of SLE [99].

In the cohort of HUVS patients with renal involvement [98], 18% were children, and in children the male to female ratio was 1:1. Renal involvement in HUVS led to ESKD in 15% and 17% of cases in adults and children, respectively. Treatment should therefore be aggressive and timely, following the indications given below for other forms of renal vasculitis in children.

Studies in familial forms have revealed that HUVS can be caused by a homozygous mutation in *DNASE1L3* [100]. The protein encoded by *DNASE1L3* is an endonuclease capable of cleaving both single- and double-stranded DNA. Individuals harboring mutations in this gene develop HUVS in infancy/childhood, have a substantial risk of developing severe organ (kidney, lung) involvement and full-blown SLE, and may require life-long immunosuppressive treatment.

Treatment and Management of Renal Vasculitis

Renal vasculitides in children are extremely rare, though they determine significant morbidity and mortality, particularly if there is diagnostic delay [101]. Therefore, conducting traditionally designed randomized clinical trials is not feasible in children, and current therapeutic strategies are based on small case series or data derived from RCTs performed in adults. Despite these limita-

tions, there have been substantial improvements in management of these conditions. This progress is related to the use of different immunosuppressive medications and newer biologic agents, and to the broader recognition of monogenic forms, which may benefit from targeted therapy. Moving forward, innovative trial design tailored to small numbers is necessary, as is a standardized approach to the management of these rare pediatric diseases. Consequently, there are now recommendations based on consensus and, where possible, on evidence, for management of these conditions. The European consensus-based recommendations on diagnosis of rare pediatric vasculitides are a successful example of this approach [6]. As described above, the AAV include GPA (formerly known as Wegener's granulomatosis), MPA, EGPA (previously referred to as Churg-Strauss syndrome) and renal-limited microscopic vasculitis, also known as pauci-immune or crescentic GN (GN). Pauci-immune GN is a fulminant, relapsing disease in children [102, 103] and is frequently associated with RPGN, characterized by clinical features of GN and rapid decline of renal function, with pathology exhibiting crescent formation affecting the majority of glomeruli. RPGN and its treatment are covered in Chap. 50 of this textbook.

A possible therapeutic approach is outlined in Table 25.6. Treatment consists of an aggressive induction treatment, aimed at switching off the fulminant inflammatory disease process, followed by a maintenance phase aimed at consolidating remission. There is no clear consensus as to when and how treatment should be discontinued. However, following induction, assessment of organ damage and of the side effects of therapy should be considered when designing a maintenance strategy that balances risks and benefits. Even in terms of induction, recent positive results from studies assessing RTX and avacopan should be considered, with the objective of minimizing long-term toxicity, such as sterility, malignancy, stunted growth and osteoporosis/aseptic necrosis, which is especially important in children. While GPA and MPA are considered separate entities, they are managed identically.

Table 25.6 AAV treatment. Modified from Pediatric Kidney Disease 2nd edition [144]

Agent	Route	Administration dosage and duration
Induction treatment		
Pulse Methylprednisolone[a]	IV	400–600 mg/m²/day (max 1000 mg/day) for 3–5 consecutive days
Prednisone[a] Prednisolone[a]	Oral	1.5–2.0 mg/kg/day (max 60 mg/day) for 4 weeks Gradually taper down over 6–12 months
Cyclophosphamide[b]	IV	Start at 500 mg/m²/day Increase monthly by 125 mg/m²/day to 750–1000 mg/m²/day (max 1000 mg/day) for 6–10 times
Cyclophosphamide	Oral	2 mg/kg/day for 2–3 months
Rituximab[c]	IV	375 mg/mg/m²/day weekly for 4 times
Plasmapheresis		Double volume on alternate day for 2 weeks
Maintenance treatment		
Azathioprine	Oral	2.0 mg/kg/day for 9 months Switch from cyclophosphamide at 3 months
Rituximab[d]	IV	Optimal dose and timing in children not available

IV intravenous

[a] Methylprednisolone pulses followed by oral prednisone or prednisolone 1.5–2.0 mg/kg/day for 4 weeks, with gradually tapering until discontinuation over 6–12 months
[b] Cyclophosphamide followed by azathioprine switching from cyclophosphamide at 3–6 months
[c] Given with pulse and oral corticosteroids
[d] No data available on use of RTX for maintenance if it has been used at induction

Induction Treatment

Cyclophosphamide and Glucocorticoids

Cyclophosphamide and glucocorticoids are well-established induction treatment of AAV. Therapy with cyclophosphamide and oral prednisone/prednisolone for 3–6 months was found to lead to clinical remission in 93% of adult patients with AAV [104], and improved remission rate from 56% to 84.7% and decreased relapse rate by approximately 50% [105]. At disease onset, given

the rapidity and severity of renal manifestations, pulse IV methylprednisolone is recommended [6] at 400–600 mg/m²/day (maximum dose 1000 mg/day) for 3–5 consecutive days. This treatment should be followed by oral prednisone/prednisolone 1.5–2.0 mg/kg of ideal body weight daily (maximum dose 60 mg/day) for 4 weeks, followed by gradual tapering over 6–12 months. Cyclophosphamide can be administered in oral or IV pulse regimens. Daily oral cyclophosphamide should start at a dose of 2 mg/kg/day and continue for 2–3 months while adjusting the dose to keep the nadir leukocyte count above 3000/mm³. When a regimen of IV pulsed cyclophosphamide is used, the initial dose should be approximately 500 mg/m² and increased monthly by 125 mg/m² to 750–1000 mg/m² (maximum dose 1000 mg/day) every 4 weeks for 6–10 doses. Cyclophosphamide should be given with adequate oral or IV hydration and with mesna, a drug which binds the cyclophosphamide metabolite which is toxic for the bladder mucosa, to minimize the risk of hemorrhagic cystitis. Subsequent doses should be adjusted depending on the 2-week post-treatment nadir leukocyte count. A RCT of IV pulse cyclophosphamide versus daily oral cyclophosphamide for induction of remission in AAV with renal involvement has been conducted [106]. This trial demonstrated that IV pulse and daily oral cyclophosphamide had similar remission rates and times to remission. Patients receiving the pulse regimen were administered approximately one-half of the cumulative dose of cyclophosphamide of the oral regimen and experienced a significantly lower rate of leukopenia for the same duration of therapy [106]. In a meta-analysis of RCTs, the pulse regimen was associated with fewer infections, increased risk of relapse, less leukopenia, and a trend toward a higher rate of requiring renal replacement therapy [107]. Because of a lower cumulative dose and a lower risk of side effects, the pulse regimen is recommended as the first line of induction therapy for pediatric pauci-immune GN. Combination therapy with oral cyclophosphamide (2 mg/kg/day) and pulse methylprednisolone followed by oral prednisolone resulted in a high remission rate (70–100%) and low mortality in pediatric ANCA-associated GN [108–110]. Thus, the duration of continuous oral cyclophosphamide should usually be limited to 3 months, with a maximum of 6 months, but whether the same duration can be applied to IV pulsed cyclophosphamide is unclear [111].

Other agents employed in remission induction include anti-TNF-α antibodies and MMF. It is now recognized that RTX is as effective as cyclophosphamide in severe or relapsing disease, particularly for those patients at risk for glucocorticoid or cyclophosphamide toxicity. PLEX and IV immunoglobulin therapy may also be used as adjuvant therapy to induce remission in more severe cases.

The only randomized study of pulse methylprednisolone is the MEPEX trial [112]. This study investigated whether the addition of PLEX to oral corticosteroids and cyclophosphamide was more effective than pulse methylprednisolone (1 g × 3) for renal recovery in patients who presented with renal failure. In this study, there was no difference in mortality and safety, but PLEX appeared more effective than pulse methylprednisolone in preserving kidney function.

Rituximab

Despite its effectiveness, the induction regimen with high-dose glucocorticoids and cyclophosphamide has significant morbidity in the long-term, which is particularly relevant in children. In a cohort of eight adults who presented with childhood-onset AAV, at a median of 19 years of follow-up, seven suffered from infections, four were infertile, two had skeletal complications, and one developed malignancy [113].

RTX is a chimeric monoclonal antibody that targets the CD20 antigen on the surface of B cells. Several case series and small studies have reported the efficacy of RTX in refractory AAV. Two randomized trials examined RTX as induction therapy for AAV. In the RITUXVAS trial, 44 patients with newly diagnosed AAV were randomized to either RTX or cyclophosphamide groups. The RTX group received four 375 mg/m² doses of RTX given weekly and IV cyclophosphamide at a dose of 15 mg/kg, 2 weeks apart for a total of two doses. The cyclophosphamide

group received 15 mg/kg of IV cyclophosphamide every 2 weeks × 3 doses, and then every 3 weeks for a maximum of 10 doses. Both groups received IV methylprednisolone, followed by oral corticosteroids. There were no significant differences in the rates of remission and serious adverse events [114]. In the RAVE trial, 197 ANCA-positive patients with either GPA or MPA were randomized to treatment with either RTX or conventional cyclophosphamide followed by azathioprine. The RTX group received four weekly doses of 375 mg/m². The cyclophosphamide group received 2 mg/kg/day orally for 3 months, followed by oral azathioprine at a dose of 2 mg/kg/day for 3 months. Both groups received 1–3 pulses of methylprednisolone (1000 mg each), followed by prednisone at a dose of 1 mg/kg/day, tapered by 5 months. At 6 months, 64% of the patients in the RTX group, compared with 53% of the patients in the cyclophosphamide–azathioprine group, experienced complete remission. There were no significant differences between the two treatment groups in the rates of complete remission, adverse events, or relapse [115]. At 12 and 18 months, 48% and 39%, respectively, of the patients in the RTX group had maintained complete remission, compared with 39% and 33%, respectively, in the cyclophosphamide–azathioprine group. There were no significant differences between the two groups in the duration of complete remission, the frequency or severity of relapses, and adverse events. This study shows that RTX is equivalent to cyclophosphamide in efficacy for the induction and maintenance of remission over 18 months [116] Following these important results obtained in adult clinical trials, the use of RTX in children with AAV is being evaluated in the Pediatric Polyangiitis Rituximab Study (PEPRS) [117]. This is an open-label study which has enrolled 25 children with newly diagnosed or relapsing GPA or MPA. They have received weekly IV RTX for 4 weeks at a dose of 375 mg/m² as well as glucocorticoids (1 mg/kg/day [max 60 mg/day]) tapered to 0.2 mg/kg/day (max 10 mg/kg/day) by 6 months. All patients received three doses of IV methylprednisolone at 30 mg/kg/day with a maximum of 1 g/day prior to the first RTX infusion.

The safety profile and pharmacokinetics were comparable to adults with GPA or MPA. No new safety signals have emerged thus far [118]. Basu et al. reported a retrospective analysis of 11 pediatric MPA patients treated with a cyclophosphamide free, RTX- and MMF-based protocol with a median follow-up period of 20.9 months [119]. Patient and renal survival at 1 year were 100%. Despite varying degrees of renal involvement at presentation, kidney function recovered in all patients, with a median eGFR of 79.5 ml/min/1.73 m^2. At last follow-up, 91% of patients were in complete remission and one (9%) child was in partial remission.

Hence, it seems reasonable to use RTX in children with severe AAV when cyclophosphamide is not available or not advisable. In terms of RTX dose, it is possible that an alternate regimen of 2 doses at 750 mg/m^2 (max 1000 mg) administered 14 days apart as in rheumatoid arthritis may be comparable to the classic regimen [77] RTX in AAV and other autoimmune disorders has been shown to induce hypogammaglobulinemia [120]: 56% of adults had IgG hypogammaglobulinemia during follow-up; IgG replacement was initiated because of recurrent infection in 4.2% of patients. No association was found between IgG levels and cumulative RTX dose.

Plasma Exchange

In severe AAV, especially with pulmonary haemorrhage or RPGN, or when the patient has significant deterioration despite an appropriate induction regimen, therapy is often augmented by PLEX, a strategy targeted towards removing the pathogenic antibodies [121–123]. Following the first positive report on PLEX in nine patients with crescentic GN, of whom five rapidly recovered renal function, [25, 124] the use of PLEX was recommended only in patients with the most severe renal disease (creatinine >500 μmol/L equivalent to >5.66 mg/dl) [125] due to the results of studies demonstrating a beneficial effect of PLEX only in dialysis-dependent patients [126, 127]. The MEPEX trial [112] compared PLEX to pulse methylprednisolone in addition to oral prednisolone and oral cyclophosphamide in patients with a new diagnosis of AAV

and serum creatinine >500 μmol/L. PLEX was associated with a significantly higher rate of kidney recovery at 3 months (69% with PLEX vs. 49% with pulse methylprednisolone), and also with a reduction in risk for progression to ESKD at 12 months. On the other hand, patient survival and the rate of severe adverse events were similar in both groups [112].

More recently, the PEXIVAS trial included all patients with a GFR <50 ml/min/1.73 m^2 and thus aimed to answer the question of whether PLEX is a good option for patients with moderate kidney function impairment. PEXIVAS showed that after a follow-up of almost 3 years routine PLEX did not provide reduce the rate of the composite outcome of ESKD or death. Taken altogether, these results indicate that PLEX should be reserved for severe cases of AAV with marked reduction in kidney function or requiring dialysis [128].

The 2021 KDIGO guidelines suggest to consider plasmapheresis for patients with refractory disease due to drug intolerance, non-adherence, concomitant morbidities, a secondary drive for vasculitis such as malignancy, drugs or infection, and true treatment failure and for patients with diffuse alveolar bleeding with hypoxemia. They recommend plasmapheresis for patients with combined AAV and anti-GBM GN, according to the proposed criteria and regimen for anti-GBM GN [129].

Mycophenolate Mofetil

Another agent which has been investigated in AAV induction as a safer, less toxic alternative to cyclophosphamide is MMF, an orally administered lymphocyte suppressive agent with short duration of action, which in small studies appeared beneficial in AAV, both in adults and in children [130, 131]. TA RCT assessed whether MMF was non-inferior to cyclophosphamide for remission induction in newly diagnosed AAV patients [132]. All patients received the same oral glucocorticoid regimen and were switched to azathioprine following remission. The primary endpoint was remission by 6 months and compliance with the tapering glucocorticoid regimen. MMF was non-inferior to cyclophosphamide for remission induction in AAV, but resulted in a higher relapse rate. Therefore, if other options are unavailable or unadvisable, MMF can be considered for induction in patients with non-severe or life-threatening AAV.

Anti-TNF Therapy

In AAV, TNF-α may have a pathogenic role, both in the formation of granulomas and in neutrophil priming, which enhances the expression of endothelial adhesion molecules on the cell surface and the capability of ANCA to stimulate neutrophil degranulation, a driver of vascular damage [77]. Etanercept, infliximab and adalimumab have been investigated in this setting with mixed results, and evidence is insufficient to recommend their use at this time [118].

Avacopan

Evidence of a role of complement, especially of C5a, a powerful anaphylatoxin which recruits neutrophils to the inflammatory site, and of the C5aR, in the pathogenesis of AAV [18] led to the use of complement inhibition with the oral C5aR antagonist avacopan. Efficacy, safety and steroid-sparing effects of avacopan in patients with GPA/MPA were shown in two phase II trials [133, 134] and a phase III trial [135]. In the phase III RCT, adult patients with AAV were randomized in a 1:1 ratio to receive oral avacopan at a dose of 30 mg twice daily or oral prednisone on a tapering schedule. All patients received either cyclophosphamide (followed by azathioprine) or RTX. The first primary end-point was remission, defined as a BVAS score of 0 at week 26 and no glucocorticoid use in the previous 4 weeks. The second primary end-point was sustained remission, defined as remission at both weeks 26 and 52. Both end-points were tested for non-inferiority and for superiority. Avacopan was non-inferior, but not superior to prednisone taper with respect to remission at week 26 and was superior to prednisone taper with respect to sustained remission at week 52. This remarkable result needs to be confirmed in a pediatric population, but suggests the possibility of a prednisone-free induction treatment for AAV.

Adjunctive Measures

The SHARE initiative European recommendations on management of pediatric vasculitides suggest the use of antiplatelet agents to prevent thrombotic complications associated with systemic vasculitis in the young [136]; antibiotic prophylaxis to prevent Pneumocystis jiroveci pneumonia at induction; osteoporosis prophylaxis with vitamin D in children treated with prednisone/methylprednisolone; and gastric protection (e.g. with protein pump inhibitors) in case of gastric pain.

Maintenance Treatment

Following induction of remission, maintenance therapy is necessary to prevent relapse. Long-term toxicity (infertility, risk of bladder cancer and lymphoproliferative disorder) makes cyclophosphamide an unattractive option for maintenance after successful induction. The CYCAZAREM trial (cyclophosphamide vs. azathioprine for early remission phase of vasculitis) found that azathioprine was as effective as continuous cyclophosphamide at maintaining remission and was associated with fewer side effects [104]. In this study, both study groups received the same induction therapy, consisting of oral cyclophosphamide and prednisolone. Once remission had been achieved, between 3 and 6 months, patients were randomly assigned to treatment with azathioprine (2 mg/kg/day) or to continued cyclophosphamide therapy (1.5 mg/kg/day), with the same dose of prednisolone (10 mg/day) up to 12 months. Subsequently, from 12 to 18 months, all patients received azathioprine (1.5 mg/kg/day) and prednisolone (7.5 mg/kg/day). The primary outcome was relapse at 18 months, and there was no difference between the groups. Once azathioprine was established as a suitable alternative therapeutic agent for maintenance, its optimal duration was not evaluated. The REMAIN study addressed this question and found that azathioprine given in association with low-dose glucocorticoids for 48 months compared to 24 months reduced the risk of relapse threefold. Moreover, the 48-month group had improved renal survival and reduced incidence of ESKD compared to the 24-month group [137]. The use of LEF in maintaining remission is less well studied, but results of 1 prematurely ended randomized study indicated that, at a dose of 30 mg/day, leflunomide was more effective than methotrexate at preventing relapse despite being associated with a higher rate of adverse events [138].

The use of MMF was evaluated in the IMPROVE study, which at a median follow-up of 39 months showed that MMF was inferior to azathioprine at preventing relapses during maintenance [139]. In this study, patients with AAV who attained remission with cyclophosphamide and prednisolone, were randomized to either MMF at a dose of 2000 mg/day or azathioprine at a dose of 2 mg/kg/day. Relapse was more common in the MMF group than in the azathioprine group. Both groups had similar adverse event rates. Therefore, azathioprine is preferred to MMF or cyclophosphamide for maintenance therapy in AAV.

Recently, the use of RTX for the maintenance of AAV has been investigated. The MAINRIT-SAN trial compared the use of repeated doses of RTX (500 mg at weeks 0 and 2, then every 6 months for 5 courses) with daily azathioprine after cyclophosphamide induction for new and relapsing patients [140]. The adult patients received azathioprine or RTX. RTX was significantly better than AZA since at 28 months major relapse had occurred in 29% of patients in the azathioprine group and in 5% of patients in the RTX group, without significant differences in severe adverse events. In considering the results of this trial, it is important to note that only a cyclophosphamide induction was used. This trial does not provide information about RTX maintenance after RTX induction. The RTX dose utilized was also different from previous trials (500 mg twice at a 14-day interval after remission is achieved, with subsequent 500 mg doses every 6 months for 5 courses), while the azathioprine dose was tapered between months 12–22, possibly to a sub-therapeutic dose [118]. The RITAZAREM trial investigated the use of RTX for the treatment of relapses in adults with AAV. RTX in conjunction with glucocorticoids demonstrated a high level of efficacy for the reinduction of remission in patients with AAV who have relapsed [141]. Seventy-nine percent and 36% had previously received cyclophosphamide and RTX, respectively. The vast majority (90%) achieved remission by 4 months. The use of RTX therefore appears promising, although not validated in a pediatric cohort, and the optimal dose and timing are not yet established.

The use of a B cell modulator, belimumab (a monoclonal antibody directed against BAFF, a B cell survival factor), has been investigated in the BREVAS study [142]. In this double-blind, placebo-controlled study, adult patients with AAV were randomized 1:1 to receive azathioprine (2 mg/kg/day), low-dose oral glucocorticoids (≤10 mg/day), and either IV belimumab (10 mg/kg) or placebo, following remission induction with RTX or cyclophosphamide along with glucocorticoids. Belimumab, although safe, did not reduce the risk of relapse of vasculitis; therefore, its use is not warranted for maintenance of AAV.

Treatment of Relapses

Relapses are not infrequent in AAV. A relapse is defined as the reactivation of vascular inflammation. It is important to assess the severity of the relapse by identifying which organs are affected. Most guidelines recommend basing treatment on what was used previously at induction and then switching (for example from cyclophosphamide to RTX or vice versa). However, if the patient responded fully to RTX at induction, it can be reasonable to repeat this therapeutic approach [143].

References

1. Jennette JC, Falk RJ, Bacon PA, et al. 2012 Revised International Chapel Hill consensus conference nomenclature of vasculitides. In: Arthritis Rheum; 2013. pp. 1–11.
2. Fries JF, Hunder GG, Bloch DA, et al. The American College of Rheumatology 1990 criteria for the classification of vasculitis: summary. Arthritis Rheum. 1990;33:1135–6.

3. Luqmani RA, Suppiah R, Grayson PC, Merkel PA, Watts R. Nomenclature and classification of vasculitis - update on the ACR/EULAR diagnosis and classification of vasculitis study (DCVAS). Clin Exp Immunol. 2011;164:11–3.
4. Ozen S, Ruperto N, Dillon MJ, et al. EULAR/ PReS endorsed consensus criteria for the classification of childhood vasculitides. Ann Rheum Dis. 2006;65:936–41.
5. Ozen S, Pistorio A, Iusan SM, et al. EULAR/ PRINTO/PRES criteria for Henoch-Schönlein purpura, childhood polyarteritis nodosa, childhood Wegener granulomatosis and childhood Takayasu arteritis: Ankara 2008. Part II: final classification criteria. Ann Rheum Dis. 2010;69:798–806.
6. Ozen S, Marks SD, Brogan P, et al. European consensus-based recommendations for diagnosis and treatment of immunoglobulin A vasculitis-the SHARE initiative. Rheumatol (United Kingdom). 2019;58:1607–16.
7. Dillon MJ, Eleftheriou D, Brogan PA. Medium-size-vessel vasculitis. Pediatr Nephrol. 2010;25:1641–52.
8. Ozen S. The changing face of polyarteritis nodosa and necrotizing vasculitis. Nat Rev Rheumatol. 2017;13:381–6.
9. Eleftheriou D, Dillon MJ, Tullus K, Marks SD, Pilkington CA, Roebuck DJ, Klein NJ, Brogan PA. Systemic polyarteritis nodosa in the young: a single-center experience over thirty-two years. Arthritis Rheum. 2013;65:2476–85.
10. Hampson LV, Whitehead J, Eleftheriou D, et al. Elicitation of expert prior opinion: application to the MYPAN trial in childhood polyarteritis nodosa. PLoS One. 2015;10(3):e0120981. https://doi.org/10.1371/journal.pone.0120981.
11. Tanaka H, Waga S, Tateyama T, Sugimoto K, Kakizaki Y, Yokoyama M. Acute tubulointerstitial nephritis following intravenous immunoglobulin therapy in a male infant with minimal-change nephrotic syndrome. Tohoku J Exp Med. 1999;189:155–61.
12. Dorval G, Lion M, Guérin S, Krid S, Galmiche-Rolland L, Salomon R, Boyer O. Immunoadsorption in Anti-GBM glomerulonephritis: case report in a child and literature review. Pediatrics. 2017; https://doi.org/10.1542/peds.2016-1733.
13. McAdoo SP, Pusey CD. Antiglomerular basement membrane disease. Semin Respir Crit Care Med. 2018;39:494–503.
14. Liou YT, Huang JL, Ou LS, Lin YH, Yu KH, Luo SF, Ho HH, Liou LB, Yeh KW. Comparison of cryoglobulinemia in children and adults. J Microbiol Immunol Infect. 2013;46:59–64.
15. Calatroni M, Oliva E, Gianfreda D, et al. ANCA-associated vasculitis in childhood: recent advances. Ital J Pediatr. 2017;43(1):1–9. https://doi.org/10.1186/s13052-017-0364-x.
16. Berden AE, Jones RB, Erasmus DD, Walsh M, Noël LH, Ferrario F, Waldherr R, Bruijn JA, Jayne DR, Bajema IM. Tubular lesions predict renal outcome in antineutrophil cytoplasmic antibody-associated glomerulonephritis after rituximab therapy. J Am Soc Nephrol. 2012;23:313–21.
17. Berden AE, Ferrario F, Hagen EC, et al. Histopathologic classification of ANCA-associated glomerulonephritis. J Am Soc Nephrol. 2010;21:1628–36.
18. Quintana LF, Kronbichler A, Blasco M, Zhao M hui, Jayne D (2019) ANCA associated vasculitis: the journey to complement-targeted therapies. Mol Immunol 112:394–398.
19. Noone DG, Twilt M, Hayes WN, Thorner PS, Benseler S, Laxer RM, Parekh RS, Hebert D. The new histopathologic classification of ANCA-associated gn and its association with renal outcomes in childhood. Clin J Am Soc Nephrol. 2014;9:1684–91.
20. Falk R, Jennette J. ANCA small-vessel vasculitis. J Am Soc Nephrol. 1997;8:314–22.
21. Haas M, Eustace JA. Immune complex deposits in ANCA-associated crescentic glomerulonephritis: a study of 126 cases. Kidney Int. 2004;65:2145–52.
22. Manenti L, Vaglio A, Gnappi E, et al. Association of serum C3 concentration and histologic signs of thrombotic microangiopathy with outcomes among patients with ANCA-associated renal vasculitis. Clin J Am Soc Nephrol. 2015;10:2143–51.
23. Villacorta J, Diaz-Crespo F, Acevedo M, Guerrero C, Campos-Martin Y, García-Díaz E, Mollejo M, Fernandez-Juarez G. Glomerular C3d as a novel prognostic marker for renal vasculitis. Hum Pathol. 2016;56:31–9.
24. Nakazawa D, Masuda S, Tomaru U, Ishizu A. Pathogenesis and therapeutic interventions for ANCA-associated vasculitis. Nat Rev Rheumatol. 2019;15:91–101.
25. Lyons PA, Rayner TF, Trivedi S, et al. Genetically distinct subsets within ANCA-associated vasculitis. N Engl J Med. 2012;367:214–23.
26. Merkel PA, Xie G, Monach PA, et al. Identification of functional and expression polymorphisms associated with risk for antineutrophil cytoplasmic autoantibody–associated vasculitis. Arthritis Rheumatol. 2017;69:1054–66.
27. Xie G, Roshandel D, Sherva R, et al. Association of granulomatosis with polyangiitis (Wegener's) with HLA-DPB1*04 and SEMA6A gene variants: Evidence grom genome-wide analysis. Arthritis Rheum. 2013;65:2457–68.
28. Lyons PA, Peters JE, Alberici F, et al. Genome-wide association study of eosinophilic granulomatosis with polyangiitis reveals genomic loci stratified by ANCA status. Nat Commun. 2019;10(1):1–3. https://doi.org/10.1038/s41467-019-12515-9.
29. Rahmattulla C, Mooyaart AL, Van Hooven D, Schoones JW, Bruijn JA, Dekkers OM, Bajema IM. Genetic variants in ANCA-associated vasculitis: a meta-analysis. Ann Rheum Dis. 2016;75:1687–92.
30. Li W, Huang H, Cai M, Yuan T, Sheng Y. Antineutrophil cytoplasmic antibody-associated

30. vasculitis update: genetic pathogenesis. Front Immunol. 2021;12:624848. https://doi.org/10.3389/fimmu.2021.624848.

31. Stegeman CA, Cohen Tervaert JW, Sluiter WJ, Manson WL, De Jong PE, Kallenberg CGM. Association of chronic nasal carriage of Staphylococcus aureus and higher relapse rates in Wegener granulomatosis. Ann Intern Med. 1994;120:12–7.

32. Popa ER, Tervaert JWC. The relation between Staphylococcus aureus and Wegener's granulomatosis: current knowledge and future directions. Intern Med. 2003;42:771–80.

33. Kain R, Exner M, Brandes R, et al. Molecular mimicry in pauci-immune focal necrotizing glomerulonephritis. Nat Med. 2008;14:1088–96.

34. Jennette JC, Falk RJ. Pathogenesis of antineutrophil cytoplasmic autoantibody-mediated disease. Nat Rev Rheumatol. 2014;10:463–73.

35. Pendergraft WF, Niles JL. Trojan horses: drug culprits associated with antineutrophil cytoplasmic autoantibody (ANCA) vasculitis. Curr Opin Rheumatol. 2014;26:42–9.

36. Graf J. Rheumatic manifestations of cocaine use. Curr Opin Rheumatol. 2013;25:50–5.

37. Fujieda M, Hattori M, Kurayama H, Koitabashi Y. Clinical features and outcomes in children with antineutrophil cytoplasmic autoantibody-positive glomerulonephritis associated with propylthiouracil treatment. J Am Soc Nephrol. 2002;13:437–45.

38. Scott J, Hartnett J, Mockler D, Little MA. Environmental risk factors associated with ANCA associated vasculitis: a systematic mapping review. Autoimmun Rev. 2020;19(11):102660. https://doi.org/10.1016/j.autrev.2020.102660.

39. Gómez-Puerta JA, Gedmintas L, Costenbader KH. The association between silica exposure and development of ANCA-associated vasculitis: systematic review and meta-analysis. Autoimmun Rev. 2013;12:1129–35.

40. Schlieben DJ, Korbet SM, Kimura RE, Schwartz MM, Lewis EJ. Pulmonary-renal syndrome in a newborn with placental transmission of ANCAs. Am J Kidney Dis. 2005;45:758–61.

41. Xiao H, Heeringa P, Hu P, Liu Z, Zhao M, Aratani Y, Maeda N, Falk RJ, Jennette JC. Antineutrophil cytoplasmic autoantibodies specific for myeloperoxidase cause glomerulonephritis and vasculitis in mice. J Clin Invest. 2002;110:955–63.

42. Little MA, Smyth CL, Yadav R, Ambrose L, Cook HT, Nourshargh S, Pusey CD. Antineutrophil cytoplasm antibodies directed against myeloperoxidase augment leukocyte-microvascular interactions in vivo. Blood. 2005;106:2050–8.

43. Xu PC, Cui Z, Chen M, Hellmark T, Zhao MH. Comparison of characteristics of natural autoantibodies against myeloperoxidase and anti-myeloperoxidase autoantibodies from patients with microscopic polyangiitis. Rheumatology. 2011;50:1236–43.

44. Roth AJ, Ooi JD, Hess JJ, et al. Epitope specificity determines pathogenicity and detectability in anca-associated vasculitis. J Clin Invest. 2013;123:1773–83.

45. Pendergraft WF, Preston GA, Shah RR, Tropsha A, Carter CW, Jennette JC, Falk RJ. Autoimmunity is triggered by cPR-3(105-201), a protein complementary to human autoantigen proteinase-3. Nat Med. 2004;10:72–9.

46. Preston GA, Pendergraft WF, Falk RJ. New insights that link microbes with the generation of antineutrophil cytoplasmic autoantibodies: the theory of autoantigen complementarity. Curr Opin Nephrol Hypertens. 2005;14:217–22.

47. Petersen HJ, Smith AM. The role of the innate immune system in granulomatous disorders. Front Immunol. 2013;4:120. https://doi.org/10.3389/fimmu.2013.00120.

48. Xiao H, Schreiber A, Heeringa P, Falk RJ, Jennette JC. Alternative complement pathway in the pathogenesis of disease mediated by anti-neutrophil cytoplasmic autoantibodies. Am J Pathol. 2007;170:52–64.

49. Schreiber A, Xiao H, Jennette JC, Schneider W, Luft FC, Kettritz R. C5a receptor mediates neutrophil activation and ANCA-induced glomerulonephritis. J Am Soc Nephrol. 2009;20:289–98.

50. Huugen D, Van Esch A, Xiao H, Peutz-Kootstra CJ, Buurman WA, Tervaert JWC, Jennette JC, Heeringa P. Inhibition of complement factor C5 protects against anti-myeloperoxidase antibody-mediated glomerulonephritis in mice. Kidney Int. 2007;71:646–54.

51. Xing GQ, Chen M, Liu G, Heeringa P, Zhang JJ, Zheng X, Jie E, Kallenberg CGM, Zhao MH. Complement activation is involved in renal damage in human antineutrophil cytoplasmic autoantibody associated pauci-immune vasculitis. J Clin Immunol. 2009;29:282–91.

52. Gou SJ, Yuan J, Chen M, Yu F, Zhao MH. Circulating complement activation in patients with antineutrophil cytoplasmic antibody-associated vasculitis. Kidney Int. 2013;83:129–37.

53. Gou SJ, Yuan J, Wang C, Zhao MH, Chen M. Alternative complement pathway activation products in urine and kidneys of patients with ANCA-associated GN. Clin J Am Soc Nephrol. 2013;8:1884–91.

54. Van Timmeren MM, Chen M, Heeringa P. Review article: Pathogenic role of complement activation in anti-neutrophil cytoplasmic auto-antibody-associated vasculitis. Nephrology. 2009;14:16–25.

55. Morgan MD, Day CJ, Piper KP, Khan N, Harper L, Moss PA, Savage COS. Patients with Wegener's granulomatosis demonstrate a relative deficiency and functional impairment of T-regulatory cells. Immunology. 2010;130:64–73.

56. Rimbert M, Hamidou M, Braudeau C, Puéchal X, Teixeira L, Caillon H, Néel A, Audrain M, Guillevin L, Josien R. Decreased numbers of blood dendritic

57. O'Dell Bunch D, McGregor JG, Khandoobhai NB, et al. Decreased CD5+B cells in active ANCA vasculitis and relapse after rituximab. Clin J Am Soc Nephrol. 2013;8:382–91.

58. Wilde B, Thewissen M, Damoiseaux J, Knippenberg S, Hilhorst M, Van Paassen P, Witzke O, Cohen Tervaert JW. Regulatory B cells in ANCA-associated vasculitis. Ann Rheum Dis. 2013;72:1416–9.

59. Krumbholz M, Specks U, Wick M, Kalled SL, Jenne D, Meinl E. BAFF is elevated in serum of patients with Wegener's granulomatosis. J Autoimmun. 2005;25:298–302.

60. Sanders JSF, Huitma MG, Kallenberg CGM, Stegeman CA. Plasma levels of soluble interleukin 2 receptor, soluble CD30, interleukin 10 and B cell activator of the tumour necrosis factor family during follow-up in vasculitis associated with proteinase 3-antineutrophil cytoplasmic antibodies: associations with disease activity and relapse. Ann Rheum Dis. 2006;65:1484–9.

61. Cabral DA, Canter DL, Muscal E, et al. Comparing presenting clinical features in 48 children with microscopic polyangiitis to 183 children who have granulomatosis with polyangiitis (Wegener's): an ARChiVe cohort study. Arthritis Rheumatol (Hoboken, NJ). 2016;68:2514–26.

62. Akikusa JD, Schneider R, Harvey EA, Hebert D, Thorner PS, Laxer RM, Silverman ED. Clinical features and outcome of pediatric Wegener's granulomatosis. Arthritis Rheum. 2007;57:837–44.

63. Bohm M, Gonzalez Fernandez MI, Ozen S, et al. Clinical features of childhood granulomatosis with polyangiitis (wegener's granulomatosis). Pediatr Rheumatol. 2014;12(1):1–5. https://doi.org/10.1186/1546-0096-12-18.

64. Iudici M, Quartier P, Terrier B, Mouthon L, Guillevin L, Puéchal X. Childhood-onset granulomatosis with polyangiitis and microscopic polyangiitis: systematic review and meta-analysis. Orphanet J Rare Dis. 2016;11:141.

65. Churg J, Strauss L. Allergic granulomatosis, allergic angiitis, and periarteritis nodosa. Am J Pathol. 1951;27:277–301.

66. Cabral DA, Uribe AG, Benseler S, et al. Classification, presentation, and initial treatment of Wegener's granulomatosis in childhood. Arthritis Rheum. 2009;60:3413–24.

67. Gendelman S, Zeft A, Spalding SJ. Childhood-onset eosinophilic granulomatosis with polyangiitis (formerly Churg-Strauss Syndrome): a contemporary single-center cohort. J Rheumatol. 2013;40:929–35.

68. Eleftheriou D, Gale H, Pilkington C, Fenton M, Sebire NJ, Brogan PA. Eosinophilic granulomatosis with polyangiitis in childhood: retrospective experience from a tertiary referral centre in the UK. Rheumatol (United Kingdom). 2016;55:1263–72.

69. Fina A, Dubus JC, Tran A, et al. Eosinophilic granulomatosis with polyangiitis in children: data from the French RespiRare® cohort. Pediatr Pulmonol. 2018;53:1640–50.

70. Luqmani RA, Bacon PA, Moots RJ, Janssen BA, Pall A, Emery P, Savage C, Adu D. Birmingham vasculitis activity score (BVAS) in systemic necrotizing vasculitis. QJM. 1994;87:671–8.

71. Mukhtyar C, Lee R, Brown D, et al. Modification and validation of the Birmingham vasculitis activity score (version 3). Ann Rheum Dis. 2009;68:1827–32.

72. Stone JH, Hoffman GS, Merkel PA, et al. A disease-specific activity index for Wegener's granulomatosis: modification of the birmingham vasculitis activity score. Arthritis Rheum. 2001;44:912–20.

73. Dolezalova P, Price-Kuehne FE, Özen S, et al. Disease activity assessment in childhood vasculitis: development and preliminary validation of the Paediatric Vasculitis Activity Score (PVAS). Ann Rheum Dis. 2013;72:1628–33.

74. Exley AR, Bacon PA, Luqmani RA, Kitas GD, Gordon C, Savage COS, Adu D. Development and initial validation of the vasculitis damage index for the standardized clinical assessment of damage in the systemic vasculitides. Arthritis Rheum. 1997;40:371–80.

75. Dolezalova P, Wilkinson N, Brogan PA, et al. SAT0286 paediatric vasculitis damage index: a new tool for standardised disease assessment. Ann Rheum Dis. 2014;73(suppl 2):696.4–97.

76. Morishita KA, Moorthy LN, Lubieniecka JM, et al. Early outcomes in children with antineutrophil cytoplasmic antibody–associated vasculitis. Arthritis Rheumatol. 2017;69:1470–9.

77. Plumb LA, Oni L, Marks SD, Tullus K. Paediatric anti-neutrophil cytoplasmic antibody (ANCA)-associated vasculitis: an update on renal management. Pediatr Nephrol. 2018;33:25–39.

78. Noone D, Yeung RSM, Hebert D. Outcome of kidney transplantation in pediatric patients with ANCA-associated glomerulonephritis: a single-center experience. Pediatr Nephrol. 2017;32:2343–50.

79. Brogan P, Eleftheriou D. Vasculitis update: pathogenesis and biomarkers. Pediatr Nephrol. 2018;33:187–98.

80. Rodero MP, Crow YJ. Type I interferonâ-mediated monogenic autoinflammation: The type I interferonopathies, a conceptual overview. J Exp Med. 2016;213:2527–38.

81. Melki I, Frémond ML. Type I interferonopathies: from a novel concept to targeted therapeutics. Curr Rheumatol Rep. 2020;22(7):1–4. https://doi.org/10.1007/s11926-020-00909-4.

82. d'Angelo DM, Di Filippo P, Breda L, Chiarelli F. Type I interferonopathies in children: an overview. Front Pediatr. 2021;9:631329. https://doi.org/10.3389/fped.2021.631329.

83. Liu Y, Jesus AA, Marrero B, et al. Activated STING in a vascular and pulmonary syndrome. N Engl J Med. 2014;371:507–18.

84. Volpi S, Insalaco A, Caorsi R, et al. Efficacy and adverse events during janus kinase inhibitor treatment of SAVI syndrome. J Clin Immunol. 2019;39:476–85.

85. Abid Q, Best Rocha A, Larsen CP, Schulert G, Marsh R, Yasin S, Patty-Resk C, Valentini RP, Adams M, Baracco R. APOL1-associated collapsing focal segmental glomerulosclerosis in a patient with stimulator of interferon genes (STING)-associated vasculopathy with onset in infancy (SAVI). Am J Kidney Dis. 2020;75:287–90.

86. Watkin LB, Jessen B, Wiszniewski W, et al. COPA mutations impair ER-Golgi transport and cause hereditary autoimmune-mediated lung disease and arthritis. Nat Genet. 2015;47:654–60.

87. Volpi S, Tsui J, Mariani M, Pastorino C, Caorsi R, Sacco O, Ravelli A, Shum AK, Gattorno M, Picco P. Type I interferon pathway activation in COPA syndrome. Clin Immunol. 2018;187:33–6.

88. Boulisfane-El Khalifi S, Viel S, Lahoche A, et al. COPA syndrome as a cause of lupus nephritis. Kidney Int Reports. 2019;4:1187–9.

89. Vece TJ, Watkin LB, Nicholas SK, et al. Copa syndrome: a novel autosomal dominant immune dysregulatory disease. J Clin Immunol. 2016;36:377–87.

90. Zhou Q, Yang D, Ombrello AK, et al. Early-onset stroke and vasculopathy associated with mutations in ADA2. N Engl J Med. 2014;370:911–20.

91. Navon Elkan P, Pierce SB, Segel R, et al. Mutant adenosine deaminase 2 in a polyarteritis nodosa vasculopathy. N Engl J Med. 2014;370:921–31.

92. Meyts I, Aksentijevich I. Deficiency of adenosine deaminase 2 (DADA2): updates on the phenotype, genetics, pathogenesis, and treatment. J Clin Immunol. 2018;38:569–78.

93. Nanthapisal S, Murphy C, Omoyinmi E, et al. Deficiency of adenosine deaminase type 2: a description of phenotype and genotype in fifteen cases. Arthritis Rheumatol. 2016;68:2314–22.

94. Ombrello AK, Qin J, Hoffmann PM, et al. Treatment strategies for deficiency of adenosine deaminase 2. N Engl J Med. 2019;380:1582–4.

95. Cooray S, Omyinmi E, Hong Y, et al. Anti-tumour necrosis factor treatment for the prevention of ischaemic events in patients with deficiency of adenosine deaminase 2 (DADA2). Rheumatology. 2021;60(9):4373–8. https://doi.org/10.1093/rheumatology/keaa837.

96. McDuffie F, Sams W, Maldonado J, Andreini P, Conn D, Samayoa E. Hypocomplementemia with cutaneous vasculitis and arthritis. Possible immune complex syndrome. Mayo Clin Proc. 1973;48:340–8.

97. Schwartz H, McDuffie F, Black L, Schroeter A, Conn D. Hypocomplementemic urticarial vasculitis. Association with chronic obstructive pulmonary disease. Mayo Clin Proc. 1982;57:231–8.

98. Ion O, Obrișcă B, Ismail G, Sorohan B, Bălănică S, Mircescu G, Sinescu I. Kidney involvement in hypocomplementemic urticarial vasculitis syndrome—a case-based review. J Clin Med. 2020;9:2131.

99. Davis M, Kirby D, Gibson L, Rogers R. Clinicopathologic correlation of hypocomplementemic and normocomplementemic urticarial vasculitis. J Am Acad Dermatol. 1998;38:899–905.

100. Özçakar ZB, Foster J, Diaz-Horta O, Kasapcopur O, Fan YS, Yalçinkaya F, Tekin M. DNASE1L3 mutations in hypocomplementemic urticarial vasculitis syndrome. Arthritis Rheum. 2013;65:2183–9.

101. Eleftheriou D, Brogan PA. Therapeutic advances in the treatment of vasculitis. Pediatr Rheumatol. 2016; https://doi.org/10.1186/s12969-016-0082-8.

102. Eleftheriou D, Dillon MJ, Brogan PA. Advances in childhood vasculitis. Curr Opin Rheumatol. 2009;21:411–8.

103. Tullus K, Marks SD. Vasculitis in children and adolescents: clinical presentation, etiopathogenesis, and treatment. Pediatr Drugs. 2009;11:375–80.

104. Jayne D, Rasmussen N, Andrassy K, et al. A randomized trial of maintenance therapy for vasculitis associated with antineutrophil cytoplasmic autoantibodies. N Engl J Med. 2003;349:36–44.

105. Nachman P, Hogan S, Jennette J, Falk R. Treatment response and relapse in antineutrophil cytoplasmic autoantibody-associated microscopic polyangiitis and glomerulonephritis. J Am Soc Nephrol. 1996;7:33–9.

106. De Groot K, Harper L, Jayne DRW, et al. Pulse versus daily oral cyclophosphamide for induction of remission in antineutrophil cytoplasmic antibody-associated vasculitis: a randomized trial. Ann Intern Med. 2009; https://doi.org/10.7326/0003-4819-150-10-200905190-00004.

107. Walters GD, Willis NS, Craig JC. Interventions for renal vasculitis in adults. A systematic review. BMC Nephrol. 2010; https://doi.org/10.1186/1471-2369-11-12.

108. Hattori M, Kurayama H, Koitabashi Y. Antineutrophil cytoplasmic autoantibody-associated glomerulonephritis in children. J Am Soc Nephrol. 2001;12:1493–500.

109. Yu F, Huang JP, Zou WZ, Zhao MH. The clinical features of anti-neutrophil cytoplasmic antibody-associated systemic vasculitis in Chinese children. Pediatr Nephrol. 2006;21:497–502.

110. Siomou E, Tramma D, Bowen C, Milford DV. ANCA-associated glomerulonephritis/systemic vasculitis in childhood: clinical features-outcome. Pediatr Nephrol. 2012;27:1911–20.

111. Radhakrishnan J, Cattran DC. The KDIGO practice guideline on glomerulonephritis: reading between the (guide)lines-application to the individual patient. Kidney Int. 2012;82:840–56.

112. Jayne DRW, Gaskin G, Rasmussen N, et al. Randomized trial of plasma exchange or high-dosage methylprednisolone as adjunctive therapy for severe renal vasculitis. J Am Soc Nephrol. 2007;18:2180–8.

113. Arulkumaran N, Jawad S, Smith SW, Harper L, Brogan P, Pusey CD, Salama AD. Long- term outcome of paediatric patients with ANCA vasculi-

113. tis. Pediatr Rheumatol. 2011;9(1):1–7. https://doi.org/10.1186/1546-0096-9-12.
114. Jones RB, Cohen Tervaert JW, Hauser T, et al. Rituximab versus cyclophosphamide in ANCA-associated renal vasculitis. N Engl J Med. 2010;363:211–20.
115. Stone JH. Rituximab versus cyclophosphamide for ANCA-associated vasculitis. J fur Miner. 2010;17:168.
116. Specks U, Merkel PA, Seo P, et al. Efficacy of remission-induction regimens for ANCA-associated vasculitis. N Engl J Med. 2013;369:417–27.
117. Brogan P, Cleary G, Hersh A, et al. Pediatric open-label clinical study of rituximab for the treatment of granulomatosis with polyangiitis and microscopic polyangiitis. Rheumatology. 2019;58(Supplement_2):kez063-044. https://doi.org/10.1093/rheumatology/kez063.044.
118. Akamine K, Punaro M. Biologics for childhood systemic vasculitis. Pediatr Nephrol. 2019;34:2295–309.
119. Basu B, Mahapatra TKS, Mondal N. Favourable renal survival in paediatric microscopic polyangiitis: efficacy of a novel treatment algorithm. Nephrol Dial Transplant. 2015;30(Suppl 1):i113–8.
120. Roberts DM, Jones RB, Smith RM, Alberici F, Kumaratne DS, Burns S, Jayne DRW. Rituximab-associated hypogammaglobulinemia: Incidence, predictors and outcomes in patients with multi-system autoimmune disease. J Autoimmun. 2015;57:60–5.
121. Jennette JC, Harrington JT, Kausz A, Narayan G, Ucci AA, Levey AS, Uhlig K, Gill J, Balakrishnan V. Rapidly progressive crescentic glomerulonephritis. Kidney Int. 2003;63:1164–77.
122. Stilmant MM, Bolton WK, Sturgill BC, Schmitt GW, Couser WG. Crescentic glomerulonephritis without immune deposits: clinicopathologic features. Kidney Int. 1979;15:184–95.
123. Noone D, Hebert D, Licht C. Pathogenesis and treatment of ANCA-associated vasculitis—a role for complement. Pediatr Nephrol. 2018;33(1):1–11. https://doi.org/10.1007/s00467-016-3475-5.
124. Lockwood CM, Pinching AJ, Sweny P, Rees AJ, Pussell B, Uff J, Peters DK. Plasma-exchange and immunosuppression in the treatment of fulminating immune-complex crescentic nephritis. Lancet. 1977;309:63–7.
125. Yates M, Watts RA, Bajema IM, et al. EULAR/ERA-EDTA recommendations for the management of ANCA-associated vasculitis. Ann Rheum Dis. 2016;75:1583–94.
126. Pusey CD, Rees AJ, Evans DJ, Peters DK, Lockwood CM. Plasma exchange in focal necrotizing glomerulonephritis without anti-GBM antibodies. Kidney Int. 1991;40:757–63.
127. Szpirt WM. Plasma exchange in antineutrophil cytoplasmic antibody-associated vasculitis-A 25-year perspective. Nephrol Dial Transplant. 2015;30:i146–9.

128. Walsh M, Merkel PA, Peh C-A, et al. Plasma exchange and glucocorticoids in severe ANCA-associated vasculitis. N Engl J Med. 2020;382:622–31.
129. Rovin BH, Adler SG, Barratt J, et al. KDIGO 2021 clinical practice guideline for the management of glomerular diseases. Kidney Int. 2021;100:S1–S276.
130. Han F, Liu G, Zhang X, Li X, He Q, He X, Li Q, Wang S, Wang H, Chen J. Effects of mycophenolate mofetil combined with corticosteroids for induction therapy of microscopic polyangiitis. Am J Nephrol. 2011;33:185–92.
131. Hu W, Liu C, Xie H, Chen H, Liu Z, Li L. Mycophenolate mofetil versus cyclophosphamide for inducing remission of ANCA vasculitis with moderate renal involvement. Nephrol Dial Transplant. 2008;23:1307–12.
132. Jones RB, Hiemstra TF, Ballarin J, et al. Mycophenolate mofetil versus cyclophosphamide for remission induction in ANCA-associated vasculitis: a randomised, non-inferiority trial. Ann Rheum Dis. 2018; https://doi.org/10.1136/annrheumdis-2018-214245.
133. Jayne DRW, Bruchfeld AN, Harper L, et al. Randomized trial of C5a receptor inhibitor avacopan in ANCA-associated vasculitis. J Am Soc Nephrol. 2017;28:2756–67.
134. Merkel PA, Niles J, Jimenez R, et al. Adjunctive treatment with avacopan, an oral C5a receptor inhibitor, in patients with antineutrophil cytoplasmic antibody–associated vasculitis. ACR Open Rheumatol. 2020;2:662–71.
135. Jayne DRW, Merkel PA, Schall TJ, Bekker P. Avacopan for the treatment of ANCA-associated vasculitis. N Engl J Med. 2021;384:599–609.
136. De Graeff N, Groot N, Brogan P, et al. European consensus-based recommendations for the diagnosis and treatment of rare paediatric vasculitides-the SHARE initiative. Rheumatol (United Kingdom). 2019;58:656–71.
137. Karras A, Pagnoux C, Haubitz M, De Groot K, Puechal X, Tervaert JWC, Segelmark M, Guillevin L, Jayne D. Randomised controlled trial of prolonged treatment in the remission phase of ANCA-associated vasculitis. Ann Rheum Dis. 2017;76:1662–8.
138. Metzler C, Miehle N, Manger K, Iking-Konert C, de Groot K, Hellmich B, Gross WL, Reinhold-Keller E. Elevated relapse rate under oral methotrexate versus leflunomide for maintenance of remission in Wegener's granulomatosis. Rheumatology. 2007;46:1087–91.
139. Hiemstra TF, Walsh M, Mahr A, et al. Mycophenolate mofetil vs azathioprine for remission maintenance in antineutrophil cytoplasmic antibody-associated vasculitis: a randomized controlled trial. JAMA. 2010;304:2381–8.
140. Guillevin L, Pagnoux C, Karras A, et al. Rituximab versus azathioprine for maintenance

in ANCA-associated vasculitis. N Engl J Med. 2014;371:1771–80.
141. Smith RM, Jones RB, Specks U, et al. Rituximab as therapy to induce remission after relapse in ANCA-associated vasculitis. Ann Rheum Dis. 2020;79:1243–9.
142. Jayne D, Blockmans D, Luqmani R, Moiseev S, Ji B, Green Y, Hall L, Roth D, Henderson RB, Merkel PA. Efficacy and safety of belimumab and azathio-prine for maintenance of remission in antineutrophil cytoplasmic antibody–associated vasculitis: a randomized controlled study. Arthritis Rheumatol. 2019;71:952–63.
143. Jariwala M, Laxer RM. Childhood GPA, EGPA, and MPA. Clin Immunol. 2020;211:108325. https://doi.org/10.1016/j.clim.2019.108325.
144. Geary D, Schaefer F. Pediatric kidney disease. 2016.

Lupus Nephritis

26

Stephen D. Marks, Matko Marlais, and Kjell Tullus

Introduction

Juvenile onset systemic lupus erythematosus (JSLE) is a lifelong, life-limiting, multi-system, autoimmune disorder, which is episodic in nature with a broad spectrum of clinical and immunological manifestations. JSLE is characterised by widespread inflammation of blood vessels and connective tissues affecting the skin, joints, kidneys, heart, lungs, nervous and other systems. There is a higher rate and more severe organ involvement in children than in adults (especially with respect to haematological and renal disease) [1–4]. Renal involvement with biopsy-proven lupus nephritis (LN) occurs in up to 80% of all cases of JSLE and is a major determinant of the prognosis. We currently have an increasing armamentarium of immunosuppressive agents that can be used to treat active disease with newer agents on the horizon. However, there is still a significant morbidity and mortality for severe disease with considerable physical and psychosocial morbidity due to the variable, and often progressive, clinical course of JSLE. This results from both the sequelae of disease activity and the side-effects of medications, including the infectious risks from over-immunosuppression, and longer-term risks with accelerated atherosclerosis [5].

There are differences between clinical diagnosis of JSLE and the utility of classification criteria of patients, which can be used in clinical trials. The American College of Rheumatology classification criteria for SLE gives 95% sensitivity and 96% specificity in clinical practice when 4 of 11 criteria are met (Table 26.1) [6, 7]. The Systemic Lupus International Collaborating Clinics (SLICC group) revised and validated the ACR classification criteria with improved methodology in order to improve clinical relevance and incorporate better understanding of the aetiopathogenesis and immunology of SLE [8]. These classification criteria have been validated in multicenter studies of children and young people with SLE [9, 10]. There has been a recent adaptation with the development of a Childhood Lupus Improvement Index (CHILI) as a tool to measure response to therapy in JSLE [11].

S. D. Marks (✉) · M. Marlais · K. Tullus
Department of Pediatric Nephrology, Great Ormond
Street Hospital for Children NHS Foundation Trust,
London, UK
e-mail: stephen.marks@gosh.nhs.uk;
matko.marlais@gosh.nhs.uk;
kjell.tullus@gosh.nhs.uk

© The Author(s), under exclusive license to Springer Nature Switzerland AG 2023
F. Schaefer, L. A. Greenbaum (eds.), *Pediatric Kidney Disease*,
https://doi.org/10.1007/978-3-031-11665-0_26

Table 26.1 American College of Rheumatology Criteria for classification of SLE

1. **Malar rash**
2. **Discoid rash**
3. **Photosensitivity**
4. **Oral ulcers**
5. **Arthritis**
6. **Serositis**
   Pleuritis
   Pericarditis
7. **Renal disorder**
   Proteinuria (>0.5 g/day) or persistently 3+
   Red blood cell casts
8. **Neurological disorder**
   Seizures
   Psychosis (after excluding other causes)
9. **Hematological disorder**
   Hemolytic anemia
   Leucopenia (<4 × 10^9/L on two occasions)
   Lymphopenia (<1.5 × 10^9/L on two occasions)
   Thrombocytopenia (<100 × 10^9/L)
10. **Immunological disorder**
    Elevated anti-double stranded DNA
    Elevated anti-Smith antibodies
    Positive antiphospholipid antibodies (previously lupus erythematosus cell tests or false positive *Treponema pallidum* immobilisation/Venereal Disease Reference Laboratory)
11. **Elevated anti-nuclear antibodies (after exclusion of drug-induced lupus)**

Epidemiology

JSLE accounts for up to 20% of all SLE cases, with epidemiological studies demonstrating a minimum incidence in a paediatric population of 0.28 per 100,000 children at risk per year [12] with a prevalence in children and adults from various epidemiological studies of between 12.0 and 50.8 per 100,000 [13–20]. However, SLE has been reported to be more common in children from China, Hong Kong and Taiwan and three times more frequent in Afro-Caribbean than Caucasian children [21, 22]. The prevalence is increased in minority ethnic backgrounds in the United Kingdom where patients were diagnosed sooner as age at diagnosis was lowest (but not age at symptom onset) in Black African/Caribbean patients compared to White Caucasians [23]. In addition, the severity of renal and neuro-

psychiatric lupus is increased in Afro-Caribbean children [24]. Asian and Afro-Caribbean children are over six times more likely to be affected when compared to Caucasian children in the United Kingdom [25]. SLE is more prevalent in females of childbearing age, possibly due to the hormonal influences, and is commoner over the age of 10 years [26, 27].

Etiopathogenesis

SLE is a multifactorial disorder with multigenic inheritance and various environmental factors implicated in its etiopathogenesis with abnormal regulation of cell-mediated and humoral immunity that lead to tissue damage. The developing immune system is immature compared to adults and the heterogeneity of the clinical manifestations probably reflects the complexity of the disease pathogenesis.

The immune system in SLE is characterised by a complex interplay between overactive B cells, abnormally activated T cells and antigen-presenting cells, which lead to the production of an array of inflammatory cytokines, apoptotic cells, diverse autoantibodies and immune complexes. They in turn activate effector cells and the complement system leading to tissue injury and damage; these are the hallmarks of the clinical manifestations [28]. Several autoantibodies against cell wall components or circulating proteins can produce specific disease manifestations. However, it is interesting that some healthy children have positive ANA titres and that 88% of adult SLE patients have autoantibodies (including ANA, anti-dsDNA and anti-Smith) present up to 9.4 years before SLE is ever diagnosed [29]. It is generally assumed that anti-dsDNA antibodies play an important role in the pathogenesis of LN. This is because an increase in anti-dsDNA titre often precedes onset of renal disease, immune deposits are present in glomeruli and eluates of glomeruli are enriched for anti-dsDNA. However, the classical concept of deposition of DNA-anti-DNA complexes inciting glomerular inflammation is questionable as free, naked, DNA is not present in the circulation and injection of these complexes hardly leads to glomerular localisation. The pathogenicity of anti-DNA has been proven with circulating immune complexes, in situ immune complexes, direct binding to renal and non-renal antigens, penetration into cells, and stimulation of cytokines in the form of immune complexes.

Neutrophil extracellular traps (NETs) are fibrous networks found in different clinical situations from infection to malignancy and from atherosclerosis to autoimmune diseases, such as SLE, where there is an imbalance between the process by which NETs are formed, called NETosis and their degradation. The key players in NETosis are neutrophils, interleukin-8 and anti-neutrophil cytoplasmic antibodies where prolonged exposure to NETs increases the change of organ damage. Neutrophils accumulate in the kidneys of patients with LN where the pathogenesis may be due to neutrophil products and low-density granulocytes [30].

Genomic and gene expression studies in patients with SLE have revealed novel gene mutations and cytokine alterations that may explain many of the features of the disease as well as the genetic susceptibility. There is a familial incidence of SLE in 12–15% of cases with a 10–20-fold increased risk of developing the disease if a sibling is affected compared to the general population (prevalence increases from 0.4% of populations up to 3.5% if there is a first degree relative with SLE) [14]. The concordance rate of SLE in monozygous twins is 24% compared with 2% in heterozygous pairs highlighting the importance of genetic (including HLA haplotypes, complement components and Fcγ receptor polymorphisms) and environmental factors in the etiology of SLE [31–34].

The genetics of SLE is now better understood with inroads made in the last decade in identification of susceptible loci, as there is a complex, multifactorial inheritance with associated environmental factors. Genetic linkage studies using microsatellite markers and single nucleotide polymorphisms have identified at least seven loci displaying significant linkage to SLE, including 1q23 (FcγRIIA, FcγRIIB, FcγRIIIA), 1q25-31, 1q41-42, 2q35-37, 4p16-15.2, 6p11-21 (MHC haplotypes), and 16q12. Genome-wide association studies have revealed further loci which are associated with susceptibility to lupus and specifically to LN [35]. New loci continue to be discovered and relate to various biological pathways associated with lupus risk, for example B-cell receptor signaling and CTLA4 co-stimulation for T-cell activation [36]. Findings from such genetics studies not only help further understanding of etiopathogenesis to develop new therapeutic options, but also may enable better diagnosis and prognostication in the future, with the publication of genetic risk scores to aid prognostication which may become applicable in future clinical practice as genetic technology advances [37].

Complement activation is involved in tissue damage with initial murine lupus models and later human studies revealing homozygous deficiencies of the components of the classical complement pathway (C1q, C1r, C1s, C2 and C4) predispose to the development of SLE. The complement system is an important part of the immune system which when dysregulated can result in the development of SLE, which occurs in 75% and 90% of patients with complete deficiencies of C4 and C1q, respectively [38]. Although initially anti-C1q was neither specific nor sensitive for SLE, in vitro testing has shown that anti-C1q is pathogenic in conjunction with complement-fixing antibodies and immune complexes with an increased prevalence in LN. Anti-C1q auto-antibodies are strongly associated with renal involvement in SLE and deposit in glomeruli together with C1q [39]. Anti-C1q antibodies are especially pathogenic in patients with SLE as they induce overt renal disease in the context of glomerular immune complex disease [40].

There are profound alterations in the B cell compartments of both children and adults with SLE [41, 42] with characteristic hypergammaglobulinemia and increased serum autoantibody titres, explaining why B cell depletion may be an effective therapy [43, 44]. In addition to autoantibodies and immune complexes, autoreactive T cells cause tissue damage in SLE with evidence of alterations in human SLE T cell signalling molecules and loss of self-tolerance [45]. Compared to healthy T cells, there are increased and accelerated signaling responses in T cells from patients with SLE with hyper-reactivity to antigenic triggers, which may be due to genetic influences [46, 47]. Many cytokines, including interferon and interleukins (IL-6, IL10, IL12 (p40) and IL-18), which are elevated in the serum of SLE patients, correlate with disease activity [48].

DNA microarray technology has helped in understanding some of the complex pathogenesis of SLE through genome-wide profiling and earlier studies using microarray analysis of peripheral blood mononuclear cells (PBMCs). There is evidence of dysregulation of inflammatory cytokines, chemokines, and immune response-related genes, as well as genes involved in apoptosis, signal transduction, and the cell cycle. Interferon (IFN)-regulated genes are highly overexpressed in the peripheral blood and kidney glomeruli, supporting a crucial role for interferon in SLE. Future studies focusing on target tissues or organs in SLE may further contribute to our understanding of the etiopathogenesis while providing new targets for therapy [49].

Type I interferons are associated with SLE and genes that are regulated by IFN-alpha are upregulated in JSLE patients, with gene deletion of the IFN-alpha/beta receptor in experimental lupus-like NZB mice resulting in reduced disease activity (although conversely, IFN-beta is a well-established treatment in multiple sclerosis). There are several underlying mechanisms of IFN-beta therapy involving cellular (decreased T cell proliferation and infiltration of leucocytes into the kidney) and humoral (decrease in IgG3 isotypes) immune responses and a reduction in nephrogenic cytokines have been identified. IFN-beta treatment of LN in MRL-Fas(lpr) mice is beneficial and suggests that IFN-beta may be a therapeutic candidate for subtypes of human SLE [50]. IFN-alpha-inducible proteins represent a novel class of autoantigens in murine lupus, and experiments suggest additional roles for IFN-alpha in SLE [51].

The increase in autoantigens in SLE may be due to impaired immune complex clearance and apoptosis. There is evidence of defective clearance of apoptotic cells in some SLE patients, due to the genetic deficiency of molecules, including complement component deficiencies, with auto-antigens undergoing structural modifications during the process of apoptosis that may induce immunogenicity [52]. The development of SLE may be attributable to genetic susceptibility with changes in the hormonal milieu, environmental, pharmaceutical and toxic agents (including crystalline silica, solvents and pesticides) [53]. However, there is also an association with infectious conditions influencing the developing immune system of children who develop SLE, including Epstein-Barr virus [54, 55].

Clinical Presentation

Children and young people with JSLE have different clinical presentations, although typically there are non-specific symptoms of being generally unwell with fatigue, malaise, lethargy, aches, pains, episodic fever, anorexia, nausea, vomiting and weight loss with a typical butterfly rash over a period of a few weeks or months. Most organ systems can be involved (Table 26.2) [56] although unusual presentations are sometimes encountered, which is why SLE has been called one of the great mimickers [57]. In view of the relatively low incidence of JSLE compared to many other paediatric

Table 26.2 Presenting symptoms of SLE

Malaise, weight loss, growth retardation	96%
Cutaneous abnormalities	96%
Hematological abnormalities	91%
Fever	84%
Lupus nephritis	84%
Musculoskeletal complaints	82%
Pleural/pulmonary disease	67%
Hepatosplenomegaly and/or lymphadenopathy	58%
Neurological disease	49%
Other disease manifestations (including cardiac, ocular, gastro-intestinal, Raynaud's phenomenon)	13–38%

Used with permission of Springer Science + Business Media from Cameron [56]

health problems, there can be a significant delay between onset of symptoms and eventual diagnosis. Pediatricians require a high index of suspicion to ensure this disease is not missed.

The majority of children with SLE present during their adolescence. From one of the largest cohort of 201 children with SLE from Toronto, Canada, 6 children (3%) presented before the age of 6 years, 41 (20%) between 6 and 10 years, 62 (31%) between 11 and 13 years and 92 between 14 and 18 years of age [58]. There was a female predominance of 80%, with a slightly higher proportion of male patients than in adulthood.

Lupus Nephritis

There is evidence of renal involvement in up to 60–80% of children and young people with SLE close to the onset of the disease [56]. In a review of the presentation of LN from different studies involving 208 children, 55% presented with nephrotic syndrome and 43% with proteinuria of lesser degrees (Table 26.3). Most children have microscopic haematuria while few (1.4%) presented with macroscopic haematuria. Fifty percent of children and young people have impaired renal function at onset while only 1.4% have acute kidney injury requiring renal replacement therapy. A small proportion will present with a rapidly progressive glomerulonephritis with biopsy-proven crescentic glomerulonephritis. Hypertension was found in 40% of children.

Table 26.3 Presenting features of lupus nephritis

Nephrotic syndrome (>3 g/day)	55%
Proteinuria (<3 g/day)	43%
Macroscopic haematuria	1.4%
Microscopic haematuria	79%
Hypertension	40%
Reduced GFR (<80 mL/min/1.73 m^2)	50%
Acute renal failure	1.4%

Used with permission of Springer Science + Business Media from Cameron [56]

Other Organ Systems

Dermatological

The butterfly or malar rash is the classical rash over the cheeks and nose with photosensitivity to sunlight. However, other rashes can be present, including maculopapular eruptions or purpuric rashes, discoid lesions, livedo reticularis, urticaria and more severe cutaneous vasculitis with ulceration, including mucosal ulceration. Hair loss and brown discolouration of the nails are common findings.

Cerebral

Neurological symptoms, including headache, migraines, seizures and mood disorders are among the most severe manifestations in SLE. There are more severe forms of cerebral lupus with ataxia, chorea, cerebrovascular accidents and deteriorating level of consciousness. The psychiatric symptoms can range from fatigue and depression to confusion, delirium, frank psychosis, hallucinations and catatonic states. Poor academic achievement is a common problem of multifactorial origin that is important to address in these children and young people [59].

Haematological

Coombs-positive haemolytic anaemia, leucopenia, thrombocytopenia and pancytopenia are common findings in children with SLE. Erythrocyte sedimentation rate (ESR) is markedly raised in most children with SLE, while high C-reactive protein (CRP) is found in only a small minority. Therefore, CRP can be helpful in differentiating between flares of lupus disease activity or an infectious complication, such as septicaemia due to the disease or treatment.

Rheumatological

Generalised pain involving the musculo-skeletal system is a very common finding in SLE patients due to myalgia and arthralgia, with severe arthritis less common.

Other Organs

All serous membranes including pleura and pericardium are frequently affected so presentation may be with dyspnoea or pleuropericardial and intermittent chest pain. Hepatosplenomegaly and lymphadenopathy are commonly found in children and young people with SLE. Growth delay is often seen in children, partly related to pubertal delay. Primary and secondary amenorrhoea are manifestations of SLE and LN, but also complications of high doses of cyclophosphamide treatment.

Antiphospholipid Syndrome

Antiphospholipid syndrome (APS) was first described in 1987 as an autoimmune disorder characterised by hypercoagulability of any blood vessel size or type of any organ with the presence of antiphospholipid antibodies [60–62]. Thromboembolism results from the involvement of larger vessels (arteries and veins), whereas thrombotic microangiopathy results from involvement of smaller vessels (capillaries, arterioles and venules). APS with anticardiolipin antibodies and/or lupus anticoagulant are found in 65% of children and young people with SLE [63]. Livedo reticularis has been documented as a marker of APS with increasing tendency to develop both venous and arterial thrombosis. Primary APS is rare in children and is unlikely to progress to SLE. APS is an independent risk factor for more severe renal disease due to microangiopathy in the kidneys and may require treatment as outlined below.

Classification Criteria

The American College of Rheumatology (ACR) classification criteria are utilised in classifying and not diagnosing patients with SLE (Table 26.1). The diagnosis of SLE is made in typical cases with classical organ involvement, elevated autoantibodies and hypocomplementaemia. However, in some cases, the initial diagnosis is more difficult due to the evolution of disease and these cases may not initially fulfil the criteria developed by ACR which have been refined for children [6, 7]. They consist of 11 different criteria of which four should be fulfilled for the diagnosis of SLE; however, meeting these criteria is not sufficient for a diagnosis of SLE because many children with other diseases can also formally match a number of these criteria.

The Systemic Lupus International Collaborating Clinics (SLICC) classification criteria for SLE was published in 2012 [8] where patients are classified if they have biopsy-proven LN with either positive ANA or anti-dsDNA antibodies or at least four criteria (at least one clinical [acute and chronic cutaneous lupus, oral or nasal ulceration, non-scarring alopecia, arthritis, serositis, renal, neurologic, haemolytic anaemia, leucopenia and thrombocytopenia] and one laboratory [ANA, anti-dsDNA, anti-Smith, anti-phospholipid antibodies, hypocomplementaemia (C3, C4, CH50) and direct Coombs test (which is not counted if haemolytic anaemia is present)] criteria and this has now been validated in children [9].

Disease Activity Scoring Systems

There are various disease activity and damage scoring systems, which are very helpful in monitoring disease activity and damage in children and adolescents with SLE with respect to both clinical long-term follow-up and scientific studies. Scales of indices of disease activity continue to evolve and include SLEDAI (Systemic Lupus

Investigations

The initial investigations of a child with suspected SLE include haematological, biochemical and immunological investigations. Further investigations are warranted depending on organ involvement so a percutaneous renal biopsy and imaging of relevant organ systems are often required.

Blood Investigations

The initial blood test should include a full blood count with a blood film, ESR and reticulocyte count. Anaemia, leucopenia and thrombocytopenia are common findings during active disease that normally improve with effective treatment. Iron studies should also be considered when there is anemia, but caution must be used in the interpretation of these in the setting of systemic inflammation. The leucocyte count, in particular the neutrophil count, should be monitored during active immunosuppressive treatment as the presence of neutropenia influences the doses of immunosuppressive therapies. However, lymphopenia is often seen with treatment and is mostly regarded as a "desired" side effect, which can sometimes be a marker of the effectiveness of treatment. ESR is a marker of disease activity, which can be clinically useful, although it is not uncommon for it to be markedly elevated even during clinical and serological remission. A direct Coombs test should be performed to look for evidence of haemolysis. Macrophage activation syndrome should be screened for in those children and young people with unexplained fever with check of ferritin, lactate dehydrogenase and consideration of bone marrow aspirate and trephine biopsy to exclude malignancy.

The biochemistry profile should include estimation of renal function with plasma creatinine and urea, serum electrolytes, bone, thyroid and liver function tests (including serum albumin), pancreatic enzymes, 25-hydroxyvitamin D levels and CRP (where sepsis is clinically suspected). Creatinine kinase may be useful if evidence of myalgia and parathyroid hormone level when there is evidence of chronic kidney disease. It is useful to calculate the estimated glomerular filtration rate using the Schwartz formula [65].

Immunology Testing

There is evidence of immune dysregulation in almost all children with SLE with positive immunological tests and anti-nuclear antibodies (ANA). ANA can sometimes be a non-specific finding but the use of anti-double-stranded DNA (dsDNA) and the extractable nuclear antibodies (ENA) and C1q levels and anti-C1q antibody testing increases the specificity (Table 26.4). The

Table 26.4 Auto-antibodies in patients with lupus nephritis

	Frequency	Specificity	Association with disease activity
Anti-dsDNA	40–90%	High	Yes
Anti-SSA/Ro	35%	Low	No
Anti-SSB/La	15%	Low	No
Anti-Sm	5–30%	High	No
Anti-C1q	80–100%	High	Yes

dsDNA double stranded DNA, *Anti-SSA/Ro* anti-Sjögren's syndrome A, *Anti-SSB/La* anti-Sjögren's syndrome B, *Anti-Sm* Anti-Smith, *Anti-C1q* Anti-complement factor C1q

pathogenic significance of these antibodies is debated and they can be found in serum sometimes several years before the development of symptoms [29]. However, it is clear that dsDNA and anti-C1q can be used to monitor disease activity, as a marker of improvement or a pending flare of disease. Anti-C1q antibodies have also been shown to predict more severe renal involvement [66]. Knowledge of patients' VZV IgG levels is important for future exposure to varicella. In some settings where the prevalence of tuberculosis is high, the Quantiferon-TB (interferon gamma release assay) may also be indicated. Antibodies against aquaporin-4 (AQP4) and myelin oligodendrocyte glycoprotein (MOG) may be helpful in patients with cerebral lupus.

Complement C3 and C4 are mostly reduced during the active phases of disease and can also be useful markers of disease activity, although some patients with inherited complement deficiencies may never normalise their serum values. Anticardiolipin antibodies and lupus anticoagulant should be regularly monitored. Hypergammaglobulinaemia is a feature of SLE and it is useful to monitor serum immunoglobulins, especially in patients treated with B-cell depletion with intravenous (IV) rituximab. It remains controversial whether hypogammaglobulinaemia should be supplemented with IV immunoglobulin if patients are free of infections. B-lymphocyte counts should be monitored in children treated with IV rituximab by measuring the number of CD19 positive cells.

Urine Investigations

Early morning urine should be regularly monitored in all children and young people with SLE with urinalysis by dipstick performed for haematuria and proteinuria. Urine microscopy is also helpful in looking for red blood cells and casts during the acute phase of LN. Some standardised measurement of proteinuria or albuminuria should be regularly followed, which in most centres is carried out by analysing an early

morning spot urine sample relating the urine excretion of protein or albumin to the urine levels of creatinine. Evidence of tubular dysfunction may help to identify LN prior to the onset of albuminuria by measuring NAG (N-acetyl-beta-D-glucosaminidase):creatinine ratio, RBP (retinol binding protein):creatinine ratio or other tubular markers [67].

Other Investigations

It is important to base treatment decisions on the histopathology of percutaneous renal biopsies as it has been shown that the severity of the renal involvement sometimes is difficult to predict from clinical symptoms and signs. Estimated or formal measurements of glomerular filtration rate should be performed when there is a clinical suspicion of impaired renal function. Even in patients with unimpaired GFR the histological findings can be significant and therefore a "normal" eGFR or serum creatinine should not be overly reassuring. Pulmonary function tests, electrocardiography, echocardiography and chest X-rays are important investigations in selected children. Electroencephalography and cerebral imaging with cranial MRI and MRA is advocated in children with neuropsychiatric evidence of cerebral lupus, when lumbar puncture examining cerebrospinal fluid may be performed in appropriate cases.

Follow-Up

Each child should at every clinic visit have a full clinical evaluation including weight, height and a disease activity score (as above). They should have their blood pressure monitored and their urine tested for proteinuria and haematuria. Regular blood tests should include full blood count, ESR, CRP, renal and liver function tests, electrolytes, C3 and C4, and autoantibodies, including dsDNA. Anticardiolipin antibodies and in particular in children treated with rituximab immunoglobulins and lymphocyte subsets should be regularly monitored. Fasting blood lipids including cholesterol, triglycerides, HDL, LDL and VLDL should be monitored at least once annually. Bone density should be measured in children with long-term daily corticosteroid therapy on a regular basis.

Histological Classification of Lupus Nephritis

The histological classification of LN was initially formatted in 1975 by the World Health Organisation (WHO) and modified in 1982 and 1995. It describes the spectrum of LN as the type and extent of renal lesion and provides information on the immunosuppression required and prognosis. There was a revision of this classification by the International Society of Nephrology (ISN) and Renal Pathology Society (RPS) Working Group after their consensus conference in 2002 in order to standardise definitions, emphasise clinically relevant lesions, and encourage uniform and reproducible reporting between centres (Table 26.5) [68, 69]. This classification facilitates clinical management by increased comprehension of the etiopathogenesis of SLE and guides the clinician with treatment decisions, protocols and clinical research. However, there is widespread variation of the timing, type and distribution of histological lesions, including immune-complex mediated vasculitis, fibrinoid necrosis, inflammatory cell infiltrate and collagen sclerosis.

Table 26.5 International Society of Nephrology and Renal Pathology Society Working Group (ISN/RPS) revised histopathological classification of lupus nephritis

1. **Minimal mesangial lupus nephritis (LN)**
   Normal glomeruli by LM, but mesangial immune deposits by IF
2. **Mesangial proliferative lupus nephritis (LN)**
   Purely mesangial hypercellularity of any degree or mesangial matrix expansion by LM with mesangial immune deposits, with none or few, isolated subepithelial or subendothelial deposits by IF or EM not visible by LM
3. **Focal lupus nephritis (LN)**
   Active or inactive focal (<50% involved glomeruli), segmental or global endo- or extracapillary GN, typically with focal, subendothelial immune deposits, with or without focal or diffuse mesangial alterations
   III (A) active focal proliferative LN
   III (A/C) active and sclerotic focal proliferative LN
   III (C) inactive sclerotic focal LN
       * Indicate the proportion of glomeruli with active and with sclerotic lesions
       * Indicate the proportion of glomeruli with fibrinoid necrosis and/or cellular crescents
4. **Diffuse segmental (IV- S) or global (IV- G) LN**
   Active or inactive diffuse (50% or more involved glomeruli), segmental or global endo- or extracapillary GN with diffuse subendothelial immune deposits, with or without mesangial alterations. This class is divided into diffuse segmental (IV-S) when at least 50% of the involved glomeruli have segmental lesions, and diffuse global (IV-G) when at least 50% of the involved glomeruli have global lesions
   IV (A) Active diffuse segmental or global proliferative LN
   IV (A/C) Diffuse segmental or global proliferative and sclerotic LN
   IV (C) Diffuse segmental or global sclerotic LN
       * Indicate the proportion of glomeruli with active and with sclerotic lesions
       * Indicate the proportion of glomeruli with fibrinoid necrosis and/or cellular crescents
5. **Membranous lupus nephritis**
   Numerous global or segmental subepithelial immune deposits or their morphologic sequelae by LM and IF or EM with or without mesangial alterations
   May occur in combination with III or IV in which case both will be diagnosed. May show advanced sclerosis
6. **Advanced sclerotic LN**
   90% or more glomeruli globally sclerosed without residual activity

ISN/RPS Classes I and II LN denote purely mesangial involvement (I, mesangial immune deposits without mesangial hypercellularity; II, mesangial immune deposits with mesangial expansion and hypercellularity), ISN/RPS Class III LN denotes focal glomerulonephritis (involving less than 50% of total number of glomeruli), with subdivisions for active and chronic lesions. ISN/RPS Class IV LN denotes diffuse glomerulonephritis (involving at least 50% of total number of glomeruli with examples in Figs. 26.1, 26.2a–d, and 26.3a–d) either with segmental (ISN/RPS Class IV-S) or global (ISN/RPS Class IV-G) involvement, and also with subdivisions for active and chronic lesions, ISN/RPS Class V denotes membranous LN (combinations of membranous and proliferative glomerulonephritis (i.e., ISN/RPS Class III and V or Class IV

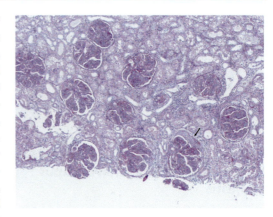

Fig. 26.1 Photomicrograph of a case of lupus nephritis demonstrating predominant diffuse endocapillary proliferative change with scattered superimposed extracapillary proliferative lesions (*Arrow*), Lupus nephritis Class IV-G (A/C) (PAS, original magnification ×100) (Used with permission of Taylor & Francis from Marks et al. [70])

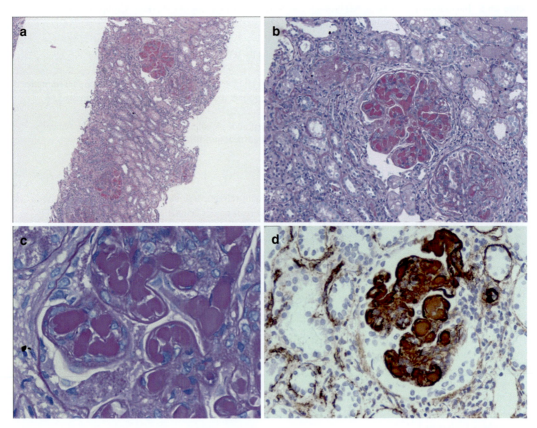

Fig. 26.2 Photomicrographs of a case of lupus nephritis presenting as apparent acute renal failure, demonstrating diffuse endocapillary proliferative change with scattered crescent formation (**a**, **b**) and extensive subendothelial deposits visualised as wire-loop and hyaline drop lesions (**b**, **c**). Immunostaining revealed a characteristic 'full-house' pattern of immunoglobulin and complement deposition. (**d**) Lupus nephritis Class IV-G (a) (PAS and immunostain, original magnifications ×40–400) (Used with permission of Taylor & Francis from Marks et al. [70])

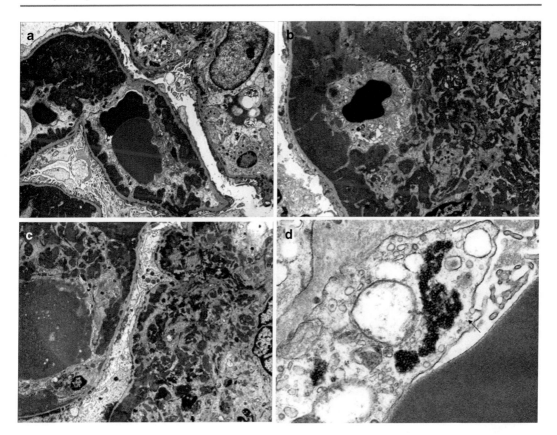

Fig. 26.3 Electron micrographs of lupus nephritis demonstrating extensive mesangial and paramesangial electron dense deposits in association with massive subendothelial deposits (**a–c**) (**a**) corresponds to the case in Fig. 26.1 and (**b, c**) correspond to the case in Fig. 26.2). In addition, some cases may demonstrate the presence of tubuloreticular inclusions. (**d**) (Used with permission of Taylor & Francis from Marks et al. [70])

and V) should be reported individually in the diagnostic line) and ISN/RPS Class VI for advanced sclerosing lesions (which now for the first time categorically states that at least 90% of glomeruli need to be globally sclerosed without residual activity). In addition, the ISN/RPS classification includes overlap cases (see Fig. 26.4a–d for an example of mixed ISN/RPS Class IV and Class V LN).

The histopathological features of LN includes the delineation of active and chronic histological lesions, which has been extensively reported in the various classification systems (Table 26.6) [71].

The active glomerular and tubulointerstitial lesions, which are potentially reversible and are scored up to 24 (with 12 denoting poor renal prognosis), include endocapillary hypercellularity, fibrinoid necrosis, karyorrhexis, cellular crescents, hyaline thrombi, wire loops (subendothelial deposits), haematoxylin bodies, leucocyte infiltration and tubulointerstitial disease with tubular atrophy and mononuclear cell infiltration. The chronic lesions are irreversible and include glomerular sclerosis, fibrous crescents, fibrous adhesions, extramembranous deposits, and tubulointerstitial disease with interstitial fibrosis and tubular atrophy.

The clinicopathological correlation of LN has been evaluated in both adults and children according to different histopathological classifications. The largest adult series investigating the clinicopathological outcomes according to the ISN/RPS classification of LN followed 60 Japanese subjects for 1–366 (mean 187) months (Fig. 26.5) [72]. The primary outcome was

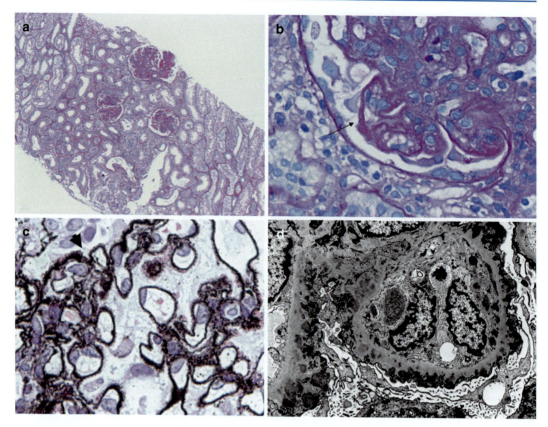

Fig. 26.4 Photomicrographs of a case of lupus nephritis presenting with nephrotic syndrome demonstrating diffuse endocapillary proliferative change with subendothelial deposits ((**a**, **b**) PAS, original magnifications ×40 and 400 respectively). In addition some glomeruli show florid 'spike' formation on silver staining (**c**) PAMS, original magnification ×400) with mesangial, subendothelial and subepithelial deposits on ultrastructural examination (**d**). Lupus nephritis, mixed Class IV and Class V changes (Used with permission of Taylor & Francis from Marks et al. [70])

Table 26.6 Activity and chronicity indices of lupus nephritis

	Activity index	Chronicity index
Glomerular	Endocapillary hypercellularity Fibrinoid necrosis Karyorrhexis Cellular crescents Hyaline thrombi Wire loops (subendothelial deposits) Haematoxylin bodies Leucocyte infiltration	Glomerular sclerosis Fibrous crescents Fibrous adhesions Extramembranous deposits
Tubulointerstitial	Mononuclear cell infiltration Tubular necrosis	Interstitial fibrosis Tubular atrophy

defined as developing end-stage kidney disease (ESKD) with secondary outcome as patients' death and/or ESKD. The primary and secondary outcomes of all subjects were 82% and 78% at 10 years, and 80% and 73% at 20 years, respectively. The primary outcome of subjects with nephrotic syndrome (n = 21 versus 39 non-nephrotic) was statistically poorer (p = 0.0007) with hazard ratio of 3.39 as the mean time of 50% renal survival was 200 ± 29 months.

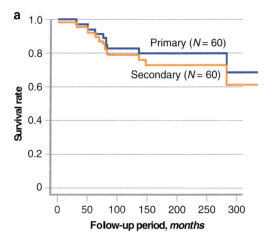 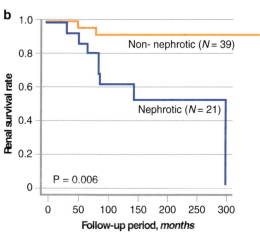

Fig. 26.5 Prognosis of lupus nephritis. The primary (ESKD) and secondary (patients' death and/or ESKD) outcomes (**a**) of 60 Japanese adult lupus nephritis subjects with and without nephrotic syndrome (**b**) at mean follow-up of 187 months (Used with permission of Nature Publishing Group from Yokoyama et al. [72])

In comparison with adult-onset SLE, there are usually less patients in the series of childhood cases of LN. There have been larger series investigating clinicopathological outcomes of 39–67 children according to the WHO classification [73] and the ISN/RPS classification of LN [74], which provide evidence that up to half of children with LN will have the most severe class (ISN/RPS Class IV or diffuse LN). The classification demonstrated that the subgroup of diffuse global sclerosing (ISN/RPS IV-G(C)) LN was associated with the worst clinical outcome [74].

Treatment

The optimal treatment of children and adolescents with SLE is provided by a multi-disciplinary team of health professionals, including a paediatric nephrologist, paediatric rheumatologist and other paediatric specialists, with a dedicated specialist nurse and members of a psychosocial team. Treatment should be guided by the most severe organ system involved.

Drug Treatment

The treatment of lupus with or without nephritis is based on evaluation of the severity of the disease. The treatment should be individually tailored depending on the presenting symptoms and severity of renal involvement, with emphasis on renal dysfunction and the degree of proteinuria. In all cases with suspected renal involvement, the histopathological grading of the renal biopsy is very helpful in deciding further treatment. Other potentially life-threatening symptoms, such as cerebral lupus should also be taken into consideration when deciding on the initial treatment. Most treatments have common or potential side-effects, which need to be considered for the individual child.

The treatment of JSLE is not based on large randomised controlled trials, but there is an increasing number of studies in adult and adolescent patients and published clinical experience in children. The recommendations below describe the most commonly used protocols for treating children with SLE. Consensus reports on the treatment of paediatric lupus have been published [75–79]. The armamentarium of immunosuppressive agents is presently developing quickly with new drugs being introduced [80], so guidelines may change in the not too distant future.

Traditionally treatment has been divided into induction therapy to gain control of acute disease and maintenance therapy to maintain control over the disease. This is a helpful approach, but it is not an uncommon clinical situation that a flare of disease activity is difficult to define.

have premature ovarian failure, which is a common consequence of CyC treatment. CyC is thus a drug that still has a place in the treatment of LN, but it is gradually being replaced by other drugs.

Rituximab

Rituximab is a humanised anti-CD20 antibody that was designed for treatment of B-cell lymphoma and in adults has been increasingly used for B-cell depletion therapy in autoimmune diseases such as rheumatoid arthritis or SLE [43]. We have used IV rituximab in over 200 children with SLE or vasculitis and published the results of our first children [44, 93]. Our patients have shown very good responses to the treatment and we have not experienced a significant increase in severe side effects.

A relatively large randomised, placebo-controlled study of IV rituximab, called the LUNAR trial, was performed in 144 adult patients with ISN/RPS Class III or IV LN [94]. The primary endpoint was the renal response at week 52. A complete response was normalisation of serum creatinine, no red blood cells (<5/hpf) in the urine and a urine protein/creatinine ratio of <1.0 mg/mg.

Only 31% of patients in the placebo group and 25% of the rituximab treated patients fulfilled these very strict criteria for a complete response. The patients that showed no response to the treatment were 43% in the rituximab and 54% in the placebo group (p = 0.18). There were more serious side effects in the placebo group: 74/100 patient years vs. 43/100 patient years in the rituximab group. Greater improvements of complement levels (p = 0.025) and antibodies to dsDNA (p = 0.007) were recorded in the rituximab group compared to placebo [95].

The negative result of this study was surprising, but several potential reasons have been postulated. Rituximab was given in addition to other treatments that in normal circumstances would have been regarded as sufficient. In addition, the endpoints were quite strict and difficult to fulfil. There are plans for further studies on rituximab with different designs. This study, along with another randomised study in lupus patients without renal involvement (the EXPLORER trial) [96], have not shown any severe side-effect profiles.

A further large case series of 164 adult patients with biopsy proven LN showed a complete response, partial response and no response in about a third of the treated patients [97]. These results, together with the paediatric case series that show a good therapeutic response, means that we continue to recommend the use of rituximab in many situations, as is becoming standard of care in ISN RPS Class III, IV and V LN as well as those with severe life-threatening disease and those patients with active disease despite standard treatment.

Different protocols have been used and our protocol involves two administrations of IV rituximab as an infusion of 750 mg/m^2 (rounded up to the nearest 100 mg with a maximum dose of 1 g) with 14 days in between. In addition, an IV dose of 100 mg methylprednisolone is given immediately prior to each rituximab infusion.

Plasma Exchange

We consider the use of plasmapheresis in very severe and refractory cases of SLE with cerebral lupus and/or crescentic glomerulonephritis, with five to ten plasma exchanges as an adjunct in some patients [81]. However, this is a controversial area and a controlled trial in adult patients with severe LN could not confirm any benefits from adding plasma exchange to the standard treatment of methylprednisolone and CyC [98], which was confirmed in a meta-analysis [99].

Intravenous Immunoglobulin

IV immunoglobulin (at a dose of 2 g/kg to a maximum of 70 g) can be useful, particularly in children with severe haematological disease. Some children benefit from regular infusions (such as every 6 weeks) (Table 26.8).

Table 26.8 Maintenance therapy of lupus nephritis

Prednisolone (oral)	0–5/10 mg alternate or every day
Mycophenolate mofetil (oral)	600 mg/m^2 twice daily (maximum of 2–3 g/day in two divided doses)
Alternatively,	
Azathioprine (oral)	2–2.5 mg/kg once daily
Hydroxychloroquine (oral)	4–6 mg/kg/day
	Normal dose 200 mg once daily

Maintenance Therapy

All cases of severe lupus require maintenance therapy for a long period, although the length of treatment is not well defined. We advocate maintenance therapy for at least 2–3 years and possibly indefinitely in many cases, especially those with active LN.

Corticosteroids

After the initial rather rapid reduction of the oral corticosteroid, the prednisolone dose should be continuously weaned; many patients may not require long-term oral corticosteroids if adequate immunosuppression is given (e.g., MMF and IV rituximab). The clinical response will decide how quickly the dose can be reduced. Long-term treatment with corticosteroids for several years is often required, although there are quite different approaches on preferred maintenance dose. Our opinion is that it is very important to reduce the dose as quickly as possible. This is important to reduce side effects, but also to improve adherence. Teenagers do not like the cushingoid appearance they develop with corticosteroids so some stop taking their medications when the acute symptoms have resolved. This can lead to non-adherence with other treatments. Our goal is to wean corticosteroids, and either t discontinue or utilize alternate day treatment at a dose in the order of 5–10 mg every other day. These doses of prednisolone should allow the child to grow normally [100].

Mycophenolate Mofetil

MMF is most likely the best choice for long-term maintenance therapy. After the 24 week induction part of the ALMS trial, 227 patients were randomised to 3 years of maintenance therapy with MMF (2 g/day) or azathioprine (2 mg/kg/day) [101]. In this study, MMF was superior to azathioprine with respect to the primary end-point, time to treatment failure; hazard ratio was 0.44 (95% CI 0.25–0.77; p = 0.003). Treatment failure occurred in 16% of the patients in the MMF group and 32% in the azathioprine group. Serious adverse events occurred in 24% of patients treated with MMF compared to 33% treated with azathioprine and the withdrawal due to adverse events was significantly higher in the azathioprine group (40% versus 25%; p = 0.02) [102].

MMF was also compared to azathioprine in the MAINTAIN trial [103]. In this study, 105 patients were treated with similar doses of azathioprine and MMF as in the maintenance phase of ALMS. There was a tendency to fewer renal flares in the MMF group, but the number of patients was not high enough for this to achieve statistical significance.

Azathioprine

Azathioprine at a dose of 2–2.5 mg/kg/day has historically been first line maintenance therapy and has a generally favourable side-effect profile. In the comparison of azathioprine or MMF used as maintenance therapy, MMF was shown to be better than azathioprine (which is the opposite of maintenance treatment of vasculitis) [102, 103]. Some centers advocate testing of thiopurine methyltransferase activity before commencement of azathioprine, but in our practice we advocate close monitoring of full blood counts [104].

Hydroxychloroquine

The use of antimalarial drugs (such as hydroxychloroquine at a dose of 4–6 mg/kg/day) should be considered for all lupus patients. It is especially helpful in children with marked skin or lung disease, lethargy and arthritis. Hydroxychloroquine also seems to reduce blood lipids and possibly the risk for later atherosclerosis. Some clinicians advocate a high dose of 10 mg/kg (up to 400 mg/day) for patients with severe lung disease. Ophthalmology referral and monitoring should take place, as there is a significant risk of retinopathy, particularly with long-term hydroxychloroquine use [105]. In the UK, national guidance suggests at least annual ophthalmology monitoring after 5 years of therapy.

Emerging Therapeutic Options

A number of new therapeutic options for SLE have emerged, with many more currently in development. Belimumab is a fully humanized monoclonal antibody targeting B-lymphocyte stimulator (BLyS) which has been licensed in a number of countries for adults and children with SLE. Adult studies have shown efficacy in SLE [106] and a recent randomized, controlled trial of belimumab in adults with LN showed an improved renal response and a lower risk of renal-related events or death when belimumab was given in addition to standard therapy alone [107]. Belimumab has also been approved for JSLE in a number of countries; the results of the ongoing Phase 2 PLUTO trial in children aged 5–17 years with SLE has shown a favorable side-effect profile with improved efficacy of belimumab compared to placebo [108].

In addition to the use of rituximab for induction therapy, there is increasing interest in its use as maintenance therapy for SLE. Currently, data are limited; a recent observational study in adults did not find any difference in relapse risk in those receiving maintenance rituximab compared to those who had a single course [109]. There may, however, be a role for maintenance rituximab particularly in adolescents or young adults with difficult to treat disease or medication adherence issues on oral treatment.

There is ongoing research into the use of other B-cell depleting monoclonal antibodies. There are reports of the use of other humanized B-cell depleting antibodies such as ofatumumab in patients with SLE. These are currently limited to case series and may be useful in certain situations such as infusion reactions or allergy to rituximab [110, 111].

There is increasing interest in the use of tacrolimus as therapy for SLE, particularly in patients with membranous (Class V) LN or with proteinuria as a predominant feature [112]. Adult studies have shown it is non-inferior to MMF, but the highest efficacy seems to come from combined tacrolimus and MMF, although many studies to date have been conducted in Asian patients so further work is needed to confirm this

in different ethnic groups [113–115]. Although there are no studies beyond case reports of tacrolimus for JSLE, its use can be considered in difficult cases and in particular with a membranous appearance on histology. A recent study on voclosporin in combination with MMF showed a superior renal response, but also higher rates of adverse events [116].

The type 1 interferon pathway has also been targeted in SLE, and the monoclonal antibody anifrolumab has recently completed phase 3 RCTs in adults, showing some efficacy in reducing composite disease activity endpoints [117]. Many other therapeutic targets are currently under investigation for SLE, and while these are currently not likely to reach children and adolescents with JSLE for some years, there is hope for many more treatment options in the future.

Treatment of Antiphospholipid Syndrome (APS)

Treatment for APS includes reducing lupus disease activity and appropriate anticoagulation treatment (such as life-long aspirin or warfarin if severe thromboembolic disease).

General Renal Management

As outlined in other parts of this book, general renal care is important in all children with renal impairment. This includes monitoring and treatment of hypertension and proteinuria; blood pressure targets are around 50th centile for age, sex and height centile and albuminuria and proteinuria should be minimised (which may be due to active disease, which requires increasing immunosuppression or chronic damage,which requires treatment with angiotensin converting enzyme inhibition or angiotensin receptor blockers). It is important to continuously evaluate renal function of these children with estimated GFR and, if appropriate, a formal GFR measurement. Supportive treatment of chronic kidney disease and ESKD is required in some of these children.

General Management

Sun Protection

All children with SLE and especially those with active skin disease should be advised to always use appropriate sunscreen and protect themselves from the sun, with regular monitoring of 25-hydroxyvitamin D levels and appropriate vitamin D supplementation.

Immunisations

Children with SLE, treated with immunosuppressive drugs, should avoid immunisation with live vaccines. Vaccination with killed vaccines should be carefully considered as they might induce a flare of the disease and also might have decreased efficacy. In the United Kingdom and in other countries, pneumococcal vaccinations are recommended for all patients likely to be on corticosteroids for more than a month.

Management of Infection

Children on immunosuppressive treatment are more susceptible to severe infections than other children and it should be emphasised to the parents and the children that they should seek medical advice early in the case of fever or symptoms of an infection.

Prognosis

In the era before treatment became available, the prognosis of patients with SLE was very poor with very few patients with a severe nephritis surviving more than 2 years [118]. The introduction of corticosteroids and immunosuppressive treatment with CyC and azathioprine made a huge impact on the long-term prognosis. Cameron showed already more than 25 years ago a general and renal survival of about 20% after 20 years [56]. He could also show that between the years 1965 and 1991 the 10-year patient survival improved from 10 to 20%.

The proportion of death from SLE improved very rapidly in high-income countries from the 1960s to the 1970s, with slower improvement thereafter. In contrast, in low and middle-income countries there was a pronounced increase in survival between 1970 and 1990 followed by a plateau or a decreased survival. There is now a significant difference in both 5- and 10-year survival between high and middle/low income countries. Five year survival estimates of 0.99 and 0.85, respectively and 10-year survival estimates of 0.97 and 0.79, respectively [119].

The proportion of children dying from their renal failure is now lower, although the prognostic factors for developing renal failure remain the same (male gender, non-Caucasian race, nephrotic syndrome at onset and severity of disease on renal biopsy [73]).

Another important measurement of success in the treatment of LN is the proportion of children achieving full renal remission. A recent German study in 79 pediatric lupus patients showed a rate at one year of complete remission of 38%, and 41% partial remission [120]. An Italian study found a rate of a complete remission of about 50% while children from South Korea showed the highest rate of complete remission at 59.7% [121, 122]. Remission was defined as normal kidney function and no proteinuria. There is thus still a need to improve long-term kidney survival. In recent years, it has also become evident that patients with SLE confront another important threat to their long-term survival due to an increased risk of atherosclerosis.

Treatment Related Complications and Mortality

In recent studies, infections have been the main cause of death, therefore suggesting that the most important short-term goal is to find therapies which are as good as current treatments but with fewer side effects. Recent comparative studies in adults showed that CyC treatment was associated with significantly more severe infections compared to treatment with azathioprine or MMF [84, 90–92]. This emphasises the importance of monitoring white cell and neutrophil counts during therapy and early treatment of infectious complications. However, infections can sometimes be difficult to differentiate from a flare of disease activity, especially in children who are in ESKD on renal replacement therapy. CRP can be used as a helpful tool in these situations as very few patients even with active lupus have raised CRP levels [56] while most children with septicaemia do.

Severe viral infections, in particular with varicella zoster virus are seen, and children exposed to the virus or with early symptoms of varicella (or more often herpes zoster virus) should be treated with aciclovir therapy to reduce the risk of generalised infection.

Growth failure is a major problem in children with lupus, which can be related to the inflammatory disease or a complication of corticosteroid treatment. Sometimes it can be difficult to differentiate between them and this is a controversial area, but it is our opinion that ongoing inflammation more often causes the growth failure than the treatment with low corticosteroid doses. Therefore, increasing immunosuppression rather than reducing treatment is often more beneficial for the growth of these children.

SLE patients have an increased risk of osteoporosis, partly caused by their long-term treatment with steroids [123]. Treatment with calcium and vitamin D supplementation is advocated by some centres, but unfortunately it seems as if the beneficial effects from that treatment only persist during the treatment [124]. However, an increased nutritional calcium intake does seem to be able to improve bone accretion over a longer time [125]. It is recommended that children with SLE should be monitored with regular bone density scans.

Children on long-term immunosuppressive treatment have an increased risk for developing malignancies, in particular skin cancers and lymphoma, and should be advised to use sun protection. Bladder cancer has been associated with the use of CyC in children with SLE [126]. A 10 year follow-up of a large cohort of 1000 adult lupus patients found that 23 developed malignancies, with breast and uterine cancers being the most common [127]. Therefore, the risk of malignancy does not seem to be excessive.

Active lupus often causes amenorrhoea and delayed puberty, whereas treatment with CyC can also reduce fertility. A study of 39 women younger than 40 years old showed that 12.5% (2 out of 16) receiving seven IV doses of CyC developed sustained amenorrhoea compared to 39% (9 out of 23) receiving 15 or more doses (with a higher risk in women older than 25 years) [128].

Thrombosis

In the aforementioned 10-year follow up of 1000 adult patients, 9.2% [129] developed thrombosis, and of the 68 patients who died, 26.5% had a thrombotic event. Thrombosis is more common in children with antiphospholipid syndrome. A 10-year follow-up of 149 children with SLE from Toronto showed that 24 were positive for lupus anticoagulant and that 13 of them experienced 21 thromboembolic events [130]. The authors emphasised the need to treat this subgroup of children with life-long anticoagulation.

Cardiovascular Disease

A Swedish registry study on 4737 patients with SLE from 1964 to 1994 showed a 16-fold increased risk of death from cardiovascular diseases [129]. Therefore, it is our new challenge to try to prevent atherosclerosis and to improve our patients' long-term survival. This increased risk for cardiovascular death is multifactorial and includes classical risk factors, such as hypertension, hyperlipidaemia and corticosteroid treatment and disease-related risk factors such as proteinuria, vasculitis, low-grade systemic inflammation, antiphospholipid syndrome and elevated levels of homocysteine [131].

Carotid plaque and coronary artery calcifications are significantly increased in lupus patients [132, 133]. Efforts to decrease atherosclerosis include good control of inflammation, aggressive treatment of hypertension and proteinuria and prevention of corticosteroid-induced obesity. A randomised placebo controlled study on treatment with atorvastatin did not significantly reduce progression of the surrogate marker for atherosclerosis, carotid intima-media thickness [134]. The active treatment did, however, reduce levels of high sensitivity CRP and total cholesterol and low-density lipoprotein. A secondary analysis suggested that atorvastatin reduced atherosclerosis progression in paediatric lupus patients with higher CRP values

[135]. Hydroxychloroquine has been shown to have a beneficial effect on the cardiovascular risk profile [136].

Adherence to Treatment

One important prognostic factor in children with LN, as in all children with chronic kidney disease, is adherence with treatment, especially during puberty. Non-adherence in adolescents is a common reason for relapse of symptoms, and may cause acute kidney injury after initially successful treatment. In such serious clinical situations, we would advocate the use of IV therapies (with rituximab treatment now our preferred option, which can be given at six-monthly intervals as maintenance treatment irrespective of peripheral CD19 counts) instead of oral treatments to ensure adherence and disease control.

Renal Replacement Therapy

The optimal therapy for patients with ESKD due to LN is renal transplantation, especially as patients seem to do equally well compared to matched controls, with less than 10% recurrence of LN and similar long-term patient and renal allograft survival [137, 138]. Patients should be in remission for 6 months prior to transplantation, and the transplant immunosuppression regimen should be standard, unless there are immunological concerns. However, it should be noted that the risk for thromboembolic complications was higher in the SLE group. Patients with SLE can have peritoneal or haemodialysis prior to transplantation, but in view of hypocomplementaemia and immunosuppression, clinicians should be wary of clinical presentation of flare of disease activity (which can be difficult to diagnose) versus infectious complications. Patients on peritoneal dialysis presenting with peritonitis should be treated with IV and intraperitoneal antibiotics.

Conclusion

The prognosis for children with SLE has improved over recent decades, with improved survival and fewer debilitating symptoms. There is, however, still a major challenge to obtain full remission of LN, which is essential for optimizing long-term kidney function. Another important challenge is to minimise treatment related mortality and morbidity. This has led to less CyC use, which has been replaced by other less toxic drugs, mainly MMF. Rituximab is now also routinely used in some centers, but further studies are needed to fully delineate its role. It is also important to find ways to reduce the burden of premature cardiovascular disease in these children.

References

1. Brunner HI, Silverman ED, To T, et al. Risk factors for damage in childhood-onset systemic lupus erythematosus: cumulative disease activity and medication use predict disease damage. Arthritis Rheum. 2002;46:436–44. https://doi.org/10.1002/art.10072.
2. Jiménez S, Cervera R, Font J, et al. The epidemiology of systemic lupus erythematosus. Clin Rev Allergy Immunol. 2003;25:3–12. https://doi.org/10.1385/CRIAI:25:1:3.
3. Rood MJ, ten Cate R, van Suijlekom-Smit LW, et al. Childhood-onset systemic lupus erythematosus: clinical presentation and prognosis in 31 patients. Scand J Rheumatol. 1999;28:222–6. https://doi.org/10.1080/03009749950155580.
4. Tucker LB, Menon S, Schaller JG, et al. Adult- and childhood-onset systemic lupus erythematosus: a comparison of onset, clinical features, serology, and outcome. Br J Rheumatol. 1995;34:866–72. https://doi.org/10.1093/rheumatology/34.9.866.
5. Schanberg LE, Sandborg C. Dyslipoproteinemia and premature atherosclerosis in pediatric systemic lupus erythematosus. Curr Rheumatol Rep. 2004;6:425–33. https://doi.org/10.1007/s11926-004-0021-4.
6. Hochberg MC. Updating the American College of Rheumatology revised criteria for the classification of systemic lupus erythematosus. Arthritis Rheum. 1997;40:1725. https://doi.org/10.1002/art.1780400928.
7. Tan EM, Cohen AS, Fries JF, et al. The 1982 revised criteria for the classification of systemic lupus erythematosus. Arthritis Rheum. 1982;25:1271–7. https://doi.org/10.1002/art.1780251101.
8. Petri M, Orbai A-M, Alarcón GS, et al. Derivation and validation of the systemic lupus international collaborating clinics classification criteria for systemic lupus erythematosus. Arthritis Rheum. 2012;64:2677–86. https://doi.org/10.1002/art.34473.
9. Sag E, Tartaglione A, Batu ED, et al. Performance of the new SLICC classification criteria in childhood systemic lupus erythematosus: a multicentre study. Clin Exp Rheumatol. 2014;32:440–4. http://www.ncbi.nlm.nih.gov/pubmed/24642380.

10. Lythgoe H, Morgan T, Heaf E, et al. Evaluation of the ACR and SLICC classification criteria in juvenile-onset systemic lupus erythematosus: a longitudinal analysis. Lupus. 2017;26:1285–90. https://doi.org/10.1177/0961203317700484.

11. Brunner HI, Holland MJ, Beresford MW, et al. American College of Rheumatology Provisional Criteria for clinically relevant improvement in children and adolescents with childhood-onset systemic lupus erythematosus. Arthritis Care Res (Hoboken). 2019;71:579–90. https://doi.org/10.1002/acr.23834.

12. Malleson PN, Fung MY, Rosenberg AM. The incidence of pediatric rheumatic diseases: results from the Canadian Pediatric Rheumatology Association disease registry. J Rheumatol. 1996;23:1981–7. http://www.ncbi.nlm.nih.gov/pubmed/8923379.

13. Fessel WJ. Systemic lupus erythematosus in the community. Incidence, prevalence, outcome, and first symptoms; the high prevalence in black women. Arch Intern Med. 1974;134:1027–35. http://www.ncbi.nlm.nih.gov/pubmed/4433183.

14. Hochberg MC. Prevalence of systemic lupus erythematosus in England and Wales, 1981–2. Ann Rheum Dis. 1987;46:664–6. https://doi.org/10.1136/ard.46.9.664.

15. Hochberg MC. Systemic lupus erythematosus. Rheum Dis Clin North Am. 1990;16:617–39. http://www.ncbi.nlm.nih.gov/pubmed/2217961.

16. Hopkinson ND, Doherty M, Powell RJ. The prevalence and incidence of systemic lupus erythematosus in Nottingham, UK, 1989–1990. Br J Rheumatol. 1993;32:110–5. https://doi.org/10.1093/rheumatology/32.2.110.

17. Hopkinson ND, Doherty M, Powell RJ. Clinical features and race-specific incidence/prevalence rates of systemic lupus erythematosus in a geographically complete cohort of patients. Ann Rheum Dis. 1994;53:675–80. https://doi.org/10.1136/ard.53.10.675.

18. Johnson AE, Gordon C, Palmer RG, et al. The prevalence and incidence of systemic lupus erythematosus in Birmingham, England. Relationship to ethnicity and country of birth. Arthritis Rheum. 1995;38:551–8. https://doi.org/10.1002/art.1780380415.

19. Nived O, Sturfelt G, Wollheim F. Systemic lupus erythematosus in an adult population in southern Sweden: incidence, prevalence and validity of ARA revised classification criteria. Br J Rheumatol. 1985;24:147–54. https://doi.org/10.1093/rheumatology/24.2.147.

20. Siegel M, Lee SL. The epidemiology of systemic lupus erythematosus. Semin Arthritis Rheum. 1973;3:1–54. https://doi.org/10.1016/0049-0172(73)90034-6.

21. Citera G, Wilson WA. Ethnic and geographic perspectives in SLE. Lupus. 1993;2:351–3. https://doi.org/10.1177/096120339300200603.

22. Symmons DP. Frequency of lupus in people of African origin. Lupus. 1995;4:176–8. https://doi.org/10.1177/096120339500400303.

23. Massias JS, Smith EM, Al-Abadi E, et al. Clinical and laboratory phenotypes in juvenile-onset systemic lupus erythematosus across ethnicities in the UK. Lupus. 2021;30(4):597–607. https://doi.org/10.1177/0961203320984251.

24. Vyas S, Hidalgo G, Baqi N, et al. Outcome in African-American children of neuropsychiatric lupus and lupus nephritis. Pediatr Nephrol. 2002;17:45–9. https://doi.org/10.1007/s004670200008.

25. Gardner-Medwin JMM, Dolezalova P, Cummins C, et al. Incidence of Henoch-Schönlein purpura, Kawasaki disease, and rare vasculitides in children of different ethnic origins. Lancet. 2002;360:1197–202. https://doi.org/10.1016/S0140-6736(02)11279-7.

26. Lahita RG. Sex hormones and systemic lupus erythematosus. Rheum Dis Clin North Am. 2000;26:951–68. https://doi.org/10.1016/s0889-857x(05)70178-2.

27. McMurray RW. Sex hormones in the pathogenesis of systemic lupus erythematosus. Front Biosci. 2001;6:E193–206. https://doi.org/10.2741/mcmurray.

28. Kyttaris VC, Katsiari CG, Juang Y-T, et al. New insights into the pathogenesis of systemic lupus erythematosus. Curr Rheumatol Rep. 2005;7:469–75. https://doi.org/10.1007/s11926-005-0054-3.

29. Arbuckle MR, McClain MT, Rubertone MV, et al. Development of autoantibodies before the clinical onset of systemic lupus erythematosus. N Engl J Med. 2003;349:1526–33. https://doi.org/10.1056/NEJMoa021933.

30. Nishi H, Mayadas TN. Neutrophils in lupus nephritis. Curr Opin Rheumatol. 2019;31:193–200. https://doi.org/10.1097/BOR.0000000000000577.

31. Deapen D, Escalante A, Weinrib L, et al. A revised estimate of twin concordance in systemic lupus erythematosus. Arthritis Rheum. 1992;35:311–8. https://doi.org/10.1002/art.1780350310.

32. Kelly JA, Moser KL, Harley JB. The genetics of systemic lupus erythematosus: putting the pieces together. Genes Immun. 2002;3(Suppl 1):S71–85. https://doi.org/10.1038/sj.gene.6363885.

33. Manderson AP, Botto M, Walport MJ. The role of complement in the development of systemic lupus erythematosus. Annu Rev Immunol. 2004;22:431–56. https://doi.org/10.1146/annurev.immunol.22.012703.104549.

34. Tsao BP. The genetics of human systemic lupus erythematosus. Trends Immunol. 2003;24:595–602. https://doi.org/10.1016/j.it.2003.09.006.

35. Chung SA, Brown EE, Williams AH, et al. Lupus nephritis susceptibility loci in women with systemic lupus erythematosus. J Am Soc Nephrol. 2014;25:2859–70. https://doi.org/10.1681/ASN.2013050446.

36. Julià A, López-Longo FJ, Pérez Venegas JJ, et al. Genome-wide association study meta-analysis identifies five new loci for systemic lupus erythematosus. Arthritis Res Ther. 2018;20:100. https://doi.org/10.1186/s13075-018-1604-1.

37. Chen L, Wang Y-F, Liu L, et al. Genome-wide assessment of genetic risk for systemic lupus erythematosus and disease severity. Hum Mol Genet. 2020;29:1745–56. https://doi.org/10.1093/hmg/ddaa030.

38. Pickering MC, Botto M, Taylor PR, et al. Systemic lupus erythematosus, complement deficiency, and apoptosis. Adv Immunol. 2000;76:227–324. https://doi.org/10.1016/s0065-2776(01)76021-x.

39. Seelen MA, Trouw LA, Daha MR. Diagnostic and prognostic significance of anti-C1q antibodies in systemic lupus erythematosus. Curr Opin Nephrol Hypertens. 2003;12:619–24. https://doi.org/10.1097/00041552-200311000-00008.

40. Trouw LA, Groeneveld TWL, Seelen MA, et al. Anti-C1q autoantibodies deposit in glomeruli but are only pathogenic in combination with glomerular C1q-containing immune complexes. J Clin Invest. 2004;114:679–88. https://doi.org/10.1172/JCI21075.

41. Odendahl M, Jacobi A, Hansen A, et al. Disturbed peripheral B lymphocyte homeostasis in systemic lupus erythematosus. J Immunol. 2000;165:5970–9. https://doi.org/10.4049/jimmunol.165.10.5970.

42. Tangye SG, Liu YJ, Aversa G, et al. Identification of functional human splenic memory B cells by expression of CD148 and CD27. J Exp Med. 1998;188:1691–703. https://doi.org/10.1084/jem.188.9.1691.

43. Leandro MJ, Cambridge G, Edwards JC, et al. B-cell depletion in the treatment of patients with systemic lupus erythematosus: a longitudinal analysis of 24 patients. Rheumatology (Oxford). 2005;44:1542–5. https://doi.org/10.1093/rheumatology/kei080.

44. Marks SD, Patey S, Brogan PA, et al. B lymphocyte depletion therapy in children with refractory systemic lupus erythematosus. Arthritis Rheum. 2005;52:3168–74. https://doi.org/10.1002/art.21351.

45. Shlomchik MJ, Craft JE, Mamula MJ. From T to B and back again: positive feedback in systemic autoimmune disease. Nat Rev Immunol. 2001;1:147–53. https://doi.org/10.1038/35100573.

46. Tsokos GC, Nambiar MP, Tenbrock K, et al. Rewiring the T-cell: signaling defects and novel prospects for the treatment of SLE. Trends Immunol. 2003;24:259–63. https://doi.org/10.1016/s1471-4906(03)00100-5.

47. Tsokos GC, Mitchell JP, Juang Y-T. T cell abnormalities in human and mouse lupus: intrinsic and extrinsic. Curr Opin Rheumatol. 2003;15:542–7. https://doi.org/10.1097/00002281-200309000-00004.

48. Gröndal G, Gunnarsson I, Rönnelid J, et al. Cytokine production, serum levels and disease activity in systemic lupus erythematosus. Clin Exp Rheumatol. 2000;18:565–70. http://www.ncbi.nlm.nih.gov/pubmed/11072595.

49. Qing X, Putterman C. Gene expression profiling in the study of the pathogenesis of systemic lupus erythematosus. Autoimmun Rev. 2004;3:505–9. https://doi.org/10.1016/j.autrev.2004.07.001.

50. Schwarting A, Paul K, Tschirner S, et al. Interferon-beta: a therapeutic for autoimmune lupus in MRL-Faslpr mice. J Am Soc Nephrol. 2005;16:3264–72. https://doi.org/10.1681/ASN.2004111014.

51. Hueber W, Zeng D, Strober S, et al. Interferon-alpha-inducible proteins are novel autoantigens in murine lupus. Arthritis Rheum. 2004;50:3239–49. https://doi.org/10.1002/art.20508.

52. Casciola-Rosen L, Andrade F, Ulanet D, et al. Cleavage by granzyme B is strongly predictive of autoantigen status: implications for initiation of autoimmunity. J Exp Med. 1999;190:815–26. https://doi.org/10.1084/jem.190.6.815.

53. Cooper GS, Parks CG. Occupational and environmental exposures as risk factors for systemic lupus erythematosus. Curr Rheumatol Rep. 2004;6:367–74. https://doi.org/10.1007/s11926-004-0011-6.

54. Incaprera M, Rindi L, Bazzichi A, et al. Potential role of the Epstein-Barr virus in systemic lupus erythematosus autoimmunity. Clin Exp Rheumatol. 1998;16:289–94. http://www.ncbi.nlm.nih.gov/pubmed/9631751.

55. Moon UY, Park SJ, Oh ST, et al. Patients with systemic lupus erythematosus have abnormally elevated Epstein-Barr virus load in blood. Arthritis Res Ther. 2004;6:R295–302. https://doi.org/10.1186/ar1181.

56. Cameron JS. Lupus nephritis in childhood and adolescence. Pediatr Nephrol. 1994;8:230–49. https://doi.org/10.1007/BF00865490.

57. Iqbal S, Sher MR, Good RA, et al. Diversity in presenting manifestations of systemic lupus erythematosus in children. J Pediatr. 1999;135:500–5. https://doi.org/10.1016/s0022-3476(99)70174-5.

58. Marks SD, Hiraki L, Hagelberg S, Silverman ED, Hebert D. Age-related renal prognosis of childhood-onset SLE. Pediatr Nephrol. 2002;17:C107.

59. Zelko F, Beebe D, Baker A, et al. Academic outcomes in childhood-onset systemic lupus erythematosus. Arthritis Care Res (Hoboken). 2012;64:1167–74. https://doi.org/10.1002/acr.21681.

60. D'Cruz DP, Khamashta MA, Hughes GRV. Systemic lupus erythematosus. Lancet. 2007;369:587–96. https://doi.org/10.1016/S0140-6736(07)60279-7.

61. Hughes GRV. Hughes syndrome (the antiphospholipid syndrome): ten clinical lessons. Autoimmun Rev. 2008;7:262–6. https://doi.org/10.1016/j.autrev.2007.11.017.

62. Uthman I, Khamashta M. Antiphospholipid syndrome and the kidneys. Semin Arthritis Rheum. 2006;35:360–7. https://doi.org/10.1016/j.semarthrit.2006.01.001.

63. Lee T, von Scheven E, Sandborg C. Systemic lupus erythematosus and antiphospholipid syndrome in children and adolescents. Curr Opin Rheumatol. 2001;13:415–21. https://doi.org/10.1097/00002281-200109000-00013.

64. Marks SD, Pilkington C, Woo P, et al. The use of the British Isles Lupus Assessment Group (BILAG) index as a valid tool in assessing disease activity in childhood-onset systemic lupus erythematosus.

64. Rheumatology (Oxford). 2004;43:1186–9. https://doi.org/10.1093/rheumatology/keh284.

65. Schwartz GJ, Muñoz A, Schneider MF, et al. New equations to estimate GFR in children with CKD. J Am Soc Nephrol. 2009;20:629–37. https://doi.org/10.1681/ASN.2008030287.

66. Marto N, Bertolaccini ML, Calabuig E, et al. Anti-C1q antibodies in nephritis: correlation between titres and renal disease activity and positive predictive value in systemic lupus erythematosus. Ann Rheum Dis. 2005;64:444–8. https://doi.org/10.1136/ard.2004.024943.

67. Marks SD, Shah V, Pilkington C, et al. Renal tubular dysfunction in children with systemic lupus erythematosus. Pediatr Nephrol. 2005;20:141–8. https://doi.org/10.1007/s00467-004-1707-6.

68. Weening JJ, D'Agati VD, Schwartz MM, et al. The classification of glomerulonephritis in systemic lupus erythematosus revisited. Kidney Int. 2004;65:521–30. https://doi.org/10.1111/j.1523-1755.2004.00443.x.

69. Weening JJ, D'Agati VD, Schwartz MM, et al. The classification of glomerulonephritis in systemic lupus erythematosus revisited. J Am Soc Nephrol. 2004;15:241–50. https://doi.org/10.1097/01.asn.0000108969.21691.5d.

70. Marks SD, Tullus K, Sebire NJ. Current issues in pediatric lupus nephritis: role of revised histopathological classification. Fetal Pediatr Pathol. 2006;25:297–309. https://doi.org/10.1080/15513810701209512.

71. Austin HA, Muenz LR, Joyce KM, et al. Prognostic factors in lupus nephritis. Contribution of renal histologic data. Am J Med. 1983;75:382–91. https://doi.org/10.1016/0002-9343(83)90338-8.

72. Yokoyama H, Wada T, Hara A, et al. The outcome and a new ISN/RPS 2003 classification of lupus nephritis in Japanese. Kidney Int. 2004;66:2382–8. https://doi.org/10.1111/j.1523-1755.2004.66027.x.

73. Hagelberg S, Lee Y, Bargman J, et al. Longterm followup of childhood lupus nephritis. J Rheumatol. 2002;29:2635–42. http://www.ncbi.nlm.nih.gov/pubmed/12465165.

74. Marks SD, Sebire NJ, Pilkington C, et al. Clinicopathological correlations of paediatric lupus nephritis. Pediatr Nephrol. 2007;22:77–83. https://doi.org/10.1007/s00467-006-0296-y.

75. Fanouriakis A, Kostopoulou M, Cheema K, et al. 2019 update of the joint European League Against Rheumatism and European Renal Association-European Dialysis and Transplant Association (EULAR/ERA-EDTA) recommendations for the management of lupus nephritis. Ann Rheum Dis. 2020;79:713–23. https://doi.org/10.1136/annrheumdis-2020-216924.

76. Groot N, de Graeff N, Avcin T, et al. European evidence-based recommendations for diagnosis and treatment of childhood-onset systemic lupus erythematosus: the SHARE initiative. Ann Rheum Dis. 2017;76:1788–96. https://doi.org/10.1136/annrheumdis-2016-210960.

77. Groot N, de Graeff N, Avcin T, et al. European evidence-based recommendations for diagnosis and treatment of paediatric antiphospholipid syndrome: the SHARE initiative. Ann Rheum Dis. 2017;76:1637–41. https://doi.org/10.1136/annrheumdis-2016-211001.

78. Groot N, de Graeff N, Marks SD, et al. European evidence-based recommendations for the diagnosis and treatment of childhood-onset lupus nephritis: the SHARE initiative. Ann Rheum Dis. 2017;76:1965–73. https://doi.org/10.1136/annrheumdis-2017-211898.

79. Bertsias GK, Tektonidou M, Amoura Z, et al. Joint European League Against Rheumatism and European Renal Association-European Dialysis and Transplant Association (EULAR/ERA-EDTA) recommendations for the management of adult and paediatric lupus nephritis. Ann Rheum Dis. 2012;71:1771–82. https://doi.org/10.1136/annrheumdis-2012-201940.

80. Tullus K. New developments in the treatment of systemic lupus erythematosus. Pediatr Nephrol. 2012;27:727–32. https://doi.org/10.1007/s00467-011-1859-0.

81. Wright EC, Tullus K, Dillon MJ. Retrospective study of plasma exchange in children with systemic lupus erythematosus. Pediatr Nephrol. 2004;19:1108–14. https://doi.org/10.1007/s00467-004-1552-7.

82. Condon MB, Ashby D, Pepper RJ, et al. Prospective observational single-centre cohort study to evaluate the effectiveness of treating lupus nephritis with rituximab and mycophenolate mofetil but no oral steroids. Ann Rheum Dis. 2013;72:1280–6. https://doi.org/10.1136/annrheumdis-2012-202844.

83. Lightstone L, Doria A, Wilson H, et al. Can we manage lupus nephritis without chronic corticosteroids administration? Autoimmun Rev. 2018;17:4–10. https://doi.org/10.1016/j.autrev.2017.11.002.

84. Chan TM, Li FK, Tang CS, et al. Efficacy of mycophenolate mofetil in patients with diffuse proliferative lupus nephritis. Hong Kong-Guangzhou Nephrology Study Group. N Engl J Med. 2000;343:1156–62. https://doi.org/10.1056/NEJM200010193431604.

85. Appel GB, Contreras G, Dooley MA, et al. Mycophenolate mofetil versus cyclophosphamide for induction treatment of lupus nephritis. J Am Soc Nephrol. 2009;20:1103–12. https://doi.org/10.1681/ASN.2008101028.

86. Isenberg D, Appel GB, Contreras G, et al. Influence of race/ethnicity on response to lupus nephritis treatment: the ALMS study. Rheumatology (Oxford). 2010;49:128–40. https://doi.org/10.1093/rheumatology/kep346.

87. Radhakrishnan J, Moutzouris D-A, Ginzler EM, et al. Mycophenolate mofetil and intravenous cyclophosphamide are similar as induction therapy for

class V lupus nephritis. Kidney Int. 2010;77:152–60. https://doi.org/10.1038/ki.2009.412.

88. Touma Z, Gladman DD, Urowitz MB, et al. Mycophenolate mofetil for induction treatment of lupus nephritis: a systematic review and meta-analysis. J Rheumatol. 2011;38:69–78. https://doi.org/10.3899/jrheum.100130.

89. Kazyra I, Pilkington C, Marks SD, et al. Mycophenolate mofetil treatment in children and adolescents with lupus. Arch Dis Child. 2010;95:1059–61. https://doi.org/10.1136/adc.2009.178608.

90. Chan T-M, Tse K-C, Tang CS-O, et al. Long-term study of mycophenolate mofetil as continuous induction and maintenance treatment for diffuse proliferative lupus nephritis. J Am Soc Nephrol. 2005;16:1076–84. https://doi.org/10.1681/ASN.2004080686.

91. Contreras G, Pardo V, Leclercq B, et al. Sequential therapies for proliferative lupus nephritis. N Engl J Med. 2004;350:971–80. https://doi.org/10.1056/NEJMoa031855.

92. Ginzler EM, Dooley MA, Aranow C, et al. Mycophenolate mofetil or intravenous cyclophosphamide for lupus nephritis. N Engl J Med. 2005;353:2219–28. https://doi.org/10.1056/NEJMoa043731.

93. Marks SD, Tullus K. Successful outcomes with rituximab therapy for refractory childhood systemic lupus erythematosus. Pediatr Nephrol. 2006;21:598–9. https://doi.org/10.1007/s00467-006-0024-7.

94. Rovin BH, Furie R, Latinis K, et al. Efficacy and safety of rituximab in patients with active proliferative lupus nephritis: the lupus nephritis assessment with rituximab study. Arthritis Rheum. 2012;64:1215–26. https://doi.org/10.1002/art.34359.

95. Furie R, Rovin B, Appel G, Kamen D, Fervenza F, Spindler A, et al. Effect of rituximab on anti-double-stranded DNA antibody and C3 levels and relationship to response: results from the LUNAR trial. 9th international congress on systemic lupus erythematosus, Vancouver, June 24–27, Poster PO2 E 22, 2010.

96. Merrill JT, Neuwelt CM, Wallace DJ, et al. Efficacy and safety of rituximab in moderately-to-severely active systemic lupus erythematosus: the randomized, double-blind, phase II/III systemic lupus erythematosus evaluation of rituximab trial. Arthritis Rheum. 2010;62:222–33. https://doi.org/10.1002/art.27233.

97. Díaz-Lagares C, Croca S, Sangle S, et al. Efficacy of rituximab in 164 patients with biopsy-proven lupus nephritis: pooled data from European cohorts. Autoimmun Rev. 2012;11:357–64. https://doi.org/10.1016/j.autrev.2011.10.009.

98. Lewis EJ, Hunsicker LG, Lan SP, et al. A controlled trial of plasmapheresis therapy in severe lupus nephritis. The Lupus Nephritis Collaborative Study Group. N Engl J Med. 1992;326:1373–9. https://doi.org/10.1056/NEJM199205213262101.

99. Flanc RS, Roberts MA, Strippoli GFM, et al. Treatment for lupus nephritis. Cochrane Database Syst Rev. 2004;CD002922. https://doi.org/10.1002/14651858.CD002922.pub2.

100. Simmonds J, Trompeter R, Calvert TTK. Does long-term steroid use influence long-term growth? Pediatr Nephrol. 2005;20:C107.

101. Wofsy D, Appel GB, Dooley M, Ginzler E, Isenberg D, Jayne D, et al. Aspreva lupus management study ALMS) maintenance results. 9th international congress on systemic lupus erythematosus, Vancouver, June 24–27, Poster PO2 E 23, 2010.

102. Dooley MA, Jayne D, Ginzler EM, et al. Mycophenolate versus azathioprine as maintenance therapy for lupus nephritis. N Engl J Med. 2011;365:1886–95. https://doi.org/10.1056/NEJMoa1014460.

103. Houssiau FA, D'Cruz D, Sangle S, et al. Azathioprine versus mycophenolate mofetil for long-term immunosuppression in lupus nephritis: results from the MAINTAIN nephritis trial. Ann Rheum Dis. 2010;69:2083–9. https://doi.org/10.1136/ard.2010.131995.

104. Ma ALT, Bale G, Aitkenhead H, et al. Measuring erythrocyte Thiopurine Methyltransferase activity in children-is it helpful? J Pediatr. 2016;179:216–8. https://doi.org/10.1016/j.jpeds.2016.08.073.

105. Melles RB, Marmor MF. The risk of toxic retinopathy in patients on long-term hydroxychloroquine therapy. JAMA Ophthalmol. 2014;132:1453–60. https://doi.org/10.1001/jamaophthalmol.2014.3459.

106. Navarra SV, Guzmán RM, Gallacher AE, et al. Efficacy and safety of belimumab in patients with active systemic lupus erythematosus: a randomised, placebo-controlled, phase 3 trial. Lancet. 2011;377:721–31. https://doi.org/10.1016/S0140-6736(10)61354-2.

107. Furie R, Rovin BH, Houssiau F, et al. Two-year, randomized, controlled trial of Belimumab in lupus nephritis. N Engl J Med. 2020;383:1117–28. https://doi.org/10.1056/NEJMoa2001180.

108. Brunner HI, Abud-Mendoza C, Viola DO, et al. Safety and efficacy of intravenous belimumab in children with systemic lupus erythematosus: results from a randomised, placebo-controlled trial. Ann Rheum Dis. 2020;79:1340–8. https://doi.org/10.1136/annrheumdis-2020-217101.

109. Cassia MA, Alberici F, Jones RB, et al. Rituximab as maintenance treatment for systemic lupus erythematosus: a multicenter observational study of 147 patients. Arthritis Rheumatol. 2019;71:1670–80. https://doi.org/10.1002/art.40932.

110. Masoud S, McAdoo SP, Bedi R, et al. Ofatumumab for B cell depletion in patients with systemic lupus erythematosus who are allergic to rituximab. Rheumatology (Oxford). 2018;57:1156–61. https://doi.org/10.1093/rheumatology/key042.

IgA Vasculitis Nephritis (Henoch-Schönlein Purpura Nephritis)

27

Jae Il Shin

Introduction

Immunoglobulin A (IgA) vasculitis, formerly called Henoch-Schönlein purpura (HSP), was first described by William Heberden [1], a London physician, in 1801 and was named after the description of the clinical entity characterized by purpura and joint pain by Johann Schönlein in 1837 [2] and of the frequent association of gastrointestinal symptoms and kidney involvement by Edouard Henoch in 1874 [3]. IgA vasculitis is the most common form of systemic vasculitis in children; it mainly affects the skin, joints, gastrointestinal tract and kidneys. IgA vasculitis is usually self-limited to 1–4 weeks, but relapses can occur. The overall prognosis of IgA vasculitis is favorable, but the long-term prognosis is dependent on the degree of renal involvement [4, 5].

Diagnostic Criteria

The American College of Rheumatology (ACR) proposed in 1990 that the presence of any 2 or more of the following criteria was required for the diagnosis of IgA vasculitis: (1) an age of less than 20 years at disease onset, (2) palpable purpura, (3) acute abdominal pain, and (4) biopsy showing granulocytes in the walls of small arterioles or venules [6]. In 2005, the diagnostic criteria for IgA vasculitis were modified by the European League Against Rheumatism/ Paediatric Rheumatology European Society (EULAR/PRES) [7]. In this new diagnostic system, the age criterion was deleted, 'predominant IgA deposition' was included in the definition of the 'biopsy' criterion, and arthritis and renal involvement were added as independent criteria [7]. Therefore, IgA vasculitis is diagnosed as follows: palpable purpura (mandatory criterion) in the presence of at least one of the following four features: (1) diffuse abdominal pain, (2) any biopsy showing predominant IgA deposition, (3) arthritis or arthralgia (acute, any joint), and (4) renal involvement (any hematuria and/or proteinuria) [7]. Skin biopsy is rarely performed to diagnose IgA vasculitis, but may be necessary in doubtful cases such as isolated purpura or atypical characteristics to differentiate from leukocytoclastic vasculitis. The latter will show no IgA deposits [7, 8].

J. I. Shin (✉)
Department of Pediatrics, Yonsei University College of Medicine, Severance Children's Hospital, Seoul, South Korea
e-mail: shinji@yuhs.ac

© The Author(s), under exclusive license to Springer Nature Switzerland AG 2023
F. Schaefer, L. A. Greenbaum (eds.), *Pediatric Kidney Disease*,
https://doi.org/10.1007/978-3-031-11665-0_27

Epidemiology

The prevalence of IgA vasculitis varies from 3.0/100,000 to 26.7/100,000 children [9, 10]. IgA vasculitis is more common in preschool aged children and in males, and there seems to be an increased frequency in autumn and winter. The pathogenesis of IgA vasculitis is unclear, but it is considered as a complex disease caused by various genetic and triggering environmental factors [9]. It is often preceded by an upper respiratory tract infection 1–3 weeks prior to the onset of symptoms. Various infectious agents, such as parvovirus B19, hepatitis B and C virus, adenovirus, Group A β-hemolytic streptococcus, staphylococcus aureus, and mycoplasma, and various drugs, vaccinations, cancers, insect bites or exposure to cold weather have been reported as triggering factors for IgA vasculitis [9, 10]. Familial cases of IgA vasculitis have also been reported [11].

Clinical Findings

Skin

Palpable purpura is the most common finding, but petechiae, maculae, papulae, urticaria, ecchymosis or bullae can also occur. Skin lesions are generally distributed symmetrically over the extensor surfaces of the lower legs (gravity or pressure-dependent areas), arms and buttocks, but trunk, face, eyelids, earlobes and genitalia can also be involved [12]. In young children, edema of the scalp, hands and feet can be observed. The skin findings usually resolve within 1–2 weeks, but persistent (>4 weeks) or relapsing skin manifestations are observed in about 25% of children with IgA vasculitis, and may be associated with the occurrence and severity of renal involvement [13–15].

Joints

Joint symptoms occur in about 80% of children with IgA vasculitis, and large joints of the lower extremities, such as the ankles and knees, are usually affected [12]. Joint pain is a frequent finding and periarticular swelling and tenderness, usually without synovial fluid effusion, may be present. Joint symptoms resolve with time without any deformity or erosions [12].

Gastrointestinal Tract

Gastrointestinal involvement is reported in about 50–70% of children with IgA vasculitis and usually presents as diffuse abdominal pain, which can be increased after meals, nausea, emesis, and bloody stools such as melaena and hematochezia [12, 16]. Gastrointestinal symptoms are caused by bowel wall edema and submucosal hemorrhage due to vasculitis. Severe gastrointestinal complications can occur, including intussusception, bowel infarction, gangrene or perforation, duodenal obstruction, massive gastrointestinal hemorrhage requiring blood transfusion, appendicitis, pancreatitis, hydrops of the gall bladder, protein losing enteropathy and formation of fistulas or strictures.

Other Nonrenal Organ Involvement

Although rare, IgA vasculitis can be complicated by various other manifestations, such as neurologic findings (obtundation, seizure, paresis, cortical blindness, chorea, ataxia and cranial or peripheral neuropathy), urologic complications (orchitis, epididymitis, and stenosing ureteritis, presenting as renal colic), carditis, myositis or intramuscular bleeding, pulmonary hemorrhage, and anterior uveitis [17]. Because some of these manifestations can be rapidly fatal, close observation and monitoring of affected patients is important.

Kidney

The incidence of renal involvement in IgA vasculitis varies from 20 to 80% in published case series [13–15]. Renal involvement includes isolated haematuria (14%), isolated proteinuria (9%), both hematuria and proteinuria (56%), nephrotic-range proteinuria (20%) and nephrotic-nephritic syndrome (1%) [15]. Hypertension may develop at the onset of disease or during recovery, even with minimal or no urinary abnormalities [18]. In a large UK primary care database of 10,405 patients with childhood-onset IgA vasculitis, there was a significantly increased risk of hypertension and stage 3–5 chronic kidney disease (CKD) compared with age-matched and sex-matched controls, although there was no evidence of association with ischaemic heart disease, cerebrovascular disease or venous thromboembolism [19]. Therefore, appropriate surveillance for hypertension and CKD in children with IgA vasculitis may be necessary, and risk factor modification could improve long-term outcomes in these patients [19].

The first urinary abnormalities are detected within 4 weeks of disease onset in 80% of children with IgA vasculitis and within the next 2 months in the remainder, although a small number of patients present with urinary abnormalities several months later or as the initial feature [20]. Minor urinary abnormalities usually resolve with time, whereas severe renal involvement such as nephrotic syndrome and acute nephritic syndrome, can progress to CKD. In a systematic review of 1133 children with IgA vasculitis observed in 12 studies, the overall incidence of long-term renal impairment (defined as persistent nephrotic syndrome, nephritis, or hypertension) was 1.8%. Permanent renal impairment occurred in none of the 65.8% children with normal urinalysis during the acute disease, in 1.6% of the 26.9% with isolated haematuria and/or proteinuria, and in 19.5% of the 7.2% patients initially presenting with nephritic or nephrotic syndrome [20].

Risk Factors for Renal Involvement

Some authors reported that an older age at onset, persistent purpura (>4 weeks), severe abdominal symptoms, decreased factor XIII (fibrin stabilizing factor) activity, and a relapsing disease pattern are significant risk factors for renal involvement in children with IgA vasculitis, and these factors were linked to each other and all indicated a severe disease course [13–15]. In addition, persistent purpura, severe abdominal symptoms, and relapse were associated with the development of significant proteinuria [14]. A recent meta-analysis showed that significant risk factors associated with renal involvement in IgA vasculitis were male gender, abdominal pain, gastrointestinal bleeding, severe abdominal pain, persistent purpura, relapse, a high white blood cell count (>15 × 10^9/L), a high platelet count (>500 × 10^9/L), elevated anti-streptolysin O (ASO) titer and decreased complement component 3 (C3) [13].

Atypical Presentation

IgA vasculitis is diagnosed clinically, but atypical presentation often causes difficulties in the diagnosis. Gastrointestinal symptoms precede the cutaneous rash in about 25% of children with IgA vasculitis, [16] and joint symptoms or scrotal pain may precede the skin rash [16]. In addition, some diseases such as systemic lupus erythematosus, microscopic polyangiitis or Crohn disease can mimic IgA vasculitis [21]. Since atypical presentation of IgA vasculitis can lead to an incorrect diagnosis, causing unnecessary therapies and procedures (e.g., appendectomy) and unfavorable outcomes, it is important to include IgA vasculitis in the differential diagnoses, although diagnosis can be very difficult in those settings.

Laboratory and Radiologic Investigations

Because IgA vasculitis is diagnosed clinically, there is no specific diagnostic test for IgA vasculitis. Recommended initial investigations are complete blood count to evaluate for anemia or leukocytosis, erythrocyte sedimentation rate to evaluate for inflammation, coagulation profile to exclude bleeding disorders, biochemical profile to screen for acute kidney injury or hypoalbuminemia, ASO titer, urine dipstick and protein/creatinine ratio to evaluate for renal involvement and tests to screen for sepsis if the diagnosis is unclear and purpura is present (e.g., blood culture for meningococcemia) [22]. Antinuclear antibody titer, anti-double stranded DNA antibody, anti-neutrophil cytoplasmic antibody (ANCA), complement levels (C3 and C4) and immunoglobulins (IgG, IgA and IgM) may also be necessary to differentiate IgA vasculitis from other vasculitides or overlapping diseases.

IgA vasculitis has a bleeding tendency due to abnormal platelet aggregation, decreased factor XIII levels by vasculitic process and increased von Willebrand factor (vWF) levels by endothelial injury despite normal platelet count and clotting factors [23, 24]. Plasma D-dimer levels can be increased [24]. A stool test for occult blood can be used to detect gastrointestinal hemorrhage.

Serum IgA levels (mostly IgA1) are increased in 50% of children with IgA vasculitis, and IgA-rheumatoid factor, IgA-containing immune complexes, IgA-fibronectin aggregates and cryoglobulins have been found [25, 26]. Serum IgE and eosinophil cationic protein (ECP) levels can be elevated, [27, 28] and C3, C4, and CH50 levels are occasionally decreased in the acute stage of disease [29]. ANCAs (c-ANCA and p-ANCA) are generally negative in IgA vasculitis except in rare cases [30, 31], but IgA-ANCA has been detected in the acute stage of disease [32, 33]. Antiphospholipid antibodies may be positive [34].

Imaging studies may be necessary to detect complications of IgA vasculitis, with selection based on the clinical picture [22]. Chest X-ray can detect pulmonary involvement; abdominal X-ray can identify ileus or perforation of the gastrointestinal tract. Renal ultrasound can detect increased echogenicity of the kidneys or hydronephrosis; abdominal ultrasound can identify thickened bowel wall or intussusception [22].

Renal Histopathologic Findings

Light Microscopy Findings

The light microscopic findings of IgA vasculitis nephritis (IgAVN) are characterized by mesangial proliferative glomerulonephritis with varying degrees of mesangial hypercellularity (Fig. 27.1a), segmental sclerosis (Fig. 27.1b) and crescents (Fig. 27.1c), similar to the predominant findings in IgA nephropathy (IgAN) [35, 36]. These glomerular changes are usually graded according to the International Study of Kidney Disease in Children (ISKDC) classification system (Table 27.1) [37]. Crescents are reportedly much more common in IgAVN than in IgAN [25] and are frequently seen in association with capillary wall destruction and endocapillary cell proliferation with subendothelial immune deposits of IgA and complement [38]. Crescents are classified as cellular, fibrocellular or fibrous. Crescents are cellular at the onset of the disease and evolve with time towards fibrous, causing global glomerulosclerosis (Fig. 27.1d).

Because the ISKDC classification does not include tubulointerstitial changes and other histologic features in IgAVN, some authors have used histopathologic scoring systems, such as activity and chronicity scores [39, 40]. Acute changes included mesangial matrix increase, mesangial hypercellularity, endothelial swelling, hyalinosis, basement membrane adhesion to Bowman's capsule, glomerular lobulations, glomerular neutrophils, fibrinoid necrosis, nuclear debris, interstitial vasculitis with leukocytoclastic reaction, tubular damage, interstitial edema and interstitial mononuclear infiltrate [39]. Chronic changes include interstitial fibrosis, tubular atrophy, fibrous crescents, global sclerosis, vascular hyalinosis and intimal hyperplasia [39]. The degree of tubulointerstitial lesions is correlated with the glomerular pathology [35].

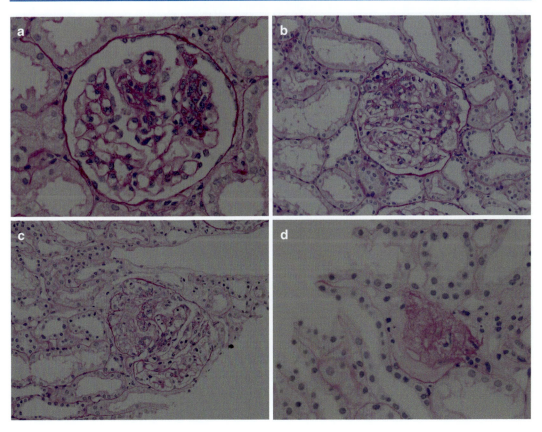

Fig. 27.1 Light microscopy findings in IgA vasculitis nephritis. (**a**) Mild mesangial cell proliferation (PAS, ×400). (**b**) Glomerulus with segmental sclerosis (PAS, ×200). (**c**) Glomerulus with cellular crescent (PAS, ×200). (**d**) Glomerulus with global sclerosis (PAS, ×400)

Table 27.1 The classification of IgA vasculitis nephritis in the International Study of Kidney Disease in Children

Grade I		Minimal alterations
Grade II		Mesangial proliferation without crescents
Grade III	IIIa	Focal mesangial proliferation or sclerosis with <50% crescents
	IIIb	Diffuse mesangial proliferation or sclerosis with <50% crescents
Grade IV	IVa	Focal mesangial proliferation or sclerosis with 50–75% crescents
	IVb	Diffuse mesangial proliferation or sclerosis with 50–75% crescents
Grade V	Va	Focal mesangial proliferation or sclerosis with >75% crescents
	Vb	Diffuse mesangial proliferation or sclerosis with >75% crescents
Grade VI		Membranoproliferative glomerulonephritis

Immunofluorescence Findings

Granular deposits of IgA (predominantly IgA1) in mesangial areas are characteristic of IgAVN (Fig. 27.2a). The IgA deposits are diffuse, in contrast to the frequent focal and segmental changes of glomeruli. C3 (Fig. 27.2b) and the alternative complement pathway components are frequently found, but the components of the classic complement pathway, such as C1q and C4, are rarely detected [38, 41]. IgA and C3 can be deposited in arterioles and capillary walls [25, 36, 38]. IgG and IgM are less frequently detected [38, 42]. Glomerular fibrin deposits (Fig. 27.2c) are more frequently found in IgAVN than in IgAN, [25, 38] and are associated with the formation of crescents.

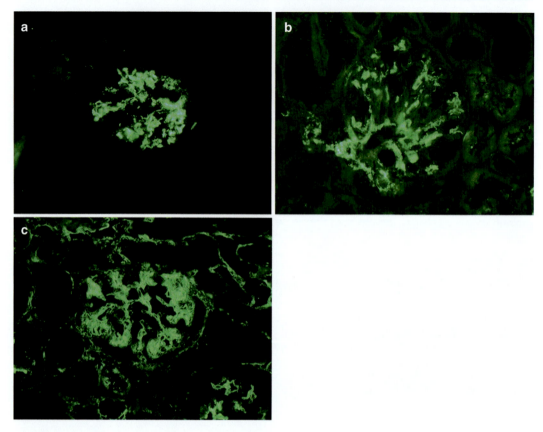

Fig. 27.2 Immunofluorescence findings in IgA vasculitis nephritis. (**a**) Mesangial IgA deposition (×100). (**b**) Mesangial C3 deposition (×200). (**c**) Mesangial fibrinogen deposition (×100)

Electron Microscopy Findings

Electron-dense deposits are mainly found in mesangial areas (Fig. 27.3a), but the deposits can be detected in subendothelial areas (Fig. 27.3b); rarely, hump-like deposits are found in subepithelial areas [25, 35, 41]. There are varying degrees of foot process effacement of visceral epithelial cells, depending on the degree of glomerular injury [25, 35, 41].

Clinicopathologic Correlations

In general, a good correlation between the severity of renal involvement and pathologic grading is observed in IgAVN and the severity of proteinuria at onset is a significant determinant of renal pathologic findings such as crescent formation, endocapillary proliferation, and tubular atrophy [43]. Proteinuria is also correlated with the ISKDC grade [44]; however, even mild to moderate proteinuria may be associated with severe morphological changes [44]. Hence, renal biopsy may be indicated, not only in patients with nephrotic syndrome, but also in those with mild proteinuria.

Although there are few reports on follow-up renal biopsies in IgAVN, there is also a generally good correlation between the clinical course and histopathologic changes [45]. IgAVN children who achieve clinical remission show a decrease in IgA deposits and regression of mesangial proliferation or crescents on follow-up renal biopsy, while those who have persistent nephritis demonstrate severe histologic findings with chronic lesions [45]. However, some reports emphasized that abnormal renal histologic findings can per-

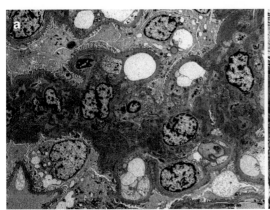
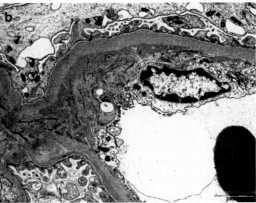

Fig. 27.3 Electron microscopy findings in IgA vasculitis nephritis. (**a**) Electron dense deposits in mesangial areas (×3000). (**b**) Electron-dense deposits in subendothelial areas (×10,000)

sist despite clinical remission [46, 47]. Algoet et al. reported that renal histologic findings were normal only in 25% of patients who had achieved complete clinical remission 5–9 years after the onset of IgA vasculitis [46]. Shin et al. also showed persistent histologic abnormalities in all patients of a IgAVN cohort after immunosuppressive treatment regardless of clinical improvement, suggesting the kidneys were not completely healed even in those with clinical remission [47].

Risk Factors for Poor Prognosis

The clinical presentation at the onset of IgAVN is predictive of long-term outcome [20]. The risk of progression to CKD was highest in IgA vasculitis children who presented with nephritic-nephrotic syndrome (45–50%) followed by those with nephrotic syndrome (up to 40%), acute nephritic syndrome (up to 15%), hematuria and non-nephrotic proteinuria (5–15%) and microscopic hematuria with or without minimal proteinuria (<5%) [20, 48]. In a systematic review, the risk of long-term renal impairment was 12 times higher in IgAVN patients with nephritic or nephrotic syndrome than in those with only abnormal urinalysis, and was 2.5 times higher in females than males [20]. Additional information is provided by very long-term outcome studies of IgAVN [49, 50]. Revisiting a cohort of IgA vasculitis patients at an average of 23 years after first manifestation, Goldstein et al. observed highly unpredictable late outcomes; 7 of 78 patients with normal urinalysis or apparent complete recovery showed active renal disease or ESRD [49]. Ronkainen et al. also showed that even patients with mild renal symptoms at the onset of IgA vasculitis have a risk for severe long-term complications [50].

Also, the clinical course during follow-up may be important to predict the prognosis [48, 51, 52]. Bunchman et al. showed that a creatinine clearance <70 mL/min/1.73 m^2 3 years after onset predicted progression to ESRD, whereas a clearance >125 mL/min/1.73 m^2 predicted normal renal function at 10-year follow-up [51]. Coppo et al. demonstrated that the risk for progression was related to increasing mean proteinuria levels during follow-up in both children and adults with IgAVN [52].

Histopathological lesions related to poor prognosis are a high grade by ISKDC, crescents in >50% of glomeruli, glomerular sclerosis or tubulointerstitial changes [48, 53, 54]. However, the initial renal biopsy may not predict the outcome of IgAVN since patients with mild histopathological disease activity (ISKDC II-III) usually receive less aggressive immunosuppressive therapy [55]. Therefore, some investigators suggested that serial biopsies might be helpful to establish the ultimate outcome in IgAVN patients with renal exacerbations [46]. A younger age at onset was an independent determinant of histological regression. The activity index at the follow-up biopsy correlated positively with changes in mesangial IgA deposits and the chronicity index at the follow-up biopsy correlated positively with the time immunosuppressive therapy was started [47]. One report suggested that the serum IgA/C3 ratio might be a useful marker for predicting serial histologic lesions of IgAVN because it correlated with the severity of renal pathology and clinical outcome in children with severe IgAVN [56].

Schärer et al., in a comprehensive multivariate analysis, demonstrated that initial renal insufficiency, nephrotic syndrome, and the severity of histological alterations (as defined by the percentage of glomeruli with crescents) are significant independent predictors of progressive renal failure in patients with IgAVN [54].

From a systematic review of 12 unselected IgA vasculitis populations, it was recommended that if the urinalysis is normal at presentation, monitoring can be limited to 6 months in patients with persistently normal urine findings [20]. However, the recommended duration of follow-up remains controversial since in individual children with normal urinalysis at onset renal involvement may still develop after several years [49, 50].

Pathogenesis

While the complete pathogenesis of IgA vasculitis remains to be elucidated, abnormalities of IgA have an important role. IgA vasculitis develops as a consequence of leukocytoclastic vasculitis due to IgA deposition in the wall of capillaries and post-capillary venules of various organs, including skin, gastrointestinal tract and the mesangium of the kidney [10, 12, 21]. Genetic predisposition, activation of complement, cytokines, autoantibodies and coagulation abnormalities are also involved in the pathogenesis of IgA vasculitis [21].

Genetic Predisposition

Although IgA vasculitis occurs mostly as sporadic cases, familial clustering has been reported [11]. Various candidate genes and genetic polymorphisms have been associated with the risk for IgA vasculitis or IgAVN [21]. These include human leukocyte antigen (HLA-A, B, B35, DRB1, DQA1), cytokines (interleukin (IL)-1ß,IL-1 receptor antagonist, IL-18, transforming growth factor (TGF)-ß), adhesion molecules (P-selectin, intracellular adhesion molecule-1), cytotoxic T-lymphocyte antigen 4, the MEFV gene (encoding pyrin, an important active member of the inflammasome), the renin-angiotensin system genes (angiotensin converting enzyme, angiotensinogen) and the C1GALT1 gene (encoding ß 1,3-galactosyltransferase, an important role in the glycosylation of the IgA1 hinge region).

Abnormalities of IgA

Elevated serum levels of IgA, principally IgA1, and circulating IgA-containing immune complexes are observed in patients with IgAVN [57, 58]. One study reported that the number of IgA-producing cells was increased in IgA vasculitis, but not in other forms of leukocytoclastic vasculitis [59]. Both increased IgA synthesis and decreased clearance have been reported as contributors to the pathogenesis of IgAVN [25]. It has been hypothesized that production of polymeric IgA by the mucosal immune system in response to various mucosally presented antigens [60] may be increased, and the reticuloendothelial system function impaired [61]. In addition, all patients with IgA vasculitis have IgA1-circulating immune complexes of small molecular mass, while only those with nephritis have additional large-molecular-mass IgA1-IgG-containing circulating immune complexes [58].

There are two subclasses of IgA (IgA1 and IgA2) and ~90% of serum IgA is IgA1. IgA1 and

IgA2 differ structurally in the hinge region of the heavy chain. IgA1, unlike IgA2, has a proline-rich hinge region composed of 5–6 O-linked glycosylation sites. An abnormal glycosylation of the IgA1 hinge region occurs in the context of a deficiency of galactose and/or sialic acid [21, 57]. Such an aberrantly glycosylated IgA1 is prone to cause IgA aggregation and may change IgA1 structure, modifying interactions with IgA receptors and matrix proteins, leading to mesangial deposition of IgA1 [21, 57]. Although no confirmed genetic loci for IgA vasculitis have been identified to date, it was recently reported that aberrant glycosylation of IgA1 is inherited in both pediatric IgAN and IgAVN [62]. However, Kiryluk et al. reported that an increase of the poorly galactosylated IgA1 O-glycoforms levels may be insufficient to cause IgAN or IgAVN because first-degree relatives had high serum levels of poorly galactosylated IgA1 O-glycoforms without any signs of either IgAN or IgAVN [62]. They suggested that a 'second hit,' such as the formation of glycan-specific IgG (and IgA) antibodies, which could form large circulating immune complexes prone to deposition, might be required to develop overt disease [62].

Activation of Complement

Activation of complement, mainly via the alternative pathway, is an important mechanism of tissue injury in IgA vasculitis. Complement components are found in skin and glomeruli, and breakdown products of complement in plasma [29, 63, 64]. C4A and C4B deficiencies have been described in patients with IgAVN, [65] and glomerular deposition of C3 and properdin has been reported in 75–100% of patients with IgAVN [66]. Activation of the lectin pathway of complement has also been demonstrated in patients with IgAVN, which might contribute to the development of advanced glomerular injury and long-term urinary abnormalities in IgAVN [64]. The lectin pathway is initiated by mannose-binding lectin (MBL). MBL also forms complexes with MBL-associated serine proteases (MASP-1, MASP-2 and MASP-3) [64]. Hisano et al. reported that MBL/MASP-1

might be associated with glomerular deposition of fibrinogen [64].

Activation of Eosinophils

Activation of eosinophils has also been proposed to contribute to the pathogenesis of IgAVN [27, 28]. Elevated plasma IgE levels were more common [27] and serum eosinophil cationic protein (ECP) levels were significantly higher in children with IgA vasculitis than in those with IgAN or healthy controls [28]. Davin et al. speculated that the IgA-containing immune complexes could enhance IgE production locally by stimulation of the dermal and intestinal mast cells and deposition of IgA immune complexes was further enhanced by a subsequent increase in local capillary permeability [27].

Cytokines and Coagulation Abnormalities

Several proinflammatory cytokines, including tumor necrosis factor (TNF)-α, IL-1β, IL-2, IL-6, IL-8, IL-17, TGF-β, and vascular endothelial growth factor, have been reported to be involved in the development of IgA vasculitis. They are likely secreted by vascular endothelial cells, thus initiating and propagating the inflammatory reaction [21].

Circulating immune complexes can cause vascular endothelial injury and coagulation abnormalities in IgA vasculitis; plasma vWF levels are elevated at the acute stage of IgA vasculitis [24]. Factor XIII activity can also be decreased during the acute stage of IgA vasculitis, possibly due to degradation of factor XIII by proteolytic enzymes from inflammatory cells [23].

Mesangial Proliferation and Crescent Formation

Once IgA-containing complexes are deposited in glomerular mesangium, various components of IgA-containing complexes, such as Fcα and Fcγ fragments, fibronectin, or C3b, can bind to their receptors on the surface of mesangial cells and trigger proliferation of mesangial cells, production of extracellular matrix and synthesis of cytokines, such as monocyte chemoattractant protein-1 and IL-8, recruiting neutrophils and monocytes [25, 36, 67–71]. Other cytokines (TNF-α, IL-1, IL-6 and TGF-β) involved in the pathogenesis of IgA vasculitis can also stimulate mesangial cells [69–71].

In addition, local complement activation and intraglomerular coagulation by mesangial fibrin deposition can destroy the glomerular basement membrane. Attraction of macrophages and proliferation of cytokine-induced epithelial cells in Bowman's space can disrupt capsular integrity, leading to interstitial fibroblast infiltration into Bowman's space, causing crescent formation [25, 36, 38, 72].

Treatment

Prevention of Nephritis in IgA Vasculitis

Corticosteroids are commonly administered in the acute stage of IgA vasculitis to reduce the severity and duration of abdominal pain or arthralgia [73]. A number of retrospective studies, randomized controlled trials (RCTs), systematic review and meta-analyses have addressed the use of corticosteroids for preventing nephritis, with conflicting results [48, 73–76]. A well-conducted, randomized, double-blind, placebo-controlled trial showed no benefit of prednisone (4-week treatment) in preventing the development of nephritis in IgA vasculitis, but observed more rapid resolution of nephritis [73]. These results might be due to the reduction of mesangial proliferation and crescent formation by prednisone [77]. In addition, another randomized, double-blind, placebo-controlled trial reported that early 2-week treatment with prednisolone did not reduce the prevalence of proteinuria 12 months after disease onset in children with IgA vasculitis [74]. Based on this evidence, the Kidney Disease Improving Global Outcome

(KDIGO) guidelines recommend not using corticosteroids to prevent nephritis in children with IgA vasculitis [78].

Although the general use of prednisone to prevent nephritis is not supported, IgA vasculitis patients with extrarenal symptoms might benefit from early treatment. Some IgA vasculitis patients cannot tolerate oral medications due to abdominal pain; in these, initial intravenous followed by oral steroid therapy could be a useful and effective therapeutic strategy [79].

Treatment of IgAVN

Treatment of IgAVN should be aimed to prevent long-term renal morbidity in patients at risk, but there have been few RCTs to establish the optimal treatment due to the rarity of severe IgAVN. Therefore, the treatment of IgAVN remains controversial.

The KDIGO Guidelines and Therapeutic Considerations in Pediatric IgAVN

The KDIGO initiative recently published guidelines on the treatment of IgAVN [78]. The guidelines suggest that IgAVN children with persistent proteinuria of >0.5–1 g/day/1.73 m^2 should be treated with angiotensin converting enzyme (ACE) inhibitors or angiotensin receptor blockers (ARB), and children with GFR >50 mL/min/1.73 m^2 and persistent proteinuria >1 g/day/1.73 m^2, after a trial of renin–angiotensin system (RAS) blockade, should receive a 6-month course of corticosteroids (same as for IgAN). For cases with >50% crescents on biopsy, the guidelines recommend steroids and cyclophosphamide. If plasma creatinine is >500 μmol/L, oral prednisone should be preceded by 3 methylprednisolone (MP) pulses, and the patient should also receive plasma exchange. These guidelines are the same as for crescentic IgAN and ANCA vasculitis, and are independent of the patient's age [78]. However, there was concern by some pediatric nephrologists that the KDIGO guidelines might delay the initiation of effective treatment and increase the long-term risk of CKD due to undertreatment of IgAVN [80]. They argued that (1) the guidelines suggested for adults and children with IgAVN are based on randomized, controlled trials performed in adults with IgAN. However, IgAVN and IgAN are different diseases and have different outcomes despite similarities; (2) it is very important to treat initial episodes adequately without delay in IgAVN, and following the KDIGO guidelines might delay a potentially more effective treatment, increase the risk of CKD progression in patients with ISKDC grade IIIa, and cause a higher cumulative exposure to immunosuppressive therapy; (3) cyclophosphamide was ineffective in the treatment of IgAVN in the randomized controlled pediatric trials of the ISKDC; and (4) the KDIGO guidelines do not suggest addition of immunosuppressive drugs to steroids in patients with <50% crescentic glomeruli, even in the presence of nephrotic syndrome and/or deterioration of GFR, but more aggressive treatments, such as MP pulses, other immunosuppressive drugs or plasma exchange, may be required in these patients [80].

There are three aspects regarding the treatment of IgAVN that warrant additional commentary. First, the highly heterogenous spontaneous evolution of IgAVN should be considered. Many children with severe proteinuria at onset achieve spontaneous remission, but some children presenting with mild proteinuria develop severe renal pathology and progress to renal failure in the long-term [44, 81]. Second, the choice of therapy should be driven by the purpose of treatment. In most glomerular diseases, proteinuria reduction is accepted as an adequate surrogate marker of renal disease remission [82]. In IgAVN, however, some long-term studies have shown that clinical remission may not uniformly translate into a favorable long-term outcome [49, 50]. One study showed a discrepancy between clinical remission and histological improvement [47]. Therefore, it may be important to induce histological regression in addition to reduction of proteinuria in treating severe IgAVN. Third, it should be considered whether treatment should be based on clinical presentation or renal pathology in IgAVN. Ronkainen et al. reported that the first renal biopsy did not predict the outcome of IgAVN. The outcome of patients with ISKDC grades II–III was worse than of those with grades IV–V, probably because the latter received more aggressive immunosuppressive treatment. The authors suggested that the treatment of IgAVN should be based on clinical presentation rather than biopsy findings [55].

Indications for Renal Biopsy

Although clear outcome-based indications for renal biopsy in IgAVN have not been established, biopsy is usually recommended in patients with (1) nephrotic syndrome, (2) nephritic syndrome, (3) decreased renal function, (4) nephrotic-range proteinuria, and (5) non-nephrotic proteinuria persisting for more than 3 months [22]. Although the utility of renal biopsy in IgAVN with persistent mild to moderate proteinuria may be controversial, Halling et al. argued for biopsy since severe morphological changes are found in some of these patients [44]. It is also important to recognize that the interval between disease onset and the time of renal biopsy may affect histopathological findings; the percentage of crescents may increase markedly within days in patients with active disease [39, 80]. Repeat renal biopsies should be considered in patients showing worsening of renal symptoms or poor response to treatment [80].

Treatment of Mild or Moderately Severe IgAVN

Patients with mild IgAVN, such as microscopic hematuria or gross hematuria of short duration, generally do not require any medications.

In IgAVN children with persistent proteinuria of 0.5–1 g/day/1.73 m^2, the KDIGO guidelines recommend the use of ACE inhibitors or ARB [78]. In a study of 31 patients with moderately severe IgAVN (ISKDC grade I–III and serum albumin >2.5 g/dL), proteinuria was reduced efficiently by RAS blockers, except a single case of a clinical relapse at one year [83]. Davin and Coppo suggested that the use of RAS blockers is appropriate in cases lacking acute inflammation and crescentic lesions, whereas delaying effective anti-inflammatory treatment may be detrimental in patients with acute inflammatory glomerular lesions [80]. This is supported by two studies: one showed that 9 of 13 patients with mild to moderate proteinuria had severe morphological changes; the second showed that 18% of patients with mild proteinuria at onset had a poor prognosis [44, 81]. Hence, a rational therapeutic approach could be as follows: in patients with non-nephrotic proteinuria and a normal serum albumin early in the course of IgAVN, monotherapy with a RAS blocker may be used for 1–2 months and the further course observed. In patients with non-nephrotic proteinuria and mildly decreased serum albumin levels at onset of IgAVN, combined oral steroids and RAS blockade may be used for 1–2 months. In patients with persistent (>2–3 months) non-nephrotic proteinuria and/or decreased serum albumin levels during the course of IgAVN despite these treatments, renal biopsy should be performed and more potent anti-inflammatory treatments considered guided by the histopathological findings. These treatments may include MP pulses, azathioprine, mycophenolate mofetil (MMF) or a calcineurin inhibitor, combined with oral steroids and RAS blockade. The beneficial effect of alternative treatments such as fish oil, rifampin or tonsillectomy on moderately severe IgAVN has not been established [48, 84].

Treatment of Severe IgAVN

Although the definition of severe nephritis in IgAVN differs among studies, it generally includes nephrotic syndrome, acute nephritic syndrome, nephrotic range proteinuria (>40 mg/ m^2/h) or proteinuria >1 g/day and histopathological lesions exceeding ISKDC grade IIIa [50]. Treatment of severe IgAVN remains controversial due to a paucity of RCTs [48, 84, 85]. Most published work relies on retrospective analyses of small cohorts with heterogenous disease severity. However, there is consensus that intense initial therapy is indicated in severe IgAVN, considering a 15% overall long-term CKD risk and well-documented unfavorable outcomes of untreated patients, reduced CKD risk following intense treatment, and worse outcomes with delayed treatment [86–89].

Oral steroids have been shown to be ineffective in severe nephritis [5, 87, 88]. Niaudet et al. suggested that intravenous MP pulses should be started early in the course of severe IgAVN before crescents become fibrous, because renal scarring by extensive glomerular damage during the acute episode may be irreversible and lead to progressive CKD [88]. Hence, in patients with very severe IgAVN, intravenous MP pulses should be initiated immediately. Oral steroids can be utilized and tapered following the MP pulses. In addition, RAS blockers can be used as an add-on therapy concurrently as a nephroprotective, proteinuria-minimizing therapy [80].

An RCT performed by the ISKDC showed no differences in outcome between oral cyclophosphamide (90 mg/m^2/day for 42 days) and supportive therapy in children with severe IgAVN [90], although retrospective case series had suggested a beneficial effect [91, 92]. A placebo-controlled, prospective study comparing cyclophosphamide plus prednisone to prednisone alone demonstrated the lack of efficacy of cyclophosphamide in adults with IgAVN [93]. In view of these negative results and the potential side effects, cyclophosphamide is not recommended in severe IgAVN [80].

Another randomized clinical trial in a limited number of children suggested that cyclosporin A was non-inferior to intravenous MP pulses in children with severe IgAVN. Resolution of nephrotic-range proteinuria was achieved within 3 months in all 11 cyclosporin-treated patients, while it was not achieved with the initial treatment of MP pulses in 6 of the 13 due to slower response [94]. Additional immunosuppressive treatment was not necessary in any of the cyclosporin-treated patients, but was needed in 6 patients treated with MP pulses [94]. Repeat renal biopsy findings performed after 2-year follow-up showed similar improvement in both treatment arms [94].

Hence, calcineurin inhibitors are an alternative first choice or follow-up therapy in patients who do not respond rapidly to intravenous MP pulses. Azathioprine, MMF or other immunosuppressive drugs can also be used, although the claim of efficacy for these drugs is based exclusively on non-randomized or uncontrolled studies [39, 40, 95–102]. In a recent meta-analysis of 9 articles, IgAVN patients treated with combined therapy (immunosuppressive agents plus steroids) demonstrated a significant increase in complete remission rates when compared with steroids alone and children seemed to benefit more from combined treatment than adults [99]. Administration of azathioprine and cyclosporin was associated with histological regression with reduced IgA deposits in severe IgAVN [40, 97, 98]. In one study, rituximab was shown to be effective for induction and maintenance of longlasting remission in adults with severe refractory IgAV with biopsy proven crescentic nephritis; 10 of the 12 patients had a complete response [100]. However, the role of rituximab in children with severe IgAVN requires additional study.

Persistence of urinary abnormalities is an ominous sign in severe IgAVN [40, 52]. Hence, in patients with persistent proteinuria after initial intensive therapy, a follow-up renal biopsy may be needed to assess the histopathological effects of initial treatment. Subsequent therapy may be guided by the extent and acute vs. chronic nature of the remaining renal lesions. If persistent active histological lesions are found, adjustment of the immunosuppressive therapy should be considered. Although rare, in persistent, severe IgAVN resistant to azathioprine late remission was induced by switching to cyclosporin or MP pulses [103, 104]. RAS blocker monotherapy is a valid approach in cases of persistent proteinuria with a high chronicity index at the follow-up renal biopsy [80]. Conversely, it should be emphasized that proteinuria can resolve spontaneously years after discontinuation of immunosuppression in patients with severe IgAVN [40, 98].

In patients presenting with impaired renal function with rapidly progressive course or crescentic IgAVN affecting more than 50% of glomeruli (ISKDC IV and V), several intensive therapies have been suggested, emphasizing that early treatment is important in achieving a successful outcome [54, 87–89, 105–112]. Plasmapheresis has been utilized for rapidly progressive IgAVN to remove circulating immune complexes, immunoglobulins and mediators of inflammation; it has been used either alone or with other immunosuppressive drugs [54, 89, 105–108]. Hattori et al. reported that plasmapheresis as the sole therapy was effective in improving the outcome of patients with rapidly progressive IgAVN, particularly if instituted early in the course of the disease [89]. Schärer et al. suggested that plasmapheresis might delay progression, albeit not prevent eventual ESRD in children with crescentic IgAVN [54]. Therefore, plasmapheresis can be utilized promptly in patients who have nephritic and nephrotic syndrome and progressive decline in kidney function associated with ISKDC IV or V, and in those who are resistant to steroids and other immunosuppressive drugs.

In addition, combinations of several drugs, including cyclophosphamide, have been tried in the setting of rapidly progressive IgAVN, although cyclophosphamide alone was not effective in treating severe IgAVN [109–112]. Öner et al. reported a beneficial effect of triple therapy (MP pulses, cyclophosphamide, dipyridamole) in 12 patients with rapidly progressive IgAVN [109]. Iijima et al. also suggested the efficacy of combined therapies (MP pulses, cyclophosphamide, heparin/warfarin, dipyridamole) in 14 patients with rapidly progressive IgAVN (ISKDC IV or V) [110].

It has been speculated that fibrinolytic urokinase treatment might decrease crescent formation by reducing glomerular fibrin deposition [72, 111, 112]. Kawasaki et al. found methylprednisolone and urokinase pulse therapy (MUPT) which includes methylprednisolone (MP) pulses, urokinase, warfarin, dipyridamole was effective in patients with rapidly progressive IgAVN [111]. Addition of cyclophosphamide to MUPT was more effective than MUPT alone in the treatment of rapidly progressive IgAVN [112].

The experimental nature of these therapeutic approaches should be emphasized. The relative efficacy of individual and combined treatments in severe and rapidly progressive IgAVN awaits demonstration in RCTs with strict inclusion

Henoch-Schönlein nephritis in children. Pediatr Nephrol. 2006;21(1):54–9.

48. Bogdanović R. Henoch-Schönlein purpura nephritis in children: risk factors, prevention and treatment. Acta Paediatr. 2009;98(12):1882–9.

49. Goldstein AR, White RH, Akuse R, Chantler C. Long-term follow-up of childhood Henoch-Schönlein nephritis. Lancet. 1992;339(8788):280–2.

50. Ronkainen J, Nuutinen M, Koskimies O. The adult kidney 24 years after childhood Henoch-Schönlein purpura: a retrospective cohort study. Lancet. 2002;360(9334):666–70.

51. Bunchman TE, Mauer SM, Sibley RK, Vernier RL. Anaphylactoid purpura: characteristics of 16 patients who progressed to renal failure. Pediatr Nephrol. 1988;2(4):393–7.

52. Coppo R, Andrulli S, Amore A, Gianoglio B, Conti G, Peruzzi L, et al. Predictors of outcome in Henoch-Schönlein nephritis in children and adults. Am J Kidney Dis. 2006;47(6):993–1003.

53. Kawasaki Y, Suzuki J, Sakai N, Nemoto K, Nozawa R, Suzuki S, et al. Clinical and pathological features of children with Henoch-Schoenlein purpura nephritis: risk factors associated with poor prognosis. Clin Nephrol. 2003;60(3):153–60.

54. Schärer K, Krmar R, Querfeld U, Ruder H, Waldherr R, Schaefer F. Clinical outcome of Schönlein-Henoch purpura nephritis in children. Pediatr Nephrol. 1999;13:816–23.

55. Ronkainen J, Ala-Houhala M, Huttunen NP, Jahnukainen T, Koskimies O, Ormälä T, et al. Outcome of Henoch-Schoenlein nephritis with nephrotic-range proteinuria. Clin Nephrol. 2003;60(2):80–4.

56. Shin JI, Park JM, Shin YH, Lee JS, Jeong HJ, Kim HS. Serum IgA/C3 ratio may be a useful marker of disease activity in severe Henoch-Schönlein nephritis. Nephron Clin Pract. 2005;101(2):c72–8.

57. Coppo R, Basolo B, Piccoli G, Mazzucco G, Bulzomì MR, Roccatello D, et al. IgA1 and IgA2 immune complexes in primary IgA nephropathy and Henoch-Schönlein nephritis. Clin Exp Immunol. 1984;57(3):583–90.

58. Levinsky RJ, Barratt TM. IgA immune complexes in Henoch-Schönlein purpura. Lancet. 1979;2(8152):1100–3.

59. Casanueva B, Rodriguez-Valverde V, Luceño A. Circulating IgA producing cells in the differential diagnosis of Henoch-Schönlein purpura. J Rheumatol. 1988;15(8):1229–33.

60. Allen A, Harper S, Feehally J. Origin and structure of pathogenic IgA in IgA nephropathy. Biochem Soc Trans. 1997;25(2):486–90.

61. Davin JC, Vandenbroeck MC, Foidart JB, Mahieu PR. Sequential measurements of the reticuloendothelial system function in Henoch-Schönlein disease of childhood. Correlations with various immunological parameters. Acta Paediatr Scand. 1985;74(2):201–6.

62. Kiryluk K, Moldoveanu Z, Sanders JT, Eison TM, Suzuki H, Julian BA, et al. Aberrant glycosylation of IgA1 is inherited in both pediatric IgA nephropathy and Henoch-Schönlein purpura nephritis. Kidney Int. 2011;80(1):79–87.

63. Garcia-Fuentes M, Martin A, Chantler C, Williams DG. Serum complement components in Henoch-Schönlein purpura. Arch Dis Child. 1978;53(5):417–9.

64. Hisano S, Matsushita M, Fujita T, Iwasaki H. Activation of the lectin complement pathway in Henoch-Schönlein purpura nephritis. Am J Kidney Dis. 2005;45(2):295–302.

65. Ault BH, Stapleton FB, Rivas ML, Waldo FB, Roy S 3rd, McLean RH, et al. Association of Henoch-Schönlein purpura glomerulonephritis with C4B deficiency. J Pediatr. 1990;117(5):753–5.

66. Evans DJ, Williams DG, Peters DK, Sissons JG, Boulton-Jones JM, Ogg CS, et al. Glomerular deposition of properdin in Henoch-Schönlein syndrome and idiopathic focal nephritis. Br Med J. 1973;3(5875):326–8.

67. Davies M. The mesangial cell: a tissue culture view. Kidney Int. 1994;45(2):320–7.

68. Oortwijn BD, Roos A, Royle L, van Gijlswijk-Janssen DJ, Faber-Krol MC, Eijgenraam JW, et al. Differential glycosylation of polymeric and monomeric IgA: a possible role in glomerular inflammation in IgA nephropathy. J Am Soc Nephrol. 2006;17(12):3529–39.

69. Chen A, Chen WP, Sheu LF, Lin CY. Pathogenesis of IgA nephropathy: in vitro activation of human mesangial cells by IgA immune complex leads to cytokine secretion. J Pathol. 1994;173(2):119–26.

70. Gómez-Guerrero C, López-Armada MJ, González E, Egido J. Soluble IgA and IgG aggregates are catabolized by cultured rat mesangial cells and induce production of TNF-alpha and IL-6, and proliferation. J Immunol. 1994;153(11):5247–55.

71. López-Armada MJ, Gómez-Guerrero C, Egido J. Receptors for immune complexes activate gene expression and synthesis of matrix proteins in cultured rat and human mesangial cells: role of TGF-beta. J Immunol. 1996;157(5):2136–42.

72. Shin JI, Park JM, Shin YH, Lee JS, Jeong HJ. Role of mesangial fibrinogen deposition in the pathogenesis of crescentic Henoch-Schonlein nephritis in children. J Clin Pathol. 2005;58(11):1147–51.

73. Ronkainen J, Koskimies O, Ala-Houhala M, Antikainen M, Merenmies J, Rajantie J, et al. Early prednisone therapy in Henoch-Schönlein purpura: a randomized, double-blind, placebo-controlled trial. J Pediatr. 2006;149(2):241–7.

74. Dudley J, Smith G, Llewelyn-Edwards A, Bayliss K, Pike K, Tizard J. Randomised, double-blind, placebo-controlled trial to determine whether steroids reduce the incidence and severity of nephropathy in Henoch-Schonlein Purpura (HSP). Arch Dis Child. 2013;98(10):756–63.

75. Weiss PF, Feinstein JA, Luan X, Burnham JM, Feudtner C. Effects of corticosteroid on Henoch-Schönlein purpura: a systematic review. Pediatrics. 2007;120(5):1079–87.
76. Hahn D, Hodson EM, Willis NS, Craig JC. Interventions for preventing and treating kidney disease in Henoch-Schonlein Purpura (HSP). Cochrane Database Syst Rev. 2015;(8):CD005128.
77. Shin JI, Lee JS. Can corticosteroid therapy alter the course of nephritis in children with Henoch-Schönlein purpura? Nat Clin Pract Rheumatol. 2008;4(3):126–7.
78. KDIGO guidelines on glomerulonephritis. Henoch–Schönlein purpura nephritis. Kidney Int. 2012;Suppl 2:218–220.
79. Shin JI, Lee SJ, Lee JS, Kim KH. Intravenous dexamethasone followed by oral prednisolone versus oral prednisolone in the treatment of childhood Henoch-Schönlein purpura. Rheumatol Int. 2011;31(11):1429–32.
80. Davin JC, Coppo R. Pitfalls in recommending evidence-based guidelines for a protean disease like Henoch-Schönlein purpura nephritis. Pediatr Nephrol. 2013;28(10):1897–903.
81. Edström Halling S, Söderberg MP, Berg UB. Predictors of outcome in Henoch-Schönlein nephritis. Pediatr Nephrol. 2010;25(6):1101–8.
82. Ruggenenti P, Schieppati A, Remuzzi G. Progression, remission, regression of chronic renal diseases. Lancet. 2001;357(9268):1601–8.
83. Ninchoji T, Kaito H, Nozu K, Hashimura Y, Kanda K, Kamioka I, et al. Treatment strategies for Henoch-Schönlein purpura nephritis by histological and clinical severity. Pediatr Nephrol. 2011;26(4):563–9.
84. Zaffanello M, Brugnara M, Franchini M. Therapy for children with henoch-schonlein purpura nephritis: a systematic review. ScientificWorldJournal. 2007;7:20–30.
85. Zaffanello M, Fanos V. Treatment-based literature of Henoch-Schönlein purpura nephritis in childhood. Pediatr Nephrol. 2009;24(10):1901–11.
86. Levy M, Broyer M, Arsan A, Levy-Bentolila D, Habib R. Anaphylactoid purpura nephritis in childhood: natural history and immunopathology. Adv Nephrol Necker Hosp. 1976;6:183–228.
87. Andersen RF, Rubak S, Jespersen B, Rittig S. Early high-dose immunosuppression in Henoch-Schönlein nephrotic syndrome may improve outcome. Scand J Urol Nephrol. 2009;43(5):409–15.
88. Niaudet P, Habib R. Methylprednisolone pulse therapy in the treatment of severe forms of Schönlein-Henoch nephritis. Pediatr Nephrol. 1998;12(3):238–43.
89. Hattori M, Ito K, Konomoto T, Kawaguchi H, Yoshioka T, Khono M. Plasmapheresis as the sole therapy for rapidly progressive Henoch-Schönlein purpura nephritis in children. Am J Kidney Dis. 1999;33(3):427–33.

90. Tarshish P, Bernstein J, Edelmann CM Jr. Henoch-Schönlein purpura nephritis: course of disease and efficacy of cyclophosphamide. Pediatr Nephrol. 2004;19(1):51–6.
91. Flynn JT, Smoyer WE, Bunchman TE, Kershaw DB, Sedman AB. Treatment of Henoch-Schönlein Purpura glomerulonephritis in children with high-dose corticosteroids plus oral cyclophosphamide. Am J Nephrol. 2001;21(2):128–33.
92. Tanaka H, Suzuki K, Nakahata T, Ito E, Waga S. Early treatment with oral immunosuppressants in severe proteinuric purpura nephritis. Pediatr Nephrol. 2003;18(4):347–50.
93. Pillebout E, Alberti C, Guillevin L, Ouslimani A, Thervet E. CESAR study group. Addition of cyclophosphamide to steroids provides no benefit compared with steroids alone in treating adult patients with severe Henoch Schönlein Purpura. Kidney Int. 2010;78(5):495–502.
94. Jauhola O, Ronkainen J, Autio-Harmainen H, Koskimies O, Ala-Houhala M, Arikoski P, et al. Cyclosporine A vs. methylprednisolone for Henoch-Schönlein nephritis: a randomized trial. Pediatr Nephrol. 2011;26(12):2159–66.
95. Bergstein J, Leiser J, Andreoli SP. Response of crescentic Henoch-Schoenlein purpura nephritis to corticosteroid and azathioprine therapy. Clin Nephrol. 1998;49:9–14.
96. Singh S, Devidayal KL, Joshi K, Minz RW, Datta U. Severe Henoch-Schönlein nephritis: resolution with azathioprine and steroids. Rheumatol Int. 2002;22:133–7.
97. Ronkainen J, Autio-Harmainen H, Nuutinen M. Cyclosporin A for the treatment of severe Henoch-Schönlein glomerulonephritis. Pediatr Nephrol. 2003;18:1138–42.
98. Shin JI, Park JM, Shin YH, Kim JH, Kim PK, Lee JS, et al. Cyclosporin A therapy for severe Henoch-Schönlein nephritis with nephrotic syndrome. Pediatr Nephrol. 2005;20:1093–7.
99. Tan J, Tang Y, Zhong Z, Yan S, Tan L, Tarun P, Qin W. The efficacy and safety of immunosuppressive agents plus steroids compared with steroids alone in the treatment of Henoch-Schonlein purpura nephritis: a meta-analysis. Int Urol Nephrol. 2019;51(6):975–85.
100. Fenoglio R, Sciascia S, Naretto C, De Simone E, Del Vecchio G, Ferro M, et al. Rituximab in severe immunoglobulin-A vasculitis (Henoch-Schonlein) with aggressive nephritis. Clin Exp Rheumatol. 2020;38 Suppl 124(2):195–200.
101. Du Y, Hou L, Zhao C, Han M, Wu Y. Treatment of children with Henoch-Schönlein purpura nephritis with mycophenolate mofetil. Pediatr Nephrol. 2012;27(5):765–71.
102. Ren P, Han F, Chen L, Xu Y, Wang Y, Chen J. The combination of mycophenolate mofetil with corticosteroids induces remission of Henoch-Schönlein purpura nephritis. Am J Nephrol. 2012;36(3):271–7.

103. Shin JI, Park JM, Lee JS, Kim JH, Kim PK, Jeong HJ. Successful use of cyclosporin A in severe Schönlein-Henoch nephritis resistant to both methylprednisolone pulse and azathioprine. Clin Rheumatol. 2006;25:759–60.

104. Shin JI, Park JM, Kim JH, Lee JS, Jeong HJ. Methylprednisolone pulse therapy by the Tune-Mendoza protocol in a child with severe Henoch-Schönlein nephritis. Scand J Rheumatol. 2006;35:162–3.

105. Kauffmann RH, Houwert DA. Plasmapheresis in rapidly progressive Henoch-Schoenlein glomerulonephritis and the effect on circulating IgA immune complexes. Clin Nephrol. 1981;16:155–60.

106. Gianviti A, Trompeter RS, Barratt TM, Lythgoe MF, Dillon MJ. Retrospective study of plasma exchange in patients with idiopathic rapidly progressive glomerulonephritis and vasculitis. Arch Dis Child. 1996;75:186–90.

107. Kawasaki Y, Suzuki J, Murai M, Takahashi A, Isome M, Nozawa R, et al. Plasmapheresis therapy for rapidly progressive Henoch-Schönlein nephritis. Pediatr Nephrol. 2004;19(8):920–3.

108. Shenoy M, Ognjanovic MV, Coulthard MG. Treating severe Henoch-Schönlein and IgA nephritis with plasmapheresis alone. Pediatr Nephrol. 2007;22:1167–71.

109. Oner A, Tinaztepe K, Erdogan O. The effect of triple therapy on rapidly progressive type of Henoch-Schönlein nephritis. Pediatr Nephrol. 1995;9:6–10.

110. Iijima K, Ito-Kariya S, Nakamura H, Yoshikawa N. Multiple combined therapy for severe Henoch-Schönlein nephritis in children. Pediatr Nephrol. 1998;12:244–8.

111. Kawasaki Y, Suzuki J, Nozawa R, Suzuki S, Suzuki H. Efficacy of methylprednisolone and urokinase pulse therapy for severe Henoch-Schönlein nephritis. Pediatrics. 2003;111:785–9.

112. Kawasaki Y, Suzuki J, Suzuki H. Efficacy of methylprednisolone and urokinase pulse therapy combined with or without cyclophosphamide in severe Henoch-Schoenlein nephritis: a clinical and histopathological study. Nephrol Dial Transplant. 2004;19:858–64.

113. Mariani LH, Bomback AS, Canetta PA, Flessner MF, Helmuth M, Hladunewich MA, et al.; CureGN Consortium. CureGN study rationale, design, and methods: establishing a large prospective observational study of glomerular disease. Am J Kidney Dis. 2019;73(2):218–229.

114. Meulders Q, Pirson Y, Cosyns JP, Squifflet JP, van Ypersele de Strihou C. Course of Henoch-Schönlein nephritis after renal transplantation. Report on ten patients and review of the literature. Transplantation. 1994;58(11):1179–86.

115. Kanaan N, Mourad G, Thervet E, Peeters P, Hourmant M, Vanrenterghem Y, et al. Recurrence and graft loss after kidney transplantation for Henoch-Schönlein purpura nephritis: a multicenter analysis. Clin J Am Soc Nephrol. 2011;6(7):1768–72.

116. Samuel JP, Bell CS, Molony DA, Braun MC. Long-term outcome of renal transplantation patients with Henoch-Schonlein purpura. Clin J Am Soc Nephrol. 2011;6(8):2034–40.

117. Thervet E, Aouizerate J, Noel LH, Brocheriou I, Martinez F, Mamzer MF, et al. Histologic recurrence of Henoch-Schonlein Purpura nephropathy after renal transplantation on routine allograft biopsy. Transplantation. 2011;92(8):907–12.

118. Van Stralen KJ, Verrina E, Belingheri M, Dudley J, Dusek J, Grenda R, Macher MA, Puretic Z, Rubic J, Rudaitis S, Rudin C, Schaefer F, Jager KJ, ESPN/ERA-EDTA Registry. Impact of graft loss among kidney diseases with a high risk of post-transplant recurrence in the paediatric population. Nephrol Dial Transplant. 2013;28:1031–8.

119. Tayabali S, Andersen K, Yoong W. Diagnosis and management of Henoch-Schönlein purpura in pregnancy: a review of the literature. Arch Gynecol Obstet. 2012;286:825–9.

Metabolic Disorders Affecting the Kidney

28

Aude Servais, Olivia Boyer, Myriam Dao, and Friederike Hörster

Introduction

Inherited diseases of metabolism are a heterogeneous group of rare diseases, most often of autosomal recessive inheritance. These include energy metabolism disorders, intoxication diseases, and abnormalities in the synthesis or catabolism of complex molecules involved in intracellular maturation (lysosomal, peroxisomal, glycosylation abnormalities, etc.).

Kidney involvement may be inaugural, or more often complicate the evolution of an already diagnosed metabolic disorder. Improved survival in patients with metabolic diseases has led to the discovery of renal features that were not apparent at the time of the initial description of the condition (e.g., methylmalonic acidemia), and extrarenal manifestations in renal or urologic diseases that were thought to be primary and isolated (e.g., cystinosis). Metabolic disorders should be considered in the presence of kidney involvement, especially when children present with extrarenal symptoms.

The renal clinical spectrum of inherited diseases of metabolism is wide:

- Fanconi syndrome (proximal tubulopathy): the proximal renal tubule is most often affected in metabolic disorders due to a very high energy expenditure.
- chronic tubulointerstitial nephropathy, resulting from acute or chronic toxic tubular epithelium injury (e.g., myoglobinuria in fatty acid oxidation defects, methylmalonic acid in methylmalonic acidemia).
- glomerular damage with proteinuria, nephrotic syndrome, hematuria and/or hypertension, due to the abnormal deposition of storage material (e.g., Fabry disease), or structural defects (e.g., glycogenosis type 1, respiratory chain defects).
- hemolytic uremic syndrome, as a result of toxic damage to endothelial cells (e.g., in methyl-malonic acidemia vitamin B12-sensitive, or cobalamin C deficiency).
- nephrocalcinosis and urinary lithiasis, resulting from a defect in the reabsorption of a specific solute (e.g., cystine in cystinuria) or from the urinary excretion of solutes accumulated

A. Servais (✉) · M. Dao
Nephrology and Transplantation Department, Reference Centre for Child and Adult Hereditary Renal Diseases (MARHEA), Necker Hospital, APHP, Paris, France
e-mail: aude.servais@aphp.fr; myriam.dao@aphp.fr

O. Boyer
Pediatric Nephrology Department, Reference Centre for Child and Adult Hereditary Renal Diseases (MARHEA), Necker Hospital, APHP, Paris, France
e-mail: olivia.boyer@aphp.fr

F. Hörster
Centre for Child and Adolescent Medicine, Division of Neuropaediatrics and Metabolic Medicine, University Hospital Heidelberg, Heidelberg, Germany
e-mail: friederike.hoerster@med.uni-heidelberg.de

© The Author(s), under exclusive license to Springer Nature Switzerland AG 2023
F. Schaefer, L. A. Greenbaum (eds.), *Pediatric Kidney Disease*,
https://doi.org/10.1007/978-3-031-11665-0_28

in the plasma (e.g., oxalate in primary hyperoxaluria).
- renal cysts as a result of developmental defects.
- urine colour abnormalities (e.g. dark or reddish in porphyria, black in alkaptonuria);
- renal consequences of rhabdomyolysis.

These pathologies can lead to chronic kidney disease (CKD) and sometimes to kidney failure requiring renal replacement therapy and kidney transplantation.

When the cause of the inherited metabolic disorder is unclear, the type of renal involvement can be suggestive (Table 28.1).

Table 28.1 Renal involvement in inherited diseases of metabolism

Clinical features	Etiologies
Proximal tubulopathy (Fanconi syndrome)	Cystinosis Mitochondriopathies Tyrosinemia type 1 CDG syndrome Fructosemia Galactosemia Glycogenosis type 1 Bickel-Fanconi syndrome Wilson disease Lowe disease Dent disease Lysinuric Protein Intolerance
Other tubular defects, chronic TIN	MMA Mitochondriopathies Glycogenosis type 1 Pyruvate carboxylase deficiency Carnitine palmitoyl transferase (CPT) type 1 deficiency Adenosine deaminase deficiency Transaldolase deficiency Fatty acid Beta-oxidation disorders Imerslund-Gräsbeck syndrome

Table 28.1 (continued)

Clinical features	Etiologies
Glomerulopathy Proteinuria, nephrotic syndrome nephrotic syndrome, haematuria and/or hypertension	Fabry disease Mitochondriopathies Glycogenosis type 1 Mucopolysaccharidosis (MPS) type 1 (Hurler) Lysinuric protein intolerance Gaucher disease LCAT (lecithine cholesterolacyl transferase) deficiency
Kidney cysts	Mitochondriopathies: Pearson syndrome Zellweger syndrome CDG syndrome Glutaric acidemia type II Smith-Lemli-Opitz syndrome

Methylmalonic Acidemia and Propionic Acidemia

Methylmalonic acidemias comprise a family of diseases which share the common feature of elevated concentration of methylmalonic acid in blood, urine and other body fluids. There are secondary forms related to vitamin B12 deficiency and different primary diseases of cobalamin metabolism and methylmalonyl-CoA mutase deficiency leading to this biochemical phenotype. It is useful to differentiate between isolated methylmalonic acidurias and combined methylmalonic acidurias, which additionally show elevated concentrations of homocysteine (Table 28.2) [1–3].

Methylmalonyl-CoA mutase is located within the metabolic pathway linking degradation of certain aminoacids (isoleucine, methionine, threonine and valine), odd-chain fatty acids and cholesterol side chains to the citric acid cycle. Propionic acidemia is caused by deficiency of propionyl-CoA carboxylase, an enzyme upstream

Table 28.2 Methylmalonic acidemia and propionic acidemia

	Gene	MIM number
Methylmalonic acidemia: isolated forms		
mut type (*mut⁰*, *mut⁻*)	MUT	#25100
cblA type	MMAA	#251100
cblB type	MMAB	#251110
cblD variant 2	MMADHC	#277410
Methylmalonic acidemia: combined forms with homocystinuria		
cblC type	MMACHC	#277400
cblD-variant 1	MMADHC	#277410
cblF type	LMBRD1	#277380
cblJ type	ABCD4	#614857
Propionic acidemia	PCCA PCCB	#606054

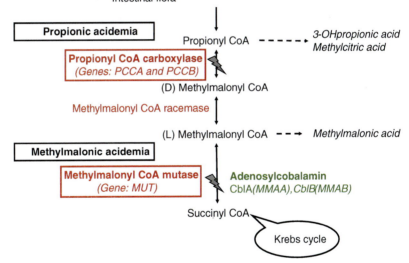

Fig. 28.1 Methylmalonic acidemia and propionic acidemia

of methylmalonyl-CoA mutase (Fig. 28.1). These diseases are the most frequent classical organoacidemias with an estimated incidence of 1:50,000 (isolated methylmalonic acidemias) and 1:150,000 (propionic acidemia). Within the group of isolated methylmalonic acidemias, most patients are affected by a complete deficiency of methylmalonyl-CoA mutase (mut⁰) [1].

Clinical Picture of Isolated Methylmalonic Acidemias

Acute manifestation is a life-threatening metabolic decompensation characterized by profound metabolic acidosis, ketosis and hyperammonemia leading to deep coma and death, if not treated adequately. Most patients manifest within the neonatal period, the others later in life. Metabolic crises are often preceded by a catabolic state, typically induced by minor infections. A severe crisis can lead to irreversible neurologic sequelae such as basal ganglia necrosis, epilepsy or mental retardation, but a growing number of patients show normal psycho-motor development. Apart from the development of chronic renal failure (see below), failure to thrive and recurrent vomiting often complicate the clinical course. Acute or chronic pancreatitis are rarer but potentially dangerous complications.

If suggestive clinical symptoms occur, the diagnostic work-up of a patient can be started by measurement of acylcarnitines in dried blood spots or directly by measurement of organic acids in urine [4]. The differential diagnosis of the several genetic defects is actually performed by molecular genetic testing, but several different genes have to be considered [4].

Disease severity differs considerably between subtypes: late onset patients who are responsive to hydroxocobalamin tend to have a better outcome if treated adequately, in contrast to patients affected by a complete deficiency of methylmalonyl-CoA mutase (mut^0) [5–7]. Synergistic impairment of different targets within mitochondrial energy metabolism by different metabolites is the key to understand the pathophysiology of these diseases as multisystem disorders [8–10].

Clinical Picture of Combined Methylmalonic Acidurias

The most common disorder in this group is *cblC* disease (more than 500 reported cases). The majority of patients has an early disease onset, which is defined as disease onset before 12 months of age. In addition to acute metabolic crisis, patients may show signs of prenatal damage (intrauterine growth retardation and/or congenital heart disease) and thrombotic microangiopathy (atypical hemolytic uremic syndrome). Visual impairment and nystagmus due to optical nerve atrophy and retinopathy are typical complications within the disease course. Patients develop a complex neurological phenotype with brain atrophy and white matter disease leading to developmental delay, psychiatric problems and peripheral neuropathy.

Elevated concentration of plasma homocysteine levels is the biochemical hallmark of the disease: usually homocysteine levels are below 50 µmol/L (depending on the individual laboratory cut-offs), but in untreated patients levels above 100 µmol/L are found. It is recommended to measure total homocysteine in blood [3]. For further diagnostic work-up, investigation of plasma amino acids to identify low levels of methionine and organic acids in urine to identify elevated levels of methylmalonic acid are recommended. To rule out deficiency, plasma levels of vitamin B12 and folate should also be investigated [3]. Molecular genetic analysis of the *cblC* gene is possible and the three most common mutations show a genotype-phenotype correlation according to early or late disease onset [3].

Kidney Involvement

Chronic kidney disease (CKD) is a common complication of MMA, manifesting in childhood in half of the patients [5, 7, 11]. It is most frequently observed in mut° and cblB phenotypes, less frequently in patients with cblA and mut− phenotypes [12]. Median age at onset varies from 6.5 to 11.9 years (range: 1.5–33 years). Twelve to fourteen percent of patients evolve to end-stage renal disease (ESRD) requiring renal replacement therapy [5, 7]. The mechanisms responsible for renal failure in MMA remain poorly understood [5, 8, 13, 14]. It has been suggested that CKD in MMA is the consequence of tubular dysfunction. The hypothesis of chronic tubulopathy is supported by experimental studies [8, 13, 14].

A recent experimental study demonstrated a link between MMA, diseased mitochondria, mitophagy dysfunction and epithelial stress in tubular renal cells [15]. However, only few clinical case reports found proximal tubulopathy or distal tubular acidosis type 2 [16–18]. Kidney biopsy studies showed severe interstitial fibrosis and tubular atrophy with ultrastructural (enlarged mitochondria in proximal tubules) and functional (loss of cytochrome C, decrease in NADPH activity) alterations [7, 13, 16, 19] (Fig. 28.2). A recent study investigated tubular functions in 13 adolescent and adult MMA patients who did not previously receive kidney and/or liver transplantation [20]. The authors confirmed the high prevalence of CKD (54% had mGFR below 60 mL/min/1.73 m^2) but they failed to demonstrate tubular involvement. No patient had complete proximal tubular syndrome. Only one patient had biological signs suggestive of incomplete proximal tubulopathy with increased β2-microglobulin excretion and renal loss of magnesium [20].

As all patients with isolated MMA, even in the moderate forms, are considered to be at risk of developing chronic kidney disease (CKD), renal function should be closely monitored. There is a risk of developing progressive kidney failure, requiring renal replacement therapy and kidney transplantation. The estimated glomerular filtration rate (eGFR) based on serum creatinine levels

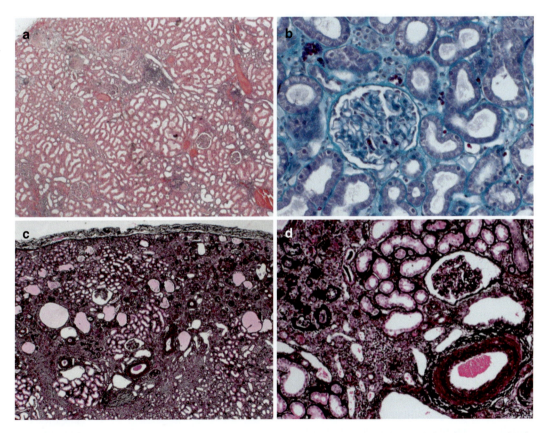

Fig. 28.2 Methylmalonic acidemia (MMA) renal biopsy. Two nephrectomy specimen procured at the time of transplantation in children with MMA at different stages of chronic kidney disease. The first specimen (**a** and **b**) shows non-specific mild tubular atrophy with interstitial fibrosis (IF/TA) and moderate inflammation within fibrotic areas (**a**) (HES staining, ×250). (**b**) Glomeruli are unremarkable and proximal tubules shows vacuoles in epithelial cells (Masson Trichrome, ×500). The second specimen (**c** and **d**) shows severe IF/TA with ischemic glomeruli (**c**) and tubular dilatations (Jones staining, ×250). Arteries display thickening of the media (**d**) (Jones staining, ×500). (Picture from M Rabant and MC Gubler)

may overestimate the actual GFR due to the low muscle mass and protein intake of patients [20]. Therefore, it is recommended to measure the GFR using "gold standard" techniques such as the inulin or iohexol clearances, when therapeutic decisions such as dialysis or transplantation are discussed.

The cumulative urinary excretion of methylmalonic acid over time (measured in repeated urine samples) correlates with the risk of CKD [5]. However, as kidney function declines, urinary methylmalonic acid is no longer a reliable marker and must be replaced by measurement of plasma methylmalonic acid. Standard medical management and follow-up of CKD follows the general therapeutic principles established in patients without inborn errors of metabolism, including monitoring of blood pressure, electrolytes, prevention and management of anemia, growth and bone disease. The experience with nephroprotective measures in the paediatric population has not been extensively studied.

In PA, a few cases of kidney failure have been reported [21].

Conservative Treatment

Isolated Methylmalonic Acidemias

The classical treatment consists of protein restricted diet (limited intake of precursor amino acids), which has to be tailored to the patients' needs and carefully monitored. L-carnitine (100 mg/kg/day) is applied to restore carnitine levels and CoA levels, bind and eliminate propionyl-CoA molecules, which are assumed to be responsible for some of the toxic metabolite effects in MMA [4]. Hydroxocobalamin is a powerful therapeutic tool in responsive patients; therefore this option has to be carefully evaluated [6]. In the recent guideline, a protocol for patients' monitoring has been proposed (Table 28.3) [4].

Combined Methylmalonic Acidurias

Experience on treatment mostly derives from cblC patients, the most common disorder. Treatment aims at normalizing plasma methionine and meth-

Table 28.3 Suggested monitoring in isolated methylmalonic acidemia and propionic acidemia according to guideline (adapted from [4])

Assessment	Frequency
Metabolic follow-up	
NH3, blood gas, lactate	Each clinic visit
Quantitative plasma amino acids (3–4 h of fasting prior to sample collection)	3–6 monthly
Methylmalonic acid in plasma (and urine if available)	3–6 monthly
Acylcarnitine profile in dried blood or plasma (propionylcarnitine and free carnitine)	3–6 monthly
Diet and nutritional status	
Diet history	Each clinic visit
Growth (weight, length or height, head circumference)	Each clinic visit
Full clinical examination	Each clinic visit
Albumin, total protein	6-monthly
Bone health (Ca, P, ALP, Mg, PTH, 25-OH vitamin D in blood; Ca, P in urine)	12-monthly
Full blood count, ferritin, folic acid, vitamin B12	12-monthly
Long-term complications	
Neurological examination with assessment of developmental milestones	Each clinic visit
Kidney function (serum creatinine, electrolytes, cystatin C, uric acid; urinary electrolytes and protein loss; GFR)	6-monthly
Pancreas function (lipase, pancreatic amylase)	6-monthly
Cardiac assessment (ECG, echocardiography)	12-monthly
Formal developmental/cognitive assessment	When clinically indicated
EEG, cerebral MRI	When clinically indicated
Ophthalmologic assessment	12-monthly
Formal hearing test	When clinically indicated

ylmalonate levels and reducing plasma total homocysteine. In severe cases levels of total homocysteine cannot be normalized, but levels between 40 and 60 μmol/L can be reached [3].

Treatment consists of hydroxocobalamine parenterally and betaine [3]. This treatment reduces homocysteine and methylmalonate levels and prevents metabolic crisis, but visual and cognitive impairment may not improve [3, 22].

Kidney and Liver Transplantation

The long-term outcome of MMA remains poor with medical treatment. Organ transplantation is an alternative, especially in case of renal failure but also as an enzyme replacement therapy. However, it remains unanswered exactly which patients should be transplanted. Liver transplantation (LT), kidney transplantation (KT), or combined liver and kidney transplantation (LKT) have been proposed for renal failure or as an enzyme replacement therapy in case of frequent metabolic decompensations, but also to prevent long-term complications [23]. Several reports emphasized the improved quality of life after LT [23].

The metabolic results after LKT are dramatically better than after KT, reducing protein restriction and improving quality of life. However, it is associated with an increased frequency of adverse events. Global patient survival after transplantation is calculated at 86–87% [23, 24], similar to non-transplanted patients and to patients receiving transplantation for other indications [24]. Mortality risk is highest within 14 days after transplantation. To decrease the mortality risk, it is recommended to ensure a stable metabolic state at time of transplantation and to have transplantation performed by an experienced transplantation team [24]. Some patients experience post-LKT neurological disorders, mainly reported in Mut0 type MMA [23, 24]. This might be due to calcineurin inhibitor toxicity [25].

Early LT may be considered to prevent years of protein deprivation and MMA toxicity and to delay the need for KT. LKT should be proposed when the measured GFR is lower than 60 mL/min/1.73 m^2 [23]. However, an isolated KT can be individually discussed.

Lysinuric Protein Intolerance

Lysinuric protein intolerance or cationic aminoaciduria is a rare autosomal recessive disorder. Affected children come to medical attention soon after weaning with failure to thrive and episodes of altered consciousness caused by hyperammonemia. This clinical picture is similar to urea cycle disorders, which are an important differential diagnosis. The disease may also present with chronic digestive symptoms and failure to thrive. Hepatosplenomegaly is often present [26]. Later, patients develop hematologic complications and bone marrow abnormalities reminding of lymphohistiocytosis or biological macrophage activation syndrome. This is accompanied by immunologic abnormalities and auto-immune manifestation. The respiratory system may also be involved by pulmonary alveolar proteinosis, which is a severe life-threatening complication.

The defect in the transporter leads to a characteristic pattern in urine amino acids, which show elevated concentrations of arginine, lysine and ornithine and low levels of these amino acids in plasma. Orotic acid in urine may also be elevated. Classically ferritin and LDH levels are elevated in plasma. Molecular genetic analysis of the *SLC7A7* gene is used to confirm the diagnosis, but there is no clear genotype-phenotype correlation [26].

Kidney Involvement

Renal involvement is described in LPI patients with both tubular and glomerular abnormalities [27]. In the first large clinical series describing kidney involvement in LPI, 74% of patients presented with proteinuria, 38% with microscopic or macroscopic hematuria and 38% with renal failure [28]. Patients may progress to ESKD [26–28]. Severe anemia and increased bleeding may be observed in these patients [28].

The majority of patients with kidney involvement have tubular dysfunction [27–29]. The most common observation is nephrocalcinosis and chronic tubulointerstitial nephritis [27, 30]. This is probably due to the accumulation of calcium phosphate in the kidney secondary to hypercalciuria and possibly to proximal tubular acidosis [27]. Hyperechogenic kidneys may be observed by renal ultrasound. Fanconi syndrome has been reported in two independent cases [31, 32].

Glomerular involvement is quite variable. Mesangial thickening can be observed [27]. Focal glomerulosclerosis, mesangial, membranous and lupus-like proliferative glomerulonephritis can also be associated with LPI [33–36]. Another striking observation is the finding of amyloidosis in the liver and in kidneys of some patients.

Treatment

To maintain metabolic control age-adapted dietary protein restriction is applied and patients have to be carefully monitored for nutritional deficiencies. Citrulline is supplemented and ammonia scavenging drugs, which are used in other urea cycle disorders, are also applied [37].

Kidney Transplantation

The disease does not prohibit treatment by transplantation. Better metabolic control is observed after transplantation.

Fabry Disease

Fabry disease is an X-linked lysosomal storage disorder caused by mutations in *GAL*, the gene that encodes the lysosomal enzyme α-galactosidase A, leading to deficient activity of this enzyme. The disease is characterized by a progressive accumulation of globotriaosylceramide (Gb-3) and related glycosphingolipids in the plasma and different cell types. Male individuals are primarily affected, but female heterozygotes may display moderate or severe disease, which is likely related to the pattern of X-chro-

mosome inactivation [38]. The disease can be divided into a severe, classical phenotype, most often seen in men without residual enzyme activity, and a generally milder non-classical phenotype. Patients with classical Fabry disease initially present with characteristic Fabry disease symptoms, such as neuropathic pain, cornea verticillata, and angiokeratoma.

Once suspected, men are diagnosed with Fabry disease if enzyme activity is below 35% of the mean and gene sequencing. The gold standard of diagnosis for females is α -Gal gene sequencing only.

The Gb3 degradation product, globotriaosylsphingosine (lysoGb3), is currently used in disease screening, but also in the determination of pathogenicity of a mutation. LysoGb3 has also been accepted as an accurate marker of disease activity [39].

Fabry Disease in Children and Adolescents

Children may present with characteristic neuropathic pain, which may lead to the diagnosis. Overt kidney involvement is rare in children, but renal histologic lesions can be demonstrated in children even before the onset of overt proteinuria and CKD [40, 41]. The natural history of Fabry nephropathy has not yet been thoroughly assessed in children [42]. Initially, glomerular hyperfiltration may mask impairment of kidney function [43]. Patients may present with microalbuminuria and proteinuria during the second or third decades, and CKD has been scarcely reported in adolescents [40–42, 44, 45].

Renal Biopsy

Renal biopsy may be performed for diagnosis in case of presentation with glomerular disease without extrarenal manifestation or for therapeutic discussion. On renal biopsy, vacuolization of podocytes and epithelial cells is a

28 Metabolic Disorders Affecting the Kidney

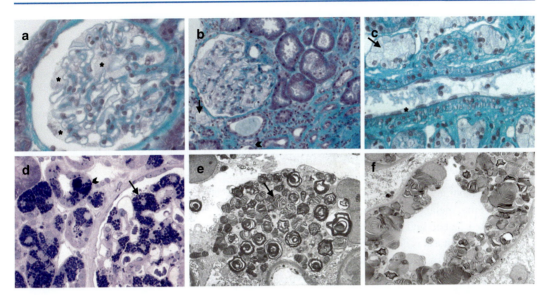

Fig. 28.3 Fabry disease renal biopsy. (**a**) Glomerulus with typical vacuolizations of podocytes (star) (Masson Trichrome ×400). (**b**) Masson Trichrome (×200) showing tubular inclusions (arrow) in distal tubules as well as peritubular capillaries inclusions (short arrow). (**c**) Vascular section showing endothelial cells inclusions (star) associated with tubules inclusions (arrow) (Masson Trichrome ×400). (**d**) Toluidine blue-stained semi-thin section showing darkly stained round inclusions in podocytes (arrow) and distal tubular cells (short arrow). (**e** and **f**) Electron microscopy showing glycosphingolipid inclusions shaped as multilamellated myelin figures in podocytes (**e**) and tubular cells (**f**). (Picture from M Rabant and MC Gubler)

characteristic histologic finding (Fig. 28.3) [46]. Tubular as well as peritubular capillaries inclusions, and endothelial cells inclusions are also observed. By electron microscopy, glycosphingolipid inclusions shaped as multilamellated myelin are found in podocytes (Fig. 28.3). Mesangial expansion, segmental and global glomerulosclerosis, tubular atrophy and interstitial fibrosis are also seen, even in early stages of the disease.

Long Term Follow-Up: Renal and Extra-Renal Complications

Long–term disease manifestations include hypertrophic cardiomyopathy, cardiac rhythm disturbances, progressive renal failure, and stroke. Non-classical Fabry disease, also referred to as late-onset or atypical Fabry disease, is characterized by a more variable disease course, in which patients are generally less severely affected and disease manifestations may be limited to a single organ.

Therapy

Treatment of Fabry disease consists of enzyme replacement therapy or chaperone molecule and adjunctive treatment, including angiotensin converting enzyme inhibitors or angiotensin receptor blockers, and analgesics. Studies have shown that enzyme therapy can delay but not always prevent some of the clinical complications of the disease. Enzyme therapy has been shown to provide the greatest benefit to patients if started early on. Antibody formation possibly also contributes to reduced therapy effect. Migalastat is a small-molecule chaperone which facilitates enzyme trafficking to lysosomes in certain mutant enzymes and can be administered orally [47, 48].

Glycogen Storage Disease (GSD) Type 1a and 1b

Glycogen Storage disease type 1 is caused by a mutation of the *G6PC* gene (GSD 1a) or *SLC37A4* gene (GSD 1b) leading to two distinct clinical subtypes. The first manifestations mostly leading to further medical work-up are hypoglycemic episodes occurring at the age of 3–6 months 3–4 h after feeding, hepatomegaly and failure to thrive. The laboratory findings (combination of hypoglycemia, metabolic acidosis, hyperuricemia, elevated lactate and triglycerides) are suggestive. The diagnosis is confirmed by molecular genetics. In GSD 1b additional neutropenia and leucocyte dysfunction render the patients susceptible to bacterial infections.

In patients with GSD I, several renal complications have been reported. Enlargement of the kidneys is the earliest finding, caused by accumulation of glycogen in the kidneys. Because of hyperuricemia, uric acid lithiasis may occur. These complications can be prevented by an optimal metabolic control with diet and by xanthine oxidase inhibitor. Another cause of lithiasis may be the decreased urinary citrate excretion together with an increased urinary calcium excretion in GSD I patients. Proximal tubular dysfunction has also been described in patients with GSD I. Hyperphosphaturia and loss of bicarbonate in urine may lead to tubular acidosis. The main renal complication is glomerular hyperfiltration and persistent proteinuria. Renal biopsies performed in three GSD I patients with persistent proteinuria showed focal segmental glomerulosclerosis [49]. These findings suggest an etiology of glomerular hyperfiltration and proteinuria similar to diabetic nephropathy.

The treatment aims at avoiding hypoglycemia by frequent carbohydrate intake. Optimal metabolic control has a renoprotective effect on the development of microalbuminuria and proteinuria. Treatment with an angiotensin converting enzyme inhibitor significantly decreases the GFR in GSD I patients with glomerular hyperfiltration and reduces proteinuria [50].

In GSD 1b bone marrow stimulation by G-CSF is often necessary [51].

References

1. Baumgartner MR, Horster F, Dionisi-Vici C, et al. Proposed guidelines for the diagnosis and management of methylmalonic and propionic acidemia. Orphanet J Rare Dis. 2014;9:130.
2. Fowler B, Leonard JV, Baumgartner MR. Causes of and diagnostic approach to methylmalonic acidurias. J Inherit Metab Dis. 2008;31(3):350–60.
3. Huemer M, Diodato D, Schwahn B, et al. Guidelines for diagnosis and management of the cobalamin-related remethylation disorders cblC, cblD, cblE, cblF, cblG, cblJ and MTHFR deficiency. J Inherit Metab Dis. 2017;40(1):21–48.
4. Forny P, Horster F, Ballhausen D, et al. Guidelines for the diagnosis and management of methylmalonic acidaemia and propionic acidaemia: first revision. J Inherit Metab Dis. 2021;44(3):566–92.
5. Horster F, Baumgartner MR, Viardot C, et al. Long-term outcome in methylmalonic acidurias is influenced by the underlying defect (mut0, mut-, cblA, cblB). Pediatr Res. 2007;62(2):225–30.
6. Horster F, Tuncel AT, Gleich F, et al. Delineating the clinical spectrum of isolated methylmalonic acidurias: cblA and mut. J Inherit Metab Dis. 2021;44(1):193–214.
7. Cosson MA, Benoist JF, Touati G, et al. Long-term outcome in methylmalonic aciduria: a series of 30 French patients. Mol Genet Metab. 2009;97(3):172–8.
8. Morath MA, Okun JG, Muller IB, et al. Neurodegeneration and chronic renal failure in methylmalonic aciduria—a pathophysiological approach. J Inherit Metab Dis. 2008;31(1):35–43.
9. Morath MA, Horster F, Sauer SW. Renal dysfunction in methylmalonic acidurias: review for the pediatric nephrologist. Pediatr Nephrol. 2013;28(2):227–35.
10. Haijes HA, Jans JJM, Tas SY, Verhoeven-Duif NM, van Hasselt PM. Pathophysiology of propionic and methylmalonic acidemias. Part 1: complications. J Inherit Metab Dis. 2019;42(5):730–44.
11. Kruszka PS, Manoli I, Sloan JL, Kopp JB, Venditti CP. Renal growth in isolated methylmalonic acidemia. Genet Med. 2013;15(12):990–6.
12. Horster F, Garbade SF, Zwickler T, et al. Prediction of outcome in isolated methylmalonic acidurias: combined use of clinical and biochemical parameters. J Inherit Metab Dis. 2009;32(5):630.
13. Manoli I, Sysol JR, Li L, et al. Targeting proximal tubule mitochondrial dysfunction attenuates the renal disease of methylmalonic acidemia. Proc Natl Acad Sci U S A. 2013;110(33):13552–7.
14. Ruppert T, Schumann A, Grone HJ, et al. Molecular and biochemical alterations in tubular epithelial cells of patients with isolated methylmalonic aciduria. Hum Mol Genet. 2015;24(24):7049–59.
15. Luciani A, Schumann A, Berquez M, et al. Impaired mitophagy links mitochondrial disease to epithelial stress in methylmalonyl-CoA mutase deficiency. Nat Commun. 2020;11(1):970.

16. Ohura T, Kikuchi M, Abukawa D, et al. Type 4 renal tubular acidosis (subtype 2) in a patient with methylmalonic acidaemia. Eur J Pediatr. 1990;150(2):115–8.
17. Wolff JA, Strom C, Griswold W, et al. Proximal renal tubular acidosis in methylmalonic acidemia. J Neurogenet. 1985;2(1):31–9.
18. D'Angio CT, Dillon MJ, Leonard JV. Renal tubular dysfunction in methylmalonic acidaemia. Eur J Pediatr. 1991;150(4):259–63.
19. Zsengeller ZK, Aljinovic N, Teot LA, et al. Methylmalonic acidemia: a megamitochondrial disorder affecting the kidney. Pediatr Nephrol. 2014;29(11):2139–46.
20. Dao M, Arnoux JB, Bienaime F, et al. Long-term renal outcome in methylmalonic acidemia in adolescents and adults. Orphanet J Rare Dis. 2021;16(1):220.
21. Shchelochkov OA, Manoli I, Sloan JL, et al. Chronic kidney disease in propionic acidemia. Genet Med. 2019;21(12):2830–5.
22. Huemer M, Baumgartner MR. The clinical presentation of cobalamin-related disorders: from acquired deficiencies to inborn errors of absorption and intracellular pathways. J Inherit Metab Dis. 2019;42(4):686–705.
23. Brassier A, Krug P, Lacaille F, et al. Long-term outcome of methylmalonic aciduria after kidney, liver, or combined liver-kidney transplantation: the French experience. J Inherit Metab Dis. 2020;43(2):234–43.
24. Molema F, Martinelli D, Horster F, et al. Liver and/or kidney transplantation in amino and organic acid-related inborn errors of metabolism: an overview on European data. J Inherit Metab Dis. 2021;44(3):593–605.
25. Molema F, Williams M, Langendonk J, et al. Neurotoxicity including posterior reversible encephalopathy syndrome after initiation of calcineurin inhibitors in transplanted methylmalonic acidemia patients: two case reports and review of the literature. JIMD Rep. 2020;51(1):89–104.
26. Mauhin W, Habarou F, Gobin S, et al. Update on lysinuric protein intolerance, a multi-faceted disease retrospective cohort analysis from birth to adulthood. Orphanet J Rare Dis. 2017;12(1):3.
27. Esteve E, Krug P, Hummel A, et al. Renal involvement in lysinuric protein intolerance: contribution of pathology to assessment of heterogeneity of renal lesions. Hum Pathol. 2017;62:160–9.
28. Tanner LM, Nanto-Salonen K, Niinikoski H, et al. Nephropathy advancing to end-stage renal disease: a novel complication of lysinuric protein intolerance. J Pediatr. 2007;150(6):631–4, 634 e1.
29. Karki M, Nanto-Salonen K, Niinikoski H, Tanner LM. Urine Beta2-microglobulin is an early marker of renal involvement in LPI. JIMD Rep. 2016;25:47–55.
30. Nicolas C, Bednarek N, Vuiblet V, et al. Renal involvement in a French Paediatric cohort of patients with lysinuric protein intolerance. JIMD Rep. 2016;29:11–7.
31. Benninga MA, Lilien M, de Koning TJ, et al. Renal Fanconi syndrome with ultrastructural defects in lysinuric protein intolerance. J Inherit Metab Dis. 2007;30(3):402–3.
32. Riccio E, Pisani A. Fanconi syndrome with lysinuric protein intolerance. Clin Kidney J. 2014;7(6):599–601.
33. DiRocco M, Garibotto G, Rossi GA, et al. Role of haematological, pulmonary and renal complications in the long-term prognosis of patients with lysinuric protein intolerance. Eur J Pediatr. 1993;152(5):437–40.
34. Parto K, Kallajoki M, Aho H, Simell O. Pulmonary alveolar proteinosis and glomerulonephritis in lysinuric protein intolerance: case reports and autopsy findings of four pediatric patients. Hum Pathol. 1994;25(4):400–7.
35. McManus DT, Moore R, Hill CM, Rodgers C, Carson DJ, Love AH. Necropsy findings in lysinuric protein intolerance. J Clin Pathol. 1996;49(4):345–7.
36. Parsons H, Snyder F, Bowen T, Klassen J, Pinto A. Immune complex disease consistent with systemic lupus erythematosus in a patient with lysinuric protein intolerance. J Inherit Metab Dis. 1996;19(5):627–34.
37. Nunes V, Niinikoski H. Lysinuric protein intolerance. In: Adam MP, Ardinger HH, Pagon RA, Wallace SE, Bean LJH, Gripp KW, et al., editors. Seattle: GeneReviews(R); 1993.
38. Germain DP, Waldek S, Banikazemi M, et al. Sustained, long-term renal stabilization after 54 months of agalsidase beta therapy in patients with Fabry disease. J Am Soc Nephrol. 2007;18(5):1547–57.
39. Cairns T, Muntze J, Gernert J, Spingler L, Nordbeck P, Wanner C. Hot topics in Fabry disease. Postgrad Med J. 2018;94(1118):709–13.
40. Gubler MC, Lenoir G, Grunfeld JP, Ulmann A, Droz D, Habib R. Early renal changes in hemizygous and heterozygous patients with Fabry's disease. Kidney Int. 1978;13(3):223–35.
41. Tondel C, Bostad L, Hirth A, Svarstad E. Renal biopsy findings in children and adolescents with Fabry disease and minimal albuminuria. Am J Kidney Dis. 2008;51(5):767–76.
42. Ramaswami U, Najafian B, Schieppati A, Mauer M, Bichet DG. Assessment of renal pathology and dysfunction in children with Fabry disease. Clin J Am Soc Nephrol. 2010;5(2):365–70.
43. Germain DP. Fabry disease. Orphanet J Rare Dis. 2010;5:30.
44. Eng CM, Fletcher J, Wilcox WR, et al. Fabry disease: baseline medical characteristics of a cohort of 1765 males and females in the Fabry registry. J Inherit Metab Dis. 2007;30(2):184–92.
45. Grunfeld JP, Lidove O, Joly D, Barbey F. Renal disease in Fabry patients. J Inherit Metab Dis. 2001;24(Suppl 2):71–4; discussion 65.
46. Fogo AB, Bostad L, Svarstad E, et al. Scoring system for renal pathology in Fabry disease: report of the International Study Group of Fabry Nephropathy (ISGFN). Nephrol Dial Transplant. 2010;25(7):2168–77.
47. Wanner C, Arad M, Baron R, et al. European expert consensus statement on therapeutic goals in Fabry disease. Mol Genet Metab. 2018;124(3):189–203.

48. Hughes DA, Nicholls K, Shankar SP, et al. Oral pharmacological chaperone migalastat compared with enzyme replacement therapy in Fabry disease: 18-month results from the randomised phase III ATTRACT study. J Med Genet. 2017;54(4):288–96.

49. Chen YT, Coleman RA, Scheinman JI, Kolbeck PC, Sidbury JB. Renal disease in type I glycogen storage disease. N Engl J Med. 1988;318(1):7–11.

50. Martens DH, Rake JP, Navis G, Fidler V, van Dael CM, Smit GP. Renal function in glycogen storage disease type I, natural course, and renopreservative effects of ACE inhibition. Clin J Am Soc Nephrol. 2009;4(11):1741–6.

51. Kishnani PS, Austin SL, Abdenur JE, et al. Diagnosis and management of glycogen storage disease type I: a practice guideline of the American College of Medical Genetics and Genomics. Genet Med. 2014;16(11):e1.

Primary Hyperoxaluria

29

Bodo B. Beck, Cristina Martin-Higueras, and Bernd Hoppe

Introduction

The **primary hyperoxalurias** (PH) are a group of rare disorders in hepatic glyoxylate metabolism that result in excessive endogenous oxalate generation, their biochemical hallmark [1–4]. The PH's *per se* are not renal diseases, but inborn errors of metabolism that usually first manifest within the kidney and genitourinary tract as recurrent urolithiasis and/or nephrocalcinosis (Fig. 29.1).

Currently, three distinctive types of PH are known. They were termed PH type 1 to 3 in the order of their identification. All are inherited in an autosomal-recessive mode and each type is caused by a single enzymatic defect in the hepatic glyoxylate metabolism that induces overproduction of oxalate [1, 2]. The level of urinary oxalate excretion describing the primary range is commonly defined as greater ≥ 1 mmol/1.73 m^2/day (normal is <0.5 mmol/1.73 m^2/day) (Tables 29.1 and 29.2).

PH type 1 (PH1) is the most frequent and most devastating PH subtype that regularly leads to end stage kidney disease (ESKD) from infancy to late adulthood. PH type 2 (PH2), which is much less frequent in Europe and North America, bears a considerable risk of chronic kidney disease (CKD) (50%) and ESKD (25%) in adulthood [6]. The third type of PH (PH3) is the second most common and, according to recent literature, also shows a certain risk of CKD (20% of patients $\geq$CKD stage 2), while ESKD has been reported in few patients [2–4, 7–10]. While PH is rare, idiopathic calcium-oxalate urolithiasis is a frequent condition that bears in comparison only a modest risk of renal impairment. However, patients with severe secondary hyperoxaluria, especially those with Crohn's disease and status post ileocecal resection, are also prone to CKD and subsequently ESKD [11].

Humans, like all mammals, cannot metabolize oxalate. Whatever amount of oxalate is produced in the organism (physiologically or at increased levels in states of primary hyperoxaluria) or absorbed from the gastrointestinal tract (physio-

B. B. Beck
Institute of Human Genetics, University of Cologne, Cologne, Germany

German Hyperoxaluria Center, Cologne/Bonn, Germany
e-mail: bodo.beck@uk-koeln.de

C. Martin-Higueras
German Hyperoxaluria Center, Cologne/Bonn, Germany

Institute of Biomedical Technologies, CIBERER, University of La Laguna, La Laguna, Spain
e-mail: cristinamh@hyperoxaluria-center.com

B. Hoppe (✉)
German Hyperoxaluria Center, Cologne/Bonn, Germany

Kindernierenzentrum Bonn, Bonn, Germany
e-mail: bernd.hoppe@knz-bonn.de;
bhoppe@hyperoxaluria-center.com

© The Author(s), under exclusive license to Springer Nature Switzerland AG 2023
F. Schaefer, L. A. Greenbaum (eds.), *Pediatric Kidney Disease*,
https://doi.org/10.1007/978-3-031-11665-0_29

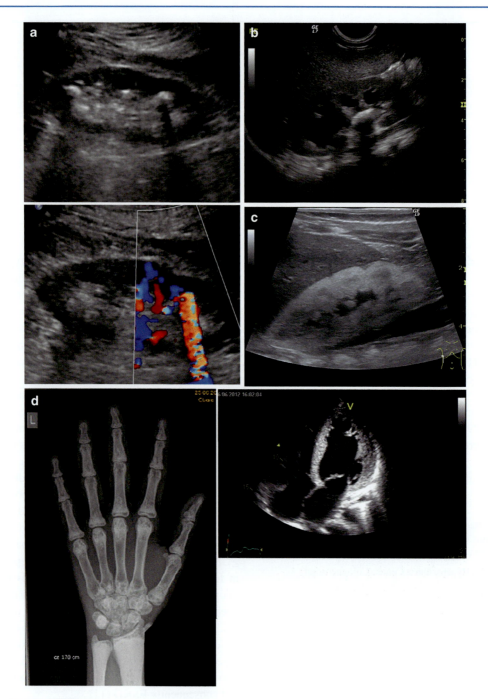

Fig. 29.1 Hallmarks of the primary hyperoxalurias. (**a**) Multiple kidney stones (with positive twinkling sign) in a 21-year-old patient with primary hyperoxaluria type 1 and recurrent stone passages. Stable kidney function with hyperhydration, vitamin B6 and alkaline citrate medication (eGFR = 80.9 mL/min). (**b**) Staghorn calculus in a 7-month-old boy with primary hyperoxaluria type 3. Repeated stone passages in the following months, now, aged 6 years, one not growing stone in the right kidney, no further stones passage. (**c**) Generalized nephrocalcinosis in a 16-month-old girl with primary hyperoxaluria type 1. (**d**) Oxalate osteopathy and cardiac manifestation of systemic oxalosis in a 24-year-old female PH1 patient. Renal replacement therapy since 5 years, plasma oxalate levels >100 μmol/L before hemodialysis. Extreme hyperechogenicity of left ventricular mass depicting severe calcium-oxalate deposition

Combined liver/kidney transplantation is the method of choice in patients with ESKD and in vitamin B6 unresponsive patients without severe systemic oxalosis. Patient and liver allograft survival following combined liver and kidney transplantation were 80% and 72% at 5 years, respectively in European registry data [21, 57]. Pre-emptive liver transplantation might be an option in patients with a more rapid decline in kidney function [136], but timing of that procedure is difficult due to the variability of the disease course. Due to mobilization and renal elimination of systemically deposited oxalate, kidney function may still deteriorate after pre-emptive liver transplantation and kidney transplantation may still become necessary [57, 61]. In patients with infantile oxalosis, sequential liver and kidney transplantation is sometimes reasonable for technical/anatomical reasons [57]. In patients with severe systemic oxalosis sequential transplantation should also be considered to avoid prompt recurrence of oxalosis within the kidney graft.

Isolated kidney transplantation was generally not recommended in PH1. There is substantial evidence that PH1 patients with isolated kidney transplantation develop renal and systemic oxalate deposition [76, 77]. Allograft oxalosis clearly limits the duration of graft function: Following isolated kidney transplantation, graft survival rates were only 46%, 28%, and 14% at 1, 3, and 5 years in PH patients, as compared to 95%, 90%, and 85% in non-PH patients [21]. By contrast, urinary and plasma oxalate normalize following combined liver and kidney transplantation. Isolated kidney transplantation might be considered in elderly patients with late onset of ESKD and a pyridoxin-sensitive genotype [137, 138]. Also, a recent report from the OxalEurope registry suggested that isolated kidney transplantation in patients with pyridoxine sensitive genotypes treated with vitamin B6 may be equivalent in long term outcome to combined transplantation procedures [139].

The advent of the RNAi therapies opens the option to reduce oxalate overproduction pharma-cologically, potentially removing the need for curative liver transplantation in patients with PH1. However, it is currently still too early to say how many patients can eventually be spared liver transplantation in the long run by RNAi therapy, comparable to those patients being sensitive to vitamin B6 medication and reduce their urinary oxalate excretion to merely normal. Long-term follow-up data will be required to address whether liver transplantation will really become obsolete and ESKD can be prevented by this therapy. Our current approach is shown in Fig. 29.4.

In the rare patients with PH2 who reached ESKD, isolated kidney transplantation has mostly been performed since the clinical picture clearly is less severe than in PH1 and liver transplantation does not truly eliminate oxalate overproduction. Although the currently followed very small group of PH2 patients with a kidney transplant show good overall graft survival, patients with oxalate related graft dysfunction, which appeared earlier than chronic rejection induced graft failure, have been described [27]. In a few PH2 cases even combined liver kidney transplantation was found to be necessary [140].

Conclusions and Outlook

The primary hyperoxalurias are challenging diseases. Diagnosis is still frequently delayed despite the availability of genetic screening as a rapid diagnostic tool. Any urolithiasis in a child should prompt an investigation of the underlying cause to treat adeuqately and not only with symptomatic empiric therapy and/or repeated stone removal procedures. This also applies to adult patients with multiple or recurrent kidney stones. The relevance of an early diagnosis for improved long-term outcomes has markedly increased with the advent of RNAi therapeutics as another effective therapy of PH1 aside vitamin B6. It may be now possible to largely prevent the hitherto dismal course of the disease, preserve kidney function and avoid liver transplantation as a curative therapy.

Further curative treatment approaches are under development. Gene therapy might be considered in patients with PH1, as new, safe and highly liver-selective vectors are becoming available which would deliver the targeted gene into the liver cells. In *AGXT* deficient mice it has already been demonstrated that PH1 can be cured with such a therapy [141]. Currently, new vector technologies are being developed since a singular gene therapy might not be sufficient in PH patients as more or less all hepatocytes must be transfected. Multiple administrations will induce immune reactions of the host, which may limit the tolerability of the procedure [142]. Induced pluripotent stem cell-derived hepatocytes, which have first been used experimentally to model human metabolic liver diseases [143], can now be generated from blood leukocytes and dermal fibroblasts of PH1 patients (hiPSC) [144, 145]. In the future, such cells could be gene-edited and used for autologous hepatocyte-like cell transplantation [146] if a proliferative advantage of the hISPC over native diseased hepatocytes can be achieved. Gene editing of the *HAO1* gene by Crispr-Cas9 has already been applied in the animal model [147].

References

1. Cochat P, Rumsby G. Primary hyperoxaluria. N Engl J Med. 2013;369:649–58.
2. Hoppe B, Beck BB, Milliner DS. The primary hyperoxalurias. Kidney Int. 2009;75:1264–71.
3. Belostotsky R, et al. Mutations in DHDPSL are responsible for primary hyperoxaluria type III. Am J Hum Genet. 2010;87:392–9.
4. Monico CG, et al. Primary hyperoxaluria type III gene HOGA1 (formerly DHDPSL) as a possible risk factor for idiopathic calcium oxalate urolithiasis. Clin J Am Soc Nephrol. 2011;6:2289–95.
5. Pitt JJ, Willis F, Tzanakos N, Belostotsky R, Frishberg Y. 4-hydroxyglutamate is a biomarker for primary hyperoxaluria type 3. JIMD Rep. 2015;15:1–6.
6. Garrelfs SF, et al. Patients with primary hyperoxaluria type 2 have significant morbidity and require careful follow-up. Kidney Int. 2019;96:1389–99.
7. Beck BB, et al. Novel findings in patients with primary hyperoxaluria type III and implications for advanced molecular testing strategies. Eur J Hum Genet. 2013;21:162–72.
8. Singh P, et al. Clinical characterization of primary hyperoxaluria type 3 in comparison with types 1 and 2. Nephrol Dial Transplant. 2022;37(5):869–75. https://doi.org/10.1093/ndt/gfab027.
9. Singh P, et al. Primary Hyperoxaluria type 3 can also result in kidney failure: a case report. Am J Kidney Dis. 2022;79(1):125–8. https://doi.org/10.1053/j.ajkd.2021.05.016.
10. Martin-Higueras C, et al. A report from the European Hyperoxaluria Consortium (OxalEurope) registry on a large cohort of patients with primary hyperoxaluria type 3. Kidney Int. 2021;100:621–35.
11. Hueppelshaeuser R, et al. Enteric hyperoxaluria, recurrent urolithiasis, and systemic oxalosis in patients with Crohn's disease. Pediatr Nephrol. 2012;27:1103–9.
12. Siener R, Ebert D, Nicolay C, Hesse A. Dietary risk factors for hyperoxaluria in calcium oxalate stone formers. Kidney Int. 2003;63:1037–43.
13. Habbig S, Beck BB, Hoppe B. Nephrocalcinosis and urolithiasis in children. Kidney Int. 2011;80:1278–91.
14. Sikora P, et al. [13C2]oxalate absorption in children with idiopathic calcium oxalate urolithiasis or primary hyperoxaluria. Kidney Int. 2008;73:1181–6.
15. Robijn S, Hoppe B, Vervaet BA, D'Haese PC, Verhulst A. Hyperoxaluria: a gut-kidney axis? Kidney Int. 2011;80:1146–58.
16. Dill H, Martin-Higueras C, Hoppe B. Diet-related urine collections: assistance in categorization of hyperoxaluria. Urolithiasis. 2022;50(2):141–8. https://doi.org/10.1007/s00240-021-01290-2.
17. Vervaet BA, Verhulst A, De Broe ME, D'Haese PC. The tubular epithelium in the initiation and course of intratubular nephrocalcinosis. Urol Res. 2010;38:249–56.
18. Mulay SR, et al. Calcium oxalate crystals induce renal inflammation by NLRP3-mediated IL-1β secretion. J Clin Invest. 2013;123:236–46.
19. Knauf F, et al. NALP3-mediated inflammation is a principal cause of progressive renal failure in oxalate nephropathy. Kidney Int. 2013;84:895–901.
20. Stokes F, et al. Plasma oxalate: comparison of methodologies. Urolithiasis. 2020;48:473–80.
21. Hoppe B. An update on primary hyperoxaluria. Nat Rev Nephrol. 2012;8:467–75.
22. Beck BB, Hoyer-Kuhn H, Göbel H, Habbig S, Hoppe B. Hyperoxaluria and systemic oxalosis: an update on current therapy and future directions. Expert Opin Invest Drugs. 2013;22:117–29.
23. Hoppe B, et al. Plasma calcium oxalate supersaturation in children with primary hyperoxaluria and end-stage renal failure. Kidney Int. 1999;56:268–74.

24. Birtel J, et al. The ocular phenotype in primary Hyperoxaluria type 1. Am J Ophthalmol. 2019;206:184–91.
25. Pfau A, et al. Assessment of plasma oxalate concentration in patients with CKD. Kidney Int Rep. 2020;5:2013–20.
26. Cochat P, et al. Primary hyperoxaluria type 1: still challenging! Pediatr Nephrol. 2006;21:1075–81.
27. Hoppe B, Langman CB. A United States survey on diagnosis, treatment, and outcome of primary hyperoxaluria. Pediatr Nephrol. 2003;18:986–91.
28. Hoppe B, Latta K, von Schnakenburg C, Kemper MJ. Primary hyperoxaluria—the German experience. Am J Nephrol. 2005;25:276–81.
29. Kopp N, Leumann E. Changing pattern of primary hyperoxaluria in Switzerland. Nephrol Dial Transplant. 1995;10:2224–7.
30. Lieske JC, et al. International registry for primary hyperoxaluria. Am J Nephrol. 2005;25:290–6.
31. Takayama T, Nagata M, Ichiyama A, Ozono S. Primary hyperoxaluria type 1 in Japan. Am J Nephrol. 2005;25:297–302.
32. van Woerden CS, Groothoff JW, Wanders RJA, Davin J-C, Wijburg FA. Primary hyperoxaluria type 1 in the Netherlands: prevalence and outcome. Nephrol Dial Transplant. 2003;18:273–9.
33. van Woerden G, Mandrile S, Hulton S, Fargue B, Beck JH. The collaborative European cohort of primary hyperoxalurias: clinical and genetic characterization with prediction of outcome at the 15th congress of the International Pediatric Nephrology Association. Pediatr Nephrol. 2010;25:1779–2004.
34. Gargah T, et al. Primary hyperoxaluria type 1 in Tunisian children. Saudi J Kidney Dis Transplant. 2012;23:385–90.
35. Kamoun A, et al. [Primary hyperoxaluria: Tunisian experience apropos of 24 pediatric cases]. Nephrologie. 1997;18:59–64.
36. Lepoutre C. Calculs multiples chez un enfant ; infiltration du parenchyme rénal par des dépôts cristallins. J Urol Medicale Chir. 1925;20:424.
37. Archer HE, Dormer AE, Scowen EF, Watts RW. Primary hyperoxaluria. Lancet. 1957;273:320–2.
38. Danpure CJ, Jennings PR, Watts RW. Enzymological diagnosis of primary hyperoxaluria type 1 by measurement of hepatic alanine: glyoxylate aminotransferase activity. Lancet. 1987;1:289–91.
39. Danpure CJ, Lumb MJ, Birdsey GM, Zhang X. Alanine:glyoxylate aminotransferase peroxisome-to-mitochondrion mistargeting in human hereditary kidney stone disease. Biochim Biophys Acta. 2003;1647:70–5.
40. Danpure CJ. Molecular aetiology of primary hyperoxaluria type 1. Nephron Exp Nephrol. 2004;98:e39–44.
41. Williams EL, et al. Primary hyperoxaluria type 1: update and additional mutation analysis of the AGXT gene. Hum Mutat. 2009;30:910–7.
42. de la Chapelle A, Wright FA. Linkage disequilibrium mapping in isolated populations: the example of Finland revisited. Proc Natl Acad Sci U S A. 1998;95:12416–23.
43. Mesa-Torres N, Tomic N, Albert A, Salido E, Pey AL. Molecular recognition of PTS-1 cargo proteins by Pex5p: implications for protein mistargeting in primary hyperoxaluria. Biomol Ther. 2015;5:121–41.
44. Zhang X, et al. Crystal structure of alanine:glyoxylate aminotransferase and the relationship between genotype and enzymatic phenotype in primary hyperoxaluria type 1. J Mol Biol. 2003;331:643–52.
45. Danpure CJ, Cooper PJ, Wise PJ, Jennings PR. An enzyme trafficking defect in two patients with primary hyperoxaluria type 1: peroxisomal alanine/glyoxylate aminotransferase rerouted to mitochondria. J Cell Biol. 1989;108:1345–52.
46. Rucktäschel R, Girzalsky W, Erdmann R. Protein import machineries of peroxisomes. Biochim Biophys Acta. 2011;1808:892–900.
47. Belostotsky R, Pitt JJ, Frishberg Y. Primary hyperoxaluria type III—a model for studying perturbations in glyoxylate metabolism. J Mol Med (Berl). 2012;90:1497–504.
48. Fargue S, Lewin J, Rumsby G, Danpure CJ. Four of the most common mutations in primary hyperoxaluria type 1 unmask the cryptic mitochondrial targeting sequence of alanine:glyoxylate aminotransferase encoded by the polymorphic minor allele. J Biol Chem. 2013;288:2475–84.
49. Coulter-Mackie MB. Preliminary evidence for ethnic differences in primary hyperoxaluria type 1 genotype. Am J Nephrol. 2005;25:264–8.
50. Lorenzo V, et al. Presentation and role of transplantation in adult patients with type 1 primary hyperoxaluria and the I244T AGXT mutation: single-center experience. Kidney Int. 2006;70:1115–9.
51. Lumb MJ, Danpure CJ. Functional synergism between the most common polymorphism in human alanine:glyoxylate aminotransferase and four of the most common disease-causing mutations. J Biol Chem. 2000;275:36415–22.
52. Fargue S, Rumsby G, Danpure CJ. Multiple mechanisms of action of pyridoxine in primary hyperoxaluria type 1. Biochim Biophys Acta. 2013;1832:1776–83.
53. Monico CG, Rossetti S, Olson JB, Milliner DS. Pyridoxine effect in type I primary hyperoxaluria is associated with the most common mutant allele. Kidney Int. 2005;67:1704–9.
54. Pirulli D, Marangella M, Amoroso A. Primary hyperoxaluria: genotype-phenotype correlation. J Nephrol. 2003;16:297–309.

55. van Woerden CS, et al. Clinical implications of mutation analysis in primary hyperoxaluria type 1. Kidney Int. 2004;66:746–52.

56. Frishberg Y, et al. Intra-familial clinical heterogeneity: absence of genotype-phenotype correlation in primary hyperoxaluria type 1 in Israel. Am J Nephrol. 2005;25:269–75.

57. Jamieson NV, European PHI Transplantation Study Group. A 20-year experience of combined liver/kidney transplantation for primary hyperoxaluria (PH1): the European PH1 transplant registry experience 1984-2004. Am J Nephrol. 2005;25:282–9.

58. Bergstralh EJ, et al. Transplantation outcomes in primary hyperoxaluria. Am J Transplant. 2010;10:2493–501.

59. Hoppe B, et al. A vertical (pseudodominant) pattern of inheritance in the autosomal recessive disease primary hyperoxaluria type 1: lack of relationship between genotype, enzymic phenotype, and disease severity. Am J Kidney Dis. 1997;29:36–44.

60. Harambat J, et al. Characteristics and outcomes of children with primary oxalosis requiring renal replacement therapy. Clin J Am Soc Nephrol. 2012;7:458–65.

61. Brinkert F, et al. Transplantation procedures in children with primary hyperoxaluria type 1: outcome and longitudinal growth. Transplantation. 2009;87:1415–21.

62. Herrmann G, Krieg T, Weber M, Sidhu H, Hoppe B. Unusual painful sclerotic plaques on the legs of a patient with late diagnosis of primary hyperoxaluria type I. Br J Dermatol. 2004;151:1104–7.

63. Lagies R, Beck BB, Hoppe B, Sreeram N, Udink Ten Cate FEA. Apical sparing of longitudinal strain, left ventricular rotational abnormalities, and short-axis dysfunction in primary hyperoxaluria type 1. Circ Heart Fail. 2013;6:e45–7.

64. Cramer SD, Ferree PM, Lin K, Milliner DS, Holmes RP. The gene encoding hydroxypyruvate reductase (GRHPR) is mutated in patients with primary hyperoxaluria type II. Hum Mol Genet. 1999;8:2063–9.

65. Cregeen DP, Williams EL, Hulton S, Rumsby G. Molecular analysis of the glyoxylate reductase (GRHPR) gene and description of mutations underlying primary hyperoxaluria type 2. Hum Mutat. 2003;22:497.

66. Van Schaftingen E, Draye JP, Van Hoof F. Coenzyme specificity of mammalian liver D-glycerate dehydrogenase. Eur J Biochem. 1989;186:355–9.

67. Baker PRS, Cramer SD, Kennedy M, Assimos DG, Holmes RP. Glycolate and glyoxylate metabolism in HepG2 cells. Am J Physiol Cell Physiol. 2004;287:C1359–65.

68. Mdluli K, Booth MPS, Brady RL, Rumsby G. A preliminary account of the properties of recombinant human glyoxylate reductase (GRHPR), LDHA and LDHB with glyoxylate, and their potential roles in its metabolism. Biochim Biophys Acta. 2005;1753:209–16.

69. Giafi CF, Rumsby G. Kinetic analysis and tissue distribution of human D-glycerate dehydrogenase/glyoxylate reductase and its relevance to the diagnosis of primary hyperoxaluria type 2. Ann Clin Biochem. 1998;35(Pt 1):104–9.

70. Knight J, Holmes RP, Milliner DS, Monico CG, Cramer SD. Glyoxylate reductase activity in blood mononuclear cells and the diagnosis of primary hyperoxaluria type 2. Nephrol Dial Transplant. 2006;21:2292–5.

71. Williams HE, Smith LH. L-glyceric aciduria. A new genetic variant of primary hyperoxaluria. N Engl J Med. 1968;278:233–8.

72. Kemper MJ, Conrad S, Müller-Wiefel DE. Primary hyperoxaluria type 2. Eur J Pediatr. 1997;156:509–12.

73. Milliner DS, Wilson DM, Smith LH. Phenotypic expression of primary hyperoxaluria: comparative features of types I and II. Kidney Int. 2001;59:31–6.

74. Wichmann G, Passauer J, Fischer R, Weise M, Gross P. A young patient with end-stage renal disease, dyspnoea, weakness, peripheral neuropathy and an unsuspected underlying disease. Nephrol Dial Transplant. 2003;18:1670–2.

75. Schulze MR, Wachter R, Schmeisser A, Fischer R, Strasser RH. Restrictive cardiomyopathy in a patient with primary hyperoxaluria type II. Clin Res Cardiol. 2006;95:235–40.

76. Del Bello A, Cointault O, Delas A, Kamar N. Primary hyperoxaluria type 2 successfully treated with combined liver-kidney transplantation after failure of isolated kidney transplantation. Am J Transplant. 2020;20:1752–3.

77. Dhondup T, Lorenz EC, Milliner DS, Lieske JC. Combined liver-kidney transplantation for primary hyperoxaluria type 2: a case report. Am J Transplant. 2018;18:253–7.

78. Rumsby G, Sharma A, Cregeen DP, Solomon LR. Primary hyperoxaluria type 2 without L-glycericaciduria: is the disease under-diagnosed? Nephrol Dial Transplant. 2001;16:1697–9.

79. Riedel TJ, et al. Structural and biochemical studies of human 4-hydroxy-2-oxoglutarate aldolase: implications for hydroxyproline metabolism in primary hyperoxaluria. PLoS One. 2011;6:e26021.

80. Williams EL, et al. The enzyme 4-hydroxy-2-oxoglutarate aldolase is deficient in primary hyperoxaluria type 3. Nephrol Dial Transplant. 2012;27:3191–5.

81. Riedel TJ, et al. 4-Hydroxy-2-oxoglutarate aldolase inactivity in primary hyperoxaluria type 3 and glyoxylate reductase inhibition. Biochim Biophys Acta. 2012;1822:1544–52.

82. Knight J, Jiang J, Assimos DG, Holmes RP. Hydroxyproline ingestion and urinary oxalate and glycolate excretion. Kidney Int. 2006;70:1929–34.

83. Cochat P, et al. Primary hyperoxaluria type 1: indications for screening and guidance for diagnosis and treatment. Nephrol Dial Transplant. 2012;27:1729–36.
84. Clifford-Mobley O, Sjögren A, Lindner E, Rumsby G. Urine oxalate biological variation in patients with primary hyperoxaluria. Urolithiasis. 2016;44:333–7.
85. Laube N, Hoppe B, Hesse A. Problems in the investigation of urine from patients suffering from primary hyperoxaluria type 1. Urol Res. 2005;33:394–7.
86. Marangella M, Petrarulo M, Vitale C, Cosseddu D, Linari F. Plasma and urine glycolate assays for differentiating the hyperoxaluria syndromes. J Urol. 1992;148:986–9.
87. Marangella M, et al. Plasma profiles and dialysis kinetics of oxalate in patients receiving hemodialysis. Nephron. 1992;60:74–80.
88. Hoyer-Kuhn H, et al. Vitamin B6 in primary hyperoxaluria I: first prospective trial after 40 years of practice. Clin J Am Soc Nephrol. 2014;9:468–77.
89. Santana A, Salido E, Torres A, Shapiro LJ. Primary hyperoxaluria type 1 in the Canary Islands: a conformational disease due to I244T mutation in the P11L-containing alanine:glyoxylate aminotransferase. Proc Natl Acad Sci U S A. 2003;100:7277–82.
90. Schouten JP, et al. Relative quantification of 40 nucleic acid sequences by multiplex ligation-dependent probe amplification. Nucleic Acids Res. 2002;30:e57.
91. Cogal AG, et al. Comprehensive genetic analysis reveals complexity of monogenic urinary stone disease. Kidney Int Rep. 2021;6:2862–84.
92. Hatch M, Freel RW, Vaziri ND. Regulatory aspects of oxalate secretion in enteric oxalate elimination. J Am Soc Nephrol. 1999;10(Suppl 1):S324–8.
93. Hatch M, Freel RW. Intestinal transport of an obdurate anion: oxalate. Urol Res. 2005;33:1–16.
94. McLaurin AW, Beisel WR, McCormick GJ, Scalettar R, Herman RH. Primary hyperoxaluria. Ann Intern Med. 1961;55:70–80.
95. Milliner DS, Eickholt JT, Bergstralh EJ, Wilson DM, Smith LH. Results of long-term treatment with orthophosphate and pyridoxine in patients with primary hyperoxaluria. N Engl J Med. 1994;331:1553–8.
96. Toussaint C. Pyridoxine-responsive PH1: treatment. J Nephrol. 1998;11(Suppl 1):49–50.
97. Monico CG, Olson JB, Milliner DS. Implications of genotype and enzyme phenotype in pyridoxine response of patients with type I primary hyperoxaluria. Am J Nephrol. 2005;25:183–8.
98. Mandrile G, et al. Data from a large European study indicate that the outcome of primary hyperoxaluria type 1 correlates with the AGXT mutation type. Kidney Int. 2014;86:1197–204.
99. Leumann E, Matasovic A, Niederwieser A. Pyridoxine in primary hyperoxaluria type I. Lancet. 1986;2:699.
100. Morgan SH, Maher ER, Purkiss P, Watts RW, Curtis JR. Oxalate metabolism in end-stage renal disease: the effect of ascorbic acid and pyridoxine. Nephrol Dial Transplant. 1988;3:28–32.
101. Edwards P, Nemat S, Rose GA. Effects of oral pyridoxine upon plasma and 24-hour urinary oxalate levels in normal subjects and stone formers with idiopathic hypercalciuria. Urol Res. 1990;18:393–6.
102. Shah GM, et al. Effects of ascorbic acid and pyridoxine supplementation on oxalate metabolism in peritoneal dialysis patients. Am J Kidney Dis. 1992;20:42–9.
103. Costello JF, Sadovnic MC, Smith M, Stolarski C. Effect of vitamin B6 supplementation on plasma oxalate and oxalate removal rate in hemodialysis patients. J Am Soc Nephrol. 1992;3:1018–24.
104. Marangella M. Transplantation strategies in type 1 primary hyperoxaluria: the issue of pyridoxine responsiveness. Nephrol Dial Transplant. 1999;14:301–3.
105. Helin I. Primary hyperoxaluria. An analysis of 17 Scandinavian patients. Scand J Urol Nephrol. 1980;14:61–4.
106. Harrison AR, Kasidas GP, Rose GA. Hyperoxaluria and recurrent stone formation apparently cured by short courses of pyridoxine. Br Med J (Clin Res Ed). 1981;282:2097–8.
107. Alinei P, Guignard JP, Jaeger P. Pyridoxine treatment of type 1 hyperoxaluria. N Engl J Med. 1984;311:798–9.
108. Gibbs DA, Watts RW. Biochemical studies on the treatment of primary hyperoxaluria. Arch Dis Child. 1967;42:505–8.
109. Holmgren G, Hörnström T, Johansson S, Samuelson G. Primary hyperoxaluria (glycolic acid variant): a clinical and genetical investigation of eight cases. Ups J Med Sci. 1978;83:65–70.
110. Musayev FN, et al. Molecular basis of reduced pyridoxine 5′-phosphate oxidase catalytic activity in neonatal epileptic encephalopathy disorder. J Biol Chem. 2009;284:30949–56.
111. Montioli R, et al. The N-terminal extension is essential for the formation of the active dimeric structure of liver peroxisomal alanine:glyoxylate aminotransferase. Int J Biochem Cell Biol. 2012;44:536–46.
112. Fodor K, Wolf J, Erdmann R, Schliebs W, Wilmanns M. Molecular requirements for peroxisomal targeting of alanine-glyoxylate aminotransferase as an essential determinant in primary hyperoxaluria type 1. PLoS Biol. 2012;10:e1001309.
113. Hopper ED, Pittman AMC, Fitzgerald MC, Tucker CL. In vivo and in vitro examination of stability of primary hyperoxaluria-associated human alanine:glyoxylate aminotransferase. J Biol Chem. 2008;283:30493–502.
114. Oppici E, et al. Biochemical analyses are instrumental in identifying the impact of mutations on holo and/or apo-forms and on the region(s) of

alanine:glyoxylate aminotransferase variants associated with primary hyperoxaluria type I. Mol Genet Metab. 2012;105:132–40.

115. Oppici E, et al. Pyridoxamine and pyridoxal are more effective than pyridoxine in rescuing folding-defective variants of human alanine:glyoxylate aminotransferase causing primary hyperoxaluria type I. Hum Mol Genet. 2015;24:5500–11.

116. Grujic D, et al. Hyperoxaluria is reduced and nephrocalcinosis prevented with an oxalate-degrading enzyme in mice with hyperoxaluria. Am J Nephrol. 2009;29:86–93.

117. Harambat J, et al. Genotype-phenotype correlation in primary hyperoxaluria type 1: the p.Gly170Arg AGXT mutation is associated with a better outcome. Kidney Int. 2010;77:443–9.

118. Latta K, Brodehl J. Primary hyperoxaluria type I. Eur J Pediatr. 1990;149:518–22.

119. Hoppe B, et al. Safety, pharmacodynamics, and exposure-response modeling results from a first-in-human phase 1 study of nedosiran (PHYOX1) in primary hyperoxaluria. Kidney Int. 2022;101(3):626–34. https://doi.org/10.1016/j.kint.2021.08.015.

120. Liebow A, et al. An investigational RNAi therapeutic targeting glycolate oxidase reduces oxalate production in models of primary hyperoxaluria. J Am Soc Nephrol. 2017;28:494–503.

121. Martin-Higueras C, Torres A, Salido E. Molecular therapy of primary hyperoxaluria. J Inherit Metab Dis. 2017;40:481–9.

122. Garrelfs SF, et al. Lumasiran, an RNAi therapeutic for primary hyperoxaluria type 1. N Engl J Med. 2021;384:1216–26.

123. Ariceta G, et al. Hepatic lactate dehydrogenase A: an RNA interference target for the treatment of all known types of primary hyperoxaluria. Kidney Int Rep. 2021;6:1088–98.

124. Lai C, et al. Specific inhibition of hepatic lactate dehydrogenase reduces oxalate production in mouse models of primary hyperoxaluria. Mol Ther. 2018;26:1983–95.

125. Allison MJ, Dawson KA, Mayberry WR, Foss JG. Oxalobacter formigenes gen. nov., sp. nov.: oxalate-degrading anaerobes that inhabit the gastrointestinal tract. Arch Microbiol. 1985;141:1–7.

126. Hatch M, et al. Oxalobacter sp. reduces urinary oxalate excretion by promoting enteric oxalate secretion. Kidney Int. 2006;69:691–8.

127. Hatch M, et al. Enteric oxalate elimination is induced and oxalate is normalized in a mouse model of primary hyperoxaluria following intestinal colonization with oxalobacter. Am J Physiol Gastrointest Liver Physiol. 2011;186:G461–9.

128. Hoppe B, et al. Effects of Oxalobacter formigenes in subjects with primary hyperoxaluria type 1 and

end-stage renal disease: a phase II study. Nephrol Dial Transplant. 2021;36(8):1464–73. https://doi.org/10.1093/ndt/gfaa135.

129. Hoppe B, et al. Oxalobacter formigenes: a potential tool for the treatment of primary hyperoxaluria type 1. Kidney Int. 2006;70:1305–11.

130. Hoppe B, et al. Efficacy and safety of Oxalobacter formigenes to reduce urinary oxalate in primary hyperoxaluria. Nephrol Dial Transplant. 2011;26:3609–15.

131. Leumann E, Hoppe B, Neuhaus T. Management of primary hyperoxaluria: efficacy of oral citrate administration. Pediatr Nephrol. 1993;7:207–11.

132. Hamm LL. Renal handling of citrate. Kidney Int. 1990;38:728–35.

133. Illies F, Bonzel K-E, Wingen A-M, Latta K, Hoyer PF. Clearance and removal of oxalate in children on intensified dialysis for primary hyperoxaluria type 1. Kidney Int. 2006;70:1642–8.

134. Hoppe B, et al. Oxalate elimination via hemodialysis or peritoneal dialysis in children with chronic renal failure. Pediatr Nephrol. 1996;10:488–92.

135. Bunchman TE, Swartz RD. Oxalate removal in type I hyperoxaluria or acquired oxalosis using HD and equilibration PD. Perit Dial Int. 1994;14:81–4.

136. Nolkemper D, et al. Long-term results of pre-emptive liver transplantation in primary hyperoxaluria type 1. Pediatr Transplant. 2000;4:177–81.

137. Saborio P, Scheinman JI. Transplantation for primary hyperoxaluria in the United States. Kidney Int. 1999;56:1094–100.

138. Monico CG, Milliner DS. Combined liver-kidney and kidney-alone transplantation in primary hyperoxaluria. Liver Transplant. 2001;7:954–63.

139. Metry EL, et al. Transplantation outcomes in patients with primary hyperoxaluria: a systematic review. Pediatr Nephrol. 2021;36:2217–26.

140. Dhondup T, Lorenz EC, Milliner DS, Lieske JC. Invited response to recurrence of oxalate nephropathy after isolated kidney transplantation for primary hyperoxaluria type 2. Am J Transplant. 2018;18:527.

141. Salido E, et al. Phenotypic correction of a mouse model for primary hyperoxaluria with adeno-associated virus gene transfer. Mol Ther. 2011;19:870–5.

142. Weigert A, Martin-Higueras C, Hoppe B. Novel therapeutic approaches in primary hyperoxaluria. Expert Opin Emerg Drugs. 2018;23:349–57.

143. Rashid ST, et al. Modeling inherited metabolic disorders of the liver using human induced pluripotent stem cells. J Clin Invest. 2010;120:3127–36.

144. Martinez-Turrillas R, et al. Generation of an induced pluripotent stem cell line (CIMAi001-A) from a compound heterozygous primary hyperoxaluria type I (PH1) patient carrying p.G170R and p.R122*

mutations in the AGXT gene. Stem Cell Res. 2019;41:101626.

145. Zapata-Linares N, et al. Generation and characterization of human iPSC lines derived from a primary Hyperoxaluria type I patient with p.I244T mutation. Stem Cell Res. 2016;16:116–9.

146. Estève J, et al. Generation of induced pluripotent stem cells-derived hepatocyte-like cells for ex vivo gene therapy of primary hyperoxaluria type 1. Stem Cell Res. 2019;38:101467.

147. Zabaleta N, et al. CRISPR/Cas9-mediated disruption of glycolate oxidase is an efficacious and safe treatment for primary hyperoxaluria type I. Mol Ther. 2018;26:384–5.

Cystinosis

30

Elena Levtchenko, Leo Monnens, and Aude Servais

Introduction

Cystinosis is an autosomal recessive disorder characterized by an accumulation of the amino acid cystine in lysosomes throughout the body. The responsible gene *CTNS* is located on the short arm of the chromosome 17 (p13) and encodes the lysosomal cystine carrier cystinosin [1, 2]. Lysosomal cystine accumulation is the hallmark of the disease.

E. Levtchenko (✉)
Division of Pediatric Nephrology, Department of Pediatrics, University Hospitals Leuven,
Leuven, Belgium

Department of Development and Regeneration,
Katholieke Universiteit (KU) Leuven,
Leuven, Belgium
e-mail: elena.levtchenko@uzleuven.be

L. Monnens
Department of Physiology, Radboud University Nijmegen Medical Centre,
Nijmegen, The Netherlands
e-mail: leo.monnens@radboudumc.nl

A. Servais
Adult Nephrology and Transplantation Department,
Centre de référence des Maladies Rénales
Héréditaires de l'Enfant et de l'Adulte, APHP, Necker Hospital, Paris, France

Inserm U1163, Imagine Institute, Paris Descartes University, Paris, France
e-mail: aude.servais@aphp.fr

Depending on the age of presentation and the degree of disease severity, three clinical forms of cystinosis are distinguished:

- Nephropathic infantile form (MIM #219800), which is the most frequent and the most severe form of the disease
- Nephropathic juvenile form (MIM #219900); synonyms: intermediate cystinosis, late-onset form, adolescent form
- Non-nephropathic adult form (MIM #219750); synonyms: benign non-nephropathic cystinosis, ocular non-nephropathic cystinosis

All three forms of the disease are caused by mutations in the *CTNS* gene and have phenotypic overlap. Unless specified otherwise, this chapter focuses on infantile nephropathic cystinosis which affects ~95% of the patients.

Historical Aspects

Cystinosis was first described as a clinical entity by the chemist Abderhalden in 1903 [3] and recognized as a main cause of generalized proximal tubulopathy, called de Toni-Debré-Fanconi syndrome in the late 1940s/early 1950s [4–6]. Real progress in the investigation of cystinosis started when amino acid chromatographic analysis allowed measuring elevated cystine concentrations in tissues of cystinotic patients [7, 8]. In the

© The Author(s), under exclusive license to Springer Nature Switzerland AG 2023
F. Schaefer, L. A. Greenbaum (eds.), *Pediatric Kidney Disease*,
https://doi.org/10.1007/978-3-031-11665-0_30

1980s it was demonstrated that cystine was stored within the lysosomes due to the impairment of cystine transport across the lysosomal membrane [9, 10]. The availability of renal transplantation and treatment with the amino thiol cysteamine dramatically improved the prognosis of cystinosis patients allowing them to survive into adulthood [11, 12]. Cloning the *CTNS* gene in 1998 was pivotal for understanding the genetic basis of the disease and performing genetic counseling of the families [1]. Moreover, the *CTNS* gene discovery opened a new chapter in studying the disease pathogenesis and searching for novel molecular therapies [13].

Epidemiology

The estimated incidence of cystinosis is 1 in 100,000–200,000 live births [2] with clustering reported in some populations [14–16]. Cystinosis affects all races, with specific hotspot mutations reported in different nations [16, 17].

Males and females are equally affected. Overall cystinosis patients account for approximately 1–2% of the pediatric end-stage renal failure population or 0.85/million of age related population [18, 19].

Genetics

Mutation Spectrum

Cystinosis is caused by mutations in the *CTNS* gene, which has been identified by positional cloning strategy [1]. *CTNS* maps to 17p13.2 (Fig. 30.1a) [1] and encodes a 367 amino acid protein, cystinosin, with a 7-transmembrane domain structure which is highly glycosylated at the N-terminus [21] (Fig. 30.1b). Cystinosin contains 2 lysosomal-targeting sequences, one situ-

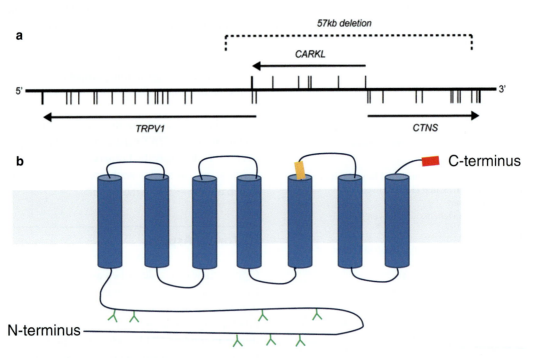

Fig. 30.1 Molecular basis of cystinosis. (**a**) The *CTNS* gene is mapped at chromosome 17p13.2 and is composed of 12 exons, with the open reading frame starting in exon 3. The *CTNS* shares promoter sequence with the *CARKL* gene. Common 57 kb deletion is the most prevalent mutation in the Northern-European population which affects *CTNS*, *CARKL* and the first two non-coding exons of the adjacent *TRPV1* gene (Used with permission of The American Physiological Society from Wilmer et al. [20]); (**b**) *CTNS* encodes lysosomal membrane protein cystinosin with seven transmembrane domain structure. Cystinosin contains two lysosomal-targeting sequences: GYDQL at C-terminus (red box), and YFPQA—in the fifth inter-transmembrane domain loop (yellow box). Y—predicted glycosylation sites

ated in its C-terminus, a tyrosine-based motif (GYDQL) and the second (YFPQA) in the fifth inter-transmembrane domain (TM) loop [21].

Mutations in *CTNS* have been detected in all three clinical forms of cystinosis, demonstrating that these forms are allelic [1, 22, 23]. The most common anomaly is a large 57 kb deletion spanning the first nine exons and a part of exon 10 of the *CTNS* gene, the upstream 5-prime region that encodes the *CARKL* (carbohydrate kinase-like) gene, and the first two noncoding exons of the *TRPV1* gene [1, 24–26]. *CARKL* encodes the enzyme sedoheptulokinase [26] and *TRPV1* encodes the protein transient receptor potential one [27]. Patients with the homozygous 57 kb deletion have increased sedoheptulose levels in tissues, serum and urine [26, 28], but no clinical disorders related to CARKL deficiency has been reported so far. Decreased sensitivity to capsaicin and altered sensation of heat due to strongly reduced activity of TRPV1 channel may account for the reported sensory alterations and thermo-regulatory deficits (such as impaired sweating) in patients carrying homozygous 57 kb deletion [27]. The common 57 kb deletion can be detected by FISH analysis, by a rapid PCR assay with the 57 kb deletion breakpoint primer sets, or by MLPA [29–31]. While being frequent in the Northern-European population, the 57 kb deletion is rare in Southern Europe and in patients originating from other ethnical groups [16].

Over 140 other mutations in *CTNS* have been reported, which include small deletions, insertions, nonsense, missense, splicing mutations, mutations in the promoter region or small genomic rearrangements (uniparental disomy on chromosome 17) [1, 16, 22, 25, 30–34].

In a recently published European cohort, 33% of patients were homozygous and 23% were heterozygous for the 57 kb deletion, and 45% had other pathogenic variants of the *CTNS* gene [35]. Missense variants, splicing variants and out-of-frame deletions were the other most frequent types of mutations. If standard analysis using PCR technique and Sanger sequencing fails to demonstrate *CTNS* mutations in patients with the clinical diagnosis of cystinosis, the *CTNS* gene transcripts analysis for detection of exon-skipping mutations should be performed [34]. Maternal heterodisomy should be suspected when no mutation is found in the father and can be detected using analysis of microsatellite markers on chromosome 17 [33].

Genotype: Phenotype Correlations

In infantile forms, individuals have severe mutations in both alleles, leading to the complete loss of cystinosin function. No differences in kidney survival and severity of the extra-renal disease between patients that inherited the 57 kb deletion in homozygous or in heterozygous state and patients with other severe pathogenic *CTNS* variants were found [35–37]. In contrast, point mutations in the *CTNS* gene that do not disrupt the open reading frame of cystinosin are more commonly associated with the late-onset phenotype and generally affect the inter-transmembrane loops or the N-terminal region [22, 23, 38–42]. In the late-onset form, patients are usually homozygous for mild mutations or compound heterozygous for a mild mutation and a severe mutation [22]. Mild mutations impair, but do not completely abolish cystine transport [43]. Moreover, the level of transport inhibition often correlates with the severity of symptoms. Some tissues might be spared in benign cystinosis due to tissue-specific splicing factors mitigating the effect of splice-site mutations in renal tissue by favoring the expression of residual normal message [23, 42, 43]. Mutations in the promoter region have also been described in patients with ocular cystinosis [25]. In addition, contrasting to almost 100% detection rate in infantile cystinosis, *CTNS* mutations are not found in all patients in late-onset forms [39, 41]. Mutations in the non-coding regions of the *CTNS*, such as the regulatory regions, may also be involved in these patients.

Pathogenesis

Following the seminal studies by Schneider et al. [7, 8], electron microscopy of lymph nodes of patients with cystinosis first suggested that cystine accumulation occurs in lysosomes [44]. The lysosomal localization of cystine was later confirmed in cystinotic leucocytes [45]. Subsequently, kinetic studies of cystine clearance from lysosomes of cystinotic leucocytes and fibroblasts provided evidence that impaired lysosomal cystine efflux represents the primary defect causing cystine accumulation in cystinosis [9, 10, 46].

The discovery of the gene defective in cystinosis allowed the functional characterization of the gene product cystinosin as a proton-driven lysosomal cystine carrier [47]. A transcript variant of the *CTNS* originating from alternative splicing of exon 12, which replaces the lysosomal targeting motif GYDQL at the C-terminus by a longer amino acid sequence (termed CTNS-LKG based on the sequence of the three last amino acids leucine (L), lysine (K), glycine (G)) shows expression in the plasma membrane, in lysosomes, in the endoplasmatic reticulum, in the Golgi apparatus, and in small intracellular vesicles [48]. In most tissues, CTNS-LKG represents 5–20% of *CTNS* transcripts with the highest expression level found in the testes [49].

The source of lysosomal cystine *in vivo* is uncertain. Because kidney proximal tubules are the first affected cells of the body, it has been suggested that the endocytosis of disulfide-reach plasma proteins with subsequent hydrolysis in lysosomes can lead to extensive cystine accumulation and early damage of proximal tubular cells. Blocking megalindriven endocytosis in a mouse model of cystinosis substantially decreased crystal formation and prevented proximal tubular atrophy, providing a proof-of-concept that the megalin pathway can be a potential therapeutic target [50]. On the other hand, inhibiting the lysosomal membrane cysteine transporter MFSD12 responsible for the import of cytosolic cysteine to the lysosomal lumen substantially decreases lysosomal cystine accumulation in fibroblasts from patients in cystinosis, pointing that cytosolic cysteine is an important source of lysosomal cystine [51].

ATP Depletion

Prior to the development of the knockout mouse model, cystine-loaded proximal tubules were used to study renal pathogenesis in cystinosis [52, 53]. Whether cystinosis causes a direct alteration of mitochondrial ATP generation remains controversial [54–56]. While studies in skin fibroblasts and immortalized proximal tubular cells derived from cystinosis patients showed overall normal ATP generating capacity and unaltered activity of Na-K ATPase [57–60], decreased mitochondrial levels of cyclic-AMP, reduced complex I and V activity and altered mitochondrial morphology and dynamics were demonstrated and point to altered mitochondrial function [61, 62] (Fig. 30.2).

Increased Apoptosis

Another pathologic mechanism involved in cystinosis is an altered regulation of cell survival and death due to enhanced apoptosis. The rate of apoptosis is increased in fibroblasts and proximal tubular cells of patients with nephropathic cystinosis compared to normal cells [63, 64].

Enhanced apoptosis has been postulated to cause the specific atrophy of renal proximal convoluted tubules adjacent to glomeruli ("swanneck" deformity), that has been demonstrated in cystinotic kidney biopsies starting from sixth month of age [65, 66]. Transcripts of proapoptotic caspase 1, caspase 4 and caspase 12 are increased in cystinotic tissues, with significant increase in caspase 3 activity being demonstrated in proximal tubular cells of cystinosis mouse model [67].

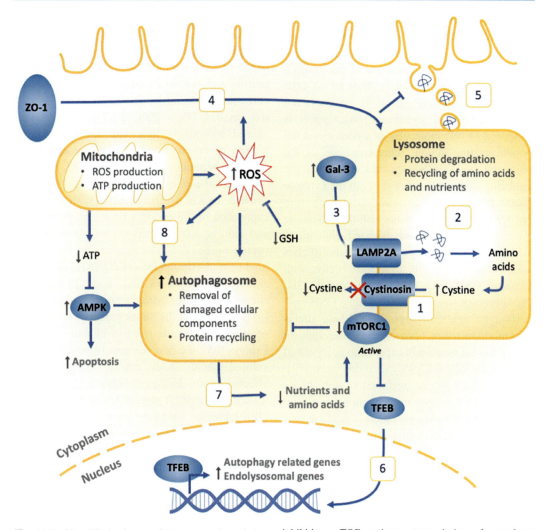

Fig. 30.2 Simplified scheme of the current knowledge on pathogenesis of cystinosis. (1) Dysfunctional cystinosin leads to the accumulation of cystine within the lumen of the lysosome. (2) Reduced protein degradation due to defective lysosomal enzyme activation. (3) Reduced chaperone-mediated autophagy leads to galectin-3 overexpression and has been associated with chronic kidney disease progression. (4) Phosphorylation of tight junction adapter protein ZO-1 results in its misrouting to endolysosomal compartments and disruption of tight junction integrity. (5) Disruption of tight junctions leads to epithelial dysfunction and dedifferentiation, repressing apical endocytic receptors and megalin/cubilin-mediated endocytosis. (6) Increased TFEB nuclear translocation by inhibiting mTOR activates transcription of autophagy related genes and can reduce cystine accumulation via increased exocytosis. (7) Reduced autophagic flux and degradation. (8) Abnormal mitophagy can lead to increased oxidative stress, further promoting epithelial dysfunction, dedifferentiation, and apoptosis. *AMPK* 5′ adenosine monophosphate-activated protein kinase, *ATP* adenosine triphosphate, *GSH* glutathione, *Gal-3* galectin-3, *LAMP2A* lysosome-associated membrane protein 2A, *mTORC1* mammalian target of rapamycin complex 1, *ROS* reactive oxygen species, *TFEB* transcription factor EB, *ZO-1* zonula occludens 1. (Reproduced with permission from Jamalpoort et al. Trends Mol Med 2021)

Altered Redox Homeostasis and Increased Oxidative Stress

Multiple studies have demonstrated that cystinosis cells are prone to oxidative stress and that the mitigation of oxidative stress is an important therapeutic target in cystinosis [68]. Cystine is composed of two molecules of cysteine and the cysteine/cystine couple represents one of the major cell thiol/disulfide systems involved in the regulation of the cell redox state. In the cytosole cystine is reduced to cysteine through electron transfer from the other major cell thiol/disulfide systems, mainly free and oxidized glutathione (GSH/GSSG) [69]. Altered GSH metabolism has been demonstrated in cystinosis cells with decreased GSH levels [58, 70], decreased GSH/GSSG ratio or inability to upregulate GSH synthesis upon oxidative stress [71]. These alterations might be a direct consequence of cystinosin dysfunction as cystinosin expression is regulated by the intracellular Cys/CySS redox state [72]. On top, mitochondrial dysfunction and altered autophagy of damaged mitochondria have been shown to increase the generation of reactive oxidative species (ROS) which can further exhaust the cellular anti-oxidative capacity and lead to cell damage [73]. Reducing lysosomal cystine accumulation with cysteamine interferes with this cascade, increases cellular glutathione levels, attenuates oxidative stress and decreases the rate of apoptosis promoting cell survival in cystinosis [60, 63, 64].

Altered Vesicle Trafficking and Cell Signaling

The fact that renal Fanconi syndrome is not fully responsive to cysteamine treatment suggested that not all cellular mechanisms of cystinosis are due to cystine accumulation and pointed to potential other functions of cystinosin [20, 68]. This hypothesis was substantiated by recent studies demonstrating that the absence of cystinosin led to alterations of cellular trafficking mechanisms, impaired cell signaling and autophagy (Fig. 30.2).

Altered vesicle movements with a predominance of slow moving lysosomes was found in murine and human cystinotic proximal tubular cells, accompanied by decreased expression of the small GTPase Rab27a [74]. In addition, altered autophagic flux was demonstrated in human cystinotic fibroblasts, proximal tubular cells and in patient kidney biopsies [75, 76].

Proximal tubular cells of the *ctns* $^{-/-}$ mouse showed signs of dedifferentiation with decreased expression of the endocytotic receptors megalin and cubilin and elevated expression of zonula occludens-1 (ZO-1)-associated nucleic acid-binding transcription factor (ZONAB) and proliferation markers PCNA and cyclin D1 characteristic of immature proximal tubular cells [77]. In line with the development of the "swanneck" lesion demonstrated in human cystinotic kidneys [65], the first segment of proximal convoluted tubules in the *ctns* $^{-/-}$ mice was first affected with lesions gradually progressing towards more distal parts of the proximal tubule [78]. Increased oxidative stress might be a link between cystinosin dysfunction and altered endocytosis as it stimulates Gα12/Src-mediated phosphorylation of tight junction protein ZO-1 and triggers a signaling cascade involving ZO-1-associated Y-box factor ZONAB, which leads to dedifferentiation of proximal tubular cells, cell proliferation and transport defects [73]. It is still a working model without explanation for decreased transport for glucose, phosphate and other small solutes.

Altered mammalian target of rapamycin (mTOR) signaling might be another potential therapeutic target in cystinosis, unrelated to cystine accumulation. While an interaction between cystinosin and Vacuolar H+—ATPase-Ragulator-Rag complex controlling mTOR has been demonstrated [79], studies of mTOR activity in cystinosis cells provided inconsistent results [80, 81]. Nevertheless, inhibiting mTOR activity by everolimus reduced the number of large lysosomes, decreases apoptosis, and activates autophagy in kidney organoids derived from *CTNS*-deficient human induced pluripotent stem cells [82]. The expression of transcription factor EB (TFEB), which inhibits mTOR activity, is reduced in cystinosis proximal tubular cells, and overexpressing TFEB improves the altered cellular phenotype [83]. Inhibiting mTOR stimulates nuclear transplocation of TFEB and can reduced cellular cystine accumulation by increasing exocytosis of cystine loaded lysosomes [68] (Fig. 30.2).

A drug-repositioning strategy combined with high-throughput screening showed that the flavonoid luteolin improves the lysosome-mediated degradation of the autophagy cargoes, restores lysosomal distribution, and stimulates endocytosis in cystinotic proximal tubular cells, opening a new therapeutic prospective in cystinosis [84].

Mechanism of Chronic Interstitial Damage

The progression of cystinotic nephropathy is characterized by the development of diffuse tubulo-interstitial lesions and fibrosis. Cystinosis is also associated with early podocyte dysfunction characterized by excessive losses of podocytes into urine and the development of glomerular proteinuria [81].

Reabsorption of excessively filtered proteins may contribute to the renal interstitial injury in analogy to other proteinuric conditions by stimulating local inflammatory response [85, 86]. Furthermore, higher circulating levels of pro-inflammatory interleukin-1β and interleukin-18 were attributed to inflammasome activation by cystine crystals [87]. Macrophage activation in the kidney is likely to contribute to the development of interstitial renal damage caused by cystine accumulation. Furthermore, studies have demonstrated an additional new role for cystinosin in inflammation through its interaction with the lectin and β-galactoside-binding protein family 21 galectin-3 (Gal-3), enhancing macrophage infiltration and CKD progression [88] (Fig. 30.2).

Clinical Presentation

Kidney Disease

Infantile nephropathic cystinosis is the most frequent cause of inherited renal Fanconi syndrome in childhood. The dysfunction of different proximal tubular transporters develops gradually after birth with aminoaciduria being present already during the first month of life [89]. Full-blown renal Fanconi syndrome characterized by excessive urinary excretion of amino acids, phosphate, bicarbonate, glucose, sodium, potassium, low molecular weight proteins and other solutes, handled in renal proximal tubules is usually present by the age of 6 months. Clinically, patients are asymptomatic at birth and develop normally until 3–6 months, when they manifest with failure to thrive, vomiting, constipation, polyuria and excessive thirst, periods of dehydration and sometimes rickets [90, 91]. Growth retardation in case of late diagnosis may reach −4 SD [90]. Renal loss of sodium and potassium can result in hyponatremia and hypokalemia, which may be life threatening. Hypouricemia, decreased plasma carnitine and medullary nephrocalcinosis related to increased calcium excretion are also observed [92, 93]. Total protein excretion can reach several grams per day and contains both low molecular weight proteins, albumin and high molecular weight proteins [85].

In untreated patients glomerular filtration declines gradually and progresses towards kidney failure before the age of 10 years [94, 95]. At start of kidney replacement therapy patients with cystinosis have better blood pressure control and lower serum phosphate levels compared to patients with end stage kidney disease (ESKD) due to other causes because of still ongoing renal Fanconi syndrome with polyuria and urinary sodium and phosphate losses [96].

Renal Pathology

The age at which the first morphological changes appear in the kidneys of patients with cystinosis is unknown. No significant renal changes were observed in the fetus [97]. Serial renal biopsies in two cystinotic patients demonstrated that the typical "swan-neck" deformity of proximal convoluted tubules appeared only after 6 months of life [65]. In a large series of kidney specimens, the most striking feature were the marked irregularities of renal tubular cells with the presence of flat cells with focal disappearance of the brush border and very large cells with a prominent and hyperchromatic cytoplasm (Fig. 30.3a) [97, 98]. Glomeruli can appear normal but most contain peculiar giant multinucleated podocytes (Fig. 30.3a) [85]. Podocyte foot process effacement seen in other proteinuric disorders is also present in cystinosis (Fig. 30.3b) [85]. Cystine crystals located in the lysosomes or in cytoplasm are seen mostly within interstitial cells and rarely within podocytes [97]. Patients with late-onset or juvenile cystinosis can demonstrate focal and segmental glomerular sclerosis (FSGS) undistinguishable from idiopathic FSGS [39].

The deterioration of kidney function is accompanied by progressive tubulo-interstitial lesions, including interstitial fibrosis, tubular atrophy and marked arteriolar thickening. The progressive glomerular damage, leading to increasing albuminuria and hematuria, consists of segmental or global collapse of the capillary tuft, accumulation of mesangial matrix material, and, observed by electron microscopy, irregular thickening of glomerular basement membrane [97].

In transplanted kidneys cystine crystals, sometimes seen at graft biopsy, have no clinical relevance as they are present in the host mononuclear cells [99].

Kidney Transplantation

Kidney transplantation is the best therapeutic option for ESKD in young patients [100]. In pediatric cohorts, the outcome of kidney transplantation in patients with cystinosis is generally better than that of other patients undergoing transplantation [96, 101–103]. In adults, a similar rate of graft survival at 5 and 10 years among patients with cystinosis and control patients has been reported [104]. Furthermore, long term graft survival is higher in patients with cystinosis compared to controls by multivariate analysis. Proximal tubular disease does not occur in the transplanted kidney because the metabolic disorder is not present in the engrafted kidney. However, retention of a native kidney can result in the persistence of renal tubular Fanconi syndrome. Renal transplantation does not correct the systemic meta-

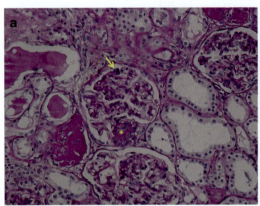
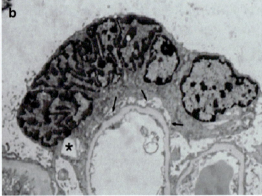

Fig. 30.3 Renal pathology in cystinosis. (**a**) Renal tissue of a 9-year-old patient with cystinosis. Some glomeruli contain giant multinucleated podocytes (yellow arrow) or show FSGS lesions (yellow asterisk). The tubules are often delineated by cuboidal cells. PAS, original magnification ×200 (Courtesy of Prof. Dr. E. Lerut, Department of Pathology, University Hospitals Leuven); (**b**) Electron microscopy of cystinotic podocyte showing multinucleation which is pathognomonic for cystinosis. Black arrows indicate podocyte foot process effacement. Black asterisk indicate cystine crystal in the cytoplasm (Used with permission of Elsevier from Wilmer et al. [85])

bolic defect of cystinosis and cystine continues to accumulate in most organs and may lead to late systemic complications.

Patients with cystinosis are at risk of developing post-transplant diabetes. However, the risk of diabetes is not increased compared with control patients [104]. Immunosuppressive maintenance treatment regimens should be equivalent between patients with or without cystinosis.

Extra-renal Involvement

Ocular Impairment

Accumulation of cystine crystals occurs in all ocular structures, including the cornea, the conjunctiva, the iris and the retina causing symptoms of photophobia, blepharospasm and other complications. The corneal crystals, pathognomonic of the disorder, are absent at birth, but generally may be visible on ophthalmological investigation from around 16 months of age in most patients with cystinosis (Fig. 30.4a). If untreated, patients develop increasingly severe photophobia, refractory blepharospasm, peripheral corneal neovascularisation and band keratopathy, eventually progressing to involvement of the posterior segment of the eye with hypopigmentary mottling of the retinal pigment epithelium, glaucoma and visual impairment [105–107].

Novel techniques such as *in vivo* confocal microscopy and anterior segment optical coherence tomography of the cornea allow not only to visualize corneal cystine crystals with high sensitivity, but also to quantify the crystals and the

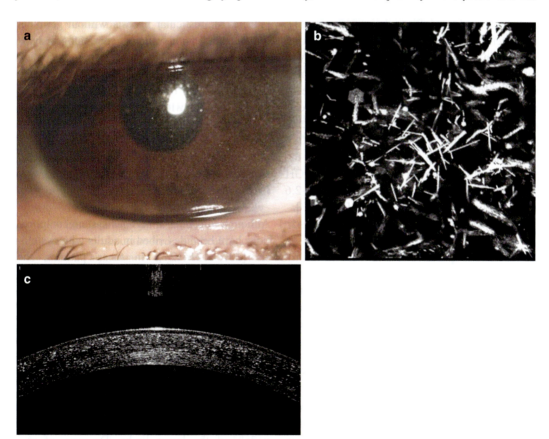

Fig. 30.4 Eye examination of cystinosis. (**a**) Slit-lamp photography of corneal cystine crystals. Corneal crystals typically appear as needle-shaped and highly reflective. (**b**) *In vivo* confocal microscopy images of crystals detected in the cornea stroma. (**c**) Anterior-Segment Optical Coherence Tomography (OCT) Z-axis: infiltration of crystals in depth of the cornea. (Courtesy of Dr Liang, Hôpital des Quinze Vingt, Paris, France)

However, nausea and vomiting are mostly caused by cysteamine treatment due to increased gastric acid secretion [141].

Hepatosplenic complications have become rare with the routine use of cysteamine [36, 37]. Liver enlargement with normal synthetic function was a frequent finding in historical cohorts, while hepatic fibrosis with portal hypertension and hypersplenism, eventually causing bleeding problems, and cholestatic liver disease due to nodular hyperplasia can still be observed. Electron microscopy showed extensive cystine crystal accumulation in Küppfer cells [110, 142, 143].

Bone Disease

Bone impairment is also described in patients with cystinosis. International recommendations concerning the management of cystinosis associated bone disease have been published in 2019 [144]. Even though the exact pathophysiology of bone impairment remains unclear, at least five distinct but complementary entities can explain it: consequences of renal Fanconi syndrome, malnutrition and copper deficiency, hormonal disturbances, myopathy, and intrinsic bone defects [144, 145]. Bone complications have a significant impact on patients' quality of life due to an increased frequency of bone pain, deformations and fractures occurring in late teenage and early adulthood [146–148].

Other Clinical Features

Diminished skin, hair and iris pigmentation is frequently observed in cystinosis patients and is explained by reduced melanin synthesis [149]. Impaired sweating has been reported in some patients. Premature skin aging is a typical feature in adult patients [150, 151].

Cystine crystals are found in the bone marrow of the patients, but has usually they have few consequences for the hematopoiesis, although some patients with bi-or pancytopenia have been reported [152, 153].

Cystinosis in Adults

Renal transplantation has transformed cystinosis from a fatal pediatric disease into a multisystem adult disease. The series of patients described in the 1990s revealed a high rate of mortality and morbidity. The main causes of death occurring before 35 years of age were aspiration, pseudobulbar palsy and uremia. The most incapacitating morbidities included blindness or severely impaired vision, and swallowing difficulties due to myopathy [122]. The long-term prognosis of patients has been substantially improved during the past two decades due to the administration of cysteamine with reduced morbidity and mortality rates [107, 133, 154], especially in patients in whom cysteamine was started before the age of 5 years [36, 37]. Transition from pediatric to adult care providers remains an area of concern due to the generally lacking expertise of internists-nephrologists with this ultra-rare disorder with historically rare survival into adulthood. Good communication between pediatric and internists-nephrologists is required to guarantee the continuation of adequate medical care [155, 156]. Management of systemic disease involvement is mandatory and requires a multi-disciplinary team.

Late Onset and Ocular Forms of Cystinosis

Less severe clinical forms of cystinosis account for less than 5% of all patients. Patients with the nephropathic late-onset form (MIM #219900) manifest with a spectrum of symptoms, varying from a milder proximal tubulopathy to apparent nephrotic syndrome, focal segmental histological lesions and generally have a slower rate of renal disease progression [2, 39, 41, 157, 158]. Cystine crystals accumulate also in the cornea and are diagnostic. In terms of the age at presentation there is probably a continuum between the infantile and the late-onset forms; however, most of the described patients were older than 10 years. Extra-renal organs may also be affected in these patients and progression towards end stage kidney disease may also occur.

Ocular non-nephropathic cystinosis (MIM #219750) affects the cornea with cystine crystal deposits causing photophobia. The kidneys, retina and other organs are clinically spared in these patients, but they do have elevated cystine leukocyte content and cystine crystals in bone marrow [23, 159]. The co-existence of the ocular form with late-onset nephropathy in the same family has been reported, warranting monitoring of kidney function in patients with ocular cystinosis [39].

Diagnosis

The diagnosis of cystinosis has to be suspected in all infants and children presenting with renal Fanconi syndrome. Other inherited and acquired forms of Fanconi syndrome should be excluded. Urine dipstick usually shows low specific gravity, overt glucosuria and mild albuminuria. Serum creatinine is generally normal in young children, unless patients are dehydrated [2].

The diagnosis is based on the measurement of elevated white blood cell (WBC) cystine levels. The isolation of polymorphonuclear (PMN) leukocytes is recommended for WBC cystine determination because cystine preferentially accumulates in this type of blood cells and not in the lymphocytes [160, 161]. It is important at a younger age when lymphocytes are the predominant cells type (up to about 60% of WBC) until the age of 5–7 years when neutrophils predominate. As leukocyte isolation and cystine measurement (by either high performance liquid chromatography or tandem mass spectrometry) require specific expertise, this analysis should

Table 30.1 Reference values for intracellular cystine

Healthy subjects	
PMN leukocytes	0.04–0.16 nmol cystine/mg protein [a]
Mixed Leukocytes	0.05–0.17 nmol cystine/mg protein [a]
Fibroblasts	0.0–0.23 nmol cystine/mg protein [a]
Patients at diagnosis	
PMN leukocytes	>2 nmol cystine/mg protein
Heterozygotes	
PMN leukocytes	0.14–0.57 nmol cystine/mg protein
Patients under cysteamine therapy	
PMN leukocytes	<1 nmol cystine/mg protein

[a]Values are provided by Laboratory of Genetic and Metabolic diseases, Radboud University Nijmegen Medical Centre, The Netherlands and presented as Percentile 5 and 95
Cystine is frequently expressed as nmol ½ cystine per mg protein. Conversion factor ½ cystine/mg protein = 2× cystine/mg protein

only be performed in specifically certified laboratories. Cystine values in healthy individuals, heterozygous subjects, patients at diagnosis and under cysteamine therapy are provided in Table 30.1. The detection of corneal cystine crystals is pathognomonic for the diagnosis in patients above the age of 1.5 years. Molecular analysis of the *CTNS* gene should be performed for confirming the diagnosis and genetic counselling of the families [162]. Including cystinosis in the list of diseases to be detected via neonatal screening programs using next generation sequencing (NGS) in on the research agenda in many countries. The feasibility of this approach and the benefit for the patients' prognosis has been demonstrated [163, 164] (Fig. 30.6).

Fig. 30.6 Proposed diagnosis algorithm for cystinosis. Other genetic, metabolic and secondary causes of renal Fanconi syndrome should be excluded (see Chap. 32 for differential diagnosis of renal Fanconi syndrome)

Clinical suspicion of cystinosis
- failure to thrive, growth retardation
- thirst, polyuria
- vomiting, constipation
- rickets
- pale skin and hair color

⇩

Serum and urine biochemistry
- hypokalemia
- hypophosphatemia
- metabolic acidosis
- hypouricemia
- aminoaciduria
- glucosuria
- proteinuria

⇒ Renal Fanconi syndrome

⇨ **Exclusion of secondary causes of renal Fanconi syndrome**
- drugs (aminoglycosides, cisplatin, ifosfamide, valproate)
- recovery of acute tubular necrosis
- infections

⇩

Making diagnosis
- determination of elevated cystine levels in WBC (preferentially PMNs)
- eye examination (corneal cystine crystals in all children > 1-2 year)

⇩

Confirmation of diagnosis
- CTNS gene analysis

⇦ **Neonatal screening**
- based on next generation sequencing (NGS)

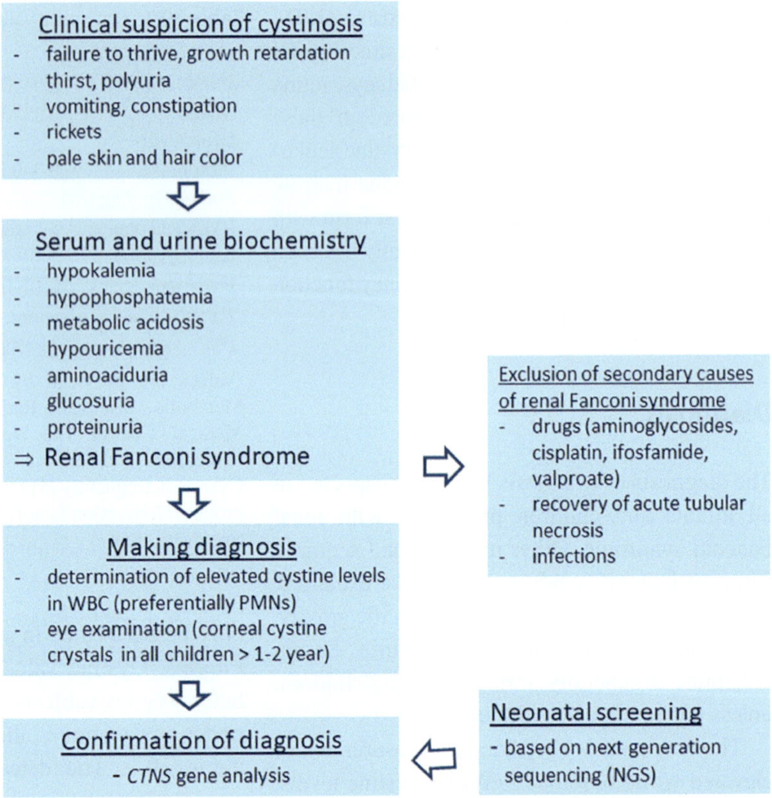

Treatment

Treatment of cystinosis includes adequate feeding, the symptomatic replacement of substances lost into urine due to renal Fanconi syndrome, hormone replacement therapy and specific cystine lowering therapy with cysteamine. Kidney replacement therapy in cystinosis patients reaching ESKD is not different compared with other underlying diseases and is beyond the scope of this chapter. Both hemodialysis and peritoneal dialysis can be successfully applied.

Feeding Recommendations

Early gastric tube placement should be considered in all children who have poor appetite or frequent vomiting [165]. Gastric tubes also facilitate administration of oral medications and fluid. Patients with frequent vomiting and gastroesophageal reflux may respond to proton pump inhibitor therapy [166]. Overall, children should receive at least 100% of the recommended dietary allowance (RDA) for their age; however, no current evidence indicates that any higher caloric intake is useful. The composition of the diet should be balanced and should include salt and fluid supplementation.

Symptomatic Therapy of Renal Fanconi Syndrome

Patients with cystinosis should have free access to water and toilet privilege, because of pronounced polyuria and polydipsia. Prolonged exposure to heat and sun should be avoided because to photophobia, and the risk of dehydration and heat stroke due to impaired sweating.

Symptomatic therapy aims to maintain fluid and electrolyte balance, to prevent rickets and to

Table 30.2 Symptomatic therapy of renal Fanconi syndrome in cystinosis

Drugs [a]	Doses
Sodium potassium citrate	
Suspension (Na 50 g = 1.2 mmol/mL, K 55 g = 1.1 mmol/mL, Citrate 33.5 g = 2.3 mmol/mL, sir Simplex ad 500 mL)	2–10 mmol K/kg/day, divided in 4 doses
Potassium citrate	
Powder (100 mg: K 37 mg = 1 mmol, Citric Acid 62 mg = 0.3 mmol)	2–10 mmol K/kg/day, divided in 4 doses
Sodium bicarbonate	
Suspension 8.4% (Na 1 mmol/mL, bicarbonate 1 mmol/mL)	2–15 mmol/kg/day, divided in 4 doses
Powder (100 mg: Na 27 mg = 1.2 mmol, bicarbonate 73 mg = 1.2 mmol)	
Potasium phosphate	
Suspension (K dihydrophosphate/K_2 hydrophosphate) 7.5 g, aqua ad 100 mL (K 39 mg = 1 mmol/ml, phosphate 18 mg = 0.6 mmol/mL	0.6–2 mmol phosphate/kg/day, divided in 4 doses
Powder (100 mg: K 52 mg = 1.3 mmol, phosphate 23 mg = 0.6 mmol)	
L-carnitine	
Suspension 100 mg/mL	20–30 mg/kg/day, divided in 3 doses
Tablets 330 mg	
Indomethacin	
Suspension 5 mg/mL	0.5–3 mg/kg/day, divided in 2–3 doses
Vitamin D	
1 alpha-hydroxycholecalciferol	0.5–2 µg/day in one dose

improve growth. An overview of frequently prescribed drugs is shown in Table 30.2. Excessive administration of phosphate, 1,25-dihydroxycholecalciferol and bicarbonate is not indicated as it may aggravate nephrocalcinosis and stimulate renal stone formation [93]. A decrease of the renal function requires adaptation of the doses.

The aim of symptomatic therapy is to maintain serum potassium levels >3 mmol/L, serum bicarbonate level 22–25 mmol/L, serum phosphate level 0.8–1.6 mmol/L with normal for age levels of alkaline phosphatases. The administration of high doses of phosphate and vitamin D can increase nephrocalcinosis. Blood for electrolyte measurements should preferentially be drawn before the next dose of electrolyte supplements as their levels fluctuate substantially during 24 h. Carnitine replacement normalizes plasma and muscular carnitine levels; however, it is not established whether carnitine administration results in improved muscular performance [167, 168]. The recommended dose of 50 mg/kg causes changes in plasma acetylcarnitine and several short and medium-chain acylcarnitines indicating oversupplementation [169]. In patients with muscular complaints lower doses of carnitine (20–30 mg/kg) might be considered, but no clinical evidence supports carnitine supplementation in all patients.

Maintaining fluid and electrolyte balance in young patients can be challenging and can be improved by the administration of indomethacin [170]. Indomethacin is a non-selective inhibitor of cyclooxygenase (Cox). The Cox-1 and Cox-2 metabolites have a direct effect on salt and water transport along the nephron. Indomethacin increases NaCl reabsorption in the medullary ascending limb and in the collecting duct and augments the antidiuretic effect of the antidiuretic hormone. These effects compensate for the proximal tubular losses [170].

The inhibition of renin-angiotensin-aldosterone system (RAAS) decreases albuminuria [171] and might improve renal function survival [112]; however, this class of drugs should be used with caution, because of the risk of hypotension and renal function decline in patients having extracellular volume and salt depletion. Concomitant administration of RAAS inhibitors and indomethacin is contra-indicated to avoid acute kidney injury. Of note, in a large European cohort of cystinosis patients no beneficial effect of RAAS inhibitors on kidney function survival could be demonstrated [35]. Long-term administration of indomethacin didn't have a detrimental effect on the kidney function [35].

Hormone Replacement Therapy

Treatment with recombinant GH improves growth in children with cystinosis, allowing them to catch-up and to maintain normal growth velocity [13]. Hence, GH therapy should be considered in children with cystinosis and subnormal growth rates even in the presence of a still normal glomerular filtration rate [109]. Levothyroxine is indicated in patients with hypothyroidism, as is insulin in case of diabetes. Testosterone supplementation should be considered in male patients with hypogonadism.

Specific Treatment with Cysteamine

Cysteamine, first introduced for the treatment of cystinosis in 1976 [172] and approved for clinical use in the 1990s, is still the only available treatment that efficiently decreases lysosomal cystine accumulation [173]. Inside lysosomes the drug reacts with cystine and breaks it into cysteine and cysteamine-cysteine mixed disulfide that can exit the lysosome via transporters other than the defective cystinosin (Fig. 30.7). Cysteamine therapy has fundamentally transformed the prognosis of the disease. In patients born between 1970 and 2000, early initiation of cysteamine delayed end stage renal disease by ~6 to 10 years [35, 36, 96, 112]. In well-treated patients in whom cysteamine was administered before the age of 2 years, renal Fanconi syndrome could be attenuated and renal function remained preserved until young adult age [36, 112, 174]. Cysteamine treatment has beneficial effects also on extra-renal symp-

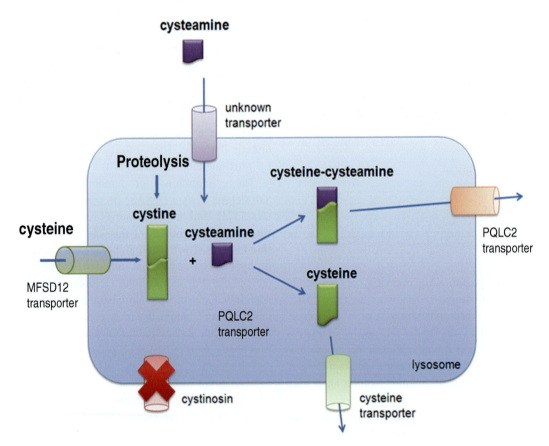

Fig. 30.7 Schematic drawing of cysteamine action in cystinotic cells. Cysteamine can enter the lysosome trough an unknown transporter. Once inside the lysosome it breaks the disulfide bond in cystine, leading to the formation of cysteine and a cysteamine-cysteine disulfide which can leave the lysosome trough the cysteine and PQLC2 transporters respectively. Lysosomal cystine is formed by the proteolytic degradation of proteins and by oxidation of cytosolic cysteine which enters lysosomes via MFSD12 transporter [51] (Used with permission of Elsevier from Besouw et al. [173])

toms of cystinosis with decreased frequencies of hypothyroidism, diabetes, myopathy, pulmonary dysfunction, swallowing difficulties, and death [36, 133, 154, 155, 175, 176]. The drug also prevents the development of visual loss due to retinopathy [105, 177].

The most widely used cysteamine salt, cysteamine bitartrate, is available as an immediate release (Cystagon®) and as a delayed release (Procysbi®) preparations. Cystagon® has to be administered every 6 h including the night period [178]. Procysbi® is a micro-spheronized enteric-coated cysteamine bitartrate with an improved pharmacokinetic profile, allowing twice daily dosing. Non-inferiority of the effect of the delayed release formulation compared to immediate-release cysteamine on WBC cystine levels has been demonstrated [179, 180]. The recommended daily dose of cysteamine is 1.3 g/m^2 of cysteamine base (or 2 g/day in patients older than 12 years). The maximum cysteamine dose should not exceed 1.95 g/m^2/day. To avoid the development of side-effects cysteamine has to be started at ~1/6 of the target dose and gradually increased over 6–8 weeks. Patients using delayed release formulation show better adherence to treatment compared with immediate release preparation ([181], see below)

WBC cystine levels are used as a biomarker to monitor the effectiveness of cystine depletion; the upper limit of asymptomatic heterozygous carries (<1 nmol ½ cystine/mg protein) is usually considered as an indication for adequate cysteamine dosing (Table 30.1). WBC cystine levels have to be measured 6 h after last dose of immediate-release cysteamine or ideally 30 min after last dose for delayed-release cysteamine, however, a pre-dose sampling is frequently performed in routine practice.

The most commonly reported side effects comprise gastro-intestinal complaints, for which the concomitant use of proton pump inhibitors is advised [141, 166] although reducing the acidity of the stomach will influence the pharmacokinetics of Procysbi®. Gastrointestinal tolerability may be improved with the slow-release cysteamine formulation [179].

Cysteamine causes disagreeable breath and sweat odor due to the conversion of cysteamine to methanethiol and dimethylsulphide [182]. This side effect may lead to significant psychosocial issues, which sometimes limit the long-term compliance with the medication especially during adolescence [181, 183].

Three cystinosis patients with lupus nephritis while receiving cysteamine were reported [173]. Eight cystinosis patients, mostly treated with high cysteamine doses, developed skin adverse events, consisting of vascular proliferative lesions on the stretchable skin surfaces, striae and severe bone and muscular pains (Fig. 30.8a, b) [184]. An abnormal morphology of dermal collagen fibers was found on EM in these patients and suggested to be caused by copper deficiency due to urinary losses that could inhibit collagen cross-linking (Fig. 30.8b) [185].

Animal studies showed an increased risk for intrauterine death, intrauterine growth retardation and fetal malformations (especially cleft palate and kyphosis) in pregnant rats given high cysteamine doses of 100 and 150 mg/kg [186]. While human teratogenicity information is lacking, FDA classified cysteamine as a category C drug based on the animal data. It is advised in female cystinosis patients to stop cysteamine administration at the diagnosis of pregnancy until the baby is born, although one normal pregnancy in a cystinosis female receiving 900 mg cysteamine per day has been reported [187].

Cysteamine Eye Drops

Corneal cystine accumulation is resistant to oral cysteamine and must be treated by topical administration of cysteamine eye drops, which dissolve corneal cystine crystals and alleviate symptoms at all ages [105, 188]. Cysteamine collyrium containing 0.55% cysteamine base needs to be administered six to ten times daily [188]. A commercial 0.44% cysteamine ophthalmic solution (Cystaran®, Sigma-Tau Pharmaceuticals, Gaithersburg, MD, USA) has been approved for clinical use in the US and should be administered 6–12 times per day. In this formulation, cyste-

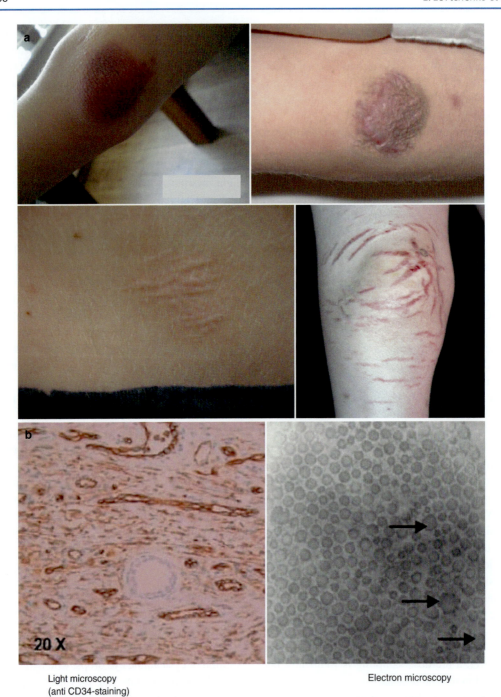

Fig. 30.8 Cutaneous signs of cysteamine toxicity. (**a**) Upper row: Bruise-like lesion at the elbow at early stage (left) and in regression (after the decrease of cysteamine dose) (right). Lower row: the lesion above lumbar vertebrae in regression, the skin is becoming loose and wrinkly (left); skin striae at the stretchable surface of the knee (right). (**b**) Skin biopsy from the elbow lesion. Left: light microscopy, anti-CD34 immuno-staining, original magnification ×20. Plump CD34-positive endothelial cells line numerous vascular structures, some of them completely developed and others with immature features. The CD34−negative sweat gland epithelium serves as negative control. Right: electron microscopy. Variability of collegan fibre caliber: focal diameter increase (arrows) (Used with permission of Elsevier from Besouw et al. [184])

amine oxidises at room temperature, necessitating cold storage. Another topical 0.55% cysteamine gel formulation (Cystadrops® Recordati Rare Diseases, Puteaux, France) for less frequent (three to four times) daily administration has been proven to be safe, efficacious and tolerable [189, 190]. The chemical stability of the formulation was improved, allowing the 0.55% cysteamine drops to be kept at room temperature for up to 7 days after opening, although refrigeration is still required for long-term storage. Eye drop administration can cause eye burning due to the low pH of the solution, especially in patients with corneal erosions. Using hydrating eye drops prior to cysteamine might improve discomfort related to cysteamine eye drop administration.

Prognosis and Future Treatments

The overall prognosis in patients with cystinosis has dramatically improved during the past decades due to the availability of renal replacement therapy and wide use of cysteamine therapy starting from the 1990s. The oldest patients with infantile cystinosis are reaching now their 50th and sometimes 60th birthday.

Although cysteamine treatment has substantially improved the prognosis of cystinosis patients, the drug offers no cure of the disease. Therefore continued efforts are undertaken to develop more definitive therapies. In a mouse model of cystinosis, allogeneic hematopoietic stem cell (HSC) transplantation significantly reduced cystine tissue content in all tested organs (by 70% in the kidney) and resulted in long-term preservation of kidney function [191, 192]. HSCs differentiate into tissue-resident macrophages forming tunneling nanotubes transferring cystinosin-bearing lysosomes into CTNS-deficient cells, even crossing tubular basement membrane. More recently, autologous HSC transplantation after *ex vivo* lentiviral *CTNS* gene transduction and subsequent injection has proven to be efficient in cystinosis mice [193]. Allogenic full HLA-matched HSC transplantation in one cystinosis patient resulted a temporary stabilization of the kidney function and demonstrated *de novo* expression of wild type cystinosin in different tissues of the recipient. The procedure, however, was complicated by therapy-resistant graft-versus-host disease with fatal outcome [194]. A clinical trial evaluating the safety and efficiency of autologous HSC transplantation after *ex vivo* gene therapy in humans is ongoing (https://clinicaltrials.gov/ct2/show/NCT03897361).

Novel pharmacological therapies targeting cystine accumulation and/or other altered pathways in cystinosis cells are currently at different stages of development and have been reviewed elsewehere [68]. It can be expected that during the next decade early diagnosis of cystinosis in pre-symptomatic patients via neonatal screening based on NGS and administration of novel thera-

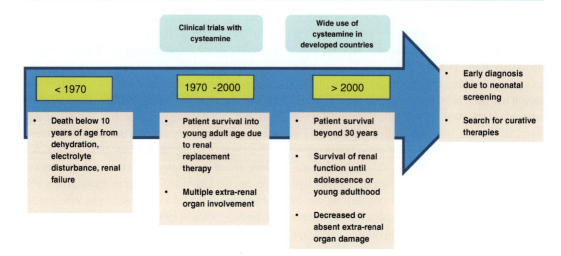

Fig. 30.9 Improved prognosis of nephropathic cystinosis. The overall prognosis of patients with cystinosis has substantially improved by the availability of renal replacement therapy allowing patients to survive into young adult age, and by wide use of cysteamine treatment prolonging renal function survival and protecting extra-renal organs. Early diagnosis in pre-symptomatic patients and the administration of novel therapies will further improve patients' survival and quality of life

pies will further improve patients survival and quality of life (Fig. 30.9).

References

1. Town M, Jean G, Cherqui S, Attard M, Forestier L, Whitmore SA, Callen DF, Gribouval O, Broyer M, Bates GP, Van't Hoff W, Antignac C. A novel gene encoding an integral membrane protein is mutated in nephropathic cystinosis. Nat Genet. 1998;18:319–24.
2. Gahl WA, Thoene JG, Schneider JA. Cystinosis. N Engl J Med. 2002;347:111–21.
3. Abderhalden E. Familiäre cystindiathese. Z Physiol Chem. 1903;38:557–61.
4. De Toni G. Remarks on the relations between renal rickets (renal dwarfism) and renal diabetes. Acta Paediatr. 1933;16:479–84.
5. Debre R, Royer P. Two cases of cystinosis with gluco-phosphate-amino renal diabetes. Arch Fr Pediatr. 1954;11:673–95.
6. Fanconi G, Bickel H. Die chronische aminoaciduria (aminosaurediabetes oder nephrotisch-glukosurischer zwergwuchs) bei der glykogenose und der cystinkrankheit. Helv Pediatr Acta. 1949;4:359–96.
7. Schneider JA, Bradley K, Seegmiller JE. Increased cystine in leukocytes from individuals homozygous and heterozygous for cystinosis. Science. 1967a;157:1321–2.
8. Schneider JA, Rosenbloom FM, Bradley KH, Seegmiller JE. Increased free-cystine content of fibroblasts cultured from patients with cystinosis. Biochem Biophys Res Commun. 1967b;29:527–31.
9. Jonas AJ, Smith ML, Schneider JA. ATP-dependent lysosomal cystine efflux is defective in cystinosis. J Biol Chem. 1982;257:13185–8.
10. Gahl WA, Bashan N, Tietze F, Bernardini I, Schulman JD. Cystine transport is defective in isolated leukocyte lysosomes from patients with cystinosis. Science. 1982a;217:1263–5.
11. Malekzadeh MH, Neustein HB, Schneider JA, Pennisi AJ, Ettenger RB, Uittenbogaart CH, Kogut MD, Fine RH. Cadaver renal transplantation in children with cystinosis. Am J Med. 1977;63:525–33.
12. Gahl WA, Reed GF, Thoene JG, Schulman JD, Rizzo WB, Jonas AJ, Denman DW, Schlesselman JJ, Corden BJ, Schneider JA. Cysteamine therapy for children with nephropathic cystinosis. N Engl J Med. 1987;316:971–7.
13. Veys KR, Elmonem MA, Arcolino FO, van den Heuvel L, Levtchenko E. Nephropathic cystinosis: an update. Curr Opin Pediatr. 2017;29(2):168–78.
14. Bois E, Feingold J, Frenay P, Briard ML. Infantile cystinosis in France: genetics, incidence, geographic distribution. J Med Genet. 1976;13:434–8.
15. Manz F, Gretz N. Cystinosis in the Federal Republic of Germany. Coordination and analysis of the data. J Inherit Metab Dis. 1985;8:2–4.
16. David D, Princiero Berlingerio S, Elmonem MA, Oliveira Arcolino F, Soliman N, van den Heuvel B, Gijsbers R, Levtchenko E. Molecular basis of cystinosis: geographic distribution, functional con-

16. sequences of mutations in the CTNS gene, and potential for repair Nephron. 2019;141(2):133–46. https://doi.org/10.1159/000495270.
17. Bertholet-Thomas A, Berthiller J, Tasic V, Kassai B, Otukesh H, Greco M, Ehrich J, de Paula Bernardes R, Deschênes G, Hulton SA, Fischbach M, Soulami K, Saeed B, Valavi E, Cobenas CJ, Hacihamdioglu B, Weiler G, Cochat P, Bacchetta J. Worldwide view of nephropathic cystinosis: results from a survey from 30 countries. BMC Nephrol. 2017;18(1):210.
18. Middleton R, Bradbury M, Webb N, O'Donoghue D, Van't Hoff W. Cystinosis. A clinicopathological conference. "From toddlers to twenties and beyond" adult-paediatric nephrology interface meeting, Manchester 2001. Nephrol Dial Transplant. 2003;18:2492–5.
19. Wühl E, van Stralen KJ, Wanner C, Ariceta G, Heaf JG, Bjerre AK, Palsson R, Duneau G, Hoitsma AJ, Ravani P. Renal replacement therapy for rare diseases affecting the kidney: an analysis of the ERA–EDTA registry. Nephrol Dial Transplant. 2014;29(suppl_4):iv1–8.
20. Wilmer MJ, Emma F, Levtchenko EN. The pathogenesis of cystinosis: mechanisms beyond cystine accumulation. Am J Physiol Renal Physiol. 2010;299:F905–16.
21. Cherqui S, Kalatzis V, Trugnan G, Antignac C. The targeting of cystinosin to the lysosomal membrane requires a tyrosine-based signal and a novel sorting motif. J Biol Chem. 2001;276:13314–21.
22. Attard M, Jean G, Forestier L, Cherqui S, Van't Hoff W, Broyer M, Antignac C, Town M. Severity of phenotype in cystinosis varies with mutations in the CTNS gene: predicted effect on the model of cystinosin. Hum Mol Genet. 1999;8:2507–14.
23. Anikster Y, Lucero C, Guo J, Huizing M, Shotelersuk V, Bernardini I, McDowell G, Iwata F, Kaiser-Kupfer MI, Jaffe R, Thoene J, Schneider JA, Gahl WA. Ocular nonnephropathic cystinosis: clinical, biochemical, and molecular correlations. Pediatr Res. 2000;47:17–23.
24. Shotelersuk V, Larson D, Anikster Y, McDowell G, Lemons R, Bernardini I, Guo J, Thoene J, Gahl WA. CTNS mutations in an American-based population of cystinosis patients. Am J Hum Genet. 1998;63:1352–62.
25. Phornphutkul C, Anikster Y, Huizing M, Braun P, Brodie C, Chou JY, Gahl WA. The promoter of a lysosomal membrane transporter gene, CTNS, binds Sp-1, shares sequences with the promoter of an adjacent gene, CARKL, and causes cystinosis if mutated in a critical region. Am J Hum Genet. 2001;69:712–21.
26. Wamelink MM, Struys EA, Jansen EE, Levtchenko EN, Zijlstra FS, Engelke U, Blom HJ, Jakobs C, Wevers RA. Sedoheptulokinase deficiency due to a 57-kb deletion in cystinosis patients causes urinary accumulation of sedoheptulose: elucidation of the CARKL gene. Hum Mutat. 2008;29:532–6.
27. Buntinx L, Voets T, Morlion B, Vangeel L, Janssen M, Cornelissen E, Vriens J, de Hoon J, Levtchenko E. TRPV1 dysfunction in cystinosis patients harboring the homozygous 57 kb deletion. Sci Rep. 2016;6:35395.
28. Wamelink MM, Struys EA, Jansen EE, Blom HJ, Vilboux T, Gahl WA, Komhoff M, Jakobs C, Levtchenko EN. Elevated concentrations of sedoheptulose in bloodspots of patients with cystinosis caused by the 57-kb deletion: implications for diagnostics and neonatal screening. Mol Genet Metab. 2011;102:339–42.
29. Bendavid A, Kleta R, Long R, Ouspenskaia M, Haddad BR, Muenke M, Gahl WA. FISH analysis of the common 57-kb deletion in cystinosis. Mol Genet Metab. 2004;81:174–5.
30. Heil SG, Levtchenko E, Monnens LA, Trijbels FJ, Van der Put NM, Blom HJ. The molecular basis of Dutch infantile nephropathic cystinosis. Nephron. 2001;89:50–5.
31. Kiehntopf M, Varga RE, Koch HG, Beetz C. A homemade MLPA assay detects known CTNS mutations and identifies a novel deletion in a previously unresolved cystinosis family. Gene. 2012;495:89–92.
32. Kiehntopf M, Schickel J, Gonne B, Koch HG, Superti-Furga A, Steinmann B, Deufel T, Harms E. Analysis of the CTNS gene in patients of German and Swiss origin with nephropathic cystinosis. Hum Mutat. 2002;20:237.
33. Lebre AS, Moriniere V, Dunand O, Bensman A, Morichon-Delvallez N, Antignac C. Maternal uniparental heterodisomy of chromosome 17 in a patient with nephropathic cystinosis. Eur J Hum Genet. 2009;17:1019–23.
34. Taranta A, Wilmer MJ, van den Heuvel LP, Bencivenga P, Bellomo F, Levtchenko EN, Emma F. Analysis of CTNS gene transcripts in nephropathic cystinosis. Pediatr Nephrol. 2010;25:1263–7.
35. Emma F, Hoff WV, Hohenfellner K, Topaloglu R, Greco M, Ariceta G, Bettini C, Bockenhauer D, Veys K, Pape L, Hulton S, Collin S, Ozaltin F, Servais A, Deschênes G, Novo R, Bertholet-Thomas A, Oh J, Cornelissen E, Janssen M, Haffner D, Ravà L, Antignac C, Devuyst O, Niaudet P, Levtchenko E. An international cohort study spanning five decades assessed outcomes of nephropathic cystinosis. Kidney Int. 2021;100(5):1112–23. S0085-2538(21)00648-7. https://doi.org/10.1016/j.kint.2021.06.019.
36. Brodin-Sartorius A, Tete MJ, Niaudet P, Antignac C, Guest G, Ottolenghi C, Charbit M, Moyse D, Legendre C, Lesavre P, Cochat P, Servais A. Cysteamine therapy delays the progression of nephropathic cystinosis in late adolescents and adults. Kidney Int. 2012a;81:179–89.
37. Brodin-Sartorius A, Tête MJ, Niaudet P, Antignac C, Guest G, Ottolenghi C, Charbit M, Moyse D, Legendre C, Lesavre P, Cochat P, Servais A. Cysteamine therapy delays the progression of

excretion pattern and renal expression of megalin and cubilin in nephropathic cystinosis. Am J Kidney Dis. 2008b;51:893–903.

86. Moreno JA, Moreno S, Rubio-Navarro A, Gomez-Guerrero C, Ortiz A, Egido J. Role of chemokines in proteinuric kidney disorders. Expert Rev Mol Med. 2014;16:e3.

87. Prencipe G, Caiello I, Cherqui S, Whisenant T, Petrini S, Emma F, De BF. Inflammasome activation by cystine crystals: implications for the pathogenesis of cystinosis. J Am Soc Nephrol. 2014;25(6):1163–9.

88. Lobry T, Miller R, Nevo N, Rocca CJ, Zhang J, Catz SD, Moore F, Thomas L, Pouly D, Bailleux A, Guerrera IC, Gubler MC, Cheung WW, Mak RH, Montier T, Antignac C, Cherqui S. Interaction between galectin-3 and cystinosin uncovers a pathogenic role of inflammation in kidney involvement of cystinosis. Kidney Int. 2019;96(2):350–62. https://doi.org/10.1016/j.kint.2019.01.029.

89. Levtchenko E, Monnens L. Development of Fanconi syndrome during infancy in a patient with cystinosis. Acta Paediatr. 2006;95:379–80.

90. Broyer M, Guillot M, Gubler MC, Habib R. Infantile cystinosis: a reappraisal of early and late symptoms. Adv Nephrol Necker Hosp. 1981;10:137–66.

91. Schneider JA, Katz B, Melles RB. Update on nephropathic cystinosis. Pediatr Nephrol. 1990;4:645–53.

92. Saleem MA, Milford DV, Alton H, Chapman S, Winterborn MH. Hypercalciuria and ultrasound abnormalities in children with cystinosis. Pediatr Nephrol. 1995;9:45–7.

93. Theodoropoulos DS, Shawker TH, Heinrichs C, Gahl WA. Medullary nephrocalcinosis in nephropathic cystinosis. Pediatr Nephrol. 1995;9:412–8.

94. Gretz N, Manz F, Augustin R, Barrat TM, Bender-Gotze C, Brandis M, Bremer HJ, Brodehl J, Broyer M, Bulla M, Callis L, Chantler C, Diekmann L, Dillon MJ, Egli F, Ehrich JH, Endres W, Fanconi A, Feldhoff C, Geisert J, Gekle D, Gescholl-Bauer B, Grote K, Gruttner R, Hagge W, Haycock CB, Hennemann H, Klare B, Leupold D, Lohr H, Michalk D, Oliveira A, Ott F, Pistor K, Rau J, Scharer K, Schindera F, Schmidt H, Schulte-Wissermann H, Verrier-Jones K, Weber HP, Willenbockel U, Wolf H. Survival time in cystinosis. A collaborative study. Proc Eur Dial Transplant Assoc. 1983;19:582–9.

95. Manz F, Gretz N. Progression of chronic renal failure in a historical group of patients with nephropathic cystinosis. European Collaborative Study on Cystinosis. Pediatr Nephrol. 1994;8:466–71.

96. Van Stralen KJ, Emma F, Jager KJ, Verrina E, Schaefer F, Laube GF, Lewis MA, Levtchenko EN. Improvement in the renal prognosis in nephropathic cystinosis. Clin J Am Soc Nephrol. 2011;6:2485–91.

97. Gubler MC, Lacoste SM, Broyer M. The pathology of the kidney in cystinosis. In: Broyer M, editor. Cystinosis. 1st ed. Paris: Elsevier; 1999. p. 42–8.

98. Lusco MA, Najafian B, Alpers CE, Fogo AB. AJKD atlas of renal pathology: cystinosis. Am J Kidney Dis. 2017;70(6):e23–4. https://doi.org/10.1053/j.ajkd.2017.10.002.

99. Spear GS, Gubler MC, Habib R, Broyer M. Dark cells of cystinosis: occurrence in renal allografts. Hum Pathol. 1989;20:472–6.

100. Dharnidharka VR, Fiorina P, Harmon WE. Kidney transplantation in children. N Engl J Med. 2014;371(6):549–58.

101. Kashtan CE, McEnery PT, Tejani A, Stablein DM. Renal allograft survival according to primary diagnosis: a report of the North American Pediatric Renal Transplant Cooperative Study. Pediatr Nephrol. 1995;9:679–84.

102. Spicer RA, Clayton PA, McTaggart SJ, Zhang GY, Alexander SI. Patient and graft survival following kidney transplantation in recipients with cystinosis: a cohort study. Am J Kidney Dis. 2015;65(1):172–3. https://doi.org/10.1053/j.ajkd.2014.07.020. Epub 2014 Sep 18.

103. Kizilbash SJ, Snyder J, Vock DM, Chavers BM. Trends in kidney transplant outcomes in children and young adults with cystinosis. Pediatr Transplant. 2019;23(8):e13572.

104. Cohen C, Charbit M, Chadefaux-Vekemans B, Giral M, Garrigue V, Kessler M, Antoine C, Snanoudj R, Niaudet P, Kreis H, Legendre C, Servais A. Excellent long-term outcome of renal transplantation in cystinosis patients. Orphanet J Rare Dis. 2015;10:90. https://doi.org/10.1186/s13023-015-0307-9.

105. Tsilou E, Zhou M, Gahl W, Sieving PC, Chan CC. Ophthalmic manifestations and histopathology of infantile nephropathic cystinosis: report of a case and review of the literature. Surv Ophthalmol. 2007;52:97–105.

106. Bishop R. Ocular complications of infantile nephropathic cystinosis. J Pediatr. 2017;183S:S19–21. https://doi.org/10.1016/j.jpeds.2016.12.055.

107. Kasimer RN, Langman CB. Adult complications of nephropathic cystinosis: a systematic review. Pediatr Nephrol. 2021;36:223–36.

108. Tsilou ET, Rubin BI, Reed GF, Iwata F, Gahl W, Kaiser-Kupfer MI. Age-related prevalence of anterior segment complications in patients with infantile nephropathic cystinosis. Cornea. 2002;21:173–6.

109. Wuhl E, Haffner D, Offner G, Broyer M, Van't Hoff W, Mehls O. Long-term treatment with growth hormone in short children with nephropathic cystinosis. J Pediatr. 2001;138:880–7.

110. Broyer M, Tete MJ, Gubler MC. Late symptoms in infantile cystinosis. Pediatr Nephrol. 1987;1:519–24.

111. van't Hoff WG, Gretz N. The treatment of cystinosis with cysteamine and phosphocysteamine in the United Kingdom and Eire. Pediatr Nephrol. 1995;9:685–9.

112. Greco M, Brugnara M, Zaffanello M, Taranta A, Pastore A, Emma F. Long-term outcome of nephropathic cystinosis: a 20-year single-center experience. Pediatr Nephrol. 2010;25:2459–67.

113. Besouw MT, Van Dyck M, Francois I, Van Hoyweghen E, Levtchenko EN. Detailed studies

114. Lucky AW, Howley PM, Megyesi K, Spielberg SP, Schulman JD. Endocrine studies in cystinosis: compensated primary hypothyroidism. J Pediatr. 1977;91(2):204–10. https://doi.org/10.1016/s0022-3476(77)80813-5.

115. Fivush B, Flick JA, Gahl WA. Pancreatic exocrine insufficiency in a patient with nephropathic cystinosis. J Pediatr. 1988;112(1):49–51. https://doi.org/10.1016/s0022-3476(88)80119-7.

116. Winkler L, Offner G, Krull F, Brodehl J. Growth and pubertal development in nephropathic cystinosis. Eur J Pediatr. 1993;152:244–9.

117. Besouw MT, Kremer JA, Janssen MC, Levtchenko EN. Fertility status in male cystinosis patients treated with cysteamine. Fertil Steril. 2010;93:1880–3.

118. Reda A, Veys K, Kadam P, Taranta A, Rega LR, Goffredo BM, Camps C, Besouw M, Cyr D, Albersen M, Spiessens C, de Wever L, Hamer R, Janssen MCH, D'Hauwers K, Wetzels A, Monnens L, van den Heuvel L, Goossens E, Levtchenko E. Human and animal fertility studies in cystinosis reveal signs of obstructive azoospermia, an altered blood-testis barrier and a subtherapeutic effect of cysteamine in testis. J Inherit Metab Dis. 2021;44(6):1393–408. https://doi.org/10.1002/jimd.12434.

119. Reiss RE, Kuwabara T, Smith ML, Gahl WA. Successful pregnancy despite placental cystine crystals in a woman with nephropathic cystinosis. N Engl J Med. 1988;319:223–6.

120. Blakey H, Proudfoot-Jones J, Knox E. Graham Lipkin Pregnancy in women with cystinosis. Clin Kidney J. 2019;12(6):855–8. https://doi.org/10.1093/ckj/sfz047. eCollection 2019 Dec.

121. Central nervous system complications in cystinosis. Broyer M, Tete MJ. In Cystinosis. Ed. M. Broyer. Elsevier. Amsterdam, Lausanne, New York, Oxford, Paris, Shannon, Tokyo. p 75–80.

122. Theodoropoulos DS, Krasnewich D, Kaiser-Kupfer MI, Gahl WA. Classic nephropathic cystinosis as an adult disease. JAMA. 1993;270:2200–4.

123. Gahl WA, Schneider JA, Thoene JG, Chesney R. Course of nephropathic cystinosis after age 10 years. J Pediatr. 1986;109(4):605–8. https://doi.org/10.1016/s0022-3476(86)80221-9.

124. Broyer M, Tête MJ, Guest G, Berthélémé JP, Labrousse F, Poisson M. Clinical polymorphism of cystinosis encephalopathy. Results of treatment with cysteamine. J Inherit Metab Dis. 1996b;19(1):65–75. https://doi.org/10.1007/BF01799350.

125. Fink JK, Brouwers P, Barton N, Malekzadeh MH, Sato S, Hill S, Cohen WE, Fivush B, Gahl WA. Neurologic complications in long-standing nephropathic cystinosis. Arch Neurol. 1989;46(5):543–8. https://doi.org/10.1001/archneur.1989.00520410077027.

126. Trauner DA, Williams J, Ballantyne AO, Spilkin AM, Crowhurst J, Hesselink J. Neurological impairment in nephropathic cystinosis: motor coordination deficits. Pediatr Nephrol. 2010;25:2061–6.

127. Trauner DA, Chase C, Scheller J, Katz B, Schneider JA. Neurologic and cognitive deficits in children with cystinosis. J Pediatr. 1988;112(6):912–4. https://doi.org/10.1016/s0022-3476(88)80214-2.

128. Viltz L, Trauner DA. Effect of age at treatment on cognitive performance in patients with cystinosis. J Pediatr. 2013;163(2):489–92. https://doi.org/10.1016/j.jpeds.2013.01.027.

129. Servais A, Saitovitch A, Hummel A, Boisgontier J, Scemla A, Sberro-Soussan R, Snanoudj R, Lemaitre H, Legendre C, Pontoizeau C, Antignac C, Anglicheau D, Funalot B, Boddaert N. Central nervous system complications in adult cystinosis patients. J Inherit Metab Dis. 2020;43(2):348–56. https://doi.org/10.1002/jimd.12164.

130. Dogulu CF, Tsilou E, Rubin B, Fitzgibbon EJ, Kaiser-Kupper MI, Rennert OM, Gahl WA. Idiopathic intracranial hypertension in cystinosis. J Pediatr. 2004;145:673–8.

131. Ehrich JH, Stoeppler L, Offner G, Brodehl J. Evidence for cerebral involvement in nephropathic cystinosis. Neuropadiatrie. 1979;10(2):128–37. https://doi.org/10.1055/s-0028-1085319.

132. Nichols SL, Press GA, Schneider JA, Trauner DA. Cortical atrophy and cognitive performance in infantile nephropathic cystinosis. Pediatr Neurol. 1990;6:379–81.

133. Gahl WA, Balog JZ, Kleta R. Nephropathic cystinosis in adults: natural history and effects of oral cysteamine therapy. Ann Intern Med. 2007;147:242–50.

134. Bava S, Theilmann RJ, Sach M, May SJ, Frank LR, Hesselink JR, Vu D, Trauner DA. Developmental changes in cerebral white matter microstructure in a disorder of lysosomal storage. Cortex. 2010;46:206–16.

135. Vester U, Schubert M, Offner G, Brodehl J. Distal myopathy in nephropathic cystinosis. Pediatr Nephrol. 2000;14(1):36–8. https://doi.org/10.1007/s004670050009.

136. Anikster Y, Lacbawan F, Brantly M, Gochuico BL, Avila NA, Travis W, Gahl WA. Pulmonary dysfunction in adults with nephropathic cystinosis. Chest. 2001;119:394–401.

137. Sonies BC, Ekman EF, Andersson HC, Adamson MD, Kaler SG, Markello TC, Gahl WA. Swallowing dysfunction in nephropathic cystinosis. N Engl J Med. 1990;323(9):565–70. https://doi.org/10.1056/NEJM199008303230903.

138. van Rijssel AE, Knuijt S, Veys K, Levtchenko EN, Janssen MCH. Swallowing dysfunction in patients with nephropathic cystinosis. Mol Genet Metab. 2019;126(4):413–5. https://doi.org/10.1016/j.ymgme.2019.01.011.

139. Scarvie KM, Ballantyne AO, Trauner DA. Visuomotor performance in children with infantile nephropathic cystinosis. Percept Mot

140. Dohil R, Carrigg A, Newbury R. A potential new method to estimate tissue cystine content in nephropathic cystinosis. J Pediatr. 2012;161:531–5.

141. Dohil R, Newbury RO, Sellers ZM, Deutsch R, Schneider JA. The evaluation and treatment of gastrointestinal disease in children with cystinosis receiving cysteamine. J Pediatr. 2003;143:224–30.

142. Klenn PJ, Rubin R. Hepatic fibrosis associated with hereditary cystinosis: a novel form of noncirrhotic portal hypertension. Mod Pathol. 1994;7:879–82.

143. Cornelis T, Claes K, Gillard P, Nijs E, Roskams T, Lombaerts R, Nevens F, Cassiman D. Cholestatic liver disease in long-term infantile nephropathic cystinosis. J Gastroenterol Hepatol. 2008;23:e428–31.

144. Hohenfellner K, Rauch F, Ariceta G, Awan A, Bacchetta J, Bergmann C, Bechtold S, Cassidy N, Deschenes G, Elenberg E, Gahl WA, Greil O, Harms E, Herzig N, Hoppe B, Koeppl C, Lewis MA, Levtchenko E, Nesterova G, Santos F, Schlingmann KP, Servais A, Soliman NA, Steidle G, Sweeney C, Treikauskas U, Topaloglu R, Tsygin A, Veys K, Vigier RV, Zustin J, Haffner D. Management of bone disease in cystinosis: statement from an international conference. J Inherit Metab Dis. 2019a;42(5):1019–29. https://doi.org/10.1002/jimd.12134.

145. Machuca-Gayet I, Quinaux T, Bertholet-Thomas A, Gaillard S, Claramunt-Taberner D, Acquaviva-Bourdain C, Bacchetta J. Bone disease in nephropathic cystinosis: beyond renal osteodystrophy. Int J Mol Sci. 2020;21(9):3109. https://doi.org/10.3390/ijms21093109.

146. Florenzano P, Ferreira C, Nesterova G, Roberts MS, Tella SH, de Castro LF, Brown SM, Whitaker A, Pereira RC, Bulas D, Gafni RI, Salusky IB, Gahl WA, Collins MT. Skeletal consequences of nephropathic cystinosis. J Bone Miner Res. 2018;33(10):1870–80. https://doi.org/10.1002/jbmr.3522.

147. Bertholet-Thomas A, Claramunt-Taberner D, Gaillard S, Deschênes G, Sornay-Rendu E, Szulc P, Cohen-Solal M, Pelletier S, Carlier MC, Cochat P, Bacchetta J. Teenagers and young adults with nephropathic cystinosis display significant bone disease and cortical impairment. Pediatr Nephrol. 2018;33(7):1165–72. https://doi.org/10.1007/s00467-018-3902-x.

148. Bacchetta J, Greco M, Bertholet-Thomas A, Nobili F, Zustin J, Cochat P, Emma F, Boivin G. Skeletal implications and management of cystinosis: three case reports and literature review. Bonekey Rep. 2016;5:828. https://doi.org/10.1038/bonekey.2016.55. eCollection 2016.

149. Chiaverini C, Sillard L, Flori E, Ito S, Briganti S, Wakamatsu K, Fontas E, Berard E, Cailliez M, Cochat P, Foulard M, Guest G, Niaudet P, Picardo M, Bernard FX, Antignac C, Ortonne JP, Ballotti R. Cystinosin is a melanosomal protein that regulates melanin synthesis. FASEB J. 2012;26:3779–89.

150. Guillet G, Sassolas B, Fromentoux S, Gobin E, Leroy JP. Skin storage of cystine and premature skin ageing in cystinosis. Lancet. 1998;352:1444–5.

151. Veys KRP, Elmonem MA, Dhaenens F, Van Dyck M, Janssen MMCH, Cornelissen EAM, Hohenfellner K, Reda A, Quatresooz P, van den Heuvel B, Boone MALM, Levtchenko E. Enhanced intrinsic skin aging in nephropathic cystinosis assessed by high-definition optical coherence tomography. J Invest Dermatol. 2019;139(10):2242–2245.e5. https://doi.org/10.1016/j.jid.2019.03.1153.

152. Abdulsalam AH, Khamis MH, Bain BJ. Diagnosis of cystinosis from a bone marrow aspirate. Am J Hematol. 2013;88:151.

153. Monier L, Mauvieux L. Cystine crystals in bone marrow aspirate. Blood. 2015;126(12):1515. https://doi.org/10.1182/blood-2015-07-656298.

154. Nesterova G, Gahl W. Nephropathic cystinosis: late complications of a multisystemic disease. Pediatr Nephrol. 2008;23:863–78.

155. Geelen JM, Monnens LA, Levtchenko EN. Follow-up and treatment of adults with cystinosis in the Netherlands. Nephrol Dial Transplant. 2002;17:1766–70.

156. Kleta R, Kaskel F, Dohil R, Goodyer P, Guay-Woodford LM, Harms E, Ingelfinger JR, Koch VH, Langman CB, Leonard MB, Mannon RB, Sarwal M, Schneider JA, Skovby F, Sonies BC, Thoene JG, Trauner DA, Gahl WA. First NIH/Office of Rare Diseases Conference on Cystinosis: past, present, and future. Pediatr Nephrol. 2005;20:452–4.

157. Hauglustaine D, Corbeel L, van Damme B, Serrus M, Michielsen P. Glomerulonephritis in late-onset cystinosis. Report of two cases and review of the literature. Clin Nephrol. 1976;6:529–36.

158. Langman CB, Moore ES, Thoene JG, Schneider JA. Renal failure in a sibship with late-onset cystinosis. J Pediatr. 1985;107:755–6.

159. Schneider JA, Wong V, Bradley K, Seegmiller JE. Biochemical comparisons of the adult and childhood forms of cystinosis. N Engl J Med. 1968;279:1253–7.

160. Smolin LA, Clark KF, Schneider JA. An improved method for heterozygote detection of cystinosis, using polymorphonuclear leukocytes. Am J Hum Genet. 1987;41:266–75.

161. Levtchenko E, de Graaf-Hess A, Wilmer M, van den Heuvel L, Monnens L, Blom H. Comparison of cystine determination in mixed leukocytes vs polymorphonuclear leukocytes for diagnosis of cystinosis and monitoring of cysteamine therapy. Clin Chem. 2004;50:1686–8.

162. Wilmer MJ, Schoeber JP, van den Heuvel LP, Levtchenko EN. Cystinosis: practical tools for diagnosis and treatment. Pediatr Nephrol. 2011;26:205–15.

163. Hohenfellner K, Bergmann C, Fleige T, Janzen N, Burggraf S, Olgemöller B, Gahl WA, Czibere L, Froschauer S, Röschinger W, Vill K, Harms E, Nennstiel U. Molecular based newborn screen-

ing in Germany: follow-up for cystinosis. Mol Genet Metab Rep. 2019b;21:100514. https://doi.org/10.1016/j.ymgmr.2019.100514.

164. Fleige T, Burggraf S, Czibere L, Häring J, Glück B, Keitel LM, Landt O, Harms E, Hohenfellner K, Durner J, Röschinger W, Becker M. Next generation sequencing as second-tier test in high-throughput newborn screening for nephropathic cystinosis. Eur J Hum Genet. 2020;28(2):193–201. https://doi.org/10.1038/s41431-019-0521-3.

165. Elenberg E, Norling LL, Kleinman RE, Ingelfinger JR. Feeding problems in cystinosis. Pediatr Nephrol. 1998;12:365–70.

166. Dohil R, Fidler M, Barshop B, Newbury R, Sellers Z, Deutsch R, Schneider J. Esomeprazole therapy for gastric acid hypersecretion in children with cystinosis. Pediatr Nephrol. 2005;20:1786–93.

167. Gahl WA, Bernardini I, Dalakas M, Rizzo WB, Harper GS, Hoeg JM, Hurko O, Bernar J. Oral carnitine therapy in children with cystinosis and renal Fanconi syndrome. J Clin Invest. 1988b;81:549–60.

168. Gahl WA, Bernardini IM, Dalakas MC, Markello TC, Krasnewich DM, Charnas LR. Muscle carnitine repletion by long-term carnitine supplementation in nephropathic cystinosis. Pediatr Res. 1993;34:115–9.

169. Besouw M, Cornelissen EAM, Cassiman D, Kluijtmans LA, van den Heuvel LP, Levtchenko E. Carnitine profile and effect of suppletion in children with renal Fanconi syndrome due to cystinosis. JIMD Rep. 2014;16:25–30.

170. Haycock GB, Al-Dahhan J, Mak RH, Chantler C. Effect of indomethacin on clinical progress and renal function in cystinosis. Arch Dis Child. 1982;57:934–9.

171. Levtchenko E, Blom H, Wilmer M, van den Heuvel L, Monnens L. ACE inhibitorenalapril diminishes albuminuria in patients with cystinosis. Clin Nephrol. 2003;60:386–9.

172. Thoene JG, Oshima RG, Crawhall JC, Olson DL, Schneider JA. Cystinosis. Intracellular cystine depletion by aminothiols in vitro and in vivo. J Clin Invest. 1976;58:180–9.

173. Besouw M, Masereeuw R, van den Heuvel L, Levtchenko E. Cysteamine: an old drug with new potential. Drug Discov Today. 2013a;18:785–92.

174. Kleta R, Bernardini I, Ueda M, Varade WS, Phornphutkul C, Krasnewich D, Gahl WA. Long-term follow-up of well-treated nephropathic cystinosis patients. J Pediatr. 2004;145:555–60.

175. Sonies BC, Almajid P, Kleta R, Bernardini I, Gahl WA. Swallowing dysfunction in 101 patients with nephropathic cystinosis: benefit of long-term cysteamine therapy. Medicine (Baltimore). 2005;84:137–46.

176. Kimonis VE, Troendle J, Rose SR, Yang ML, Markello TC, Gahl WA. Effects of early cysteamine therapy on thyroid function and growth in nephropathic cystinosis. J Clin Endocrinol Metab. 1995;80:3257–61.

177. Tsilou ET, Rubin BI, Reed G, Caruso RC, Iwata F, Balog J, Gahl WA, Kaiser-Kupfer MI. Nephropathic cystinosis: posterior segment manifestations and effects of cysteamine therapy. Ophthalmology. 2006;113:1002–9.

178. Levtchenko EN, van Dael CM, de Graaf-Hess AC, Wilmer MJ, van den Heuvel LP, Monnens LA, Blom HJ. Strict cysteamine dose regimen is required to prevent nocturnal cystine accumulation in cystinosis. Pediatr Nephrol. 2006b;21:110–3.

179. Langman CB, Greenbaum LA, Sarwal M, Grimm P, Niaudet P, Deschenes G, Cornelissen E, Morin D, Cochat P, Matossian D, Gaillard S, Bagger MJ, Rioux P. A randomized controlled crossover trial with delayed-release cysteamine bitartrate in nephropathic cystinosis: effectiveness on white blood cell cystine levels and comparison of safety. Clin J Am Soc Nephrol. 2012;7:1112–20.

180. Langman CB. Quality of life is improved and kidney function preserved in patients with nephropathic cystinosis treated for 2 years with delayed-release cysteamine bitartrate. J Pediatr. 2014;165(3):528–33.e1.

181. Gaillard S, Roche L, Lemoine S, Deschênes G, Morin D, Vianey-Saban C, Acquaviva-Bourdain C, Ranchin B, Bacchetta J, Kassai B, Nony P, Bodénan E, Laudy V, Rouges C, Zarrabian S, Subtil F, Mercier C, Cochat P, Bertholet-Thomas A. Adherence to cysteamine in nephropathic cystinosis: a unique electronic monitoring experience for a better understanding. A prospective cohort study: CrYSTobs. Pediatr Nephrol. 2021;36(3):581–9.

182. Besouw M, Blom H, Tangerman A, de Graaf-Hess A, Levtchenko E. The origin of halitosis in cystinotic patients due to cysteamine treatment. Mol Genet Metab. 2007;91:228–33.

183. Ariceta G, Lara E, Camacho JA, Oppenheimer F, Vara J, Santos F, Muñoz MA, Cantarell C, Gil Calvo M, Romero R, Valenciano B, García-Nieto V, Sanahuja MJ, Crespo J, Justa ML, Urisarri A, Bedoya R, Bueno A, Daza A, Bravo J, Llamas F, Jiménez Del Cerro LA. Cysteamine (Cystagon) adherence in patients with cystinosis in Spain: successful in children and a challenge in adolescents and adults. Nephrol Dial Transplant. 2015;30(3):475–80. https://doi.org/10.1093/ndt/gfu329.

184. Besouw MT, Bowker R, Dutertre JP, Emma F, Gahl WA, Greco M, Lilien MR, McKiernan J, Nobili F, Schneider JA, Skovby F, van den Heuvel LP, Van't Hoff WG, Levtchenko EN. Cysteamine toxicity in patients with cystinosis. J Pediatr. 2011;159:1004–11.

185. Besouw MT, Schneider J, Janssen MC, Greco M, Emma F, Cornelissen EA, Desmet K, Skovby F, Nobili F, Lilien MR, De PA, Malfait F, Symoens S, van den Heuvel LP, Levtchenko EN. Copper deficiency in patients with cystinosis with cysteamine toxicity. J Pediatr. 2013b;163:754–60.

186. Beckman DA, Mullin JJ, Assadi FK. Developmental toxicity of cysteamine in the rat: effects on embryofetal development. Teratology. 1998;58:96–102.
187. Haase M, Morgera S, Bamberg C, Halle H, Martini S, Dragun D, Neumayer HH, Budde K. Successful pregnancies in dialysis patients including those suffering from cystinosis and familial Mediterranean fever. J Nephrol. 2006;19:677–81.
188. Gahl WA, Kuehl EM, Iwata F, Lindblad A, Kaiser-Kupfer MI. Corneal crystals in nephropathic cystinosis: natural history and treatment with cysteamine eyedrops. Mol Genet Metab. 2000;71:100–20.
189. Labbe A, Baudouin C, Deschenes G, Loirat C, Charbit M, Guest G, Niaudet P. A new gel formulation of topical cysteamine for the treatment of corneal cystine crystals in cystinosis: the Cystadrops OCT-1 study. Mol Genet Metab. 2014;111:314–20.
190. Liang H, Labbé A, Baudouin C, Plisson C, Giordano V. Long-term follow-up of cystinosis patients treated with 0.55% cysteamine hydrochloride. Br J Ophthalmol. 2021;105(5):608–13. https://doi.org/10.1136/bjophthalmol-2020-316450.
191. Syres K, Harrison F, Tadlock M, Jester JV, Simpson J, Roy S, Salomon DR, Cherqui S. Successful treatment of the murine model of cystinosis using bone marrow cell transplantation. Blood. 2009;114:2542–52.
192. Yeagy BA, Harrison F, Gubler MC, Koziol JA, Salomon DR, Cherqui S. Kidney preservation by bone marrow cell transplantation in hereditary nephropathy. Kidney Int. 2011;79:1198–206.
193. Harrison F, Yeagy BA, Rocca CJ, Kohn DB, Salomon DR, Cherqui S. Hematopoietic stem cell gene therapy for the multisystemic lysosomal storage disorder cystinosis. Mol Ther. 2013;21:433–44.
194. Elmonem MA, Veys K, Oliveira Arcolino F, Van Dyck M, Benedetti MC, Diomedi-Camassei F, De Hertogh G, van den Heuvel LP, Renard M, Levtchenko E. Allogeneic HSCT transfers wild-type cystinosin to nonhematological epithelial cells in cystinosis: first human report. Am J Transplant. 2018;18(11):2823–8. https://doi.org/10.1111/ajt.15029.

The Kidney in Sickle Cell Disease

31

Jeffrey Lebensburger and Cristin Kaspar

Sickle cell disease (SCD) is the most common inherited red blood cell disorder in the United States, impacting approximately 100,000 Americans and 1 in 365 African American births [1]. SCD is most prevalent in sub-Saharan Africa due to its protective inheritance against malaria. About 1000 children are born in Africa each day with SCD [2]. Some Hispanic and Indian populations have also been identified with up to 40% of residents having at least one sickle gene mutation.

The sickle cell mutation causes a hydrophobic valine to replace a hydrophilic glutamic acid in the sixth amino acid position of the β-globin protein. This mutation allows polymerization of hemoglobin S in the deoxyhemoglobin state. Two inherited β-globin sickle cell mutations result in the diagnosis of hemoglobin SS (HbSS). Different mutations in one of the β-globin subunits cause other forms of SCD. These include mutations that lead to no beta globin synthesis (β0 thalassemia) or minimal globin synthesis (β+ thalassemia) as well as other mutations, including hemoglobin C (HbC). The most prevalent, severe forms of SCD are HbSS and hemoglobin Sβ0 (HbSβ0) thalassemia; these genotypes are referred to as sickle cell anemia (SCA) and occur in about 70% of SCD patients. Other genotypes usually have less severe disease, and include hemoglobin Sβ+ (HbSβ+) thalassemia and hemoglobin SC (HbSC).

Sickle cell trait, which occurs in 1 in 13 African Americans, has been studied for its association with progressive kidney disease in adults, hematuria, renal papillary necrosis, and pyelonephritis during pregnancy. Sickle cell trait is associated with the rare cancer, renal medullary carcinoma. Patients with sickle cell trait do not have a significant pediatric clinical disease course due to the protective effect of one normal β-globin gene. Therefore, patients with sickle cell trait do not have SCD and, aside from counseling, do not receive follow-up care by a pediatric hematologist.

Hyposthenuria, Renal Papillary Necrosis, and Nocturnal Enuresis

Hyposthenuria

Pathophysiology: The development of hyposthenuria and renal papillary necrosis begin with sickling of the red blood cells in the vasa recta, leading to marked vascular changes. Necropsy studies have demonstrated almost complete destruction of the vasa recta and medullary

---

J. Lebensburger (✉) · C. Kaspar
The University of Alabama at Birmingham, Birmingham, AL, USA

Children's Hospital of Richmond at VCU, Pediatric Nephrology, Richmond, VA, USA
e-mail: jlebensburger@peds.uab.edu;
cristin.kaspar@vcuhealth.org

© The Author(s), under exclusive license to Springer Nature Switzerland AG 2023
F. Schaefer, L. A. Greenbaum (eds.), *Pediatric Kidney Disease*,
https://doi.org/10.1007/978-3-031-11665-0_31

capillaries in patients with SCA as compared to a reduced number of vasa recta in patients with sickle cell trait and HbSC disease [3]. These findings may be related to the impact of the hyperosmolar environment of the kidney on red cell rheology. In vitro models have demonstrated that sickle red blood cells exposed to even mildly hypertonic environments (sodium levels of 141 mEq/L) experience a delay in transit time, an increase in red cell rigidity and an increase in red cell adherence to vascular walls [4]. The renal medulla is an extremely hypertonic, hyperosmotic environment (800–1200 mOsm/kg) relative to the milder in vitro environments studied, which likely contributes to the more pronounced pathophysiologic changes seen in vivo. In addition, the renal medulla is a relatively hypoxic environment. Sickle red blood cells are stable in normoxia, but hemoglobin S begins to polymerize during the hypoxic state. Finally, acidic environments promote sickling of RBCs. Therefore, the combination of hypertonicity, hypoxia, and the acidotic environment in the renal medulla causes sickling of red blood cells within the vasa recta, with subsequent ischemic and reperfusion injury.

Epidemiology: A diminished urine concentrating ability is a well-established complication in patients with SCD [5–8]. The prevalence of hyposthenuria increases with disease severity (SCA > HbSC disease > sickle cell trait) [9, 10]. Urine concentration defects are first noted in infants and toddlers with SCA. In the baseline analysis of the BABY HUG study of children with SCA, only 30% of infants concentrated their urine >500 mOsm/kg, and only 13% of infants concentrated their urine >2 times their serum osmolality [11]. Of note, infants whose urine osmolality was >500 mOsm/kg after fluid deprivation had higher mean fetal hemoglobin concentrations, and the urine osmolality correlated with glomerular filtration rate (GFR).

Treatment: The BABY HUG study treated infants with 24 months of hydroxyurea, which increases fetal hemoglobin, versus placebo. While treatment with hydroxyurea for 24 months did not affect GFR, it did result in a significantly higher mean urine osmolality (495 mOsm/kg hydroxyurea vs. 452 mOsm/kg placebo) and a higher percentage of infants with a urine osmolality >500 mOsm/kg after fluid deprivation [12]. Murine models also suggest that a higher percentage of fetal hemoglobin and higher hemoglobin levels are associated with less severe concentrating defects [13]. Thus, hydroxyurea may decrease the urine concentrating defect early in life in SCA patients. Chronic transfusion therapy may also improve hyposthenuria [5, 6, 14]. However, preventing hyposthenuria is not an indication for initiating chronic transfusion; it is restricted to patients with increased risk of a poor central nervous system outcome or a very severe clinical course.

Interventions to prevent hyposthenuria should be initiated early in life. Red blood cell transfusions before the age of 10 years are effective in reversing hyposthenuria, but this reversibility was lost when initiated after the first decade [3, 5]. In a study of HbSC patients with a mean age of 11 years, hydroxyurea treatment for 12 months did not improve urinary concentrating ability [15]. This contrasts with the BABY HUG study and suggests loss of reversibility in older children.

Renal Papillary Necrosis

Another complication resulting from destruction of the renal vasculature is renal papillary necrosis. The pathophysiology is likely due to the renal medullary environment that promotes a higher level of sickling of red blood cells. It is believed that occlusion of the blood supply causes ischemia-induced necrosis of the renal medulla and papillae. This necrosis initiates subclinical and clinical hematuria. Pathology studies in SCD patients identified papillary necrosis in about one-third, most often located in the tips of the papillae [16]. Hematuria is secondary to changes in the permeability of the vasculature that allows red cell leakage into the collecting system.

Epidemiology: In radiologic studies, 30–75% of SCD patients have evidence of papillary necrosis [17–19]. Studies in Africa suggest 2% of patients will develop symptomatic renal papillary necrosis [20]. Risk factors for renal papillary necrosis are female sex, older age, more severe anemia and hypertension. Renal papillary necrosis is more common in the left kidney.

Diagnosis: While renal papillary necrosis is a common etiology of hematuria in pediatric patients with SCD, a standard diagnostic workup for hematuria should be performed on initial presentation. Since hemoglobinuria may cause a positive urine dipstick result, microscopic evaluation of the urine is necessary to confirm hematuria. SCD patients should also have a complete blood count (CBC) and creatinine to identify acute changes in hemoglobin and kidney function. Patients should be queried regarding other acute symptoms of SCD, prior history of hematuria, and medication use.

Several diagnostic imaging techniques can be considered in the initial evaluation of hematuria in a SCD patient. Ultrasound, which does not require contrast and is readily available, will identify hydronephrosis, and may provide evidence for a kidney stone as a cause of hematuria. A renal mass suggesting renal medullary carcinoma is more often identified in patients with sickle cell trait than SCA [21]. Findings on ultrasound suggestive of renal papillary necrosis include filling defects and necrosed papillae in cavities [22]. However, ultrasound is not the optimal imaging for identifying renal papillary necrosis. Most patients require a contrast evaluation, including intravenous urography, retrograde pyelography, or CT with contrast [23]. Intravenous urography and retrograde pyelography have less radiation exposure than CT [23]. Findings on a contrast study will often demonstrate filling defects of the renal calyx, including deformities of the renal papillae (hooks, spurs) and a blunted calyx [22].

Treatment: Some cases of hematuria due to papillary necrosis will be mild, painless, and self-resolve; other cases may require therapy. There are no guidelines addressing the efficacy of supportive care or when patients should be admitted to the hospital for care. Treatment may include intravenous (IV) fluids, analgesia, bedrest, alkalization, and low-dose aminocaproic acid [24, 25]. Patients who develop severe anemia require transfusion. Surgical interventions such as papillary tamponade, shunt placement, or nephrectomy are rarely indicated unless a pediatric patient is experiencing severe, persistent, life-threatening hemorrhage [16, 26].

The goal of fluid therapy is to ensure adequate hydration and to maintain high urine output. For mild cases, aggressive oral hydration as an outpatient is sufficient. For more severe cases, IV fluids can be prescribed in either outpatient day hospital settings or inpatient units. Patients can be administered fluids at maintenance to 1.5 times maintenance with or without a loop diuretic to further ensure adequate urinary output [27]. Since acidosis promotes sickling, adding base to the IV fluids to create a more alkaline environment to reduce sickling is theoretically appealing; however, there are no trials demonstrating benefit in SCD patients with papillary necrosis [28]. Bedrest may reduce the risk for dislodging of clots. Clinicians should closely monitor for the development of respiratory symptoms or fluid overload in patients receiving higher rates of IVF and/or suggested bedrest. Analgesia is used in patients with painful hematuria. If patients presenting with painless hematuria progress to painful hematuria, additional imaging may be required to evaluate new obstructive disease due to blood clots. Low dose aminocaproic acid at 20–50 mg/kg IV or po every 8 or 12 h has been used in severe cases as well as lower maintenance oral dosing [24, 25, 29]. SCD is a hypercoagulable state so close monitoring for new clot formation or ureteral obstruction should occur when using aminocaproic acid. Transfusion therapy can improve the anemia and reduce the concentration of sickle red blood cells, which should reduce sickling. In very severe cases, exchange transfusion may be used to significantly reduce the concentration of sickle cells, often to a sickle cell concentration of less than 30%. Reducing the sickle cell concentration may not treat the acute complication, but may allow more rapid recovery and prevent early recurrence of another renal injury.

Nocturnal Enuresis

Epidemiology: Primary nocturnal enuresis (PNE) is bedwetting that occurs in an individual who has never been dry at night, and is usually not associated with daytime wetting symptoms. PNE affects approximately 15% of children aged 5 years in the general population, and spontaneously remits at a rate of 15% per year [30]. The prevalence of PNE in SCD is much higher; children with SCD aged 14–17 years old were five times more likely to have PNE than controls [31–35]. Similar to the general population, PNE is more common in males, younger children and children with a positive family history of PNE [31–35]. Children with SCA and PNE are more likely to have sleep-disordered breathing [36]. In a study of 8-year-old Jamaican children, the prevalence of enuresis was 52% for boys and 38% for girls with HbSS disease, and 10% for boys and 20% for girls with HbSC disease. The prevalence of PNE in HbSS disease was significantly more common than HbSC disease or controls, but there was no significant difference between HbSC disease and controls. There was no significant difference by sex [37].

Risk Factors: PNE in HbSS disease has been attributed to hyposthenuria and polyuria. However, in a study comparing HbSS patients with and without enuresis, there was no difference in urinary concentrating ability or overnight urine volume [38]. However, the bladder capacity corrected to body surface area was lower, and the ratio of overnight urine volume divided by bladder capacity was higher in enuretic compared to non-enuretic children. A high prevalence of daytime symptoms of overactive bladder was also present in those with nocturnal enuresis and SCA [34]. These results suggest that hyposthenuria-induced polyuria may not be the primary cause of PNE in HbSS disease. In addition to urinary tract pathology, an association has been identified between sleep disordered breathing and PNE [36].

Therapy: Several pharmacological and behavioral therapies have been identified to treat patients with PNE in the general populations [39]. However, there are no controlled trials demonstrating benefit in children with SCD. One prospective study of 10 patients with SCD treated with desmopressin reported improvement in six patients [32]. Hence, the evidence for pharmacologic treatment is inadequate, and thus the focus of therapy is watchful waiting and bed-wetting alarms in some patients [40].

Albuminuria

Epidemiology: Fifty to seventy percent of adults with SCA have albuminuria in large cross-sectional studies [41–43]. Children with SCD develop albuminuria around 5–10 years of age and the prevalence increases throughout adolescence. The reported prevalence of albuminuria in cross-sectional pediatric SCA studies is 20–40% [44–46]. There is a need for longitudinal data on the natural history of the progression of kidney disease and development of end-stage kidney disease (ESKD) among pediatric patients with albuminuria as they transition into adulthood [47].

Pathology: Patients with SCA develop albuminuria due to either direct glomerular injury or impaired tubular reabsorption of albumin. In adults with SCD, glomerular complications include glomerular hypertrophy, focal segmental glomerulosclerosis, and membranoproliferative glomerulonephritis [48]. Kidney pathologic data was reported from 36 pediatric patients that underwent renal biopsy for proteinuria or low estimated GFR (eGFR) [49]. The majority had glomerular hypertrophy. In addition, the majority of the biopsies had mesangial hypercellularity and/or increased mesangial matrix. All patients in this cohort with mesangial hypercellularity, had proteinuria, including 88% with nephrotic range proteinuria. Eleven of the 36 patients had focal segmental glomerulosclerosis, six of the 11 also had global sclerosis. Five patients had membranoproliferative glomerulonephritis. On electron microscopy, more than 50% of biopsies had podocyte effacement, and a quarter had mesangial deposits. This study supports the importance of nephrology evaluation of children with SCD and significant proteinuria or decreased GFR.

Impaired tubular reabsorption of albumin may also contribute to albuminuria independent of glomerular disease in patients with SCA. Some albumin is normally filtered at the glomerulus and then reabsorbed by receptor-mediated endocytosis by megalin and cubilin in the proximal tubule [50]. However, internalization of albumin is subject to competition from many other proteins. Importantly in SCD, hemoglobin dimers can also be reabsorbed in the proximal tubule. In preclinical models, the addition of oxyhemoglobin to proximal tubule cells significantly reduced albumin uptake [51]. As SCD patients have daily variations in the amount of hemolysis consequent hemoglobinuria, it is plausible that albuminuria may vary depending on the amount of hemolysis. Studies have demonstrated that a single urine sample with albuminuria may not represent persistent albuminuria [47, 52]. While free hemoglobin or heme reuptake may lead to non-glomerular albuminuria, the uptake of free heme by the proximal tubule may induce pathologic changes and kidney disease progression, as described in the section on acute kidney injury.

Risk factors: Older age is a risk factor for albuminuria in SCD [43, 47]. Inheritance of two apolipoprotein L1 (APOL1) risk alleles, which are common in people of African descent, is associated with increased risk of albuminuria and CKD in SCD [53, 54]. Albuminuria in SCD patients with two APOL1 risk alleles begins in the first decade of life [44]. Serum hemoglobin is inversely related to risk of albuminuria [45, 55–57]. Patients with severe anemia in their second year of life are more likely to develop albuminuria earlier in life [45]. There is inconsistent data on the association of albuminuria with leukocytosis, hemolytic markers (lactate dehydrogenase), and blood pressure [46, 58–61].

Similar to diabetes, hyperfiltration is a risk factor for albuminuria in SCD. In cross-sectional studies, there are conflicting results on the association of eGFR with albuminuria [55, 62, 63]. A large, prospective, pediatric cohort evaluated the impact of hyperfiltration on progression of albuminuria; patients with hyperfiltration in the first decade of life were more likely to develop albuminuria at an earlier age [64]. Patients that developed albuminuria had a significant increase in eGFR prior to developing albuminuria while patients without albuminuria did not experience a significant rise in eGFR during the first decade of life. Adult data also suggests that hyperfiltration is associated with albuminuria [65].

Diagnosis: The National Heart, Lung, and Blood Institute (NHLBI) guidelines recommend screening for albuminuria by age 10 years, with annual screening thereafter [66]. Patients with a positive screening result should have a first morning test for albuminuria (albumin/creatinine ratio [ACR] >30 mg/g), with referral to a kidney specialist if positive. If a first morning void is not available or feasible, scheduling patients for an early morning appointment to obtain a second morning void may be of benefit. This second urine measurement is important as patients with SCD experience intermittent albuminuria, but may not have persistent albuminuria. About 25–50% of SCA patients with ACR <100 mg/g do not have persistent albuminuria; patients with ACR >100 mg/g are more likely to have persistent albuminuria [47, 67].

Albuminuria can begin prior to 10 years of age; therefore, some centers may begin screening for albuminuria earlier than 10 years of age [44, 64]. This is especially relevant in patients with two APOL1 risk alleles since almost 25% of these patients with SCD develop albuminuria prior to age 10 years.

The presence of severe albuminuria (ACR >300 mg/g) in SCD is less likely in pediatric patients than adults. As severe albuminuria is a rare complication in children with SCA, patients presenting with severe albuminuria require a complete diagnostic workup for proteinuria.

Treatment: The therapeutic approach in patients with SCD and albuminuria focuses on traditional modifiers of SCD and interventions to reduce hyperfiltration.

SCD Modifying Therapies: All patients with SCA should be offered hydroxyurea, a daily oral therapy, starting at 9 months of age regardless of clinical complications [66]. Therefore, patients that have progressed to albuminuria should be encouraged to begin hydroxyurea or improve adherence if nonadherence is present.

struggle to determine whether a decline in eGFR during the study is related to an improvement in renal function back to baseline, the beginning of a progressive decline in renal function to CKD, or regression to the mean among participants with higher eGFR at one time point. Long-term pediatric research is vital to determine whether a change in eGFR represents a benefit or risk.

Progressive CKD, End-Stage Kidney Disease, and Mortality

It is important to monitor pediatric patients with SCA for progression from glomerular hypertrophy with elevated GFR to CKD with decreased GFR due to sclerosis and fibrosis [80]. CKD in SCA is an independent risk factor for early death [100]. The management of CKD in SCD is similar to other patients with CKD, including control of hypertension and proteinuria with an ACEI or ARB. Currently, there are no FDA-approved medications for the specific treatment of sickle cell nephropathy.

Renal Replacement Therapy: The average age of initiation of renal replacement therapy (RRT) in SCD patients is 40–45 years [101–103]. Patients with SCD are currently a small minority of U.S. dialysis patients, but this population is expected to grow as overall life expectancy improves [104]. A longitudinal cohort study of SCA patients published in 1991 reported that the median survival of patients requiring dialysis was a mere 4 years [105]. In a more contemporary study (2005–2009), the hazard ratio for mortality among SCD patients with ESKD was 2.8 (95% CI 2.31–3.38) compared to those without SCD as the primary cause of renal failure, and 26.3% of incident SCD ESKD patients died within the first year of dialysis [101].

SCD patients are less likely than other ESKD patients to have a functioning arteriovenous fistula at the time of hemodialysis initiation, an important quality metric tied to improved RRT survival [103]. SCD patients on RRT experience greater rates of bacteremia and sepsis, atrial flutter and fibrillation, congestive heart failure exacerbations, and major hemorrhage than other

ESKD patients [103]. SCD patients on RRT have more RBC transfusions than other RRT patients. SCD patients not receiving erythropoietin stimulating agents (ESAs) have the highest transfusion burden, while those treated with ESAs and hydroxyurea have the lowest transfusion burden [103]. The 2019 ASH guidelines recommend that hydroxyurea and ESAs be used in combination to promote fetal hemoglobin production. Clinicians should use a lower hemoglobin threshold (<10 g/dL) when prescribing this combination therapy as higher hemoglobin levels, especially with higher HbS percentage, may be associated with increased SCD complications [77].

Renal Transplantation: For those with advanced CKD, the ASH evidenced-based guidelines suggests referral for renal transplant. As SCD is associated with chronic inflammation, the guidelines suggest judicious use of corticosteroids in post-transplant protocols due to the risk for vaso-occlusive pain with the increase in WBCs that accompanies steroid use [77]. Referral rates for transplantation for SCA patients are lower than other ESKD patients, even after adjusting for covariates [102]. One potential explanation for this disparity may be related to historical data reporting high rates of complication and poor graft survival in SCD patients. An analysis of the U.S. Renal Data System data from 1984–1996 showed that SCA patients and other renal transplant recipients have similar 1-year cadaveric graft survival [106]. Recipients had higher rates of 3-year graft loss (RR 1.60) and a significantly higher adjusted mortality rate at 1 year (RR 2.95) and 3 years (RR 2.82) compared to non-SCA transplant recipients [106]. However, more recent data (2000–2011 compared to 1988–1999) showed that 6-year survival among SCA recipients improved in the more recent era compared to the early era (78% versus 55.7%, p < 0.001) [107]. While the 6-year patient survival was still significantly lower than non-SCA recipients (HR for mortality 2.03, 95% CI 1.31–3.16), it was equal to that of black diabetic transplant recipients [107].

An additional concern that may hinder referral for renal transplantation is the perceived risk of alloimmunization if blood transfusion is required in anemic SCD transplant recipients. It is not surprising, given the lifetime exposure to RBC transfusions, that a greater proportion of SCA renal transplant recipients had allosensitization, with panel reactive antibodies >20% [107]. One retrospective multicenter study compared the proportion of *de novo* donor specific antibodies (DSAs) and graft survival among SCD renal transplant recipients who received regular automated exchange blood transfusions (EBT) pre or post renal transplant versus those who did not receive regular EBT [108]. Goals for EBT were to maintain hemoglobin >9 g/dL, to reduce HbS to <30%, and to reduce sickling-related complications. The median number of red blood cell units transfused per year was 37 and 8 in the EBT and non-EBT group, respectively. Overall, patient survival, graft survival, and graft function were superior in those who were on EBT, and the proportion of patients who developed *de novo* DSAs was not different (20% and 21%) between the groups. In addition, the incidence of rejection was lower in those on EBT (28% vs 54%). These data, while limited by sample size, indicate that blood transfusions peri-transplant are effective, safe and lead to improved outcomes in the SCA renal transplant population.

SCA patients with advanced CKD should therefore be counseled on the shortened graft survival and increased complication rates expected after transplantation, but should not be restricted from renal transplant access. Moreover, they should receive blood transfusions as needed pre or post transplantation.

Acute Kidney Injury

Patients with SCD may be at increased risk for acute kidney injury (AKI) due to high use of nephrotoxic medications and hemolysis causing proximal tubule injury from free heme and hemoglobin exposure [51, 109]. Acute pain events are a leading cause of hospitalization in children with SCD and repeated acute pain events can progress to chronic pain. Aggressive and early pain management is important, and many centers utilize individualized pain plans

for home and during hospitalizations [110]. These pain plans often include non-steroidal anti-inflammatory medications (NSAIDs) during home pain events and inpatient IV ketorolac as adjunctive therapy to opioids [111–113]. The 2014 NIH guidelines provide a moderate recommendation for the use of NSAIDs for mild to moderate pain in the absence of contraindications [110]. The 2019 ASH guidelines suggest a short course of NSAIDs in addition to opioids for acute pain management based on a low certainty of evidence [113]. The ASH guidelines remark that patients with known risk for renal toxicity should be identified as the mild potential benefit to NSAIDs for pain may not outweigh the risks associated with NSAID use. One concern with these guidelines is that pediatric patients may utilize a significant amount NSAIDs without appropriate monitoring of kidney function or fluid intake. Rarely, a single dose of ketorolac in the absence of volume depletion may precipitate irreversible renal failure [114].

In addition to acute pain events, infections may lead to use of nephrotoxic medications in SCD patients, who are increased risk for infection with pneumococcus and other encapsulated bacteria [115–117]. Patients may receive vancomycin or other nephrotoxic antibiotics for acute chest syndrome, fever, sepsis, or skin infections. It is important to consider the pros and cons of nephrotoxic medications given the potential long-term exposure and underlying risk of developing sickle cell nephropathy; monitoring of kidney function is needed when patients with SCD are at risk of AKI from nephrotoxins, volume depletion or infection.

When pediatric SCD patients are admitted for pain events or acute chest syndrome, AKI, when defined as an increase in creatinine occurs in 10–20% [118–120]. Risk factors for AKI in these studies include ketorolac exposure and an acute drop in hemoglobin, which probably reflects increased hemolysis and tubular exposure to free heme and hemoglobin. In another study using coding data, 1.4% of hospitalized SCD patients develop AKI, with risk factors including HbSS genotype, older age and greater number of total hospitalizations [121].

Adult studies of SCD patients demonstrate a higher incidence of AKI during hospitalization than described in children [122]. In a prospective study of adult SCD patients observed for a median of 5.5 years, 46% developed AKI [122]. Patients with AKI were older, had lower hemoglobin levels, higher white blood cell counts, and higher use of vancomycin. Moreover, genetic variants of heme catabolism (HMOX1) were independently associated with the development of AKI. Finally, adults with AKI were likely to develop CKD sooner, with the highest risk associated with more severe AKI.

Tubular Abnormalities and Acidification Defects

Along with defects in urinary concentrating ability (see above), SCD patients have well-described defects in other tubular functions, including urinary acidification and potassium excretion. SCA patients have an incomplete distal renal tubular acidosis as evidenced by decreased urine acidification in response to a systemic acid load [10, 123]. In one study, 42% of adult SCA patients had a metabolic acidosis [124]. Defects in acid excretion are associated with poor outcomes. In one adult study, the lowest tertile of urinary ammonia excretion increased the risk of ESKD [125]. Acidification of the urine was impaired in 52% of adults SCD patients, and was associated with older age, higher serum uric acid, increased hemolysis, lower eGFR, and lower serum bicarbonate [121]. Poor urinary ammonium excretion, as a measure of acid excretion, is associated with poor urinary concentrating ability [121].

SCA patients also have impaired potassium excretion [126]. In this study, patients had a normal renin-aldosterone axis and normal GFR, but had impaired potassium excretion, urine acidification and urinary concentrating ability, indicating that a severe distal tubular dysfunction is present in SCA patients despite preservation of glomerular function.

In one study of 24 children without decreased GFR, 75% had hyperphosphatemia, but serum calcium was normal [127]. Seventy-nine percent of participants had elevated FGF-23 levels, which is the expected physiologic response to hyperphosphatemia and would be expected to increase renal phosphate excretion. However, patients had evidence of impaired phosphate excretion, suggesting t that SCA patients have a proximal tubular resistance to FGF-23 before evidence of GFR decline.

Hypertension

A meta-analysis conducted for the 2014 NHLBI guidelines demonstrated that patients with HbSS genotype have lower diastolic and systolic blood pressures than healthy children. A large cohort study developed 90th percentile curves for children with SCD [128]. Hence, it may be appropriate to use SCD-specific blood pressure (BP) tables when evaluating BP in children with SCD.

There is an association in SCD patients between elevated BP and higher hemoglobin values [128, 129]. Hypertension in SCD patients has been associated with increased risk of acute stroke, although causality has not been established [128, 130]. Finally, data suggests that there is a direct correlation between higher blood pressure and increased mortality [128].

SCD patients have a high prevalence of masked hypertension and "white coat" hypertension in studies using 24-h ambulatory blood pressure monitoring (ABPM). Patients with SCA have only moderate concordance between in-clinic blood pressure and ABPM, with 25–33% having masked hypertension and 60% having white coat hypertension [61, 90, 131–133]. This may explain why some studies of in-clinic BP did not find a correlation between albuminuria and hypertension while there was an association when using ABPM [90, 132, 133]. Hence, since ABPM is the gold standard for measurement of BP, it is especially important to follow the American Academy of Pediatrics Guidelines and perform ABPM prior to initiation of antihypertensive treatment in SCD patients. Screening for masked hypertension may be appropriate in children with SCD and evidence of kidney disease. Patients identified with nocturnal hypertension or abnormal nocturnal dipping may have an increased risk for more rapid annual decline in GFR, albuminuria, and silent cerebral infarcts [61, 90, 131–133].

The ASH evidence-based guidelines for the management of SCD patients recommends a lower BP goal (<130/80) than the usual goal in adults without additional co-morbidities (<140/90) [77]. This strong recommendation was based on a moderate certainty in the evidence. The guidelines did not address BP management in children, and thus there are no recommendations to have a lower BP goal in SCD patients than in healthy children. Hence, BP management in children with SCD should follow the guidelines for healthy children.

References

1. Hassell KL. Population estimates of sickle cell disease in the U.S. Am J Prev Med. 2010;38:S512–21.
2. Piel FB, Patil AP, Howes RE, et al. Global distribution of the sickle cell gene and geographical confirmation of the malaria hypothesis. Nat Commun. 2010;1:104.
3. Statius van Eps LW, Pinedo-Veels C, de Vries GH, et al. Nature of concentrating defect in sickle-cell nephropathy. Microradioangiographic studies. Lancet. 1970;1:450–2.
4. Carden MA, Fay ME, Lu X, et al. Extracellular fluid tonicity impacts sickle red blood cell deformability and adhesion. Blood. 2017;130:2654–63.
5. Itano HA, Keitel HG, Thompson D. Hyposthenuria in sickle cell anemia: a reversible renal defect. J Clin Invest. 1956;35:998–1007.
6. Cochran RT Jr. Hyposthenuria in sickle cell states. Arch Intern Med. 1963;112:222–5.
7. Perillie PE, Epstein FH. Sickling phenomenon produced by hypertonic solutions: a possible explanation for the hyposthenuria of sicklemia. J Clin Invest. 1963;42:570–80.
8. Kunz HW, Pratt EL, Mellin GW, et al. Impairment of urinary concentration in sickle cell anemia. Pediatrics. 1954;13:352–6.
9. Schlitt L, Keitel HG. Pathogenesis of hyposthenuria in persons with sickle cell anemia or the sickle cell trait. Pediatrics. 1960;26:249–54.
10. Badr M, El Koumi MA, Ali YF, et al. Renal tubular dysfunction in children with sickle cell haemoglobinopathy. Nephrology (Carlton). 2013;18:299–303.
11. Miller ST, Wang WC, Iyer R, et al. Urine concentrating ability in infants with sickle cell disease: baseline data from the phase III trial of hydroxyurea (BABY HUG). Pediatr Blood Cancer. 2010;54:265–8.
12. Alvarez O, Miller ST, Wang WC, et al. Effect of hydroxyurea treatment on renal function parameters: results from the multi-center placebo-controlled BABY HUG clinical trial for infants with sickle cell anemia. Pediatr Blood Cancer. 2012;59:668–74.
13. Lebensburger JD, Pestina TI, Ware RE, et al. Hydroxyurea therapy requires HbF induction for clinical benefit in a sickle cell mouse model. Haematologica. 2010;95:1599–603.
14. Statius van Eps LW, Schouten H, La Porte-Wijsman LW, et al. The influence of red blood cell transfusions on the hyposthenuria and renal hemodynamics of sickle cell anemia. Clin Chim Acta. 1967;17:449–61.
15. Iyer R, Baliga R, Nagel RL, et al. Maximum urine concentrating ability in children with Hb SC disease: effects of hydroxyurea. Am J Hematol. 2000;64:47–52.
16. Mostofi FK, Vorder Bruegge CF, Diggs LW. Lesions in kidneys removed for unilateral hematuria in sickle-cell disease. AMA Arch Pathol. 1957;63:336–51.
17. Pandya KK, Koshy M, Brown N, et al. Renal papillary necrosis in sickle cell hemoglobinopathies. J Urol. 1976;115:497–501.
18. Odita JC, Ugbodaga CI, Okafor LA, et al. Urographic changes in homozygous sickle cell disease. Diagn Imaging. 1983;52:259–63.
19. Eckert DE, Jonutis AJ, Davidson AJ. The incidence and manifestations of urographic papillary abnormalities in patients with S hemoglobinopathies. Radiology. 1974;113:59–63.
20. Madu AJ, Okoye AE, Ajuba IC, et al. Prevalence and associations of symptomatic renal papillary necrosis in sickle cell anemia patients in south-eastern Nigeria. Niger J Clin Pract. 2016;19:471–4.
21. Alvarez O, Rodriguez MM, Jordan L, et al. Renal medullary carcinoma and sickle cell trait: a systematic review. Pediatr Blood Cancer. 2015;62:1694–9.
22. Sutariya HC, Pandya VK. Renal papillary necrosis: role of radiology. J Clin Diagn Res. 2016;10:TD10–2.
23. Henderickx M, Brits T, De Baets K, et al. Renal papillary necrosis in patients with sickle cell disease: how to recognize this 'forgotten' diagnosis. J Pediatr Urol. 2017;13:250–6.
24. Gabrovsky A, Aderinto A, Spevak M, et al. Low dose, oral epsilon aminocaproic acid for renal papillary necrosis and massive hemorrhage in hemoglobin SC disease. Pediatr Blood Cancer. 2010;54:148–50.
25. Black WD, Hatch FE, Acchiardo S. Aminocaproic acid in prolonged hematuria of patients with sicklemia. Arch Intern Med. 1976;136:678–81.
26. Kiryluk K, Jadoon A, Gupta M, et al. Sickle cell trait and gross hematuria. Kidney Int. 2007;71:706–10.
27. Zadeii G, Lohr JW. Renal papillary necrosis in a patient with sickle cell trait. J Am Soc Nephrol. 1997;8:1034–9.
28. Meyersfield SA, Morganstern SL, Seery W, et al. Medical management of refractory hematuria in sickle-cell trait. Urology. 1976;8:112–3.

29. Baldree LA, Ault BH, Chesney CM, et al. Intravenous desmopressin acetate in children with sickle trait and persistent macroscopic hematuria. Pediatrics. 1990;86:238–43.
30. Arda E, Cakiroglu B, Thomas DT. Primary nocturnal enuresis: a review. Nephrourol Mon. 2016;8:e35809.
31. Esezobor CI, Akintan P, Nwaogazie U, et al. Enuresis in children and adolescents with sickle cell anaemia is more frequent and substantially different from the general population. PLoS One. 2018;13:e0201860.
32. Figueroa TE, Benaim E, Griggs ST, et al. Enuresis in sickle cell disease. J Urol. 1995;153:1987–9.
33. Barakat LP, Smith-Whitley K, Schulman S, et al. Nocturnal enuresis in pediatric sickle cell disease. J Dev Behav Pediatr. 2001;22:300–5.
34. Portocarrero ML, Portocarrero ML, Sobral MM, et al. Prevalence of enuresis and daytime urinary incontinence in children and adolescents with sickle cell disease. J Urol. 2012;187:1037–40.
35. Ekinci O, Celik T, Unal S, et al. Nocturnal enuresis in sickle cell disease and thalassemia major: associated factors in a clinical sample. Int J Hematol. 2013;98:430–6.
36. Lehmann GC, Bell TR, Kirkham FJ, et al. Enuresis associated with sleep disordered breathing in children with sickle cell anemia. J Urol. 2012;188:1572–6.
37. Readett DR, Morris JS, Serjeant GR. Nocturnal enuresis in sickle cell haemoglobinopathies. Arch Dis Child. 1990;65:290–3.
38. Readett DR, Morris J, Serjeant GR. Determinants of nocturnal enuresis in homozygous sickle cell disease. Arch Dis Child. 1990;65:615–8.
39. Neveus T, Eggert P, Evans J, et al. Evaluation of and treatment for monosymptomatic enuresis: a standardization document from the International Children's Continence Society. J Urol. 2010;183:441–7.
40. Wolf RB, Kassim AA, Goodpaster RL, et al. Nocturnal enuresis in sickle cell disease. Expert Rev Hematol. 2014;7:245–54.
41. Drawz P, Ayyappan S, Nouraie M, et al. Kidney disease among patients with sickle cell disease, hemoglobin SS and SC. Clin J Am Soc Nephrol. 2016;11:207–15.
42. Asnani MR, Reid ME. Renal function in adult Jamaicans with homozygous sickle cell disease. Hematology. 2015;20:422–8.
43. Guasch A, Navarrete J, Nass K, et al. Glomerular involvement in adults with sickle cell hemoglobinopathies: prevalence and clinical correlates of progressive renal failure. J Am Soc Nephrol. 2006;17:2228–35.
44. Zahr RS, Rampersaud E, Kang G, et al. Children with sickle cell anemia and APOL1 genetic variants develop albuminuria early in life. Haematologica. 2019;104:e385–7.
45. Aban I, Baddam S, Hilliard LM, et al. Severe anemia early in life as a risk factor for sickle-cell kidney disease. Blood. 2017;129:385–7.

46. King L, MooSang M, Miller M, et al. Prevalence and predictors of microalbuminuria in Jamaican children with sickle cell disease. Arch Dis Child. 2011;96:1135–9.
47. Niss O, Lane A, Asnani MR, et al. Progression of albuminuria in patients with sickle cell anemia: a multicenter, longitudinal study. Blood Adv. 2020;4:1501–11.
48. Maigne G, Ferlicot S, Galacteros F, et al. Glomerular lesions in patients with sickle cell disease. Medicine (Baltimore). 2010;89:18–27.
49. Zahr RS, Yee ME, Weaver J, et al. Kidney biopsy findings in children with sickle cell disease: a Midwest Pediatric Nephrology Consortium study. Pediatr Nephrol. 2019;34:1435–45.
50. Dickson LE, Wagner MC, Sandoval RM, et al. The proximal tubule and albuminuria: really! J Am Soc Nephrol. 2014;25:443–53.
51. Eshbach ML, Kaur A, Rbaibi Y, et al. Hemoglobin inhibits albumin uptake by proximal tubule cells: implications for sickle cell disease. Am J Physiol Cell Physiol. 2017;312:C733–40.
52. Lebensburger JD, Miller ST, Howard TH, et al. Influence of severity of anemia on clinical findings in infants with sickle cell anemia: analyses from the BABY HUG study. Pediatr Blood Cancer. 2012;59:675–8.
53. Saraf SL, Shah BN, Zhang X, et al. APOL1, alpha-thalassemia, and BCL11A variants as a genetic risk profile for progression of chronic kidney disease in sickle cell anemia. Haematologica. 2017;102:e1–6.
54. Ashley-Koch AE, Okocha EC, Garrett ME, et al. MYH9 and APOL1 are both associated with sickle cell disease nephropathy. Br J Haematol. 2011;155:386–94.
55. Hamideh D, Raj V, Harrington T, et al. Albuminuria correlates with hemolysis and NAG and KIM-1 in patients with sickle cell anemia. Pediatr Nephrol. 2014;29:1997–2003.
56. Becton LJ, Kalpatthi RV, Rackoff E, et al. Prevalence and clinical correlates of microalbuminuria in children with sickle cell disease. Pediatr Nephrol. 2010;25:1505–11.
57. McBurney PG, Hanevold CD, Hernandez CM, et al. Risk factors for microalbuminuria in children with sickle cell anemia. J Pediatr Hematol Oncol. 2002;24:473–7.
58. Aygun B, Mortier NA, Smeltzer MP, et al. Glomerular hyperfiltration and albuminuria in children with sickle cell anemia. Pediatr Nephrol. 2011;26:1285–90.
59. McPherson ME, Hutcherson D, Olson E, et al. Safety and efficacy of targeted busulfan therapy in children undergoing myeloablative matched sibling donor BMT for sickle cell disease. Bone Marrow Transplant. 2011;46:27–33.
60. Youssry I, Makar S, Fawzy R, et al. Novel marker for the detection of sickle cell nephropathy: solu-

60. ble FMS-like tyrosine kinase-1 (sFLT-1). Pediatr Nephrol. 2015;30:2163–8.

61. Becker AM, Goldberg JH, Henson M, et al. Blood pressure abnormalities in children with sickle cell anemia. Pediatr Blood Cancer. 2014;61:518–22.

62. McPherson Yee M, Jabbar SF, Osunkwo I, et al. Chronic kidney disease and albuminuria in children with sickle cell disease. Clin J Am Soc Nephrol. 2011;6:2628–33.

63. Gurkan S, Scarponi KJ, Hotchkiss H, et al. Lactate dehydrogenase as a predictor of kidney involvement in patients with sickle cell anemia. Pediatr Nephrol. 2010;25:2123–7.

64. Lebensburger JD, Aban I, Pernell B, et al. Hyperfiltration during early childhood precedes albuminuria in pediatric sickle cell nephropathy. Am J Hematol. 2019;94:417–23.

65. Vazquez B, Shah B, Zhang X, et al. Hyperfiltration is associated with the development of microalbuminuria in patients with sickle cell anemia. Am J Hematol. 2014;89:1156–7.

66. Yawn BP, Buchanan GR, Afenyi-Annan AN, et al. Management of sickle cell disease: summary of the 2014 evidence-based report by expert panel members. JAMA. 2014;312:1033–48.

67. Zahr RS, Hankins JS, Kang G, et al. Hydroxyurea prevents onset and progression of albuminuria in children with sickle cell anemia. Am J Hematol. 2019;94:E27–9.

68. Ware RE. How I use hydroxyurea to treat young patients with sickle cell anemia. Blood. 2010;115:5300–11.

69. Wang WC, Ware RE, Miller ST, et al. Hydroxycarbamide in very young children with sickle-cell anaemia: a multicentre, randomised, controlled trial (BABY HUG). Lancet. 2011;377:1663–72.

70. Lebensburger J, Johnson SM, Askenazi DJ, et al. Protective role of hemoglobin and fetal hemoglobin in early kidney disease for children with sickle cell anemia. Am J Hematol. 2011;86:430–2.

71. Bartolucci P, Habibi A, Stehle T, et al. Six months of hydroxyurea reduces albuminuria in patients with sickle cell disease. J Am Soc Nephrol. 2016;27:1847–53.

72. Alvarez O, Montane B, Lopez G, et al. Early blood transfusions protect against microalbuminuria in children with sickle cell disease. Pediatr Blood Cancer. 2006;47:71–6.

73. Coates TD, Wood JC. How we manage iron overload in sickle cell patients. Br J Haematol. 2017;177:703–16.

74. Ataga KI, Kutlar A, Kanter J, et al. Crizanlizumab for the prevention of pain crises in sickle cell disease. N Engl J Med. 2017;376:429–39.

75. Vichinsky E, Hoppe CC, Ataga KI, et al. A phase 3 randomized trial of Voxelotor in sickle cell disease. N Engl J Med. 2019;381:509–19.

76. Niihara Y, Miller ST, Kanter J, et al. A phase 3 trial of l-glutamine in sickle cell disease. N Engl J Med. 2018;379:226–35.

77. Liem RI, Lanzkron S, Coates TD, et al. American Society of Hematology 2019 guidelines for sickle cell disease: cardiopulmonary and kidney disease. Blood Adv. 2019;3:3867–97.

78. Foucan L, Bourhis V, Bangou J, et al. A randomized trial of captopril for microalbuminuria in normotensive adults with sickle cell anemia. Am J Med. 1998;104:339–42.

79. Aoki RY, Saad ST. Enalapril reduces the albuminuria of patients with sickle cell disease. Am J Med. 1995;98:432–5.

80. Falk RJ, Scheinman J, Phillips G, et al. Prevalence and pathologic features of sickle cell nephropathy and response to inhibition of angiotensin-converting enzyme. N Engl J Med. 1992;326:910–5.

81. Fitzhugh CD, Wigfall DR, Ware RE. Enalapril and hydroxyurea therapy for children with sickle nephropathy. Pediatr Blood Cancer. 2005;45:982–5.

82. Haymann JP, Hammoudi N, Stankovic Stojanovic K, et al. Renin-angiotensin system blockade promotes a cardio-renal protection in albuminuric homozygous sickle cell patients. Br J Haematol. 2017;179:820–8.

83. Kasztan M, Fox BM, Speed JS, et al. Long-term endothelin-a receptor antagonism provides robust renal protection in humanized sickle cell disease mice. J Am Soc Nephrol. 2017;28:2443–58.

84. Kutlar A, Pollock J, Meiler SE, et al. Phase-I study of ETA receptor antagonist Ambrisentan in sickle cell disease. Blood. 2019;134:617.

85. Aloni MN, Ngiyulu RM, Ekulu PM, et al. Glomerular hyperfiltration is strongly correlated with age in Congolese children with sickle cell anaemia. Acta Paediatr. 2017;106:819–24.

86. Bodas P, Huang A, O'Riordan MA, et al. The prevalence of hypertension and abnormal kidney function in children with sickle cell disease -a cross sectional review. BMC Nephrol. 2013;14:237.

87. Ephraim RK, Osakunor DN, Cudjoe O, et al. Chronic kidney disease is common in sickle cell disease: a cross-sectional study in the Tema metropolis, Ghana. BMC Nephrol. 2015;16:75.

88. Kaspar CDW, Beach I, Newlin J, et al. Hyperuricemia is associated with a lower glomerular filtration rate in pediatric sickle cell disease patients. Pediatr Nephrol. 2020;35:883–9.

89. Lebensburger JD, Aban I, Hilliard LM, et al. Hyperuricemia and abnormal nocturnal dipping impact glomerular filtration rate in patients with sickle cell anemia. Am J Hematol. 2021;96(5):E143–6.

90. Lebensburger JD, Cutter GR, Howard TH, et al. Evaluating risk factors for chronic kidney disease in pediatric patients with sickle cell anemia. Pediatr Nephrol. 2017;32:1565–73.

91. Aygun B, Mortier NA, Smeltzer MP, et al. Hydroxyurea treatment decreases glomerular hyper-

filtration in children with sickle cell anemia. Am J Hematol. 2013;88:116–9.

92. Quinn CT, Saraf SL, Gordeuk VR, et al. Losartan for the nephropathy of sickle cell anemia: a phase-2, multicenter trial. Am J Hematol. 2017;92:E520–8.

93. Yee ME, Lane PA, Archer DR, et al. Losartan therapy decreases albuminuria with stable glomerular filtration and permselectivity in sickle cell anemia. Blood Cells Mol Dis. 2018;69:65–70.

94. Yee MEM, Lane PA, Archer DR, et al. Estimation of glomerular filtration rate using serum cystatin C and creatinine in adults with sickle cell anemia. Am J Hematol. 2017;92:E598–9.

95. Arlet JB, Ribeil JA, Chatellier G, et al. Determination of the best method to estimate glomerular filtration rate from serum creatinine in adult patients with sickle cell disease: a prospective observational cohort study. BMC Nephrol. 2012;13:83.

96. Lebensburger JD, Gossett J, Zahr R, et al. High bias and low precision for estimated versus measured glomerular filtration rate in pediatric sickle cell anemia. Haematologica. 2021;106(1):295–8.

97. Xu JZ, Garrett ME, Soldano KL, et al. Clinical and metabolomic risk factors associated with rapid renal function decline in sickle cell disease. Am J Hematol. 2018;93:1451–60.

98. Derebail VK, Ciccone EJ, Zhou Q, et al. Progressive decline in estimated GFR in patients with sickle cell disease: an observational cohort study. Am J Kidney Dis. 2019;74:47–55.

99. Derebail VK, Zhou Q, Ciccone EJ, et al. Rapid decline in estimated glomerular filtration rate is common in adults with sickle cell disease and associated with increased mortality. Br J Haematol. 2019;186:900–7.

100. Platt OS, Brambilla DJ, Rosse WF, et al. Mortality in sickle cell disease. Life expectancy and risk factors for early death. N Engl J Med. 1994;330:1639–44.

101. Abbott KC, Hypolite IO, Agodoa LY. Sickle cell nephropathy at end-stage renal disease in the United States: patient characteristics and survival. Clin Nephrol. 2002;58:9–15.

102. Viner M, Zhou J, Allison D, et al. The morbidity and mortality of end stage renal disease in sickle cell disease. Am J Hematol. 2019;94:E138–41.

103. McClellan AC, Luthi JC, Lynch JR, et al. High one year mortality in adults with sickle cell disease and end-stage renal disease. Br J Haematol. 2012;159:360–7.

104. Boyle SM, Jacobs B, Sayani FA, et al. Management of the dialysis patient with sickle cell disease. Semin Dial. 2016;29:62–70.

105. Powars DR, Elliott-Mills DD, Chan L, et al. Chronic renal failure in sickle cell disease: risk factors, clinical course, and mortality. Ann Intern Med. 1991;115:614–20.

106. Ojo AO, Govaerts TC, Schmouder RL, et al. Renal transplantation in end-stage sickle cell nephropathy. Transplantation. 1999;67:291–5.

107. Huang E, Parke C, Mehrnia A, et al. Improved survival among sickle cell kidney transplant recipients in the recent era. Nephrol Dial Transplant. 2013;28:1039–46.

108. Willis JC, Awogbade M, Howard J, et al. Outcomes following kidney transplantation in patients with sickle cell disease: the impact of automated exchange blood transfusion. PLoS One. 2020;15:e0236998.

109. Ofori-Acquah SF, Hazra R, Orikogbo OO, et al. Hemopexin deficiency promotes acute kidney injury in sickle cell disease. Blood. 2020;135:1044–8.

110. Yawn BP, Buchanan G, Hassell K. Management of patients with sickle cell disease—reply. JAMA. 2015;313:91–2.

111. Han J, Saraf SL, Lash JP, et al. Use of anti-inflammatory analgesics in sickle-cell disease. J Clin Pharm Ther. 2017;42:656–60.

112. Cacciotti C, Vaiselbuh S, Romanos-Sirakis E. Pain management for sickle cell disease in the pediatric emergency department: medications and hospitalization trends. Clin Pediatr (Phila). 2017;56:1109–14.

113. Brandow AM, Carroll CP, Creary S, et al. American Society of Hematology 2020 guidelines for sickle cell disease: management of acute and chronic pain. Blood Adv. 2020;4:2656–701.

114. Simckes AM, Chen SS, Osorio AV, et al. Ketorolac-induced irreversible renal failure in sickle cell disease: a case report. Pediatr Nephrol. 1999;13:63–7.

115. Bala N, Chao J, John D, et al. Prevalence of bacteremia in febrile patients with sickle cell disease: meta-analysis of observational studies. Pediatr Emerg Care. 2021;37(12):e1695–700.

116. Baskin MN, Goh XL, Heeney MM, et al. Bacteremia risk and outpatient management of febrile patients with sickle cell disease. Pediatrics. 2013;131:1035–41.

117. Sirigaddi K, Aban I, Jantz A, et al. Outcomes of febrile events in pediatric patients with sickle cell anemia. Pediatr Blood Cancer. 2018;65:e27379.

118. Baddam S, Aban I, Hilliard L, et al. Acute kidney injury during a pediatric sickle cell vaso-occlusive pain crisis. Pediatr Nephrol. 2017;32:1451–6.

119. Lebensburger JD, Palabindela P, Howard TH, et al. Prevalence of acute kidney injury during pediatric admissions for acute chest syndrome. Pediatr Nephrol. 2016;31:1363–8.

120. Oakley J, Zahr R, Aban I, et al. Acute kidney injury during parvovirus B19-induced transient aplastic crisis in sickle cell disease. Am J Hematol. 2018.

121. Cazenave M, Audard V, Bertocchio JP, et al. Tubular acidification defect in adults with sickle cell disease. Clin J Am Soc Nephrol. 2020;15:16–24.

122. Saraf SL, Viner M, Rischall A, et al. HMOX1 and acute kidney injury in sickle cell anemia. Blood. 2018;132:1621–5.

123. Silva Junior GB, Liborio AB, Vieira AP, et al. Evaluation of renal function in sickle cell disease patients in Brazil. Braz J Med Biol Res. 2012;45:652–5.

124. Maurel S, Stankovic Stojanovic K, Avellino V, et al. Prevalence and correlates of metabolic acidosis among patients with homozygous sickle cell disease. Clin J Am Soc Nephrol. 2014;9:648–53.

125. Vallet M, Metzger M, Haymann JP, et al. Urinary ammonia and long-term outcomes in chronic kidney disease. Kidney Int. 2015;88:137–45.

126. DeFronzo RA, Taufield PA, Black H, et al. Impaired renal tubular potassium secretion in sickle cell disease. Ann Intern Med. 1979;90:310–6.

127. Raj VM, Freundlich M, Hamideh D, et al. Abnormalities in renal tubular phosphate handling in children with sickle cell disease. Pediatr Blood Cancer. 2014;61:2267–70.

128. Pegelow CH, Colangelo L, Steinberg M, et al. Natural history of blood pressure in sickle cell disease: risks for stroke and death associated with relative hypertension in sickle cell anemia. Am J Med. 1997;102:171–7.

129. Wolf RB, Saville BR, Roberts DO, et al. Factors associated with growth and blood pressure patterns in children with sickle cell anemia: silent cerebral infarct multi-center clinical trial cohort. Am J Hematol. 2015;90:2–7.

130. DeBaun MR, Sarnaik SA, Rodeghier MJ, et al. Associated risk factors for silent cerebral infarcts in sickle cell anemia: low baseline hemoglobin, sex, and relative high systolic blood pressure. Blood. 2012;119:3684–90.

131. Strumph K, Hafeman M, Ranabothu S, et al. Nocturnal hypertension associated with stroke and silent cerebral infarcts in children with sickle cell disease. Pediatr Blood Cancer. 2021;68:e28883.

132. Ranabothu S, Hafeman M, Manwani D, et al. Ambulatory hypertension in pediatric patients with sickle cell disease and its association with end-organ damage. Cureus. 2020;12:e11707.

133. Shatat IF, Jakson SM, Blue AE, et al. Masked hypertension is prevalent in children with sickle cell disease: a Midwest Pediatric Nephrology Consortium study. Pediatr Nephrol. 2013;28:115–20.

Diabetic Kidney Disease

32

Allison B. Dart

Introduction to Diabetic Kidney Disease

While diabetic nephropathy is the most common cause of end-stage kidney disease (ESKD) in adults in many countries [1, 2], it has become increasingly relevant to children and adolescents. Traditionally, the chronic kidney disease (CKD) associated with diabetes in adults has been termed diabetic nephropathy in both type 1 and type 2 subtypes. As the clinical phenotype of kidney complications associated with diabetes has broadened, the term diabetic kidney disease (DKD) is increasingly utilized. It has been defined as CKD, with diabetes being partially involved in the pathogenesis of the kidney disease. DKD in adults can include diabetic nephropathy, ischemic nephropathy, hypertensive nephrosclerosis, and non-diabetic kidney disease, with multiple entities possible in the same patient [3]. In general, the natural history of DKD is similar in adult type 1 and type 2 diabetes

populations. In children, the natural history and pathology of kidney complications in the diabetes subtypes is quite different. Currently, DKD is used to describe the kidney complications in all youth with diabetes. Important differences in DKD associated with youth onset type 1 and type 2 diabetes will be outlined in each section. This chapter will outline the clinical risk factors, natural history, pathology, and treatment of DKD.

Epidemiology of Diabetes in Children

Youth onset diabetes, defined as disease onset prior to 18 years of age, is an important clinical problem in children and adolescents, with an increasing incidence of both type 1 and type 2 diabetes in the last 20 years [4, 5]. While type 1 diabetes is the most common endocrine condition in children, the proportion of children with type 2 is increasing, especially in disadvantaged populations and minority ethnic groups, including children of African, Arab, Asian, Hispanic, and Indigenous descent [6]. The increasing prevalence of obesity in children is an important cause; however, most important are the social determinants of health such as poverty, colonization and systemic racism that are driving the increased risk of chronic disease in disadvantaged populations [7, 8].

A. B. Dart (✉)
Section of Nephrology, Department of Pediatrics and Child Health, University of Manitoba,
Winnipeg, MB, Canada

Children's Hospital Research Institute of Manitoba (CHRIM), The Diabetes Research Envisioned and Accomplished in Manitoba (DREAM) Theme of the Children's Hospital Research Institute of Manitoba,
Winnipeg, MB, Canada
e-mail: adart@hsc.mb.ca

© The Author(s), under exclusive license to Springer Nature Switzerland AG 2023
F. Schaefer, L. A. Greenbaum (eds.), *Pediatric Kidney Disease*,
https://doi.org/10.1007/978-3-031-11665-0_32

The unadjusted estimated incidence of type 1 diabetes and type 2 diabetes in the United States (US) between 2002–2003 and 2011–2012 increased annually by 1.4% and 7.1%, respectively [9]. Overall, 87% of youth with diabetes in North America have type 1 diabetes [10], but type 2 diabetes accounts for up to 50% of cases in some clinical settings [11]. The incidence of type 1 diabetes is now 1–3 per 100,000 per year in South America, China and other Asian countries; 10–20 per 100,000 in South European countries and the US; and 30–60 per 100,000 in Scandinavia [12, 13]. In North America, the prevalence of type 2 diabetes is 12.5 cases per 100,000 and the prevalence of diabetes in youth overall is now up to 0.8% [14, 15].

Clinical Risk Factors for Diabetic Kidney Disease

The most well-characterized and clinically important risk factors for DKD are glycemic control and hypertension. Additional risk factors include hyperlipidemia, smoking, duration of diabetes, and post-pubertal status. More common in youth with type 2 diabetes are risk factors for non-diabetic kidney disease, such as in-utero exposure to diabetes and obesity, which affect nephron endowment, and an increased risk of immune-mediated kidney disease, such as IgA nephropathy, in Indigenous and Asian populations [16, 17].

Hyperglycemia is a consistent and important determinant of renal injury. The Diabetes Control and Complications Trial (DCCT) [18] and the UK Prospective Diabetes Study (UKPDS) [19] evaluated intensive glycemic control vs. conventional regimens and provided clear evidence that optimized glycemic control was associated with improved long-term kidney health. In the DCCT study, the 9-year risk of microalbuminuria was reduced by 34% and macroalbuminuria by 56% in the intensive therapy group when compared with standard therapy. The intensive therapy group also had improved long-term outcomes with respect to estimated glomerular filtration rate (eGFR) [20].

However, target glycemic control is often very difficult to achieve in adolescents. Many observational studies have reported hemoglobin A1c (HbA1c) levels well above the recommended <7% [21, 22]. There are important psychological factors related to adolescence that make adherence to the complex care regimens of diabetes management unattainable. There is also increasing recognition of mental health co-morbidities that both affect adolescents ability to self-manage their chronic disease [23].

Hypertension has also been consistently identified as an important modifiable risk factor for DKD in type 1 diabetes [24]. Youth onset type 2 diabetes studies that included 24 h ABPM data also support the importance of this clinical risk factor [25, 26]. Additional risk factors include duration of diabetes, and post-pubertal status [27]. Hyperlipidemia and smoking have also been associated with an increased risk of albuminuria [28, 29]. Obesity is common in youth with type 2 diabetes; however, it has not independently been shown to increase the risk of DKD early in the disease course [30].

Natural History

The natural history of DKD has 5 stages: glomerular hyperfiltration with a period of subclinical morphological changes; onset of albuminuria; progressive increases in albumin excretion; declining GFR; and ultimately ESKD (Table 32.1). The period of glomerular hyperfiltration is fairly consistent, but its pathogenicity is controversial [31]. Following this period, albuminuria starts to manifest, which once consistent, is considered the first clinical marker of DKD [3]. Historically, thresholds for microalbuminuria, and macroalbuminuria were described, but these thresholds are no longer recommended; albuminuria should be evaluated as a continuous outcome.

Traditionally, DKD developed in 25–35% of patients with type 1 diabetes, but typically manifested 10–20 years after diagnosis [32]. In modern adolescent cohorts, persistent albuminuria occurs in 0.7–9.2% of youth with type 1 diabetes

Table 32.1 Typical stages of diabetic kidney disease

	Clinical feature	Typical timeline after diagnosis
Hyperfiltration	eGFR >140 mL/min/1.73 m^2	0–<5 years
Albuminuria (Incipient Nephropathy)	UAE 30–300 mg/day ACR > 30 mg/g	5–15 years
Progressive albuminuria (Overt Nephropathy)	Increasing UAE >300 mg/day Declining eGFR	10–20 years
Progressive nephropathy (Chronic Kidney Disease)	Declining eGFR	15–25 years
End Stage Kidney Disease	eGFR <15 mL/min/1.73 m^2	>20 years

UAE Urinary Albumin Excretion, *ACR* Albumin:Creatinine Ratio, *eGFR* estimated Glomerular Filtration Rate

[29, 33] and 5.1–30.5% of youth with type 2 diabetes [25, 34]. Indigenous youth are at particularly high risk of early onset albuminuria and progression of CKD [30, 34–36]. This may reflect the important impact of developmental risk factors in this population. Autopsy studies have identified larger and fewer glomeruli in Indigenous adults, especially in individuals exposed to diabetes in pregnancy [37] and living in remote locations [38].

DKD is generally slowly progressive, typically taking 5 years to progress through each stage, with a decrease in GFR manifesting after many years of progressive albuminuria. GFR generally starts to decrease after more severe albuminuria has developed. Early in the course, the GFR decreases by 1–2 mL/min/1.73 m^2/year, but this can accelerate to 5–10 mL/min/1.73 m^2/year subsequently [3]. Once more severe albuminuria has developed, rates of progression are very high (cumulative risk of ESKD are 24.4%, 43% and 52% at 5, 10 and 15 years) [39].

With modern therapy, however, rates of ESKD have improved. Long-term, 30-year follow-up from the DCCT trial has shown nephropathy in only 9% of the trial cohort 30 years after diagnosis, and only 2% require kidney replacement therapy [40]. Similarly, a Swedish study reported a rate of persistent albuminuria of only 8.9% at

25 years, presumed to be secondary to improvement in glycemic control [41]. Studies in which glycemic control remains suboptimal continue to show high rates of kidney complications [42].

Rates of progression in youth with type 2 diabetes are much higher. Long-term follow-up of Indigenous youth from Canada and Australia with type 2 diabetes have shown rates of ESKD up to 50% [30, 43]. The modern type 2 diabetes cohorts are only now reaching young adulthood; therefore, more knowledge regarding eGFR trajectories in this population will be available [44, 45].

Ultimately, individuals with type 1 [46] and type 2 [47] diabetes that develop kidney disease are at increased risk of mortality; hence, prevention and delay of progression of kidney disease are very important.

Pathophysiology

The mechanisms proposed to contribute to hyperfiltration in diabetes include up-regulation of sodium-glucose cotransporter-2 (SGLT-2) in the proximal tubule due to the higher load of glucose. Up-regulation of SGLT-2, which co-transports sodium and glucose back into the circulation, decreases distal sodium delivery to the macula densa, thereby promoting renin release, and thus over-activation of the renin-angiotensin-aldosterone system (RAAS) [48]. Glomerular hypertrophy also leads to an increased filtration surface area. Additionally, abnormal vascular control decreases afferent glomerular arteriolar resistance and increases efferent glomerular resistance, ultimately causing an increase in renal blood flow [49].

Metabolic factors are also important, including advanced glycation end products (AGEs), which are thought to increase production of reactive oxygen species; stimulate intracellular molecules such as protein kinase C and NF-kB; and activate growth factors, including TGF-B and vascular endothelial growth factor. These factors, along with hemodynamic changes, contribute to podocyte injury, oxidative stress, inflammation and, ultimately, fibrosis.

Exacerbating factors in youth with type 2 diabetes may include a decreased functional nephron mass, as well as a higher prevalence of immune-mediated glomerular diseases [16]. Adults with diabetes may have hypertensive nephrosclerosis or ischemic nephropathy from atherosclerotic changes, either overlapping with traditional DKD or on their own.

Biomarkers

Albuminuria is the most established biomarker of early kidney disease, but there is a subset of patients that develop progressive CKD in the absence of proteinuria [50, 51]. This suggests that albuminuria may not identify all patients with DKD. There are several potential additional biomarkers that are predictive of progressive kidney disease. These include uric acid, tumor necrosis factor receptors, markers of oxidative stress and profibrotic cytokines [52], but their role in clinical practice is not defined.

Pathology

The typical pathological changes in DKD include mesangial matrix expansion, glomerular basement membrane thickening, diffuse or nodular glomerulosclerosis, and ultimately tubulointerstitial inflammation and fibrosis (Fig. 32.1). Biopsy studies in youth with type 1 diabetes between 1.5 and 5 years after diabetes onset show early pathological changes [53–55].

Pathologic classification of diabetic nephropathy has been divided into four hierarchical glomerular lesions [56]. Class I is defined by isolated glomerular basement membrane thickening and only mild changes on light microscopy. Class II includes mild (IIa) and severe (IIb) mesangial expansion. Class III includes nodular sclerosis (Kimmelstiel-Wilson lesions) in at least one glomerulus. Class IV, advanced diabetic glomerulosclerosis, includes glomerulosclerosis in more that 50% of glomeruli, along with lesions from Classes I-III. Interstitial and vascular lesions including interstitial fibrosis and tubular atrophy (IFTA) and arteriolar hyalinosis and arteriosclerosis develop concomitantly.

Biopsy findings in youth with type 2 diabetes often occur early in the disease course, but have frequently shown features other than typical diabetic nephropathy [57]. In Canadian First Nation children with type 2 diabetes, histologic changes included enlarged glomeruli; focal, mild hyaline arteriolosclerosis; and focal and mild glomerular basement membrane thickening (Fig. 32.2). Additional findings included immune complex deposition, and focal segmental or global glomerulosclerosis [57]. Most adults with type 2 diabetes exhibit typical DKD [58]; however, the prevalence of non-diabetic kidney disease varies (3–82.9%), with IgA nephropathy being a common finding, occurring in 3–59% of biopsies in a meta-analysis [17].

Kidney biopsy may therefore be indicated if a patient's course is not following the expected natural history of DKD in order to identify alternative causes of albuminuria or decreased eGFR. Non-diabetic kidney is more likely in patients with diabetes if there is nephrotic range proteinuria with a disease duration of <5 years; persistent hematuria suggestive of an immune-mediated process; rapidly progressive proteinuria or renal insufficiency; or a family history of non-diabetic kidney disease, [3] and may be an indication for kidney biopsy. The absence of retinopathy has been utilized as a criterion for biopsy is adult populations, but the association between retinopathy and DKD in youth with type 2 diabetes is unknown.

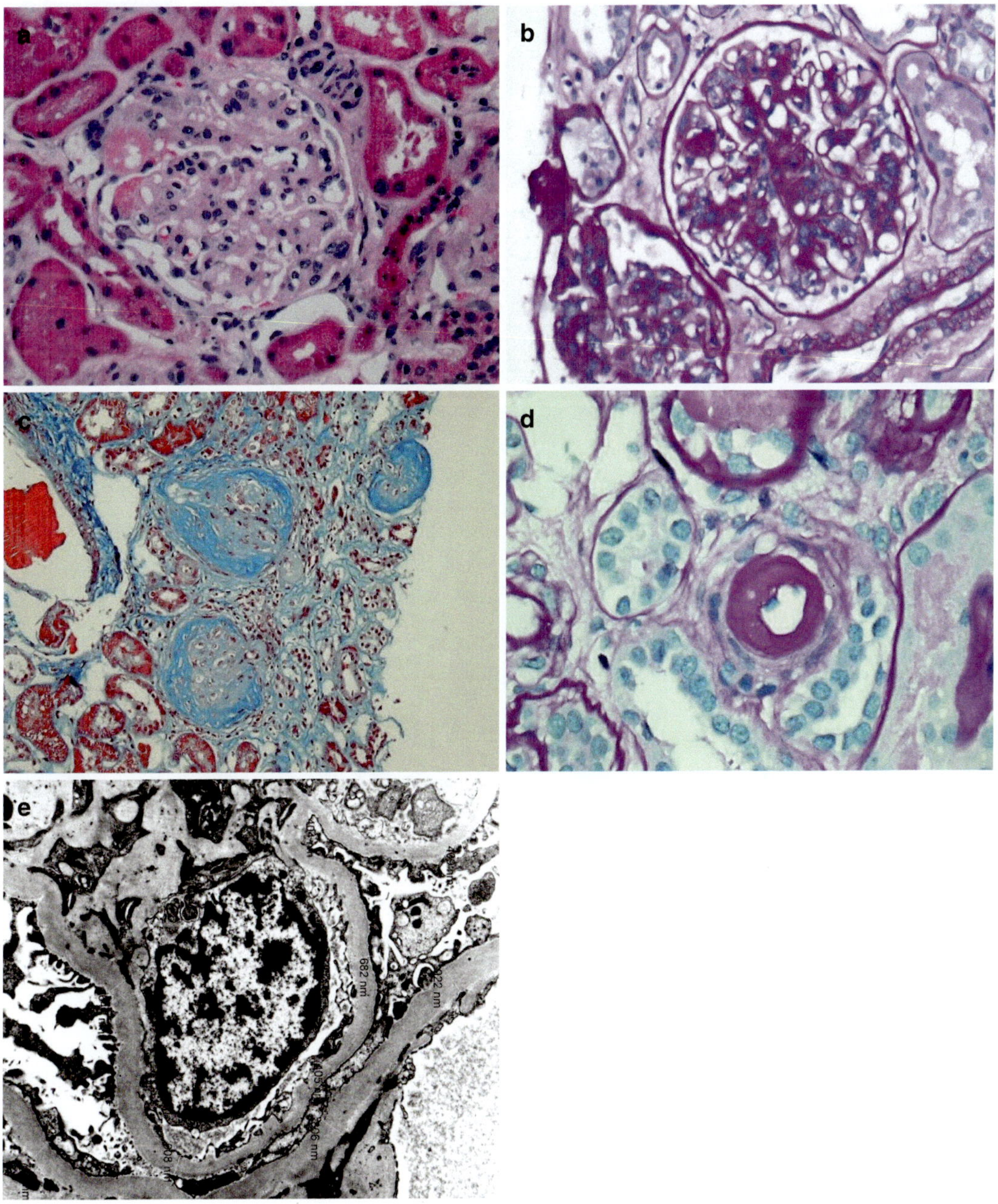

Fig. 32.1 Kidney pathology in an adolescent with type 1 diabetes for 10 years with poor glycemic control showing characteristic features of diabetic kidney disease. (**a**) Hematoxylin + Eosin [H+E] stain showing diffuse diabetic glomerulosclerosis with mesangial matrix expansion and secondary focal segmental glomerulosclerosis and hyalinosis. (**b**) Periodic acid-Schiff [PAS] stain showing moderate mesangial matrix expansion. (**c**) Trichrome stain showing three globally sclerosed glomeruli and associated severe tubular atrophy and interstitial fibrosis. (**d**) PAS stain showing nodular hyaline arteriolosclerosis. (**e**) Electron micrograph showing diffuse glomerular basement membrane thickening (>600 nm) and patchy epithelial cell foot process effacement. (*Images courtesy of Dr. Ian Gibson, University of Manitoba*)

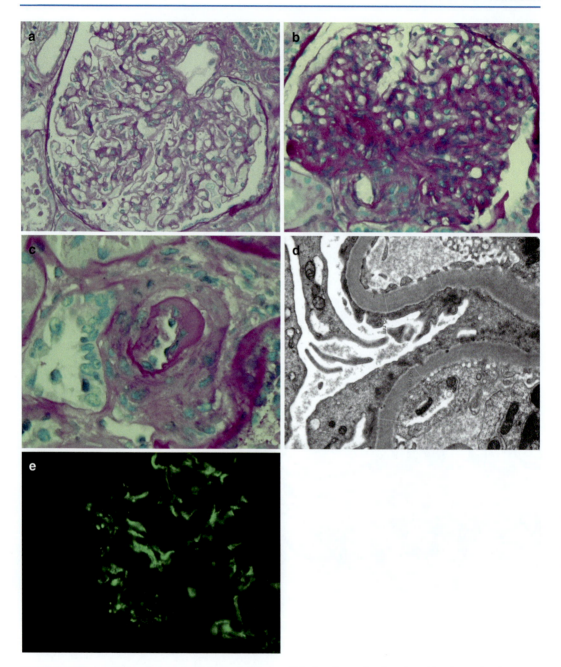

Fig. 32.2 Kidney pathology in a youth with type 2 diabetes and albuminuria. (**a–c**) Light microscopy (Periodic acid-Schiff stain), (**d**) Electron microscopy. (**e**) Immunofluorescence. Findings include (**a**) Glomerular hypertrophy; (**b**) Hilar focal segmental glomerulosclerosis; (**c**) Nodular arteriolar hyalinosis; (**d**) Early diffuse diabetic glomerulosclerosis with glomerular basement membrane thickening up to 500 nm; (**e**) Mesangial staining for IgA indicating co-existent non-proliferative IgA nephropathy. (*Images courtesy of Dr. Ian Gibson, University of Manitoba*)

Screening and Monitoring

Albuminuria

Yearly screening for albuminuria is recommended when patients with type 1 diabetes are at least 11 years of age and have had 5 years of diabetes [59] and at diagnosis for youth with type 2 diabetes [60]. Random urines are acceptable as initial screening tests. However, a first morning urine or overnight urine collection is required to confirm the diagnosis of non-orthostatic albuminuria if the random sample is abnormal [2]. The confirmation of persistent albuminuria also requires albuminuria in 2/3 samples at least 1 month apart over a 6-month time period [61]. Thresholds for albuminuria differ slightly across consensus guidelines. The Diabetes Canada urine albumin:creatinine ratio (ACR) threshold for albuminuria is >2 mg/mmol in adults with DKD (equivalent to a 24 h albumin excretion >30 mg/day) [3]; the American Diabetes Association utilizes an ACR threshold of 30 mg/g (3.39 mg/mmol); and the International Society for Pediatric and Adolescent Diabetes ACR threshold is >3.5 mg/mmol for males and >2.5 mg/mmol for females. KDIGO utilizes an ACR threshold of >3 mg/mmol [61]. Limitations of this test are false positives due to the high prevalence of orthostatic proteinuria in adolescents and intercurrent illness causing transient albuminuria. In addition, reduction in kidney function in the absence of albuminuria occurs in a subset of patients with DKD [62].

Glomerular Filtration Rate

Annual measurement of creatinine to determine the eGFR is also recommended, although the best equation for estimating eGFR in this population is unknown. As many youth have hyperfiltration, elevated eGFRs are quite common. For youth with type 1 diabetes, options for eGFR include the CKiD equation [63], with or without the addition cystatin C, or other cystatin C based equations if cystatin C is available [64]. Equations utilized in the youth onset type 2 diabetes population include the Zappitelli equation [65, 66] and the iCARE study equation, which was developed and validated in an Indigenous population in Canada [67]. All existing formulas have limitations, and therefore should be interpreted with caution.

Blood Pressure

Blood pressure should be measured at each healthcare encounter. Based on the American Academy of Pediatrics clinical practice guidelines, blood pressure is considered elevated at a threshold of >90th percentile for age, sex and height or >120/80 in adolescents >13 years of age. Hypertension is defined as >95th percentile for age, sex and height or>130/80 in adolescents >13 years of age. In addition, routine performance of 24-h ambulatory blood pressure is strongly recommended in children with diabetes to assess hypertension severity and to evaluate circadian blood pressure patterns [68].

Lipids

Screening for dyslipidemia is recommended after stabilization of hyperglycemia in children with type 1 diabetes after age 11. As fasting lipid profiles are not always feasible, non-fasting screening is acceptable. If abnormal, a fasting sample should be obtained [69].

Treatment

Preventive strategies should be considered early in the disease course of diabetes. Intervention during childhood and adolescence prevents or delays complications [70]. Specific treatment targets for DKD include glycemic and blood pressure control. Optimization of glycemic control is critical for preventing or delaying albuminuria and progression in youth with both types of diabetes. The target HbA1c and blood pressure is the same for both types of diabetes: HbA1c <7% and the blood pressure <90th percentile for age, sex and height or <130/80 in adolescents >13 years.

Blood Sugar Control

Treatment with insulin is required in youth with type 1 diabetes. Pharmacologic therapy approved for youth with type 2 diabetes includes insulin or metformin [60]. Efforts to address lifestyle related risk factors for diabetes, especially in patients with type 2 diabetes, include healthy eating, with a diet high in vegetables, fruits, whole grains, fiber, legumes, plant-based proteins, unsaturated fats, and nuts, with few processed meats, refined carbohydrates and sweetened beverages; light and vigorous exercise; and adequate sleep quality and quantity [60]. Specific recommendations include 60 min of daily moderate-to-vigorous physical activity, screen time limited to no more than 2 h per day, limiting sitting, and time spent indoors [71]. Team-based, multidisciplinary care, including nutrition specialists, to support patients with these recommendations is critical. In addition, the screening and treatment of mental health co-morbidities is essential [25, 72]. It is important, however, to provide counselling to patients that is non-judgmental, and considers the social context of the individual, the impact of food insecurity [73] and access to safe places to be active [74]. Many youth with type 2 diabetes confront stigma, which can significantly add to the challenges of managing a chronic disease [75]. Healthcare providers have a responsibility to educate themselves about systemic barriers that families confront, and to focus less on individual behavior strategies and blame.

Smoking Cessation

Implementation of strategies to promote smoking prevention or cessation is also important [76].

Lipid Management

The intervention for hyperlipidemia depends on the severity of the problem. An LDL cholesterol >2.6 mmol/L warrants a low fat diet and increased exercise. An LDL >3.4 mmol/L is the threshold for initiation of a statin in children over age 10, with a target of <2.6 mmol/L [69].

Hypertension Management

The first line medications for the treatment of hypertension and albuminuria are RAAS inhibitors, including angiotensin-converting enzyme inhibitors (ACEi) and angiotensin receptor blockers (ARBs). Many intervention studies in adults have documented decreased progression of albuminuria and attenuated decline of GFR with these therapies [77, 78]. These drugs are safe and effective in children with CKD [79]. The AdDIT trial, which randomized youth with type 1 diabetes in the upper tertile of ACR to an ACEi, a statin or both, did not identify a significant effect on albuminuria progression over 2–4 years [33]. Hence, initiation of these medications prior to the onset of hypertension or albuminuria is not recommended.

Combinations of ACEs and ARBs have been associated with safety concerns, including increased risk of acute kidney injury and hyperkalemia [80], and are therefore not recommended. Side effects of ACEi include hyperkalemia, cough, and a decrease in eGFR. They should be avoided if eGFR <30 mL/min/1.73 m^2. Monitoring of serum creatinine and potassium is indicated within 2 weeks of starting the medication. In addition, due to the potential teratogenicity in pregnancy, pre-conception counselling in postmenarchal girls is essential [81].

Novel Therapies

SGLT2 inhibitor trials, including The Canagliflozin and Renal Events in Diabetes with Established Nephropathy Clinical Evaluation (CREDENCE) trial, have demonstrated improved

32 Diabetic Kidney Disease

glycemic control, weight loss, and renal protection in adults with type 2 diabetes [82]. Randomized trials which include adolescents with type 2 diabetes are ongoing. These drugs are associated with an increased risk of euglycemic diabetic ketoacidosis; therefore, they likely warrant significant caution in adolescents. Guidelines now consider SGLT2 inhibitors standard of care for adults with type 2 diabetes [83]. They have the potential to significantly delay DKD progression in adolescents if safety is demonstrated.

Glucagon-like peptide-1 agonists have been studied and approved by the United States Food and Drug Administration in children and adolescents with type 2 diabetes [84]. The potential kidney benefits, beyond glycemic control, are not fully understood. Newer studies are also focusing on AGE inhibitors, metabolic memory resulting from epigenetic changes from hyperglycemia, and incretin-related drugs for their effects on renal outcomes [85] (Table 32.2).

Table 32.2 Screening, risk factors and treatment of diabetic kidney disease in youth with type 1 and type 2 diabetes

	Type 1 diabetes	Type 2 diabetes
Timing of screening	11 years with 2–5 years diabetes duration	At diagnosis
Screening method	Random urine for albumin:creatinine ratio annually Serum creatinine and/or Cystatin C for calculation of eGFR annually	
Follow-up screening	If random urine ACR 30mg/g to align or 3mg/mmol then collect 2–3 first am urine samples over the next 6 months, at least 1 month apart	
Risk factors	Hyperglycemia Hypertension Lipid abnormalities Smoking Duration of diabetes Post-pubertal status	Hyperglycemia Hypertension Minority ethnicity Socioeconomic factors
Treatment	Diet and exercise, smoking cessation Angiotensin converting enzyme inhibitors or angiotensin receptor blockers for persistent urine ACR 30mg/g or 3mg/mmol and/or blood pressure >130/80	

Table 32.2 (continued)

	Type 1 diabetes	Type 2 diabetes
Targets	HbA1c <7% Blood pressure <130/80 >13 years or <90th percentile for age, sex, height <13 years	
Treatment considerations	Multidisciplinary teams Mental health assessment and treatment	

eGFR estimated glomerular filtration rate, *ACR* albumin:creatinine ratio, *HbA1c* glycosylated hemoglobin A1c

References

1. Corr. 2016 CORR statistics: treatment of end-stage organ failure in Canada, 2005 to 2014. 2016.
2. Tuttle KR, Bakris GL, Bilous RW, Chiang JL, de Boer IH, Goldstein-Fuchs J, et al. Diabetic kidney disease: a report from an ADA consensus conference. Am J Kidney Dis. 2014;64(4):510–33.
3. Diabetes Canada Clinical Practice Guidelines Expert Committee, McFarlane P, Cherney D, Gilbert RE, Senior P. Chronic kidney disease in diabetes. Can J Diabetes. 2018;42 Suppl 1:S201–9.
4. Mayer-Davis EJ, Lawrence JM, Dabelea D, Divers J, Isom S, Dolan L, et al. Incidence trends of type 1 and type 2 diabetes among youths, 2002-2012. N Engl J Med. 2017;376(15):1419–29.
5. DIAMOND Project Group. Incidence and trends of childhood type 1 diabetes worldwide 1990–1999. Diabet Med. 2006;23(8):857–66.
6. Dabelea D. The accelerating epidemic of childhood diabetes. Lancet. 2009;373(9680):1999–2000.
7. Maple-Brown LJ, Graham S, McKee J, Wicklow B. Walking the path together: incorporating indigenous knowledge in diabetes research. Lancet Diabetes Endocrinol. 2020;8(7):559–60.
8. Brave Heart MY, DeBruyn LM. The American Indian holocaust: healing historical unresolved grief. Am Indian Alsk Native Ment Health Res. 1998;8(2):56–78.
9. Mayer-Davis EJ, Dabelea D, Lawrence JM. Incidence trends of type 1 and type 2 diabetes among youths, 2002–2012. N Engl J Med. 2017;377(3):301.
10. Dabelea D, Mayer-Davis EJ, Saydah S, Imperatore G, Linder B, Divers J, et al. Prevalence of type 1 and type 2 diabetes among children and adolescents from 2001 to 2009. JAMA. 2014;311(17):1778–86.
11. Divers J, Mayer-Davis EJ, Lawrence JM, Isom S, Dabelea D, Dolan L, et al. Trends in incidence of type 1 and type 2 diabetes among youths—selected counties

11. and Indian reservations, United States, 2002–2015. MMWR Morb Mortal Wkly Rep. 2020;69(6):161–5.

12. Norris JM, Johnson RK, Stene LC. Type 1 diabetes-early life origins and changing epidemiology. Lancet Diabetes Endocrinol. 2020;8(3):226–38.

13. Dabelea D, Hamman RF, Knowler WC. Diabetes in youth. In: Cowie CC, Casagrande SS, Menke A, Cissell MA, Eberhardt MS, et al., editors. Diabetes in America. Bethesda; 2018.

14. Menke A, Casagrande S, Cowie CC. Prevalence of diabetes in adolescents aged 12 to 19 years in the United States, 2005–2014. JAMA. 2016;316(3):344–5.

15. Menke A, Casagrande S, Cowie CC. US trends for diabetes prevalence among adults—reply. JAMA. 2016;315(7):705–6.

16. Narva AS. The spectrum of kidney disease in American Indians. Kidney Int Suppl. 2003;(83):S3–S7.

17. Fiorentino M, Bolignano D, Tesar V, Pisano A, Biesen WV, Tripepi G, et al. Renal biopsy in patients with diabetes: a pooled meta-analysis of 48 studies. Nephrol Dial Transplant. 2017;32(1):97–110.

18. Diabetes Control and Complications Trial Research Group, Nathan DM, Genuth S, Lachin J, Cleary P, et al. The effect of intensive treatment of diabetes on the development and progression of long-term complications in insulin-dependent diabetes mellitus. N Engl J Med. 1993;329(14):977–86.

19. Intensive blood-glucose control with sulphonylureas or insulin compared with conventional treatment and risk of complications in patients with type 2 diabetes (UKPDS 33). UK Prospective Diabetes Study (UKPDS) Group. Lancet. 1998;352(9131):837–853.

20. Diabetes Control and Complications Trial (DCCT)/ Epidemiology of Diabetes Interventions and Complications (EDIC) Study Research Group. Intensive Diabetes treatment and cardiovascular outcomes in type 1 diabetes: the DCCT/EDIC study 30-year follow-up. Diabetes Care. 2016;39(5):686–93.

21. Carino M, Elia Y, Sellers EA, Curtis J, McGavock J, Scholey J, Hamilton J, Clarson C, Pinto T, Hadjiyannakis S, Martens L, Samaan C, Ho J, Nour M, Panagiotopoulos C, Jetha M, Gabbs M, Mahmud F, Wicklow B, Dart A. A comparison of clinical and social characteristics of Canadian youth living with type 2 and type 1 diabetes. Can J Diabetes. 2021;45(5):428–35.

22. Dabelea D, Stafford JM, Mayer-Davis EJ, D'Agostino R Jr, Dolan L, Imperatore G, et al. Association of type 1 diabetes vs type 2 diabetes diagnosed during childhood and adolescence with complications during teenage years and young adulthood. JAMA. 2017;317(8):825–35.

23. Ducat L, Rubenstein A, Philipson LH, Anderson BJ. A review of the mental health issues of diabetes conference. Diabetes Care. 2015;38(2):333–8.

24. Mogensen CE. Progression of nephropathy in long-term diabetics with proteinuria and effect of initial anti-hypertensive treatment. Scand J Clin Lab Invest. 1976;36(4):383–8.

25. Dart AB, Wicklow B, Blydt-Hansen TD, Sellers EAC, Malik S, Chateau D, et al. A holistic approach to risk for early kidney injury in indigenous youth with type 2 diabetes: a proof of concept paper from the iCARE cohort. Can J Kidney Health Dis. 2019;6:2054358119838836.

26. Eppens MC, Craig ME, Cusumano J, Hing S, Chan AK, Howard NJ, et al. Prevalence of diabetes complications in adolescents with type 2 compared with type 1 diabetes. Diabetes Care. 2006;29(6):1300–6.

27. Donaghue KC, Marcovecchio ML, Wadwa RP, Chew EY, Wong TY, Calliari LE, et al. ISPAD clinical practice consensus guidelines 2018: microvascular and macrovascular complications in children and adolescents. Pediatr Diabetes. 2018;19(Suppl 27):262–74.

28. Shah AS, Dabelea D, Talton JW, Urbina EM, D Agostino RB Jr, Wadwa RP, et al. Smoking and arterial stiffness in youth with type 1 diabetes: the SEARCH cardiovascular disease study. J Pediatr. 2014;165(1):110–6.

29. Maahs DM, Snively BM, Bell RA, Dolan L, Hirsch I, Imperatore G, et al. Higher prevalence of elevated albumin excretion in youth with type 2 than type 1 diabetes: the SEARCH for Diabetes in Youth study. Diabetes Care. 2007;30(10):2593–8.

30. Dart AB, Sellers EA, Martens PJ, Rigatto C, Brownell MD, Dean HJ. High burden of kidney disease in youth-onset type 2 diabetes. Diabetes Care. 2012;35(6):1265.

31. Tonneijck L, Muskiet MH, Smits MM, van Bommel EJ, Heerspink HJ, van Raalte DH, et al. Glomerular hyperfiltration in diabetes: mechanisms, clinical significance, and treatment. J Am Soc Nephrol. 2017;28(4):1023–39.

32. An Y, Xu F, Le W, Ge Y, Zhou M, Chen H, et al. Renal histologic changes and the outcome in patients with diabetic nephropathy. Nephrol Dial Transplant. 2015;30(2):257–66.

33. Marcovecchio ML, Chiesa ST, Armitage J, Daneman D, Donaghue KC, Jones TW, et al. Renal and cardiovascular risk according to tertiles of urinary albumin-to-creatinine ratio: the adolescent type 1 diabetes cardio-renal intervention trial (AdDIT). Diabetes Care. 2018;41(9):1963–9.

34. TODAY Study Group. Rapid rise in hypertension and nephropathy in youth with type 2 diabetes: the TODAY clinical trial. Diabetes Care. 2013;36(6):1735–41.

35. Hill K, Ward P, Grace BS, Gleadle J. Social disparities in the prevalence of diabetes in Australia and in the development of end stage renal disease due to diabetes for Aboriginal and Torres Strait Islanders in Australia and Maori and Pacific Islanders in New Zealand. BMC Public Health. 2017;17(1):802.

36. Pavkov ME, Bennett PH, Knowler WC, Krakoff J, Sievers ML, Nelson RG. Effect of youth-onset type 2 diabetes mellitus on incidence of end-stage renal

36. disease and mortality in young and middle-aged Pima Indians. JAMA. 2006;296(4):421–6.
37. Tran S, Chen YW, Chenier I, Chan JS, Quaggin S, Hebert MJ, et al. Maternal diabetes modulates renal morphogenesis in offspring. J Am Soc Nephrol. 2008;19(5):943–52.
38. Hoy WE, Samuel T, Mott SA, Kincaid-Smith PS, Fogo AB, Dowling JP, et al. Renal biopsy findings among indigenous Australians: a nationwide review. Kidney Int. 2012;82(12):1321–31.
39. Rosolowsky ET, Skupien J, Smiles AM, Niewczas M, Roshan B, Stanton R, et al. Risk for ESRD in type 1 diabetes remains high despite renoprotection. J Am Soc Nephrol. 2011;22(3):545–53.
40. Diabetes Control and Complications Trial/Epidemiology of Diabetes Interventions and Complications (DCCT/EDIC) Research Group, Nathan DM, Zinman B, Cleary PA, et al. Modern-day clinical course of type 1 diabetes mellitus after 30 years' duration: the diabetes control and complications trial/epidemiology of diabetes interventions and complications and Pittsburgh epidemiology of diabetes complications experience (1983–2005). Arch Intern Med. 2009;169(14):1307–16.
41. Bojestig M, Arnqvist HJ, Hermansson G, Karlberg BE, Ludvigsson J. Declining incidence of nephropathy in insulin-dependent diabetes mellitus. N Engl J Med. 1994;330(1):15–8.
42. Rossing P, Rossing K, Jacobsen P, Parving HH. Unchanged incidence of diabetic nephropathy in IDDM patients. Diabetes. 1995;44(7):739–43.
43. Wang Z, Hoy WE. Remaining lifetime risk for developing end stage renal disease among Australian Aboriginal people with diabetes. Diabetes Res Clin Pract. 2014;103(3):e24–6.
44. Zeitler P. Progress in understanding youth-onset type 2 diabetes in the United States: recent lessons from clinical trials. World J Pediatr. 2019;15(4):315–21.
45. Dart AB, Wicklow BA, Sellers EA, Dean HJ, Malik S, Walker J, et al. The improving renal complications in adolescents with type 2 diabetes through the REsearch (iCARE) cohort study: rationale and protocol. Can J Diabetes. 2014;38(5):349–55.
46. Groop PH, Thomas MC, Moran JL, Waden J, Thorn LM, Makinen VP, et al. The presence and severity of chronic kidney disease predicts all-cause mortality in type 1 diabetes. Diabetes. 2009;58(7):1651–8.
47. Afkarian M, Sachs MC, Kestenbaum B, Hirsch IB, Tuttle KR, Himmelfarb J, et al. Kidney disease and increased mortality risk in type 2 diabetes. J Am Soc Nephrol. 2013;24(2):302–8.
48. Anderson S, Brenner BM. Pathogenesis of diabetic glomerulopathy: hemodynamic considerations. Diabetes Metab Rev. 1988;4(2):163–77.
49. Hostetter TH. Hyperfiltration and glomerulosclerosis. Semin Nephrol. 2003;23(2):194–9.
50. Krolewski AS. Progressive renal decline: the new paradigm of diabetic nephropathy in type 1 diabetes. Diabetes Care. 2015;38(6):954–62.
51. Macisaac RJ, Jerums G. Diabetic kidney disease with and without albuminuria. Curr Opin Nephrol Hypertens. 2011;20(3):246–57.
52. Macisaac RJ, Ekinci EI, Jerums G. Markers of and risk factors for the development and progression of diabetic kidney disease. Am J Kidney Dis. 2014;63(2 Suppl 2):S39–62.
53. Osterby R. Morphometric studies of the peripheral glomerular basement membrane in early juvenile diabetes. I. Development of initial basement membrane thickening. Diabetologia. 1972;8(2):84–92.
54. Mauer SM, Steffes MW, Ellis EN, Sutherland DE, Brown DM, Goetz FC. Structural-functional relationships in diabetic nephropathy. J Clin Invest. 1984;74(4):1143–55.
55. Brito PL, Fioretto P, Drummond K, Kim Y, Steffes MW, Basgen JM, et al. Proximal tubular basement membrane width in insulin-dependent diabetes mellitus. Kidney Int. 1998;53(3):754–61.
56. Tervaert TW, Mooyaart AL, Amann K, Cohen AH, Cook HT, Drachenberg CB, et al. Pathologic classification of diabetic nephropathy. J Am Soc Nephrol. 2010;21(4):556–63.
57. Sellers EA, Blydt-Hansen TD, Dean HJ, Gibson IW, Birk PE, Ogborn M. Macroalbuminuria and renal pathology in first nation youth with type 2 diabetes. Diabetes Care. 2009;32(5):786–90.
58. Osterby R, Gall MA, Schmitz A, Nielsen FS, Nyberg G, Parving HH. Glomerular structure and function in proteinuric type 2 (non-insulin-dependent) diabetic patients. Diabetologia. 1993;36(10):1064–70.
59. Diabetes Canada Clinical Practice Guidelines Expert Committee, Wherrett DK, Ho J, Huot C, Legault L, Nakhla M, et al. Type 1 diabetes in children and adolescents. Can J Diabetes. 2018;42 Suppl 1:S234–46.
60. Diabetes Canada Clinical Practice Guidelines Expert Committee, Panagiotopoulos C, Hadjiyannakis S, Henderson M. Type 2 diabetes in children and adolescents. Can J Diabetes. 2018;42 Suppl 1:S247–54.
61. Kidney Disease Improving Global Outcomes CKDWG. KDIGO 2012 clinical practice guideline for the evaluation and management of chronic kidney disease. 2013;3:1.
62. MacIsaac RJ, Tsalamandris C, Panagiotopoulos S, Smith TJ, McNeil KJ, Jerums G. Nonalbuminuric renal insufficiency in type 2 diabetes. Diabetes Care. 2004;27(1):195–200.
63. Schwartz GJ, Munoz A, Schneider MF, Mak RH, Kaskel F, Warady BA, et al. New equations to estimate GFR in children with CKD. J Am Soc Nephrol. 2009;20(3):629–37.
64. Larsson A, Malm J, Grubb A, Hansson LO. Calculation of glomerular filtration rate expressed in mL/min from plasma cystatin C values in mg/L. Scand J Clin Lab Invest. 2004;64(1):25–30.
65. Bjornstad P, Laffel L, Lynch J, El Ghormli L, Weinstock RS, Tollefsen SE, et al. Elevated serum uric acid is associated with greater risk for hypertension and diabetic kidney diseases in obese adolescents with type 2 diabetes: an observational analysis

66. Zappitelli M, Parvex P, Joseph L, Paradis G, Grey V, Lau S, et al. Derivation and validation of cystatin C-based prediction equations for GFR in children. Am J Kidney Dis. 2006;48(2):221–30.
67. Dart AB, McGavock J, Sharma A, Chateau D, Schwartz GJ, Blydt-Hansen T. Estimating glomerular filtration rate in youth with obesity and type 2 diabetes: the iCARE study equation. Pediatr Nephrol. 2019;34(9):1565–74.
68. Flynn JT, Kaelber DC, Baker-Smith CM, Blowey D, Carroll AE, Daniels SR, et al. Clinical practice guideline for screening and management of high blood pressure in children and adolescents. Pediatrics. 2017;140(3):e20171904.
69. de Ferranti SD, de Boer IH, Fonseca V, Fox CS, Golden SH, Lavie CJ, et al. Type 1 diabetes mellitus and cardiovascular disease: a scientific statement from the American Heart Association and American Diabetes Association. Diabetes Care. 2014;37(10):2843–63.
70. DCCT/EDIC Research Group, de Boer IH, Sun W, Cleary PA, Lachin JM, Molitch ME, Steffes MW, Zinman B. Intensive diabetes therapy and glomerular filtration rate in type 1 diabetes. N Engl J Med. 2011;365(25):2366–76.
71. Piercy KL, Troiano RP, Ballard RM, Carlson SA, Fulton JE, Galuska DA, et al. The physical activity guidelines for Americans. JAMA. 2018;320(19):2020–8.
72. Buchberger B, Huppertz H, Krabbe L, Lux B, Mattivi JT, Siafarikas A. Symptoms of depression and anxiety in youth with type 1 diabetes: A systematic review and meta-analysis. Psychoneuroendocrinology. 2016;70:70–84.
73. Power EM. Conceptualizing food security or aboriginal people in Canada. Can J Public Health. 2008;99(2):95–7.
74. Bell HS, Odumosu F, Martinez-Hume AC, Howard HA, Hunt LM. Racialized risk in clinical care: clinician vigilance and patient responsibility. Med Anthropol. 2019;38(3):224–38.
75. Wicklow B, Dart A, McKee J, Griffiths A, Malik S, Quoquat S, Bruce S. First nations adolescents experiences living with type 2 diabetes: a focus group study. Can Med Assoc J. 2021;193(12):E403–9.
76. Harvey J, Chadi N, Canadian Paediatric Society, Adolescent Health Committee. Preventing smoking in children and adolescents: recommendations for practice and policy. Paediatr Child Health. 2016;21(4):209–21.
77. Lewis EJ, Hunsicker LG, Bain RP, Rohde RD. The effect of angiotensin-converting-enzyme inhibition on diabetic nephropathy. The Collaborative Study Group. N Engl J Med. 1993;329(20):1456–62.
78. Brenner BM, Cooper ME, de Zeeuw D, Keane WF, Mitch WE, Parving HH, et al. Effects of losartan on renal and cardiovascular outcomes in patients with type 2 diabetes and nephropathy. N Engl J Med. 2001;345(12):861–9.
79. ESCAPE Trial Group, Wuhl E, Trivelli A, Picca S, Litwin M, Peco-Antic A, et al. Strict blood-pressure control and progression of renal failure in children. N Engl J Med. 2009;361(17):1639–50.
80. Fried LF, Emanuele N, Zhang JH, Brophy M, Conner TA, Duckworth W, et al. Combined angiotensin inhibition for the treatment of diabetic nephropathy. N Engl J Med. 2013;369(20):1892–903.
81. Bullo M, Tschumi S, Bucher BS, Bianchetti MG, Simonetti GD. Pregnancy outcome following exposure to angiotensin-converting enzyme inhibitors or angiotensin receptor antagonists: a systematic review. Hypertension. 2012;60(2):444–50.
82. Heerspink HJ, Desai M, Jardine M, Balis D, Meininger G, Perkovic V. Canagliflozin slows progression of renal function decline independently of glycemic effects. J Am Soc Nephrol. 2017;28(1):368–75.
83. Kidney Disease: Improving Global Outcomes Diabetes Work Group. KDIGO 2020 clinical practice guideline for diabetes management in chronic kidney disease. Kidney Int. 2020;98(4S):S1–S115.
84. Tamborlane WV, Barrientos-Perez M, Fainberg U, Frimer-Larsen H, Hafez M, Hale PM, et al. Liraglutide in children and adolescents with type 2 diabetes. N Engl J Med. 2019;381(7):637–46.
85. Yamazaki T, Mimura I, Tanaka T, Nangaku M. Treatment of diabetic kidney disease: current and future. Diabetes Metab J. 2021;45(1):11–26.

Disordered Hemostasis and Renal Disorders

33

Sara Rodriguez-Lopez, Verna Yiu,
Stephanie Carlin, and Leonardo R. Brandão

Hemostasis

Hemostasis constitutes a physiologic response of the human body to injury regulated by the dynamic equilibrium between pro-coagulant and natural anticoagulant mechanisms. An inherited and/or acquired defect in any of those pro- or anticoagulant forces may "tip the clotting balance", resulting in either bleeding or excessive hypercoagulability.

Endothelial cells are one of the major components of the hemostatic system, covering the vascular structures and having a primordial anticoagulant role when the body is in a steady state. However, after an endothelial injury occurs, a process entitled primary hemostasis ensues, where platelets play a major role towards thrombus formation particularly under high shear stress

S. Rodriguez-Lopez (✉) · V. Yiu
Division of Nephrology, Department of Pediatrics, Alberta Health Services/University of Alberta, Edmonton, AB, Canada
e-mail: sara7@ualberta.ca; verna.yiu@ualberta.ca

S. Carlin
Department of Pharmacy, Hamilton Health Sciences, Hamilton, ON, Canada
e-mail: carlins@hhsc.ca

L. R. Brandão
Department of Pediatrics, The Hospital for Sick Children, Toronto, ON, Canada

Dalla Lana School of Public Health, University of Toronto, Toronto, ON, Canada
e-mail: leonardo.brandao@sickkids.ca

forces (e.g., arterial circulatory component). Secondly, in conjunction with the now activated platelets and their newly exposed negatively charged phospholipid (PL) membranes, the coagulation factors that are circulating in a non-active state are activated in sequence to promote the formation of an insoluble thrombus, which will ultimately anchor the platelet plug to the newly formed wound site, preventing excessive bleeding. The steps summarized above are part of the accepted model that integrates the hemostatic response, entitled the "cellular model" of the coagulation cascade [1]. The mechanisms of the second wave, called secondary hemostasis, are counterbalanced by the progressively increased activation of natural anticoagulant pathways, which will ultimately tailor down the formation of insoluble thrombus in an attempt to restrain its growth to the wound site. Additionally, the fibrinolytic system will also help contain the newly formed thrombus to the wound site by promoting a local thrombolytic effect to digest thrombus formed in excess (Fig. 33.1). Moreover, noncoagulation components in blood, such as red blood cells (RBC) and white blood cells (WBC), also have a contributory role in the hemostatic system. Understanding normal hemostasis is helpful and necessary to explain the pathophysiology of hemorrhage and thrombosis in patients with renal diseases.

© The Author(s), under exclusive license to Springer Nature Switzerland AG 2023
F. Schaefer, L. A. Greenbaum (eds.), *Pediatric Kidney Disease*,
https://doi.org/10.1007/978-3-031-11665-0_33

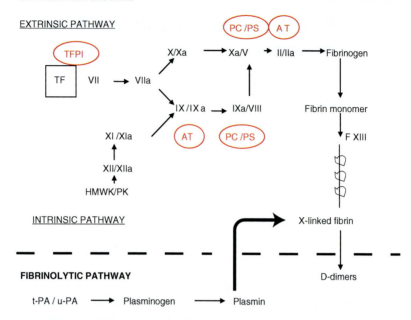

Fig. 33.1 The coagulation cascade and the fibrinolytic pathway. *Red*: natural coagulation inhibitors; *black*: pro-coagulant system: *bold*: fibrinolytic pathway. *PC* protein C, *PS* protein S, *AT* antithrombin, *TFPI* tissue factor pathway inhibitor, *TF* tissue factor, *VII* factor VII, *VIIa* activated factor VII, *X* factor X, *Xa* activated factor X, *V* factor V, *II* prothrombin, *IIa* thrombin, *IX* factor IX, *IXa* activated factor IX, *FXIII* factor XIII, *XII* factor XII, *XIIa* activated factor XII, *HMWK* high molecular weight kininogen, *PK* pre-kallikrein, *X-linked* cross linked, *t-PA* tissue plasminogen activator, *u-PA* urokinase

Primary Hemostasis

Vessel Wall

When a vessel wall is damaged, many different pro-coagulant components of the hemostatic system are activated to generate a clot (i.e., thrombus). The release of cytokines leading to vasoconstriction and activation of the local endothelial cells occurs immediately after injury. This process is a result of the neurogenic reflex when endothelin, a vasoconstrictive agent, is released from endothelial cells in a process that sustains hemostasis for an initial short period of time [2]. Additionally, serotonin, a substance which is released from dense granules of activated platelets, and thromboxane A2 (TXA2), a derivative of platelet membrane PL metabolism, stimulate smooth muscles of the vessel wall and augment the process of vasoconstriction [3].

Endothelium

Endothelial cells have a great influence on hemostasis because of their interaction with all parts of the hemostatic system. Endothelial cells produce several important substances directly or indirectly related to the hemostatic processes: [2, 3]

- Vasoactive substances
  - Nitric oxide (NO) and prostacyclin (PGI2), which are both potent vasodilators.
  - Heparan sulfates, a group of "heparin-like" compounds that prevent the initiation phase of the coagulation cascade.
- Pro-coagulant activation
  - Von Willebrand factor (VWF).
  - Coagulation cascade: tissue factor (TF) and factor VIII (FVIII).
- Anticoagulation mechanisms

(a) Natural anticoagulant pathways
- Protein C (PC)
- Protein S (PS)
- Thrombomodulin (TM)
- Endothelial PC receptor (EPCR).
- Tissue factor pathway inhibitor (TFPI).
(b) Fibrinolytic system
- Tissue-type plasminogen activator (t-PA)
- Urinary type plasminogen activator (u-PA).
- Plasminogen activator inhibitor type 1 (PAI-1).

In addition, the disruption of endothelial cells at the site of vascular injury exposes subendothelial matrix, which is an activator of platelets and of the coagulation system [3–5].

Platelets

Platelets are disc-like, anucleated cells generated by megakaryocytes in the bone marrow that have a major role in primary hemostasis. After the exposure of subendothelial matrix, circulating platelets adhere to the injured site in a process called "platelet adhesion." This first step of platelet activation results from the interaction between several glycoprotein (GP) complexes expressed by the platelet surface (e.g., GP Ib/IX/V, GP Ia/IIa and GP VI), with the subendothelial matrix. For instance, the complex named GP Ib/IX/V interacts with VWF under high shear conditions as the VWF molecule unfolds, exposing the domains which will bind to the GP complex expressed by the platelet membrane, promoting the platelet to vessel wall interaction that leads to adherence of platelets to subendothelial matrix. In addition, GP Ia/IIa and GP VI adhere directly to collagen fibers in subendothelial matrix [5, 6].

After platelet adhesion, platelet activation occurs rapidly. During this process, the many pro-coagulant substances contained within platelet granules are released, including calcium (Ca^{++}) and ADP from dense granules, FV, FXI, FXIII, VWF, platelet factor-4 (PF4) and other substances from alpha granules, all ultimately leading to further activation of other platelets. During this second step of platelet activation, platelets also change their shapes by remodeling their platelet cytoskeleton, to fully spread with pseudopodia and expose important platelet membrane PL, phosphatidylserine and phosphatidylethanolamine [4]. This process further increases the amount of activated platelet surface area, which is necessary for the next step of secondary hemostasis [4, 7].

The major platelet GP activated during this step is GP IIb/IIIa, which works with fibrinogen under low shear flow and VWF under high shear flow to promote platelet-platelet interactions, also known as platelet aggregation. Several agonists, such as ADP, collagen, arachidonic acid and thrombin at the damaged vessel wall, also play a role on specific receptors in this process [4, 5].

Secondary Hemostasis

The secondary hemostatic wave combines serial proteolytic reactions to activate coagulation proteins (i.e., coagulation factors), culminating in the formation of an insoluble fibrin clot (Fig. 33.1). Postulated in 1964, the original waterfall cascade model of coagulation is still helpful to explain the in vitro phenomenon evaluated by screening coagulation tests, namely the prothrombin time (PT) for the extrinsic pathway and the activated partial thromboplastin time (APTT) for the intrinsic pathway of the coagulation cascade [7, 8]. Coagulation factors are most often synthesized in the liver, and can be classified by their functions into a few distinct groups as follows: contact factors (include prekallikrein, high-molecular-weight kininogen, FXII and FXI), extrinsic tenase complex (comprises TF and activated FVIIa), intrinsic tenase complex (consists of both FVIIIa and FIXa), prothrombinase complex (includes FXa and FVa), thrombin (FIIa) (activates fibrinogen and FXIII, which stabilizes fibrin), and fibrinogen and factor XIII (FXIII), which work together to form a fibrin clot.

Anticoagulation System

There are three major systems of proteins that counteract the coagulation system by inactivating coagulation proteins.

(a) *Antithrombin* (AT; formerly known as ATIII) inhibits mainly FIIa and FXa. In addition, it also inactivates FIXa, FXIa and FXIIa. The liver synthesizes AT, which potentiates unfractionated heparin anticoagulant power by 1000-fold.
(b) *TFPI* inactivates the extrinsic tenase complex. TFPI is released from endothelial cells and platelets.
(c) *PC, PS and TM* work together to inhibit FVa and FVIIIa. After being released from endothelium and activated by thrombin, TM combines with TM receptor and EPCR to form a complex with PC. Then activated PC (APC) is released from the complex and works with PS to inhibit target factors. Both PC and PS are vitamin K-dependent enzymes and synthesized by the liver [2–7].

Fibrinolytic System

The fibrinolytic system is a complex system that lyses or "digests" fibrinogen and non-cross linked and cross-linked fibrin. There are many proteins involved in the fibrinolytic system [9] and these include:

(a) *Plasminogen, t- PA and u- PA* work together to lyse a clot.
(b) *α 2 - antiplasmin (α 2–AP)* is synthesized in the liver and inactivates plasmin by forming a 1:1 ratio complex.
(c) *α 2 - macroglobulin (α 2–M)* is a four-polypeptide protease that can inhibit plasmin and tPA.
(d) *Thrombin-activatable fibrinolytic inhibitor (TAFI)* is synthesized by the liver and activated by thrombin and plasmin. It inhibits fibrinolysis by cleaving some parts of fibrin, which prevent fibrin degradation by plasmin.

The final products of fibrinolysis are called fibrin degradation products (FDP), which consist of different-sized lysed fibrin-derived fragments. One of the FDP- laboratory tests, which is commonly used in clinical practice, is called D-dimer.

Other Components

(a) *Red Blood Cells (RBCs)*: in normal blood flow conditions, RBCs circulate in the central part of the flow within vessels while platelets flow along the vessel wall [4]. This blood rheology facilitates platelets reaching injured sites quicker. Patients with decreased red cell mass lose this mechanism, potentially having impaired platelet function. Nonetheless, hemolytic anemias may cause a hypercoagulable state leading to an increased risk for thromboembolic events (TEs) by other mechanisms [10].
(b) *White Blood Cells (WBCs)*: an extremely high number of WBC causes hyperviscosity of the blood and can result in thromboembolism in leukemic patients. In addition, monocytes can be activated and express TF in some specific conditions, contributing to thrombus formation [11].
(c) *Neutrophil Extracellular Traps (NETs):* an original defense mechanism by neutrophils and leukocytes to extrude their DNA and protein components (e.g., histones) to trap and kill pathogenic microorganisms, which can lead to pathogenic thrombosis [12].

Age-Appropriate Development of Hemostasis (Developmental Hemostasis)

Hemostasis evolves from the fetal period, starting at 10 weeks of gestational age.

Primary Hemostasis

(a) Vessel wall and endothelial cells: increased levels of glycosaminoglycans in the vessel walls of neonates promote antithrombotic property by working with AT, while increased levels of VWF and large VWF multimers from endothelial cells counteract this effect [13].

(b) Platelets: there is no difference in platelet numbers between healthy neonates and children. Conversely, the platelet count in preterm neonates can be lower than term neonates due to several factors. Platelets in full-term neonates express a lower quantity of specific receptors on the platelet surface. The response to several agonists may also be less pronounced in comparison to the response found in adult platelets. However, these observations suggestive of a likely platelet function defect in neonates is counterbalanced by a higher red cell mass, mean corpuscular volume (MCV), higher circulating VWF level and a higher proportion of large VWF multimers [14].

Secondary Hemostasis

At birth, the levels of vitamin K-dependent factors (prothrombin, FVII, FIX and FX), contact factors and FV are lower than in adults. In contrast, FVIII, VWF and TF levels are higher than in adults during the first 6 months of life, subsequently decreasing [15–18]. The levels of fibrinogen and FXIII are similar from birth to adulthood [15, 17, 18]. However, a study of endogenous thrombin potential (ETP) showed almost two-times higher levels in adults compared to children less than 5 years of age [18].

Anticoagulation System

At birth, the levels of AT and TFPI are lower than circulating adult levels. The same finding applies for PC and PS [15, 17, 18]. PS gradually increases to adult levels at 6 months of age; whereas, for PC circulating levels reach adult values only after 11 years of age [16].

Thrombolytic System

The levels of plasmin, PAI-1 and α_2-AP are lower at birth than in adults. In contrast, t-PA and α_2-M are much higher at birth than in adults. Most of the fibrinolytic proteins reach adult levels within 5 days of life, except plasminogen, which increases to adult levels at 6 months of age, and α_2-M, which is still elevated until the second to third decade of life. The level of u-PA measured in neonates remains controversial [8, 15].

Ultimately, healthy neonates and infants do not bleed spontaneously when challenged during birth despite their distinct platelet-related laboratory testing results. Likewise, despite having lower circulating levels of many of the natural anticoagulant pathways, neonates, infants, and children have an incidence of thrombosis that is much lower than the one reported in adults [19]. Moreover, venous thrombotic events in neonates and infants are almost invariably provoked. This contrast between laboratory and clinical findings highlights some of the limitations of current laboratory testing, as well as the yet unraveled aspects of developmental hemostasis.

Bleeding in Renal Disease

Uremic Coagulopathy

The association between uremia and bleeding was first described in 1764 by GB Morgagni. In 1836, Richard Bright published on 100 cases of patients with albuminous urine and also noted the connection between purpura and uremia. The observation that bleeding in uremic patients occurs despite having normal clotting factors led to the supposition that the primary abnormality must be within the platelet system [20]. Despite many theories and suppositions, the exact etiology of uremic coagulopathy remains poorly understood.

Clinical Manifestations

The occurrence of bleeding in uremia is twofold higher in those with chronic kidney disease (CKD) and has been widely reported [20–22]. This includes potential bleeding in many locations, including the skin and mucosa, the gastrointestinal tract, the retroperitoneum, ocular tissues, genitourinary system, and intracranial. There are potential risks of bleeding during surgery or post-operatively and from venipuncture and renal biopsy sites. Pleural and pericardial hemorrhagic effusions have also been described. Most of these reports have been in the adult population with only a few scattered reports of increased bleeding risk in uremic children [20]. Whether the adult risks of bleeding can be extrapolated to children is a question that is still unanswered, given the developmental hemostatic differences.

Pathogenesis

The levels and function of coagulation factors are normal in patients with CKD [23]. From these data, it is assumed that platelet dysfunction is primarily responsible for the increased bleeding risk due to uremia. When placed into normal plasma, uremic platelets demonstrate normal function, implying that causative factors are present in the surrounding uremic plasma. However, research has found that there are both intrinsic and extrinsic platelet abnormalities that result in the uremic coagulopathy.

Intrinsic Platelet Abnormalities

In CKD and uremia, the content of ADP and serotonin is reduced in the platelet granules. This is felt to be either an acquired storage pool defect or a defect in secretory mechanisms [23]. Cyclic adenosine monophosphate (cAMP) has been reported to be increased in CKD, which can affect the mobilization of calcium in response to stimulus and, ultimately, platelet activation. It may be through an imbalance among ADP, serotonin and cAMP that results in platelet activation defects. Other defects include low levels of GP Ib/V/IX in association with elevated levels of glycocalicin, a proteolytic byproduct released by GP Ib/V/IX when damaged on the platelet surface [24]. Thromboxane A2 levels, generated from free arachidonic acid, are also low in uremia and result in poor platelet adhesion and aggregation [25].

Platelet contractility defects may be another factor contributing to platelet dysfunction by reducing its mobility and secretory capacity [26]. In uremic states, platelets have deficient cytoskeletal proteins, such as α-actin and tropomyosin, with the abnormalities becoming more pronounced after activation by thrombin.

Platelet: Vessel Wall Abnormalities

Levels of VWF and fibrinogen are normal in uremic states [22, 23]. There is normal surface expression of the platelet receptor GP Ib/V/IX, although the total levels of GP Ib/V/IX have been found to be suboptimal [24]. It has also been shown that there is impaired binding of VWF to GP 1b/V/IX and that this results in lower levels of TXA2 and ADP, both necessary to stabilize hemostatic plugs [27]. Another noted abnormality is reduced binding capacity of VWF and fibrinogen to GP IIb/IIIa, resulting in reduced platelet adhesion to injured endothelium. This may be secondary to receptor blockade by fibrinogen, or through substances that are dialyzable, as dialysis improves this anomaly.

Other extrinsic factors that might come into play include platelets and prostaglandins [28–30]. Anemia in CKD may influence platelet function through changes in laminar blood flow, as previously noted. A reduction in hematocrit can change platelet travel from where it is normally at the periphery of a blood vessel to the central part where erythrocytes traverse. Reduced contact with vessel wall results in stimulation of platelet ADP release and activation of PGI-1, which reduces platelet activity. Prostaglandin-I2 (PGI2) is a vasodilator released by endothelial cells and inhibits platelet function through its action on adenylyl cyclase and its modulating effects on cAMP and calcium mobilization within platelets. Although several studies have shown increased production of PGI2 in endothelium of uremic models, blockage of PGI2 production does not result in improved coagulation, thereby suggesting that there are other factors that are involved in platelet dysfunction in renal failure. Vasoactive substances like nitric oxide are increased in CKD, which can further inhibit platelet function.

Circulating uremic toxins may also play a role in uremic coagulopathy. Substances such as urea, creatinine, phenol, phenolic acids and guanidino-succinic acid (GSA) have all been investigated for their potential effects on platelet function [24]. GSA inhibits the second wave of ADP-induced platelet aggregation. This is further supported by the observation that dialysis can partially correct these defects.

Finally, platelet number and volume are both reduced in uremia [30]. Platelet numbers are lower in uremia when compared to healthy controls, although they are rarely less than 80×10^9/L. The reduction in platelet volume can further reduce the amount of circulating platelet mass, resulting in ineffectual platelet contact with injured endothelium.

Treatment

Treatment for uremic coagulopathy in the past was based on its ability to normalize the prolonged bleeding time (BT) observed in uremic patients. However, BT has no in vivo correlation with risk of bleeding, so that treatment should only be directed towards active cases of bleeding in the setting of uremia. There is also limited evidence that prophylactic treatment reduces the bleeding risk [31]. Treatment should therefore be utilized if there is active bleeding and includes dialysis, erythropoietin, desmopressin (DDAVP), estrogens, and cryoprecipitate [27, 28, 32–34]. DDAVP should be the first line of therapy in a bleeding uremic patient [27]. Discussion here will focus around the use of DDAVP in settings where there is a significant history of clinical bleeding.

DDAVP was first utilized for its anti-diuretic properties until it was discovered in the 1970s to have hemostatic properties [35]. Infusions of DDAVP increase VWF, factor VIII coagulant activity, ristocetin co-factor and tissue plasminogen activator. The rise of coagulation factors is rapid, likely related to release of endogenous reserves rather than new synthesis. DDAVP may also promote the glycoprotein transmembrane proteins, including VWF and GP IIb/IIIa.

Administration of DDAVP:

- Administered via intravenous, subcutaneous, or intranasal routes.
- The maximal effect on clotting factor levels occurs at 30 min, lasting up to 6 h, with an intravenous dose of 0.3 μg/kg (to a maximum of 20 μg/dose infused in 20–50 mL of normal saline over 15–30 min).
- With subcutaneous dosing, the levels peak at 1–2 h.
- For intranasal administration, a dose of 300 μg is comparable to 0.2 μg/kg intravenous dose. Use one single spray in one nostril (150 μg) if <12 years/50 kg; 1 puff per nostril (300 μg) if ≥12 years/50 kg.
- Tachyphylaxis occurs after the first dose due to depletion of FVIII and vWF endothelial stores.
- Adverse effects of DDAVP include facial flushing, headache, hypotension, tachycardia, water retention, hyponatremia and seizures (uncommon but higher incidence in children less than 5 years of age). Hypotonic solutions should be administered with caution in children who have received DDAVP.
- DDAVP should not be used in children <3 years, or in cases of polydipsia, unstable angina, or congestive heart failure because of its antidiuretic effects.

Conjugated estrogens improve the BT in uremia by increasing platelet responsiveness [32]. There have been no reports of its use in children, although adult studies recommend a dosage of 0.6 mg/kg/day given intravenously daily for 4–5 days. Effects start within 6 h and can last for up to 2 weeks after an intravenous course. It can also be given as an oral dose, but the effect is shorter, lasting up to 5 days. Side effects include hypertension, fluid retention and raised liver transaminases.

Cryoprecipitate is rich in factor VIII, vWF, fibrinogen and factor XIII, but has the risks of blood borne infections and anaphylaxis [36].

Clotting in Renal Disease

Thrombotic Manifestations of Nephrotic Syndrome

Epidemiology

Nephrotic syndrome (NS) is a hypercoagulable state with a predisposition to the development of thromboembolic events [37–42]. With effective treatments for inducing remission, thromboembolism (TE) is much less common now in children as compared to adults with an overall incidence of 3% versus 25%, respectively [43–46]. TE seems to be more likely in adolescents [46], in children with congenital NS (incidence around 10%) [47, 48], and in secondary NS, such as NS associated with vasculitis (incidence around 17%) [46]. Membranous nephropathy or a histologically similar process (e.g. class V SLE nephritis) seems to confer the highest risk, where the incidence of TE approaches that seen in adults (25%) [46]. A correlation between infection and TE has also been observed [49].

Venous TE (VTE) is the predominate form of thromboembolic disease in children with NS, accounting for 97% of the cases in a large, retrospective study [46]. In that study, arterial disease was encountered in only 0.3% of subjects. Commonly affected areas for VTE include: deep venous system within the lower limbs, inferior vena cava, renal vein, hepatic veins, and sagittal and transverse sinovenous vessels. Arterial thromboses can involve any artery, including femoral, mesenteric and intracardiac [39, 41, 46]. Finally, TE tend to occur early in the course of the disease (usually <3 months from onset) [38].

Pathogenesis

The prothrombotic tendencies in nephrotic patients have been attributed to a number of factors including state of hydration and hyperviscosity, imbalance between clotting factors and thrombophilic proteins, increase in platelets and platelet activation, abnormalities of the fibrinolytic system and use of medications [38, 40].

Antithrombin (AT; formerly known as ATIII) is an endogenous anticoagulant that was first documented to be low in NS in 1976, with confirmation in subsequent studies [37–39]. In these studies, AT had a strong correlation with plasma albumin levels and a negative correlation with urinary protein excretion, suggesting that one of the mechanisms resulting in low AT levels is due to its loss in the urine [50]. Subsequent remission of the nephrotic syndrome results in normalization of AT levels. Data on other *in vivo* anticoagulants have not been conclusive, although the majority of studies suggest that PC, PS, and tissue factor pathway inhibitor are all elevated during acute nephrotic relapses, but functionality may be reduced [37, 42, 51–53]. This might exert a protective effect against thrombosis and might explain why children have fewer thromboembolic events than adults with NS.

Platelets have been found to be higher in number and more active in children with NS. Studies suggest improved platelet availability due to their higher numbers and increased exposure of the normally albumin-bound arachidonic acid leading to thromboxane A2 activation and subsequent platelet aggregation [42, 54]. Hyperlipidemia may also promote platelet aggregation, based on the simple observation that treatment with lipid lowering agents decreases platelet hyperaggregability in NS [55].

The fibrinolytic system is also speculated to influence the risk of thromboembolic events in NS. Lower levels of plasminogen and tissue-type plasminogen activator (tPA) results in diminished fibrinolytic activity. This may be accentuated by hypoalbuminemia since albumin is a cofactor for binding plasminogen to fibrin [37, 42, 46, 56].

The use of corticosteroids has been reported to be associated with hypercoagulability [57, 58]. Mechanisms responsible include increase in coagulation factors and reduction in fibrinolysis.

Finally, children with congenital nephrotic syndrome are at higher risk of TE, which may be explained in part by a disease-specific pathophysiology. In addition, they are unlikely to achieve NS remission and are thus hypercoagulable for a longer time-frame, and they more often require the use of a central venous catheter (CVC), which is a well-known risk factor for TE.

Prevention and Treatment

Non-pharmacologic strategies to limit the risk of VTE include regular ambulation, adequate hydration, and avoidance of CVCs whenever possible [59].

The use of prophylactic anticoagulation to prevent TE in children with NS is controversial, due in part to the lack of randomized trials to determine the efficacy and safety of such an approach [60]. Despite the lack of robust evidence, some authors have suggested prophylactic strategies for children based on risk factors, severity markers, or coagulation abnormalities. Among these strategies, some authors have recommended aspirin prophylaxis in some circumstances [59, 61, 62]. Others propose AT replacement by administration of AT concentrates [40, 63].

Once TE has developed, clinical management is similar to that utilized in patients without NS, starting with heparinization [64]. In this case (i.e., severe AT deficiency), treatment with AT concentrate may be necessary as heparinoids are dependent on AT for their mechanism of action. However, the optimal target level of AT to achieve an adequate anticoagulant effect in children with NS is unclear. Both plasma-derived and recombinant AT are clinically available [65].

Renal Vein Thrombosis

Although renal vein thrombosis (RVT) is the most common non-catheter related thrombosis in the newborn period, few long-term outcome studies have been carried out [66–71]. Most RVTs present in the first month, with 70% presenting in the first week of life. It affects twice as many males and there is a left sided predominance. The clinical features of RVT are variable and include hematuria, oliguria-anuria, hypertension, decreased renal function, palpable flank mass and thrombocytopenia. Doppler ultrasound may show a decrease in amplitude or absence of venous signal, abnormal flow patterns in a number of renal venous branches or evidence of venous collateral development. The etiology of RVT in most cases is unknown. There is speculation about decreased levels of naturally occurring anticoagulants and fibrinolytic compounds leading to the thrombotic event [71]. Risk factors reported for the development of RVT include prematurity, maternal diabetes mellitus (either type 1 or gestational), pathologic states associated with thrombosis (e.g., shock, dehydration, perinatal asphyxia, polycythemia, cyanotic heart disease), sepsis, umbilical venous catheterization, conjoined twins, and inherited prothrombotic abnormalities [69, 72, 73]. However, the prevalence of these disorders has not been studied in a cohort of patients with neonatal RVT.

The sequelae of RVT reported in the literature include death (5%), glomerular disease (3–100%), tubular dysfunction (9–47%), hypertension (9–100%), and evidence of renal scarring or atrophy (27–100) [66–71]. Performance of multicentre, randomized clinical trials is required to investigate the safety and efficacy of treatment for RVT and to determine the long-term outcomes.

Renal Artery Thrombosis

In neonates, renal artery thrombosis (RAT) occurs as a result of umbilical arterial cannulation, with a low incidence of symptomatic cases (1–3%) [74]. In older children, RAT is most commonly associated with renal transplant and occurs at the site of vascular anastomosis. It has also been reported in patients placed on ventricular assist devices [75].

Risk factors for RAT in kidney transplant recipients include cadaver donor source, pretransplant peritoneal dialysis, more than five pre-transplant blood transfusions, cold ischemia time >24 h, type of immunosuppression, and prior renal transplant [76–79]. There are no studies on the treatment of RAT determining the safety and efficacy of embolectomy, fibrinolysis or anticoagulation. If RAT associated with renal transplant is diagnosed, embolectomy or fibrinolytic/anticoagulation therapy should be considered in the absence of contraindications (bleeding) to attempt to save the graft [80].

Renal Vascular Thrombosis in Renal Transplantation

Graft failure secondary to renal vascular thrombosis in the most recent report of NAPRTCS is noted to be high at 10.7% in the transplant era of 2008–2017 [81].

Different from RAT predisposing factors, risk factors for renal vascular thrombosis include underlying renal disease, pre-existing thrombotic history, abnormal anatomy, young donor, recipient age (<5 years) and donor-recipient size mismatch [76, 82–85]. Thrombophilia may also be a potential risk factor for thrombosis and early graft loss, but conclusions are not definitive [86, 87]. Therefore, some programs screen all patients for genetic and acquired thrombophilic disorders before transplantation, while others selectively screen high risk patients, such as those with a personal or family history of thrombosis.

Outcomes of graft thrombosis are not favorable and preventative strategies are crucial, including a proper history and identification of risk factors for thrombosis. Evidence for routine heparinization of all patients post-transplantation is not conclusive. Some authors suggest selective heparinization only for higher risk groups, such as small patients (<20 kg) or those with confirmed inherited thrombophilia [87–93]. The type and duration of anticoagulation prophylaxis to prevent thrombosis is also unclear. Some centres use unfractionated heparin while others use low molecular weight heparin, sometimes followed by aspirin, for various durations of time [87, 91, 92]. The effect of using anticoagulation prophylaxis on the incidence of thrombosis and graft survival in the pediatric population is unknown. Any potential benefits of heparin must be closely balanced with the risks of bleeding, which was shown to be increased in some groups using that approach [87, 90, 91].

Hemolytic Uremic Syndrome and Coagulation

Although hemolytic uremic syndrome (HUS) is reviewed in detail elsewhere (Chaps. 24 and 25), because HUS is a pro-coagulant state, it is pertinent to review this feature of the disease here. The HUS triad of hemolytic anemia, thrombocytopenia and renal involvement underscore the primary abnormality with this entity, which is related to a procoagulant state initiated by endothelial injury [72]. In the presence of Shiga toxin, up-regulation occurs of the chemokine stromal cell-derived factor-1 (SDF-1), which is found in kidney, spleen, lung, liver, brain, heart, and muscle. This chemokine activates a pathway that enhances platelet activation induced by thrombin, thereby resulting in platelet aggregation [73, 94]. Shiga toxin also inhibits prostacyclin production and increase thromboxane A2 release from endothelial cells, thereby favoring platelet aggregation. Inhibition of SDF-1 normalized platelets in vivo and prevented formation of platelet strings [95].

The procoagulant state of HUS is evidenced by the formation of microthrombi throughout the systemic circulation. Subclinical thrombogenesis occurs prior to the clinical onset of HUS, with elevation of markers of thrombin activation (increase in prothrombin fragments 1 + 2 and thrombin-antithrombin complexes) [73]. In the normal state, levels of thrombin activation markers are negligible. Tissue factor (TF), expressed on mononuclear and endothelial cells and an initiator of the coagulation cascade leading to thrombin generation, has been found to be upregulated by Shiga toxin. Blockade of thrombin activity with lepirudin prevented lethal Shiga toxin effects in greyhounds, suggesting that Shiga toxin may mediate injury via thrombin activation.

The thrombocytopenia in HUS is also intertwined in this process and is due to a consumptive process with platelet deposition in the microthrombi [94]. The platelets are activated with degranulation as evidenced by reduction in intracellular levels of β-thromboglobulin and impaired aggregation in vitro. Other evidence of platelet activation includes increase in platelet microparticles and platelet derived factors including platelet factor-4, β-thromboglobulin, and P-selectin. The resultant effect is the formation of platelet aggregates through binding of fibrinogen leading to thrombus formation.

Fibrinolysis has been suggested to be depressed in the setting of HUS, adding to the prothrombotic state [73, 94]. However, studies are conflicting as to whether indications of depressed fibrinolysis, such as elevated levels of plasminogen activator inhibitor type 1 (PAI-1), support this finding [95].

Finally, other evidence of vascular and complement activation includes increases terminal complement complex, *Fas*-ligand and soluble *Fas*, interleukin-1 receptor antagonist, transforming growth factor, platelet activating factor, degraded VWF multimers and numerous plasma factors as previously noted [95–97]. All of these changes support an enhanced thrombogenic state.

Diagnosis of Thromboembolism

Deep vein thrombosis (DVT) and pulmonary embolism (PE) are the two major categories of venous thrombotic events (VTE), both notably prevalent in the adult population [98]. In the USA, approximately 160,000–240,000 cases of DVT are diagnosed every year [99]. In children, VTE was initially thought to be extremely rare. International pediatric thrombosis registries were instrumental in changing this perception by characterizing the higher prevalence of VTE in hospitalized pediatric patients. Moreover, registries described peaks of thrombotic events during infancy and adolescence [100]. Pediatric VTE is commonly associated with several different underlying conditions (e.g., congenital heart defects, cancer, systemic lupus erythematosus), as well as treatment-related prothrombotic risk factors (e.g., CVCs, steroids, asparaginase). In comparison to adults, unprovoked VTE is uncommon in children. VTE occurs in 1:200 individuals admitted to pediatric tertiary care facilities [101, 102].

Importantly, thrombotic events in children are also associated with a significant thrombus-related morbidity and mortality, and affect children with a variety of underlying conditions [103]. For example, patients with nephrotic syndrome are at increased risk of developing DVT, particularly RVT and PE [50, 104]. RVT can be associated with several clinical complications including chronic renal tubular dysfunction and hypertension [105], whereas PE has an associated mortality rate of approximately 9% [106]. Therefore, prompt investigation of children, either under clinical suspicion or at risk for VTE development, is vital to decrease VTE-related short and long-term complications.

DVT can present with symptoms such as pain or swelling of the affected limb [107]. However, thrombotic events in children are commonly not accompanied by signs and symptoms, given that they are usually secondary to the placement of a CVC [108]. In those instances, their clinical presentation usually occurs in a sub-acute manner, when partial obstruction of the venous territory caused by the CVC and thrombus is counterbalanced by collateral vessel development. Moreover, CVC-related DVT in children is very prevalent in the upper venous system, where the mild findings of limb swelling can also be interpreted as line-related infection, leading to under-recognition of those events. Hence, to diagnose VTE in children imaging studies are required. A summary of the various imaging modalities used for the diagnosis of VTE in children is listed in Table 33.1.

The most common radiological modality utilized to diagnose DVT, the ultrasound Doppler (USD), is very sensitive for the detection of lower limb DVT. However, this imaging modality is not as sensitive for the diagnosis of upper limb DVT in children, especially for events located within the intrathoracic territory, as USD relies on vessel compressibility to confirm the presence of an intraluminal thrombus [109]. Therefore, a composite of USD and venogram has been suggested as the best way to diagnose upper extremity DVT in children. The role of computerized tomography (CT) and magnetic

Table 33.1 Summary of imaging studies for diagnosis of TE

Types of TE	Imaging	Advantages	Disadvantages
Deep vein thrombosis of limbs [95, 107–110]	Venography	Gold standard, ability to quantify venous obstruction and identify collateral veins	Invasive procedure, technical experience, cost, contrast media-related side effects, exposure to radiation, inter-radiologist interpretation discrepancy (up to 16%)
	Doppler ultrasound sensitivity 94% and specificity 98% (adults)	Noninvasive procedure, readily available, possible for bedside evaluation	Inter-variation between operators, difficulty to test in patients with obesity, edema, trauma, burns and casts, less sensitive for upper limb DVT especially for intrathoracic vessels
	CT venography sensitivity 100% and specificity 96% (adults)	Minimally invasive procedure, less radiation exposure, well tolerated contrast media	High technical demand, cost, not readily available, radiation and contrast exposure
	MR venography sensitivity 100% and specificity 96–100% (adults)	Minimally invasive procedure, well tolerated contrast media	High technical demands, cost, not readily available, requirement for anesthesia in young children
Pulmonary embolism [98, 107–111]	Pulmonary angiography	Gold standard	Same as venography for DVT of limbs; mortality of ~1% in adults
	Ventilation/perfusion (V/Q) scan sensitivity 31% and specificity 97% for high-probability scan (adults)	Less radiation exposure	Not convenient for young children due to the requirement of cooperation of patients
	CT pulmonary angiography sensitivity 69% and specificity 69% (adults)	Same as CT venography for DVT of limbs	Same as CT venography for DVT of limbs
	MR pulmonary angiography sensitivity 78% and specificity 99% (adults)	Same as MR venography for DVT of limbs	Same as MR venography for DVT of limbs
	Echocardiography for RV free wall hypokinesis sensitivity 77% and specificity 94% (adults)	Same as ultrasound for DVT of limbs	Unable to detect mild degree of PE, same as ultrasound for DVT of limbs
Renal vein thrombosis [107, 108, 111, 112]	Ultrasound high sensitivity	Same as ultrasound for DVT of limbs	Inter-variation between operators, bowel gas obscuring abdominal findings
	CT venography sensitivity almost 100% and specificity almost 100% (adults)	Findings not affected by bowel gas, same as CT venography for DVT of limbs	Same as CT venography for DVT of limbs
	MR venography sensitivity 94–96% and specificity 100% (adults)	Findings not affected by bowel gas, same as MR venography for DVT of limbs	Same as MR venography for DVT of limbs
Portal vein thrombosis [107, 108, 113–115]	Doppler ultrasound sensitivity 70–90%, specificity 99% and negative predictive value 98% (adults)	Same as ultrasound for DVT of limbs	Same as ultrasound of renal vein thrombosis
	CT venography	Able to show varices and hepatic parenchyma, same as CT venography for renal vein thrombosis	Same as CT venography for DVT of limbs
	MR venography	Able to show varices and hepatic parenchyma, same as MR venography for renal vein thrombosis	Same as MR venography for DVT of limbs

CT computerized tomography, *DVT* deep vein thrombosis, *MR* magnetic resonance
Data from: Young [107] and Monagle [108]

resonance imaging to diagnose upper extremity DVT in children is evolving.

Besides imaging studies, laboratory biomarkers have also been used in the diagnosis of adults with VTE. Most commonly, a normal D-dimer is used to rule out thrombotic events. To further improve the use of D-dimer testing, clinical predictive rules were instituted. They stratify patients into low, moderate or high clinical suspicion groups, which further improve the positive and negative pre-imaging predictive values of D-dimer.

The sensitivity of D-dimer for the diagnosis of VTE in adult patients is around 90% [116] and the specificity around 49–78% [117, 118]. For example, a normal D-dimer may have a negative predictive value as high as 99% to exclude VTE in patients who have a low pretest clinical likelihood [118]. Conversely, the low specificity of D-dimer testing for the diagnosis of VTE may be due to the fact that D-dimer levels are usually influenced by several factors, particularly underlying diseases such as recent major surgery, trauma, cancer, pregnancy, disseminated intravascular coagulation and end-stage liver disease [119, 120].

The three most comprehensive pediatric studies to date have shown disappointing results regarding the performance of D-dimer testing as a diagnostic tool for DVT in children. A retrospective chart evaluated children with suspected VTE that had D-dimer testing done within 72 h of imaging. The researchers identified 33 patients; 26 diagnosed with acute VTE, 6 unchanged chronic VTE, and 1 without VTE. D-dimer levels were significantly higher in patients with acute VTE compared to the remaining patients (77% sensitivity; 71% specificity) [121]. Conversely, another study evaluated 132 patients referred for CT pulmonary angiography to rule out PE: 88% of the patients with PE and 87% of those without PE had a positive D-dimer result, thus showing that D-dimer positivity did not show a significant relationship with the presence of PE [122]. The third study examined the role of the Wells score, which has been validated for the stratification of adults at risk for PE, as a potential tool to risk stratify children investigated for PE. The Wells score used in combination with D-dimer testing

did not differentiate children with or without PE [123], illustrating that pediatric-specific tools will be required to improve the use of D-dimer.

Thrombophilia Work Up

Thrombus formation results from a dynamic balance between pro- and anticoagulant forces; more specifically, from several different pro- and anticoagulant factors involved in the generation or inhibition of thrombin formation.

Thrombophilia refers to conditions, either inherited or acquired, that increase the risk of thrombus formation. Patients identified with an inherited or acquired thrombophilia may be predisposed to sustain a thrombotic event. However, having one isolated thrombophilia trait rarely leads to an immediate VTE.

A little more than a decade ago, the International Society on Thrombosis and Haemostasis (ISTH) published a position statement suggesting that thrombophilia investigation should occur in a stratified manner in all pediatric patients with an objectively documented VTE. However, the epidemiology of VTE in children has evolved, demonstrating that underlying conditions and/or acquired risk factors other than thrombophilia are usually present in children with VTE, rendering the role of thrombophilia as a potential causal risk factor less relevant [124].

We now understand that laboratory investigation of a child with a recently diagnosed with VTE is rarely justified. Moreover, acute VTE may also affect the circulating levels of many of the natural anticoagulant factors [e.g., PC, PS, AT], adding to the reasoning of why thrombophilia evaluation should not be performed at the time of initial VTE diagnosis [124]. Furthermore, except in extremely rare instances, thrombophilia work-up results do not change the choice of antithrombotic intensity or duration [125, 126]. Those rare instances include newborns with purpura fulminans, as its recognition requires prompt PC or PS replacement in addition to anticoagulation [125]. Similarly, children with unprovoked VTE, who may have higher recurrence rates than provoked VTE, particularly if associated with lupus anticoagulant antibodies, PC, PS or AT

Table 33.2 The summary of thrombophilic risks in children

Thrombophilic risks	Prevalence in the general population [129]	OR (95% CI) for first onset VTE in children [128]	OR (95% CI) for recurrent VTE in children [128]	Acquired conditions related to abnormal thrombophilic tests [124]
Congenital thrombophilic risks				
Antithrombin deficiency—AT activity[a]	0.02%	8.73 (3.12–24.42)	3.37 (1.57–7.20)	Acute thrombosis, nephrotic syndrome, complex congenital heart disease, L-asparaginase therapy, liver disease, heparin therapy
Protein C deficiency—PC activity[a]	0.2%	7.75 (4.48–13.38)	2.53 (1.30–4.92)	Acute thrombosis, nephrotic syndrome, complex congenital heart disease, liver disease, warfarin therapy
Protein S deficiency—total and free PS antigen[a]	0.03–0.3%	5.77 (3.07–10.85)	3.76 (1.57–7.20)	Acute thrombosis, nephrotic syndrome, complex congenital heart disease, liver disease, warfarin therapy, inflammation, pregnancy
Factor V Leiden (G1691A)—genetic test[a]	3–7%	3.56 (2.57–4.93)	0.77 (0.40–1.45)	–
Prothrombin G20210A—genetic test[a]	0.7–4%	2.63 (1.61–4.29)	2.15 (1.12–4.10)	–
Lipoprotein (a)[a]	–	4.50 (3.19–6.35)	0.84 (0.50–1.40)	Inflammation, nephrotic syndrome
Acquired thrombophilic risks				
Antiphospholipid antibodies (persistent)[b] [33]—lupus anticoagulant[a]—anticardiolipin antibodies[a]—anti beta-2 glycoprotein I antibodies [33]	1–8% 5% 3.4%	4.9 (2.20–10.90)	–	Infection

AT antithrombin, *CI* confidence interval, *OR* odds ratio, *PC* protein C, *PS* protein S

[a] Level I laboratory testing for thrombophilia in pediatric patients on behalf of the Subcommittee for Perinatal and Pediatric Thrombosis of the Scientific and Standardization Committee of the International Society on Thrombosis and Haemostasis (ISTH) [130]

[b] Persistent means that at least one of the three tests were positive twice with at least 12 weeks between the repeated testing

deficiencies [127], may also benefit from an initial laboratory work-up [125].

The results of a meta-analysis enumerating the thrombotic risk for first onset and recurrent VTE of the most common thrombophilia traits in children [127, 128] are summarized in Table 33.2.

Treatment

When a patient is diagnosed with VTE, treatment with antithrombotic agents, including antiplatelet, anticoagulant or thrombolytic agents is usually considered. The goal of using anticoagulant drugs is to prevent progression of acute TE, whereas in thrombolytic therapy the goal is to lyse the thrombus in cases where the patient has a life-, limb-, or organ-threatening condition.

The guidelines of antithrombotic treatment in children published by the American College of Chest Physician [125], the British Committee for Standard in Haematology [126], and the American Society of Hematology [131] are the main available references regarding anticoagulant therapy in children. However, most recommendations are not based on randomized controlled trials due to the limitation in the number of studies in children. The following text summarizes those recommendations regarding the most commonly used agents.

33 Disordered Hemostasis and Renal Disorders

Unfractionated heparin (UFH) or heparin is a glycosaminoglycan which forms a complex with AT, enhancing the inhibitory effect of AT against both activated factors X (FXa) and factor II (FIIa, e.g., thrombin) [132]. Moreover, this complex can also inhibit FIXa, FXIa and FXIIa [133]. Due to higher volume of distribution and physiologically low AT in infants [125, 126], the dose of heparin required for anticoagulation in infants is higher than the one required in children aged more than 1 year (Table 33.3). The anticoagulant effects of heparin can be monitored by the activated partial thromboplastin time (aPTT) or the anti-FXa assay [127]. Because of its short half-life, around 30 min in children, heparin is rapidly cleared from the body after discontinuation and its effect can be fully reversed by protamine sulfate [134].

Low molecular weight heparin (LMWH) is derived from unfractionated heparin after it is chemically fragmented into smaller molecular sizes. Whereas UFH contains polysaccharide chains from 5 to 40 kDa with at least 18 repeats of pentasaccharide sequences that bind to AT, conferring on the molecule its most potent anticoagulant effects (e.g., protease activity inhibition of activated coagulation FII (thrombin) and FX [anti-IIa and anti-Xa inhibition]), LMWH has chains with an average molecular weight between 4 and 5 kDa that still contain enough pentasaccharide sequences to retain anti-IIa and anti-Xa activity, depending on the LMWH length [132]. Overall, because of its reduced molecular size, LMWH inhibits FXa more effectively than thrombin. Similar to what occurs with unfractionated heparin, the dose requirements for LMWH are also age-dependent (Tables 33.4 and 33.5). Infants younger than 2 months need higher doses than older children. Because the kidney excretes LMWH, patients who have decreased

Table 33.3 Unfractionated heparin dosing

Loading dose: 50–75 units/kg, IV, over 10 min					
Maintenance dose:	≤1 year of age: 28 units/kg/h				
	>1 year of age: 20 units/kg/h				
aPTT (s)	Anti-Xa (units/mL)	Bolus (units/kg)	HOLD (min)	Rate change	Repeat aPTT
<50	<0.1	50	0	Increase 10%	4 h
50–59	0.1–0.34	0	0	Increase 10%	4 h
60–85	0.35–0.7	0	0	0	24 h
86–95	0.71–0.89	0	0	Decrease 10%	4 h
96–120	0.9–1.20	0	30	Decrease 10%	4 h
>120	>1.20	0	60	Decrease 10%	4 h

Table 33.4 Low molecular weight heparin (enoxaparin) dosing

	Age ≤ 2 months	Age > 2 months–18 years
Initial treatment dose	1.75 mg/kg/dose SC q12h	1 mg/kg/dose SC q 12 h
Initial prophylactic dose	0.75 mg/kg/dose SC q12h	0.5 mg/kg/dose SC q12h
	or 1.5 mg/kg/dose SC q24h	or 1 mg/kg/dose SC q24h

Table 33.5 Low molecular weight heparin (enoxaparin) adjustment

Anti-Xa (units/kg)	HOLD	Dose change	Repeat anti-Xa
<0.35	No	Increase 25%	4 h post next dose
0.35–0.49	No	Increase 10%	4 h post next dose
0.5–1.0	No	0	1×/week; 4 h post morning dose
1.01–1.5	No	Decrease 20%	4 h post morning dose
1.6–2.0	3 h	Decrease 30%	Trough level prior to next dose; and then
			4 h post morning dose
>2.0	Yes (until level < 0.5)	Decrease 40%	Trough level prior to next dose, until
			Level < 0.5, and then 4 h post
			Morning dose

kidney function should be monitored with the anti-FXa assay carefully to prevent drug retention [132]. While there are several formulations of LMWH available, enoxaparin is the one most commonly used. Unlike heparin, LMWH is only partially reversed by protamine sulfate [134].

Warfarin is an oral vitamin-K antagonist that inhibits the carboxylation of the vitamin K-dependent FII, FVII, FIX and FX by blocking the activity of the enzyme vitamin K epoxide reductase complex subunit 1 (VKORC1) in the vitamin K cycle [135]. Therefore, the production of carboxylated factors, which are the active forms of these coagulation proteins, is depleted.

The effect of warfarin can be reversed by vitamin K. To date, oral vitamin K inhibitors constitute the main class of oral anticoagulants widely used in children (Table 33.6). However, there are limitations for using warfarin in children: the drug level, which is monitored by international normalization ratio (INR), can be affected by many foods and other drugs; it takes a longer time than heparin or LMWH for patients to reach a therapeutic drug level; no liquid preparation is available; and its use is not recommended in infants [125, 126].

A summary of conventional anticoagulation in children is shown in Table 33.7.

Table 33.6 Warfarin loading doses (days 2–4)

	0.2 mg/kg PO, daily; maximum 5 mg	
Loading dose	0.1 mg/kg; with liver dysfunction, Fontan procedure, or severe renal impairment	
INR	1.1–1.3	Repeat initial loading dose
INR	1.4–3.0	50% of initial loading dose
INR	3.1–3.5	25% of initial loading dose
INR	>3.5	Hold until INR <3.5, then restart at 50% less than previous dose

Table 33.7 Conventional anticoagulant in children

	Heparin	Enoxaparin	Warfarin
Route of administration	Intravenous	Subcutaneous	Oral
Treatment dose	Bolus 75–100 units/kg/dose then: Age less than 1 year: 28 units/kg/dose Age 1 year and more: 20 units/kg/dose	Age less than 2 months: 1.75 mg/kg/dose Age 2 months and more: 1 mg/kg/dose	0.2 mg/kg/dose
Administration interval for treatment dose	Bolus followed by continuous infusion	Every 12 h	Once daily
Target range	Anti-FXa for heparin 0.35–0.70 U/mL APTT which correlates to anti-FXa at therapeutic level	Anti-FXa for enoxaparin 0.5–1.0 U/mL	INR 2.0–3.0
Half-life	30 min	6 h	42 h
Anti-thrombin dependence	Yes	Yes	No
Antidote	Protamine	Protamine (partial)	Vitamin K
Elimination	Renal	Renal	Liver
Bleeding risk	1.5–24%	0.8–5% (major bleeding)	0.05–12.2%/year (major bleeding)
Other complications	Heparin-induced thrombocytopenia (HIT) (0.3–1.0%) Osteoporosis (rare)	No report of HIT and osteoporosis in children	Warfarin- induced skin necrosis (0.01–0.1%) Hair loss (rare) Tracheal calcification (rare)

Data from Chalmers et al. [125]; Paul et al. [126]; and Young [134]

Table 33.8 Anticoagulation duration in children

VTE type	Neonates	Infants	Childhood	Level of evidence
CNS	0–6 months	0–6 months	3–12 months	2C
Non-CNS				
Provoked[a], symptomatic	6 weeks–3 months	6 weeks–3 months	3 months	2C
Unprovoked, symptomatic	6–12 months	6–12 months	6–12 months	2C

VTE venous thromboembolism, *CNS* central nervous system

Data from Monagle [80] and Monagle [64]

[a] Provoked includes central venous catheter (CVC)-related events. In those instances, if the CVC remains *in situ* after the end of anticoagulation, prophylaxis until the catheter is removed is recommended (please, see Table 33.4 for doses)

Adults with provoked VTE are treated for 3 months, while anticoagulation in unprovoked VTE is typically indefinite [136–138]. In children, anticoagulation duration is summarized in Table 33.8

Heparin-induced thrombocytopenia (HIT) is a clinical-laboratory entity where an immunological response against heparin and platelet factor-4 creates a hypercoagulable state. HIT is suspected when patients who receive heparin develop thrombocytopenia within 5–10 days after heparin treatment accompanied by a new episode or progression of TE.

Three additional major groups of anticoagulants are used in current adult practice with a high clinical suspicion of HIT: direct thrombin inhibitors (DTI, parenteral: bivalirudin and argatroban), indirect FXa inhibitor (parenteral: fondaparinux), and a direct FXa inhibitor (parenteral: danaparoid).

Bivalirudin, argatroban, and danaparoid can be used for children requiring hemodialysis who develop HIT, but most dosing recommendations have been extrapolated from the adult literature. There are only a few studies including children on hemodialysis or continuous renal replacement therapy with HIT [139–144]. The available pediatric doses that have been reported derive mostly from children undergoing surgery under cardiopulmonary bypass (CPB) who had also been diagnosed with HIT [145–150]. Of note, bivalirudin or argatroban can be monitored by the activated partial thromboplastin time (aPTT), which can be confounded in patients with disseminated intravascular coagulation (DIC), liver dysfunction, or a lupus anticoagulant. In such instances, danaparoid or fondaparinux may be preferred

[151–154]. The summary of parenteral anticoagulants available for treatment of HIT in children requiring hemodialysis is shown in Table 33.9.

New oral anticoagulants (NOAC), or direct oral anticoagulants (DOAC), including the DTI dabigatran etexilate and the direct anti-Xa inhibitors apixaban, betrixaban, edoxaban, and rivaroxaban, have been approved in adult patients. Recently, rivaroxaban has also been approved by the Food and Drug Administration and Health Canada for the treatment of acute VTE in children, and dabigatran has been approved by the European Medicines Agency. A summary of the NOAC/DOAC under investigation in children is listed in Table 33.10.

Thrombolytic therapy is used when immediate thrombus lysis is required, such as life-, limb- or organ threatening scenarios. Pulmonary embolism accompanied by hypotension (massive PE), extensive or progressive DVT of a lower limb, bilateral RVT, or failure of treatment with conventional anticoagulants are examples of pediatric cases when this therapy should be considered [155, 156]. Tissue plasminogen activator (tPA) has been the drug of choice in children [155] and is the recommended agent by the American College of Chest Physician, the British Committee for Standard in Haematology [125, 126], and the American Society of Hematology to be used for thrombolytic therapy in neonates and children. However, the risk of major bleeding can be as high as 11–18% and intracerebral hemorrhage has been reported in up to 1.5% of pediatric patients who receive this therapy. Therefore, some patients might not be ideal candidates for this type of treatment. Contraindications for thrombolytic therapy

Table 33.9 Anticoagulants that can be used for treatment of HIT in children requiring hemodialysis

	Fondaparinux	Bivalirudin [145, 147, 148]	Argatroban [145, 148–150]	Danaparoid [144, 145]
Route of administration	Subcutaneous	Intravenous	Intravenous	Intravenous
Treatment dose	0.1 mg/kg/dose, x1, and reassess subsequent doses based on anti-Xa levels	Loading dose 0.5–1.0 mg/kg, then continuous infusion 2.5 mg/kg/h	Loading dose 75–250 μg/kg, then continuous infusion with 0.1–24 μg/kg/min (average dose 1–5 μg/kg/min)	1000 U plus 30 U/kg in patients aged <10 years and 1500 plus 30 U/kg in patients aged 10–17 years, then subsequent dose adjusted by anti-Xa
Half-life	17–21 h	25–34 min	39–60 min	Approximately 25 h
Target range	0.5–1 U/mL peak level 3 h post-dose	ACT >200–400 s or APTT ratio 1.5–2 times of baseline	ACT >200–400 s or APTT ratio 1.5–2 times of baseline	Anti-Xa <0.3 U/mL pre-dialysis If anti-Xa 0.3–0.5 U/mL, then decrease dose by 250 U If anti-Xa >0.5 U/mL, then hold next dose
Elimination	Renal	Intravascular proteolysis	Liver	Renal
Antidote	None	None	None	None

Table 33.10 Direct oral anticoagulant use in children

	Dabigatran	Rivaroxaban	Apixaban	Edoxaban	Betrixaban
Evidence in pediatrics	Yes (phase 3)	Yes (phase 3)	No (study ongoing)	No (study ongoing)	No
Mechanism of action	Direct thrombin inhibitor	Xa inhibitor	Xa inhibitor	Xa inhibitor	Xa inhibitor
Bioavailability	3–7%	Almost complete when administered with a meal	~50%	62%	34%
Time to peak concentration	1 h; delayed by food	2–4 h	3–4 h	1–2 h	3–4 h
Protein binding	35%	92–95%	87%	55%	60%
Half-life	12–17 h (prolonged in renal dysfunction)	5–9 h	8–15 h	10–14 h	19–27 h
Renal clearance (unchanged)	80%	36%	27%	50%	11%
PGP substrate	Yes	Yes	Yes	Yes	Yes
CYP3A4 substrate	No	Yes (~18%)	Yes (~25%)	No (<4%)	No (<1%)
Administration considerations	Do not open capsules; swallow whole	Administer with a meal (or up to 2 h after)	N/A	N/A	Administer with food
Usual effect on coagulation parameters at therapeutic doses	Increased dilute thrombin time and often increased aPTT. May increase PT	Increased anti-Xa and often increased PT. May increase aPTT	Increased anti-Xa. May increase PT and aPTT	Increased anti-Xa and PT. May increase aPTT	Increased anti-Xa. May increase PT and aPTT
Reversal agent	Idarucizumab (no published pediatric data; study ongoing). Partially removed by dialysis.	Prothrombin complex concentrate (limited pediatric data) or andexanet alfa (no pediatric data)	Prothrombin complex concentrate (very limited pediatric data) or andexanet alfa (no pediatric data)	Prothrombin complex concentrate (very limited pediatric data) or andexanet alfa (no pediatric data)	Prothrombin complex concentrate (very limited pediatric data) or andexanet alfa (no pediatric data)

include any type of previous operation within 10 days prior to therapy, severe asphyxia within 7 days prior to therapy, an invasive procedure within 3 days of therapy, seizures within 48 h of therapy, preterm newborns with gestational age less than 32 weeks and patients who are bleeding and are unable to maintain a platelet count >50–100 × 10^9/L and fibrinogen >1.0 g/L [155, 156].

There are two methods to administer thrombolytic therapy in children: systemic thrombolysis and catheter-directed thrombolysis. Two types of dosage of systemic thrombolysis have been published in children: high dose tPA, with doses ranging between 0.1 and 0.6 mg/kg/h for 6 h, and low dose tPA, with doses ranging between 0.01 and 0.06 mg/kg/h for 4–48 h. Even though lower doses have been claimed to have a lower incidence of therapy-associated bleeding [155, 156], the American College of Chest Physician recommends a dose of 0.5 mg/kg/h for 6 h [126].

For catheter-directed tPA therapy, there have been no randomized trials and very few prospective pediatric series in children [157]. Even though the risk of major bleeding is potentially smaller and the efficacy higher in patients who are treated with this modality (dose reduction of tPA to 0.015–0.2 mg/kg/h), there have been no comparisons regarding efficacy and safety in children [155, 156]. Currently, the use of catheter-directed thrombolysis in children depends on center availability, local protocol, and level of complexity of care delivered.

In summary, in the last decade, there has been tremendous progress in the recognition and care of children affected by VTE, which includes children with underlying renal conditions.

Conclusion

Children with renal disease may have disordered hemostasis, resulting in a risk of either bleeding or clotting. Normal hemostasis in children must be understood by the clinician in order to determine whether, in a child with renal disease, therapeutic intervention to prevent abnormal bleeding or clotting is prudent. Unfortunately, there are few properly designed studies in children with renal disease providing guidelines for best prac-

tice relating to diagnosis and treatment of disordered hemostasis.

Acknowledgments We would like to acknowledge the past contributions of the late Dr. Patricia Massicotte and Mary Bauman for their work in the original chapter published in the first edition, for which some of the content was utilized for this current chapter.

References

1. Mann KG. Thrombin generation in hemorrhage control and vascular occlusion. Circulation. 2011;124(2):225–35.
2. Lyonel IG. Endothelium. In: Lyonel IG (ed) Mechanisms in hematology, 3rd ed. 2002. pp. 393–402.
3. Israels S. Platelet structure and function. In: Lyonel IG (ed) Mechanisms in hematology, 3rd ed. 2002. pp. 369–392.
4. Hoffman M. Remodeling the blood coagulation cascade. J Thromb Thrombolysis. 2003;16(1–2):17–20.
5. Rumbaut RE, Thiagarajan P. Platelet-vessel wall interactions in hemostasis and thrombosis. San Rafael: Morgan & Claypool Life Sciences; 2010. p. 13–22.
6. Adams RL, Bird RJ. Review article: coagulation cascade and therapeutics update: relevance to nephrology. Part 1: overview of coagulation, thrombophilias and history of anticoagulants. Nephrology (Carlton). 2009;14(5):462–70.
7. Davie EW. A brief historical review of the waterfall/cascade of blood coagulation. J Biol Chem. 2003;278(51):50819–32.
8. Renne T, Schmaier AH, Nickel KF, Blomback M, Maas C. In vivo roles of factor XII. Blood. 2012;120(22):4296–303.
9. Albisetti M. The fibrinolytic system in children. Semin Thromb Hemost. 2003;29(4):339–48.
10. Mosesson MW. Fibrinogen and fibrin structure and functions. J Thromb Haemost. 2005;3(8):1894–904.
11. Ataga KI. Hypercoagulability and thrombotic complications in hemolytic anemias. Haematologica. 2009;94(11):1481–4.
12. Martinod K, Wagner DD. Thrombosis: tangled up in NETs. Blood. 2014;123(18):2768–76.
13. Van Cott EM, Grabowski EF. Vascular hemostasis in flowing blood in children. Semin Thromb Hemost. 1998;24(6):583–90.
14. Sola-Visner M. Platelets in the neonatal period: developmental differences in platelet production, function, and hemostasis and the potential impact of therapies. Hematology Am Soc Hematol Educ Program. 2012;2012:506–11.
15. Andrew M, Paes B, Milner R, Johnston M, Mitchell L, Tollefsen DM, Castle V, Powers P. Development of the human coagulation system in the healthy premature infant. Blood. 1988;72(5):1651–7.

16. Andrew M, Vegh P, Johnston M, Bowker J, Ofosu F, Mitchell L. Maturation of the hemostatic system during childhood. Blood. 1992;80(8):1998–2005.
17. Kuhle S, Male C, Mitchell L. Developmental hemostasis: pro- and anticoagulant systems during childhood. Semin Thromb Hemost. 2003;29(4):329–38.
18. Monagle P, Barnes C, Ignjatovic V, Furmedge J, Newall F, Chan A, De Rosa L, Hamilton S, Ragg P, Robinson S, Auldist A, Crock C, Roy N, Rowlands S. Developmental haemostasis. Impact for clinical haemostasis laboratories. Thromb Haemost. 2006;95(2):362–72.
19. Rosendaal FR. Thrombosis in the young: epidemiology and risk factors. A focus on venous thrombosis. Thromb Haemost. 1997;78(1):1–6.
20. Davidovich E, Schwarz Z, Davidovitch M, Eidelman E, Bimstein E. Oral findings and periodontal status in children, adolescents and young adults suffering from renal failure. J Clin Periodontol. 2005;32(10):1076–82.
21. Parikh AM, Spencer FA, Lessard D, Emery C, Baylin A, Linkletter C, Goldberg RJ. Venous thromboembolism in patients with reduced estimated GFR: a population-based perspective. Am J Kidney Dis. 2011;58(5):746–55.
22. Pavord S, Myers B. Bleeding and thrombotic complications of kidney disease. Blood Rev. 2011;25(6):271–8.
23. Casonato A, Pontara E, Vertolli UP, Steffan A, Durante C, De Marco L, Sartorello F, Girolami A. Plasma and platelet von Willebrand factor abnormalities in patients with uremia: lack of correlation with uremic bleeding. Clin Appl Thromb Hemost. 2001;7(2):81–6.
24. Kaw D, Malhotra D. Platelet dysfunction and end-stage renal disease. Semin Dial. 2006;19(4):317–22.
25. Mezzano D, Tagle R, Panes O, Perez M, Downey P, Munoz B, Aranda E, Barja P, Thambo S, Gonzalez F, Mezzano S, Pereira J. Hemostatic disorder of uremia: the platelet defect, main determinant of the prolonged bleeding time, is correlated with indices of activation of coagulation and fibrinolysis. Thromb Haemost. 1996;76(3):312–21.
26. Di Minno G, Martinez J, McKean ML, De La Rosa J, Burke JF, Murphy S. Platelet dysfunction in uremia. Multifaceted defect partially corrected by dialysis. Am J Med. 1985;79(5):552–9.
27. Escolar G, Diaz-Ricart M, Cases A. Uremic platelet dysfunction: past and present. Curr Hematol Rep. 2005;4(5):359–67.
28. Hedges SJ, Dehoney SB, Hooper JS, Amanzadeh J, Busti AJ. Evidence-based treatment recommendations for uremic bleeding. Nat Clin Pract Nephrol. 2007;3(3):138–53.
29. Leung N. Hematologic manifestations of kidney disease. Semin Hematol. 2013;50(3):207–15.
30. Gaarder A, Jonsen J, Laland S, Hellem A, Owren PA. Adenosine diphosphate in red cells as a factor in the adhesiveness of human blood platelets. Nature. 1961;192:531–2.
31. Radhakrishnan S, Chanchlani R, Connolly B, Langlois V. Pre-procedure desmopressin acetate to reduce bleeding in renal failure: does it really work? Nephron Clin Pract. 2014;128(1–2):45–8.
32. Sloand JA, Schiff MJ. Beneficial effect of low-dose transdermal estrogen on bleeding time and clinical bleeding in uremia. Am J Kidney Dis. 1995;26(1):22–6.
33. Cases A, Escolar G, Reverter JC, Ordinas A, Lopez-Pedret J, Revert L, Castillo R. Recombinant human erythropoietin treatment improves platelet function in uremic patients. Kidney Int. 1992;42(3):668–72.
34. Gonzalez J, Bryant S, Hermes-DeSantis ER. Transdermal estradiol for the management of refractory uremic bleeding. Am J Health Syst Pharm. 2018;75(9):e177–83.
35. Lethagen S. Desmopressin (DDAVP) and hemostasis. Ann Hematol. 1994;69(4):173–80.
36. Triulzi DJ, Blumberg N. Variability in response to cryoprecipitate treatment for hemostatic defects in uremia. Yale J Biol Med. 1990;63(1):1–7.
37. Singhal R, Brimble KS. Thromboembolic complications in the nephrotic syndrome: pathophysiology and clinical management. Thromb Res. 2006;118(3):397–407.
38. Mehls O, Andrassy K, Koderisch J, Herzog U, Ritz E. Hemostasis and thromboembolism in children with nephrotic syndrome: differences from adults. J Pediatr. 1987;110(6):862–7.
39. Hoyer PF, Gonda S, Barthels M, Krohn HP, Brodehl J. Thromboembolic complications in children with nephrotic syndrome. Risk and incidence. Acta Paediatr Scand. 1986;75(5):804–10.
40. Citak A, Emre S, Sairin A, Bilge I, Nayir A. Hemostatic problems and thromboembolic complications in nephrotic children. Pediatr Nephrol. 2000;14(2):138–42.
41. Lilova MI, Velkovski IG, Topalov IB. Thromboembolic complications in children with nephrotic syndrome in Bulgaria (1974–1996). Pediatr Nephrol. 2000;15(1–2):74–8.
42. Barbano B, Gigante A, Amoroso A, Cianci R. Thrombosis in nephrotic syndrome. Semin Thromb Hemost. 2013;39(5):469–76.
43. Orth SR, Ritz E. The nephrotic syndrome. N Engl J Med. 1998;338(17):1202–11.
44. Schlegel N. Thromboembolic risks and complications in nephrotic children. Semin Thromb Hemost. 1997;23(3):271–80.
45. Eddy AA, Symons JM. Nephrotic syndrome in childhood. Lancet. 2003;362(9384):629–39.
46. Kerlin BA, Blatt NB, Fuh B, Zhao S, Lehman A, Blanchong C, Mahan JD, Smoyer WE. Epidemiology and risk factors for thromboembolic complications of childhood nephrotic syndrome: a Midwest Pediatric Nephrology Consortium (MWPNC) study. J Pediatr. 2009;155(1):105–10, 110.e101.
47. Mahan JD, Mauer SM, Sibley RK, Vernier RL. Congenital nephrotic syndrome: evolution of

medical management and results of renal transplantation. J Pediatr. 1984;105(4):549–57.

48. Hamed RM, Shomaf M. Congenital nephrotic syndrome: a clinico-pathologic study of thirty children. J Nephrol. 2001;14(2):104–9.

49. Carpenter SL, Goldman J, Sherman AK, Selewski DT, Kallash M, Tran CL, Seamon M, Katsoufis C, Ashoor I, Hernandez J, Supe-Markovina K, D'Alessandri-Silva C, DeJesus-Gonzalez N, Vasylyeva TL, Formeck C, Woll C, Gbadegesin R, Geier P, Devarajan P, Smoyer WE, Kerlin BA, Rheault MN. Association of infections and venous thromboembolism in hospitalized children with nephrotic syndrome. Pediatr Nephrol. 2019;34(2):261–7.

50. Suri D, Ahluwalia J, Saxena AK, Sodhi KS, Singh P, Mittal BR, Das R, Rawat A, Singh S. Thromboembolic complications in childhood nephrotic syndrome: a clinical profile. Clin Exp Nephrol. 2014;18(5):803–13.

51. Elidrissy AT, Abdurrahman MB, Bahakim HM, Jones MD, Gader AM. Haemostatic measurements in childhood nephrotic syndrome. Eur J Pediatr. 1991;150(5):374–8.

52. al-Mugeiren MM, Gader AM, al-Rasheed SA, Bahakim HM, al-Momen AK, al-Salloum A. Coagulopathy of childhood nephrotic syndrome—a reappraisal of the role of natural anticoagulants and fibrinolysis. Haemostasis. 1996;26(6):304–10.

53. Yermiahu T, Shalev H, Landau D, Dvilansky A. Protein C and protein S in pediatric nephrotic patients. Sangre (Barc). 1996;41(2):155–7.

54. Anand NK, Chand G, Talib VH, Chellani H, Pande J. Hemostatic profile in nephrotic syndrome. Indian Pediatr. 1996;33(12):1005–12.

55. Yashiro M, Muso E, Shio H, Sasayama S. Amelioration of hypercholesterolaemia by HMG-CoA reductase inhibitor (pravastatin) improved platelet hyperaggregability in nephrotic patients. Nephrol Dial Transplant. 1994;9(12):1842–3.

56. Loscalzo J. Venous thrombosis in the nephrotic syndrome. N Engl J Med. 2013;368(10):956–8.

57. Patrassi GM, Sartori MT, Livi U, Casonato A, Danesin C, Vettore S, Girolami A. Impairment of fibrinolytic potential in long-term steroid treatment after heart transplantation. Transplantation. 1997;64(11):1610–4.

58. Llach F. Hypercoagulability, renal vein thrombosis, and other thrombotic complications of nephrotic syndrome. Kidney Int. 1985;28(3):429–39.

59. Raffini L, Trimarchi T, Beliveau J, Davis D. Thromboprophylaxis in a pediatric hospital: a patient-safety and quality-improvement initiative. Pediatrics. 2011;127(5):e1326–32.

60. Glassock RJ. Prophylactic anticoagulation in nephrotic syndrome: a clinical conundrum. J Am Soc Nephrol. 2007;18(8):2221–5.

61. Gargah T, Abidi K, Nourchene K, Zarrouk C, Lakhoua MR. [Thromboembolic complications of childhood nephrotic syndrome]. Tunis Med. 2012;90(2):161–165.

62. Hodson E. The management of idiopathic nephrotic syndrome in children. Paediatr Drugs. 2003;5(5):335–49.

63. Zaffanello M, Brugnara M, Fanos V, Franchini M. Prophylaxis with AT III for thromboembolism in nephrotic syndrome: why should it be done? Int Urol Nephrol. 2009;41(3):713–6.

64. Monagle P, Chalmers E, Chan A, de Veber G, Kirkham F, Massicotte P, Michelson AD. Antithrombotic therapy in neonates and children: American College of Chest Physicians evidence-based clinical practice guidelines (8th edition). Chest. 2008;133(6 Suppl):887S–968S.

65. Kerlin BA, Haworth K, Smoyer WE. Venous thromboembolism in pediatric nephrotic syndrome. Pediatr Nephrol. 2014;29(6):989–97.

66. Goldenberg NA. Long-term outcomes of venous thrombosis in children. Curr Opin Hematol. 2005;12(5):370–6.

67. Marks SD, Massicotte MP, Steele BT, Matsell DG, Filler G, Shah PS, Perlman M, Rosenblum ND, Shah VS. Neonatal renal venous thrombosis: clinical outcomes and prevalence of prothrombotic disorders. J Pediatr. 2005;146(6):811–6.

68. Winyard PJ, Bharucha T, De Bruyn R, Dillon MJ, van't Hoff W, Trompeter RS, Liesner R, Wade A, Rees L. Perinatal renal venous thrombosis: presenting renal length predicts outcome. Arch Dis Child Fetal Neonatal Ed. 2006;91(4):F273–8.

69. Brandao LR, Simpson EA, Lau KK. Neonatal renal vein thrombosis. Semin Fetal Neonatal Med. 2011;16(6):323–8.

70. Kosch A, Kuwertz-Broking E, Heller C, Kurnik K, Schobess R, Nowak-Gottl U. Renal venous thrombosis in neonates: prothrombotic risk factors and long-term follow-up. Blood. 2004;104(5):1356–60.

71. Kuhle S, Massicotte P, Chan A, Mitchell L. A case series of 72 neonates with renal vein thrombosis. Data from the 1-800-NO-CLOTS registry. Thromb Haemost. 2004;92(4):729–33.

72. Chandler WL, Jelacic S, Boster DR, Ciol MA, Williams GD, Watkins SL, Igarashi T, Tarr PI. Prothrombotic coagulation abnormalities preceding the hemolytic-uremic syndrome. N Engl J Med. 2002;346(1):23–32.

73. Karpman D, Papadopoulou D, Nilsson K, Sjogren AC, Mikaelsson C, Lethagen S. Platelet activation by Shiga toxin and circulatory factors as a pathogenetic mechanism in the hemolytic uremic syndrome. Blood. 2001;97(10):3100–8.

74. Seibert JJ, Northington FJ, Miers JF, Taylor BJ. Aortic thrombosis after umbilical artery catheterization in neonates: prevalence of complications on long-term follow-up. AJR Am J Roentgenol. 1991;156(3):567–9.

75. Poudel A, Neiberger R. Enlarged and echogenic kidneys while on a pediatric ventricular assist device. J Extra Corpor Technol. 2013;45(4):248–50.

76. Smith JM, Stablein D, Singh A, Harmon W, McDonald RA. Decreased risk of renal allograft thrombosis associated with interleukin-2 receptor antagonists: a report of the NAPRTCS. Am J Transplant. 2006;6(3):585–8.

77. Harmon WE, Stablein D, Alexander SR, Tejani A. Graft thrombosis in pediatric renal transplant recipients. A report of the North American Pediatric Renal Transplant Cooperative Study. Transplantation. 1991;51(2):406–12.

78. Massicotte-Nolan P, Glofcheski DJ, Kruuv J, Lepock JR. Relationship between hyperthermic cell killing and protein denaturation by alcohols. Radiat Res. 1981;87(2):284–99.

79. Proesmans W, van de Wijdeven P, Van Geet C. Thrombophilia in neonatal renal venous and arterial thrombosis. Pediatr Nephrol. 2005; 20(2):241–2.

80. Monagle P, Chan A, Massicotte P, Chalmers E, Michelson AD. Antithrombotic therapy in children: the seventh ACCP conference on antithrombotic and thrombolytic therapy. Chest. 2004;126(3 Suppl):645S–87S.

81. Chua A, Cramer C, Moudgil A, Martz K, Smith J, Blydt-Hansen T, Neu A, Dharnidharka VR, NAPRTCS Investigators. Kidney transplant practice patterns and outcome benchmarks over 30 years: the 2018 report of the NAPRTCS. Pediatr Transplant. 2019;23(8):e13597.

82. Singh A, Stablein D, Tejani A. Risk factors for vascular thrombosis in pediatric renal transplantation: a special report of the North American Pediatric Renal Transplant Cooperative Study. Transplantation. 1997;63(9):1263–7.

83. McDonald RA, Smith JM, Stablein D, Harmon WE. Pretransplant peritoneal dialysis and graft thrombosis following pediatric kidney transplantation: a NAPRTCS report. Pediatr Transplant. 2003;7(3):204–8.

84. Ponticelli C, Moia M, Montagnino G. Renal allograft thrombosis. Nephrol Dial Transplant. 2009;24(5):1388–93.

85. Donati-Bourne J, Roberts HW, Coleman RA. Donor-recipient size mismatch in paediatric renal transplantation. J Transp Secur. 2014;2014:317574.

86. Luna E, Cerezo I, Collado G, Martinez C, Villa J, Macias R, Garcia C, Cubero JJ. Vascular thrombosis after kidney transplantation: predisposing factors and risk index. Transplant Proc. 2010;42(8):2928–30.

87. Kranz B, Vester U, Nadalin S, Paul A, Broelsch CE, Hoyer PF. Outcome after kidney transplantation in children with thrombotic risk factors. Pediatr Transplant. 2006;10(7):788–93.

88. Dick AA, Lerner SM, Boissy AR, Farrell CE, Alfrey EJ. Excellent outcome in infants and small children with thrombophilias undergoing kidney transplantation. Pediatr Transplant. 2005;9(1):39–42.

89. Rodricks N, Chanchlani R, Banh T, Borges K, Vasilevska-Ristovska J, Hebert D, Patel V, Lorenzo AJ, Parekh RS. Incidence and risk factors of early surgical complications in young renal transplant recipients: a persistent challenge. Pediatr Transplant. 2017;21(7).

90. Broyer M, Gagnadoux MF, Sierro A, Fischer AM, Niaudet P. Preventive treatment of vascular thrombosis after kidney transplantation in children with low molecular weight heparin. Transplant Proc. 1991;23(1 Pt 2):1384–5.

91. Nagra A, Trompeter RS, Fernando ON, Koffman G, Taylor JD, Lord R, Hutchinson C, O'Sullivan C, Rees L. The effect of heparin on graft thrombosis in pediatric renal allografts. Pediatr Nephrol. 2004;19(5):531–5.

92. Esfandiar N, Otukesh H, Sharifian M, Hoseini R. Protective effect of heparin and aspirin against vascular thrombosis in pediatric kidney transplants. Iran J Kidney Dis. 2012;6(2):141–5.

93. Kim JK, Chua ME, Teoh CW, Lee MJ, Kesavan A, Hebert D, Lorenzo AJ, Farhat WA, Koyle MA. Assessment of prophylactic heparin infusion as a safe preventative measure for thrombotic complications in pediatric kidney transplant recipients weighing <20 kg. Pediatr Transplant. 2019;23(6):e13512.

94. Petruzziello-Pellegrini TN, Yuen DA, Page AV, Patel S, Soltyk AM, Matouk CC, Wong DK, Turgeon PJ, Fish JE, Ho JJ, Steer BM, Khajoee V, Tigdi J, Lee WL, Motto DG, Advani A, Gilbert RE, Karumanchi SA, Robinson LA, Tarr PI, Liles WC, Brunton JL, Marsden PA. The CXCR4/CXCR7/SDF-1 pathway contributes to the pathogenesis of Shiga toxin-associated hemolytic uremic syndrome in humans and mice. J Clin Invest. 2012;122(2):759–76.

95. Van Geet C, Proesmans W, Arnout J, Vermylen J, Declerck PJ. Activation of both coagulation and fibrinolysis in childhood hemolytic uremic syndrome. Kidney Int. 1998;54(4):1324–30.

96. Tarr PI. Basic fibroblast growth factor and Shiga toxin-O157:H7-associated hemolytic uremic syndrome. J Am Soc Nephrol. 2002;13(3):817–20.

97. Kremer Hovinga JA, Heeb SR, Skowronska M, Schaller M. Pathophysiology of thrombotic thrombocytopenic purpura and hemolytic uremic syndrome. J Thromb Haemost. 2018;16(4):618–29.

98. Goldhaber SZ, Bounameaux H. Pulmonary embolism and deep vein thrombosis. Lancet. 2012;379(9828):1835–46.

99. Grosse SD. Incidence-based cost estimates require population-based incidence data. A critique of Mahan et al. Thromb Haemost. 2012;107(1):192–3; author reply 194–195.

100. Andrew M, David M, Adams M, Ali K, Anderson R, Barnard D, Bernstein M, Brisson L, Cairney B, DeSai D, et al. Venous thromboembolic complications (VTE) in children: first analyses of the Canadian Registry of VTE. Blood. 1994;83(5):1251–7.

101. Raffini L, Huang YS, Witmer C, Feudtner C. Dramatic increase in venous thromboembolism in

children's hospitals in the United States from 2001 to 2007. Pediatrics. 2009;124(4):1001–8.

102. Anderson FA Jr, Wheeler HB, Goldberg RJ, Hosmer DW, Patwardhan NA, Jovanovic B, Forcier A, Dalen JE. A population-based perspective of the hospital incidence and case-fatality rates of deep vein thrombosis and pulmonary embolism. The Worcester DVT study. Arch Intern Med. 1991;151(5):933–8.

103. Monagle P, Adams M, Mahoney M, Ali K, Barnard D, Bernstein M, Brisson L, David M, Desai S, Scully MF, Halton J, Israels S, Jardine L, Leaker M, McCusker P, Silva M, Wu J, Anderson R, Andrew M, Massicotte MP. Outcome of pediatric thromboembolic disease: a report from the Canadian childhood thrombophilia Registry. Pediatr Res. 2000;47(6):763–6.

104. Zaffanello M, Franchini M. Thromboembolism in childhood nephrotic syndrome: a rare but serious complication. Hematology. 2007;12(1):69–73.

105. Lau KK, Stoffman JM, Williams S, McCusker P, Brandao L, Patel S, Chan AK, Canadian Pediatric T, Hemostasis N. Neonatal renal vein thrombosis: review of the English-language literature between 1992 and 2006. Pediatrics. 2007;120(5):e1278–84.

106. Biss TT, Brandao LR, Kahr WH, Chan AK, Williams S. Clinical features and outcome of pulmonary embolism in children. Br J Haematol. 2008;142(5):808–18.

107. Young G. Diagnosis and treatment of thrombosis in children: general principles. Pediatr Blood Cancer. 2006;46(5):540–6.

108. Monagle P. Diagnosis and management of deep venous thrombosis and pulmonary embolism in neonates and children. Semin Thromb Hemost. 2012;38(7):683–90.

109. Male C, Kuhle S, Mitchell L. Diagnosis of venous thromboembolism in children. Semin Thromb Hemost. 2003;29(4):377–90.

110. Huisman MV, Klok FA. Diagnostic management of acute deep vein thrombosis and pulmonary embolism. J Thromb Haemost. 2013;11(3):412–22.

111. Brandao LR, Labarque V, Diab Y, Williams S, Manson DE. Pulmonary embolism in children. Semin Thromb Hemost. 2011;37(7):772–85.

112. Zhang LJ, Wu X, Yang GF, Tang CX, Luo S, Zhou CS, Ji XM, Lu GM. Three-dimensional contrast-enhanced magnetic resonance venography for detection of renal vein thrombosis: comparison with multidetector CT venography. Acta Radiol. 2013;54(10):1125–31.

113. Williams S, Chan AK. Neonatal portal vein thrombosis: diagnosis and management. Semin Fetal Neonatal Med. 2011;16(6):329–39.

114. Parikh S, Shah R, Kapoor P. Portal vein thrombosis. Am J Med. 2010;123(2):111–9.

115. Rodriguez-Luna H, Vargas HE. Portal vein thrombosis. Curr Treat Options Gastroenterol. 2007;10(6):435–43.

116. Brill-Edwards P, Lee A. D-dimer testing in the diagnosis of acute venous thromboembolism. Thromb Haemost. 1999;82(2):688–94.

117. Wells P, Anderson D. The diagnosis and treatment of venous thromboembolism. Hematology Am Soc Hematol Educ Program. 2013;2013:457–63.

118. Yamaki T, Nozaki M, Sakurai H, Kikuchi Y, Soejima K, Kono T, Hamahata A, Kim K. Combined use of pretest clinical probability score and latex agglutination D-dimer testing for excluding acute deep vein thrombosis. J Vasc Surg. 2009;50(5):1099–105.

119. Hunt BJ. Bleeding and coagulopathies in critical care. N Engl J Med. 2014;370(22):2153.

120. Stein PD, Hull RD, Patel KC, Olson RE, Ghali WA, Brant R, Biel RK, Bharadia V, Kalra NK. D-dimer for the exclusion of acute venous thrombosis and pulmonary embolism: a systematic review. Ann Intern Med. 2004;140(8):589–602.

121. Strouse JJ, Tamma P, Kickler TS, Takemoto CM. D-dimer for the diagnosis of venous thromboembolism in children. Am J Hematol. 2009;84(1):62–3.

122. Lee EY, Tse SK, Zurakowski D, Johnson VM, Lee NJ, Tracy DA, Boiselle PM. Children suspected of having pulmonary embolism: multidetector CT pulmonary angiography—thromboembolic risk factors and implications for appropriate use. Radiology. 2012;262(1):242–51.

123. Biss TT, Brandao LR, Kahr WH, Chan AK, Williams S. Clinical probability score and D-dimer estimation lack utility in the diagnosis of childhood pulmonary embolism. J Thromb Haemost. 2009;7(10):1633–8.

124. Raffini L. Thrombophilia in children: who to test, how, when, and why? Hematology Am Soc Hematol Educ Program. 2008:228–235.

125. Chalmers E, Ganesen V, Liesner R, Maroo S, Nokes T, Saunders D, Williams M, British Committee for Standards in Haematology. Guideline on the investigation, management and prevention of venous thrombosis in children. Br J Haematol. 2011;154(2):196–207.

126. Monagle P, Chan AKC, Goldenberg NA, Ichord RN, Journeycake JM, Nowak-Gottl U, Vesely SK. Antithrombotic therapy in neonates and children: antithrombotic therapy and prevention of thrombosis, 9th ed: American College of Chest Physicians evidence-based clinical practice guidelines. Chest. 2012;141(2 Suppl):e737S–801S.

127. Kenet G, Aronis S, Berkun Y, Bonduel M, Chan A, Goldenberg NA, Holzhauer S, Iorio A, Journeycake J, Junker R, Male C, Manco-Johnson M, Massicotte P, Mesters R, Monagle P, van Ommen H, Rafini L, Simioni P, Young G, Nowak-Gottl U. Impact of persistent antiphospholipid antibodies on risk of incident symptomatic thromboembolism in children: a systematic review and meta-analysis. Semin Thromb Hemost. 2011;37(7):802–9.

128. Young G, Albisetti M, Bonduel M, Brandao L, Chan A, Friedrichs F, Goldenberg NA, Grabowski

E, Heller C, Journeycake J, Kenet G, Krumpel A, Kurnik K, Lubetsky A, Male C, Manco-Johnson M, Mathew P, Monagle P, van Ommen H, Simioni P, Svirin P, Tormene D, Nowak-Gottl U. Impact of inherited thrombophilia on venous thromboembolism in children: a systematic review and meta-analysis of observational studies. Circulation. 2008;118(13):1373–82.

129. Middeldorp S. Is thrombophilia testing useful? Hematology Am Soc Hematol Educ Program. 2011;2011:150–5.

130. Manco-Johnson MJ, Grabowski EF, Hellgreen M, Kemahli AS, Massicotte MP, Muntean W, Peters M, Nowak-Gottl U. Laboratory testing for thrombophilia in pediatric patients. On behalf of the Subcommittee for Perinatal and Pediatric Thrombosis of the Scientific and Standardization Committee of the International Society of Thrombosis and Haemostasis (ISTH). Thromb Haemost. 2002;88(1):155–6.

131. Monagle P, Cuello CA, Augustine C, Bonduel M, Brandao LR, Capman T, Chan AKC, Hanson S, Male C, Meerpohl J, Newall F, O'Brien SH, Raffini L, van Ommen H, Wiernikowski J, Williams S, Bhatt M, Riva JJ, Roldan Y, Schwab N, Mustafa RA, Vesely SK. American Society of Hematology 2018 guidelines for management of venous thromboembolism: treatment of pediatric venous thromboembolism. Blood Adv. 2018;2(22):3292–316.

132. Davenport A. Review article: low-molecular-weight heparin as an alternative anticoagulant to unfractionated heparin for routine outpatient haemodialysis treatments. Nephrology (Carlton). 2009;14(5):455–61.

133. Garcia DA, Baglin TP, Weitz JI, Samama MM. Parenteral anticoagulants: antithrombotic therapy and prevention of thrombosis, 9th ed: American College of Chest Physicians evidence-based clinical practice guidelines. Chest. 2012;141(2 Suppl):e24S–43S.

134. Young G. New anticoagulants in children: a review of recent studies and a look to the future. Thromb Res. 2011;127(2):70–4.

135. Vear SI, Stein CM, Ho RH. Warfarin pharmacogenomics in children. Pediatr Blood Cancer. 2013;60(9):1402–7.

136. Kearon C, Ginsberg JS, Anderson DR, Kovacs MJ, Wells P, Julian JA, Mackinnon B, Demers C, Douketis J, Turpie AG, Van Nguyen P, Green D, Kassis J, Kahn SR, Solymoss S, Desjardins L, Geerts W, Johnston M, Weitz JI, Hirsh J, Gent M, Investigators S. Comparison of 1 month with 3 months of anticoagulation for a first episode of venous thromboembolism associated with a transient risk factor. J Thromb Haemost. 2004;2(5):743–9.

137. Kearon C, Gent M, Hirsh J, Weitz J, Kovacs MJ, Anderson DR, Turpie AG, Green D, Ginsberg JS, Wells P, MacKinnon B, Julian JA. A comparison of three months of anticoagulation with extended anticoagulation for a first episode of idio-

pathic venous thromboembolism. N Engl J Med. 1999;340(12):901–7.

138. Ortel TL, Neumann I, Ageno W, Beyth R, Clark NP, Cuker A, Hutten BA, Jaff MR, Manja V, Schulman S, Thurston C, Vedantham S, Verhamme P, Witt DM, Florez ID, Izcovich A, Nieuwlaat R, Ross S, Schünemann HJ, Wiercioch W, Zhang Y, Zhang Y. American Society of Hematology 2020 guidelines for management of venous thromboembolism: treatment of deep vein thrombosis and pulmonary embolism. Blood Adv. 2020;4(19):4693–738.

139. Gay BE, Raz HR, Schmid HR, Beer JH. Long-term application of lepirudin on chronic haemodialysis over 34 months after heparin-induced thrombocytopenia. Nephrol Dial Transplant. 2007;22(6):1790–1.

140. Gajra A, Vajpayee N, Smith A, Poiesz BJ, Narsipur S. Lepirudin for anticoagulation in patients with heparin-induced thrombocytopenia treated with continuous renal replacement therapy. Am J Hematol. 2007;82(5):391–3.

141. Tsu LV, Dager WE. Bivalirudin dosing adjustments for reduced renal function with or without hemodialysis in the management of heparin-induced thrombocytopenia. Ann Pharmacother. 2011;45(10):1185–92.

142. Delhaye C, Maluenda G, Wakabayashi K, Ben-Dor I, Collins SD, Syed AI, Gonzalez MA, Gaglia MA, Torguson R, Xue Z, Suddath WO, Satler LF, Kent KM, Lindsay J, Pichard AD, Waksman R. Safety and in-hospital outcomes of bivalirudin use in dialysis patients undergoing percutaneous coronary intervention. Am J Cardiol. 2010;105(3):297–301.

143. Link A, Girndt M, Selejan S, Mathes A, Bohm M, Rensing H. Argatroban for anticoagulation in continuous renal replacement therapy. Crit Care Med. 2009;37(1):105–10.

144. Neuhaus TJ, Goetschel P, Schmugge M, Leumann E. Heparin-induced thrombocytopenia type II on hemodialysis: switch to danaparoid. Pediatr Nephrol. 2000;14(8–9):713–6.

145. Chan VH, Monagle P, Massicotte P, Chan AK. Novel paediatric anticoagulants: a review of the current literature. Blood Coagul Fibrinolysis. 2010;21(2):144–51.

146. Knoderer CA, Knoderer HM, Turrentine MW, Kumar M. Lepirudin anticoagulation for heparin-induced thrombocytopenia after cardiac surgery in a pediatric patient. Pharmacotherapy. 2006;26(5):709–12.

147. Gates R, Yost P, Parker B. The use of bivalirudin for cardiopulmonary bypass anticoagulation in pediatric heparin-induced thrombocytopenia patients. Artif Organs. 2010;34(8):667–9.

148. Almond CS, Harrington J, Thiagarajan R, Duncan CN, LaPierre R, Halwick D, Blume ED, Del Nido PJ, Neufeld EJ, McGowan FX. Successful use of bivalirudin for cardiac transplantation in a child with heparin-induced thrombocytopenia. J Heart Lung Transplant. 2006;25(11):1376–9.

149. Young G, Boshkov LK, Sullivan JE, Raffini LJ, Cox DS, Boyle DA, Kallender H, Tarka EA, Soffer

J, Hursting MJ. Argatroban therapy in pediatric patients requiring nonheparin anticoagulation: an open-label, safety, efficacy, and pharmacokinetic study. Pediatr Blood Cancer. 2011;56(7):1103–9.

150. Potter KE, Raj A, Sullivan JE. Argatroban for anticoagulation in pediatric patients with heparin-induced thrombocytopenia requiring extracorporeal life support. J Pediatr Hematol Oncol. 2007;29(4):265–8.

151. Warkentin TE. Anticoagulant failure in coagulopathic patients: PTT confounding and other pitfalls. Expert Opin Drug Saf. 2014;13(1):25–43.

152. Shen X, Wile R, Young G. FondaKIDS III: a long-term retrospective cohort study of fondaparinux for treatment of venous thromboembolism in children. Pediatr Blood Cancer. 2020;67(8):e28295.

153. Wahby KA, Riley LK, Tennenberg SD. Assessment of an extended interval Fondaparinux dosing regimen for venous thromboembolism prophylaxis in critically ill patients with severe renal dysfunction using Antifactor Xa levels. Pharmacotherapy. 2017;37(10):1241–8.

154. Warkentin TE. Heparin-induced thrombocytopenia in critically ill patients. Semin Thromb Hemost. 2015;41(1):49–60.

155. Albisetti M. Thrombolytic therapy in children. Thromb Res. 2006;118(1):95–105.

156. Williams MD. Thrombolysis in children. Br J Haematol. 2010;148(1):26–36.

157. Goldenberg NA, Branchford B, Wang M, Ray C Jr, Durham JD, Manco-Johnson MJ. Percutaneous mechanical and pharmacomechanical thrombolysis for occlusive deep vein thrombosis of the proximal limb in adolescent subjects: findings from an institution-based prospective inception cohort study of pediatric venous thromboembolism. J Vasc Interv Radiol. 2011;22(2):121–32.

Printed by Printforce, the Netherlands